Textbook of Anaesthesia

For Churchill Livingstone

Commissioning Editor: Gavin Smith
Project Controller: Sarah Lowe
Copy Editors: Holly Regan-Jones, Liz Graham
Cover Design: Keith Kail
Index: Hilary Tarrant

Textbook of Anaesthesia

Edited by

A. R. Aitkenhead BSc MD FRCA

Professor of Anaesthesia, University Department of Anaesthesia,
Queen's Medical Centre, Nottingham, UK

G. Smith BSc(Hons) MD FRCA

Professor of Anaesthesia, University Department of Anaesthesia,
University of Leicester, Leicester, UK

THIRD EDITION

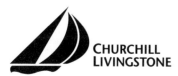

CHURCHILL
LIVINGSTONE

NEW YORK EDINBURGH LONDON MADRID MELBOURNE SAN FRANCISCO TOKYO 1996

CHURCHILL LIVINGSTONE
Medical Division of Pearson Professional Limited

Distributed in the United States of America by Churchill
Livingstone Inc., 650 Avenue of the Americas, New York, N.Y.
10011, and by associated companies, branches and
representatives throughout the world.

First published 1985
Second Edition 1990
Third Edition 1996

Standard Edition ISBN 0443 050562
International Edition ISBN 0443 051135

British Library Cataloguing in Publication Data
A catalogue record for this book is available from the British Library.

Library of Congress Cataloging in Publication Data
A catalog record for this book is available from the Library of Congress.

Medical knowledge is constantly changing. As new information
becomes available, changes in treatment, procedures, equipment and
the use of drugs become necessary. The editors/authors/contributors
and the publishers have, as far as it is possible, taken care that the
information given in this text is accurate and up to date. However,
readers are strongly advised to confirm that the information,
especially with regard to drug usage, complies with the latest
legislation and standards of practice.

The
publisher's
policy is to use
paper manufactured
from sustainable forest

Printed in the UK by BPC Consumer Books, Ltd.

Preface

The first edition of this book was intended to satisfy the needs of the new recruit into anaesthesia during the first 1–2 years in the specialty. In addition, it was hoped that it might provide suitable reading for anaesthetists studying for the (then) new Part 1 FFARCS examinations (later Part 1 FRCA), the European Diploma of Anaesthesiology, or equivalent examinations in other parts of the world. The response to the first edition was very encouraging, and it clearly proved useful not only to the intended audience but also to a wider readership including medical practitioners in rural areas or under-developed countries, and non-medical staff involved full-time in anaesthesia.

The success of the first edition stimulated us to produce a second edition, in which we undertook major revisions of several chapters, and introduced new chapters dealing with basic sciences and some additional clinical fields encountered frequently by trainee anaesthetists. The second edition also proved to be very popular, and this has prompted us to compile a third edition.

In this edition, we have invited new authors to contribute approximately one-third of the chapters in the book. This is not a reflection of the quality of the contributions of the previous authors, to whom we are very grateful; our intentions are simply to ensure that fresh minds are applied to the subject matter, and to avoid the risks which can be associated with asking authors merely to update their contributions. In future editions, it is our aim to pursue a similar policy with the remaining chapters. However, we are grateful to the authors of these chapters for the quality of the revisions which they have made in this edition. We are also indebted to the many reviewers and readers of the book who have provided helpful comments, which we have tried to address.

The publication of this edition coincides with the introduction of the new Primary FRCA examination. This book is not intended to provide comprehensive coverage of the syllabus of that examination, although, like the syllabus, it does embrace principles of physiology and pharmacology as well as clinical anaesthesia.

The astute observer will note that we have omitted the chapter on anatomy which opened the first two editions. Whilst useful, this chapter was not sufficiently comprehensive and we felt that its inclusion might undervalue the importance of this subject, especially to trainees.

As with previous editions, we are grateful to all of our contributors for allowing us to undertake widespread revision of manuscripts in an attempt to obtain uniformity of style. We are indebted again to our publishers, Churchill Livingstone, who have allowed extensive revisions of the proofs in order to accommodate very recent advances, particularly in relation to newly introduced drugs. Our gratitude must be recorded to Mrs Alice Whyte in Nottingham and Mrs Karen Marden in Leicester for substantial secretarial work.

We hope that this text will prove as popular as the first two editions, and will be used by trainees as a practical guide in the operating theatre and as the foundation of their theoretical training. It may be valuable also as an 'aide memoire' for teachers in anaesthesia, and may be appropriate reading for undergraduates who undertake an elective period of training in anaesthesia, for anaesthetic and recovery rooms nurses, for operating department practitioners and for nurse anaesthetists.

Nottingham and
Leicester, 1996

A. R. Aitkenhead
G. Smith

Contributors

Alan Aitkenhead BSc MD FRCA
Professor of Anaesthesia, University Department of Anaesthesia, Queen's Medical Centre, Nottingham, UK

Douglas S. Arthur MB ChB FRCA
Consultant Anaesthetist, Royal Hospital for Sick Children, Yorkhill, Glasgow, UK

David B. Barnett MD FRCP
Professor of Clinical Pharmacology, University of Leicester Medical School, Leicester, UK

David G. Bogod MB BS FRCA
Consultant Anaesthetist, City Hospital, Nottingham, UK

Beverley J. Collett MB BS FRCA
Consultant, Department of Anaesthesia, Leicester Royal Infirmary, Leicester, UK

David R. Derbyshire MB ChB FRCA
Consultant, Department of Anaesthesia, Warwick General Hospital, Warwick, UK

Howard Fee MD PhD FRCA
Professor of Anaesthesia, Department of Anaesthetics, The Queen's University of Belfast, Whitla Medical Building; Consultant Anaesthetist, Royal Victoria and Musgrove Park Hospitals, Belfast, UK

David Fell MB ChB FRCA
Consultant Anaesthetist, Department of Anaesthesia, Leicester Royal Infirmary, Leicester, UK

Ian S. Grant MB ChB FRCP(Edin-Glasg) FRCA
Consultant Anaesthetist and Medical Director, Intensive Therapy Unit, Western General Hospital, Edinburgh, UK

Christopher D. Hanning BSc MB BS FRCA
Consultant, Department of Anaesthesia, Leicester General Hospital, Leicester, UK

Greg Hobbs BM BS DipRACOG FRCA
Senior Lecturer, University Department of Anaesthesia, University Hospital, Queen's Medical Centre, Nottingham, UK

Stephen A. Hudson BPharm MPharm MRPharmS
Professor of Pharmaceutical Care, Department of Pharmaceutical Sciences, School of Pharmacy, University of Strathclyde, Glasgow, UK

Jennifer M. Hunter MB ChB FRCA
Reader in Anaesthesia, University of Liverpool, Royal Liverpool University Hospital, Liverpool, UK

Gareth W. Jones BSc MB BS MRCP FRCA
Consultant Anaesthetist, Department of Anaesthesia, Leicester Royal Infirmary, Leicester, UK

Michael J. Jones BSc MB ChB MRCP FRCA
Consultant Anaesthetist, Glenfield General Hospital, Leicester, UK

Jeremy A. Langton MB BS FRCA
Consultant, Department of Anaesthesia, Derriford Hospital, Plymouth, UK

Alastair Lee BSc MB ChB FRCA
Consultant, Department of Anaesthetics and
Intensive Care Unit, Royal Infirmary, Edinburgh,
UK

Stephen D. Logan BSc(Hons) PhD
Professor of Neuroscience, Department of
Biomedical Sciences, Marischal College,
University of Aberdeen, Aberdeen, UK

Rosemary MacDonald PhD FRCA
Formerly Consultant Obstetric Anaesthetist, St
James's University Hospital, Leeds; Postgraduate
Dean (Yorkshire), Department of Postgraduate
Medical Education, Ward H, Seacroft Hospital,
Leeds, UK

John M. V. Nicoll FFA(SA)
Consultant Anaesthetist, Department of
Anaesthesia, University Hospital, Nottingham,
UK

Graham R. Nimmo MD MRCP(UK) FFARCSI
Consultant Physician, Emergency Medicine and
Intensive Care, Western General Hospital,
Edinburgh, UK

Timothy O'Carroll MB BS FRCA
Consultant Anaesthetist, Department of
Anaesthesia, Leicester Royal Infirmary, Leicester,
UK

David G. Raitt MB ChB FRCA DA
Consultant Anaesthetist and Clinical Director,
Department of Anaesthesia, Leicester General
Hospital, Leicester, UK

Charles S. Reilly MD FRCA
Professor of Anaesthesia, Department of Surgical
and Anaesthetic Sciences, University of Sheffield,
Royal Hallamshire Hospital, Sheffield, UK

Guy S. Routh MB BS FRCA
Consultant Anaesthetist, Cheltenham General
Hospital, Cheltenham, Gloucestershire, UK

David J. Rowbotham MD MRCP FRCA FFARCSI
Professor of Anaesthesia and Pain Management,
University Department of Anaesthesia, Leicester
Royal Infirmary, Leicester, UK

Colin J. Runcie MB ChB MRCP FRCA
Consultant Anaesthetist, Department of
Anaesthesia, Western Infirmary, Glasgow, UK

Peter J. Simpson MD FRCA
Consultant Anaesthetist, Frenchay Hospital,
Bristol; Senior Clinical Lecturer in Anaesthetics,
University of Bristol, Bristol, UK

Graham Smith BSc(Hons) MD FRCA
Professor of Anaesthesia, Department of
Anaesthesia, University of Leicester, Leicester,
UK

John Thorburn FRCA FRCP(Glas)
Consultant Anaesthetist, Queen Mother's
Hospital, Yorkhill, Glasgow, UK

J. Gordon Todd MB ChB FRCA
Consultant Anaesthetist, West Glasgow Hospitals
University NHS Trust, Western Infirmary,
Glasgow, UK

Douglas A. B. Turner MB ChB FRCA
Consultant Anaesthetist, Department of
Anaesthesia, Leicester Royal Infirmary; Honorary
Clinical Lecturer, University of Leicester;
Clinical Head of Service, Critical Care Services,
Leicester Royal Infirmary, Leicester, UK

Mairlys Vater MB BCh FRCA
Consultant Anaesthetist, Derby City General
Hospital, Derby, UK

Peter G. M. Wallace MB ChB FRCA
Consultant Anaesthetist, Western Infirmary,
Glasgow, UK

John Walls MB ChB FRCP
Professor of Nephrology, Department of
Nephrology, Leicester General Hospital,
Leicester, UK

Malcolm J. H. Wellstood-Eason MB ChB FRCA
Consultant, Department of Anaesthesia,
Leicester Royal Infirmary, Leicester, UK

John A. W. Wildsmith MD FRCA
Professor of Anaesthesia, Department of
Anaesthesia, Ninewells Hospital and Medical
School, Dundee, UK

Sheila M. Willatts MD FRCA FRCP
Clinical Reader in Anaesthesia, University of
Bristol, Bristol, UK

J. Keith Wood FRCP FRCPE FRCPath
Consultant Haematologist, Leicester Royal
Infirmary, Leicester, UK

David A. Zideman QHP(c) BSc MB BS FRCA
Consultant and Honorary Senior Lecturer,
Department of Anaesthesia, Hammersmith
Hospital, London, UK

Contents

1. Respiratory physiology

The principal purpose of the respiratory system is the exchange of oxygen and carbon dioxide between the blood and the respired gas. It has secondary roles in the control of acid base balance, the metabolism of hormones and the removal of compounds and particulate matter, taking advantage of its position as the only organ which receives the entire cardiac output.

Breathing is the most obvious attribute of the respiratory system and the sequence of events in a normal breath in the upright posture will be outlined as a basis for further consideration.

A BREATH

Initiation of a breath starts in the inspiratory neurones of the respiratory centre in the floor of the fourth ventricle. As expiration ends, increasing neuronal traffic develops in the descending motor neurones of the lateral and ventral columns which synapse with the anterior horn cells of the nerves supplying the respiratory muscles. As the muscles start to contract, muscle spindles sense the load and adjust anterior horn cell activity to achieve the required force.

The diaphragm is the main muscle of respiration and contraction of the inverted J shaped fibres causes it to descend with a consequent decrease in intrapleural pressure. Simultaneously, the dilator muscles of the upper airway (alae nasi, tensor palatini, palatoglossus, myoglossus, posterior cricoarytenoid) constrict, opening the airway and resisting the developing subatmospheric collapsing force. The strap muscles and the intercostal muscles also contract, stabilizing the upper chest, preventing it from being indrawn and aiding the expansion of the lower rib cage by the 'bucket handle' movement of the ribs.

The increasing subatmospheric intrapleural pressure expands the lung and dilates the intrathoracic airways. Air is drawn through the nose, where it is warmed and humidified, through the pharynx, larynx, trachea and bronchi until it reaches the terminal bronchioles. The increase in total cross-sectional area of the airways is so great at this point that little further mass movement of gas occurs and transfer of gas to and from the alveoli is by diffusion. The distance is less than 5 mm and takes less than 1 s to reach equilibrium.

The inspired air is not distributed evenly around the lung but is directed preferentially to those areas which are best perfused, the dependent areas of the lung. Final matching of blood flow and gas exchange is achieved by the mechanism of hypoxic pulmonary vasoconstriction (HPV).

Oxygen diffuses from the terminal bronchioles, through the respiratory bronchioles and alveolar sacs into the alveoli. It then diffuses across the alveolar epithelium, basement membranes, capillary endothelium, plasma and red cell membrane before combining with haemoglobin. Carbon dioxide diffuses in the reverse direction.

As inspiration proceeds, increasing afferent neuronal traffic from stretch receptors in the lungs, rib cage and muscles, coupled with increasing feedback from the inspiratory neurones themselves, ultimately inhibits the inspiratory neurones so that inspiration ceases.

Expiration then generally proceeds passively with the stored elastic energy in the lung and chest wall providing the force to overcome the resistance to airflow through the bronchial tree and upper airway. As lung volume decreases to the functional residual capacity (FRC), activity in the expiratory neurones decreases and increases in the inspiratory neurones, heralding the start of the next breath.

CONTROL OF RESPIRATION

Respiration is regulated by the respiratory neurones (often known as the respiratory centre) to maintain homoeostasis. Arterial carbon dioxide tension (Pa_{CO_2}) is regulated at about 5.3 kPa (40 mmHg) and thus under normal circumstances the main determinant of the minute ventilation ($\dot{V}$) is the production of carbon dioxide ($\dot{V}_{CO_2}$) which in turn is determined by the metabolic activity of the body and the energy source. Ventilation is greater on a carbohydrate based diet (respiratory quotient (RQ) = 1.0) than a fat based diet (RQ = 0.7) as the energy produced per unit of CO_2 evolved is greater with the latter.

Respiration is modified by many other factors, particularly from higher centres in the brain including the cortex. The pattern of respiration is modulated by speech and ingestion of food and drink. The anticipation of exercise as well as the activity itself increases respiration. The respiratory centre also balances the depth of respiration (tidal volume (V_t)) against the rate so that the least energy is spent on breathing ($\dot{V}_{O_2 resp}$). Increases in the elastic work of breathing (e.g. pulmonary oedema or fibrosis) tend to increase the respiratory rate whereas increases in the resistive work (e.g. asthma) tend to increase V_t.

Respiration is influenced also by the Pa_{CO_2}, the arterial pH and the Pa_{O_2}, the former two via the central chemoreceptors and the latter via the peripheral chemoreceptors.

Central control

The central chemoreceptors lie in the floor of the fourth ventricle and are either the neurones responsible for generation of the respiratory rhythm or are closely related to them. The cells are responsive to changes in the interstitial fluid pH and their sensitivity to changes in Pa_{CO_2} is in part due to the poor buffering of cerebrospinal fluid (CSF) compared with blood. The response is very rapid and injection of blood with an increased Pa_{CO_2}

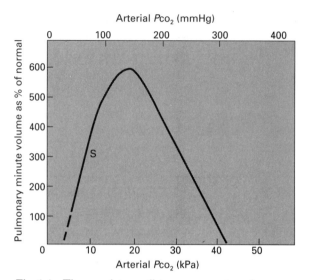

Fig. 1.1 The complete ventilatory response to carbon dioxide. Only the straight portion of the ascending limb has been determined in man and the slope, s, is used to quantify the response.

into the carotid artery of an experimental animal during inspiration results in an augmentation of that breath. The change in $\dot{V}$ with Pa_{CO_2} is approximately linear up to a Pa_{CO_2} of about 12 kPa (90 mmHg) and averages about 15 litre.min^{-1}.kPa^{-1} (Fig. 1.1).

Peripheral chemoreceptors

The peripheral chemoreceptors are located in the carotid and aortic bodies. They are best regarded as sensors of oxygen delivery as they respond to both a decrease in Pa_{O_2} and in blood flow rate. The carotid bodies effectively monitor the oxygen supply to the brain, the organ most easily damaged by hypoxaemia. The mechanism is probably similar to the central chemoreceptors in that the sensor cells respond to changes in pH. The ventilatory response to hypoxaemia is shown in Figure 1.2 and, if the Pa_{CO_2} is kept constant, changes exponentially with Pa_{O_2}. The response is linear when oxygenation is expressed as oxyhaemoglobin saturation (Sa_{O_2}). The response is much greater if Pa_{CO_2} increases at the same time.

Respiratory reflexes

Cough

A cough is one means of removing unwanted

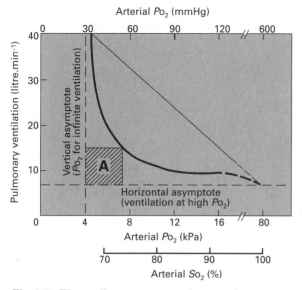

Fig. 1.2 The ventilatory response to hypoxaemia, expressed as Pa_{O_2} (heavy line) and as Sa_{O_2} (light line).

material from the respiratory tract. It complements the mucociliary escalator which clears small particulate matter. A cough may be induced voluntarily but is normally spontaneous from stimulation of receptors in the airways. It comprises a maximal inspiration followed by a forced expiration against a closed glottis, when intrathoracic pressures may reach $80\ cmH_2O$. The larynx then opens allowing expiration to occur at maximum velocity. The increased intrathoracic pressure causes dynamic compression of the bronchi, thus further increasing the velocity of expired air, often approaching the speed of sound and creating shear forces which detach the mucus from the mucosa. A wave of dynamic compression sweeps from the smaller to the larger bronchi as the cough progresses.

An effective cough thus requires three elements: an adequate inspired volume, adequate expiratory power and a functioning glottis. Absence of any of these elements leads to impaired coughing and retention of secretions.

Laryngospasm

Laryngospasm is, phylogenetically, a very primitive reflex and is intended to protect the lungs from inhalation of noxious substances. It is in-

duced by stimulation of both chemical and touch receptors above and below the glottis. The reflex is less vigorous in the elderly.

Arousal

The ability to arouse from sedation or sleep in response to apnoea, airway obstruction or the need to cough is an important respiratory response. It is obtunded during normal sleep and by sedative and analgesic drugs such as morphine and may be a major contributory factor in postoperative respiratory complications.

MECHANICS OF RESPIRATION

The respiratory system may be regarded as a collapsible elastic sac (the lungs) surrounded by a semirigid cage (the thorax) with a piston at one end (the diaphragm) supplied through a branching set of semirigid tubes (the airway and bronchial tree). The volume of the system at rest is a balance between the tendency of the lungs to collapse, the thorax to expand and the position of the diaphragm.

Lung volumes

The total volume of the respiratory system (total lung capacity (TLC)) when fully expanded by voluntary effort is about 3–6 litres in the average adult and is related more to height than weight. It can be divided into the parts that participate in gas exchange (alveolar volume) and those that do not (dead space). The alveolar volume may be divided also into that which can be measured at the lips (vital capacity (VC)) and that which remains in the lung after a maximal expiration (residual volume (RV)) (Fig. 1.3). These volumes change little with body position, unlike the volume left in the lungs after a normal expiration (functional residual capacity (FRC)). The FRC is influenced by body position, being greatest in the upright position and least when lying head downwards, the changes being mostly due to movement of the diaphragm. The closing capacity (CC) is that volume of the lung where small airways in the dependent parts of the lung begin to collapse during expiration. Normally CC is less than FRC

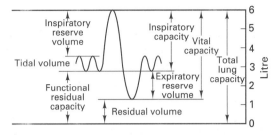

Fig. 1.3   The static lung volumes in a normal 70 kg adult male.

Table 1.1   Factors influencing the functional residual capacity (FRC).

Factors decreasing FRC
  Increasing age
  Posture – supine
  Anaesthesia – intraoperative
  Abdominal and thoracic surgery – postoperative
  Pulmonary fibrosis
  Pulmonary oedema
  Obesity
  Abdominal swelling – pregnancy, tumour, ascites
  Thoracic cage distortion
  Reduced muscle tone

Factors increasing FRC
  Increased intrathoracic pressure – PEEP, CPAP
  Emphysema
  Asthma

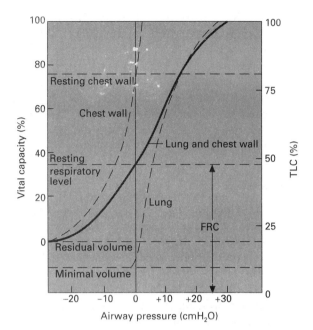

Fig. 1.4   The compliance curves of the lungs, chest wall and total respiratory system. The latter is obtained by adding the individual curves. The FRC is a balance between the lung and chest wall.

but greater than RV. This can be demonstrated by expiration to RV which is inevitably followed by a sigh to re-expand collapsed lung. CC increases with age and FRC is decreased by a number of factors (Table 1.1) and if CC is greater than FRC, dependent parts of the lung collapse during normal tidal breathing resulting in hypoxaemia.

The volumes described above are obtained by slow breathing so that airway resistance is not important. For clinical evaluation of patients, dynamic lung volumes are more useful such as the forced vital capacity (FVC) and the forced expiratory volume in the first second (FEV_1). The limiting factor in a forced expiration is the dynamic compression of the intrathoracic airways by the raised intrathoracic pressure.

Compliance

Both the lungs and the chest wall require a distending force, usually expressed as volume change per unit of distending pressure (compliance) ($ml.cmH_2O^{-1}$) and are both approximately 200 $ml.cmH_2O^{-1}$. The compliance of the whole respiratory system (100 $ml.cmH_2O^{-1}$) is clearly less than the individual components and is derived by adding the reciprocals ($1/200 + 1/200$). The compliance curve of the lung is shown in Figure 1.4. The compliance is approximately linear over most of the range but is less when the lung is small and nearly fully inflated. The former is due to the added force needed to expand collapsed areas of the lung and overcome surface tension effects and the latter is due to the elastic fibres in the lung reaching their limit.

The lung exhibits hysteresis, i.e. the compliance differs during inflation and deflation. This is due to the effect of alveolar surfactant and is absent if the lung is inflated with a fluid.

Surfactant

If the alveoli are regarded as a series of interconnected bubbles then the normal surface tension effects would ensure that the smaller bubbles emptied into the larger. However, the presence of a surface active material, dipalmitoyl lecithin, secreted by the type II alveolar cells, ensures that this does not occur. As the alveolus decreases in size, the concentration of surfactant in the surface layer of fluid increases, thus effectively reducing the surface tension. Collapsed lung and small airways have no air–liquid interface and thus additional force is required to open those areas.

Resistance

The flow of air into and out of the lungs is opposed by the frictional resistance of the airways and to a lesser extent by the inertia of the gas. The type of flow is important, with laminar flow offering less resistance than transitional or turbulent flow. Laminar flow occurs at low flow rates and in the smaller bronchi. In the larger airways and at branches in the bronchial tree, transitional and turbulent flow may occur.

Laminar flow rate ($\dot{V}$) is related to driving pressure (δP) by Poiseuille's equation:

$$\dot{V} = \frac{\delta P \pi r^4}{8 \eta L}$$

where r is the radius of the tube, L its length and η the viscosity of the gas. Note that the radius of the tube is critical, a halving of the tube diameter reducing the flow by a factor of 16 for the same δP, an important factor in paediatric practice.

Airway resistance is related to lung volume, decreasing as the lung expands. It is also related to bronchomotor tone and the thickness of the mucosal layer.

MATCHING OF VENTILATION AND PERFUSION

As noted earlier, the purpose of the lungs is to exchange gases by bringing the inspired gas into contact with pulmonary capillary blood. Under normal circumstances, the distributions of ventilation and blood flow are nearly perfectly matched. The main determinant of the distribution of perfusion is gravity which is not under bodily control and thus the changes necessary to ensure matching with changes in posture predominantly occur in the distribution of ventilation.

Distribution of perfusion

The distribution of blood flow within the lungs is largely influenced by gravity with the dependent portions of the lung being best perfused. In the erect posture three distinct zones may be described (Fig. 1.5). In the upper zone, alveolar pressure exceeds both pulmonary arterial and venous pressures and there is no flow. This zone does not occur under normal conditions but may occur in the presence of hypovolaemia and with increased alveolar pressure. In the middle zone alveolar pressure is exceeded by pulmonary artery pressure but is greater than pulmonary venous pressure. In the lower zone, both pulmonary arterial and venous pressures exceed alveolar pressure. In both these latter zones flow increases in the more dependent areas.

Within the substance of the lung, the pulmonary arteries divide and subdivide following the lobar pattern of the bronchi. The pulmonary capillaries form a dense network around the alveoli. The nuclei of the endothelial cells and supportive collagen fibres are arranged so that they are on the opposite side to the alveoli and gas diffusion occurs through the thinned service wall which comprises just the flattened epithelial and endothelial cells and their fused basement membranes (Fig. 1.6). A red cell traverses two or three alveoli in its passage through the lung.

Diffusion of CO_2 and oxygen is very rapid and under normal circumstances saturation of the

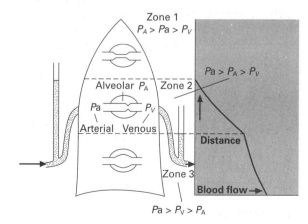

Fig. 1.5 Pressure flow relationships in different parts of the lung in the erect posture. The three zones are described in the text. (Redrawn from West et al 1964.)

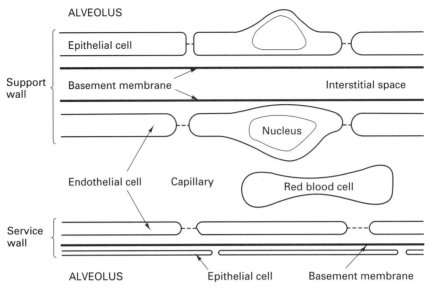

Fig. 1.6 Cross-section of the alveolar wall.

haemoglobin with oxygen is complete before the red cell is halfway through its journey.

Distribution of ventilation

Several factors ensure that the inspired gas is directed towards the dependent parts of the lungs. The major factor is the compliance of the different parts of the lung. A pressure gradient exists from the top to the bottom of the pleural space due to the weight of the lung such that it is less negative at the base compared with the apex. The different parts of the lung are thus on different parts of the compliance curve (Fig. 1.7). When inspiration occurs the *change* in pleural pressure, typically about 5 cmH_2O for an average V_t, is the same for all parts of the lung but results in a greater increase in volume in the dependent parts of the lung than the non-dependent parts.

Hypoxic pulmonary vasoconstriction

The mechanisms outlined above are very effective at matching blood flow and gas exchange but the local fine tuning is achieved by a local reflex vasoconstriction in the supplying pulmonary artery in response to alveolar hypoxaemia. This mechanism is of minor importance in the normal lung but very important in the presence of disease such as

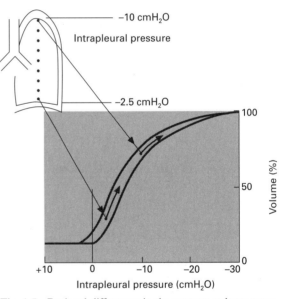

Fig. 1.7 Regional differences in the pressure volume curve of the lung. The same change in pressure causes a greater change in volume at the base of the lung compared with the apex.

pneumonia or during one-lung anaesthesia for thoracic surgery.

Dead space, $\dot{V}/\dot{Q}$ matching and shunt

In ideally ventilated and perfused lung the ratio

between alveolar ventilation and perfusion ($\dot{V}/\dot{Q}$) is 1.0. If ventilation exceeds perfusion the ratio is >1 and if perfusion is absent = ∞. Conversely if perfusion exceeds ventilation the $\dot{V}/\dot{Q}$ ratio is <1 and if ventilation is absent = 0. The former condition comprises part of the dead space and the latter comprises part of the intrapulmonary shunt.

Dead space

The dead space of the respiratory system is that part which does not participate in gas exchange. It comprises the anatomical dead space, the upper airway and tracheobronchial tree down to the respiratory bronchioles and the physiological dead space, those parts of the lung whose $\dot{V}/\dot{Q}$ ratio is >1. The anatomical dead space is about 150 ml in the average adult and may be reduced by a tracheal tube. The more useful measure is the ratio of dead space (V_d) to tidal volume (V_t).

The volume of CO_2 expired in a single breath is the product of V_t and the mixed expired concentration ($F\bar{E}_{CO_2}$). This is comprised of gas from the alveoli (V_A) whose CO_2 concentration is the same as arterial blood and the dead space which contains no CO_2. Gas concentrations can be converted into partial pressure if the barometric pressure is known. V_A is equal to V_t-V_d and thus:

$$V_t \times P\bar{E}_{CO_2} = (V_t-V_d) \times Pa_{CO_2}$$

This can be rearranged to give Bohr's equation:

$$\frac{V_d}{V_t} = \frac{Pa_{CO_2} - P\bar{E}_{CO_2}}{Pa_{CO_2}}$$

The ratio is about 0.3 under normal circumstances over a wide range of tidal volume from 50 ml to 1.5 l. At greater tidal volumes, dead space is greater than the anatomical because of dilatation of the airways and by increased ventilation of the upper parts of the lung where the $\dot{V}/\dot{Q}$ ratio is >1. When tidal volume is less than the anatomical dead space, the apparent dead space is reduced by the tendency of the gas flow in the airway to be axial. The gas adjacent to the wall of the airway moves very little, thus decreasing the effective diameter of the airway.

Shunt

The oxygen tension in the arterial blood (Pa_{O_2})

is less than that in the alveolus (PA_{O_2}). This difference ($PA_{O_2} - Pa_{O_2}$) is due to the diffusion gradient across the alveolar capillary membrane, dilution of the pulmonary capillary blood by blood which has bypassed the lungs (bronchial circulation, Thebesian veins and cardiac anomalies) and which has come from areas of the lung with a $\dot{V}/\dot{Q}$ ratio of <1. For convenience the different causes of an A–a difference can be aggregated and the lung regarded as perfect but with a proportion of the cardiac output ($\dot{Q}_t$) bypassing or shunting past the lungs ($\dot{Q}_s$). The ratio $\dot{Q}_s/\dot{Q}_t$ (virtual shunt fraction) is derived in a similar way to the Bohr equation:

$$\frac{\dot{Q}_s}{\dot{Q}_t} = \frac{Cc'_{O_2} - Ca_{O_2}}{Cc'_{O_2} - C\bar{v}_{O_2}}$$

where Cc'_{O_2}, Ca_{O_2}, $C\bar{v}_{O_2}$ are the oxygen content (ml/100 ml^{-1} blood) of end pulmonary capillary, arterial and mixed venous blood respectively. The concept of virtual shunt, which normally is less than 4% of cardiac output, is useful in critically ill patients.

GAS EXCHANGE AND CARRIAGE

Oxygen is utilized and CO_2 is produced in the mitochondria. This section describes the means by which the gases are transported to and from the atmosphere to the cells.

Oxygen

Oxygen cascade

The oxygen cascade (Fig. 1.8) is a convenient method for demonstrating the steps in the concentration gradient for oxygen between the atmosphere and the mitochondria.

The partial pressure of oxygen in the inspired air (PI_{O_2}) is about 21 kPa (160 mmHg) and is influenced by barometric pressure (P_B) and the fractional concentration of oxygen (FI_{O_2}) (0.21).

$$PI_{O_2} = P_B \times FI_{O_2}$$

The inspired gas is 'diluted' by the presence of water vapour and as it is fully saturated the reduction is determined by:

$$PI_{O_2(sat)} = (P_B - P_{H_2O}) \times FI_{O_2}$$

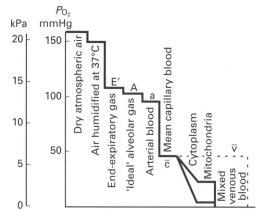

Fig. 1.8 The oxygen cascade.

Where P_{H_2O} is the saturated vapour pressure of water at 37°C (normally 6.3 kPa, 47 mmHg).

The inspired gas is further 'diluted' by the addition of carbon dioxide and the removal of oxygen in the alveolus. With a normal diet, slightly less CO_2 is produced than oxygen is consumed (respiratory quotient (RQ) < 1.0) and the alveolar oxygen tension (P_{AO_2}) is given by the alveolar air equation:

$$P_{AO_2} = P_{IO_2} - \frac{P_{ACO_2}}{RQ}$$

As noted above, the difference between the P_{ACO_2} and the P_{aCO_2} is very small and the latter term may be substituted into the equation. This is an important equation; for example, it enables the effect of changing the minute ventilation (hyper- and hypoventilation) on P_{aO_2} to be determined.

The relationship between alveolar ventilation ($\dot{V}_A$) and P_{ACO_2} is shown in Figure 1.9 and is exponential. Thus a doubling of $\dot{V}_A$ results in a halving of P_{ACO_2} and a halving of $\dot{V}_A$ results in a doubling of P_{ACO_2}. If this change is entered into the alveolar air equation then the relationship between $\dot{V}_A$ and P_{AO_2} shown in Figure 1.9 becomes apparent. Two curves are shown, the lower for an F_{IO_2} of 0.21 and the upper for an F_{IO_2} of 0.3. It can be seen that hypoxaemia develops rapidly as $\dot{V}_A$ decreases but is readily corrected by a small increase in F_{IO_2} while hyperventilation results in little increase in P_{AO_2}.

Oxygen then diffuses from the alveolus to the red cell where it binds with haemoglobin.

Haemoglobin

Each 100 ml of blood contains about 20 ml of oxygen, almost all of which is carried on the haemoglobin. Oxygen is poorly soluble in blood (0.023 ml.100 ml^{-1} blood.kPa^{-1} (0.003 ml.100 ml^{-1}

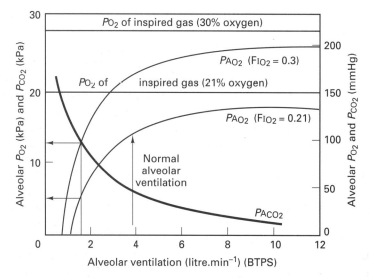

Fig. 1.9 The effect of changing alveolar ventilation on P_{ACO_2} (heavy line) and on P_{AO_2} (light lines). The effect of increasing the F_{IO_2} from 0.21 to 0.3 on P_{AO_2} is also shown.

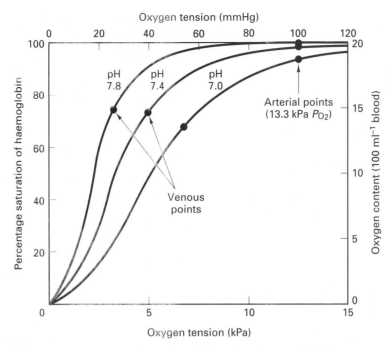

Fig. 1.10 The oxyhaemoglobin dissociation curves for normal adult haemoglobin at normal pH and with acidosis and alkalosis.

blood.$mmHg^{-1}$)). The oxygen content of blood (C_{O_2}) is thus:

$$C_{O_2} \text{ (ml.100 ml}^{-1} \text{ blood)} = 0.023 \times P_{O_2} \text{ (kPa)} + (1.34 \times Hb \text{ (g.dl}^{-1}) \times S_{O_2} \text{ (\%)}/100$$

where S_{O_2} is the oxyhaemoglobin saturation. Each molecule of Hb can carry four molecules of oxygen, the relationship between P_{O_2} and S_{O_2} being the familiar sigmoid shape of the oxyhaemoglobin dissociation curve (Fig. 1.10). The normal Pa_{O_2} is about 13 kPa (100 mmHg) and Sa_{O_2} is 97% while the mixed venous values ($P\bar{v}_{O_2}$ and $S\bar{v}_{O_2}$) are 6 kPa (45 mmHg) and 75% respectively. Note that increasing the Pa_{O_2} above normal has little effect on arterial oxygen content because of the poor solubility of oxygen and thus the venous point changes little even if 100% oxygen is respired. $P\bar{v}_{O_2}$ is determined by the balance between oxygen supply and demand. Thus an increased demand (e.g. shivering) or decreased supply (e.g. cardiogenic shock) reduces $P\bar{v}_{O_2}$ while a decreased utilization (e.g. cyanide poisoning) or excessive supply (e.g. sepsis) increases it.

The position of the curve is best described by the P_{50}, the P_{O_2} at which the Hb is 50% saturated

(3.6 kPa, 27 mmHg). Several factors can influence the curve. An increase in temperature, P_{CO_2}, hydrogen ion concentration (decrease in pH) and concentration of 2,3-diphosphoglycerate all shift the curve to the right while a decrease in these factors shifts the curve to the left. Displacement of the curve to the right (acidosis) slightly decreases the affinity for oxygen in the lungs but increases the availability of oxygen in the tissues. Conversely, displacement to the left (alkalosis) slightly increases uptake in the lungs but renders the tissues hypoxic in order to achieve the same oxygen extraction. A small shift of the curve with pH and P_{CO_2} occurs under normal physiological conditions in the lungs and tissues to facilitate oxygen transport and is known as the Bohr effect.

The final part of the diffusion pathway for oxygen is from the haemoglobin to the mitochondria where the P_{O_2} is only 0.5–3 kPa (4–23 mmHg).

The oxygen stores of the body are limited to about 1500 ml of which about 750 ml is combined with Hb, 500 ml in the lungs and 250 ml combined with myoglobin. A glance at the oxyhaemoglobin dissociation curve shows that only about half the oxygen attached to Hb is available and almost none of that attached to myoglobin and thus the available stores in the event of apnoea are less than 1000 ml or 4 min at the normal $\dot{V}_{O_2}$ of 250 ml.min^{-1}. If cardiac arrest occurs, the stores in the lungs are unavailable and as the brain has no oxygen stores, unconsciousness occurs within 10 s. Preoxygenation with 100% oxygen increases the stores to about 4500 ml and thus increases the potential duration of apnoea at least fourfold.

Carbon dioxide

Carbon dioxide passes in a reverse cascade from mitochondria to atmosphere. It is much more water soluble than oxygen and diffuses more readily. Carbon dioxide is mostly carried in the blood as bicarbonate ion (HCO_3^-):

$$CO_2 + H_2O \Leftrightarrow H_2CO_3 \Leftrightarrow H^+ + HCO_3^-$$

The first part of the reaction is inherently slow and is catalysed by carbonic anhydrase which is found in the red cells. The hydrogen ion is buffered by protein, predominantly reduced haemoglobin (Haldane effect) and the HCO_3^- diffuses into the red cell in exchange for chloride (Hamburger shift). The reverse occurs in the lungs as CO_2 is eliminated.

EFFECTS OF ANAESTHESIA ON RESPIRATION

The depressant effect of anaesthetic drugs on respiration has been known since the earliest days when the depth, character and rate of respiration were recognized as valuable clinical signs to the depth of anaesthesia.

Control of respiration

The volatile and intravenous anaesthetic agents and the opioid analgesics all depress respiration and decrease the responsiveness to CO_2. The response is not uniform, the opioids characteristically reducing respiratory rate while some of the volatile agents such as trichlorethylene may increase it. Hypoxic ventilatory drive is similarly impaired by the volatile agents in low concentrations.

Other respiratory responses such as the arousal response to airway obstruction and cough are reduced during anaesthesia. The pattern of respiration during anaesthesia tends to be regular without the intermittent sighs seen during wakefulness.

Mechanics of respiration

The induction of anaesthesia results in a reduction in the FRC of about 0.5 litre, probably due to cranial displacement of the diaphragm. This effect is greatest after neuromuscular blockade. The thoracic contribution to inspiration also diminishes and expiratory abdominal muscle activity increases, giving the characteristic pattern often seen during anaesthesia with spontaneous respiration.

Matching of ventilation and perfusion

Induction of anaesthesia does not affect the distribution of perfusion except that the increased intrathoracic pressure of mechanical ventilation may reduce cardiac output and increase or create the zone in the lung where alveolar pressure exceeds pulmonary arterial pressure, thus increasing dead space.

The distribution of ventilation is impaired during spontaneous respiration and worsened with mechanical ventilation when there is a reduction in the ventilation to the dependent parts of the lung. Atelectasis develops in the dependent areas. Hypoxic pulmonary vasoconstriction is abolished by low concentrations of volatile agents and the overall effect is to increase both dead space and shunt in the anaesthetized patient. Pa_{CO_2} is usually increased and Pa_{O_2} usually decreased during general anaesthesia and it is thus conventional to administer a gas mixture with an $F_{I_{O_2}}$ of about 0.3 during anaesthesia.

Gas exchange and carriage

Gas exchange is impaired during anaesthesia as outlined above and oxygen carriage may be impaired by the reduced cardiac output. However, the reduced metabolic rate tends to compensate for the reduced oxygen delivery. By reducing the Pa_{CO_2} hyperventilation reduces oxygen delivery by shifting the oxyhaemoglobin dissociation curve to the left (see above). The associated vasoconstriction further impairs tissue oxygenation.

Increased oxygen consumption

Shivering commonly occurs in the postoperative period causing a marked increase in oxygen consumption. Cardiac output cannot always increase to meet the demand and mixed venous oxygen tension decreases. This increases the impact of intrapulmonary shunting due to atelectasis and $\dot{V}/\dot{Q}$ mismatching and worsens arterial oxygenation and sets up a 'vicious circle'.

Second gas effect

Under normal circumstances only oxygen is taken up from the lungs and there is no net uptake of nitrogen. When a second gas which is absorbed rapidly, such as nitrous oxide, is introduced into the lungs then the uptake of that gas has the effect of 'concentrating' the gases remaining in the alveoli. The effect on oxygen is of no clinical importance but the increase in concentration of volatile anaesthetic agents speeds the induction of anaesthesia.

The reverse occurs when the administration of nitrous oxide is stopped. The elimination of the gas 'dilutes' the alveolar gases and may result in significant hypoxaemia unless the $F_{I_{O_2}}$ is increased. This effect lasts for about 5 min after discontinuation of the nitrous oxide.

NON-RESPIRATORY FUNCTIONS

Acid–base balance

Maintenance of a normal arterial pH is important for cellular function and the respiratory system provides a means for rapid adjustment by controlling the elimination of an important acid, carbonic acid.

Rearrangement of the equation for the buffering of CO_2 given above gives the familiar Henderson–Hasselbach equation. It can be seen that alterations to the Pa_{CO_2} affect the pH.

$$pH = pK + \frac{[HCO_3^-]}{s \times Pa_{CO_2}}$$

A decrease in plasma pH stimulates the respiratory centre via the central chemoreceptors, increasing alveolar ventilation and reducing Pa_{CO_2}. This is well shown in diabetic ketoacidosis where the patient is usually found to be hyperventilating, demonstrating respiratory compensation for a metabolic acidosis.

The reverse occurs during a metabolic alkalosis when Pa_{CO_2} increases. Metabolic compensation also occurs for chronic changes in the respiratory component of acid base balance. With a chronic reduction in Pa_{CO_2}, for example following an ascent to high altitude when the reduced Pa_{O_2} has stimulated respiration, there is increased renal loss of bicarbonate ion thus restoring the pH towards normal. Conversely, when Pa_{CO_2} is chronically increased with respiratory failure, the kidney retains bicarbonate to maintain the balance.

Metabolic

The lungs have many of the enzyme systems found in the liver but as their metabolic mass is considerably less, their contribution to overall drug metabolism is small. Nevertheless, they have considerable synthetic and metabolic functions.

Synthesis

Surfactant is synthesized by the type II alveolar cells and is necessary for the stability of the alveoli (see above). Coagulation factors, including heparin and various components of the pulmonary defence mechanisms, are also produced and are discussed below.

Metabolism

The best known metabolic function of the lung is the conversion of angiotensin I, which is inactive, to the active angiotensin II. Several other hormones are also inactivated by passage through the lung, including noradrenaline, serotonin, bradykinin, prostaglandins and leukotrienes.

The cytochrome P-450 general oxidative system is active in the lung and several largely basic drugs are metabolized to some extent. However, the contribution is generally small in comparison with the liver.

Filtration

Any particulate matter, including thrombi, released

into the venous system passes to the lungs. The theoretical pore size of the lung as a filter is about 70 μm although in practice, much large particles can traverse the lungs, presumably through arteriovenous connections.

The lung possesses active proteolytic systems for dissolving fibrin clots and the endothelium contains plasmin activator which converts plasminogen to plasmin. It is also rich in heparin and thromboplastin and presumably plays a role in the regulation of coagulation.

Pulmonary defence mechanisms

Inhaled air contains particles of dust and airborne bacteria and viruses. The respiratory system contains several defence mechanisms to protect the lower airways and alveoli. The primary defence is the nose with its lining of mucus-producing ciliated epithelium. The turbinates ensure turbulence thus avoiding streaming of the inhaled air. The nasal mucosa becomes engorged and secretes extra mucus in response to inhaled irritants, as every hayfever sufferer knows. The tracheobronchial tree is also lined with ciliated epithelium and equipped with mucus glands. The cilia sweep the mucus coat with the entrapped particles towards the pharynx where it is swallowed with the saliva. Coughing (see above) also contributes.

Cellular mechanisms

Pulmonary macrophages are found throughout the airways and alveoli. They phagocytose inhaled particles and microorganisms, producing several proteases to kill the bacteria. The lung contains α_1-antitrypsin to inactivate the proteases and prevent damage to itself. The macrophages also lead to the release of highly reactive oxygen compounds, including the superoxide radical. Superoxide dismutase is produced in the lung to prevent damage from these compounds. IgA is secreted in pulmonary mucus and contributes to the killing of microorganisms.

FURTHER READING

Nunn J F 1993 Nunn's applied respiratory physiology, 4th edn. Butterworths, London
West J B, Dollery C T, Naimark A 1964 Distribution of blood flow in isolated lung: relation to vascular and alveolar pressures. J Appl Physiol 19: 713–724
West J B 1985 Respiratory physiology – the essentials, 3rd edn. Williams & Wilkins, Baltimore
West J B 1985 Ventilation, blood flow and gas exchange, 4th edn. Blackwell Scientific Publications, Oxford

2. Cardiovascular physiology

The purpose of the cardiovascular system is the delivery of oxygen and nutrients to the organs and the removal of metabolites. It also acts as the conduit for cells of the immune system and hormones.

The cardiovascular system may be considered under two major headings: the peripheral circulation, which adjusts blood flow to individual tissues, and the heart which generates the sum of the individual flows.

PERIPHERAL CIRCULATION

Under normal physiological conditions, blood flow through an organ is determined by its metabolic requirements and is independent of perfusion pressure (autoregulation). Blood flow per unit mass of tissue varies widely from organ to organ both in the basal resting state and at maximum flow (Fig. 2.1). Disease states, such as hypovolaemia and sepsis, and drug therapy, including anaesthesia, may interfere with autoregulatory mechanisms resulting in excessive or inadequate perfusion.

Blood flow rate is determined by the driving pressure (the difference between mean arterial pressure, MAP, and mean venous pressure, MVP), and the resistance to that flow.

$$\text{Flow} = \frac{\text{MAP} - \text{MVP}}{\text{Resistance}}$$

Resistance to blood flow is determined by three

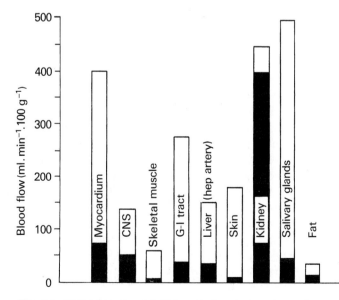

Fig. 2.1 Blood flow at rest (solid portion) and at maximum flow rate (total height) in various organs.

factors: calibre and length of the vessels, viscosity of blood and nature of the flow (turbulent or laminar).

Flow profile

In the absence of irregularities of the vessel wall (e.g. resulting from atheroma), flow in blood vessels is laminar. The relationship between driving pressure and flow under such conditions is expressed by the Hagen–Poiseuille formula:

$$\dot{Q} = \frac{\delta P \pi r^4}{8 \eta L}$$

where $\dot{Q}$ is the flow rate, r the radius of the vessel and L its length. δP is the driving pressure and η the blood viscosity. This relationship holds true only for steady flow of Newtonian fluids, i.e. those whose viscosity is independent of flow rate. These conditions do not apply to the cardiovascular system, where flow is pulsatile and blood viscosity is determined by flow rate. It is thus an over-simplification, but illustrates the critical role of the vessel radius in determining flow rate, since the relationship is to the fourth power of the radius.

Viscosity

Blood is a mixture of solutes (e.g. electrolytes and proteins) and particles (e.g. cells and chylomicrons). At low flow rates, the cells tend to aggregate, thus increasing viscosity. The subject is further complicated by the tendency of cells to concentrate in the centre of the blood vessel where the velocity is greatest. The haematocrit is therefore lowest at the periphery of the lumen where the velocity is lowest. Thus blood tends to act much more as a Newtonian fluid in vivo than in vitro. The tendency of erythrocytes to concentrate in the centre of a vessel results in a lower haematocrit in blood which enters side branches. This process is known as plasma skimming and has obvious implications for flow rate and oxygen delivery.

Anaemia reduces oxygen carrying capacity and results in an increase in blood flow to maintain oxygen delivery. The increased flow rate is facilitated by reduced viscosity secondary to the reduced erythrocyte count. Clinically, there is little effect on cardiac index until the haemoglobin concentra-

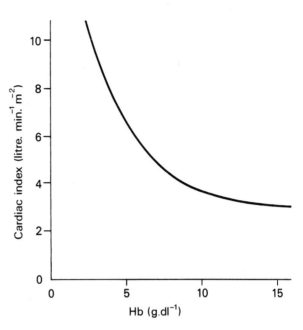

Fig. 2.2 Relationship between haemoglobin concentration and cardiac index in chronic anaemia.

tion decreases below 10 g.dl^{-1} (Fig. 2.2), the usually accepted lower limit for routine anaesthesia.

Volatile anaesthetic agents increase blood viscosity by increasing the rigidity of the erythrocyte membrane. However, the effect is slight in comparison with the effect of anaemia and has no significant effect on tissue blood flow rates.

Control of the peripheral circulation

Blood flow through the capillary beds is controlled by local mechanisms and, under normal circumstances, cardiac output adjusts to meet the total flow required. Regulatory mechanisms ensure that the perfusion pressure (arterial pressure) is maintained irrespective of changes in total flow and posture. During periods of stress, e.g. hypovolaemia, the regulatory mechanisms override local control to maintain the blood supply of essential organs including the brain, heart and kidney. These organs also possess autoregulation, i.e. a constant blood flow despite changes in perfusion pressure.

The capillary bed (Fig. 2.3)

Capillaries are composed of a single layer of endothelial cells which permit free exchange of

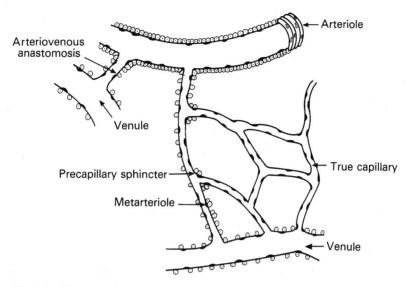

Fig. 2.3 Diagrammatic representation of the microcirculation.

nutrients and metabolites between tissues and blood. Not all capillaries are open at any one time and there are generally preferred routes through which blood flows predominantly. The density of capillaries in tissue is dependent upon the maximum oxygen consumption and the oxygen delivery. Capillary density increases as a response to arterial hypoxaemia.

In many tissues, there are also direct arteriovenous anastomoses. In the skin, these facilitate heart loss by increasing tissue flow rate without affecting capillary perfusion.

Control of flow through capillaries is effected by contraction and relaxation of the smooth muscle of the metarterioles and the precapillary sphincters. A number of metabolic factors including oxygen, ATP, nitric oxide and hydrogen ions have been shown to affect capillary flow but the exact mechanism has not been elucidated.

Local regulation of flow by metabolites controls the distribution of blood flow within an organ, in addition to total flow.

Control of the systemic circulation

The systemic circulation is controlled by mechanisms which determine the distribution of blood flow according to priority rather than local needs, the maintenance of an adequate perfusion pressure and the adjustment of cardiac output by variations in the capacity of the circulation.

Arteriolar diameter

The calibre of the arterioles and precapillary sphincters determines blood flow to the peripheral circulation. The calibre depends upon the inherent tone of the smooth muscle, the activity of the autonomic nervous system, circulating hormones and the local concentration of metabolites (Fig. 2.4).

Inherent tone

Smooth muscle generally exhibits spontaneous contraction in the absence of other stimuli and this is the likely source of inherent tone. Mechanical stretching of the muscle by pulsatile internal pressure may also initiate contractions. In general, those tissues with the least sympathetic innervation have the greatest inherent tone. For example, vessels in skeletal muscle, brain and myocardium have a high tone whereas those in skin have a low inherent tone.

Some years ago it was shown that the ability of a blood vessel to react depended upon the presence of an intact endothelium. Recent work (Searle & Sahab 1992) has shown that a number of factors including shear stress from blood flow,

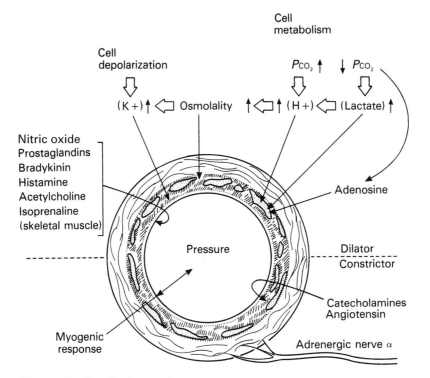

Fig. 2.4   Factors affecting vascular tone.

catecholamines, acetylcholine, serotonin and hypoxia act through a calcium dependent enzyme which converts l-arginine to nitric oxide (NO) within the endothelial cells. The nitric oxide diffuses to the vascular smooth muscle where it induces relaxation by conversion of cyclic GMP to cyclic AMP. Studies with inhibitors of NO synthase have resulted in hypertension, suggesting that the vascular smooth muscle is under a tonic vasodilator influence as well as a tonic vasoconstrictor influence.

Autonomic nervous system (Chs 4 and 12)

Sympathetic adrenergic (Fig. 2.5). The adrenergic sympathetic fibres are the predominant pathway whereby the systemic circulation is controlled. The vasomotor areas in the medulla send descending fibres to the preganglionic cells in the thoracolumbar segment of the spinal cord. The preganglionic fibres synapse with postganglionic fibres in the ganglia of the sympathetic chain from which postganglionic fibres travel to vascular

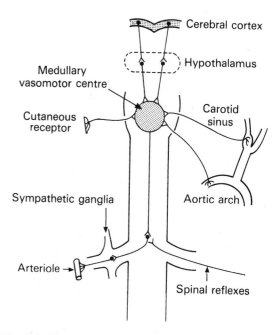

Fig. 2.5   The vasomotor centre.

smooth muscle. Noradrenaline is the transmitter which acts on the α_1 receptors on the vascular smooth muscle. The activity of the vasomotor centres is influenced by afferent impulses from many sensory areas including baroreceptors, chemoreceptors and skin and from higher centres in the cortex and hypothalamus. The preganglionic cells in the spinal cord may also be influenced directly by higher centres and by reflex activity at spinal level.

The vasomotor centre is active continuously, resulting in a resting tone in vascular smooth muscle. Increased sympathetic activity does not affect all tissues equally. Tissues with the highest intrinsic vascular tone respond less well than those with a lower tone (Fig. 2.6). Thus with increased adrenergic sympathetic activity there is redistribution of blood from skin, muscle and gut to brain, heart and kidney.

Sympathetic cholinergic. Activation of sympathetic cholinergic fibres results in vasodilatation in skeletal muscle. These fibres are represented centrally in the cerebral cortex and are involved in the anticipatory response to exercise, the 'fight or flight' reaction. Stimulation of the appropriate area of the brain results in redistribution of blood flow from skin and viscera to skeletal muscle.

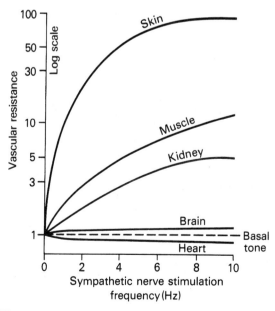

Fig. 2.6 The effect of sympathetic nervous stimulation on vascular resistance in various organs.

Vascular smooth muscle in skeletal muscle, heart and liver also possesses β2 adrenergic receptors which have a vasodilator effect.

Dopaminergic receptors. Dopamine is a precursor of noradrenaline and has been shown to have a vasodilator effect on splanchnic and renal vessels mediated through specific receptors. This response is useful pharmacologically but the physiological role of such receptors is unclear.

Humoral control. Adrenaline and noradrenaline are released by the adrenal medulla and from adrenergic nerve endings. Their concentrations may increase dramatically during stress but they probably contribute little to cardiovascular control. Their prime role may be in the metabolic response to stress.

Angiotensin II is a potent vasopressor produced by the conversion of angiotensinogen by renin. Renin is released from the juxtaglomerular apparatus of the kidney in response to a reduction in systemic arterial pressure. Angiotensin II probably plays little part in acute regulation of the circulation but, by increasing the secretion of aldosterone, leads to retention of sodium and hence an increase in circulating volume.

Metabolic control

A number of metabolites influence the calibre of blood vessels, including CO_2, K^+ and H^+. Adenosine, bradykinin and prostaglandins are among the chemicals known to cause vasodilatation. It is likely that different tissues respond more readily to some compounds than others.

Induced hypocapnia resulting from hyperventilation results is generalized vasoconstriction and reduction in tissue blood flow which may be deleterious.

Hypoxia results in vasodilatation in all parts of the circulation except the pulmonary vessels, where vasoconstriction occurs. The vasodilatation is countered by reflex vasoconstriction mediated by the sympathetic nervous system resulting from stimulation of the chemoreceptors. This acts as a protective mechanism to increase blood flow to the brain.

Autoregulation

Blood flow through many organs remains almost

constant over a wide range of perfusion pressure. In man, this phenomenon is most marked in the renal and cerebral circulations. The mechanism is unclear, although accumulation or washout of vasodilator metabolites seems a likely explanation. Alterations in the intrinsic tone of vascular smooth muscle have also been proposed.

Measurement of blood flow

The measurement of blood flow in absolute terms through tissues is technically difficult. However, the relationship between flow and oxygen consumption is of more importance. If the imbalance is severe, organ failure occurs and this may be manifest in oliguria, clouding of consciousness, etc. Clinically, it is useful to assess flow in the organ which is most accessible, the skin. Clinical assessment of skin flow by capillary refill may be supplemented by the measurement of the gradient between core temperature and skin temperature, which is normally less than 5°C. Mixed venous oxygen tension may provide a global assessment of the adequacy of tissue perfusion. Normal mixed venous oxygen tension is 6 kPa and values below 3.7 kPa are associated with a poor prognosis. The value must be interpreted with care particularly in the presence of arteriovenous shunting of blood, when the value may be elevated despite tissue hypoxia.

The adequacy of gut mucosal perfusion can be assessed from the indirect measurement of its pH (pHi). Values less than 7.2 are indicative of mucosal ischaemia and are useful prognostic indicators (Gutierrez et al 1992).

Capacitance vessels

The veins contain approximately 80% of the blood volume (Fig. 2.7). Venoconstriction and dilatation adjust the capacity of the circulation to maintain a balance with the blood volume, for example during hypovolaemia (see below) and with changes in posture. Impairment of venoconstriction by disease or drugs, e.g. antihypertensive agents, leads to a reduction in cardiac output and hypotension on standing (postural hypotension).

The calibre of the veins is adjusted by changes in sympathetic activity, mediated both by nervous

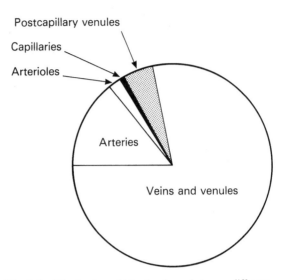

Fig. 2.7 Distribution of blood volume between different parts of the circulation.

and humoral stimulation. The postcapillary venules are also sensitive to local concentrations of metabolites in the same manner as the precapillary sphincters.

Control of arterial pressure

Systemic arterial pressure is controlled closely in order to maintain the driving pressure necessary for tissue perfusion. The normal values vary with age and sex (Table 2.1) in addition to physiological changes including sleep. It must be stressed that although systemic arterial pressure may be measured readily the readings obtained should be interpreted with care. A normal or even elevated arterial pressure is no guarantee of adequate tissue perfusion. Mean arterial pressure (MAP) may be calculated from the formula:

$$\text{MAP} = \text{diastolic arterial pressure} + \frac{\text{pulse pressure}}{3}$$

Its value is determined by the product of cardiac output (CO) and total systemic peripheral resistance (TPR).

$$\text{MAP} = \text{CO} \times \text{TPR}$$

Traditionally, the units of TPR have been expressed as dyne.s.cm^{-5} and more recently as N.s.m^{-5} (1 dyne.s.cm^{-5} = 100 N.s.m^{-5}).

Table 2.1 Changes in arterial pressure, cardiac output and peripheral vascular resistance with age

| Age (years) | Arterial pressure (mmHg) | | Blood flow | | Peripheral vascular resistance** | |
	Systolic/diastolic	Mean	Cardiac index* (litre.min^{-1}.m^{-2})	Cardiac output (litre.min^{-1})	(mmHg.litre^{-1}.min^{-1})	(dyne.s.cm^{-5})
10	100/65	75	4.0	4.8	15	1150
20	110/70	85	3.7	6.7	12	950
30	115/75	90	3.4	6.1	14	1100
40	120/80	92	3.2	5.8	15	1200
50	125/82	95	3.0	5.4	17	1300
60	130/85	98	2.8	5.0	19	1500
70	135/88	102	2.6	4.7	21	1650
80	140/90	105	2.5	4.5	22	1800

* Assuming a body surface area of 1.2 m^2 at age 10 and 1.8 m^2 thereafter
** Assuming a CVP of 5 mmHg

$$TPR \text{ (dyne.s.cm}^{-5}) = \frac{MAP \text{ (mmHg)}}{CO \text{ (litre.min}^{-1})} \times 80$$

Thus, if MAP = 100 mmHg and CO = 5 litre.min^{-1}, TPR = 1600 dyne.s.cm^{-5}.

Mean arterial pressure is thus a balance between cardiac output and resistance to flow posed by the vascular beds.

Neurones in the medulla receive and integrate afferent impulses from the baroreceptors, chemoreceptors, skin, muscle and viscera and from higher centres, the hypothalamus and cortex. Classically these neurones have been described as a discrete vasomotor centre but it is now thought that they are distributed in several regions of the medulla. Activity in these neurones leads to increased vasoconstrictor tone and thus an increased arterial pressure, provided that cardiac output does not decrease.

Baroreceptors

Arterial baroreceptors are located in the carotid sinus and the wall of the aortic arch. The nerve endings are not sensitive to pressure but to deformation of the arterial wall (stretch receptors). Stimulation of the baroreceptors leads to reflex reduction in vasoconstrictor and venoconstrictor tone and to bradycardia. Arterial pressure is thus reduced by diminution of both total peripheral resistance and cardiac output. Conversely a reduction in baroreceptor activity leads to vaso- and venoconstriction and increased heart rate.

Other cardiovascular reflexes

The chemoreceptors located in the carotid and aortic bodies respond to hypoxaemia and, to a lesser extent, hypoperfusion. Chemoreceptor stimulation results in a general increase in cardiovascular sympathetic activity, increasing systemic arterial pressure.

A large number of stretch receptors have been described in the heart and great vessels but their role is unclear. Stimulation of receptors in the atria increases sympathetic activity, thus aiding the increase in cardiac output which results from increased atrial pressure. Other atrial receptors appear to be responsible for regulation of blood volume by influencing ADH release and thus water balance.

Assessment of baroreceptor responses

The blood pressure response to change in posture is a useful guide to the ability of a patient to respond to cardiovascular stress. This is of importance in patients with autonomic neuropathy (e.g. diabetics) and those receiving vasodilator drugs.

The Valsalva manoeuvre, a forced expiration against a closed glottis resulting in increased intrathoracic pressure and decreased venous return, is a convenient clinical assessment also. In the normal individual, arterial pressure is maintained by a combination of tachycardia and vasoconstriction during the period of increased intrathoracic pressure (Fig. 2.8). On release of the raised

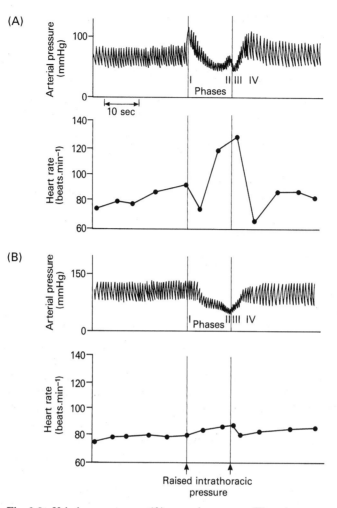

Fig. 2.8 Valsalva manoeuvre: (**A**) normal response; (**B**) patient with impaired cardiovascular control. See text for details.

intrathoracic pressure there is transient hypertension and bradycardia until the vasoconstriction is reversed. The heart rate response is easiest to detect and may be measured at the bedside.

The baroreceptors may be tested also by external stimulation or by inducing a transient increase in arterial pressure by administration of a short acting vasopressor, e.g. noradrenaline. These latter tests are more suitable for research than for clinical evaluation.

THE HEART

Anatomy

The heart comprises four chambers: the right and

left ventricles, which generate the energy to propel the blood around the pulmonary and systemic circulations respectively, and the atria which serve as reservoirs for blood and as accessory pumps to augment ventricular filling. Uncompensated loss of atrial activity, e.g. atrial fibrillation, reduces cardiac output by approximately 35%.

Cardiac muscle has properties intermediate between those of skeletal and smooth muscle. It has cross-striations similar to those of skeletal muscle and, in common with smooth muscle, exhibits spontaneous rhythmic contractions acting as a single unit or syncitium. The muscle fibres are arranged in an interdigitating spiral fashion to form the two ventricles. The left ventricle, which

(A) Right ventricular ejection

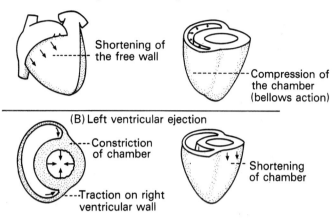

Shortening of the free wall

Compression of the chamber (bellows action)

(B) Left ventricular ejection

Constriction of chamber

Shortening of chamber

Traction on right ventricular wall

Fig. 2.9 Ventricular contraction. Note influence of left ventricular contraction on the right ventricle.

performs approximately six times as much work as the right, has a much thicker wall and is conical in shape. The right ventricular wall is thinner and applied to the left ventricular wall (Fig. 2.9). The ventricular and atrial muscle fibres are inserted into a fibrous framework at the atrioventricular junction which provides an attachment also for the cardiac valves.

The cardiac valves ensure that blood flows only from atria to ventricles to arterial systems. The aortic and pulmonary valves act passively, opening in response to a pressure gradient between ventricle and artery and closing when the gradient reverses. The tricuspid and mitral valves are prevented from bulging back into the atria during ventricular systole by the papillary muscles and their chordae tendineae.

The conducting system (Fig. 2.10) comprises fibres of specialized muscle cells and is responsible for the initiation and spread of cardiac contraction. The sinoatrial (SA) node lies in the wall of the right atrium close to the superior vena cava. An impulse originating here sweeps through the atria, leading to atrial systole, and activates the atrioventricular (AV) node. The AV node is continuous with the AV bundle (bundle of His)

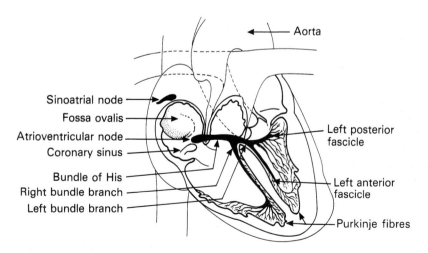

Aorta

Sinoatrial node
Fossa ovalis
Atrioventricular node
Coronary sinus
Bundle of His
Right bundle branch
Left bundle branch

Left posterior fascicle

Left anterior fascicle

Purkinje fibres

Fig. 2.10 The cardiac conducting system.

which pierces the fibrous septum separating atria and ventricles. The AV bundle runs through the ventricular septum and divides into right and left bundles which supply their respective ventricles.

Electrophysiology of the heart

A normal heart beat is initiated by cells of the SA node. The wave of contraction passes around the atria through the AV node and bundle to the ventricles. Cells of the conducting system (pacemaker cells) exhibit spontaneous depolarization resulting from a relative permeability to sodium ions (Fig. 2.11). At a threshold of −50 mV a sudden sharp depolarization occurs which is propagated to other cells, initiating a heart beat. The rate of spontaneous depolarization is fastest in the SA node which thus has the fastest intrinsic rate and

normally determines heart rate. Inhibition of higher parts of the system may result in other cells, for example in the AV node or ventricles, acting as pacemaker at their own slower intrinsic rates. The heart rate is determined by the rate of spontaneous depolarization which is increased by sympathetic activity and decreased by vagal activity. Extreme vagal activity may halt spontaneous depolarization, resulting in asystole until an impulse is generated by a pacemaker cell further down the system (vagal escape).

The initiation of the action potential is caused by a sudden increase in permeability to Na^+ and consequent influx. The membrane potential then starts to decrease rapidly due to outflow of K^+ and is then maintained at a plateau lasting approximately 200 ms (in contrast to 1–2 ms in skeletal muscle) due to inward movement of Ca^{++} ions.

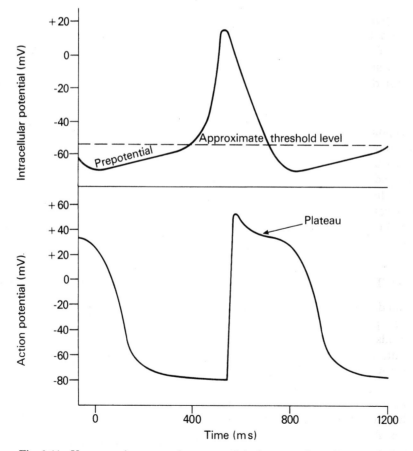

Fig. 2.11   Upper panel: transmembrane potential of a pacemaker cell; heart rate 75 beats.min^{-1}. Lower panel: cardiac muscle action potential.

Cardiac muscle is inexcitable during this period and thus cannot be tetanized. Repolarization is due to further outflow of K^+.

Excitation–contraction coupling

Ca^{++} ions are the link between the action potential and muscle contraction. The arrival of an action potential releases Ca^{++} ions from the sarcoplasmic reticulum which binds to the troponin C and activates the actin–myosin interaction leading to contraction. Further calcium comes from the inward movement during the plateau phase of the action potential and prolongs and enhances the contraction. The force of contraction is proportional to the concentration of free intracellular Ca^{++}.

The electrocardiogram (ECG)

Electrical currents generated by cardiac muscle during depolarization and repolarization are reflected in changes of electrical potential at the skin. The magnitude and polarity of the potential at a particular point depends upon the mass of muscle contracting and upon its orientation. The P wave reflects atrial depolarization, the QRS complex ventricular depolarization and the T wave ventricular repolarization.

The ECG reflects the electrical activity of the heart and it may indicate rate and rhythm in addition to some indication of myocardial damage. It does not reflect the adequacy of mechanical contraction. Normal complexes may be observed in the absence of mechanical activity.

The cardiac cycle (Fig. 2.12)

A heartbeat is initiated by spontaneous depolarization of an SA node pacemaker cell. A wave of depolarization spreads over the atria, which contract. At this point, the atrioventricular valves are open and the ventricles are filling under the pressure of the venous return; the pulmonary and aortic valves are held closed by the pressure gradient between pulmonary artery or aorta and their respective ventricles. Atrial contraction augments ventricular filling as diastole nears its end. The wave of depolarization passes through the AV

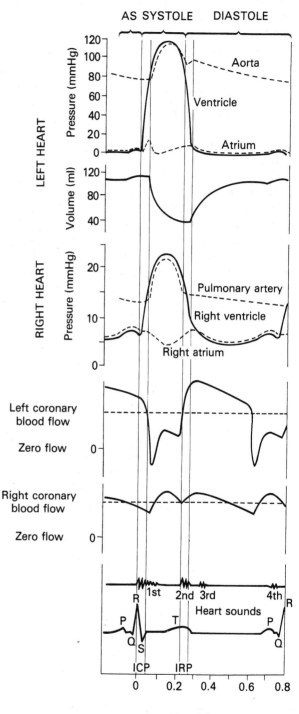

Fig. 2.12 The cardiac cycle. ICP = isometric contraction period. IRP = isometric relaxation period. AS = atrial systole.

node, along the AV bundle and spreads over the ventricles from apex to AV ring. Ventricular contraction (systole) follows. As ventricular pressure increases, the AV valves close and a phase of isometric contraction (i.e. increasing tension without shortening) begins. The aortic and pulmonary valves open as ventricular pressures exceed aortic and pulmonary arterial pressures and the ejection phase commences. Atrial repolarization occurs during early systole and the atria refill with blood as they relax. Spontaneous depolarization begins in the SA node.

Towards the end of systole, ventricular repolarization occurs and the ventricles relax. The pulmonary and aortic valves close as pulmonary arterial and aortic pressures exceed the respective ventricular pressures, marking the end of systole. The closure of the AV valves and aortic and pulmonary valves is audible as the first and second heart sound respectively. The aortic valve normally closes before the pulmonary, splitting the second sound. Aortic valve closure is seen as the dicrotic notch on the aortic pressure waveform.

Relaxation is isometric until ventricular pressure is less than atrial pressure when the AV valves open and ventricular filling begins. Filling continues passively until the SA node initiates a further cardiac cycle. At a normal heart rate of 70 beats.min^{-1}, a cardiac cycle occupies about 850 ms, of which approximately 220 ms is systole. Increased heart rates are accomplished almost entirely by a reduction in the duration of diastole (and ventricular filling). Thus, the atrial contribution to ventricular filling becomes proportionately more important as heart rate increases.

The passage of cardiac catheters and the interpretation of the waveforms is possible only if the cycle of events and their temporal relationship is understood clearly. Figure 2.12 summarizes these events. Normal intracardiac pressures and oxygen tensions are shown in Figure 2.13.

Coronary circulation (Fig. 2.14)

The myocardium is supplied by two coronary arteries, the right and left, which supply their respective ventricles. There is often a degree of overlap in the areas supplied but there is little communication between the two vessels. The

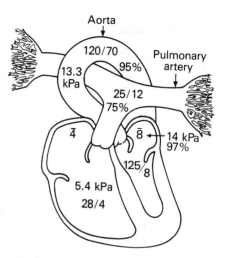

Fig. 2.13 Cardiovascular pressures, oxygen tensions and saturations.

arteries run over the surface of the heart giving off branches which penetrate the myocardium to supply the capillary beds. Venous drainage from the left ventricle passes via the coronary sinus into the right atrium; that from the right passes via the anterior cardiac vein also into the right atrium. In addition, a small proportion of the coronary flow (3–5%) drains directly into the ventricles through the Thebesian veins.

The normal coronary blood flow at rest is approximately 250 ml.min^{-1} (80 ml.min^{-1} per 100 g of tissue) and may increase fivefold during maximal exercise (Fig. 2.1). Myocardial oxygen consumption is approximately 11 ml.min^{-1}.100 g^{-1} compared with skeletal muscle at 8 ml.min^{-1}.100 g^{-1}. Coronary venous Po$_2$ is very low (approximately 4 kPa (30 mmHg)) and oxygen extraction is near maximal. Thus increased oxygen consumption must be accommodated by increased flow or an increase in myocardial efficiency. If increased flow cannot be achieved, increased extraction may result in tissue hypoxia. This feature of the coronary circulation is illustrated by the response to anaemia; if the oxygen carrying capacity of blood is halved (Hb 7 g.dl^{-1}) and cardiac output is doubled then myocardial blood flow should *quadruple* if myocardial hypoxia is to be avoided.

The coronary circulation is unique in that blood flows principally during diastole because the intramyocardial vessels are compressed during systole (Fig. 2.14). Increased heart rate shortens diastole

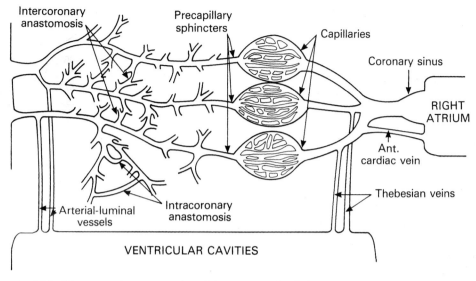

Fig. 2.14 Diagrammatic representation of the coronary circulation.

and may thus impair myocardial blood supply if flow rate cannot increase during diastole. The intramyocardial pressure is greatest in the subendocardial region and least at the epicardium. An increased intraventricular pressure during diastole, as may occur during sudden hypertension, has a greater effect on flow through the subendocardial vessels and may result in subendocardial ischaemia.

Coronary blood flow is determined predominantly by myocardial metabolic activity. Although there are sympathetic nerve fibres to the heart, changes in myocardial oxygen demand induced by sympathetic stimulation override the local vascular effects of the catecholamines. Although autoregulation occurs in the coronary circulation, this phenomenon may be difficult to demonstrate in vivo because of the changes in myocardial oxygen demand that accompany changes in perfusion pressure.

Cardiac output

Cardiac output ($\dot{Q}$) is the product of stroke volume (SV) and heart rate (HR).

$$\dot{Q} = SV \times HR$$

In a normal 70 kg man at rest, SV = 70 ml, HR = 70 beats.min^{-1} and $\dot{Q}$ = 5 litre.min^{-1}. In order to compare the cardiac output of patients of different size, the cardiac output per square metre of body surface area is often calculated. This is termed cardiac index (CI). For example, surface area = 1.7 m^2 in a 70 kg man, and:

$$CI = \frac{5}{1.7} = 3 \, \text{litre.min}^{-1}.\text{m}^{-2}$$

Control of cardiac output

The cardiac output is determined by the metabolic requirements of the body and over a period of time it equals the venous return (Fig. 2.15). The outputs of the two ventricles must also be identical. A consistent difference of 1 ml between the right and left ventricular stroke volumes at a heart rate of 70 beats.min^{-1} would lead to an imbalance of 1 litre in only 14 min. The balancing of venous return and cardiac output, and of right and left ventricular outputs, is an intrinsic property of the myocardium and occurs even in a denervated heart with a fixed rate. If this were not so, cardiac transplantation would be impossible and patients with cardiac pacemakers could not exercise.

In 1915, Starling stated the relationship between the force of cardiac contraction and muscle fibre length thus: 'The law of the heart is thus the same as the law of muscular tissue generally, that the

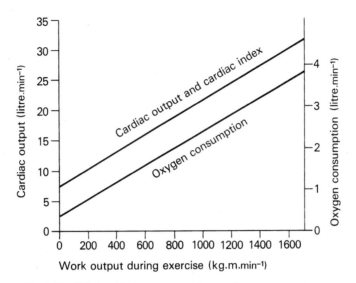

Fig. 2.15   Relationship between exercise, cardiac output and oxygen consumption.

energy of contraction, however measured, is a function of the length of the muscle fibre'. This intrinsic property of cardiac muscle enables the heart to balance venous return and cardiac output and the outputs of right and left ventricles. This mechanism alone compensates for increases in venous return of 200–300% above resting values. Further increases in venous return are met by increases in contractility of the muscle fibres and heart rate. These changes are mediated by the autonomic nervous system.

The mechanism is best understood if the effect of an increase in activity in a muscle group is considered. Increased metabolism in muscle leads to locally induced vasodilatation and increased blood flow. The increased flow rate increases venous return, which distends the right atrium and ventricle. The resulting increased force of contraction increases right ventricular stroke volume which leads to left ventricular distension. This in turn causes increased left ventricular stroke volume and an increase in cardiac output if heart rate remains constant. The increased cardiac output is maintained until reduced muscle metabolism leads to vasoconstriction, reversing the process. If the vasodilatation is sufficient to reduce peripheral vascular resistance, arterial pressure decreases transiently. Baroreceptor activity diminishes and vasoconstriction and increases in heart

rate and contractility occur, as a result of increased sympathetic activity. The increased heart rate and contractility lead to a further increase in cardiac output. In the case of muscular exercise, increased sympathetic activity may occur before the increase in venous return as the cerebral cortex 'anticipates' the activity.

Cardiac contractility

The force of contraction is determined by the initial fibre length (Frank–Starling mechanism) and by the ability of the cardiac muscle to contract at a given initial fibre length (contractility). These relationships are illustrated usually as a curve relating force of contraction to fibre length (Fig. 2.16), changes in contractility being shown as displaced but parallel curves.

Starling's law, as stated above, is almost impossible to validate in man because the two parameters (force of contraction and fibre length) cannot be measured directly. Consequently, parameters such as stroke volume, speed of contraction, maximum rate of rise of ventricular pressure, peak ventricular pressure, ejection fraction (stroke volume/end-diastolic volume) and stroke work (SV × [MAP – MVP]) have been used. All these parameters are indirect measures of the force of contraction and must be interpreted with care.

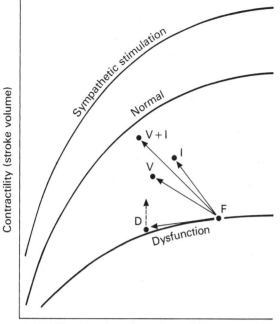

Fig. 2.16 Starling's law of the heart and changes in myocardial contractility. Letters and arrows signify effects of different treatments in cardiac failure. I = inotropic drugs; V = vasodilator drugs; V + I = combined use; D = diuretics. Broken arrow indicates that ventricular function may improve later.

For example, a leaking mitral valve results in a reduction in forward stroke volume despite an increase in left ventricular work.

Similarly, alternative parameters have been used to reflect initial fibre length. End-diastolic volume and pressure have been used widely. End-diastolic pressures, particularly right and left atrial pressures, require careful interpretation as the change in pressure with a given volume change depends upon the compliance of the chamber. Thus the pressure change in a stiff ventricle is greater than in a flabby ventricle for the same volume change.

Ventricular function curves based on the indirect parameters mentioned above are useful clinically in plotting the response to treatment but may be of limited value in determining deviations from normality.

Sympathetic stimulation is the most significant extrinsic factor which increases myocardial contractility. The effect may be induced by neuronal activity or by circulating endogenous or exogenous catecholamines. Both heart rate and contractility increase, with a parallel effect on cardiac output and myocardial oxygen consumption.

Calcium ions increase contractility, as do digoxin and insulin as well as all the sympathomimetic amines. Conversely, contractility is reduced by β-adrenergic blocking drugs, antiarrhythmic agents, the majority of general anaesthetics (see below) and an elevated extracellular potassium ion concentration.

Control of heart rate

Heart rate is determined by the rate of spontaneous depolarization of the sinoatrial node. The resting heart rate is approximately 75 beats.min^{-1} and increases to 110 beats.min^{-1} after total denervation, indicating the importance of inhibitory vagal parasympathetic activity. Thus cardiac acceleration may be achieved either by a decrease in vagal activity or an increase in sympathetic activity.

Increases in heart rate occur largely as a result of shortening of diastole. Excessive increases in heart rate impair ventricular diastolic filling such that stroke volume and cardiac output decrease.

Similarly, cardiac output decreases if an increasing stroke volume is unable to compensate for a decreasing heart rate. In a normal heart, cardiac output is unimpaired between 40 and 150 beats.min^{-1} although this range may be reduced considerably by disease.

Assessment of cardiac function

The best clinical indication of cardiac function is the state of the peripheral circulation. Simple methods of assessment, as discussed previously, are often adequate and should be employed before more invasive techniques are contemplated.

Ventricular filling pressures

The pressure in the central veins (CVP) is equated with the right ventricular end-diastolic pressure. The pressure measured depends on venous return, the ability of the heart to respond, the state of filling of the circulation and venous tone. Because CVP measurement is influenced by many factors and because the value noted depends

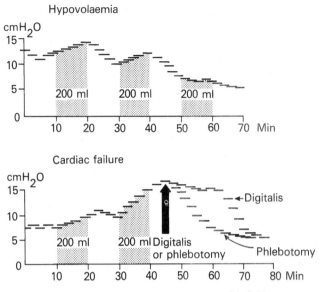

Fig. 2.17 Changes in central venous pressure with fluid replacement. Upper panel: hypovolaemia in a young patient. Lower panel: cardiac failure. See text for details.

critically on the zero point chosen, isolated readings are of little value. With any control system, the maximum information can be obtained by observing the effect of small perturbations. Thus the response of the CVP to small fluid challenges is more valuable than single readings. This is illustrated in Figure 2.17, where the upper panel illustrates the course of a young traumatized hypovolaemic patient who, with vigorous sympathetic activity, has induced such venoconstriction that CVP is elevated. Fluid challenges decrease the CVP as cardiac output increases and vasodilatation occurs. In contrast, the lower panel illustrates a patient with cardiac impairment. Fluid challenges produce a sustained elevation of CVP which on the second occasion exceeds the ability of the heart to respond and active intervention is required.

In the examples given above, it is assumed that right and left ventricular function is comparable and that changes in CVP reflect changes in left atrial pressure (LAP) both in direction and magnitude. Clinically, there is often a marked disparity between the function of the two ventricles and left ventricular filling pressures must be measured more directly. This is achieved usually by floating into the pulmonary artery a balloon tipped catheter which is then wedged in a branch (see Ch. 20).

Since there is no flow through that segment of the pulmonary circulation, the pressure at the tip of the catheter (PCWP) equilibrates to a value close to LAP.

Cardiac output

The measurement of cardiac output is useful as part of an overall assessment of the circulation. Isolated measurements are of little value. For example, a cardiac output of 5 litre.min^{-1} indicates excellent function after myocardial infarction but indicates failure in severe sepsis or major burns. Again, this measurement is most useful in assessing the response to therapy. The standard method of measurement is the Fick principle, namely that oxygen consumption ($\dot{V}_{O_2}$) equals the arteriovenous oxygen content difference $(A - V)C_{O_2}$ multiplied by cardiac output:

$$\dot{Q} = \frac{\dot{V}_{O_2}}{(A - V)\, C_{O_2}} = \frac{250\ ml.min^{-1}}{5\ ml.dl^{-1}} = 5\ litre.min^{-1}$$

This method is time consuming and has been replaced in clinical use by thermal or dye dilution methods. The principal of these techniques is that a bolus of indicator is injected into blood entering the heart, where it mixes in the venous return.

The concentration of indicator is measured downstream and plotted against time. As the mass of indicator is known, integration of the concentration curve may be used to derive the volume in which the indicator was distributed, the cardiac output. Cold glucose solution, the indicator in the thermal technique, is injected into the right atrium and the decrease in blood temperature is sensed in the pulmonary artery by a thermistor, which is incorporated into a balloon tipped catheter. Estimations may be repeated at frequent intervals.

CARDIOVASCULAR RESPONSE TO DISEASE AND ANAESTHESIA

Hypovolaemia (Fig. 2.18)

Hypovolaemia is a common clinical problem. It is a result of imbalance between the blood volume and the capacity of the circulation and causes impaired tissue perfusion. It may be caused by loss of fluid, e.g. haemorrhage, or excessive vasodilatation, e.g. high spinal anaesthesia.

Loss of fluid reduces venous return, decreasing right atrial filling pressure and thus cardiac output. The resulting hypotension is countered by the baroreceptors, which increases heart rate and induce vaso- and venoconstriction. These measures maintain arterial pressure and minimize the de-

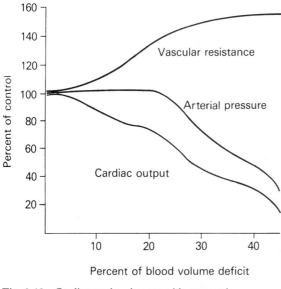

Fig. 2.18 Cardiovascular changes with progressive hypovolaemia.

crease in cardiac output. Cardiac output is redistributed away from skin, muscles and viscera and blood flow is maintained to heart and brain. Arterial pressure is maintained usually until approximately 20% of the blood volume is lost and cardiac output has diminished by 30%; thereafter it decreases progressively. Any drug which attenuates vasoconstriction or tachycardia, for example anaesthetic agents or β-blockers, results in earlier hypotension.

Increased ADH and aldosterone secretion retain water and sodium, compensating for the fluid loss in the longer term. Reduction in capillary pressure results in translocation of fluid from the extracellular space into the circulation as a result of the oncotic pressure of plasma, further compensating for the hypovolaemia.

Severe or prolonged reduction in perfusion may lead to organ failure, for example renal failure. In addition, accumulation of tissue metabolites and absorption of endotoxin from the bowel may result in vasodilatation, overcoming the vasoconstriction and exacerbating the hypotension. This phase was previously termed 'irreversible shock' and represents clinically the phase when simple fluid replacement is inadequate to restore a normal circulation.

The initial management of hypovolaemia consists of replacement with the appropriate fluid. It is important that fluid is not given blindly but that a cycle of assessment, therapy, reassessment, further therapy and so on is initiated to ensure optimum replacement.

Cardiac failure

The heart may fail as a pump for many reasons, e.g. ischaemia, trauma, drugs and sepsis. As the ventricles fail, stroke volume is reduced and baroreceptor activity increased. The resulting venoconstriction increases ventricular filling pressures and initial myocardial fibre length and restores stroke volume towards normal. The reduced cardiac output results also in fluid retention. Eventually the myocardial fibres are unable to generate any further increase in contractility and cardiac output diminishes rapidly. Venous pressures become so high that pulmonary and/or peripheral oedema occur.

Management of cardiac failure may be approached in three ways: optimization of ventricular filling pressures, enhancement of contractility and reduction of cardiac work. A reduction of filling pressure is necessary in most patients in right or left ventricular failure. This may be achieved by diuretics, venesection or venodilator drugs. Contractility may be enhanced by a variety of drugs (see above) but usually at the expense of increased myocardial oxygen consumption. Cardiac work is determined by the volume of blood pumped (cardiac output) and the resistance against which it is pumped (vascular resistance). The former is reduced already but reduction of the latter with vasodilators may enhance cardiac performance considerably. Such treatment must be given with care as excessive vasodilatation may result in severe hypotension and impairment of perfusion of vital organs including the heart itself. Filling pressures are often reduced by vasodilatation and may require adjustment.

Once again the need for a cycle of assessment therapy and reassessment is emphasized. Figure 2.16 shows the effect of various therapies on ventricular function.

Anaesthesia

All anaesthetic agents depress myocardial function in the isolated heart, but clinically the depressant effect may be countered or exacerbated so that the resultant effects on cardiac output may vary greatly (see Ch. 8).

Sympathetic activity

Ether, cyclopropane and ketamine increase sympathetic activity, with maintenance of cardiac output during light anaesthesia. In contrast, halothane and enflurane depress sympathetic activity leading to reduced contractility and peripheral vasodilatation. Halothane also enhances parasympathetic activity, resulting in bradycardia.

Ventilation

Artificial ventilation of the lungs may reduce venous return by increasing mean intrathoracic pressure. However, lighter planes of anaesthesia are usually used when IPPV is employed and this may offset the reduction in cardiac output.

Changes in Pa_{CO_2} may have profound effects. Hypercapnia increases cardiac output by sympathetic stimulation and by peripheral vasodilatation. However, hypercapnia may induce ventricular arrhythmias in the presence of volatile anaesthetics, e.g. halothane. Hypocapnia induces peripheral vasoconstriction, increased vascular resistance and thus a reduction in cardiac output. Arterial pressure is usually maintained.

Surgical stimulation

Surgical stimulation results generally in increased sympathetic activity, counteracting the depressant effects of anaesthesia. Variations in arterial pressure with anaesthesia and surgical stimulation are often more pronounced in elderly or hypertensive patients. Some surgical stimuli, e.g. distension of viscera or traction on peritoneum, may induce vasodilatation and bradycardia, reducing arterial pressure and cardiac output.

Other drugs

Several drugs, e.g. opioids and muscle relaxants, cause peripheral vasodilatation by direct action on the vessels, histamine release or ganglion blockade. These actions may be unwelcome in some circumstances, while in others they may be used deliberately to induce arterial hypotension.

Subarachnoid and extradural anaesthesia

Subarachnoid and extradural anaesthesia block the sympathetic outflow and cause arteriolar and venous dilatation. Bradycardia results also if the cardiac fibres are involved (T1–T4). In general, the circulation is well maintained provided that arterial pressure is prevented from decreasing excessively by the judicious use of volume replacement and vasopressors.

FURTHER READING

Ahumda G G (ed) 1988 Cardiovascular pathophysiology.
Oxford University Press, Oxford
Gutierrez G et al 1992 Gastric intramucosal pH as a
therapeutic index of tissue oxygenation in critically ill
patients. Lancet 339, 195–199

Levick J R 1991 An introduction to cardiovascular
physiology. Butterworths, London
Searle N, Sahab P 1992 Endothelial vasomotor regulation
in health and disease. Canadian Journal of Anaesthesia
39, 838–857

3. Outlines of renal physiology

The kidney plays a vital role in maintaining homoeostasis. It safeguards the stable internal environment necessary for each of the cellular components to function efficiently, despite a variable fluid and solute intake by the organism as a whole. Homoeostasis is achieved by a combination of complex processes:

1. Excretion of the waste products of metabolism.
2. Production of hormones which influence other organs in the body.
3. Control of the extracellular fluid (ECF). This influences indirectly the intracellular composition in terms of volume, osmolality and acid–base status.

Before discussing the various components and functions of the kidney, it is necessary to consider briefly the body fluids and their compartments.

BODY FLUIDS AND COMPARTMENTS

Total body water in man is approximately 60% of total body weight, i.e. 42 litres of water for a 70 kg man. In females, total body water is approximately 10% less, because of the greater proportion of fat than in males; fat cells have a lower water content than other cells of the body. The water is distributed in various spaces or compartments.

Intracellular fluid

This is the largest water compartment in the body, representing two-thirds of total body water (approximately 28 litres).

Extracellular fluid

This constitutes the remaining one-third of total body water (14 litres) and may be subdivided further into two compartments:

1. Intravascular, i.e. within the plasma (4 litres).
2. Interstitial. This fluid (approximately 11 litres in volume) is outside the intravascular compartment and serves to 'bathe' individual cells.

The composition of the various fluids differs with the requirements of each compartment (Table 3.1). Sodium is the main cation in the extracellular compartment, whereas potassium is the principal cation of the intracellular compartment. This is achieved by the different permeability of cell membranes for some cations; the cell membrane is approximately 50 times more permeable to potassium than to sodium. Intracellular protein carries a negative charge which attracts the positively charged potassium ions. Most importantly, however, the sodium pump extrudes sodium actively from the cell in exchange for potassium with the use of the enzyme Na-K-ATPase.

The water content of plasma is 93%; the

Table 3.1 Composition and volume of body fluids according to compartment

	Intravascular (Plasma) 4 litres	Interstitial 10 litres	Intracellular 28 litres
Sodium (mmol.litre^{-1})	142	142	10
Potassium (mmol.litre^{-1})	5	5	150
Chloride (mmol.litre^{-1})	103	113	10
Bicarbonate (mmol.litre^{-1})	25	26	10
Protein (g.litre^{-1})	60–80	0	25
Osmolality (mosmol.kgH$_2$O^{-1})	285	285	285

remainder comprises proteins, lipids and other large molecular weight substances. Therefore, the actual value for sodium concentration in intravascular water should be approximately 153 mmol.litre^{-1}. In clinical practice, if the proportion of water is reduced, e.g. by large increases in protein, lipid or glucose concentration, the plasma sodium value is spuriously lowered; this is termed pseudohyponatraemia.

Cell membranes are permeable to water and there is a continual flux of fluid among the different body compartments at different rates of exchange. Two main mechanisms are responsible for these fluid shifts:

1. Osmotic pressure. Osmotic pressure is the pressure exerted by the number of particles in a solution. Osmolality, the usual term used in clinical practice, is defined as the number of milliosmoles per kg of water (mosmol.kg^{-1}). Ions, being in greater abundance, exert a greater osmotic pressure. For example, 1 mmol of sodium chloride exerts an osmotic pressure of 2 mosmol, as each molecule is composed of 1 sodium and 1 chloride ion. Although of a larger molecular mass, proteins exert less osmotic pressure. Water moves freely across a semipermeable membrane and does so from an area of low osmolality to one of higher osmolality, i.e. the increase in osmotic pressure attracts water. This movement continues until the osmotic pressure is equal on both sides of the membrane. This mechanism is in effect between the intracellular and interstitial compartments. As shown in Table 3.1, the osmolality in the three compartments is identical. Any increase in intracellular osmolality increases water transport into the cell, thereby increasing its volume, and vice versa.

2. Hydrostatic pressure. This is the main mechanism for fluid movement across a capillary bed from the intravascular to the interstitial compartment. Figure 3.1 shows the various pressures exerted as the hydrostatic pressure decreases from 32 mmHg at the arterial end to 12 mmHg at the venous end of the capillary. The oncotic pressure exerted by plasma proteins represents a constant 'negative' pressure that draws fluid into the capillary. Thus, fluid moves out of the capillary at the arterial end and is withdrawn at the venous end. These hydrostatic pressures are known as Starling's forces. There is a small interstitial pressure, estimated to be approximately 2–5 mmHg, although it appears to have little or no effect on this mechanism unless the capillary, which may be damaged by some pathological process, leaks protein into the interstitium. If this occurs, then the interstitial pressure is increased and the existing balance of forces altered.

Renal blood flow

Before considering renal blood flow, it is necessary to understand the gross anatomy of the kidney.

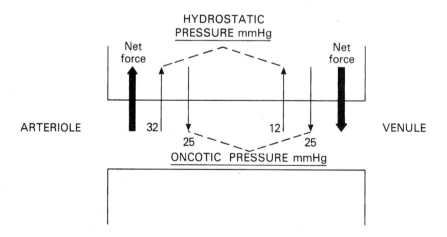

Fig. 3.1 Hydrostatic forces across a capillary wall (Starling's forces).

There are two populations of nephrons in the mammalian kidney:

1. *Cortical.* These nephrons (approximately 85% in man) lie within the cortex of the kidney and have short loops of Henle which dip only into the outer medulla.

2. *Juxtamedullary.* These nephrons, which constitute the remaining 15% in man, lie in the juxtamedullary area of the cortex, and are distinguished from their outer cortical neighbours by having long loops of Henle entering the inner medulla to participate in the diluting and concentrating mechanisms of the kidney.

The blood supply to the kidney is from the renal artery, which, having entered the renal pelvis, divides into a number of interlobar arteries. These further divide into the arcuate arteries and supply the small interlobular arteries from which the glomerular vessels arise. Each glomerulus is supplied by a single afferent arteriole which branches into a network throughout the glomerulus. It then reforms into a single vessel, the efferent arteriole. The efferent arteriole in turn forms branches around the proximal tubule (pars recta) and around the loop of Henle to form the vasa recta. It is possible for the efferent arteriole from one glomerulus to form the vasa recta of an adjacent tubule. The mesh of vessels then reforms into a single vessel which drains into the interlobular vein and thence to the renal vein.

Considering its size in relation to other organs of the body, the kidney is unique in receiving an extremely high blood flow (approximately 20–25% of cardiac output). This amounts to 500–600 $ml.min^{-1}$ to each kidney. Such a flow rate is necessary to carry sufficient oxygen for the high energy requirements of tubular processes, especially sodium reabsorption.

Renal plasma flow (RPF) may be measured using the Fick principle:

$$RPF = \frac{U_x V}{RA_x - RV_x}$$

where U_x = urine concentration of a substance x

V = urine volume

RA_x = renal artery concentration of the substance

RV_x = renal vein concentration of the substance

The commonest substance used is *para*-aminohippuric acid (PAH) which is cleared almost completely in one passage through the kidney. It is both filtered by the glomerulus and secreted by the renal tubule. In this instance, RV_x should be negligible and, as there is no extrarenal clearance of PAH, the expression may be modified as follows:

$$RPF = \frac{U_{PAH} V}{P_{PAH}} \quad ml.min^{-1}$$

where V = urine volume in $ml.min^{-1}$

U_{PAH} = urine PAH concentration in $mg.ml^{-1}$

P_{PAH} = plasma PAH concentration in $mg.ml^{-1}$

Renal blood flow (RBF) may be calculated by adjusting the RPF for the haematocrit:

$$RBF = \frac{RPF}{1 - Hct} \quad ml.min^{-1}$$

where Hct = haematocrit

As only 90% of PAH is extracted by the human kidney, the clearance of PAH (C_{PAH}) underestimates RPF by approximately 10%. In order to improve the accuracy of measurement it is possible to estimate RPF from the disappearance curve of intravenously injected ^{131}I-labelled PAH, eliminating the potential error introduced by timed urine collections.

The extrinsic control of RBF is influenced by the sympathetic nerve outflow from T4 to L2. Increases in sympathetic tone such as those produced by haemorrhage, shock, pain, cold or severe exercise produce vasoconstriction.

Some hormones (adrenaline, noradrenaline, antidiuretic hormone (vasopressin) in large non-pharmacological doses, serotonin and angiotensin) also reduce renal blood flow.

Within the kidney, RBF is redistributed to various anatomical areas. This has been demonstrated in animals using radioactive labelled tracers or microspheres and in man by the injection of radiolabelled inert agents (such as xenon or krypton) and measurement of their rate of disappearance over the kidney. From such studies in man, it has been shown that the cortex receives approximately $500 \text{ ml.min}^{-1}.100 \text{ g}^{-1}$, the outer medulla receives approximately $100 \text{ ml.min}^{-1}.100 \text{ g}^{-1}$ and the inner medulla only $20 \text{ ml.min}^{-1}.100 \text{ g}^{-1}$. The lower medullary flow rate is necessary for the working of the counter-current mechanism.

There are two other properties that confer distinguishing features on the renal circulation. The first is that the mean glomerular capillary pressure is maintained at 45 mmHg, which is approximately 20 mmHg more than other capillary networks in the body. This is necessary for glomerular filtration (see below). The mean peritubular capillary pressure is only 15 mmHg and lower than intratubular pressure, thereby enhancing tubular reabsorption.

The second feature is autoregulation, which occurs in the cortex but not in the medulla and allows constant blood flow when renal perfusion pressure is altered. It is an intrinsic property of the renal vasculature, i.e. it is independent of nerves or hormones, and occurs over a range of systolic arterial pressure from 90–180 mmHg. Over this range glomerular filtration rate (GFR) parallels RPF, but glomerular filtration ceases when systolic arterial pressure decreases below 60 mmHg. The effects of autoregulation are achieved by changes in resistance in the afferent and efferent arterioles. When arterial pressure decreases, there is relative vasodilatation of the afferent arteriole and vasoconstriction of the efferent arteriole. This results in an increase in the fraction of plasma filtered (filtration fraction) and glomerular filtration is maintained. If arterial pressure increases, the vasoconstriction occurs in the afferent arteriole, with the opposite effects on filtration fraction.

The autoregulatory mechanism may be dampened by vasodilator drugs which act on smooth muscle vasculature, e.g. acetylcholine, dopamine, prostaglandins and the calcium channel blockers.

The exact mechanism of autoregulation is still a matter of debate. Originally it was believed to result either from mechanical factors, i.e. skimming of red blood cells and an increase in blood viscosity within the renal vasculature, or a response to overall increase in intrarenal pressure generated by changes in systemic arterial pressure. Current evidence now favours the 'myogenic theory' which states that the increase in smooth muscle contraction is produced by an increase in the intraluminal pressure or in the tangential tension of the vascular wall. The role of locally generated vasoactive substances, e.g. angiotensin II, remains controversial.

Glomerular filtration

The process of glomerular filtration allows $180 \text{ litre.24 h}^{-1}$ or 120 ml.min^{-1} of fluid and solutes to pass through the glomerular capillaries via the endothelial fenestrations, the glomerular capillary basement membrane and the pedicles of the podocyte into Bowman's space. The fluid which enters the proximal tubule from Bowman's space is an ultrafiltrate of plasma, i.e. it is virtually protein-free. Small amounts of albumin pass through the glomerular basement membrane but are reabsorbed almost entirely in the proximal tubule so that the final urinary concentration of albumin is less than 120 mg.24 h^{-1}. The ease with which solutes pass through the glomerular basement membrane depends on their size, charge and possibly shape.

The filtering process is extremely efficient for substances of low molecular weight, i.e. the ratio of solute concentration between the plasma within the glomerular capillary and the fluid in Bowman's capsule is 1. As molecular weight increases, the amount of filtered solute decreases until a cut-off point at a molecular weight of 70 000 is reached, above which no further molecules pass. It should be noted that this range allows for a small quantity of albumin (molecular weight 69 000) to be filtered. The constituents of the glomerular basement membrane are mainly negatively charged sialoproteins which repel the negatively charged protein particles in plasma. It has been demonstrated that dextrans, with a molecular weight similar to some small proteins but with no charge, pass through the glomerular basement membrane 10–20% more efficiently. There is also some evidence that changes in molecular shape may facilitate the passage of some molecules through the membrane.

The forces required to drive glomerular filtration are similar to the Starling forces across capillary networks elsewhere in the body, although of a greater magnitude. The mean arterial pressure in the glomerular capillary is 45 mmHg compared with 20 mmHg elsewhere. As discussed previously, this is a result of the presence of a second resistance vessel, the efferent arteriole. Also, this pressure remains relatively constant over a wide range of systolic arterial pressure as a result of the process of autoregulation. Glomerular filtration rate (GFR) is a product of the forces driving filtration minus the forces opposing filtration and may be expressed thus:

$$GFR \propto (P_{CAP} + \pi_{BC}) - (P_{BC} + \pi_{CAP})$$

where P_{CAP} = hydrostatic pressure in the glomerular capillary
  P_{BC} = hydrostatic pressure in Bowman's capsule
  π_{BC} = oncotic pressure in Bowman's capsule
  π_{CAP} = oncotic pressure in glomerular capillary.

However, as π_{BC} is negligible, i.e. ultrafiltrate is virtually protein-free, the relationship may be rewritten:

$$GFR \propto P_{CAP} - P_{BC} - \pi_{CAP}$$

To convert this relationship into an equation, the slaving coefficient (K_f), i.e. the resistance to flow across the glomerular basement membrane, is introduced:

$$GFR = K_f (P_{CAP} - P_{BC} - \pi_{CAP})$$

Measurement of glomerular filtration rate

The measurement of GFR is one of the commonest assessments of renal function in clinical practice. It is measured by determining the clearance of a substance which is filtered by the glomerulus but not reabsorbed or secreted by the renal tubule. The polyfructose inulin (MW 5000) is such a substance. Using the standard clearance formula:

$$C_{IN} = \frac{U_{IN}V}{P_{IN}} = 120 \text{ ml.min}^{-1}$$

where C_{IN} = inulin clearance in ml.min^{-1}
  U_{IN} = inulin concentration in urine (mg.ml^{-1})
  P_{IN} = inulin concentration in plasma (mg.ml^{-1})
  V = urine volume (ml.min^{-1}).

There are two major disadvantages to this technique. Firstly, as inulin does not occur naturally in the body, it is necessary to infuse inulin intravenously to achieve a steady plasma level. To overcome this, it is customary to measure creatinine clearance using plasma creatinine, a product of muscle metabolism. There is a slight diurnal variation of plasma creatinine levels and creatinine is secreted by the renal tubules at very low GFRs; however, creatinine clearance values are adequate for clinical practice and relate reasonably closely to inulin clearance.

The other disadvantage is the accuracy of timed urine collections. As with measurement of RPF, it is possible to use a radioactive-labelled substance to measure GFR. Chromium-labelled ethylene diamine tetracetic acid (^{51}Cr-EDTA) is injected intravenously and the disappearance rate calculated from blood samples obtained at 2 and 4 hours after injection. This avoids urine collection, may be standardized for body surface area (as should all measurements of GFR) and may be used as an accurate reference method.

Filtration fraction

Although RPF is quite large, only a proportion is filtered and that proportion is called the filtration fraction (FF). It is derived as follows:

$$FF = \frac{GFR}{RPF} = \frac{C_{IN}}{C_{PAH}} = \frac{120 \text{ ml.min}^{-1}}{600 \text{ ml.min}^{-1}} = 0.2 \ (20\%)$$

FF may alter as a result of autoregulation. For example, if RBF decreases there is an increase in efferent arteriolar vasoconstriction and FF increases in order to maintain glomerular filtration.

Tubular function

The role of the renal tubule is to modify the volume and composition of the glomerular filtrate according to the needs of the organism. This is an enormous task. 180 litres of filtrate are produced per day and it is necessary to reduce this volume by 99% to achieve a final 24-h urine volume of approximately 1.8 litres. Similarly, approximately 25 000 mmol of sodium are filtered per day, the vast majority of this being reabsorbed to provide a urinary output of 100 to 200 mmol.24 h^{-1}. In

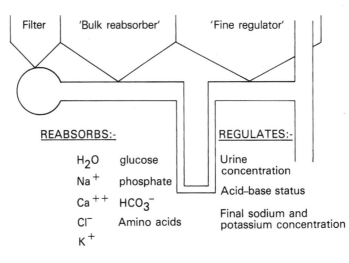

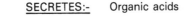

SECRETES:- Organic acids

Fig. 3.2 Simple schema of tubular function.

addition, the kidney conserves other filtered substances that are essential for the maintenance of homoeostasis, e.g. glucose, bicarbonate, phosphate, etc. The renal tubule is responsible also for excretion of waste products of ingestion or metabolism, e.g. potassium, urea, creatinine, etc. The final regulation of acid–base status and of the concentration or dilution of the urine are also performed along the renal tubule.

Although each nephron acts as a single unit, it is possible, for ease of understanding, to divide tubular function into the individual portions of the tubule, i.e. proximal tubule, loop of Henle, distal tubule and collecting tubule. In simple terms, the proximal tubule may be considered the 'bulk reabsorber' and the remainder, the 'fine regulator' (Fig. 3.2).

Proximal tubule

In many ways, the proximal tubule is considered the bulk reabsorber as it is responsible for reducing the volume of glomerular filtrate by 80%. Seventy per cent of sodium and chloride, 90% of calcium, bicarbonate and magnesium, and 100% of glucose, phosphate and amino acids are reabsorbed during their passage through the proximal tubule. The fluid entering the proximal

tubule from Bowman's space has a composition similar to that of plasma except for the absence of protein (see Table 3.1). As the reabsorptive process is isosmotic, the osmolality remains identical at the beginning and end of the proximal tubule (290 mosmol.kg^{-1}). The main ion to be reabsorbed in terms of concentration, energy requirements and its effect on other reabsorptive processes is sodium.

Sodium reabsorption. Sodium is reabsorbed through the proximal tubular cell both passively and actively.

Passive reabsorption. There are two forms of passive reabsorption for sodium:

1. Chemical. The intracellular sodium concentration in the proximal tubular cell is 30 mmol.litre^{-1}. This is considerably less than the concentration of 140 mmol.litre^{-1} in the tubular fluid. Sodium travels down the chemical gradient from the lumen to the cell.

2. Electrical. The potential difference within the tubular cell is –70 mV. This creates an electrical gradient for the positively charged sodium ions to travel from the lumen into the cell. Chloride, although negatively charged, travels with sodium in linked transport.

Active transport. When sodium is within the

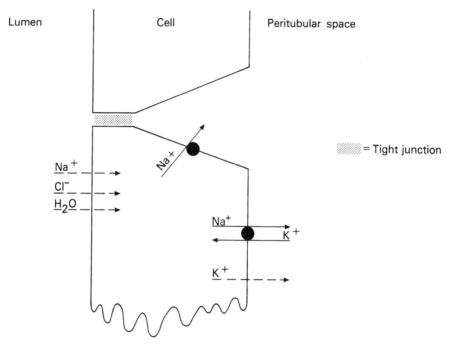

Fig. 3.3 Sodium transport through a proximal tubular cell.

cell it is pumped out (actively) in two directions. The first is into the intercellular space behind the so-called 'tight junction' (Fig. 3.3). This is an active energy-requiring pump which appears to be Na-K-ATPase independent. The effect of increased sodium concentration in the intercellular space is to increase the osmolality and thus water passes from the cell into that space. The sodium and water within the intercellular space are then available for reabsorption by the peritubular capillary. In conditions of extracellular fluid expansion, the tight junction may open and sodium flows together with water from the intercellular space into the tubular lumen (back flow).

There is a second sodium pump situated on the contraluminal surface of the tubular cell. This is an Na-K-ATPase-dependent pump which exchanges sodium for potassium. Potassium, however, is freely permeable through the cell wall and may diffuse passively out again into the peritubular space. Again, the sodium in the peritubular space is available for reabsorption into the peritubular capillary.

The movement of sodium, chloride and water into the peritubular capillary is governed by Starling's forces. The driving forces are hydrostatic pressure in the peritubular space and capillary oncotic pressure; the opposing forces are capillary hydrostatic pressure and oncotic pressure in the peritubular space. However, as peritubular space oncotic pressure in negligible and the peritubular space hydrostatic pressure is small, the main controlling factor is peritubular oncotic pressure. The sodium, chloride and water which are not taken up into the peritubular capillary re-enter the tubular lumen via the tight junction, i.e. there is an increase in back flow.

Having described the mechanisms of sodium reabsorption within the proximal tubular cell it is necessary also to consider sodium reabsorption and excretion by the kidney as a whole. As previously stated, the daily fractional excretion of sodium (the amount of sodium excreted in the final urine relative to the filtered load of sodium) remains relatively constant at approximately 1–2%. Filtered load (expressed in $mmol.min^{-1}$) is the product of GFR and plasma sodium concentration. However, the sodium intake varies and various mechanisms are required to cope with states of relative hypo- and hypervolaemia. Three main mechanisms are responsible:

1. Glomerulotubular balance. Glomerular filtration rate remains relatively constant despite changes in systemic arterial pressure because of the autoregulatory mechanism. However, small changes in GFR produce large changes in the filtered load of sodium. When these occur, sodium reabsorption must alter in order to prevent large alterations in final sodium excretion. The anatomical arrangement of the peritubular capillaries, originating from the efferent arteriole, provides the ideal situation for a compensatory mechanism. When GFR decreases there is a decrease in filtration fraction. This reduces the normally occurring increase in peritubular capillary oncotic pressure which in turn decreases reabsorption of sodium, chloride and water from the peritubular space. Conversely, if GFR increases, there is an increase in filtration fraction, a greater increase in peritubular capillary oncotic pressure and enhanced reabsorption. This mechanism is known as 'glomerulotubular balance'.

2. Aldosterone. Aldosterone has its main site of action in the distal tubule and is considered later.

3. Third factor. It has been known for over 20 years that when blood of a volume-expanded animal is perfused into a normal animal, avoiding volume expansion in the recipient, there is a modest increase in fractional sodium excretion, despite unchanged renal haemodynamics. This phenomenon has been demonstrated in both isolated perfused kidneys and denervated kidneys and has led to the postulate that during volume expansion there is secretion of a so-called 'natriuretic factor' (see 'atrial natriuretic peptide', p. 44). The opposing view to the natriuretic factor is that all changes occurring during volume expansion may be explained by 'physical forces', e.g. changes in plasma proteins and therefore peritubular capillary oncotic pressure.

The possibility that redistribution of intrarenal blood flow exerts an influence on overall sodium balance has yet to be evaluated fully. It is known that in cardiac failure, when a state of positive sodium balance occurs from increased sodium reabsorption, blood flow is directed away from the short outer cortical nephrons (salt-losing) and directed to the longer juxtamedullary nephrons (salt-retaining). It is not known if a similar modified mechanism plays a significant role in daily sodium balance.

Rate-limited tubular transport

As shown in Figure 3.2, glucose, phosphate, bicarbonate and amino acids are reabsorbed almost totally in the proximal renal tubule. The mode of reabsorption differs from that described for sodium, chloride and water. The basic mechanism, as obtained in a titration study, is shown in Figure 3.4 using glucose as the example. During such a study the plasma glucose concentration is increased slowly, avoiding extracellular fluid volume expansion. Plasma and urinary glucose concentrations and GFR are measured. As the plasma glucose concentration increases, glucose appears in the urine when the point of the renal threshold for glucose has been reached. This occurs when the plasma glucose concentration is approximately 10 mmol.litre^{-1} in man. The tubular reabsorption of glucose continues to increase with increments in plasma glucose concentration until a plateau is reached when no further increase in glucose reabsorption rate can be achieved despite an increase in the filtered load of glucose. At that point, the transport mechanisms for glucose reabsorption by the tubular cells have been saturated. Thereafter, glucose excretion increases in parallel with the filtered load of glucose as plasma glucose concentration increases. The 'plateau' at which maximal glucose reabsorption occurs is termed 'the tubular maximal reabsorption for glucose' (Tm_g). In man the value is 20 mmol.min^{-1}. It should be noted from Figure 3.4 that the point at which glucose reabsorption reaches its maximum is not a fine 'cut-off' but a small curve entitled 'splay'. Splay is caused by the heterogeneity of the nephron population in respect of glucose reabsorption. Some nephrons reabsorb maximally at a lower plasma glucose concentration than other nephrons within the kidney. A large splay is the cause of one type of renal glycosuria.

The same mechanism applies for phosphate reabsorption in the proximal tubule although this

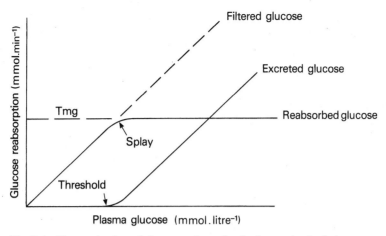

Fig. 3.4 The mechanism of glucose reabsorption in the proximal tubule.

differs slightly from glucose in that the excretion of phosphate follows the filtered load more closely and the Tm for phosphate is much lower (0.125 mmol.min^{-1}). The Tm for bicarbonate is approximately 3–3.5 mmol.min^{-1} but may be altered by hydrogen ion secretion. There are five identified individual transport processes for the different groups of amino acids but their reabsorptive kinetics are similar to that of glucose. The reabsorption of sulphate in the proximal tubule follows a similar pattern. Many of the above substances share a cotransport system with sodium. It is known that when proximal tubular reabsorption of sodium decreases with an increased fractional excretion of sodium, Tm is decreased for glucose, phosphate and bicarbonate.

The mechanism of bicarbonate transport through the tubular cell (Fig. 3.5) is of particular importance because of its role in the renal regulation of acid–base balance. This mechanism may be summarized in three equations:

$$NaHCO_3 \rightleftharpoons Na^+ + HCO_3^- \quad (1)$$

$$HCO_3^- + H^+ \rightleftharpoons H_2CO_3 \underset{\text{ANHYDRASE}}{\overset{\text{CARBONIC}}{\rightleftharpoons}} H_2O + CO_2 \quad (2)$$

$$H_2O + CO_2 \underset{\text{ANHYDRASE}}{\overset{\text{CARBONIC}}{\rightleftharpoons}} H_2CO_3 \rightleftharpoons H^+ + HCO_3^- \quad (3)$$

Bicarbonate enters the tubular lumen as sodium bicarbonate and dissociates into bicarbonate (a relatively impermeable anion) and sodium (1). The sodium passes into the cell in exchange for

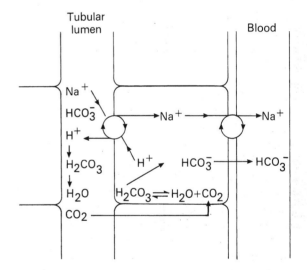

Fig. 3.5 Bicarbonate reabsorption in the proximal tubule.

a hydrogen ion. The hydrogen ion combines with bicarbonate in the tubular lumen to form carbonic acid. The enzyme carbonic anhydrase, present on the brush border of the proximal tubular cell, splits carbonic acid into carbon dioxide and water (2), both of which are freely permeable and enter the tubular cell. Here, intracellular carbonic anhydrase reforms carbonic acid which in turn dissociates into free hydrogen and bicarbonate ions (3). The bicarbonate ion passes through the basal cell membrane into the peritubular space and is available for reabsorption by the peritubular capillary. The hydrogen ion can be extruded from the cell in exchange for sodium and the cycle repeated. The enzyme carbonic anhydrase participates in both the dissociation and formation of carbonic acid depending on its site of action.

Another substance to be reabsorbed in the proximal tubule is uric acid. This is a small molecule which is filtered freely and over 90% is reabsorbed in the proximal tubule. However, uric acid homoeostasis is regulated by secretion of uric acid in the distal tubule. Anther small molecule which is filtered freely is urea and approximately 50% of the filtered load is reabsorbed passively in the proximal tubule, the remainder passing down into the distal tubule to participate in the osmolar regulatory mechanisms of the inner medulla.

In addition to hydrogen ions, some other substances such as organic acids and bases are secreted (i.e. moved from the peritubular capillary into the tubular lumen) in the proximal tubule. These include a number of drugs, e.g. penicillin, PAH. The secretory processes may be either active or passive and some have tubular maximal secretory capacities.

The loop of Henle, distal tubule and collecting tubule (Fig. 3.6)

The tubular fluid entering the loop of Henle is isosmotic and finally leaves the collecting duct as urine varying in volume, osmolality and composition according to the needs of the body. The fine regulatory mechanisms are situated in this portion of the nephron. The loops of Henle of the juxtamedullary nephrons dip deeply into the medulla whereas the collecting tubules of all nephrons pass through the medulla. There is an increase in osmolality from the cortex to the medulla; this is essential for the concentration and dilution of tubular fluid. The main mechanism for this is the counter-current multiplier situated in the loop of Henle (Fig. 3.6).

Counter-current mechanism

The loop of Henle consists of a thin descending limb and a thin first part followed by thick upper part of the ascending limb. The volume of fluid entering the loop of Henle is approximately 15%

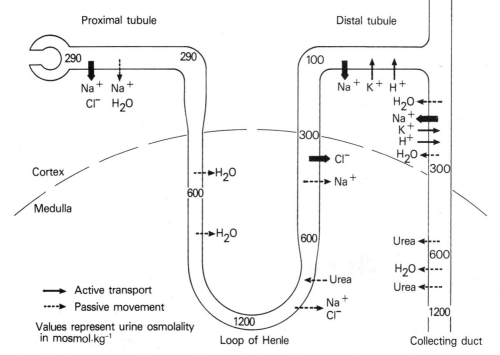

Fig. 3.6 Concentration of glomerular filtrate in the loop of Henle and collecting tubule.

of the glomerular filtrate and only one-third of this leaves the cortical part of the collecting tubule. The tubular fluid enters the loop with an osmolality of 290 mosmol.kg^{-1} and leaves at 100 mosmol.kg^{-1}. The loop is the active part (a counter-current multiplier) and the vasa recta surrounding the loop of Henle are the counter-current exchanger. Two main transport processes are responsible for the work of the counter-current mechanism:

1. *Sodium and water reabsorption.* The thick ascending part of the loop is impermeable to water but both sodium and chloride are transported into the interstitium. Although this is an active transport process there is much debate as to whether sodium or chloride is transported actively. Current opinion favours chloride, with sodium moving by a cotransport mechanism (see above). This results in an increase in the osmolality of the interstitium ranging from 300 mosmol.kg^{-1} in the cortex to 1200 mosmol.kg^{-1} at the tip of the loop. The descending limb is freely permeable to water, sodium and chloride and all three move into the interstitium. Fluid enters the descending limb at an osmolality of 290 mosmol.kg^{-1} and the osmolality increases slowly until it is equivalent to that at the tip of the loop, i.e. 1200 mosmol.kg^{-1}. On passing up the ascending limb, sodium and chloride are removed but water is retained and the osmolality decreases from 1200 to 100 mosmol.kg^{-1}.

The vasa recta play an important role in this osmolar transport. Although there is no active transport present in these vessels, water and solutes are freely permeable. The osmolality of blood entering the vasa recta is the same as that of the fluid entering the descending limb, i.e. 290 mosmol.kg^{-1}, and slowly increases to 1200 mosmol.kg^{-1} as it passes down to the tip of the loop. This is achieved by the passage of water and solutes across its surface. The blood flow is significantly slower in the lower parts of the vasa recta, thus improving the efficiency of this exchange. As the vasa recta move from the medullary tip back towards the cortex, the same process occurs and the osmolality is returned to 290 mosmol.kg^{-1}. As a consequence of the low flow rate in these vessels, oxygen content and energy requirements are markedly reduced.

2. *Urea recycling.* Urea, a waste product of protein metabolism, contributes up to 50% of the osmolality of the medullary interstitium. Because it is a small molecule it is filtered freely at the glomerulus and approximately half is reabsorbed during passage through the proximal tubule. As the tubular fluid passes down the descending limb the urea concentration is increased, firstly by the passage of water out of the descending limb and secondly at the tip of the loop by the addition of urea, which moves freely from the medullary interstitium, an area of high urea concentration. The high concentration of urea at the tip of the medulla is achieved by the collecting tubule. The cortical part of the collecting tubule is impermeable to urea but permeable to water, resulting in an increase in urea concentration within the tubule. However, in the medullary portion of the collecting tubule, both water and urea pass into the interstitium. Hence, urea is recycled through the medulla and plays an important part in maintaining the high medullary osmolality essential for the counter-current mechanism.

Sodium–potassium exchange

More than 90% of filtered potassium is reabsorbed in the proximal tubule and potassium which appears in the final urine is secreted in the distal tubule by a transport process coupled loosely to active sodium transport. As sodium is reabsorbed from the tubular lumen, a negative potential is created within the lumen which allows potassium to move passively down an electrochemical gradient. In this region, hydrogen ions are secreted also and compete with potassium to a degree dependent on the acid–base status. The control of sodium reabsorption in the distal tubule is primarily hormonal and controlled probably via the renin–angiotensin system.

Renin–angiotensin system

The renin–angiotensin system is an important part of the complex mechanism responsible for controlling extracellular fluid volume, the other 'effector' parts being plasma proteins (see above) and osmolar control (see below). Renin is a proteolytic enzyme secreted from the juxtaglomerular apparatus situated in the afferent arteriole. The secretion of renin is a matter of some debate. It has been suggested that a baroreceptor mechanism situated in the afferent arteriole detects a decrease in renal blood flow and responds by increasing renin production. The alternative hypothesis is that changes in sodium concentration in the distal tubule are detected by the macula densa situated in the early part of the distal tubule, increases in sodium concentration causing an increase in renin secretion. However, there is conflicting evidence on this latter point. The renin acts on an α_2 plasma protein (angiotensinogen) and splits off a decapeptide, angiotensin I. A converting enzyme found both in plasma and various tissues of the body, including lung, converts angiotensin I to angiotensin II. This agent has three main actions. It is a potent vasopressor which may act on the glomerular arterioles and thereby contribute to glomerulotubular balance. It has a direct action on the brain, stimulating the thirst centre. Of most importance is its effect of stimulating secretion of aldosterone from the zona glomerulosa of the adrenal gland. Plasma aldosterone levels are affected also by the plasma potassium concentration, an increase in potassium reducing the aldosterone concentration. The converse occurs with plasma sodium concentration, i.e. a decrease in plasma sodium increases aldosterone. The main action of aldosterone is to increase sodium reabsorption in the distal tubule. Potassium and/or hydrogen ions are then secreted into the tubule in exchange for reabsorbed sodium. The renin–angiotensin system has its own feedback control, angiotensin II suppressing further secretion of renin.

Atrial natriuretic peptide (ANP)

In recent years, there has been great interest in a 28-amino acid peptide which is found in the atria of most mammalian species. The peptide is released in response to atrial stretching either by increased right or left atrial pressure or by an elevated central venous pressure. ANP has a dual effect on renal function. Firstly, it increases GFR by decreasing afferent arteriolar resistance and increasing efferent arteriolar resistance. Secondly, there are direct effects on tubular function, although these are more controversial. In essence, ANP produces a decrease in proximal tubular sodium reabsorption and an alteration in sodium handling in the ascending loop of Henle and in the inner medullary collecting tubule. The net effect of these alterations is a marked natriuresis accompanied by a diuresis with increased excretion of phosphate, magnesium, calcium and, to a lesser extent, potassium. In addition, ANP interacts with other renal hormones, decreasing renin and aldosterone secretion. Its final place in the control of extracellular fluid volume has yet to be established but it may occupy a pivotal role.

Renal regulation of acid–base balance

The distal tubule participates both qualitatively and quantitatively in acid–base control. As described previously the majority (up to 80%) of filtered bicarbonate is reabsorbed in the proximal tubule and the remainder by the distal tubule. The absorptive mechanism for bicarbonate reabsorption in the distal tubule is similar to that of the proximal tubule, namely the formation and dissociation of carbonic acid by the enzyme carbonic anhydrase. Conversely, although there is some hydrogen ion secretion in the proximal tubule, the bulk is secreted in the distal tubule.

Hydrogen ions are excreted in the final urine in combination with either ammonia or phosphates. Approximately 60 mmol of hydrogen ions are excreted per day, of which two-thirds are combined with ammonia (NH_3) to form ammonium ion (NH_4^+) and one-third with sodium phosphate salts, often referred to as titratable acids (TA).

Ammonia (NH_3) is generated within the tubular cell mainly from the metabolism of the amino acid glutamine. When glutamine is converted to either glutamate or α-ketoglutarate, which enters the citric acid cycle, a free ammonia molecule is generated. This is freely permeable through the cell wall and passes down the concentration gradient into the tubular lumen. Here it combines with free hydrogen ions to form NH_4^+. This hydrophilic anion is unable to re-enter tubular cells and so is excreted in the urine.

The remaining one-third of hydrogen ions are excreted when combined with phosphate. Disodium hydrophosphate enters the distal tubule and dissociates. One sodium ion is reabsorbed, leaving a negatively charged molecule. The positive hydrogen ion in the tubular lumen combines to form sodium dihydrophosphate which is excreted in the final urine.

Hydrogen ions for both ammonium and TA formation come from intracellular dissociation of carbonic acid and the net effect is the intracellular generation of a bicarbonate ion which passes through the basal border of the cell into the peritubular capillary. The amount of hydrogen ion secretion and bicarbonate regeneration depends predominantly on the acid–base status. The total hydrogen ion secretion may be expressed by the following formula:

$$\text{Total H}^+ \text{ excretion} = \text{NH}_4^+ \text{ excretion} + \text{TA excretion} - \text{HCO}_3 \text{ excretion}$$

Osmolar regulation

By the time the glomerular filtrate enters the collecting tubule, its original volume has been reduced to 5% and when it leaves the collecting tubule it is reduced to 1%. Final urine volumes depend in part on the extracellular fluid volume and its regulation via sodium excretion and in part on the regulation of plasma osmolality. The osmolar regulation system has a detector (osmoreceptors), a messenger (antidiuretic hormone, ADH) and an effector (the collecting tubule).

The osmoreceptors situated in the hypothalamus detect changes in plasma osmolality, the major contribution being from plasma sodium. An increase in plasma osmolality stimulates the synthesis of ADH (vasopressin) in the supraoptic nuclei of the hypothalamus. The hormone is an octapeptide (8-arginine vasopressin) which passes along the nerve fibres to the posterior pituitary. After appropriate stimulation, the hormone is released from storage granules in the posterior pituitary and secreted into the systemic circulation. Its action on the peritubular cell membrane is to increase the permeability of water; this involves activation of the cyclic 3′,5′-AMP system. Water is then reabsorbed from the collecting tubule and passes into the peritubular capillary to return the plasma osmolality to normal and reduce the urine volume. The reverse situation occurs if plasma osmolality decreases. ADH secretion ceases and the collecting tubule becomes impermeable to water; more

water is excreted, urine volume increases and plasma osmolality increases towards normal levels. By this mechanism, it is possible that urine osmolality may vary from a hypotonic urine with a minimum value of approximately 60 mosmol.kg^{-1} to a maximal value of 1200 to 1400 mosmol.kg^{-1}. It should be noted that the final osmolality of hypertonic urine is equivalent to the tonicity at the tip of the renal medulla. ADH also increases the amount of urea reabsorbed in the cortical part of the collecting tubule, thereby contributing to the counter-current mechanism by increasing medullary tip osmolality.

It is possible to estimate the action of ADH by determining the amount of water excreted or reabsorbed compared with the amount of solutes excreted. Osmolar clearance (C_{osm}), an expression of solute excretion, is determined by using the standard clearance formula:

$$C_{osm} = \frac{U_{osm} \, V}{P_{osm}}$$

where U_{osm} = osmolar clearance in ml.min^{-1}
P_{osm} = plasma osmolality in mosmol.kg^{-1}
V = urine excretion rate in ml.min^{-1}.

If urine is dilute, i.e. hypotonic, V is greater than C_{osm}. The difference is termed free water clearance (C_{H_2O}) and may be expressed as follows:

$$C_{H_2O} = V - C_{osm}$$

where C_{H_2O} = free water clearance in ml.min^{-1}.

Conversely, if urine is concentrated, i.e. hypertonic, more water is reabsorbed and C_{osm} becomes greater than V. Free water clearance then becomes negative.

Another way of explaining negative free water clearance is to consider that water is being reabsorbed, i.e. solute-free water reabsorption, and may be expressed as follows:

$$V = C_{osm} - T^c_{H_2O}$$
$$\text{or, } T^c_{H_2O} = C_{osm} - V$$

where $T^c_{H_2O}$ = solute-free water reabsorption in ml.min^{-1}.

By varying the amount of water reabsorbed in the collecting tubule and influencing the plasma sodium concentration it may be seen that osmolar regulation plays a vital part in controlling body fluid status. The two systems, i.e. osmolar regulation and volume regulation, are interrelated and in considering overall fluid balance it is not possible to dissociate the two.

In summary, the kidney plays a vital role in maintaining the 'milieu interieur'. It does so by variable adjustments of glomerular filtration rate, tubular reabsorption and secretion to produce a final urine which varies in volume, composition and acid–base status.

FURTHER READING

Bevan D R 1994 Renal function. In: Nimmo W S, Rowbotham D J, Smith G (eds) Anaesthesia, 2nd edn. Blackwell Scientific Publications, Oxford, p 272–290

Innes A, Catto G R D 1994 Renal failure. In: Nimmo W S, Rowbotham D J, Smith G (eds) Anaesthesia, 2nd edn. Blackwell Scientific Publications, Oxford, p 1771–1792

4. Physiology of the nervous system

STRUCTURE AND FUNCTION

The function of the human nervous system is the acquisition of information from the external environment and its computation to produce an integrated response. The central nervous system (CNS) comprises the brain and spinal cord. The peripheral nervous system is composed of 43 pairs of nerves which contain afferent sensory fibres conducting impulses to the CNS from the periphery, and efferent motor fibres conducting in the reverse direction. There are 10^9–10^{12} neurones, each surrounded by neuroglial cells, in the CNS. These cells are of two types:

1. Oligodendrocytes, which form myelin.
2. Microglia, which phagocytose degenerating neurones.

The physiology of the nervous system is related intimately to membrane physiology and cell excitation. Excitability results from specialization of excitable cell membranes. The intracellular environment is controlled by cell membranes which exhibit selective permeability by virtue of channels or pores in the membrane. Excitable membranes undergo rapid reversible changes in permeability to some charged molecules or ions. At a pressure receptor the membrane ionic permeability alters in response to mechanical deformation, and flow of ions occurs across the membrane.

A cell membrane is composed of lipids and protein (Fig. 4.1). Phospholipid forms the major part of the cell membrane, which may be considered as a bilayer arranged such that a polar head is located on the outside of the cell membrane and one or two hydrocarbon chains, which are hydrophobic, constitute the inner part of the bilayer. Cell membrane proteins are composed of chains of amino acids with different side chains, either hydrophilic or hydrophobic, which by folding can 'hide' their hydrophobic amino acids on the interior.

A lipid bilayer is very impermeable to small ions; consequently, cell membrane permeability resides

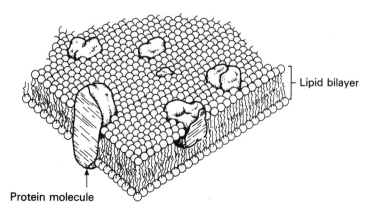

Fig. 4.1 Structure of the cell membrane.

in the membrane proteins. The proteins confer specific ionic permeability on the membrane whilst only a small part of the membrane appears to be directly involved in ion flow.

Membrane protein as ion pump

Ion movement across a cell membrane can occur against the electrochemical gradient and is therefore active. Membrane proteins which achieve active transport are termed ion pumps. All cell membranes contain a sodium pump (Fig. 4.2). Ionic permeability is of two types:

1. Constant resting ionic permeability to ions including potassium (K^+) and chloride (Cl^-), which is not affected by physiological stimuli.
2. Non-constant permeability, which changes rapidly due to the action of a stimulus on an appropriate membrane protein.

Permeability is 'gated' by the stimulus. This is a characteristic of excitable membranes.

Several possibilities exist for the actual transport of an ion across the cell membrane. A protein may act as a carrier and ferry the ion across, or it may span the bilayer and produce a pore (Fig. 4.3). The latter mechanism produces much more rapid transport.

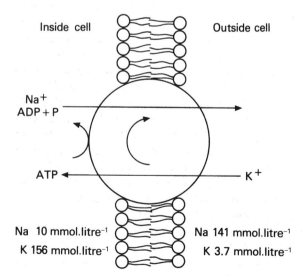

Fig. 4.2 The sodium pump. Na = Sodium; K = potassium; ADP = adenosine diphosphate; ATP = adenosine triphosphate.

Na 10 mmol.litre^{-1}
K 156 mmol.litre^{-1}

Na 141 mmol.litre^{-1}
K 3.7 mmol.litre^{-1}

Inside cell

Outside cell

Na$^+$
ADP + P

ATP

K$^+$

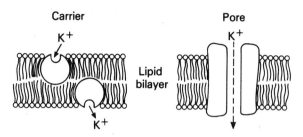

Fig. 4.3 Mechanisms of ion transport by proteins.

Electrochemical gradient

This is a measure of the force driving a specific ion into or out of the cell. It comprises an electrical component, which is the potential difference between the inside and outside of the cell (−60 mV). The chemical gradient is a simple concentration gradient. In certain conditions, these two components may oppose and cancel each other out, at which point the ion is in electrochemical equilibrium across the membrane and the Nernst equation applies. This is dependent upon the unequal distribution of ions across membranes. If permeability to sodium (Na^+) and Cl^- is assumed to be zero at the resting potential of biological membranes, then:

$$V = \frac{RT}{F} \log_e \frac{K_o^+}{K_i^+}$$

where: V = potential difference, R = the gas constant, F = Faraday's constant, T = temperature, K_o^+ = concentration of K^+ in extracellular fluid (ECF), and K_i^+ = concentration of K^+ in intracellular fluid (ICF).

Nerve impulse and conduction

Characteristic changes in membrane potential on passage of a nerve impulse constitute an action potential. The passage of a stimulating current to this nerve axon produces first a stimulus artefact and then an action potential (Fig. 4.4).

Action potential

This is an all-or-none phenomenon. The least stimulus strength required to produce an action potential is termed the threshold stimulus. The transient reversal of the membrane potential pro-

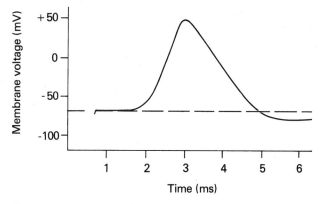

Fig. 4.4 The action potential.

pagates along an axon at constant velocity in a non-decremental manner. The refractory period is the period during which a second stimulating current does not elicit a second action potential. The absolute refractory period occurs immediately after the initial stimulus and lasts for approximately the same duration as the action potential itself. At this time, it is not possible to initiate a new impulse. Thereafter, the relative refractory period requires an increased threshold to initiate an impulse.

In the giant squid axon the resting membrane potential (−60 mV) is close to the Nernst potential for K^+ and results from selective permeability to K^+ in the axon membrane.

A change in resting potential is produced by changes in external and internal K^+ concentration. The resting potential is the result of two factors:

1. Ionic gradients produced by the sodium pump.
2. Selective permeability of the resting axon to K^+ with respect to Na^+.

As an action potential passes, the axon membrane becomes active and the membrane voltage is reversed from negative to positive. This corresponds to depolarization with an overshoot up to +40 mV. The action potential results from an increase in membrane conductance to Na^+, resulting in an increase in membrane potential towards the Nernst potential for Na^+. Thus, if the external Na^+ concentration decreases, the action potential becomes smaller in amplitude and eventually is reduced to zero. Selective block of Na^+ ion current can be produced experimentally with tetrodotoxin

and of K^+ with tetraethylammonium. Such studies show that the following events occur:

1. The sodium channel is opened rapidly by depolarization of membrane voltage and closes slowly (inactivates) even if depolarization is maintained. The open phase is always transient.
2. The potassium channel is slowly opened by depolarization of the membrane and does not close during the short time-scale of the action potential, i.e. there is late outward K^+ current whilst depolarization is maintained.

A threshold stimulus produces an all-or-nothing response. The Na^+ channel is opened by membrane depolarization; Na^+ ions pass through into the axon to produce more depolarization, thereby opening more channels and further increasing Na^+ ion influx and outward flux of K^+, which resists depolarization. Na^+ channels do not open until the membrane voltage has changed by 20 mV from the resting potential. Inactivated Na^+ channels take a few milliseconds to become functional again and therefore are not opened again by immediate depolarization. These are the underlying events of the refractory period. The increase in K^+ conductance always tends to increase K^+ ion current, which resists any change of membrane voltage away from the resting level.

Propagation of impulse (Fig. 4.5). Large axons have high conduction velocities. For fibres of a given diameter, conduction is greatly increased by myelination. Axons from 1 to 25 μm in diameter are myelinated; those less than 1 μm are unmyelinated. Nerve fibres have a structure

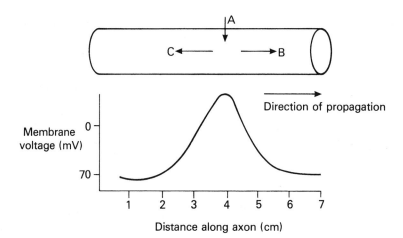

Fig. 4.5 Local circuit theory of impulse propagation. A = Influx of Na$^+$ ions at active membrane; B, C = current flow. B propagates the impulse; C finds the membrane refractory.

akin to a shielded electrical cable, in other words a central conducting core with insulation and an external conducting area which is ECF. In vertebrate myelinated fibres, a Schwann cell lays down myelin in concentric layers. Between neighbouring segments of myelin there is a very narrow gap termed the node of Ranvier, which is less than 1 μm wide; here no obstacle exists between the axon membrane and the ECF. This accounts for conduction occurring in a saltatory manner. The myelin sheaths act as high-resistance barriers to current flow and excitation occurs only at the nodes of Ranvier. Thus, the impulse is propagated from node to node.

Repetitive stimulation of nerve fibres induces an increase in their size. This is the basis of experimental spinal cord stimulation techniques in the treatment of conditions such as chronic pain, and in patients with multiple sclerosis and bladder dysfunction.

The synapse

A synapse occurs where the membranes of two excitable cells are closely apposed to allow transmission of information. The transmitter is usually chemical, is released in a controlled amount by the cell and diffuses rapidly to bind to a receptor site on the second cell, where it produces rapid changes in ion flux. Presynaptic fibres divide into numerous fine branches, producing presynaptic

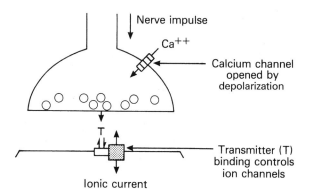

Fig. 4.6 Chemical synapse transmission.

knobs. A single anterior horn cell may receive 30 000 knobs from a large number of axons. The presynaptic membrane releases transmitter from synaptic vesicles into a synaptic cleft, 20–25 nm in width, to the postsynaptic membrane (Fig. 4.6).

Transmission of information across a synapse is usually undirectional and involves a time delay. In the spinal motor neurone, this amounts to 0.4 ms. A knowledge of total delay in a reflex pathway is useful in determining the number of synapses involved. Synapses operate in a graded fashion which allows the neurone to carry out integration and sifting of information.

Enzymes break down the transmitter after release, thereby reducing its duration of action at the postsynaptic membrane.

Control of transmitter release

The arrival of an action potential produces depolarization of the terminal membrane, which opens voltage-sensitive calcium ion (Ca^{++}) channels, resulting in flux of Ca^{++} into presynaptic areas. This in turn stimulates transient exocytosis of the transmitter into the synaptic gap, where it diffuses rapidly to specific protein-binding sites (receptors) on the postsynaptic membrane. Ionic currents through these sites then alter the membrane potential of the postsynaptic cell in a direction determined by the ion selectivity of the channels concerned. Depolarization causes excitation, and hyperpolarization results in inhibition.

The postsynaptic membrane channels are gated by specific chemical stimuli. In the absence of nerve stimulation, miniature end-plate potentials (MEPPs) occur; these are produced by arrival of single transmitter vesicles. A propagative end-plate potential requires 100 transmitter vesicles. At the neuromuscular junction, one impulse produces 100 vesicles, each containing 50 000 molecules of acetycholine (ACh). Of the 5 000 000 transmitter molecules released, only 100 000 open a postsynaptic channel, but this is sufficient to cause 10 000 000 000 Na^+ ions to enter muscle in 1 ms. Both excitatory and inhibitory postsynaptic potentials can be recorded intracellularly. Presynaptic inhibition may also occur from inhibitory terminals situated on excitatory presynaptic nerve endings; stimulation of these terminals reduces the amount of neurotransmitter released.

It is well-known that antibiotics may interfere with neuromuscular conduction, often by decreasing end-plate transmitter. High concentrations of magnesium (Mg^{++}) and some antibiotics decrease evoked release of ACh. Postjunctional effects include receptor or end-plate ion channel blockade. There is considerable variability between antibiotics in their neuromuscular blocking mechanisms. Aminoglycosides, polymyxin and tetracyclines produce neuromuscular block by a combination of pre- and postjunctional effects.

Information is processed by nerve networks by two basic mechanisms:

1. *Spatial summation*. This occurs when stimulation of two afferent nerves together produces a response which neither alone can elicit. Both synapses may be excitatory for that particular nerve.

2. *Temporal summation*. Stimulation of the same nerve twice in rapid succession produces a response where a single stimulus elicits none.

There are also electrical synapses (e.g. in the retina) and synapses at which transmitter release is controlled by graded depolarizations.

Neurotransmitters

Neurotransmitters are of three main types (amino acids, monoamines and peptides) which are present in widely differing concentrations. Synaptic transmission is more complex than simple transfer of excitation or inhibition from presynaptic neurone to the postsynaptic cell. There is a great range of synaptic connections, and the possibility of chemical coding exists. Axoaxonal synapses may regulate the amount of transmitter released from presynaptic terminals; other inputs may trigger very long-lasting postsynaptic events (lasting for minutes) and therefore control the excitability of a target cell, rather than directly controlling its firing.

Fast chemical signalling in the CNS. Amino acids are fast neurotransmitters in the CNS. L-glutamate (Glu) and L-aspartate (Asp) act at excitatory synapses and γ-aminobutyric acid (GABA) and glycine (Gly) act at inhibitory synapses.

Fast excitatory transmitters. Glutamate is the most important excitatory transmitter in the CNS. It acts on at least three types of receptor, two of which are coupled to ion channels (ionotropic receptors) and one coupled to second messenger-producing systems (metabotropic receptors). The ionotropic receptors are named after specific agonists γ-amino-3-hydroxy-5-methyl-4-isoxazole propionate (AMPA) and *N*-methyl-D-aspartate (NMDA; Table 4.1). The AMPA receptor is linked to an ion channel that is permeable to both Na^+ and K^+ ions, whereas the NMDA receptor, in addition to permitting flow of Na^+ and K^+, is also permeable to calcium ions. This receptor is usually blocked at the resting membrane potential with magnesium which is removed from the channel by depolarization due to activation of

Table 4.1   Excitatory amino acid receptors

	Ionotropic		Metabotropic
Other agonists	AMPA Glutamate Kainate	NMDA Glutamate Aspartate	ACPD Glutamate Quisqualate Ibotenate
Antagonists	Nitro-quinoxalines	APV MK 801 (Dizocilpine) Dissociative anaesthetics such as ketamine Magnesium	Phenylglycines

AMPA = γ-amino-3-hydroxy-5-methyl-4-isoxazole propionate; NMDA = N-methyl-D-aspartate; ACPD = (1S,3R)-1-aminocyclopentane-1,3-dicarboxylic acid; APV = 2-amino-5-phosphonopentanoic acid.

AMPA receptors or other excitatory receptors. The channel can also be blocked by dissociative anaesthetics such as ketamine. The metabotropic receptors are coupled to different intracellular second-messenger systems and can lead to changes in intracellular calcium and activation of protein kinase C via hydrolysis of phosphatidylinositol 4,5 biphosphate (the PI system) or to activation of adenylate cyclase to alter cyclic adenosine monophosphate (cAMP) levels.

L-glutamate is widely distributed in the CNS and has been implicated in sensory processing, motor control and higher cortical functions, including memory and learning. Moreover, in neurological or pathological conditions such as stroke, anoxia or epilepsy, these transmitters are believed to have key roles, and drugs that antagonize their effects have great therapeutic potential.

Inhibitory amino acids. GABA is the main inhibitory neurotransmitter in the CNS, and acts at almost one-third of all synapses. There are two main GABA receptors: GABA_A and GABA_B. GABA_A receptors are associated with chloride channels and the receptor contains modulatory sites to which benzodiazepines and barbiturates can bind to enhance the actions of GABA (Fig. 4.7). The GABA_B receptor is linked to a potassium channel. Glycine predominates as the inhibitory transmitter in the spinal cord.

Diffuse regulatory systems: monoamines. These are associated with diffuse neural pathways, mainly in the brain stem. Much of the monoamine release may be at non-synaptic sites.

Neuropeptides. Virtually all peptide hormones of the endocrine and neuroendocrine systems also exist in distinct systems of the CNS. Active peptides released from endocrine and neural tissue are called regulatory peptides. They are capable of producing an effect by acting as hormones, local regulators or neurotransmitters, or a combination of all of these. Vasoactive intestinal peptide (VIP), which acts as a neurotransmitter, is one example. Enteric nerves containing peptides belong to a non-adrenergic, non-cholinergic subdivision of the autonomic nervous system. The spinal cord contains a very large number of regulatory peptides, including substance P, VIP, enkephalin and neuropeptide Y.

Membrane receptor function in anaesthesia

Most hormones and drugs produce effects by binding to cell recognition sites termed receptors. A receptor is an integral membrane protein which is recognized selectively by a precise hormone or neurotransmitter termed a ligand (Fig. 4.8). A

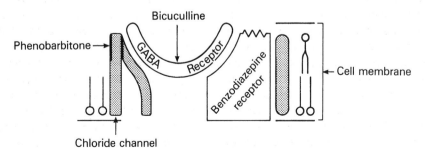

Fig. 4.7 γ-Aminobutyric acid (GABA) receptor, benzodiazepine receptor and chloride channel.

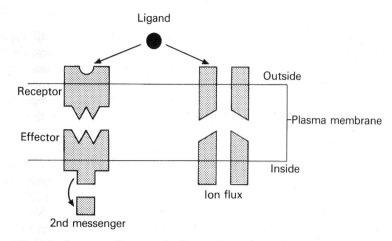

Fig. 4.8 Receptor-effector mechanisms: release of second messenger or promotion of ion flux.

ligand is an agonist if it activates a receptor to transduce a response, or an antagonist when the substance interacts with a receptor causing it to remain inactive and, by occupying the receptor, diminishes or aborts the effect of an agonist. The interaction between ligand and receptor is specific, reversible, saturable and a high-affinity binding process. Binding is followed by alterations in metabolic events within the cell, e.g. ion flux, which produce the characteristic physiological effect.

Receptor types have been purified in recent years using affinity chromatography, photoaffinity labelling and radioligand techniques. Positron emission tomography allows quantitative imaging of muscarinic, cholinergic, opioid and benzodiazepine receptors. Radioactive tracer molecules can be incorporated into substrates such as glucose or into a drug, and become bound to receptors so that serial images can be obtained from different areas of the brain. Such techniques allow measurement of regional oxygen metabolism, assist the differential diagnosis of coma and are useful in cases of epilepsy if surgery is being considered.

Adrenergic receptors. Agonists at β-adrenoceptors in order of potency include isoprenaline, adrenaline, noradrenaline and dopamine. β_1-Receptors are found in the heart and are equally sensitive to adrenaline and noradrenaline. β_2-Receptors are found in smooth muscle and are more sensitive to adrenaline than to noradrenaline. The effects are mediated by intracellular cAMP, the second messenger, which activates protein kinases. Thus the β-adrenergic agonist–receptor complex couples to adenylate cyclase (the effector molecule) which is then activated, and catalyses synthesis of cAMP; this is subsequently hydrolysed by phosphodiesterase.

α-Adrenoceptors mediate control of smooth muscle in the vasculature of the uterus and gastrointestinal tract. The order of potency of agonists is: adrenaline, noradrenaline, isoprenaline. There are two classes of α-receptor (Fig. 4.9); α_1-receptors are postsynaptic and mediate constriction of smooth muscle. These are blocked selectively by prazosin and phenoxybenzamine. α_2-Receptors are presynaptic and mediate feedback inhibition of further neurotransmitter release by noradrenaline. These receptors are blocked selectively by yohimbine. α_2-Receptors are also found on platelets, where they mediate aggregation. Methoxamine and phenylephrine are selective α_1-agonists. There are at least two subtypes of presynaptic α_2-adrenoreceptors involved in noradrenaline release. Clonidine, an α_2-agonist, inhibits central sympathetic activity, producing sedation and a reduced requirement for anaesthetic agents.

Within the CNS, adrenaline is found in small groups of cells in the pons and medulla which project to the hypothalamus and brain stem and to the nucleus tractus solitarius, which may be important in central arterial pressure control. Noradrenaline is found in all areas of the brain

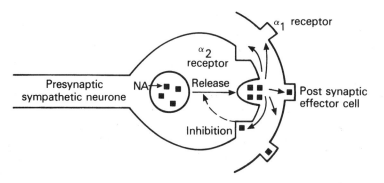

Fig. 4.9 Types of α-adrenergic receptors. NA = Noradrenaline.

and spinal cord, with a high density in the hypothalamus. Experimentally, noradrenaline in low doses enhances the response to excitatory amino acids, but in high doses it inhibits these responses. Adrenergic receptors in central and peripheral neurones are coupled to G proteins linked to adenylate cyclase. Activation of β-adrenoreceptors increases cAMP production via G_s (stimulatory) protein and activation of α-receptors decreases cAMP via G_i (inhibitory) protein. Dexmedetomidine is a selective α_2-adrenoreceptor agonist with similar sedative effects to clonidine, and exerts its effects by inhibiting conductance through a G_i protein-modulated potassium channel.

Dopamine receptors. Dopamine receptors occur in basal ganglia, the substantia nigra, corpus striatum and the limbic system. In the basal ganglia, dopamine is antagonistic to ACh. Absence of dopamine is an important aetiological factor in Parkinsonism. In the hypothalamus, dopamine is concerned with release of prolactin. Dopamine suppresses prolactin secretion and dopamine antagonists (e.g. metoclopramide) increase hyperprolactinaemia.

A dopaminergic system connects the limbic cortex, basal ganglia and hypothalamus and is concerned with behaviour. This system is involved in the pathogenesis of schizophrenia (phenothiazines block dopamine receptors). Dopaminergic fibres are found in the chemoreceptor trigger zone; stimulation produces nausea and vomiting. Dopaminergic and sympathomimetic receptors have been identified in the coronary, renal, cerebral and mesenteric vessels. Dopamine receptors also occur on the presynaptic membrane of post-

ganglionic sympathetic nerves and sympathetic ganglia where their physiological role is unclear.

Acetylcholine. ACh is found in motor neurones of the spinal cord and cranial nerve motor nuclei, where it acts as a *fast* chemical transmitter for neuromuscular transmission. In intrinsic pathways in the CNS, it probably acts as a modulator in basal ganglia, the hippocampus, and the diffuse ascending pathways to the cortex, and may represent what was known as the ascending reticular activating system. ACh probably plays an important part in cortical arousal and electroencephalographic (EEG) changes of rapid eye movement (REM) sleep. The effects of ACh are terminated by hydrolysis by cholinesterase. Its peripheral effects may be classified into two types:

1. Muscarinic effects at postganglionic parasympathetic fibres.
2. Nicotinic effects at sympathetic and parasympathetic ganglia and the neuromuscular junction.

Muscarinic cholinergic receptors in the intestine stimulate electrolyte transport by acting directly on the enterocyte, whereas nicotinic agonists act indirectly to augment absorption by stimulating release of intermediary neurotransmitters.

Denervation of skeletal muscle enhances its sensitivity to ACh by development of a diffuse distribution of ACh receptors over post-junctional surfaces. Administration of suxamethonium in these circumstances results in severe hyperkalaemia.

Histamine receptors. H_1-Receptors are responsible for contraction of smooth muscle (e.g. in the gut, and bronchi). H_2-Receptors stimulate acid secretion by the stomach and increase heart rate. These H_2 effects are not prevented by H_1-antihistamines, but by H_2-receptor blockers such as cimetidine and ranitidine. The vascular effects of histamine are mediated by both types of receptor. In some instances, H_1 and H_2 have opposing actions, e.g. H_1 produces pulmonary vasodilatation. Both H_1-and H_2-receptors occur in the brain.

5-Hydroxytryptamine (5-HT, serotonin). This has been isolated from the brain stem, many forebrain sites and the dorsal horns of the spinal cord. It may represent one of the descending control pathways which modulate sensitivity of the spinal cord to pain input from the periphery, and therefore plays a key role in mediating analgesic actions of morphine and related opioid analgesics. In the forebrain, this system may be responsible for control of sleep and waking, central temperature regulation and control of aggressive behaviour.

Benzodiazepines. Although not endogenous substances, these drugs act at specific synapses in the CNS (including the spinal cord) at which GABA is the transmitter. Benzodiazepines selectively facilitate GABA action at synapses. Aminophylline may reverse diazepam sedation by its adenosine-blocking effect at GABA receptors. Adenosine is as potent a CNS-depressant mediator as GABA, and may have an amplifying effect on the GABA–receptor complex. Flumazenil is a benzodiazepine antagonist. Benzodiazepines exert their effects via a GABA–benzodiazepine receptor–chloride channel complex (Fig. 4.7), which may also mediate anxiety, and which is enclosed in the lipid bilayer of cell membranes.

Neurotransmitters in disease

Anxiety probably involves many neurotransmitters including GABA, 5-HT, noradrenaline and dopamine. There are strong indications that central monoamine metabolism is disturbed in endogenous depression, and that the disturbance is causal. Tricyclic antidepressants inhibit the presynaptic uptake of 5-HT and noradrenaline (Fig. 4.10). All antidepressants facilitate synaptic activity of amines; however, tricyclic antidepressants also block cholinergic receptors. The anticholinesterase physostigmine can relieve manic symptoms.

In patients with *affective disorders*, cholinergic receptor density is increased. In schizophrenia, catecholamine activity may worsen symptoms. Neuroleptic drugs administered in small doses dramatically reverse amphetamine-induced psychoses; amphetamine induces schizophrenic exacerbations. This provides further support for the concept of a dopaminergic abnormality in schizophrenia. Some symptoms of schizophrenia are reduced by naloxone, suggesting that opioid peptides (e.g. enkephalins) are involved, although naloxone also blocks GABA receptors. The brain of patients who have died with Alzheimer's disease contains reduced concentrations of choline acetyltransferase, noradrenaline, GABA and somatostatin, although the most severe abnormality is a cholinergic deficit.

Epilepsy. A binding site for phenytoin, which interacts with the GABA/chloride inophore benzodiazepine complex and an endogenous compound which binds to this site have been

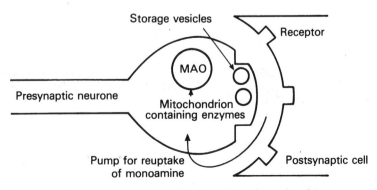

Fig. 4.10 Tricyclic antidepressants inhibit presynaptic uptake of 5-hydroxytryptamine and noradrenaline. MAO = Monoamine oxidase.

isolated from the brain. It is thought that one or more components of the GABA inhibitory system may be concerned with maintenance of a normal state (Fig. 5.12). It may be that in epilepsy there is a lower threshold for seizure, but inhibitory systems within the brain terminate the seizure. Drugs which increase GABA in the CNS are useful in the control of epilepsy.

Hepatic encephalopathy. This may result from increased concentrations of false neuro-transmitters such as octopamine and 5-HT, which replace the normal dopamine and noradrenaline. GABA is produced in the gut by bacterial action on protein and may lead to coma by passing through the blood–brain barrier in liver failure. The number of binding sites for GABA, glycine and benzodiazepines on postsynaptic neurones is increased in acute liver failure; present data suggest that this mechanism is the most important contributor to hepatic encephalopathy. The benzodiazepine antagonists reverse hepatic en-cephalopathy temporarily. The hypersensitivity to benzodiazepines in patients with hepatic en-cephalopathy may be explained by an increase in the free drug concentration.

Asthma. In this condition, there is reduced β-adrenergic, and increased cholinergic and α-adrenergic, responsiveness.

Generally, treatment of disease states with agonists produces alterations in receptor density and desensitization, probably mediated via cAMP. In the case of β-adrenergic receptors, this is effected by phosphorylation. Abrupt discontinua-tion of a β-blocking drug such as propranolol may produce hypersensitivity to catecholamines, and may precipitate angina or myocardial infarction.

Many intracellular events require release of a neurotransmitter, the action of which depends subsequently on activation of calmodulin by calcium binding. There are huge numbers of cir-cuits, transmitters and coupled reactions within the CNS. A number must act simultaneously to produce co-ordinated CNS responses.

The sensory system

Detection of mechanical stimuli

Peripheral receptors exist in excitable tissues. Skin receptors appreciate touch, cold, warmth and pain, and deeper receptors appreciate pressure and proprioception. There are large numbers of different receptors and end-organs and, although end-organs are specialized for one form of sensa-tion, the quality of sensation does not depend on the type of stimulus arousing it. Information is transmitted to the CNS by varying the frequency and patterns of action potentials. There is often extensive branching of axons and a single fibre may be said to have a peripheral receptive field.

Adaptation

A sustained, mechanical stimulus produces only a transient response, i.e. there is processing of infor-mation at receptor level, so that the brain is not constantly informed of an unchanging stimulus.

Mechanical transduction

This consists of transfer of a mechanical stimulus through accessory structures to the nerve terminal itself. A graded electrical response is then pro-duced equivalent to the generator or receptor potential, with initiation of an action potential.

A generator potential is produced by a mechani-cal stimulus and is a transient depolarization of the nerve terminal membrane, independent of the ion channels. The potential appears to be created by the nerve terminal itself and the important stimulus is distortion of the terminal.

Modalities of cutaneous sensation

There are four main modes of cutaneous sen-sation: touch, cold, warmth and pain. Tactile receptors are shown in Figure 4.11. Pain regis-tered by stimulation of the skin has a pricking, itching quality and is well-localized. The pain threshold may be increased by one-third by dis-tracting the subject's attention and reduced by half in sunburnt skin. The first sensation of pain arises abruptly and is carried by moderately large fibres, conducting impulses at 10 m.s^{-1}. The sec-ond sensation is slower and of a burning nature, probably being carried by unmyelinated fibres. Pain nerve endings are distributed in a punctate fashion independent of the end-organs concerned with touch and temperature. Sensations from

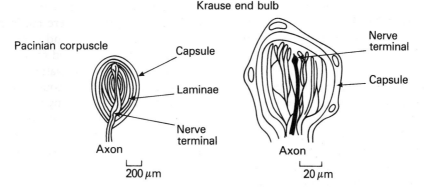

Fig. 4.11   Tactile receptors. Pacinian corpuscles are subcutaneous structures with a receptive field of 100 mm² which respond to vibration (40–600 Hz). Krause end-bulbs are found in the dermis and respond to vibration (10–200 Hz) and movement from a field of 2 mm². They are concerned with the spatial and intensity aspects of touch.

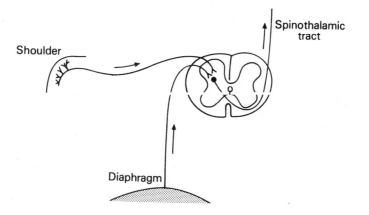

Fig. 4.12   Referred pain; irritation of the diaphragm is felt in the shoulder tip. Nerves from these areas synapse with common neurones in the spinal cord.

viscera and vessels travel in autonomic nerves and are often projected to a definite position on the surface of the body with the corresponding dermatome (referred pain; Fig. 4.12).

Spinal cord pathways

These may be divided into afferent (sensory), motor, cerebellar and autonomic.

Sensory afferent

Impulses arise in muscles, tendons, joints or skin. Dorsal root sensory ganglia and cranial nerve ganglia comprise primary neurones whose periph-eral processes run with spinal nerves and whose central processes run into the cord. Some dorsal root fibres on entering the cord pass directly to motor neurones, constituting a monosynaptic re-flex arc. Others synapse with cells in the dorsal horn of the grey matter and influence ventral horn cells by a reflex arc involving several neurones. The majority, however, form synapses with dorsal horn cells, cells in thoracic nuclei, the base of the dorsal horn or the nuclei gracilis and cuneatus (Fig. 4.13).

The second-order neurone fibres cross to the opposite side and end in the ventrolateral nucleus of the thalamus, where they synapse with third-order sensory neurones, the fibres of which pass

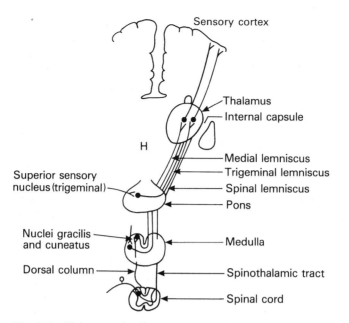

Fig. 4.13 Major somatic afferent sensory pathways. H = Hypothalamus.

through the posterior end of the internal capsule to the postcentral gyrus of the cerebral cortex. There are two major sensory systems:

1. The dorsal column-medial lemniscus system, which conducts proprioception, fine touch, vibration and some autonomic fibres.
2. The spinothalamic tracts; crude touch and pressure are conducted along the anterior spinothalamic tract, and pain and temperature in the lateral spinothalamic tract.

Both the sensory systems decussate before they reach the sensory cortex. The dorsal column system decussates in the medulla and the lateral spinothalamic tract close to its site of entry in the cord.

Descending control of sensory pathways is by efferent nerves acting at synaptic junctions of the relay nuclei of the ascending pathways, e.g. the dorsal horn, dorsal column and thalamic nuclei. These may be either facilitatory or inhibitory.

In the medulla, the two spinothalamic tracts blend to form the spinal lemniscus which is closely associated with corresponding fibres from the fifth cranial nerve. The thalamus acts as a relay station for sensory pathways. Ultimately, somato-sensory impulses from one side of the body are represented on the contralateral cerebral cortex. Removal of the cerebral cortex results in the thalamus undertaking crude appreciation of sensation. The sensory cortex is responsible for perception of sensation, including the full appreciation of pain.

Motor efferent

Lower motor neurones (LMNs) are anterior horn cells of the spinal cord grey matter and some cranial nerve nuclei whose axons innervate voluntary muscle. Upper motor neurones run from the cortex or brain stem to LMNs and comprise the pyramidal and extrapyramidal tracts which are concerned with control of movement.

The pyramidal tract (Fig. 4.14) originates mainly in the precentral gyrus of the cerebral cortex and runs first to cranial nerve nuclei (corticonuclear fibres) and then to the anterior columns of the spinal cord (corticospinal fibres). As these fibres descend from the cortex they traverse the internal capsule in an orderly arrangement. Most corticonuclear fibres cross the midline in the brain stem, terminating in the motor cranial nerve nuclei (cranial nerves III–VII, IX and X). Some uncrossed fibres remain and the tract

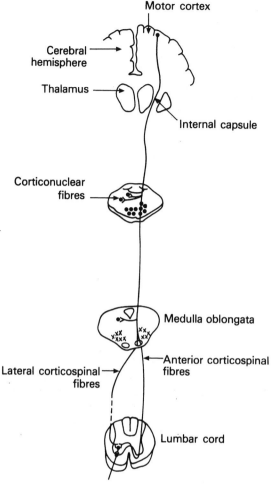

Fig. 4.14 The pyramidal tract.

continues through the pons in a dispersed fashion. Fibres become grouped together in a pyramid on the ventral aspect of the medulla oblongata. In the lower half of the medulla, 90% of fibres cross to the opposite side to descend in the posterior part of the lateral columns as the lateral pyramidal tract. A few fibres pass down on the same side in the anterior white column as the ventral pyramidal tract. A lesion of pyramidal fibres above the decussation produces a contralateral paralysis of voluntary muscles, impairing especially precise movements of the distal aspect of the limbs.

The extrapyramidal system is chiefly concerned with regulation of muscle tone, and influences posture and more stereotyped movements. It comprises a series of tracts connecting various areas of cerebral cortex, subcortical nuclei and brain stem nuclei. These tracts descend to the lower brain stem and spinal cord to influence LMNs through intermediate neurones.

Descending extrapyramidal tracts include the rubrobulbar and reticulospinal (Fig. 4.15). These accompany the pyramidal tracts to interneurones in the cord. Both systems influence the final common pathways (LMNs), which are also influenced reflexly by sensory impulses.

The net result of extrapyramidal activity is inhibitory, so that lesions in the midbrain nuclei associated with this system may result in increased postural tone, and spasticity with uncontrolled tremors or movement. Two other descending pathways influence motor activity — the tectospinal and vestibulospinal tracts. These two tracts account for the influence of stimuli from the eye and the ear produced by movement.

Cerebellar pathways

Afferent and efferent pathways traverse via the cerebellar peduncles. The afferent pathways contain information from muscle spindles, Golgi tendon organs and other proprioceptors, and reach the cerebellum in three main ascending pathways in each half of the spinal cord — the posterior and anterior spinocerebellar tracts and the posterior external arcuate fibres.

Efferent fibres from Purkinje cells in the cerebellar cortex ultimately traverse the superior cerebellar peduncles and cross to the opposite side in the lower half of the midbrain, ending mainly in the contralateral red nucleus. They project to the cerebral cortex, brain stem, reticular, vestibular and the other nuclei.

Autonomic pathways

The sympathetic system. This is a two-neurone system; preganglionic sympathetic fibres have their cells of origin in the lateral horns of the grey matter in segments T1 to L2, and fibres leave the cord with motor nerves via the ventral nerve root. Preganglionic fibres pass to the sympathetic trunk which runs from the superior cervical ganglion down to the pelvis. Postganglionic fibres arise from these ganglia and usually join spinal nerves. Those to the head accompany the carotid

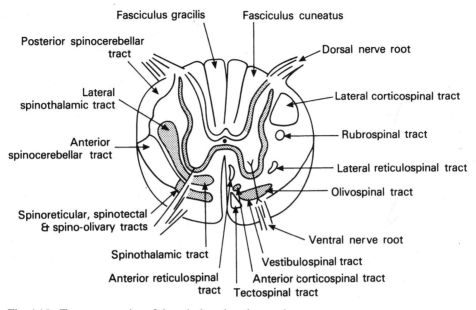

Fig. 4.15 Transverse section of the spinal cord to show major nerve tracts.

artery. Sympathetic fibres to the gut do not relay in the sympathetic trunk, but in midline ganglia in front of the aorta (coeliac, superior and inferior mesenteric plexuses). The functions of the sympathetic nerves are described in Chapter 12.

Parasympathetic system. This comprises a craniosacral outflow via cranial nerves III, VII, IX and X, and S2–4. The actions are described in Chapter 12 and Table 12.1.

Central representations. Integration of autonomic and somatic activity maintains stable internal conditions despite a changing environment. CNS areas concerned with autonomic activity include nuclei in the hypothalamus around the third ventricle, particularly the supraoptic, paraventricular, dorsal and ventral medial hypothalamic, posterior hypothalamic and mamillary. There is close association with the frontal lobes and the posterior pituitary. The hippocampal circuit (hippocampus, fornix, mamillary body, anterior thalamic nuclei, cingulate gyrus, hippocampus) represents a continuous relationship between the cortex, thalamus, hypothalamus and hippocampus and is influenced by pathways ascending from the spinal cord and brain stem and descending from the cortex. This area is involved in reactions which are often the result of somatic and emotional interactions (nausea, flushing) and with

memory. The hypothalamus is also important in temperature regulation, the sleep/wake rhythm, and endocrine and cardiovascular systems. Autonomic afferent fibres ascend through the cord and brain stem with somatosensory pathways to the hypothalamus, which acts as a relaying and redistributing centre from which impulses are projected onwards to the thalamus and frontal cortex.

Cranial nerves

These arise from the base of the brain. Cranial nerve I, the olfactory, is a special visceral afferent nerve, conveying impulses from the olfactory area of the nasal mucous membrane, and traverses the cribriform plate of the ethmoid to the olfactory bulbs on the orbital surface of the frontal lobe.

Cranial nerve II, the optic nerve, is a special sensory afferent nerve carrying visual impulses from the retina to the optic chiasma.

Cranial nerve III, the oculomotor, is a general sensory afferent and efferent nerve and constitutes the most important motor supply to extrinsic voluntary and intrinsic eye muscles.

The trochlear nerve (IV), is a general sensory afferent and efferent nerve and the only nerve to arise from the dorsal aspect of the brain stem. It supplies the superior oblique muscle.

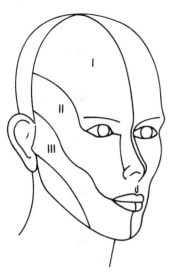

Fig. 4.16 Cutaneous divisions of the fifth nerve.
I = Ophthalmic; II = maxillary; III = mandibular.

Nerve V, the trigeminal nerve, is a general sensory afferent and special visceral efferent nerve, concerned with facial sensation. It also supplies the muscles of mastication. Its cutaneous distribution (Fig. 4.16) is of great clinical importance in the management of trigeminal neuralgia. This nerve may be involved together with cranial nerves VII and VIII in a tumour arising in the cerebello-pontine angle, e.g. an acoustic neuroma.

The abducent nerve (VI) is a general somatic afferent and efferent nerve, supplying the lateral rectus muscle. It has the longest intracranial course and may be damaged in conditions which raise intracranial pressure.

Nerves III, IV and VI can be tested by comparing eye movements and examining for ptosis and diplopia.

Cranial nerve VII (facial) is a general and special visceral afferent and efferent nerve, which provides the main motor nerve supply to the face.

Cranial nerve VIII, the auditory, is a special afferent nerve, concerned with hearing and equilibrium, which may be tested by audiometry and caloric testing.

The glossopharyngeal nerve (IX) is a general and special visceral afferent and efferent nerve, which subserves one-third of taste and provides the motor supply to the pharynx.

Cranial nerve X, the vagus, is the major motor nerve to the viscera, palate and vocal cords and supplies most sensory modalities. Its function may be tested by examination of palatal movement, the voice and the ability to cough.

Nerve XI, the spinal accessory, is a general and special visceral efferent nerve, which supplies the sternomastoid and the upper part of the trapezius muscle.

The hypoglossal nerve (XII) is a general somatic afferent and efferent nerve which is motor to the tongue.

Because of the close proximity of the last four cranial nerves, they may be involved together in pathological lesions, producing a weak, hoarse voice, nasal speech, difficulty in swallowing and regurgitation with an aspiration pneumonia. This constitutes a bulbar palsy and the airway should be protected.

Brain stem and midbrain function

The functions of the brain stem are crucial to the concept of brain stem death. An understanding of these functions requires some knowledge of the anatomy of the area.

Medulla (Fig. 4.17)

1. Motor pathways are stimulated ventrally. Corticospinal fibres traverse the internal capsule via the genu. They are situated medially in the cerebral peduncle, crossing the midline to supply the relevant cranial nerves of the opposite side. The motor nucleus of V, controlling the muscles of mastication, derives only half its innervation from the opposite hemisphere, i.e. there is bilateral innervation. Nerve VII has similar innervation for the forehead muscles, but the muscles of the lower face are mainly innervated by crossed fibres. Cranial nerve nuclei are situated in the dorsal areas of the medulla.

2. Sensory pathways constitute the intermediate layer of the brain stem. The gracile and cuneate nuclei are situated in the dorsal medulla. Spino-thalamic sensation is closely associated with descending sympathetic pathways. The trigeminal sensory system is very complex. Information from the side of the face enters the brain stem in the fifth nerve at the level of the mid-pons. Fibres

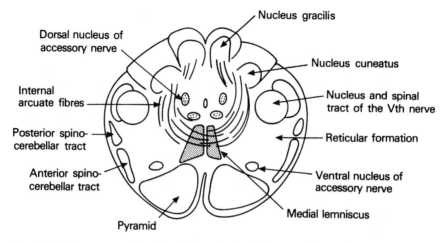

Fig. 4.17 Transverse section of medulla at the level of sensory decussation.

concerned with the corneal reflex and touch decussate to the opposite side. Pain and temperature fibres descend parallel to the descending nucleus of the fifth nerve, relay to the opposite side in the lower medulla and become the secondary ascending tract of the fifth nerve adjacent to the medial lemniscus.

3. The brain stem contains cranial nerve nuclei of cranial nerves III–XII.

4. Control of ventilation, heart rate and blood pressure reside within the medulla; the so-called vital centres are concerned with the automatic reflex control of the heart, lungs and circulation. Afferent fibres originate in highly specialized visceral receptors (e.g. the carotid sinus and receptor cells within the medulla itself) which are responsive, for example, to arterial carbon dioxide tension (Pa_{CO_2}). Groups of neurones in the floor of the fourth ventricle project downwards to synapse with anterior horn cells supplying the respiratory muscles. Control of swallowing, coughing and vomiting is also integrated in the medulla.

5. The fourth ventricle is situated within the brain stem.

Pons

A major feature of the pons is its peduncular connections. The medial lemniscus is the continuation upwards of the dorsal column sensory system.

Midbrain (Fig. 4.18)

This lies between the cerebrum and the pons. It contains the cerebral peduncles and the tectum. The cerebral aqueduct runs through the midbrain and connects the third and fourth ventricles. The tectum contains the colliculi and receives some retinal fibres via the optic cortex and ascending fibres from the cord. It is responsible for co-ordination of input from the auditory areas of the temporal cortex and cervical cord. The colliculi are also responsible for visual, auditory and vestibular reflexes.

The cerebral peduncles consist of a ventral aspect (which becomes continuous with the internal capsule), the substantia nigra and a dorsal tegmentum. The corticonuclear, corticospinal and corticopontine fibres traverse the ventral aspect. The periaqueductal grey matter contains nuclei of cranial nerves III and IV and the mesencephalic nucleus of V. The red nucleus, which is an important relay station in paths between cerebellum, corpus striatum and spinal cord, is situated in the tegmentum.

The reticular formation

This constitutes the central core of the brain stem, projecting widely to the limbic system and cortex with many ascending connections. Stimulation activates the cortex, initiating an arousal reaction, i.e. this area is responsible for generating the

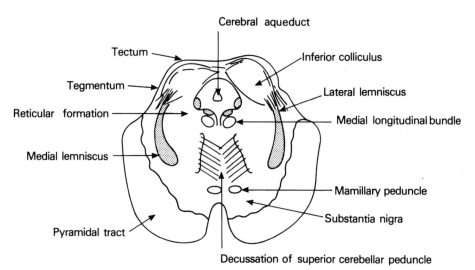

Fig. 4.18   Transverse section of midbrain at the level of inferior colliculi.

capacity for consciousness. Attention and circadian rhythms are also dependent upon the correct functioning of the reticular formation.

Brain stem function tests

1. Activity of nerves II to XII may be tested individually to permit localization of a lesion.

2. All motor information from the cortex to the spinal cord and all sensory information in the opposite direction is transmitted through the brain stem. Although spinal reflexes may be active when the brain stem is destroyed, there should be no abnormal posture, either decorticate (flexed forearms and extended legs) or decerebrate (extended hyperpronated forearms and extended legs), nor trismus.

3. Control of ventilation. In the absence of brain stem activity there is apnoea. Loss of vasomotor control also occurs.

4. Brain stem reflexes.

a. *Oculocephalic.* In the absence of brain stem function, when the head is rotated to one side and held there for 3–4 s and then rotated through 180° in the opposite direction, the head and eyes move together. In a patient with damaged cerebral hemispheres and an intact brain stem, there is deviation of the eyes to the opposite side as the head is rotated, followed by realignment of the eyes with the head.

b. *Vestibulo-ocular.* If the clear, external auditory canal is irrigated with ice-cold saline and the brain stem is intact, there is nystagmus. When the brain stem is totally destroyed there are no eye movements.

The cerebral cortex

The surface anatomy of the cerebral cortex with underlying functions is illustrated in Figure 4.19. The dominant hemisphere is that opposite the dominant hand in right-handed individuals, but variable in those who are left-handed. If the dominant hemisphere is destroyed early in life, then the other may slowly but incompletely assume intellectual functions. The cerebral cortex is concerned with higher intellectual functions (memory, learning and language); in humans, three major areas are involved:

1. Frontal, in front of the motor cortex.
2. Temporal, between the superior temporal gyrus and limbic cortex.
3. Parieto-occipital, between the sensory and visual cortex.

These areas have complex connections from the thalamus, to each other and to the deeper cortex.

Coning

Brain swelling may cause part of a cerebral

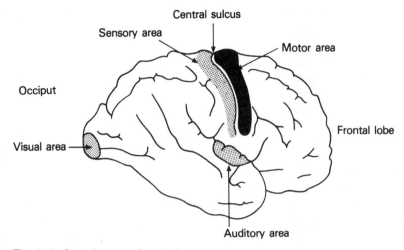

Fig. 4.19   Lateral aspect of cerebral cortex.

hemisphere, usually the temporal lobe, to become impacted under the falx cerebri or tentorial hiatus. Any expanding supratentorial lesion, e.g. middle meningeal haemorrhage, forces the medial aspect of the temporal lobe into the tentorial hiatus. Compression of the cerebral peduncle and oculomotor nerve causes ipsilateral pupillary dilatation with contralateral hemiparesis. Later, brain stem compression produces apnoea.

An expanding posterior fossa lesion may push the cerebellum into the tentorial hiatus. Medullary coning from high intracranial pressure forces

the medulla and cerebellar tonsil down into the foramen magnum, and is rapidly fatal because of compression of the respiratory and vasomotor centres.

Cerebrospinal fluid (CSF)

CSF is formed by secretory cells of the choroid plexus which project into the lateral and third ventricles (Fig. 4.20). CSF then flows via the third ventricle through the aqueduct and fourth ventricle to escape by two lateral foramina of Luschka

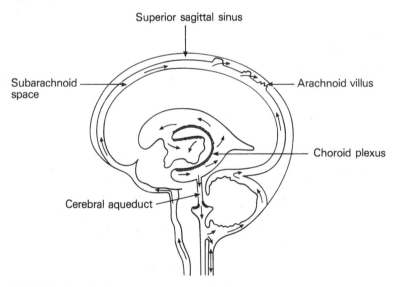

Fig. 4.20   The circulation of cerebrospinal fluid.

and the median foramen of Magendie into the subarachnoid space around the brain and spinal cord.

The total volume of CSF is approximately 140 ml in the adult; approximately 50% is intracranial, and the remainder occupies the spinal canal. CSF is produced at a rate of 0.3–0.5 ml.min^{-1}.

Production must match absorption to prevent an increase in pressure. Obstruction to the flow of CSF increases pressure, with dilatation of the ventricles upstream from the obstruction.

Resorption is mainly into the venous system via arachnoid villi, which are areas where the arachnoid invaginates into large venous sinuses. If the CSF pressure is less than venous pressure, the vacuoles collapse. Some CSF is also probably absorbed around spinal nerves into spinal veins and through the ependymal lining of the ventricles. CSF acts as a cushion between the skull and the brain. It may accommodate some change in brain volume by displacement into the lumbar region. In conditions producing cerebral atrophy, there is an increase in CSF volume.

CSF is a clear, colourless liquid of specific gravity 1005, with fewer than 5 lymphocytes per mm^3 and pH 7.33 (Table 4.2). It is produced from plasma, probably by a combination of secretion and ultrafiltration. The high concentration of chloride arises because carbon dioxide passes into glial cells where, by the action of carbonic anhydrase, it is hydrated to carbonic acid. Resulting bicarbonate ions are exchanged for chloride which passes into the CSF against a concentration gradient. CSF is slightly hypertonic; Na$^+$ and Mg^{++} ions are actively transported into CSF. Lipophilic substances pass readily from blood to brain, but dissociated hydrophilic substances pass only very slowly.

Table 4.2 Composition of plasma and cerebrospinal fluid

	Plasma (mmol.litre^{-1})	Cerebrospinal fluid (mmol.litre^{-1})
Urea	2.5–6.5	2.0–7.0
Glucose (fasting)	3.0–5.0	2.5–4.5
Sodium	136–148	144–152
Potassium	3.8–5.0	2.0–3.0
Calcium	2.2–2.6	1.1–1.3
Chloride	95–105	123–128
Bicarbonate	24–32	24–32
Protein	60–80 g.litre^{-1}	200–400 mg.litre^{-1}

The blood–brain barrier (Fig. 4.21) is composed of a lipid membrane of capillary walls, the endothelial cells of which are joined by tight junctions around the entire periphery of each cell. Solutes at higher concentration in the ECF of the brain diffuse into CSF and are carried into blood at the arachnoid villi. Some substances are transported actively by cells of the choroid plexus from CSF into blood.

CSF proteins are derived by filtration of plasma, from brain interstitial fluid and brain cells, and from cells of the CSF compartment itself. They may reflect abnormalities of the filtration mechanism, of barrier function, brain metabolism or activities of the CSF. Electrophoresis is used for investigation of neurological conditions such as multiple sclerosis, Guillain–Barré syndrome and neurosyphilis.

PAIN

Pain is a combination of severe discomfort, fear,

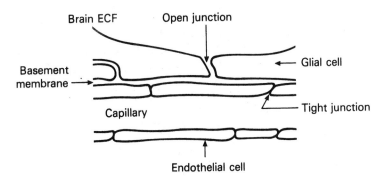

Fig. 4.21 Blood–brain barrier. ECF = Extracellular fluid.

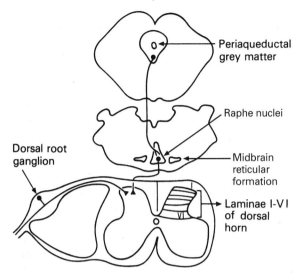

Fig. 4.22   Pain pathways.

autonomic changes, reflex activity and suffering. Peripheral nerve endings are stimulated by pressure, temperature and inflammatory substances such as prostaglandins, leukotrienes, peptides and amines.

Pain is transmitted by unmyelinated peripheral afferent fibres which terminate in the substantia gelatinosa (lamina II) of the dorsal horn (Fig. 4.22) and smaller, myelinated afferents which terminate in the nucleus proprius (lamina V). Spinothalamic fibres arise at this layer. In 1952, Rexed showed that cells of the grey matter of the spinal cord were arranged in nine laminae, I to IX, from the dorsal to the ventral cord, with the 10th lamina lying around the central zone. Lamina I comprises the marginal zone, laminae II the substantia gelatinosa, and laminae IV–VI the nucleus proprius. Small myelinated fibres activated by pinprick and hot and cold receptors terminate here. Laminae VII and VIII correspond to the nucleus intermedius, and give rise to spinoreticular fibres. Lamina IX is the ventral horn, and the output from this constitutes the ventral root.

Nociceptive impulses activate nerve fibres which stimulate the substantia gelatinosa and nucleus proprius, and large myelinated axons of the dorsal column fibres. Two physiological types of nociceptive sensory transmission have been demonstrated: wide dynamic range or multireceptive neurones and nociceptive-specific neurones. Primary nociceptive C afferents contain both L-glutamate and substance P in their dorsal horn terminals and both are released on painful stimulation. L-glutamate binds to post-synaptic receptors mediating fast excitatory responses and also to NMDA receptors, which mediate longer-term effects.

Pain transmission occurs by segmental collaterals from the dorsal column fibres which synapse in lamina IV. These exert an inhibitory influence on transmission of impulses from the substantia gelatinosa, with a reduction in painful sensation. Descending impulses control sensory input by direct and indirect modulation at every level of the brain stem and spinal cord, including the dorsal horn of the cord where they form part of the gate control mechanism. It is known that pain may be suppressed by stress, hypnosis, electrical stimulation and trance-like euphoria.

The gate control theory of pain (Fig. 4.23) was originally developed by Melzack and Wall in 1965. They postulated that large-diameter A fibres (Aβ), small-diameter A fibres (Aδ) and C fibres are all activated during noxious stimulation of peripheral receptors. At cord level, a gate exists which, under specific circumstances, opens to permit pain stimuli to pass through to higher centres. Small nerve fibre stimulation opens the gate, and large nerve fibre stimulation closes it by depression or facilitation of synaptic transmission. Two possible mechanisms of afferent synaptic inhibition have been described: via a glycine transmitter site and via a GABA site with a longer latency.

In post-herpetic neuralgia the pain results from

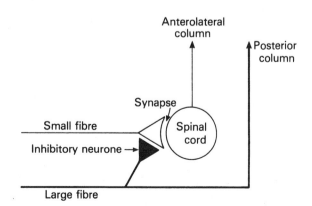

Fig. 4.23   Gate control mechanism.

loss of large fibres. In polyneuropathy, there is a relative increase in the small fibres without an increase in pain, i.e. selective inhibition of supraspinal origin, which can shut down transmission from nociceptors, leaving mechanoreceptor conduction almost unimpaired.

Recent studies show that tissue injury disrupts the normal specialization in the CNS and alters processing of afferent stimuli. Facilitation occurs and stimuli which do not normally cause pain generate pain or hyperalgesia, leading to development of spontaneous pain. An increase in excitatory, or decrease in inhibitory, inputs may be involved. These observations led to speculation that pre-emptive analgesia may reduce postoperative pain.

Endogenous opioids and pain

The opioid molecule is stereospecific, which supports the concept of specific binding sites. Sites of opioid receptors in the spinal cord include the marginal zone and substantia gelatinosa of the dorsal horn and the descending spinal trigeminal nucleus. At higher levels they are found in the palaeospinothalamic pain pathway and limbic system related to emotional behaviour. They are also found in the gut.

In 1975, two related pentapeptides — methionine and leucine enkephalin (Met-enk and Leu-enk) — were isolated from brain. These had sequence homology with β-endorphin, a pituitary peptide. Subsequent studies have identified a family of opioid peptides, sharing some common sequences and widely distributed through the CNS. Parallel studies on the distribution of binding sites for opioid drugs suggest that these peptides play an important role in mediating analgesia.

There are several subclasses of opioid receptor, including μ, δ and κ. The spinal distribution of μ opioid receptors parallels that of enkephalins. The μ receptors are those most likely to be associated with pain pathways. A descending projection from neurones of the periaqueductal grey matter via the midbrain raphe nuclei and reticular formation is responsible for stimulus-produced analgesia and opioid analgesia.

Other neuropeptides, including substance P and calcitonin gene-related peptide (CGRP) may be concerned with noxious inputs into the spinal cord.

Transmission from substance P-containing primary afferents is blocked by morphine or enkephalin and pretreatment with naloxone prevents this. Lofentanil, a potent long-acting opioid, inhibits release of substance P from both central and peripheral terminals of primary afferents. The inhibitory enkephalinergic synapses are probably activated by segmental collaterals of large myelinated primary afferents of the dorsal columns, explaining the value of transcutaneous and dorsal column stimulation in pain relief.

The binding characteristics of opioid analgesics, such as receptor affinity and speed of binding, account for differences in analgesic properties and may explain sequential analgesia. For example, the partial agonist buprenorphine possesses stronger affinity for the μ receptor than does morphine, and with increasing dosage may initially reverse morphine-induced analgesia and ventilatory depression before causing these effects itself in high doses.

Descending control pathways in unmyelinated and serotoninergic neurones from the raphe nuclei are closely related anatomically to enkephalinergic neurones. It seems probable, therefore, that both systems are concerned with pain suppression. Deafferentation pain after spinal cord injury may be relieved by extradural administration of clonidine. This suggests that a noradrenergic system may be involved in transmission of pain. Intrathecal administration of midazolam depresses nociceptive sympathetic reflexes, an effect mediated perhaps through a non-opioid GABA mechanism. Chemical mediators such as prostaglandins seem to amplify pain transmission at the hypothalamic level.

MECHANISMS OF GENERAL ANAESTHESIA

The underlying mechanisms of general anaesthesia (a reversible loss of awareness and pain sensation) still await complete elucidation.

The well-known correlation between anaesthetic potency and lipid-solubility indicates that anaesthetics have a hydrophobic mechanism of

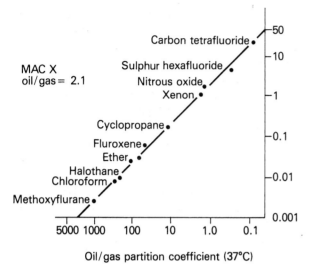

MAC X
oil/gas = 2.1

Fig. 4.24 Correlation of anaesthetic potency (minimum alveolar concentration; MAC) with oil/gas partition coefficient. Standard deviations are omitted.

action. Originally developed in 1901 by H H Meyer and E Overton as the lipid-solubility theory, this is illustrated in Figure 4.24 as the correlation of anaesthetic potency (minimum alveolar concentration; MAC) with oil/gas partition coefficient. The oil/gas partition coefficient increases with decreasing temperature, and MAC decreases to maintain the constant relationship.

Against this is the aqueous theory of anaesthetic action suggested by the relationship between anaesthetic partial pressure and the composition pressure of the gas hydrates (clathrates) formed by anaesthetics. It was suggested that anaesthetics affect water molecules in such a way as to reduce the conductance in the brain, perhaps by expanding the lipid membrane to occlude its microchannels. However, some potent volatile agents do not form clathrates under the relevant conditions. Some anaesthetics, e.g. fluorocarbons, do not fit this correlation and there is no mechanism for the additivity of anaesthetic potencies. Therefore the lipid region of the cell membrane or the hydrophobic region of protein molecules is most likely to be the site of a common anaesthetic mechanism.

Pressure reversal and the critical volume hypothesis

If mice are placed in a pressure chamber and anaesthetized with halothane, the addition of helium to the chamber to increase the pressure to 50 atmospheres allows the mice to wake up, although the partial pressures of halothane and oxygen are unaltered. In addition, high pressure reverses anaesthetic-induced depression of the evoked cortical response (see p. 73). The critical volume hypothesis proposes that there is a critical hydrophobic molecular site which is expanded by an anaesthetic and contracted by pressure. The percentage reduction in anaesthetic potency is linearly related to the total increase in pressure and the slope is the same for all agents. However, at very high pressures, this relationship no longer pertains and, in addition, not all agents behave in the same way at high pressure.

Anaesthetic action on cell membranes

Anaesthetics may block conduction by preventing channels opening, altering the Na^+ flux or by favouring the inactive state. Any agent which chronically depolarizes a membrane favours the inactive state, preventing channels opening. However, K^+ channels may be blocked completely and an action potential may still be produced. Anaesthetic agents have variable effects on sodium, potassium and calcium channels and there is some correlation between lipid-solubility and sodium blocking ability.

Role of conduction block in anaesthesia

General anaesthetics may act by reducing synaptic transmission whilst the impulse in presynaptic terminals remains unimpaired. There are two possible mechanisms:

1. Anaesthetic agents may, by inducing chronic depolarization, reduce the amount of transmitter release per impulse by a mechanism similar to presynaptic inhibition. This may be mediated by a specific effect of anaesthetics on Ca^{++} entry.

2. Anaesthetics may interfere with the movement of the vesicle to, and its fusion with, the postsynaptic membrane.

There is strong evidence that anaesthetics inhibit the depolarization-induced secretion of neurotransmitter from nerve endings by inhibiting calcium influx through voltage-gated calcium channels.

Depression of the postsynaptic response

It is highly likely that this occurs in the anaesthetized patient. There is some evidence that anaesthetics may be selective for a specific type of synapse. Ketamine decreases synaptic transmission selectively at terminals of excitatory neurones. It preferentially depresses responses in the NMDA subtype of glutamate receptor. In contrast, methohexitone enhances synaptic inhibition mediated by GABA. Such specific effects on particular synaptic processes do not support a common mechanism of anaesthesia but anaesthetics as a group do not affect the function of GABA-activated chloride conductance at concentrations in the clinical range. In the invertebrates, volatile general anaesthetics preferentially depress excitatory rather than inhibitory transmission.

The critical volume hypothesis should permit temperature reversal of anaesthesia, but this is difficult to test. There is considerable variation of pressure reversal characteristics among the intravenous anaesthetics and this does not support the critical volume hypothesis for a single site of action for all anaesthetic agents. Consequently, the concept of a multisite expansion hypothesis has been developed by Halsey (1979).

Multisite expansion hypothesis

Much of this is controversial but the hypothesis may be summarized as follows:

1. General anaesthesia may be produced by the expansion of more than one molecular site; the sites may have different physical properties.
2. The physical properties of the molecular sites may be influenced by the presence of anaesthetics or pressure.
3. The molecular sites have a finite size and limited degree of occupancy.
4. Pressure need not necessarily act at the same site as the anaesthetic.
5. Molecular sites for anaesthesia are not perturbed by a decrease in temperature in a manner analogous to an increase in pressure.

Lipids in membranes move and rotate within the bilayer and influence the activity of proteins which control ionic and neurotransmitter fluxes. Perhaps the presence of a general anaesthetic in the membrane increases the movement of lipid and is associated with an increase in its volume. This might effect conformational changes in the protein. The Na^+ channel protein requires an annulus of lipid in the more solid gel state to allow activity (i.e. the open state). Anaesthetics fluidize lipid, causing protein to relax into the inactive (closed-channel) state. Other studies suggest that anaesthetic agents increase the thickness of the lipid bilayer so that the protein pore cannot expand the membrane adequately.

Protein change

Nuclear magnetic resonance studies of volatile anaesthetic agents on haemoglobin have provided the first evidence that anaesthetic agents interact with hydrophobic pockets within proteins at sites which appear to behave as bulk solvents. Conformational changes are then transmitted and detected in non-hydrophobic areas of the protein. Conformational changes specific to an individual anaesthetic have been observed in the same protein.

Sensorimotor modulation systems

Anaesthetic action on sensorimotor modulation systems switches off excitation and turns on inhibition such that messages between the periphery and brain are blocked mainly at thalamic level, with loss of motor control. Loss of consciousness occurs by a mechanism similar to an exaggerated sleep state. The number of synapses in such pathways is irrelevant but the degree of supraspinal modulation of postsynaptic membrane excitation is important.

Somatosensory evoked responses in animals show four effects of anaesthetics. The older anaesthetics, and those currently used for induction and maintenance of general anaesthesia, act by impeding transmission of information to the cerebral cortex at the level of thalamic relay nuclei, and impede the onward transmission of information to the cerebral cortex. The second group, represented by propofol and etomidate, act by blocking the access of information to the cortex. The third group (the benzodiazepines) and the fourth (the α_2-agonists) disrupt the transmission of sensory information at thalamic and cortical level, which distorts the coherence of cellular responses at these two sites.

Miscellaneous

It is well-known that inhalation agents produce dose-dependent toxic effects, such as depression of cell multiplication, mitotic abnormalities and reduced synthesis of DNA with perhaps mutagenic and carcinogenic effects. These may be related to anaesthetic mechanisms.

Other areas of study have included the effect of anaesthetic agents on the microtubules which give rigidity to cytoplasm. These are rings of protein molecules bound longitudinally. Cold and hydrostatic pressure both reversibly depolymerize these microtubular proteins, and produce narcosis. There remains the possibility that general anaesthetics reversibly depolymerize microtubular proteins by binding to non-polar sites on globular proteins.

Proton pump leak theory

Anaesthetic agents increase leakiness in presynaptic vesicles; this reduces pH gradients, and in turn affects the release and uptake of neurotransmitter. This concept is dependent primarily on intracellular pH. Cooling and high pressure reduce proton pump activity and neurotransmitter concentration. Anaesthetic effects of high concentrations of carbon dioxide (30%) in animals are not related to lipid-solubility but to a direct action on intracellular pH. Complete anaesthesia occurs at a CSF pH of 6.7. Changes of ECF calcium concentration affect cell surface potential in a similar manner to addition of anaesthetic agents such as chloroform. Thus, it is possible that modulation of surface potential by variation in ECF composition is important for the function of excitable cells.

Summary

Anaesthetics do expand one or more sites with hydrophobic solubility characteristics. Lipid and protein sites on the membrane, and synaptic transmission, are affected. The most susceptible function is the release and interaction of neurotransmitters, and the most vulnerable synapses are those in the ventrolateral thalamus.

NEUROPHYSIOLOGICAL INVESTIGATIONS

Background activity of the brain may be recorded from the intact skull by scalp electrodes which may be unipolar or bipolar, the latter measuring the potential difference fluctuations between two electrodes. The EEG (Fig. 4.25) is a continuous recording of the immediate electrical responses from the underlying brain and represents excitatory and inhibitory postsynaptic potentials in the larger dendrites of neurones of the superficial cortex.

In the resting adult, with the eyes closed, the most prominent component is α rhythm (8–13 Hz, 50 μV amplitude), recorded best in the parieto-occipital region. β Activity is 18–30 Hz, of lower voltage, and is mainly found over the frontal region. θ Activity occurs in children at 4–7 Hz and is composed of large regular waves. δ Activity is very slow (less than 4 Hz). If the eyes are open, fast, irregular low-voltage activity occurs with no dominant frequency. This is termed α block or desynchronization, and occurs with any form of sensory stimulation.

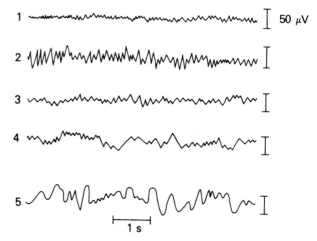

Fig. 4.25 Electroencephalogram. 1 = Excited; 2 = relaxed; 3 = drowsy; 4 = asleep; 5 = deep sleep.

Deep sleep induces large, irregular δ waves interspersed with α-like activity. REM or paradoxical sleep occurs with rapid low-voltage irregular EEG activity, resembling arousal. Wakening during this period is associated with reports of dreaming. REM periods occur approximately every 50 min and occupy a total of 20% of the young adult's normal sleep time. They are associated with a marked reduction in skeletal muscle tone. Repeated awakening during REM sleep produces anxiety and irritability with an increased percentage of REM sleep in subsequent undisturbed nights.

Characteristic changes in the EEG occur in anaesthesia and other forms of coma. Increasing depth of anaesthesia with more potent agents produces slowing of the basic frequency of activity with a progressive increase in amplitude. Periods of isoelectricity appear, interspersed with bursts of activity. This is known as burst suppression. With progressive depth of anaesthesia, there is increasing distance between bursts, resulting finally in an isoelectric line.

Characteristic changes with spike formation in the EEG occur during epilepsy. Hypoxaemia produces an acute increase in the amplitude of the EEG initially and then a marked reduction in amplitude, with the appearance of slow waves as hypoxaemia worsens.

There are problems with using the EEG to monitor the brain continuously. These are related largely to the cumbersome equipment, problems of interpretation and interference from other electrical equipment. The unprocessed EEG is still used by some anaesthetists in cerebrovascular surgery, including carotid artery surgery, as an indication of cerebral ischaemia, when it shows a good correlation with cerebral blood flow.

Processed EEG techniques

These offer no improvements in diagnostic sensitivity, but are simpler to use and clarify the display of information. Such techniques may be of limited value in evaluation of a complex situation, e.g. hypoxic changes occurring during hypothermia. There are numerous reports of the relationship between the processed EEG and anaesthetic depth, indicating that small changes are detectable which would be missed in the absence of processing.

Cerebral function monitor (CFM)

This compresses all frequency and amplitude information in the EEG into a single value. It uses two parietal electrodes, the signal from which is passed through a wide-band frequency filter to remove frequencies of less than 2 Hz and more than 15 Hz (to reduce artefact and interference). The signal is amplified, rectified, integrated and compressed to produce a slow-running chart recording as a line, the height (above baseline) of which indicates total power (Fig. 4.26). Un-

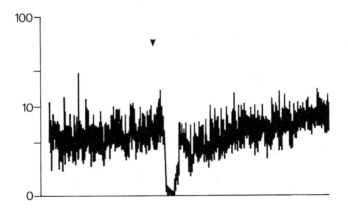

Fig. 4.26 Cerebral function monitor. This trace shows interruption of the circulation at the arrow, causing a transient absence of cerebral activity.

dulations reflect fluctuations in power from one moment to the next; upward movement indicates increased activity. The machine also monitors electrode impedance to detect artefacts from incorrect function of the electrodes.

Such a monitor requires supplementing at regular intervals by a full EEG because of the loss of information by processing. The main objection to the CFM is that the record is neither one of frequency nor amplitude but a mixture of the two. However, it does permit continuous monitoring of electrical activity.

The cerebral function analysing monitor (CFAM) produces a more detailed analysis of the EEG waveform and its frequency distribution (Fig. 4.27). The percentage of weighted activity of the α, β, θ and δ bands is displayed; this overcomes some of the objections to the loss of information which occurs with the standard CFM. Both muscle activity and electrode impedance are displayed continuously. Anaesthetics such as nitrous oxide

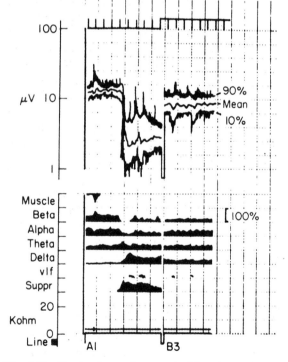

Fig. 4.27 Simulated trace from cerebral function analysing monitor, showing mean, 10th and 90th centiles of overall electroencephalogram amplitude distribution, and a display of relative distribution of activity in the β, α, θ and δ frequencies.

produce a significant reduction in amplitude and a tendency towards lower frequencies on the CFAM.

Power spectrum analysis

This technique retains all information from the original EEG. Analysis of the EEG occurs as follows:

1. The EEG is digitized at frequent intervals, known as epochs (2–16 s).

2. The epoch of data is subjected to Fourier analysis, separating the total EEG waveform into a number of component sine waves of different amplitudes, the sum of which is equal to the original waveform, i.e. conversion into a number of standard waves for easy comparison.

3. The power spectrum is calculated by squaring the amplitudes of each individual frequency component, and displayed for each epoch graphically, so that patterns may be identified by examination of a number of epochs in succession. If epochs are short (2–4 s), this constitutes almost a continuous monitor.

Advantages
1. All information is retained and small changes may be identified readily.
2. Each frequency band may be considered separately so that changes in one part of the spectrum cannot balance out changes elsewhere, as occurs with the CFM.
3. Generation of the power spectrum minimizes baseline drift by converting all low-frequency components (0.05–0.50 Hz) to a single point.
4. Predictable changes may be detected; for example, during halothane anaesthesia, there is less power at high frequencies and increased low-frequency activity.

The currently available Berg analyser has the facility to switch from compressed data to raw data. It uses two pairs of electrodes and displays each hemisphere separately.

A rapid-response graphical display is essential because one of the main advantages of this technique is the vast amount of data generated (2000 data points per minute for each EEG channel processed). The output consists of a graph of relative power versus frequency at each epoch of the analysis (Fig. 4.28). Time is presented vertically to produce a three-dimensional graph, with a hill-and-valley appearance. Hills constitute those frequencies making a large contribution and valleys occur at frequencies containing less power. The points behind the hill are not printed.

Disadvantages

1. High-amplitude activity obscures subsequent lower-amplitude activity at the same frequency.

2. Both time and power are displayed vertically and therefore output requires a two-dimensional *XY* plotter. Another technique for displaying power spectrum of the EEG uses density modulation, which produces a grey-scale display.

Power spectrum techniques can detect differences between the two hemispheres and monitor changes during cerebral sedation techniques. Such therapy may require reduction in EEG activity to the level of burst suppression or reduction of activity in the CFM to 5 μV.

The CFM is the simplest automated EEG processor for intraoperative use, but is less sensitive than the multilead EEG for detection of focal ischaemia. The CFM can discriminate between severe global cerebral ischaemia and hypoxia or hypotension, and to some extent indicates depth of anaesthesia. Gross anaesthetic overdose and severe global hypoperfusion are detectable. The CFM has proved useful in predicting the outcome of severe coma; patients with activity greater than 10 μV have survived, whereas all those with less than 3 μV died.

Evoked potentials

Electrical events occurring in the cortex after stimulation of the sense organs may be detected by an exploring electrode over primary receiving areas for that sense. Evoked potential recordings constitute a non-invasive, objective and repeatable supplement to clinical examination. Uses include assessment of functional integrity of specific cortical areas and pathways within the CNS. Visual, auditory and somatosensory evoked potentials are widely used in diagnosis. In order to detect the low amplitudes involved, an electronic averaging technique must be used to exclude the larger-amplitude background electrical noise, composed largely of EEG activity, with some non-neuronal electrical activity.

The signal varies with body size, position of the applied stimulus, conduction velocity of axons, number of synapses, location of neural generators of the evoked potential (EP) component (i.e. either cortex or brain stem) and the presence of pathology.

Clinical applications of evoked potentials

1. *Multiple sclerosis*. As demyelination increases, complete conduction block occurs at lower temperatures. Subclinical lesions can be detected by the combined use of auditory, visual and somatosensory EPs which show an abnormality in 80% of patients with a definite history.

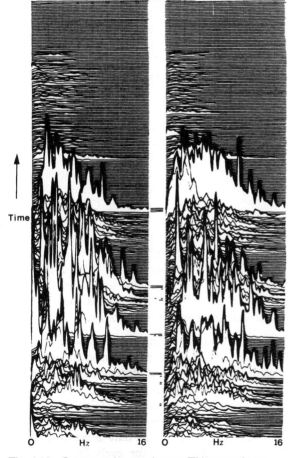

Fig. 4.28 Compressed spectral array. This trace shows fitting followed by electrical silence in a patient with meningoencephalitis.

2. *Other demyelinating diseases*. In demyelination, dissociation may occur of the EP peak latency and amplitude abnormalities. Latency prolongation with preservation of amplitude results from axon demyelination, but a reduction in peak amplitude occurs as more fibres die.

3. *Intracranial tumours*. EPs may be used in intraoperative monitoring of involvement of specific neural pathways. Auditory brain stem EPs have been used in the early diagnosis of posterior fossa tumours where there is an inverse relationship between operability and detectability for acoustic neuromas.

4. *Head injury*. Somatosensory EPs are sensitive to hypoxia and ischaemia. With a reduction in cerebral blood flow, there is a reduction in amplitude of somatosensory EPs, but the waveform is unchanged. Compressive lesions, e.g. subdural haematoma, increase the latency of the waveform. The number of wave peaks recognized in a finite period of time correlates well with outcome, but not with computed tomographic scan findings (i.e. gives information on functional rather than anatomical lesions).

5. *Disease of, and surgery to, the spinal cord and brachial plexus*. During surgery to the spinal cord, extradural motor EPs can be monitored and are relatively unaffected by anaesthetic drugs.

6. *Investigation of apnoea in preterm infants*. Auditory brain stem EP conduction time is longer in babies with apnoea than in those without, at similar post-conception ages, suggesting that apnoea may be related to neural function in the brain stem.

Central conduction time (CCT)

This is the time delay between an action potential generated in the brain stem and the first cortical potential recordable (normally less than 6.4 ms). Other times are also described, for example, the dorsal column to cortex conduction time. CCT is independent of body size and peripheral nerve conduction velocity and is probably also independent of body temperature and barbiturate concentrations. Changes result from cortical dysfunction, abnormal synaptic delay in the thalamus or cortex (or both) and slowed axonal conduction. CCT at 10 and 35 days correlates well with outcome in head injury. Changes in brain electrical activity vary with cerebral blood flow, and CCT has been used as an index of reduction of cerebral blood flow in subarachnoid haemorrhage. It may also be used as a monitor of developing ischaemia in association with surgery for subarachnoid haemorrhage.

For prediction of outcome in severe head injury, multimodality EPs are more accurate than clinical neurological signs, or the Glasgow coma scale.

Nuclear magnetic resonance (NMR)

Nuclei of atoms with an odd number of protons or neutrons absorb or emit electromagnetic radiation when placed in a magnetic field. Hydrogen (protons), phosphorus ^{31}P, sodium ^{23}Na and carbon ^{13}C nuclei have been studied; ^{31}P spectroscopy is used to measure concentrations of adenosine triphosphate, phosphocreatine (PCr) and intracellular pH in muscle and neonatal brain metabolism. Repeated examinations, e.g. of tumour PCr, can indicate progression or remission of disease.

NMR imaging uses information on differences in relaxation times of nuclei. The contrast between grey and white matter in the brain is readily apparent, and excellent delineation is provided of pathologies such as demyelination and tumours in inaccessible sites. In the evaluation of lesions produced by multiple sclerosis or vascular lesions, findings are not pathognomonic but must be assessed, as with all ancillary investigation techniques, together with clinical signs. As with computed tomographic scanning, contrast enhancement may be used. The hazards associated with NMR are discussed on page 505.

Near-infrared spectrophotometry

Indices of cerebral oxygenation and haemodynamics may be quantified by this technique. Concentrations of oxygenated and reduced haemoglobin, oxidized cytochromes and total haemoglobin, together with cerebral blood volume and changes in cerebral blood flow, can be measured and displayed instantaneously. Striking changes have been observed in babies with cerebral oedema after birth trauma.

Some clinical aspects of neurophysiology may

be investigated quantitatively, e.g. Glasgow coma scale. The increasing sophistication of peripheral nerve stimulators now makes it possible to monitor nerve conduction during neuromuscular blockade; this technique is discussed in Chapter 11. Electrodiagnostic procedures such as nerve conduction velocity and electromyography are useful investigations of neuromuscular disorders, but are beyond the scope of this chapter.

CEREBRAL CIRCULATION

The circle of Willis comprises an arterial circle at the base of the brain, supplied by the two internal carotid and two vertebral arteries. In humans, there is almost no anastomosis between the internal and external carotid arteries but stenosis of one supplying vessel to the circle of Willis may be accommodated by an anastomotic collateral flow from other supplies. The branches of these four arteries communicate with each other over the surface of the cortex. Watershed areas between areas of major vessel supply are those most likely to suffer in hypoxia and ischaemia. Venous drainage is into sinuses which also receive CSF from arachnoid villi.

Cerebral blood flow

In dealing with the damaged brain, there are many circumstances in which it is important to obtain information on both global and regional blood flow. Autoregulation of cerebral blood flow and manipulation of intracranial pressure are discussed in Chapter 37. These two important aspects are therefore not considered further here.

FURTHER READING

Angel A 1993 How do anaesthetics work? Current Anaesthesia and Critical Care 4: 37–45
Dahl J B, Kehlet H 1993 The value of pre-emptive analgesia in the treatment of postoperative pain. British Journal of Anaesthesia 70: 434–439
Diuzewski A R, Halsey M J, Simmonds A C 1983 In: Baum H, Gergely J, Fauberg B L (eds) Molecular aspects of medicine 6. Pergamon Press, Oxford, p 459
Greenburg R P, Ducker T P 1982 Evoked potentials in clinical neurosciences. Journal of Neurosurgery 56: 1
Hagbarth K-E 1983 Microelectric exploration of human nerves: physiological and clinical implications. Journal of the Royal Society of Medicine 76: 7
Halsey M J, Prys-Roberts C, Strunin L 1993 (eds) Symposium on cellular and molecular aspects of anaesthesia. British Journal of Anaesthesia 71: 1–163
Hendry B 1981 Membrane physiology and cell excitation. Croom Helm, London

Levy W J, Shapiro H M, Maruchak G, Meathe E 1980 Automated EEG processing for intraoperative monitoring. Anesthesiology 53: 223
Marshall B E 1981 Clinical implications of membrane receptor function in anesthesia. Anesthesiology 55: 160
Maze M, Tranquilli W 1991 Alpha-2 adrenoreceptor agonists. Defining the role in clinical anesthesia. Anesthesiology 74: 581–605
Mitchell J D 1983 Nerve conduction studies and electromyography. Hospital Update 9: 443, 829
Pallis C, Harley D H 1995 ABC of brainstem death, 2nd edition. BMJ Publishing Group.
Pocock G, Richards C D 1991 Cellular mechanisms in general anaesthesia. British Journal of Anaesthesia 66: 116–128
Price D D 1991 Normal and abnormal pain mechanisms. Current Opinion in Anaesthesiology 4: 696–700

5. Maternal and neonatal physiology

The ability of nature to ensure continuation of the species is illustrated by the changes in maternal homeostasis associated with pregnancy. Hormonal changes after ovulation initiate the physiological preparation for pregnancy. Following conception, an increased blood volume is circulated ahead of the metabolic demands of the developing feto-placental unit. Safe parturition is effected by the complementary changes in coagulation and fibrinolysis. Maternal physiology returns to normal remarkably quickly following parturition.

PHYSIOLOGY OF PREGNANCY

Progesterone

The hormone progesterone could be considered the most important physiological substance in pregnancy. It is initially secreted in increasing amounts during the second half of the menstrual cycle to prepare the woman for pregnancy. Following conception, the corpus luteum ensures adequate blood levels until placental secretion is adequate. The most important physiological role of progesterone is its ability to relax smooth muscle. All other physiological changes stem from this pivotal function (Fig. 5.1).

Haematological and haemodynamic changes

The increase in blood volume from 60–65 to 80–85 ml.kg^{-1} is mainly due to an expansion of plasma volume which starts shortly after conception and implantation, and is maximal at 30–32 weeks (Fig. 5.2). Red cell volume increases linearly but not as much as plasma volume. Haemoglobin concentration falls from 14 to 12 g.dl^{-1} (Table 5.1). Thus the haematocrit also falls.

Although erythrocyte production is increased due to the stimulus of erythropoietin, the red cell count is usually reduced to approximately 3.8×10^{12} litre^{-1}. Mean cell volume increases and the cells become more spherical. There is no significant change in platelets or lymphocytes, although cell-mediated immunity is depressed. A neutrophilia increases the white cell count to 9×10^9 litre^{-1} by the third trimester, peaking to 40×10^9 litre^{-1} during labour. Haematological changes return to normal by the sixth day after delivery. The erythrocyte sedimentation rate is increased. Blood viscosity decreases to assist the hyperdynamic circulation.

The development of the pulmonary artery catheter with the facility for measurement of cardiac output by thermodilution has led to central haemodynamic assessment of critically ill mothers. Interpretation of abnormal physiological variables is easier if based on a sound knowledge of the changes in normal pregnancy. Many of the early studies on cardiac output were performed before the full significance of aortocaval compression was appreciated. Modern technology has led to a reassessment of the haemodynamic changes in pregnancy (Table 5.2).

The increase in blood volume is accompanied by an increase in cardiac output (Fig. 5.1) within the first 10–12 weeks by approximately 1.5 litre.min^{-1}. By the third trimester, cardiac output has increased by about 44% as a result of significant increases in heart rate (17%) and stroke volume (27%).

During labour, cardiac output may double, especially with the expulsive efforts of the second

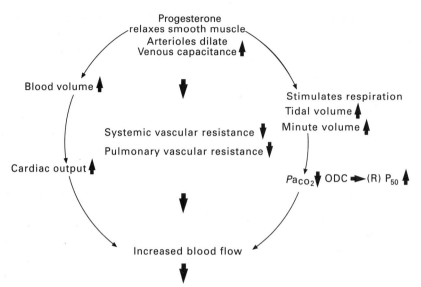

Fig. 5.1 Summary of the main actions of progesterone — it establishes the maternal physiological adaptation to pregnancy. Pa_{CO_2} = Arterial carbon dioxide tension; ODC = oxyhaemoglobin dissociation curve; P_{50} = partial pressure of oxygen when haemoglobin is 50% saturated at pH 7.4 and temperature 37°C; HCO_3^- = bicarbonate.

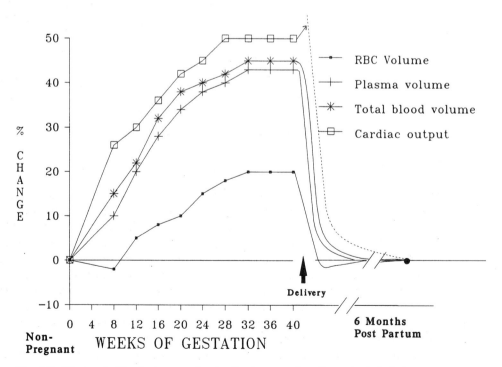

Fig. 5.2 Changes in blood, plasma and red cell volumes and cardiac output, during pregnancy.

Table 5.1 Haematological changes associated with pregnancy

Variable	Non-pregnant	Pregnant
Haemoglobin	14 g.dl^{-1}	12 g.dl^{-1}
Haematocrit	0.40–0.42	0.31–0.34
Red cell count	4.2×10^{12} litre^{-1}	3.8×10^{12} litre^{-1}
White cell count	6.0×10^9 litre^{-1}	9×10^9 litre^{-1}
Erythrocyte sedimentation rate	10	58–68

Table 5.2 Haemodynamic changes in pregnancy

Variable	Non-pregnant	Pregnant
Cardiac output (litre.min^{-1})	4.3 ± 0.9	6.2 ± 1.0
Heart rate (beat.min^{-1})	71 ± 10	83 ± 10
Systemic vascular resistance (dyn.cm.s^{-5})	1530 ± 520	1210 ± 266
Pulmonary vascular resistance (dyn.cm.s^{-5})	119 ± 47	78 ± 22
Colloid oncotic pressure (mmHg)	20.8 ± 1.0	18.0 ± 1.5
Central venous pressure (mmHg)	3.7 ± 2.6	3.6 ± 2.5
Pulmonary capillary wedge pressure (mmHg)	6.3 ± 2.1	7.5 ± 1.8

Data from Clark et al (1989).

stage. There is a further increase in the immediate post-delivery period due to autotransfusion at delivery. This is the most dangerous time for the mother with intrinsic cardiac disease or a rigid vascular system, as occurs in pre-eclamptic toxaemia.

Despite the increased blood volume and hyperdynamic circulation, the pulmonary capillary wedge pressure (PCWP) and central venous pressure do not rise because of the relaxant effect of progesterone on the smooth muscle of arterioles and veins. There is a significant decrease in systemic (21%) and pulmonary vascular resistance (34%). These decreases permit the increased blood volume to be accommodated at normal vascular pressures. Although the stroke volume increases, the PCWP does not rise because the left ventricle dilates.

The decrease in colloid oncotic pressure is due to the fact that the increase in plasma volume is in the water rather than the colloid component. The colloid oncotic pressure–PCWP gradient decreases significantly; consequently, the pregnant woman is more prone to develop pulmonary oedema if there is either a change in capillary permeability or an increase in cardiac preload.

The heart enlarges due to increases in both myocardial thickness and the volume of the chambers. It is raised by the elevated diaphragm and rotated forwards, the apex beat being moved upwards and laterally. On X-ray, the upper border of the heart is straightened, and pulmonary vascularity is increased. There are also changes in the heart sounds; the first sound is frequently split and a third sound is common. A systolic ejection murmur is usual and an innocent diastolic murmur with the third heart sound may occur. Electrocardiogram (ECG) changes comprise left axis deviation, flattened or inverted T waves and occasionally ST depression. Cardiac arrhythmias can occur; these include atrial and ventricular extrasystoles. Supraventricular tachycardia is the commonest arrhythmia.

In essence, a large heart pumps a larger blood volume more quickly through an enlarged and expanding vascular bed which provides a low resistance to less viscous blood.

Despite the reductions in haemoglobin concentration and red cell mass, the physiological changes are geared to maximize oxygen transport to the placenta and eliminate carbon dioxide from the developing fetus.

Arterial and venous pressures

There is little change in systolic arterial pressure but a marked fall in diastolic pressure, lowest at mid-pregnancy. Pregnant women who lie supine may suffer from aortocaval compression. The blood pressure decreases because the gravid uterus compresses the inferior vena cava to reduce venous return, and therefore cardiac output. The aorta is also frequently compressed, so that femoral arterial pressure may be lower than brachial arterial pressure.

Venous pressure in the arms is not increased, but pressures in the femoral and other leg veins increase throughout pregnancy. This is due to obstruction by the weight of the uterus on the iliac veins and inferior vena cava, hence the propensity for development of varicose veins.

Haematinics. Iron absorption increases from 5–10% to 40% by late pregnancy. Routine iron supplementation is not necessary in women with adequate nutrition and a singleton pregnancy.

Folate requirements increase. Folic acid is actively transported by the placenta even when there is folate deficiency. Fetal deformity, premature delivery and antepartum haemorrhage are all associated with folate deficiency. Folate supplements are thought to prevent neural tube defects.

Vitamin B_{12} levels decrease in pregnancy because there is preferential transfer to the fetus. Vitamin B_{12} deficiency is associated with infertility and intrauterine death. Strict vegans require B_{12} supplementation during pregnancy.

Regional blood flow

There is an increased blood flow to various organs, especially the uterus and placenta, from 85 to 500 ml.min^{-1} (Fig. 5.3). Uterine blood flow is reduced during aortocaval compression or maternal hypotension from other causes.

Renal blood flow is increased by about 400 ml.min^{-1}. By 10–12 weeks, glomerular filtration rate (GFR) has increased by 50% and remains at that level until delivery. Twenty-four-hour creatinine clearance is elevated: serum creatinine and urea concentrations decrease. Sodium balance is maintained because tubular reabsorption of water and electrolytes increases in proportion to the GFR and the effects of the mineralocorticoids. Glycosuria often occurs because of decreased tubular reabsorption and the increased load. Increased levels of aldosterone, cortisol and human placental lactogen contribute to the changes in renal function. The renal pelvis, calyces and ureters all dilate due to the action of progesterone and intermittent obstruction from the uterus, especially on the right.

Liver blood flow is *not* increased. Serum concentrations of total proteins, especially albumin, are reduced in blood, further reducing plasma

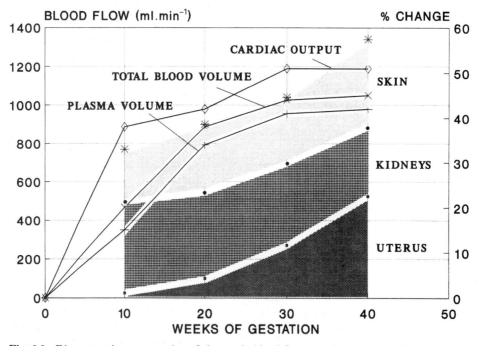

Fig. 5.3 Diagrammatic representation of changes in blood flow to various organs during pregnancy, along with percentage changes in cardiac output, and blood and plasma volumes.

oncotic pressure. Serum alkaline phosphatase concentration is increased by a factor of 2–4 but the major source of this enzyme is the placenta (50%). The increase in liver alkaline phosphatase concentration may be due to injuries to the canalicular membrane. Concentrations of aspartate aminotransferase (AST) and alanine aminotransferase (ALT) are only slightly altered in pregnancy; an increase in concentrations of these enzymes indicates liver dysfunction. Serum lipids and cholesterol concentrations are markedly increased. Plasma cholinesterase concentration decreases by 30%. This is probably only clinically significant in women who are heterozygous for an abnormal gene or who have had plasmapheresis for Rhesus isoimmunization.

Blood flow to the nasal mucosa is increased. Nasal intubation may be associated with epistaxis.

There is a great increase in blood flow to the skin, resulting in warm, clammy hands and feet. The purpose of this vasodilatation, along with that in the nasal mucosa, is to dissipate heat from the metabolically active fetoplacental unit.

Respiratory changes

Respiratory function undergoes several important modifications (Table 5.3), also as a result of the action of progesterone. The larger airways dilate and airway resistance decreases. The transverse and anteroposterior diameters of the thorax increase *early* in pregnancy. Chest wall compliance and total lung compliance decrease, by about 30%. This enables the mechanical component of

Table 5.3 Changes in respiratory function in pregnancy

Variable	Non-pregnant	Term pregnancy
Tidal volume ↑	450 ml	650 ml
Respiratory rate	16 min^{-1}	16 min^{-1}
Vital capacity	3200 ml	3200 ml
Inspiratory reserve volume	2050 ml	2050 ml
Expiratory reserve volume ↓	700 ml	500 ml
Functional residual capacity ↓	1600 ml	1300 ml
Residual volume ↓	1000 ml	800 ml
Pa_{O_2} slightly ↑	11.3 kPa	12.3 kPa
Pa_{CO_2} ↓	4.7–5.3 kPa	4 kPa
pH slightly↑	7.40	7.44

Pa_{O_2} = Arterial oxygen tension; Pa_{CO_2} = arterial carbon dioxide tension.

ventilation to facilitate the increase in tidal volume (from the 10th to the 12th week) and the minute volume (50%). Progesterone exerts a stimulant action on the respiratory centre and carotid body receptors.

Forced expiratory volume in one second (FEV$_1$) and peak expiratory flow rate (PEFR) are unaffected.

Anatomical dead space is unchanged (until late pregnancy, when upper airway oedema may effect a reduction) but physiological dead space increases. The dead space/tidal volume (V_D/V_T) ratio is unchanged, as is the alveolar–arterial oxygen difference $P(A–a)_{O_2}$, although alveolar ventilation is increased by 20% at term.

Alveolar hyperventilation leads to a low arterial carbon dioxide tension (Pa_{CO_2}) during the second and third trimesters. The significance of the low Pa_{CO_2} is apparent when gas exchange in the placenta is considered.

The functional residual capacity (FRC) is reduced by about 300 ml at term due to the enlarged uterus. The residual volume is also reduced by 20–30%. This substantial reduction, combined with the increase in tidal volume, results in large volumes of inspired air mixing with a smaller volume of air in the lungs. The composition of alveolar gas can be altered with unusual rapidity; inhalational induction of anaesthesia is rapid but alveolar and arterial hypoxia also develop more rapidly during apnoea or airway obstruction. In normal pregnancy, closing volume does not intrude into tidal volume.

Oxygen consumption ($\dot{V}_{O_2}$) increases gradually from 200 to 250 ml.min^{-1} at term (up to 500 ml.min^{-1} in labour). Carbon dioxide production parallels oxygen consumption. Rapid desaturation occurs during apnoea at term. Pulse oximetry demonstrates this phenomenon with alarming clarity during difficult intubation. Desaturation occurs even more rapidly in women with multiple pregnancies and in morbidly obese pregnant women, illustrating the combined effect of increased oxygen consumption, decreased mechanical effectiveness of ventilation and an even lower FRC.

Arteriovenous oxygen difference is smaller in early pregnancy because the increase in cardiac output occurs before the increase in oxygen consumption. The average non-pregnant level is not achieved until the third trimester (i.e. oxygen-carrying capacity more than compensates for increased oxygen demand). Although the haemoglobin concentration is reduced, compensatory changes in the oxyhaemoglobin dissociation curve mean that the term physiological anaemia of pregnancy is a misnomer.

Blood gases, acid–base balance and the oxyhaemoglobin dissociation curve

By the 12th week of pregnancy, Pa_{CO_2} may be as low as 4.1 kPa (Pa_{CO_2} gradually reduces during the premenstrual phase of the menstrual cycle). Progesterone also enhances the response of the respiratory centre to carbon dioxide; for every 0.13 kPa increase in Pa_{CO_2}, the pregnant woman increases ventilation by about 6 litre.min^{-1} (2 litre.min^{-1} in non-pregnant subjects). The respiratory alkalosis is accompanied by a decrease in plasma bicarbonate concentration due to renal excretion (base excess decreases from 0 to −3.5 mmol.litre^{-1}). Arterial pH does not change significantly. Peripheral venous pH is higher because of the increase in peripheral blood flow. Progesterone also increases the concentration of carbonic anhydrase B in red cells, which tends to decrease Pa_{CO_2} independently of any change in ventilation.

The oxyhaemoglobin dissociation curve is shifted to the right because the increase in red cell 2,3-diphosphoglycerate (2,3-DPG) concentration outweighs the effects of a low P_{CO_2} and high pH, both of which normally shift the curve to the left. The P_{50} increases from about 3.5 to 4.0 kPa. Thus, oxygen delivery and carbon dioxide transport to and from the tissues (i.e. the fetoplacental unit) are enhanced. Changes in respiratory variables are shown in Table 5.3.

Gastrointestinal changes

These also stem from the effects of progesterone on smooth muscle. Gastrointestinal motility decreases.

A reduction in lower oesophageal sphincter pressure occurs before the enlarging uterus exerts its mechanical effects (an increase in intragastric pressure and a decrease in the gastro-oesophageal angle). These mechanical effects are greater when there is multiple pregnancy, hydramnios or morbid obesity. A history of heartburn denotes a lax gastro-oesophageal sphincter.

Placental gastrin increases gastric acidity. This, along with the sphincter pressure changes, makes regurgitation and inhalation of acid gastric contents more likely to occur during pregnancy.

It is now thought that gastric emptying, as measured by paracetamol absorption, is not delayed during pregnancy. However, it is delayed during labour until 18 h after delivery. Pain, anxiety and systemic opioids (including extradural administration of opioids) aggravate gastric stasis.

The effects of labour on gastric emptying coupled with the mechanical changes cause the labouring woman to be at risk of regurgitation of gastric acid until approximately 18 h following delivery.

Haemostatic mechanisms in pregnancy

As placental separation takes place following parturition, a blood flow of 500–800 ml.min^{-1} must be arrested within a few seconds or serious blood loss will occur. Arrest of bleeding depends on the complex interaction of the three components of haemostasis:

1. *Vasoconstriction.* In the placental bed, this is mainly dependent on myometrial retraction. Prostacyclin is an unstable prostaglandin synthesized by blood vessels. It is a vasodilator and potent inhibitor of platelet aggregation, protecting the vessel wall from platelet deposition. Prostacyclin concentrations increase in pregnancy. It is synthesized in increasing quantities by the placenta and the uterus as pregnancy advances. Umbilical cord arteries also produce prostacyclin.

2. *Formation of an adequate platelet plug at the site of injury.* Platelets have a key role in the maintenance of vascular integrity and in blood coagulation. Platelet count and function (i.e. aggregation) remain unchanged in normal pregnancy. Platelets produce thromboxane A_2 (TXA_2), which causes vasoconstriction and platelet aggregation. There is a balance between production of prostacyclin by vessel walls and of thromboxane by platelets. This dynamic equilibrium controls the tendency of the platelets to aggregate. Increased prostacyclin production in pregnancy helps to promote

increased blood flow to the fetoplacental unit. The fetus is able to maintain a low arterial pressure in the umbilical arteries despite a high cardiac output.

In pre-eclampsia, the TXA_2/prostacyclin ratio is altered so that there is vasoconstriction and platelet aggregation. This leads to poor placental blood flow.

3. *Activation of the clotting cascade.* Blood becomes hypercoagulable and fibrinolytic activity is reduced. Although these changes prevent excessive blood loss at delivery, they predispose the pregnant woman to two apparently opposing hazards: haemorrhage and thrombosis.

Changes in clotting factors (Table 5.4)

In the intrinsic pathway, factor VIII concentration doubles; in the extrinsic pathway, factor VII concentration increases 10-fold. In the common pathway, factor X and fibrinogen concentrations increase (this alters the negative surface charge on red cells which form rouleaux, and increases the erythrocyte sedimentation rate). Concentrations of factors II and V rise in early pregnancy and then decrease steadily. Concentrations of antithrombin IIIa and factors XI and XIII decrease because of consumption at the placental site due to low-level coagulation with fibrin deposition (5–10% total circulating fibrinogen). Bleeding time, prothrombin time and partial thromboplastin time remain within normal limits.

Plasma fibrinogen concentration increases from the 12th week to twice that in the non-pregnant

Table 5.4 Coagulation changes in late pregnancy

Fibrinogen increased from 2.5 (non-pregnant value) to 4.6–6.0 g.litre^{-1}
Factor II slightly increased
Factor V slightly increased
Factor VII increased 10-fold
Factor VIII increased — twice non-pregnant state
Factor IX increased
Factor X increased
Factor XI decreased 60–70%
Factor XII increased 30–40%
Factor XIII decreased 40–50%
Antithrombin IIIa decreased slightly
Plasminogen activator reduced
Plasminogen inhibitor increased
Fibrinogen-stabilizing factor falls gradually to 50% of non-pregnant value

state. A progressive inhibition of fibrinolysis occurs from 11 to 12 weeks. Plasminogen remains unchanged, plasminogen activator activity decreases and the concentrations of the inhibitors (antiplasmin and macroglobulin) increase, leading to delayed fibrinolysis, especially in late pregnancy. The hypercoagulable state of the blood and the reduced fibrinolytic activity represent a compensatory response to local utilization of fibrin and are advantageous for haemostasis at placental separation.

The epidural and subarachnoid spaces

The volume of the vertebral canal is finite. An increase in volume of contents of one compartment reduces the compliance of the other compartments and increases the pressures throughout.

In pregnancy, the epidural veins are dilated by the action of progesterone. These valveless veins of Bateson form collaterals and become engorged due to aortocaval compression, during a uterine contraction or secondary to raised intrathoracic or intra-abdominal pressure, e.g. coughing, sneezing or expulsive efforts of parturition. The dose of local anaesthetic for extradural analgesia or extradural/subarachnoid anaesthesia is reduced by about one-third for the following reasons:

1. Spread of local anaesthetic in either the subarachnoid or epidural space is more extensive due to the reduced volume.

2. Progesterone-induced hyperventilation leads to a low Pa_{CO_2} and a reduced buffering capacity; thus, local anaesthetic drugs remain as free salts for longer.

3. Pregnancy itself produces antinociceptive effects. The onset of nerve block is more rapid, and human peripheral nerves have been shown to be more sensitive to lignocaine during pregnancy. Increased plasma and cerebrospinal fluid (CSF) progesterone concentrations may contribute towards the reduced excitability of the nervous system. There may also be interaction of local anaesthetic and spinal opioid systems, e.g. intrathecal naltrexone reduces pregnancy-induced antinociception in rats.

4. Increased pressure in the epidural space facilitates diffusion across the dura and produces higher concentrations of local anaesthetic in CSF.

5. Venous congestion of the lateral foramina decreases loss of local anaesthetic along the dural sleeves.

In pregnancy, the epidural pressure is slightly positive, and becomes negative a few hours after delivery. During contractions, the pressure may rise by 0.2–0.8 kPa and become very high (2.0–5.9 kPa) in the second stage of labour. Since the spread of local anaesthetics is exaggerated during contractions, top-ups should not be administered at that time.

In the sitting position, both the epidural and CSF pressures are higher, the dura bulges and inadvertent dural puncture is more likely. The spread of solutions injected while sitting may be more extensive.

The CSF pressure increases from about 2.2 to 3.8 kPa during contractions and 6.9 kPa in second stage.

Even if precautions are taken to prevent it, intermittent aortocaval compression always occurs in association with maternal movement. Consequently, the epidural veins become intermittently and unpredictably engorged; this prompted Harrison (1987) to state that there is a 'complex dynamic equilibrium of forces which exist between the vertebral canal, the contents of the extradural region and the dural sac'. Anaesthetists may use these clinical phenomena to advantage.

Summary

There is a hyperdynamic circulation of an increased blood volume to the placenta. The metabolic changes effected by the respiratory system encourage haemoglobin to give up its oxygen and take up carbon dioxide. The kidneys rapidly filter the increased blood volume but maintain homeostasis.

Relaxed arterioles and venous capacitance vessels accommodate the increased blood volume. The increase in plasma volume with a reduction in serum albumin concentration reduces colloid osmotic pressure. Blood viscosity is reduced, which assists blood flow to all organs vital for the metabolic support of the pregnancy (e.g. liver) and preparation for nutrition of the newborn (e.g. breast).

The effect of the changes in blood volume

and dilatation of epidural veins is also reflected in the altered physiology of the epidural and subarachnoid spaces which change the pharmacological profile of extradural and subarachnoid analgesia and anaesthesia. Obstetric anaesthetists occasionally use CSF surges consequent upon aortocaval compression to increase the height of a block.

THE PLACENTA

The placenta (Figs 5.4–5.6) is both a vital barrier and a vital link between maternal and fetal circulations. It also has hormonal and immunological functions.

The placenta consists of maternal and fetal tissue — the basal and chorionic plates, separated by the intervillous space. The structures which enable the placenta to function arise from these plates.

The basal plate comprises the following structures:

1. The decidua basalis, forming the placental bed. Decidual septa arise from this layer. These septa do not reach the chorionic plate but greatly increase the surface area exposed to the intervillous space.

2. Decidua capsularis, overlying the fetus.

3. Decidua parietalis — a parietal layer which fuses with the amnion to form the amniochorionic membrane containing liquor.

The decidua basalis contains the final branch of the uterine vasculature — the spiral arteries. These end-arteries open into the intervillous space. The spiral arteries have no smooth muscle.

Chorionic villi are formed from the chorionic plate. The fertilized ovum, i.e. the blastocyst, is firmly attached to the endometrium via an outer layer of cells (the trophoblast) which proliferates into an inner layer (cytotrophoblast) and an outer layer (syncytiotrophoblast). Both layers arborize to form chorionic villi dipping into the intervillous space. Initially cuboidal, these cells become flatter with increased arborization. Microvilli enhance their surface area, facilitating transfer of gases and other substances.

The chorionic villi containing branches of the umbilical vein and artery are bathed by maternal

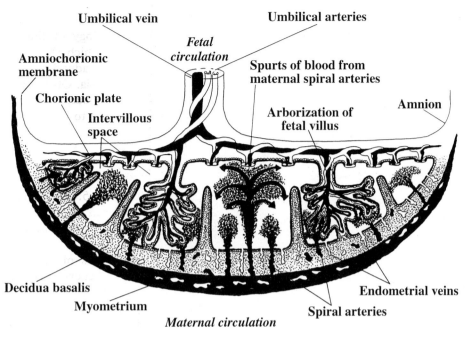

Fig. 5.4 The placenta.

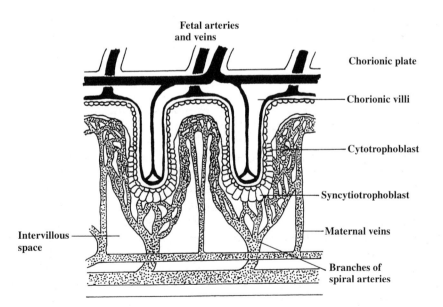

Fig. 5.5 Maternal and fetal blood vessels in the placenta. Chorionic villi are seen dipping down into the maternal circulation. Maternal vessels either envelop a chorionic villus or release spurts of blood directly into the intervillous space. The two circulations are separated by two layers of cells. These cells have microvilli and present a huge surface area for exchange of gases and essential nutrients.

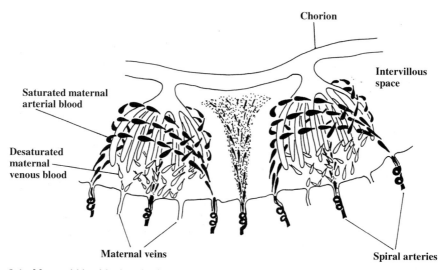

Fig. 5.6 Maternal blood bathes the fetal vessels in the chorionic villi. Some maternal blood will circle the fetal villi before draining into the maternal veins; some will enter the centre of a villus, and disperse laterally before draining; some will be ejected from spiral arteries directly into the intervillous space.

blood from the spiral arteries (Figs 5.5 and 5.6). These either release spurts of blood into the intervillous space or wind round the chorionic villi. Thus the two circulations are separated by two layers of cells — the cytotrophoblast and the syncytiotrophoblast.

Placental blood flow

Fetal well-being depends on an adequate placental blood flow. At term, the uterine blood flow is approximately 500 ml.min^{-1}, of which 70–90% is distributed to the placenta.

The smooth muscle in the spiral arteries disappears during placentation, thus providing a low resistance to the driving pressure of the maternal cardiac output, which forces blood into the intervillous space.

Placental blood flow depends on the balance between the perfusion pressure across the intervillous space and the resistance of the spiral arteries. Placental perfusion is therefore reduced by changes in cardiac output (e.g. haemorrhage) or uterine hypertonicity (e.g. overstimulation by Syntocinon).

Intervillous pressure is increased by intrauterine (i.e. amniotic fluid) pressure and by increased venous pressure (e.g. aortocaval compression).

$$\text{Placental blood flow} = \frac{\text{uterine arterial pressure} - (\text{intrauterine pressure} + \text{uterine venous pressure})}{\text{intrinsic resistance of spiral arteries} + \text{extrinsic resistance (myometrial tone)}}$$

The normal fetus can tolerate a 50% reduction in uteroplacental blood flow, because there is good circulatory reserve.

Functions of the placenta

Hormonal

Placental syncytiotrophoblasts secrete human chorionic gonadotrophin (hCG). hCG production commences in very early pregnancy, increases at a remarkable rate, peaks at 8–10 weeks, and declines until a few weeks before term when secretion starts to rise again. The rapid rise in early pregnancy is to stimulate the corpus luteum to secrete progesterone to maintain the viability of the pregnancy. No obvious biological function for hCG in late pregnancy has yet been defined.

Human placental lactogen (hPL) concentration increases from 0.3 µg.litre^{-1} at 10–14 weeks to 5.4 µg.litre^{-1} by 35–38 weeks. It increases lipolysis, inhibits gluconeogenesis and prevents glucose uptake by maternal tissues (i.e. an anti-insulin effect). hPL can be considered as a metabolic signal by which the fetus obtains nutrients.

Oestrogens. Four oestrogens are secreted: oestrone, oestradiol, oestriol and oestetrol. The role of oestrogens in pregnancy is not entirely clear, although their effect on the breast and the uterus are obvious. They also play a part in fetal development.

Progestogens. Progesterone is the most important hormone in this group and the physiological effects are necessary for the initiation and maintenance of maternal adaptation to pregnancy. Its role in late pregnancy has not been elucidated.

Other hormones. The placenta secretes alkaline phosphatase, cystine aminopeptidase and a number of other protein hormones. Their role in the physiology of pregnancy is not yet clear.

Immunological

The placenta modifies the immune systems of both mother and fetus so that the fetus is not rejected. The mechanism by which this occurs is poorly understood. Modification of the maternal immune system may be the cause of the rapid spread of some cancers during pregnancy and the rapidity with which some viral disorders become life-threatening, e.g. chickenpox with pneumonitis.

Transport of respiratory gases

This is the most important function of the placenta. Gas exchange between mother and fetus takes place in the intervillous space and is governed by the laws of diffusion, aided by the different oxygen affinities of maternal and fetal haemoglobins. Fetal haemoglobin (HbF) has a much higher affinity for oxygen than does adult haemoglobin (HbA). The high affinity of HbF is explained partly by diminished binding of 2,3-DPG in the central cavity which is formed by the gamma chains. Thus 2,3-DPG cannot facilitate release of oxygen in the placenta; HbF can carry more oxygen than can HbA.

The oxyhaemoglobin dissociation curve (ODC) of HbF is to the left of that for HbA. As the oxygen tension decreases on the normal oxygen cascade,

HbA unloads 4.7 ml of oxygen from each 100 ml of blood, whereas HbF unloads only 3.0 ml of oxygen. However, between an oxygen tension of 2.0 kPa (fetal tissue) and 4.5 kPa (placenta), HbF loads 10.3 ml of oxygen to each 100 ml of blood, compared with 8.8 ml for HbA. The loading–unloading advantages of HbF are at *low* oxygen tensions.

The sequence of events in placental gas transfer is best considered in the following steps:

1. Fetal blood gives up carbon dioxide.
2. Fetal blood becomes more alkaline.
3. Fetal ODC shifts further to the left, increasing oxygen affinity.
4. Fetal carbon dioxide diffuses across to maternal blood.
5. Maternal pH decreases.
6. Maternal ODC shifts to the right (Bohr effect).
7. Oxygen release is facilitated.
8. Oxygen taken up by left-shifted fetal ODC (double Bohr effect).
9. Within the placenta, HbF becomes more acidic with oxygenation.
10. HbF releases carbon dioxide (Haldane effect).
11. HbA becomes less acidic as it becomes increasingly deoxygenated.
12. HbA binds more carbon dioxide (double Haldane effect).
13. Carbon dioxide enters maternal cells.
14. HCO_3^- is formed and exchanged for chloride (reversed Hamburger phenomenon).
15. A fetomaternal diffusion gradient is maintained.
16. Maternal blood has carbonic anhydrase.
17. Therefore maternal blood has higher carbon dioxide binding power.

In the intervillous space, the diffusion gradient for oxygen is approximately 4.0 kPa and for carbon dioxide approximately 1.3 kPa.

Placental exchange of oxygen is mainly regulated by a change in oxygen affinities of HbA and HbF caused principally by altered hydrogen ion and carbon dioxide concentrations on both sides of the placenta.

Without the double Bohr and double Haldane effects, the diffusion gradients or placental blood flow would have to be considerably increased to maintain the same efficiency of gas transfer.

Placental transfer of drugs

Drugs cross the placenta by simple diffusion of un-ionized molecules. Fick's law of diffusion applies. The rate is directly proportional to the maternofetal concentration gradient and the area of the placenta available for transfer, and inversely proportional to placental thickness. Lipid-solubility, degree of ionization and protein binding all affect placental transfer, as do the dose and route of administration along with absorption, distribution and metabolism in the mother.

Lipid-solubility. The placental membrane is freely permeable to lipid-soluble substances which undergo flow-dependent transfer. Since the rate of transfer depends on the concentration gradient of the drug across the membrane and blood flow on either side, maternal hypotension reduces placental blood flow and consequently transfer of lipid-soluble drugs.

Hydrophilic substances. The placental membrane carries an electrical charge; ionized molecules with the same charge are repelled while those with the opposite charge are retained within the membrane. The rate of this permeability-dependent transfer is inversely proportional to molecular size. Size limitation for polar substances begins at molecular weights between 50 and 100 Da. Ions diffuse much more slowly. Factors affecting the degree of ionization alter the rate of transfer.

Maternal pH. This alters ionization of a partially ionized drug. The maternal–fetal pH gradient also affects transfer. The degree of ionization of acidic drugs is greater on the maternal side and less on the fetal side. The converse applies for basic drugs.

Protein binding. A dynamic equilibrium exists between bound (unavailable) and unbound (available) drug. Protein binding is pH-dependent, e.g. acidosis reduces protein binding of local anaesthetics. Reduced albumin concentration increases the proportion of unbound drug. Many basic drugs are bound to α_1-glycoprotein which is present in much lower concentrations in the fetus.

THE FETUS

The fetus has adapted to life in a hypoxic environment, surviving the 'valley of the shadow of birth' and quickly adjusting to extrauterine life.

Fetal circulation (Fig. 5.7). Oxygenated blood in the umbilical vein divides into two branches passing though the ductus venosus and the portal sinus. The ductus venosus enters the inferior vena cava, bypassing the liver. The portal sinus supplies the left lobe of the liver. The blood in the right atrium divides into two streams. The main stream enters the left atrium via the foramen ovale, and is carried ultimately to the head, brain and heart, via the left ventricle and aorta.

A smaller stream, along with superior vena caval blood, enters the right ventricle. The right ventricle is dominant, ejecting 66% of the combined ventricular output. Blood in the right ventricle enters the pulmonary artery, but the high pulmonary vascular resistance ensures that blood is shunted to the aorta via the ductus arteriosus. Mixing of saturated and desaturated blood takes place, and this blood supplies the lower body of the fetus and enters the umbilical arteries. The low systemic vascular resistance of the placenta aids shunting away from the fetal lungs. The fetus has a high cardiac output (160 ml.kg^{-1}) and operates a hierarchy of circulation.

1. Non-negotiable: brain, heart, lung tissue.
2. Negotiable: liver, gut, spleen, kidney.
3. Expendable: bone, muscles, skin.

The non-negotiable blood flow is unreactive to α- and β-stimulation and very sensitive to changes in partial pressures of oxygen and carbon dioxide (Po_2, Pco_2) and pH; the negotiable and expendable circulations are sensitive to neurogenic and hormonal influences.

Fetal lung. Pulmonary circulation is essentially a high-pressure, low-flow circuit with little blood volume. The adult lung is essentially a low-pressure, high-flow circuit which also acts as a reservoir for the left ventricle. In the fetal lung, the vasomotor responses are greater and the large arteriolar muscle mass confers high resistance. There are very few autonomic nerve endings and the pulmonary blood flow is less sensitive to neurogenic and endocrine stimuli.

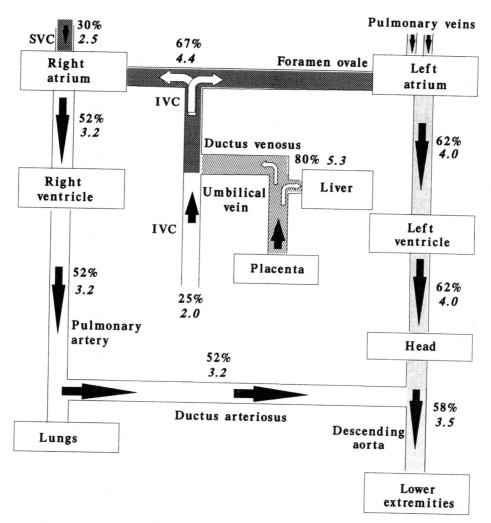

Fig. 5.7 Fetal circulation showing oxygen saturation (So_2; %) and oxygen tension (Po_2; kPa) in different parts of the circulation. SVC = Superior vena cava; IVC = inferior vena cava.

Surfactant. Although the respiratory function of the lungs is performed by the placenta before birth, blood supply to the fetal lung is much greater than to the adult lung because alveolar cells are metabolically very active. They manufacture surfactant, a complex glycoprotein which confers stability on alveoli. Surfactant is manufactured from 28 weeks' gestation.

Effects of drugs on the fetus. These effects depend on fetal distribution, metabolism and excretion; for example, polar substances cross the placenta slowly, but once they reach the fetus, they are rapidly excreted into the amniotic fluid. Lipophilic substances are transferred quickly,

but it can take up to 40 min for equilibration to occur.

The first breath and changes in circulation

The instant the umbilical cord is cut, the fetus becomes physiologically and legally an independent and separate individual. The events may be summarized as follows:

1. During delivery, the chest wall is squeezed.
2. Recoil of the chest wall assists expansion of the lungs against forces of surface tension; the FRC reaches 75% of its ultimate volume in a few minutes.

3. Within a few breaths, the fetal Pa_{O_2} of 2–3.5 kPa becomes the neonatal Pa_{O_2} of 9–13 kPa.

4. As the lungs expand, pulmonary vascular resistance decreases, and pulmonary capillaries and post-alveolar vessels dilate. Arteriolar constriction decreases because of increasing alveolar P_{O_2}; pulmonary blood flow increases.

5. Right atrial pressure decreases below left atrial pressure. There is functional closure of the foramen ovale.

6. Clamping the umbilical cord increases systemic vascular resistance, which helps to maintain left atrial pressure.

7. Closure of the foramen ovale means that blood from the venae cavae enters the pulmonary circulation.

8. The rapid increase in pulmonary blood flow is assisted by the developing low pulmonary vascular resistance.

9. Flow through the ductus arteriosus is gradually reduced; this, along with a rising Pa_{O_2}, leads to closure of the ductus.

In the first hour, there may be bi-directional shunting through the ductus but the right-to-left flow gradually decreases. There is a *transitional* circulation until the adult circulatory pattern is irreversibly developed.

Effects of drugs on the neonate

Many studies use the ratio of maternal vein to umbilical vein concentration which indicates only the situation at delivery and gives little information regarding the effects or distribution of the drug in the neonate. The distribution is different because of the anatomical and physiological organization of the fetal circulation; for example, drugs accumulate in the liver because of the umbilical venous flow to the liver, and are metabolized before distribution. The relatively high extracellular fluid volume explains the large volumes of distribution of local anaesthetics and relaxants. In addition, fetal plasma contains less α_1-glycoprotein and albumin at term, which affects protein binding of drugs, particularly local anaesthetics. Many hepatic enzyme systems are immature; for example, the hydroxylating pathway is not developed. Renal function in the neonate is immature, and urinary elimination of drugs is reduced.

Inhalational anaesthetics diffuse readily, but provided that the induction–delivery interval is short, the fetus is minimally affected. Neonatal elimination is dependent on ventilation.

Neuromuscular blocking drugs, which are quaternary ammonium compounds and fully ionized, cross the placenta very slowly. Fetomaternal ratios at delivery are very low. Only prolonged administration of a relaxant, e.g. in the intensive care unit, might lead to neonatal paralysis. Bolus doses of suxamethonium are safe.

Thiopentone is highly lipid-soluble, weakly acidic and 75% protein-bound. It crosses the placenta rapidly, is detectable in the umbilical vein within 30 s and reaches its peak level within 1 min. At delivery, the umbilical venous concentration is approximately equal to maternal venous concentration. Neonatal concentration falls much more slowly than that of the mother. Since thiopentone crosses the placenta so rapidly, it is impossible to deliver the baby before significant transfer has taken place. The longer the induction–delivery interval, the higher is the neonatal/maternal ratio, suggesting that ongoing transfer of the drug to the fetus in utero occurs. If the dose does not exceed 4 mg.kg^{-1}, no significant fetal central nervous system depression occurs. However, repeated doses do lead to depression; one-third of the original dose can return the neonatal level to that following the original dose. Widespread clinical use testifies to the safety of thiopentone.

Propofol is highly protein-bound, neutral and lipophilic. It is less readily transferred than thiopentone. Provided that the dose is < 5 mg.kg^{-1}, the neonate should not suffer drug-induced central nervous system depression.

Diazepam is a most sinister agent. It is a non-polar compound which is bound to albumin, but the fetomaternal ratio may reach 2. The neonate may suffer from respiratory depression, hypotonia, poor thermoregulation and raised bilirubin concentrations. Prolonged maternal diazepam administration should be avoided, if possible.

Opioids are mainly weak bases bound to α_1-glycoprotein. Pethidine depresses all aspects of neurobehaviour in the neonate. Fetomaternal ratios rise to exceed 1 after 2–4 h. Neonatal elimination is slower, resulting in prolongation of the effects. Fentanyl is highly lipid-soluble and albumin-bound, and rapidly crosses the placenta. Apgar scores are low following intravenous fentanyl. Epidural administration of fentanyl along with bupivacaine has also led to consistently lower Apgar scores.

Alfentanil is less lipophilic but more protein-bound to α_1-glycoprotein. Fetomaternal ratios are low and at Caesarean section are more related to fetomaternal α_1-glycoprotein levels. Theoretically, Apgar and neurobehavioural scores should be less affected.

Sufentanil is principally bound to α_1-glyco-protein. Therefore it should be the best opioid additive for epidural analgesia. However, a dose-related reduction in both Apgar and neuro-behavioural scores has been observed.

Assessment of effects of drugs on the neonate

The Apgar score is not sensitive enough to detect neurobehavioural changes. The Brazelton neo-natal assessment score is the basis of neonatal neurobehavioural assessment systems.

1. Early neonatal neurobehavioural scale (ENNS). This is based on the neonate's ability to adapt to the environment and depends on tests of habituation, reflexes, tone, placing, alertness, finalized by a general assessment of the neonate's behaviour. Although better than an Apgar score, it is very subjective.

2. Neurological and adaptive capacity score (NACS). This was introduced to assess the effects of medication in labour, perinatal asphyxia and birth trauma. It includes response and habituation to sound and light, consolability, active and pas-sive tone, primary reflexes, finalized by a general assessment.

Drugs produce a generalized motor depression. Birth trauma or asphyxia may lead to unilateral or upper-body hypotonia.

The long-term significance of transient neuro-behavioural changes is difficult to assess.

Lactation and drugs in obstetric anaesthesia

Women are encouraged to breast-feed. Oestrogen and progesterone stimulate mammary develop-ment during pregnancy. These hormones inhibit prolactin. This inhibition ceases at delivery. Suck-ling triggers lactation and stimulates the release of more prolactin and oxytocin, both of which promote production of milk.

Many women wish to suckle their infant imme-diately following delivery and are encouraged to do so. The anaesthetist is therefore required to know whether the drugs used for obstetric anaes-thesia and analgesia are secreted in the milk and, if so, whether they are likely to have an adverse effect either on the process of lactation itself, or on the neonate.

The maternal concentration of drug presented to the breast varies with dose, route of adminis-tration, volume of distribution, lipid-solubility, ionization and protein binding. Lipid-soluble drugs enter by passive diffusion.

The physicochemical properties of a drug which determine transfer into the milk are pKa, the par-tition coefficient and molecular weight. The pH of human milk is 7.09. Therefore weak acids are less easily transferred than weak bases.

Human breast milk consists of an emulsion of fat in water, with lactose and protein in the aqueous phase. The total amount of drug con-tained in the milk depends on binding to milk protein, partition into milk lipid and the quantity which remains unbound in the aqueous phase, e.g. lipid-soluble drugs such as diazepam are con-centrated in milk lipid. The dose of drug delivered to the neonate from the milk varies with the volume ingested. The higher gastric pH, different gastrointestinal flora and delayed gastric emptying of the neonate all influence drug absorption.

Opioids. Morphine appears safe with conven-tional administration. Patient-controlled analgesia may increase maternal plasma concentration. As yet, adverse effects on neonates have not been reported. With pethidine, however, neuro-behavioural depression has been noted. Short-acting opioids such as fentanyl and alfentanil, even by continuous epidural infusion, are safe.

Non-steroidal anti-inflammatory drugs. The non-steroidal anti-inflammatory drugs keto-rolac and diclofenac are safe. The neonate has immature biotransformation and excretory path-ways. Aspirin should be avoided because high concentrations have been observed following a single oral dose. Neonates are at risk of developing Reye's syndrome.

Thiopentone and propofol. These appear to be safe when used to induce anaesthesia for Caesarean section.

Diazepam. Diazepam and its metabolites are excreted in breast milk. As with placental transfer, there is the possibility of adverse effects on the neonate, especially with continuous administration.

The amounts of lignocaine and bupivicaine excreted in breast milk are small.

The physiological changes of pregnancy are exaggerated in multiple pregnancy. The success of assisted conception means that obstetric anaesthetists care for more women with twins, triplets and quadruplets.

The obstetric anaesthetist must understand maternal adaptation to pregnancy in order to manipulate physiological changes following general anaesthesia or regional analgesia and anaesthesia in such a way that the condition of the neonate at delivery is optimized.

The success of colleagues in other specialties now enables many more women with chronic disease processes to achieve pregnancy. The obstetric anaesthetist requires an understanding of the pathophysiological changes associated with the disease process and their interaction with the changes consequent upon pregnancy. Anaesthetists have a great contribution to make to the successful outcome which more women now expect and should achieve.

FURTHER READING

Clark S L, Cotton D B, Lee W et al 1989 Central hemodynamic assessment of normal term pregnancy. American Journal of Obstetrics and Gynecology 161: 1439–1442

Harrison G R 1987 A model of the extradural space and a reappraisal of the extradural space pressure. British Journal of Anaesthesia 59: 1177–1180

Hytten F E, Chamberlain G 1992 Clinical physiology in obstetrics, 2nd edn. Blackwell Scientific Publications, Oxford

James F M III, Wheeler A S, Dewan D M (eds) 1988 Obstetric anesthesia. The complicated patient, 2nd edn. Davies, Philadelphia

Lee J J, Rubin A P 1993 Breast feeding and anaesthesia. Anaesthesia 48: 616–625

Letski E A 1985 Coagulation problems during pregnancy. In: Lind T (ed) Current reviews in obstetrics and gynaecology, no. 10. Churchill Livingstone, Edinburgh

Macdonald R (ed) 1978 Scientific basis of obstetrics and gynaecology, 2nd edn. Churchill Livingstone, Edinburgh

Reynolds F 1991 Placental transfer of drugs. Current Anaesthesia and Critical Care 2.2: 108–116

Smith C A, Nelson N M (eds) 1976 The physiology of the newborn infant. Charles C Thomas, Springfield, Illinois

6. Haematology

Surgery and anaesthesia make heavy demands on departments of haematology and blood transfusion. Consultation between the anaesthetist and haematologist should be frequent both in the operating theatre and intensive therapy unit if the provision of, for example, appropriate blood products and the correct investigation of the bleeding patient are to proceed smoothly and expeditiously.

ANAEMIA

Anaemia is present when the red cell mass (the erythron) is reduced below the reference range for the patient's age and sex. There are many causes and these are classified conventionally as:

1. *Blood loss* which may be acute or chronic.
2. *Failure of erythropoiesis* resulting from, for example, inadequate supplies to the bone marrow of nutrients: iron, vitamin B_{12}, folate, some hormones or protein. Erythropoiesis may be impaired by bone marrow infiltration in leukaemia or other malignant disease. Anaemia of chronic disorders is the term used for the secondary anaemias of chronic inflammation, infection and malignant disease (when the marrow is not infiltrated). Such anaemia is also seen in rheumatoid arthritis and chronic renal failure.
3. *Shortened red cell lifespan.* The haemolytic anaemias are subdivided into:

   a. inherited, e.g. hereditary spherocytosis, sickle cell anaemia and some red cell enzyme defects;
   b. acquired, e.g. autoimmune haemolytic anaemia, paroxysmal nocturnal haemoglobinuria and drug-induced haemolysis.

Alternative classifications are possible and forms of anaemia may be allocated to more than one category. Thus, chronic blood loss produces negative iron balance with eventual failure of erythropoiesis from iron deficiency. Pernicious anaemia is an erythropoietic failure resulting from lack of correct digestion of vitamin B_{12}, but red cell precursors and mature red cells in this disease have a shortened life span.

Anaemia is demonstrated by the measurement of the amount of haemoglobin in a known volume of blood. Haemoglobin concentration is reported as grams per decilitre $(g.dl^{-1})$ or grams per litre $(g.litre^{-1})$. Anaemia is said to be present in an adult male if the haemoglobin concentration is less than 13.5 $g.dl^{-1}$ (135 $g.litre^{-1}$) and in an adult female if less than 11.5 $g.dl^{-1}$ (115 $g.litre^{-1}$). In the first year of life the haemoglobin concentration decreases from 13.5–19.5 $g.dl^{-1}$ at birth to 9.5 $g.dl^{-1}$ at one month to attain levels at 12 months close to those of female adults. In pregnancy, haemoglobin levels should not decrease below 11.5 $g.dl^{-1}$ if iron and/or folate are not deficient.

Modern electronic blood counting equipment provides accurate red cell indices in addition to haemoglobin estimation and these provide guidance on the type of anaemia before resort to further investigation. It is worth noting that the commonest form of anaemia worldwide is that due to iron deficiency.

With the notable exception of acute blood loss, reduction in red cell mass is accompanied by an increase in plasma volume, thus preserving blood volume. The mechanism for this is not clear but it is one of the compensatory mechanisms adopted during anaemia of any duration. Of equal importance is a shift of the oxygen dissociation curve to the right through increased synthesis of 2,3-diphosphoglycerate (2,3-DPG) in the red cell via the Embden–Meyerhof pathway of anaerobic glycolysis and the Rapaport–Luebering shunt. Increases in 2,3-DPG render the haemoglobin molecule less avid for oxygen at any given partial pressure and improve tissue oxygenation. Two remaining compensatory mechanisms in anaemia are an increase in cardiac stroke volume and an increase in heart rate.

In acute blood loss, red cells and plasma are lost together, such that in the first few hours haemoglobin and haematocrit measurements change little and cannot be used to estimate blood loss. Surgeons have always attributed much importance to the haematocrit but in continued acute bleeding the haemoglobin and haematocrit move in parallel. Haemodilution is complete by 24–48 h if transfusion of red cells is not carried out.

HAEMOGLOBINOPATHIES

The haemoglobinopathies are a complex and diverse series of inherited abnormalities of globin chain synthesis. The thalassaemias are characterized by absent or reduced production of the affected globin chain whilst the other chains which make up the haemoglobin molecule are structurally normal. In the haemoglobinopathies the affected chain, usually the beta or alpha chain, has an amino acid substitution which, if it affects the structure or function of the haemoglobin molecule as a whole, may produce clinical effects.

β-Thalassaemia

β-Thalassaemia, in which β-globin chain synthesis is impaired, is classified into three clinical grades.

1. *β-Thalassaemia trait (thalassaemia minor)* is the heterozygous state and produces little clinical effect. There may be slight anaemia and the condition may be mistaken for iron deficiency. In pregnancy the haemoglobin may fall below the reference range.

2. *Thalassaemia intermedia*, as the name implies, is associated with more marked anaemia than thalassaemia trait and is generally caused by double heterozygosity or homozygosity of less severe β-thalassaemia genes. Occasionally, patients may require transfusions of red cells.

3. *Thalassaemia major (Cooley's anaemia)* is the homozygous inheritance of severe β-thalassaemia genes. β-chain production is reduced or absent, thus impairing the synthesis of adult haemoglobin. Without blood transfusion the condition is generally fatal in the early years of childhood and even with regular transfusion support patients may not live beyond their early twenties as a result of iron overload. Long-term iron chelation therapy may prevent transfusional iron overload and bone marrow transplantation may be considered.

α-Thalassaemia

α-Thalassaemia is a genetically variegate disorder which ranges in severity from fetal death in utero in the homozygous form to a mild hypochromic disorder in the heterozygous form. Patients with three of the four α-chain genes deleted suffer HbH disease of intermediate severity and some require transfusion with red cells.

Haemoglobinopathies

More than 100 haemoglobin variants have been described but only one has significant global clinical impact – haemoglobin S. Ten per cent of patients of African extraction carry the S gene. It is also seen in Italy, Greece, Arabia and the Indian subcontinent. Haemoglobin S has valine substituted for glutamine in position 6 of the β-globin chain and this confers physical differences on the haemoglobin molecule with profound clinical consequences in homozygotes. Haemoglobin S becomes insoluble at oxygen tensions in the venous range (5–5.5 kPa) and crystallizes, imposing a sickle-cell shape on the red cell. The sickled red cell is rigid and does not pass easily through capillaries, leading to occlusion, tissue infarction and the pain which is characteristic of clinical episodes known as crises. Red cell survival is reduced greatly and homozygous patients invariably have anaemia (6–10 g.dl⁻¹) and jaundice. Heterozygotes are almost asymptomatic and their red cells sickle only when oxygen tensions are unphysiologically low (2 kPa). Sickle haemoglobin may be demonstrated rapidly in patients' blood using a commercial kit, e.g. Sickledex (Ortho Diagnostics). The presence or absence of haemoglobin S should be established before anaesthesia in all patients of affected ethnic groups by haemoglobin electrophoresis. It may be necessary to electively pretransfuse homozygotes or consider exchange transfusion to raise the percentage of haemoglobin A compared with haemoglobin S. Clearly it is essential to maintain good oxygenation of the homozygous patient pre-, intra- and postoperatively and consideration should be given to oxygen therapy for 24 h after anaesthesia. Postoperative infarctive episodes may occur even with the most meticulous attention to detail. Sickling is enhanced by low blood pH, high red cell 2,3-DPG, stasis, dehydration and increased plasma osmolality.

HAEMOSTASIS AND FIBRINOLYSIS

The haemostatic mechanism

There are three principal components: platelets, coagulation and what may be termed limiting mechanisms including fibrinolysis. These may be altered individually or collectively in disease to produce haemostatic failure. Investigation of the bleeding patient should include all three components.

Platelets

Primary haemostasis depends on the presence of adequate functional platelet numbers (Fig. 6.1).

Contact between the platelet and collagen in the presence of von Willebrand's factor (vWf) initiates the arachadonic acid pathway, resulting in the release of ADP from platelet dense granules. ADP induces exposure of fibrinogen receptors on the platelet surface, allowing fibrinogen to bind platelets into aggregates. Strands of fibrin truss platelets and red cells into the platelet plug.

The normal whole-blood platelet count is 150–400 $\times$ 10^9 litre^{-1}. The lower limit of 'normal', or reference range, depends upon the method used for their quantitation but a platelet count below 100 $\times$ 10^9 litre^{-1} is considered to be thrombocytopenia. The risk of haemostatic failure increases as the platelet count decreases and when levels below

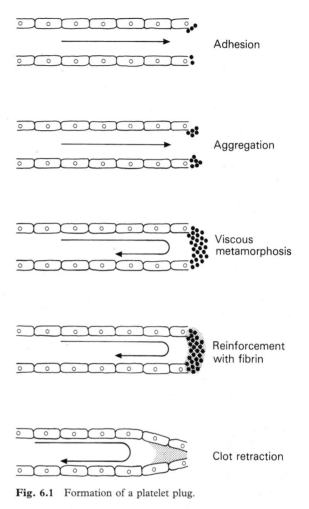

Fig. 6.1 Formation of a platelet plug.

Labels (top to bottom): Adhesion; Aggregation; Viscous metamorphosis; Reinforcement with fibrin; Clot retraction

30 $\times$ 10^9 litre^{-1} are reached spontaneous bleeding may occur. Bleeding is precipitated if there is local pathology, e.g. peptic ulcer, or if there is a surgical wound. Thrombocytopenic bleeding occurs less at a particular platelet count if the low platelet numbers result from peripheral destruction with a functional bone marrow (e.g. autoimmune thrombocytopenia) than if platelet production is impaired, for example in bone marrow disorders (e.g. leukaemia or myeloma).

For adequate primary haemostasis the platelets should also function normally. In comparison to the rare inherited platelet functional disorders, drug-induced platelet metabolic damage occurs more commonly. Non-steroidal anti-inflammatory drugs (NSAIDs) impair prostaglandin synthetic pathways by inhibition of the enzyme cyclo-oxygenase. Aspirin (acetylsalicylic acid) is the prime example and its effect on measured in vitro function of platelets lasts up to 14 days. Other therapeutic agents affecting platelet function include sulphinpyrazone, dipyridamole and dextran. Drug-induced platelet dysfunction may cause bleeding in the face of adequate platelet numbers and patients should be encouraged to discontinue the drug, preferably 2 weeks before major surgery, particularly with respect to the NSAIDs. Uraemia is accompanied by acquired platelet dysfunction which may be corrected by dialysis. Platelets in the myeloproliferative disorders including some leukaemias may function poorly.

Stored whole blood for transfusion contains few viable platelets; after storage for only 3 days, platelet recovery in vivo is only 20%. Thus, in massive transfusion (replacement of the patient's blood volume in less than 24 h by stored allogeneic blood), platelet numbers decline progressively but rarely decrease below 50×10^9 litre^{-1} even when twice the patient's blood volume has been transfused.

Platelet function in vivo is measured best by the template bleeding time carried out by haematology staff according to strict methodology. This should not be undertaken unless platelet numbers have been shown to be normal or bleeding is out of proportion to platelet numbers and coagulation is demonstrably normal. Careful examination of the patient reveals clues to thrombocytopenia: petechial purpura particularly below the knee, blood-filled blisters in the mouth and fundal haemorrhages. In the patient in theatre, oozing at the operation and venepuncture sites acts as an indicator. The strategy of platelet transfusion is described below.

Coagulation

The second phase of haemostasis involves the coagulation proteins (Table 6.1) which stabilize the haemostatic plug provided by the platelets. Central to this is the production of thrombin (Fig. 6.2) from prothrombin by the action of activated factor X. Thrombin cleaves fibrinogen to form fibrin. Two pathways lead to the conversion of prothrombin and are composed of linked proteolytic enzymes which act first as substrates and

Table 6.1 International nomenclature of clotting factors

Factor	Synonym
I	Fibrinogen
II	Prothrombin
III	Tissue thromboplastin
IV	Calcium ions
V	Labile factor
VII	Stable factor
VIII	Antihaemophilic factor (AHF)
IX	Christmas factor
X	Stuart–Prower factor
XI	Plasma thromboplastin antecedent (PTA)
XII	Contact factor, Hageman factor
XIII	Fibrin stabilizing factor
Prekallikrein	Fletcher factor
High molecular weight kininogen	Fitzgerald factor

then as activated enzymes. The first pathway is intrinsic (all components circulate in plasma). Its first component is the contact factor XII which requires an exposed subendothelial surface for its activation. A series of reactions involving coagulation factors and cofactors culminates in the prothrombin–thrombin reaction. Extrinsic coagulation joins the cascade at the pivotal factor X and requires tissue juices for its inception. Activated by thrombin, factor XIII stabilizes the fibrin polymer by cross-linkages between amino acids in adjacent fibrin strands.

Limiting factors

The third set of reactions serves to inhibit the unbridled extension of thrombus and vessel occlusion. Firstly, as the vessel relaxes, returning blood flow dilutes activated clotting proteins and mechanically discourages extension of the plug. Vascular endothelial cells secrete prostacyclin, a powerful inhibitor of platelet aggregation. Circulating inhibitors neutralize clotting intermediates, the most important being antithrombin (AT). New vitamin K dependent inhibitors of coagulation have been described. They are protein C and its cofactor S. AT regulates factor Xa and thrombin (IIa) whereas protein C and protein S

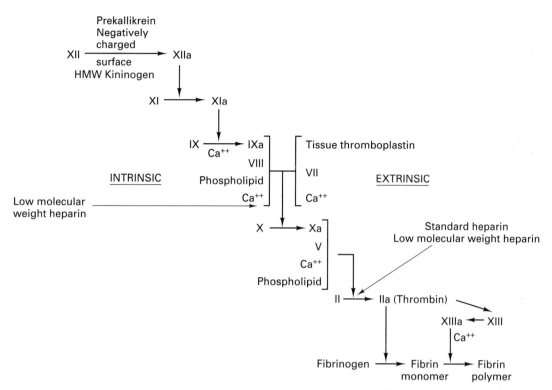

Fig. 6.2 Intrinsic and extrinsic coagulation pathways: 'a' indicates activation of the factor concerned. Phospholipid is provided by platelets and plasma. The actions of standard and low molecular weight heparin are indicated.

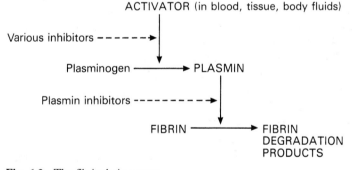

Fig. 6.3 The fibrinolytic system.

regulate factors VIII and V. Inherited individual deficiencies of these three proteins are now well recognized and present with thrombotic events.

The fibrinolytic system (Fig. 6.3) is also of great importance. Plasmin (the active enzyme of fibrinolysis) cleaves fibrin and fibrinogen and is derived from an inactive precursor, plasminogen. Activator of plasminogen is released from damaged endothelial cells and activated factor XII also

converts plasminogen. Both plasminogen and activator bind to fibrin. Thus fibrinolysis has similar triggers to coagulation. The resulting fibrin fragments (fibrin degradation products, FDP) are both anticoagulant and interfere with fibrin polymerization.

The interaction of and balance between coagulation and fibrinolysis are essential in maintaining vessel integrity and patency after injury. Risk factors for venous thromboembolism are well recognized; important amongst these is the hyper-coagulability that follows surgery and anaesthesia. Surgeons are increasingly employing various prophylactic strategies to prevent this complication.

DISSEMINATED INTRAVASCULAR COAGULATION (DIC)

This is also referred to as *consumption coagulopathy*, which suggests the pathogenesis. Essentially, the process represents the inappropriate triggering of the coagulation cascade in flowing blood by specific disease processes. There is considerable variation in severity, ranging from the coagulo-pathy as the predominant clinical manifestation (with haemostatic failure) to merely a laboratory sign of the underlying disease with no clinical haemostatic lesion. Some possible causes are listed in Table 6.2.

The principal laboratory findings are produced by the consumption of platelets during intra-vascular coagulation with reduction of fibrinogen and elevation of FDP in the serum as secondary (physiological) fibrinolysis breaks down throm-bus. Thrombocytopenia, hypofibrinogenaemia and elevation of serum FDP are thus the hall-marks of DIC. Scrutiny of the blood film may reveal red cell distortion or fragmentation if there is associated microangiopathy.

As the majority of clotting tests rely on the

fibrinogen–fibrin reaction as the end-point, the prothrombin time, partial thromboplastin time and thrombin time are prolonged as a result of the anticoagulant effect of FDP and consumption of other coagulation factors (II, V, VIII). DIC which is associated with endotoxaemia and endothelial damage tends to have more profound thrombo-cytopenia. There is some suggestion that in severe DIC there is, in addition, an induced platelet functional defect. DIC is inevitable to some degree where there is tissue damage (particularly the brain), hypotension, shock and poor organ perfusion.

Variants of the syndrome (with similar labora-tory findings) may occur with localized extra-vascular consumption (e.g. placental abruption) and localized intravascular consumption (e.g. thrombotic thrombocytopenic purpura). Occa-sionally, primary pathological fibrinolysis (PF) occurs without the microthrombosis seen in DIC, e.g. in neoplasia. Laboratory tests are not dis-similar to DIC but the platelet count tends to be higher. Differentiation of the commoner DIC from the less common PF rests on a careful clinical assessment and informed interpretation of addi-tional laboratory tests, which may require haemato-logical advice.

The management of DIC depends on clinical rather than laboratory severity. Whatever the de-gree of DIC, the first principle is an attempt to alleviate the underlying cause. In septicaemia, the infection should be treated vigorously along conventional lines, and in hypovolaemic shock with DIC, adequate blood volume expansion is required. After successful treatment, most pa-tients with DIC settle spontaneously and only in those with significant and continuing coagulation failure is there a need to repair the haemostatic mechanism with blood components. The ap-proach to each patient depends on clinical circum-stances and laboratory results but treatment may include the administration of fresh frozen plasma (FFP), cryoprecipitate (fibrinogen, factor VIII and fibronectin), platelets and heparin (rarely). Advice should be sought from the haematologist.

Table 6.2 Clinical associations of disseminated intravascular coagulation

Release of tissue thromboplastin	Eclampsia
	Placental abruption
	Fetal death in utero
	Amniotic fluid embolism
	Disseminated malignancy including acute leukaemia
	Head injury
	Burns
Infection	Malaria
	Bacteria, especially Gram-negative
	Viruses
Miscellaneous	Incompatible blood transfusion
	Extracorporeal circulation
	Antigen–antibody complexes
	Fat embolism
	Pulmonary embolism
	Shock

THE BLEEDING PATIENT

The anaesthetist and surgeon are confronted not

infrequently with a patient who is known to have a pre-existing haemostatic defect and the haematologist is asked if the patient is either fit for surgery or can be rendered operable.

Inherited coagulation abnormalities

These comprise classical haemophilia (haemophilia A) arising from coagulation factor VIII deficiency, Christmas disease (haemophilia B) from deficiency of factor IX (and clinically identical to classical haemophilia) and von Willebrand's disease from absence of part of the factor VIII molecule. Other inherited coagulation factor deficiencies occur but are uncommon.

The bleeding manifestations in the haemophilias are related directly to the degree of deficiency. The patient with severe classical haemophilia, with coagulation factor VIII levels of less than 1% (0.01 iu.ml^{-1}) of average normal, bleeds spontaneously, particularly into joints. In those with higher levels (1 to 3% of average normal) spontaneous bleeding is less common. In those moderately affected (3–16%), spontaneous bleeding is uncommon. The least affected group (16–40%) may remain undiagnosed until late in life. However, any haemophiliac patient whatever grade of severity bleeds excessively if challenged by trauma or by surgery and an occasional patient is diagnosed initially under those circumstances.

For surgery to proceed safely, the concentration of the appropriate factor must be raised to, and maintained at, a haemostatic level. The manner in which this is achieved depends on the type of surgery envisaged, the native factor level in the plasma, the half-life of the factor concerned after infusion, the type of factor concentrate available and the number of days to healing (which in turn depends on the procedure which has been performed). With the availability of factor VIII and IX concentrates, surgery of any type may now be contemplated safely. Six per cent of severe haemophiliacs develop antibodies to factor VIII, making management much more difficult. Surgery of any type, however minor, should be carried out only in designated haemophilia centres which have the staff, technical facilities and experience to supervise the haemostatic management of such patients. In the emergency situation, advice should be sought from the haematologist at the nearest designated centre.

About one quarter of previously treated haemophiliacs in the UK have antibody to human immunodeficiency virus (HIV) in their serum; the percentage in each haemophiliac population depends on geographical location and previous treatment policy. These infection rates are related to the previous use of contaminated blood products. Heat treatment and other biological and chemical manipulations of both National Health Service and commercial factor concentrates have interrupted this trend.

The anticoagulated patient

A more commonly encountered problem is that of the orally anticoagulated patient who presents as an emergency requiring surgical intervention within a short time. Although some major surgery may be carried out in the orally anticoagulated patient, surgeons are generally reluctant to proceed without at least partial reversal of anticoagulation.

The anticoagulant drug of choice in the United Kingdom is warfarin sodium and maintenance dose ranges from 3 to 10 mg daily. This prolongs the prothrombin time to 2–4 times normal (the therapeutic range). This is reported as the International Normalized Ratio (INR). Phytomenadione (vitamin K$_1$) may be used (i.v.) to reverse the warfarin lesion. It should be noted that if an excess is given, it may render the patient refractory to further warfarinization for days or weeks. The dose of vitamin K in warfarin induced and serious haemorrhage is 5 mg but in the therapeutically anticoagulated patient about to undergo surgery, doses of 0.5 to 1.0 mg are sufficient and the INR will return to the target range within 24 h. Reversal may take up to 12 h and cannot be hastened by a larger dose. If the planned surgery cannot be delayed until vitamin K reversal is achieved the most widely available material is fresh frozen plasma (FFP). Up to 1 litre may be required and its effect measured by further INRs. Group O and Group A FFP is available. Alternatively vitamin K dependent coagulation factor concentrates may be used (prothrombin complex concentrate – PCC) containing factors II, IX and X at a dose of 50 u/kg body weight of factor IX if full reversal is required. Factor VII concentrate may be used in addition if available.

It is unwise to fully reverse anticoagulation in patients with prosthetic heart valves and advice should be sought from a cardiothoracic unit.

Liver disease

Hepatocellular disease (cirrhosis or acute liver failure) results in diminished synthesis of vitamin K-dependent clotting factors (II, VII, IX and X) and fibrinogen, producing a laboratory lesion similar to that resulting from oral anticoagulants. In addition, these patients may be thrombocytopenic and clear FDP from the plasma at a reduced rate. Recourse to vitamin K, FFP, cryoprecipitate and platelet support may be required.

HEPARIN

Heparin is a potent, naturally occurring anticoagulant which is isolated commercially from animal intestinal mucous membranes. Bearing a strong negative charge, it interferes with the thrombin–fibrinogen reaction and potentiates the physiological antagonist of activated clotting factors, antithrombin (Fig. 6.2). It is given i.v., continuously, at a dose of 24–48 000 units per 24 h (for deep vein thrombosis). It is possible that the administration of similar doses intermittently but subcutaneously may produce the plasma concentration of heparin required for treatment of deep venous thrombosis or pulmonary embolus. Its action is immediate and if given by bolus it has a half-life of only 40 to 80 min. It has now gained wide acceptance in some but not all forms of major surgery as a successful means of preventing postoperative venous thromboembolism. For this indication, the dose by the s.c. route is 5000 units 8- or 12-hourly given for 7 to 10 days. Low molecular weight heparins are now widely available and are as safe as standard heparins for the prevention of venous thromboembolism. They are administered once daily. All heparins may cause thrombocytopenia.

If a patient who is therapeutically heparinized requires emergency surgery, cessation of the infusion may suffice because of the short half-life of the drug. The laboratory test of choice to monitor adequacy of full heparinization is the partial thromboplastin time with kaolin (PTTK or APTT) which should be 1.5 to 2.5 times prolonged compared with the control time. This desired ratio may differ between laboratories. Prior to emergency surgery in the heparinized patient, recourse to the PTTK may indicate that there is little risk of bleeding if the test is prolonged less than 1.5:1. Reversal of heparin in an emergency may be achieved using protamine sulphate given by slow i.v. injection at a dose of 1 mg per 100 units of heparin. Not more than 50 mg of protamine sulphate should be given because, in addition to side effects of flushing, bradycardia and hypotension, it is itself an anticoagulant.

PLATELET THERAPY

Unlike red cells, platelets have an inconveniently short shelf-life. Whereas red cells in citrate–phosphate dextrose with adenine have a safe storage life of 35 days, platelets in the same anticoagulant are only satisfactory when given to the recipient within 4 days of donation. This places obvious constraints on the supply of viable platelets to hospitals by transfusion centres. Platelets are supplied usually as concentrates, i.e. platelet-rich plasma (PRP) (produced from low g spun freshly donated blood) spun down again and much of the supernatant plasma removed. Platelet concentrates are stored at 22°C with agitation.

The indications for platelet transfusion remain controversial. In patients with e.g. acute leukaemia, who (because of both bone marrow disease and cytotoxic chemotherapy) are producing no endogenous platelets, the debate centres on the need for prophylactic versus therapeutic platelet transfusions. Because of rapid development of platelet antibodies, leukaemia centres are tending to limit prophylaxis to specific situations when the risk of haemorrhage is high, e.g. during serious infective episodes, and opting to treat other haemorrhagic episodes vigorously as they occur. Seventy per cent of patients develop platelet-destroying alloantibodies after repeated transfusions.

In surgical practice, as a general rule, significant bleeding should not occur if platelet numbers are greater than 100×10^9 litre^{-1}. Below 30×10^9 litre^{-1}, bleeding may be anticipated. Between 30 and 100×10^9 litre^{-1}, operative and postoperative oozing depends on the nature of the surgical procedure and the aetiology of the thrombocytopenia.

In autoimmune thrombocytopenia (e.g. idiopathic thrombocytopenic purpura) patients in whom medical treatment has failed may be referred for splenectomy with very low platelet counts. They do not require platelet transfusion for two reasons. Firstly, therapeutic platelets would be of short survival, being cleared by the same immune mechanism which is causing the patient's thrombocytopenia. Secondly, following the tying of the splenic pedicle, platelet counts may increase rapidly, ensuring adequate intra- and postoperative haemostasis. However, the local regional transfusion centre should be notified of the elective splenectomy in order that platelets might be furnished at relatively short notice if required.

If surgery is to be covered with platelet transfusions, the standard dose is 4 units per square metre of body surface, a unit being the platelets from a single donation. Currently, platelets are not crossmatched but where possible ABO and Rh D compatible platelets should be chosen. This dose may need to be given twice on the day of surgery and half of the first dose at least 60 min preoperatively. Further twice-daily doses on the first and succeeding postoperative days may be required and the need for further platelets should be assessed on the patient's progress and demonstration of normal coagulation proteins if haemostasis is not total. Satisfactory post-transfusion increments in the platelet count should be demonstrated if bleeding continues to be troublesome.

In DIC from any cause, platelet transfusions are rarely needed but should be given if platelet consumption has been documented as severe and haemorrhage is a clinical problem. In the massively transfused patient with haemostatic failure, platelets may be required if thrombocytopenia is unusually low (less than 50×10^9 litre^{-1}) and the coagulation mechanism is not judged to be at fault on laboratory testing.

BLOOD TRANSFUSION

The ABO blood groups first described in 1901 by Landsteiner and the Rhesus system described by Landsteiner and Weiner in 1940 together form the important blood group systems for those practising blood transfusion primarily at the bedside. However, there are many other clinically important blood group systems which are the more immediate concern of the blood transfusion laboratory staff. Problems relating to these groups are normally resolved by the laboratory before blood products are issued as compatible for use in the patient.

ABO groups

In the United Kingdom, 47% of persons are group O, 42% group A, 8% group B and 3% group AB. Patients, and thus donors, have these percentage distributions (Table 6.3). Proportions vary elsewhere in the world mainly from increased gene frequency of B. ABO blood group substances may be found also on leucocytes and platelets and 77% of persons secrete ABO blood group substances in body fluids. ABO antibodies are said to be naturally occurring, that is they are a constant feature of the system in all persons and do not arise as a result to exposure to A or B blood group substances at some time during life. Although A and B blood group substances appear in red cells early in fetal development, the corresponding antibodies appear only after birth at 3–6 months of age and are present in greatest strength at the age of 10 years. After the early months of life, anti-A and anti-B are present invariably in the serum when the red cells lack the corresponding antigen. Table 6.3 shows the old rationale, now outmoded, for the designation of group O persons as 'universal donors', because

Table 6.3 Distribution of ABO blood groups in the United Kingdom, their red cell antigens and antibodies

	%	RBC antigen	Serum	
O	47	—	Anti-A Anti-B	'Universal donor'
A	42	A	Anti-B	
B	8	B	Anti-A	
AB	3	A + B	—	'Universal recipient'

Rhesus D positive 85%
Rhesus D negative 15%

they lack group A and B substances in their red cells, and persons of group AB as 'universal recipients' as their serum does not contain either anti-A or anti-B. ABO antibodies are predominantly IgM and thus do not cross the placenta. An occasional person, usually group O, may have 'immune' anti-A (or less commonly, anti-B), an IgG molecule capable of crossing the placenta and active at 37°C. Such persons are called 'dangerous' donors and are screened at transfusion centres. If pregnant with a group A (or B) fetus, ABO maternofetal incompatibility may ensue with haemolytic disease of the newborn.

Whenever possible, blood transfusion laboratories try to provide blood of the same ABO group as the recipient. If a patient of group AB requires an emergency transfusion of more than a few units, further AB units may be unavailable and A blood is used, being likely to be more plentiful than B. If ABO compatible blood is unavailable for a group B patient, group O is used with suitable preceding compatibility tests.

ABO incompatible transfusion accidents are the most serious of the transfusion incompatibilities and have significant morbidity and mortality. Properly conducted routine compatibility techniques detect such problems in vitro and they occur only if there has been an error of patient identification or sample identification. Most accidents of this type result from clerical errors.

Rhesus groups

Shortly after the discovery of the Rhesus groups it was recognized that some haemolytic transfusion reactions and haemolytic disease of the newborn (erythroblastosis fetalis) resulted from incompatibilities in this system. In bedside blood transfusion practice, the Rh D antigen is the most important of the Rhesus antigens. Units of blood or blood products labelled Rh D positive may also be positive for C and E antigens. Units labelled Rh D negative may, however, be positive for antigens C and E unless additionally labelled C D E negative. Colour coded ABO and Rh D labels are no longer used. The Rhesus factors are inherited in a 'packet', one from each parent, each 'packet' containing one of each pair of alleles, C, D, E. The commonest genes are CDe (gene frequency 0.41)

and cde (0.39) followed by cDE (0.14). The other genes are much less common.

Antibodies of clinical significance occur in the Rhesus system and these rarely occur naturally, i.e. they are formed as the result of exposure to Rhesus antigens which the patient does not possess naturally. The commonest circumstance is the bearing of a Rh D positive fetus by a Rh D negative woman. The most common antibody is anti-D and at least two pregnancies are required. The national (UK) programme for prevention of Rhesus immunization in pregnancy has reduced the incidence of this. Such antibodies are detected readily in compatibility tests but, if undetected, may result in an immediate transfusion reaction or at best, impaired survival of the transfused cells.

Other blood groups

The known number of blood group antigens is increasing constantly, usually because of the discovery first of the corresponding antibody. Many are of little clinical significance. Ability to react at 37°C and specificity characterize those antibodies in recipient serum which necessitate the provision of red cells lacking the corresponding antigen. Of greatest importance are, in order of frequency, Kell, Duffy, Kidd, Ss and Lewis. Of all clinically significant alloantibodies, 83% are in the Rhesus system (Table 6.4).

Storage and preservation of blood

Until recently, blood for transfusion was collected

Table 6.4 Percentage frequency of clinically important 37°C alloantibodies detected in recipients

Anti-D	61
Anti-C (± D)	11
Anti-E	7
Anti-Kell	6
Anti-c	4
Anti-Duffy	2.2
Anti-Kidd	0.9
Anti-e	0.5
Anti-Ss	0.04
Others (Lewis included)	7

into ACD (acid citrate dextrose solution containing trisodium citrate, citric acid and dextrose) which acted both as an anticoagulant and red cell preservative. This was superseded in some parts of the world in the 1970s by CPD (citrate phosphate dextrose) in which the addition of sodium dihydrogen phosphate raised the pH of the solution and improved red cell survival in vivo. The duration of storage considered suitable with an anticoagulant is such that, on the last day of storage, 70% of red cells are recoverable in the circulation at 24 h after transfusion and subsequently have a normal survival pattern. In this context red cell survival is related to cellular levels of ATP. The addition of adenine to CPD assists maintenance of ATP levels and this preferred anticoagulant–preservative, known as CPD-A, enables the shelf life of stored blood to be increased to 35 days compared with 21 days for ACD and standard CPD. Storage of red cells for transfusion should be at 2–6°C in a blood bank refrigerator. Resort to other domestic-type refrigerators is hazardous because of the risk of inadequate thermostatic control leading to the possibility of freezing of blood and lysis of red cells on warming in the event of equipment failure. Ministry of Health-type insulated boxes maintain precooled red cells for transfusion at a satisfactory temperature, when used with ice inserts, for up to 24 h.

At appropriate storage temperatures, bacterial replication in blood is inhibited and red cell glycolysis is slowed with some preservation of 2,3-DPG levels. The prime function of the erythrocyte is delivery of oxygen to the tissues and this is dependent on red cell levels of 2,3-DPG. In ACD, red cells lose 40% and 90% of 2,3-DPG at 1 and 2 weeks respectively with a resulting shift to the left of the oxygen dissociation curve. In CPD, 2,3-DPG is better maintained (20% loss at 2 weeks) but slightly less so in CPD-A. Whatever the storage medium, however, levels of 2,3-DPG return to normal in 6–24 h after transfusion.

Blood grouping and compatibility tests

Elective grouping is now being undertaken more commonly using automated apparatus suited to large batches. This process may take up to half a day. In the emergency situation, if the patient's group is not known it can be ascertained within 5–10 min of receipt of the samples.

There is incomplete agreement as to what constitutes the ideal crossmatching test system to ensure compatibility between donor red cells and patient's serum. Essential components include a test at room temperature to detect the important ABO incompatibilities between donor and patient and two or more tests at 37°C to detect Rh and other alloantibodies in the patient's serum which would result in a transfusion reaction and reduced red cell survival. The clinically important antibodies are shown in Table 6.4. The introduction of low ionic strength saline (LISS) to replace ordinary saline as a red cell suspension medium has resulted in incubation times being greatly reduced and an acceptable 30 min crossmatch is now a reality.

Trends towards the elective screening of all patients' sera for irregular antibodies simultaneously with automated grouping may soon obviate the need for any crossmatching technique. This would ensure that once a patient had been shown to be free of alloantibodies to blood group antigens, blood of appropriate ABO and Rh group would simply be selected and given without matching (and the resultant time delays).

More recently the introduction of commercial gel-based technology is revolutionizing grouping, antibody screening and compatibility testing.

Red cell concentrates ('packed cells', plasma-reduced cells)

In the UK, regional transfusion centres issue a minority of units as whole blood and an increasing proportion is distributed as red cell concentrates. Some red cell concentrates are suspended in plasma. These are produced by the removal of 150–200 ml of citrated plasma from the final donated volume of 510 ml (450 ml blood + 60 ml of CPD-A anticoagulant–preservative). This fresh, platelet-rich plasma is used for production of platelet concentrates and as raw material for blood component manufacture. An increasing proportion of donations has a much greater percentage of plasma removed and replaced by a preservative solution as a suspension medium. The additive used in the UK is SAGM (saline, adenine, glucose, mannitol). Both types of red cell concentrate are produced in sterile closed plastic blood-bag systems and have the same shelf-life as whole blood.

Cryoprecipitate is manufactured from some freshly donated units and results in a unit of whole blood with an almost normal amount of plasma but labelled 'cryoprecipitate poor'.

Many hospital blood bank laboratories now provide the first two units of blood for surgery as red cell concentrates. These have a high haematocrit and are more viscous than whole blood. The volume of red cell concentrates is 380–410 ml.

Donations of blood in the UK have been tested for HIV antibody since 1985 and for antibody to hepatitis C virus since 1991. This is in addition to hepatitis B surface antigen and syphilis. For selected recipients donations may be screened for cytomegalovirus (CMV).

Future developments may include the manufacture of artificial blood in the form of oxygen-carrying plasma volume expander solutions.

Transfusion reactions

In addition to the haemolytic transfusion reactions referred to above there are other types of reaction which may interfere with the completion of transfusion of blood or blood components. About 2% of all transfusions are followed by some form of reaction and three-quarters of these are febrile reactions. These latter result from antibodies to white cells in the HLA system. Such reactions may be accompanied by rigors, hypotension, dyspnoea, occasionally cyanosis, nausea and vomiting. It is worth remembering that the symptoms and signs of any form of transfusion reaction may be obscured or abolished by general anaesthesia. Fever after platelet transfusion in patients with platelet alloantibodies is less common but platelet preparations are always contaminated by white cells. Prevention of reactions to white cells includes the transfusion of buffy coat-poor blood, washing of red cells or the use of white cell filters at the bedside.

Milder anaphylactic reactions are associated frequently with urticaria (weals or hives) and very occasionally with flushing, dyspnoea and hypo-

Table 6.5 Complications of blood transfusion

Transmission of disease, e.g. viral hepatitis, syphilis, malaria, HIV

Bacterial contamination

Pyrogenic reactions

Incompatibility reactions

Haemolytic reactions

Allergic reactions

Citrate toxicity

Hypothermia

Hyperkalaemia

Metabolic acidosis

Circulatory overload

Air embolism

Microaggregate embolism

tension and are thought to result from reaction between IgA in the transfused blood and anti-IgA in the recipient. Less commonly, other antibodies may be implicated in an atopic subject.

Non-immunological reactions to stored blood include induced hypothermia from transfusion of large volumes of cold blood and citrate toxicity in similar circumstances. Other consequences are air embolism, transfusion of particulate matter from transfusion equipment and reactions to cellular debris in blood, for example 'postperfusion' lung. Some complications of blood transfusion are listed in Table 6.5.

Plasma volume expanders

In acute hypovolaemia plasma volume expanders are frequently used while blood is being prepared. Transfusion is often started with electrolyte solutions but continued with volume expanders.

Three non-human source materials are in use.

Gelatins

In these preparations, bovine gelatin is modified to produce an average molecular weight of 30 000–35 000. The two available products, polygeline (Haemaccel) and succinylated gelatin (Gelofusine), have a pH, colloid osmotic pressure and viscosity similar to those of plasma. Their half-lives are approximately 4 h. They have a shelf-life at ambient temperatures of up to 8 years. Occasionally, rapid infusion, particularly in a normovolaemic patient, may result in the release of vasoactive substances which cause rash, hypotension and tachycardia; these may be managed by antihistamines and/or hydrocortisone and the infusion should be discontinued. Gelatin solutions do not interfere with blood grouping or compatibility testing and renal function is not impaired.

The two preparations differ in their electrolyte content. Polygeline must not be allowed to mix with citrated blood products as it has a high calcium content (6.25 mmol.litre^{-1}). Gelofusine contains little potassium (0.4 mmol.litre^{-1}). No more than 1–1.5 litres of gelatin solution should be transfused before blood is available.

Dextrans

Dextran 70 injection BP (6% dextran) is most frequently employed in 5% glucose or in 0.9% saline. The average molecular weight of the material is 70 000. Dextrans should not be administered to patients with renal impairment, severe congestive heart failure or thrombocytopenia. The dextrans are believed to interfere with the haemostatic mechanism if transfused in large quantity and cause difficulty with grouping and compatibility tests in the laboratory by promotion of rouleaux. This is less of a problem with the introduction to blood transfusion laboratories of gel technology. No acutely bleeding patient should receive more than 1.5 litre and, as unpredictable anaphylactic reactions may occur with erythema, bronchospasm, urticaria and hypotension, the patient should be observed carefully during the first few minutes of the infusion. If such a reaction occurs, the infusion should be stopped immediately and resuscitation measures instituted.

Etherified starch

This plasma volume expander is an artificial colloid derived from amylopectin and closely resembles glycogen. Its average molecular weight is 200–450 000 and its infusion results in an expansion of plasma volume slightly in excess of the volume infused. Plasma volume expansion is maintained for at least 24 h. Contraindications and side effects are similar to those of dextran 70. No more than 1 litre should be given.

Human albumin solution

This material, known previously as plasma protein fraction, is prepared from donor plasma both by the Bio-Products Laboratory of the National Blood Transfusion Service and by the pharmaceutical industry. It contains protein (principally albumin), 45 g.litre^{-1} in saline. It is heat-treated and present evidence suggests that this inactivates hepatitis-producing agents. It has a 3-year shelf-life (away from light). It is remarkably free from adverse effects.

The Bio-Products Laboratory material remains in short supply and hospitals frequently supplement stocks from commercial sources.

The relative net prices of these volume expanders (September 1994) for one unit are: succinylated gelatin £4.01; polygeline £3.71; dextran 70 in saline £4.45; starch £12.18 and commercial human albumin £30.00.

FURTHER READING

Bloom A L, Thomas D P 1987 Haemostasis and thrombosis, 2nd edn. Churchill Livingstone, Edinburgh
Contreras M (ed) ABC of Transfusion, 2nd edn. BMJ Publishing Group, London
Hardisty R M, Weatherall D J (eds) 1993 Blood and its disorders, 2nd edn. Blackwell Scientific Publications, Oxford
Herxheimer A (ed) 1987 Plasma substitutes. Drug and Therapeutics Bulletin 25: 10, 37
Hoffbrand A V, Pettit J E 1993 Essential haematology, 3rd edn. Blackwell Scientific Publications, Oxford
Mollison P L, Engelfriet C P, Contreras M 1992 Blood transfusion in clinical medicine, 9th edn. Blackwell Scientific Publications, Oxford
Petz L D, Swisher S M N (eds) 1989 Clinical practice of transfusion medicine, 2nd edn. Churchill Livingstone, Edinburgh
Serjeant G R 1992 Sickle cell disease, 2nd edn. Oxford University Press, Oxford
Weatherall D J, Clegg J B 1981 Thalassaemia syndromes, 3rd edn. Blackwell Scientific Publications, Oxford

7. Principles of pharmacology

HOW DO DRUGS ACT?

Drugs have an effect because of their physico-chemical properties, activity at receptors on the cell surface, inhibition of enzyme systems or influence on synthesis of nucleic acid.

Physicochemical properties

Sodium citrate neutralizes acid and is given frequently to aid prevention of pneumonitis after inhalation of gastric contents. Chelating agents act by combining with metal ions, reducing their toxicity and enhancing elimination, usually in the urine. Such drugs include desferrioxamine (iron, aluminium), dicobalt edetate (cyanide toxicity), sodium calcium edetate (lead) and penicillamine (copper, lead).

Receptors

A receptor is a complex structure on the cell mem-brane which can bind selectively with endogenous compounds or drugs and transduce this chemical signal into the initiation of change within the cell. In order to do this, the receptor may be linked with ion channels or second messenger systems (e.g. cyclic adenosine monophosphate, cyclic guanosine monophosphate, inositol triphosphate) depending on its type. Considerable advances have been made recently in our understanding of the function and structure of receptors and many types and subtypes have been identified.

A compound which binds to a receptor and changes intracellular function is called an agonist. The classical dose–response relationship of an agonist is shown in Figure 7.1. As the concentration of agonist increases, a maximum effect (C_{max}) is reached as the receptors in the preparation become saturated. Conventionally, log dose is plotted against effect resulting in a sigmoid curve which is approximately linear between 20% and 80% of C_{max} (Fig. 7.1B). Three agonists are shown

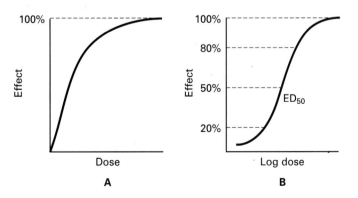

Fig. 7.1 (**A**) The effect of an agonist peaks when all the receptors are occupied. (**B**) A semilog plot produces a sigmoid curve which is linear between 20% and 80% effect. ED_{50} is the dose which produces 50% of maximum effect.

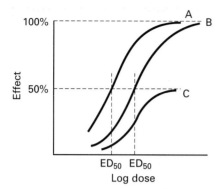

Fig. 7.2 Agonist B has a similar dose–response curve to A but is displaced to the right. A is more potent than B (smaller ED_{50}) but has the same efficacy. C is a partial agonist which is less potent than A and B and less efficacious (maximum effect 50% of A and B).

in Figure 7.2. Agonist A produces 100% effect at a lower concentration than agonist B. Therefore, compared with A, agonist B is less potent but has similar efficacy. Drug C is termed a partial agonist as C_{max} is only 50% of that of A or B. Buprenorphine is a partial agonist (at the μ opioid receptor), as are some of the β-blockers with intrinsic activity, e.g. oxprenolol, pindolol, acebutalol.

Antagonists combine selectively with the receptor but produce no effect. They can interact with the receptor in a reversible or irreversible fashion. In the presence of a reversible antagonist, the dose response curve is shifted to the right but C_{max} remains unaltered (Fig. 7.3A). Examples of this

include the displacement of acetylcholine from the nicotinic receptors by non-depolarizing muscle relaxants, 5-hydroxytryptamine (5-HT) by $5-HT_3$ antagonist in the gut wall and chemoreceptor trigger zone and endogenous catecholamines by α- and β-blockers.

An irreversible or non-competitive antagonist shifts the dose–response curve to the right also but with increasing concentrations reduces C_{max} (Fig. 7.3B). This phenomenon is observed more frequently in enzyme systems where the antagonist combines chemically and inactivates the enzyme. However, some antagonists dissociate very slowly indeed from receptor sites and produce irreversible antagonism similar to that shown in Figure 7.3B. This is described also as irreversible competitive antagonism. For example, the α_1-blocker phenoxybenzamine, used in the preoperative preparation of patients with phaeochromocytoma, has a long duration of action resulting from the formation of stable chemical bonds between drug and receptor.

Drugs acting on enzymes

Drugs may act by inhibiting the action of an enzyme or competing for its endogenous substrate. Reversible inhibition is the mechanism of action of allopurinol (xanthine oxidase), aminophylline (phosphodiesterase) and captopril (angiotensin converting enzyme). Irreversible enzyme

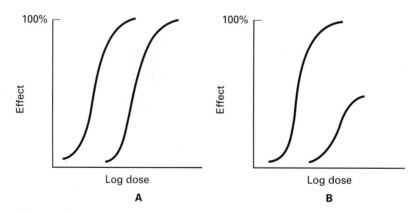

Fig. 7.3 (**A**) The dose–response curve of an agonist is displaced to the right in the presence of a reversible antagonist. There is no change in maximum effect but the ED_{50} is increased. (**B**) The dose–response curve is displaced to the right also in the presence of an irreversible antagonist but the maximum effect is reduced.

inhibition occurs when a stable chemical bond is formed between drug and enzyme, resulting in prolonged or permanent inactivity, e.g. omeprazole (gastric hydrogen-potassium ATPase), aspirin (prostaglandin synthetase) and organophosphorus compounds (cholinesterase).

Neostigmine inhibits acetylcholinesterase in a reversible manner but, in fact, the mechanism of action is more akin to that of an irreversible drug as the enzyme is carbamylated by the formation of covalent chemical bonds.

Nucleic acid synthesis

Drugs may act at sites within the cell and have effects on the synthesis of protein by stimulating the production of messenger RNA via steroid receptors on the cell nucleus. Consequently, drugs acting in this manner, e.g. corticosteroids, have a slow speed of onset.

The blood–brain barrier and placenta

Most drugs used in anaesthetic practice must cross the blood–brain barrier in order to reach their site of action. The brain is protected from most potentially toxic agents by tightly overlapping endothelial cells which surround the capillaries and interfere with passive diffusion. Enzyme systems are present in the endothelium which can metabolize many potential toxins also. Consequently, only relatively small molecules which are highly lipid soluble, such as intravenous and volatile anaesthetic agents, opioids and local anaesthetics, have access to the central nervous system (CNS). Morphine has a profound effect but takes some time to reach its site of action because of its relative water solubility. Highly ionized drugs, e.g. muscle relaxants, glycopyrronium, do not cross the blood–brain barrier.

The chemoreceptor trigger zone is situated in the area postrema near the base of the 4th ventricle and, although within the brain, is not protected by the blood–brain barrier. The capillary endothelial cells are not bound tightly and allow relatively free passage of large and small molecules into this area. This is an important afferent limb of the vomiting reflex and stimulation of this area by toxins or drugs in the blood or cerebrospinal fluid

often lead to vomiting. Many antiemetics act at this site.

The transfer of drugs across the placenta is of considerable importance in obstetric anaesthesia. In general, all drugs which affect the CNS cross the placenta and affect the fetus. Highly ionized drugs, e.g. muscle relaxants, pass across less readily.

Plasma protein binding

Many drugs are bound to proteins in the plasma. This is important as only the unbound portion of the drug is available for diffusion to its site of action. Changes in protein binding may have significant effects on the active unbound concentration of a drug and therefore its actions.

Albumin is the most important protein in this regard and is responsible mainly for the binding of acidic and neutral drugs. Globulins, especially α_1-glycoprotein, bind mainly basic drugs. If a drug is highly protein bound (> 80%) any change in plasma protein concentration, or displacement of the drug by another with similar binding properties, may have clinically significant effects. Plasma albumin may be decreased in the elderly and neonates and in the presence of malnutrition, liver, renal and cardiac failure and malignancy. α_1-glycoprotein is decreased during pregnancy and in the neonate but may be increased in the postoperative period and other conditions such as infection, trauma, burns and malignancy.

METABOLISM

Most drugs are lipid soluble and many are metabolized in the liver into more ionized compounds which are inactive pharmacologically and excreted by the kidney. However, metabolites may be active and some examples are given in Table 7.1. The liver is not the only site of metabolism. For example, suxamethonium and mivacurium are metabolized by plasma cholinesterase, esmolol by erythrocyte esterases and, in part, dopamine by the kidney and prilocaine by the lungs.

A substance is termed a *prodrug* if it is inactive in the form in which it is administered, pharmacological effects being dependent on the formation of active metabolites. Examples of this include

Table 7.1 Active metabolites

Drug	Metabolite	Action
Morphine	Morphine-6-glucuronide	Potent μ opioid receptor agonist
Pethidine	Nor-pethidine	Epileptogenic
Diazepam	Desmethyldiazepam Temazepam Oxazepam	Sedative
Atracurium	Laudanosine	Epileptogenic
Pancuronium	3-Hydroxypancuronium	Relaxant

chloral hydrate (trichlorethanol), methyldopa (methyl-noradrenaline) and prednisone (prednisolone). Midazolam is ionized and water soluble at an acid pH in the ampoule; after intravenous injection the molecule becomes lipid soluble.

Drugs undergo two types of reactions during metabolism: phase I and phase II. Phase I reactions include reduction, oxidation and hydrolysis. Drug oxidation occurs in the smooth endoplasmic reticulum, primarily by the cytochrome P-450 enzyme system. This system, and other enzymes, can perform reduction reactions also; a phenomenon of particular importance in the mechanism of halothane toxicity. Hydrolysis is a common phase I reaction in the metabolism of ester and amide drugs.

Phase II reactions involve conjugation of a metabolite or the drug itself with an endogenous substrate. Conjugation with glucuronic acid is a major metabolic pathway but others include acetylation, methylation and conjugation with sulphate and glycine.

Enzyme induction and inhibition

Some drugs may enhance the activity of enzymes responsible for drug metabolism, particularly the cytochrome P-450 enzymes and glucuronyl transferase. Such drugs include phenytoin, barbiturates, ethanol, steroids and inhalational anaesthetic agents.

Enzyme inhibition has been described above as a method of drug action. However, drugs with other mechanisms of action can also interfere significantly with enzyme systems. For example, etomidate inhibits the synthesis of cortisol and aldosterone; an effect which probably explains the increased mortality which has been reported with its use as a sedative agent in critically ill patients. Cimetidine is a potent enzyme inhibitor and can prolong the elimination of drugs such as diazepam, propranolol, oral anticoagulants, phenytoin and intravenous lignocaine.

DRUG EXCRETION

Ionized compounds, with a low molecular weight, are excreted mainly by the kidneys. Most drugs diffuse passively into the proximal renal tubules by the process of glomerular filtration but some are secreted actively, e.g. penicillins, aspirin, many diuretics, morphine, lignocaine and glucuronides. Ionization is a significant barrier to reabsorption at the distal tubule. Consequently, basic drugs are excreted more efficiently in acid urine and acidic compounds in alkaline urine.

Some drugs and metabolites, particularly those with larger molecules (MW > 400), are excreted in the bile, e.g. glycopyrronium, vecuronium, alcuronium, pancuronium and the metabolites of morphine and buprenorphine.

PHARMACOKINETIC PRINCIPLES

An understanding of the basic principles of pharmacokinetics is an important aid to the safe use of drugs in anaesthesia and intensive care. Pharmacokinetics is an attempt to fit observed changes in plasma concentration of drugs into mathematical equations which then enable prediction. Derived values describing volume of distribution (Vd), clearance (Cl) and half-life ($t_{\frac{1}{2}}$) may give an indication of the likely properties of a drug. However, even in healthy individuals of the same sex, weight and age, there may be significant interpatient variability which makes prediction very difficult. Values quoted are usually the mean of several observations and it is of great value to note the standard deviation or range.

Volume of distribution

Volume of distribution is a good example of the abstract nature of pharmacokinetics; it is not a real volume but merely a concept which helps us understand what we observe. Nevertheless, it is a very useful concept which enables us to predict certain properties of a drug and also calculate other pharmacokinetic values.

Imagine that a patient, receiving an intravenous dose of an anaesthetic induction agent, is in fact a bucket of water and that the drug is distributed evenly throughout the water immediately after injection. The volume of water represents the initial Vd. It can be calculated easily:

$$C_0 = \frac{Dose}{Vd} \qquad (1)$$

where C_0 = initial concentration.

Therefore:

$$Vd = \frac{Dose}{C_0} \qquad (2)$$

A more accurate measurement of Vd is possible during constant rate infusion when the distribution of the drug in the tissues has time to equilibrate; this is termed volume of distribution at steady-state (V^{ss}).

Drugs which remain in the plasma and do not pass easily to other tissues have a large C_0 and therefore a small Vd. Relatively ionized drugs, e.g. muscle relaxants, or drugs highly bound to plasma proteins often have a small Vd. Drugs with a large Vd are often lipid soluble and therefore penetrate and accumulate in tissues outside the plasma. Most induction agents, for example, have large volumes of distribution and the values for some drugs are greater than total body volume (a reminder of the abstract nature of pharmacokinetics). Large Vd values are observed often for drugs highly bound to proteins outside plasma (e.g. local anaesthetics, digoxin).

Several factors can affect initial Vd and therefore C_0 on bolus injection. Patients who are dehydrated or have lost blood have a significantly greater plasma C_0 after normal doses of intravenous induction agent, increasing the likelihood of severe side-effects, especially hypotension. Neonates have a significantly greater volume of extracellular fluid compared with adults and water soluble drugs, e.g. muscle relaxants, tend to have a greater Vd. Factors affecting plasma protein binding (see above) may affect Vd also.

Finally, Vd can give some indication as to the relative speed of drug elimination. A large Vd may be associated with a relatively slow decline in plasma concentrations; this relationship is expressed below in a useful pharmacokinetic equation.

Clearance

Clearance is defined as the volume of blood or plasma from which the drug is removed completely in unit time. Drugs can be eliminated from the blood by the liver, kidney or occasionally other routes (see above). The relative proportion of hepatic and renal clearance of a drug is important. Most drugs used in anaesthetic practice are cleared predominantly by the liver but some rely on renal clearance. Excessive accumulation of a drug occurs in patients in renal failure if its renal clearance is significant. For example, morphine is metabolized primarily in the liver and this is not affected significantly in renal impairment. However, the active metabolite morphine-6-glucuronide is excreted predominantly by the kidney; this accumulates and is responsible for the toxic effects often observed in these patients.

As with Vd, clearance may suggest likely properties of a drug. For example, if clearance is greater than hepatic blood flow, factors other than hepatic metabolism must account for its total clearance. Values greater than cardiac output may indicate metabolism in the plasma (e.g. suxamethonium). Clearance is an important, but not the only, factor affecting $t_{1/2}$ and steady-state plasma concentrations achieved during constant rate infusions (see below).

Elimination half-life

The administration of a drug is influenced considerably by its plasma $t_{1/2}$ as this often reflects duration of action. It is important to remember that $t_{1/2}$ is influenced not only by clearance but also Vd.

$$t_{1/2} \propto \frac{Vd}{Cl} \qquad (3)$$

or

$$t_{1/2} = constant \frac{Vd}{Cl}$$

The constant in this equation = the natural logarithm of 2 (ln 2), i.e. 0.693

Therefore:

$$t_{\frac{1}{2}} = 0.693 \frac{Vd}{Cl} \qquad (4)$$

Half-life often reflects the duration of action but not if the drug acts irreversibly (e.g. some non-steroidal anti-inflammatory agents, omeprazole, phenoxybenzamine) or if active metabolites are formed (e.g. morphine, diazepam).

So far, we have considered metabolic or elimination $t_{\frac{1}{2}}$ only. The initial decrease in plasma concentrations after administration of many drugs, e.g. induction agents, occurs primarily because of redistribution into extracorporeal tissues. Therefore, the simple relationship between elimination $t_{\frac{1}{2}}$ and duration of action does not apply (see below, two compartmental models).

Calculating $t_{\frac{1}{2}}$, Vd and clearance

We shall calculate these values for a drug after intravenous bolus administration and regular blood sampling for plasma concentration measurements. In this example, we assume that the drug remains in the plasma and is removed only by metabolism, e.g. a one compartmental model. After achieving C_0, plasma concentration (C_p) declines in a simple exponential manner as shown

in Figure 7.4A. If the natural log of the concentrations is plotted against time (semi-log plot) a straight line will be produced (Fig. 7.4B). The gradient of this line is the elimination rate constant k, which may be related to $t_{\frac{1}{2}}$ in the following equation:

$$k = \frac{\ln 2}{t_{\frac{1}{2}}} \qquad (5)$$

We can calculate Vd using equation (2) and then clearance from equation (4). C_p can be predicted at any time from the equation shown in the figure.

Clearance can be derived also by calculation of the area under the concentration-time curve extrapolated to infinity (AUC_∞) and substituting in the following equation.

$$Cl = \frac{Dose}{AUC_\infty} \qquad (6)$$

Two compartmental models

The body is not, of course, a single homogeneous compartment but the mathematics describing the real situation of, for example, 20 compartments are extremely complex. However, plasma concentrations of many drugs behave approximately as if they were distributed in two or three compartments. Applying these mathematical models is a reasonable compromise.

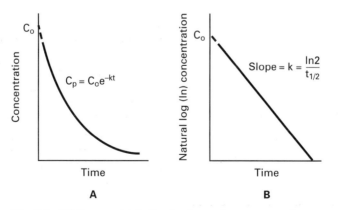

Fig. 7.4 (**A**) Exponential decline in plasma drug concentration (C_p) in a one compartmental model. The equation predicts C_p at any time (t). (**B**) Semilog plot enables easy calculation of elimination rate constant (k) and $t_{\frac{1}{2}}$. ln = natural logarithm of 2 (0.693). Extrapolation of this line enables C_0 and AUC_∞ to be derived easily.

Let us consider a two compartmental model; one compartment may be thought of as representing the plasma and the other, the rest of the body. When an intravenous bolus is injected into this system C_p decreases because of an exponential decay resulting from elimination and another exponential decay resulting from redistribution into the tissues. Therefore, when C_p is plotted against time, the curve may be described by a biexponential equation. If plotted on a semilogarithmic plot (Fig. 7.5), two straight lines can be identified. Their gradients are the elimination rate constant dependent on elimination and that dependent on redistribution.

Redistribution kinetics are not only of theorectical interest because it is often the decline in C_p resulting from redistribution which is responsible for the cessation of an observed effect of a drug; intravenous induction agents and *initial* doses of fentanyl are good examples of this.

Calculating the separate pharmacokinetic values is easy; one curve is simply subtracted from the other. Consider Figure 7.5. The elimination curve is back extrapolated to time 0 to give the theoretical C_0 for the elimination part of the equation (A). From this, the elimination half-life $t_{1/2}^\beta$ can

be calculated using the simple equations described above in the one compartmental model. This extrapolated curve is now subtracted from the original to give the decline caused by redistribution from which $t_{1/2}^\alpha$ can be obtained. The equation for C_p at any time is therefore:

$$C_p = Ae^{-\alpha t} + Be^{-\beta t}$$

where α and β are the redistribution and elimination rate constants respectively and A and B are the C_0 from the derived redistribution and elimination curves.

Some drugs, e.g. propofol, are best fitted to a triexponential, three compartmental model which reveals half-lives for two processes of redistribution ($t_{1/2}^\alpha$ and $t_{1/2}^\beta$) and one for elimination ($t_{1/2}^\gamma$).

METHODS OF DRUG ADMINISTRATION

Oral

The oral route of drug administration is important in modern anaesthetic practice, e.g. premedication, analgesia after minor surgery. It is often necessary also to continue concurrent medication during the perioperative period, e.g. antihypertensives, antianginal medication. It is therefore important to appreciate the factors involved in the absorption of oral medication.

The formulation of tablets or capsules is very precise as their consistent dissolution is necessary before absorption can take place. The rate of absorption, and therefore effect of the drug, may be influenced significantly by this factor. Most preparations dissolve in the acidic gastric juices and the intact drug is absorbed in the upper intestine. However, some drugs are broken down by acids (e.g. omeprazole, benzylpenicillin) or are irritant to the stomach (e.g. aspirin, phenylbutazone) and can be given as enteric coated preparations. Drugs given in solution are often absorbed more rapidly but this may induce nausea or vomiting immediately after anaesthesia.

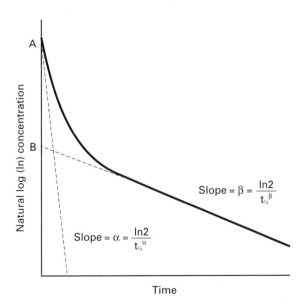

Fig. 7.5 Semilog plot of a two compartmental model. α = rate constant for exponential decay resulting from redistribution, β = rate constant for exponential decay resulting from elimination.

Gastric emptying

Most drugs are absorbed only when they have left the stomach and, if gastric emptying is delayed, absorption is affected. Furthermore, if oral

Table 7.2 Causes of delayed gastric emptying

Physiological
  Pain
  Anxiety
  Pregnancy (in some patients)

Pathological
  GI tract obstruction/acute abdomen
  Acute gastroparesis:
    gastroenteritis
    ketoacidosis
    electrolyte imbalance
    hypercalcaemia
    migraine
  Diabetes
  Polymyositis, dermatomyositis
  Systemic sclerosis

Pharmacological
  Opioids
  Partial & mixed opioid agonists:
    buprenorphine
    pentazocine
    meptazinol
    nalbuphine
  Nefopam
  Anticholinergics:
    atropine, hyoscine
    antihistamines
    phenothiazines
    tricyclic antidepressants
  Sympathomimetics:
    isoprenaline
    salbutamol
  Dopamine
  Alcohol

medication is given continuously during periods of impaired emptying, it may accumulate in the stomach, only to be delivered to the small intestine en masse when gastric function returns, resulting in overdose. Table 7.2 describes the factors which delay gastric emptying; many are common in anaesthetic practice.

Any factor increasing upper intestinal motility, e.g. prokinetic drugs such as metoclopramide, reduces the time available for absorption and reduces total bioavailability (i.e. amount of drug absorbed).

First-pass effect

Before entering the systemic circulation, the drug must pass through the portal circulation and, if metabolized extensively by the liver or even the gut wall, absorption may be reduced significantly, i.e. first-pass effect. For example, compared with intramuscular administration, significantly larger doses of oral morphine are required for the same effect. Other drugs susceptible to first-pass metabolism include pethidine, dopamine, isoprenaline, propranolol and glyceryl trinitrate.

Lingual and buccal

This is a useful method of administration if the drug is lipid soluble and passes the oral mucosa with relative ease. First-pass metabolism is avoided. Glyceryl trinitrate and buprenorphine are available as sublingual tablets and morphine as a buccal preparation. Fentanyl lollipops for premedication in children have been described but interest in this novel approach has waned, in part as a result of ethical considerations.

Intramuscular

This is still a popular route of administration in anaesthesia. It may avoid the problems associated with large initial plasma concentrations after rapid intravenous administration, is devoid of first-pass effects and can be administered relatively easily. However, absorption may be unpredictable, some preparations are particularly painful and irritant, e.g. diclofenac, and complications include damage to nervous and vascular tissue and inadvertent intravenous injection. An important disadvantage is the often intense patient dislike of injections, particularly in children.

Administration of postoperative analgesia by this route is still used frequently and the variation in absorption can be great. For example, peak plasma concentrations of morphine may occur at any time from 5 to 60 min after intramuscular administration, an important factor in the failure of this method to produce good reliable analgesia.

Subcutaneous

Absorption is very susceptible to changes in skin perfusion and tissue irritation may be a significant problem. It may be expected that this route of administration has little place in anaesthetic practice. However, it is used in several centres for providing postoperative pain relief, particularly in children, and has the advantage that difficult intravenous access is not required. A small cannula is placed subcutaneously during anaesthesia which can be replaced, if necessary, with relative ease. Even patient controlled analgesia (PCA) (see below) has been used effectively by this route. Prophylactic heparin is, of course, administered subcutaneously.

Intravenous

Bolus

The majority of drugs used in anaesthetic practice are given intravenously as boluses and the pharmacokinetics of this have been described in some detail above. The major disadvantage of this method is that overdosage can occur readily, particularly with drugs with narrow therapeutic indexes and large interpatient pharmacodynamic and pharmacokinetic variations (i.e. most drugs used in anaesthetic practice). After administration, the dose cannot be retrieved. It is an important general rule, therefore, that all drugs administered intravenously should be given slowly. Manufacturers' recommendations in this regard are often surprising; for example, a 10 mg dose of metoclopramide should be given over 1–2 min.

Only two factors have a major influence on the maximum plasma concentration achieved during a bolus intravenous injection: speed of injection and cardiac output. An elderly, sick or hypovolaemic patient undergoing intravenous induction of anaesthesia is likely, therefore, to suffer significant side-effects if the drug is given at the same speed as to a normal, healthy patient.

Infusion

Drugs may be given by constant-rate infusion, a method used frequently for neuromuscular blocking agents, opioids and many drugs administered to patients in intensive care units. Plasma concentrations achieved during infusions can be described by a simple wash-in exponential curve (Fig. 7.6). The only factor influencing time to reach steady-state concentration is $t_{1/2}$, i.e. maximum concentration is achieved after approximately 4–5 half-lives. Therefore, this method of administration is best suited to drugs with short

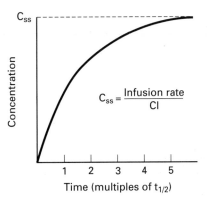

Fig. 7.6 Plasma concentrations during a constant-rate intravenous infusion against time expressed as multiples of $t_{1/2}$. C_{ss} = concentration at steady state, Cl = clearance.

half-lives such as glyceryl trinitrate, adrenaline, dopamine and alfentanil. However, in practice, it is often used for drugs such as morphine. Assuming a morphine $t_{1/2}$ of 4 h, it will be 24 h before steady-state concentration is reached. Therefore, vigilant observation is required with this method of delivery, especially if active metabolites are involved; in this example, morphine-6-glucuronide.

There is a simple equation describing the concentration achieved at steady state during a constant-rate infusion; this is based on the principle that, at steady state, the amount of drug cleared from the plasma is equal to that delivered.

$$\text{Rate of infusion} = \text{Cl} \times C_{ss} \qquad (7)$$

where C_{ss} = concentration at steady state.
Many pathological conditions reduce drug clearance and may therefore result in unexpectedly large plasma concentrations during infusions. Half-life does not influence C_{ss}, only how quickly it is achieved.

Patient controlled analgesia

The use of PCA for the treatment of postoperative pain has become widespread. The patient titrates opioid delivery to requirements by pressing a button on a PCA device which results in the delivery of a small bolus dose. A lock-out time is set also which will not allow another bolus to be delivered until the previous dose has had time to have an effect. There is an enormous interpatient variability in the pharmacodynamics and pharmacokinetics of opioids; PCA is able to allow for this and produce superior analgesia (see Ch. 24).

Rectal

This technique avoids the problems of first-pass metabolism and the need for injections. It is used in children (paracetamol, diclofenac) and adults (diclofenac) for postoperative analgesia. The rectal preparation of diclofenac is particularly useful as the intramuscular route is painful. Morphine can be given rectally also.

Transdermal

Drugs with a high lipid solubility and potency may be given by this route. The pharmacological properties of glyceryl trinitrate render it ideal for this technique. Transdermal hyoscine is used for travel sickness and increasingly for postoperative nausea and vomiting. Fentanyl transdermal delivery systems are effective in the treatment of pain, particularly in patients with terminal cancer.

It may take some time before a steady-state plasma concentration is achieved and many devices incorporate large amounts of drug in the adhesive layer in order to provide a loading dose which reduces this period. At steady state, transdermal delivery has several similarities to intravenous infusions. However, on removing the adhesive patch, plasma concentrations may decline relatively slowly because of a depot of drug in the surrounding skin; this occurs with transdermal fentanyl systems.

Inhalation

The delivery of inhaled volatile anaesthetics is discussed below but other drugs may be given by this route, especially bronchodilators and steroids. Atropine and adrenaline are absorbed if injected into the bronchial tree and this offers a route of administration in emergencies if no other method of delivery is possible. Opioids such as fentanyl and diamorphine have been given as nebulized solutions but this technique is not routine.

Extradural

This is a common route of administration in anaesthetic practice. The extradural space is very vascular and significant amounts of drug may be absorbed systemically, even if any vessels are avoided by the needle or cannula. Opioids diffuse across the dura to act on spinal opioid receptors but much of their action when given extradurally results from systemic absorption. Complications include subdural haematoma and infection and inadvertent dural puncture with consequent headache or spinal administration of the drug.

Spinal

When given spinally, drugs have free access to the neural tissue of the spinal cord and small doses have profound rapid effects; an advantage and also disadvantage of the method. Protein binding is not a significant factor as CSF protein concentration is relatively low.

DRUG INTERACTIONS

There are three basic types of drug interactions; examples are listed in Table 7.3.

Pharmaceutical

In this type of interaction, drugs, often mixed in the same syringe or infusion bag, react chemically with adverse results. For example, mixing suxamethonium with thiopentone (pH 10–11) hydrolyses the former, rendering it inactive. Before mixing drugs data should be sought on their compatibility. Another anaesthetic example of pharmaceutical interaction is the reaction of trichlorethylene with soda lime producing the toxic compound dichloracetylene.

Pharmacokinetic

Absorption of a drug, particularly if given orally, can be affected by other drugs. We have discussed already pharmacological factors affecting gastric emptying (Table 7.2). Interference with protein binding (see above) is a common cause of drug interaction. We have discussed drug metabolism

Table 7.3 Examples of drug interaction in anaesthesia

Type	Drugs	Effect
Pharmaceutical	Thiopentone/suxamethonium	Inactivation of suxamethonium
	Ampicillin/glucose or lactate solutions	Reduced potency
	Blood/dextrans	Rouleaux formation Crossmatching difficulties
	Trichlorethylene/soda lime	Toxic dichloroacetylene
Pharmacokinetic	Opioids/many drugs	Reduced oral absorption
	Cimetidine/lignocaine	Reduced clearance
	Barbiturates/warfarin	Reduced anticoagulation
	Neostigmine/ester local anaesthetics	Prolonged action of local anaesthetic
Pharmacodynamic	Benzodiazepines opioids/volatiles	Reduced MAC
	Volatiles/muscle relaxants	Enhanced relaxation
	Naloxone/morphine	Reversal (receptor antagonism)
	Neostigmine/muscle relaxants	Reversal
	Volatile/N_2O	Reduced MAC

in some detail and there are many potential sites in this process where interaction can occur, e.g. competition for enzyme systems, enzyme inhibition or induction. Finally drugs can affect the elimination of each other; in this case inhibition is the likely result.

Pharmacodynamic

This is the most frequent type of interaction seen in anaesthetic practice. It may be adverse, e.g. increased respiratory depression with opioids and volatile agents, or advantageous, e.g. reversal of muscle relaxation with neostigmine. The understanding of the many subtle pharmacodynamic interactions in modern anaesthesia accounts for the difference in the quality of anaesthesia and recovery associated with the experienced compared with the novice anaesthetist.

VOLATILE ANAESTHETIC AGENTS

Mechanism of action

The mechanism of action of volatile anaesthetic agents is at present unknown and is one of the greatest mysteries in modern pharmacology. A full discussion of the many and varied theories is outside the scope of this text. Potency is, in gen-

eral, related to lipid solubility (Meyer–Overton relationship, Table 7.4) and this has given rise to the concept of volatile agents dissolving in the lipid cell membrane in a non-specific manner disrupting membrane function and thereby influencing the structure and function of proteins, e.g. ion channels, within the lipid membrane. However, there is some evidence that volatile agents may produce their effect by combining specifically and directly with membrane proteins.

Potency

Potency is defined classically in terms of minimum alveolar concentration (MAC). A MAC is the

Table 7.4 MAC in oxygen and lipid solubility (expressed as oil/gas solubility coefficient)

Agent	MAC (%)	Oil/gas solubility coefficient
N_2O	105	1.4
Desflurane	7	18.7
Ether	1.9	65
Enflurane	1.68	98
Isoflurane	1.15	97
Halothane	0.78	220
Trichlorethylene	0.17	960

alveolar concentration of a volatile agent that produces no movement in 50% of spontaneously breathing patients after skin incision. MAC is inversely related to lipid solubility (Table 7.4).

Onset of action

When considering onset of action of volatile agents, there is a fundamental difference compared with intravenous agents. Effects of non-volatile drugs are related to plasma or tissue concentrations; this is not so with volatile agents. Of importance in this case is the partial pressure of the agent, not the concentration. Therefore, if a volatile agent is highly soluble in blood, the partial pressure increases slowly as large amounts will dissolve in the blood. Consequently, onset of anaesthesia is slow with agents soluble in blood and rapid with agents which are relatively insoluble. The same applies to recovery from anaesthesia. Table 7.5 lists the most commonly used volatile agents (in order of speed of onset) and their relative blood/gas solubilities. Ether and trichlorethylene are not available now in the UK for anaesthesia but are included as they illustrate the point and are still used in some countries.

Alveolar partial pressure (P_A) is assumed to be equivalent to cerebral artery partial pressure and therefore depth of anaesthesia. At a fixed inspired partial pressure (P_I), the rate at which P_A approaches P_I is related to speed of onset of effect (Fig. 7.7). This is rapid with agents of low blood solubility, e.g. N_2O, and relatively slow with more soluble agents, e.g. halothane.

Clearly, solubility of the agent in blood is a major determinant of the speed of onset of

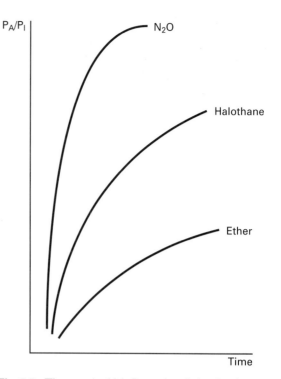

Fig. 7.7   The rate at which P_A reaches P_I is related to speed of induction of anaesthesia. Agents insoluble in blood equilibrate more rapidly.

anaesthesia but other factors can have significant effects. The rate of delivery of the agent to the alveolus is important; therefore increasing P_I by adjusting the vaporizer (a factor limited by irritant effects on the airway in spontaneously breathing patients), reducing apparatus dead space and increasing alveolar ventilation increase speed of induction of anaesthesia. If cardiac output is reduced, relatively less agent is removed from the alveolus and P_A increases towards P_I more rapidly. Consequently, induction of anaesthesia is more rapid in patients with reduced cardiac output and vice-versa. Both rate of delivery and cardiac output have particularly significant effects with agents that are relatively blood soluble; less so with insoluble agents, e.g. N_2O.

Ventilation perfusion mismatch can reduce speed of induction, an effect more significant in agents of low solubility. For example, if one lung is collapsed, i.e. perfused but not ventilated, increasing ventilation or inspired concentration of agents such as halothane will help to compensate. However, this is not the case for N_2O.

Table 7.5   Solubility of volatile agents in blood (expressed as blood/gas solubility coefficients).

Agent	Blood/gas solubility coefficient
Desflurane	0.42
N_2O	0.47
Isoflurane	1.4
Enflurane	1.9
Halothane	2.3
Trichlorethylene	9.0
Ether	12.0

FURTHER READING

Calvey T N, Williams N E 1991 Principles and practice of pharmacology for anaesthetists, 2nd edn. Blackwell Scientific Publications, Oxford

Wood M, Wood A J J 1990 Drugs and anaesthesia, 2nd edn. Williams & Wilkins, Baltimore

Mueller R A, Lundberg D B A 1992 Manual of drug interactions for anesthesiology, 2nd edn. Churchill Livingstone, New York

8. Inhalational anaesthetic agents

Volatile and gaseous anaesthetic agents remain popular for maintenance of anaesthesia and, under some circumstances, for induction of anaesthesia. In many situations, it is appropriate to use a mixture of 66% N_2O in oxygen and a small concentration of a volatile agent to maintain anaesthesia, although for reasons discussed below there are occasions when an anaesthetist might wish actively to avoid the use of nitrous oxide.

PROPERTIES OF THE IDEAL INHALATIONAL ANAESTHETIC AGENT

1. It should have a pleasant odour, be non-irritant to the respiratory tract and allow pleasant and rapid induction of anaesthesia.

2. It should possess a low blood/gas solubility, which permits rapid induction of and rapid recovery from anaesthesia.

3. It should be chemically stable in storage and should not interact with the material of anaesthetic circuits or with soda lime.

4. It should be neither flammable nor explosive.

5. It should be capable of producing unconsciousness with analgesia and preferably some degree of muscle relaxation.

6. It should be sufficiently potent to allow the use of high inspired oxygen concentrations when necessary.

7. It should not be metabolized in the body, should be non-toxic and should not provoke allergic reactions.

8. It should produce minimal depression of the cardiovascular and respiratory systems and should not interact with other drugs used commonly during anaesthesia, e.g. pressor agents or catecholamines.

9. It should be completely inert and eliminated completely and rapidly in an unchanged form via the lungs.

None of the inhalational anaesthetic agents approaches the standards required of the ideal agent.

Minimum alveolar anaesthetic concentration

MAC is the minimum alveolar concentration of an anaesthetic at 1 atmosphere absolute that prevents movement of 50% of the population to a standard stimulus. Anaesthesia is related to the partial pressure of an inhalational agent in brain rather than its percentage concentration in alveoli, but the term MAC has gained widespread acceptance as an index of anaesthetic potency as it is measured. It can be applied to all inhalational anaesthetics and it permits comparison of different agents. However, it represents only one point on a dose–response curve; 1 MAC of one agent is equivalent in anaesthetic potency to 1 MAC of another, but it does not follow that the agents are equipotent at 2 MAC. Nevertheless, in general terms, 0.5 MAC of one agent in combination with 0.5 MAC of another approximates to 1 MAC in total.

The MAC values for the anaesthetic agents quoted in Appendix II on page 733 were determined experimentally in humans (volunteers) breathing a mixture of the agent in oxygen. MAC values vary under the following circumstances:

1. MAC is reduced in the presence of premedication agents.

2. MAC is reduced in the presence of nitrous oxide.

3. MAC may change in some disease states, e.g. an increase in thyrotoxicosis and a decrease in myxoedema.

4. MAC is increased in the presence of pyrexia.

5. Sympathoadrenal stimulation induced, for example, by hypercapnia is associated with an increase in MAC. Thus, estimation of MAC in an individual requires stabilization of factors such as the end-tidal CO_2 concentration.

6. MAC decreases with advancing age. MAC is higher in infants and neonates than in adults and declines with advancing years. For halothane, MAC is almost 1.1% in the neonate, 0.95% in the infant, 0.9% at 1–2 years, 0.75% at 40 years and 0.65% at 80 years.

7. Drugs which affect release of CNS neurotransmitters affect MAC. MAC values are increased in the presence of ephedrine, amphetamine or iproniazid and decreased by reserpine, methyldopa, pancuronium and clonidine.

8. MAC changes with atmospheric pressure, as anaesthetic potency is related to partial pressure. For example, MAC for enflurane is 1.68% (1.66 kPa) at a pressure of 1 atmosphere absolute (ata), but 0.84% (still 1.66 kPa) at 2 ata.

Individual anaesthetic agents

Physical and pharmacological properties of the inhalational anaesthetic agents are summarized in Appendix II (p. 733). The structural formulae of the agents discussed in this chapter are shown in Fig. 8.1.

AGENTS IN OCCASIONAL USE

Diethyl ether

Because of its flammability, the use of ether has been abandoned in Western countries, but it remains an agent of widespread use in underdeveloped countries. It therefore warrants a brief description in this text.

It is a colourless, highly volatile liquid with a characteristic smell. In air it forms a mixture which burns with a blue flame; in oxygen-enriched mixtures, it forms an explosive combination. In air, the flammability range of ether is 1.9–48% but in oxygen the range is 2.0–82%.

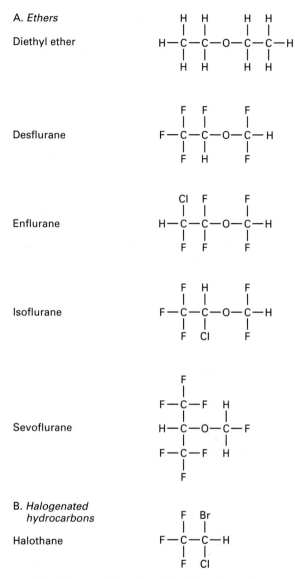

Fig. 8.1　Structural formulae of inhalational anaesthetic agents.

Ether is decomposed by air, light and heat, the most important products being acetaldehyde and ether peroxide. It should be stored in a cool environment in opaque containers.

Uptake and distribution

Ether has a relatively high blood/gas solubility coefficient of 12 and thus the rate of equilibration of alveolar with inspired concentrations is slow.

In addition, ether is irritant to the respiratory tract and so the inspired concentration must be increased slowly. The net effect is that induction of anaesthesia is prolonged; recovery is also slow.

Central nervous system

In common with all general anaesthetic agents, there is depression of the cortex, resulting in loss of higher inhibitions initially, followed by depression. Because induction of anaesthesia with ether is so slow, the classical stages of anaesthesia are seen; these are described in detail on page 324 and in Figure 19.2.

Depression of the respiratory centre precedes that of the vasomotor centre. Ether anaesthesia is associated with stimulation of the sympatho-adrenal system and increased levels of circulating catecholamines which offset the direct myocardial depressant effect of the drug.

Respiratory system

Ether is irritant to the respiratory tract and provokes coughing, breath-holding and profuse secretions from all mucus-secreting glands, including the salivary glands and those of the bronchial and respiratory tracts. Premedication with atropine or hyoscine is therefore essential.

Ether stimulates ventilation and minute volume is maintained with increasing depth of anaesthesia until surgical anaesthesia is achieved; thereafter, there is a gradual diminution in alveolar ventilation as plane 4 of stage 3 is approached (Fig. 19.2). Arterial carbon dioxide tensions of approximately 4 kPa occur commonly during ether anaesthesia; Pa_{CO_2} does not increase above normal until alveolar ether concentrations of 6% are reached.

Laryngeal spasm is not uncommon during induction with ether, but during established anaesthesia there is dilatation of the bronchi and bronchioles; at one time, the drug was recommended for treatment of bronchospasm.

Cardiovascular system

In vitro, ether is a direct myocardial depressant, but during light planes of clinical anaesthesia there is usually little change in cardiac ouput, arterial pressure or peripheral resistance. However, in patients who are receiving β-blocking or ganglion blocking drugs, or in combination with sub-arachnoid or extradural anaesthesia, the indirect sympathoadrenal stimulant effects of ether are obviated and myocardial depression may become clinically evident. In deep planes of anaesthesia, cardiac output decreases as a result of myocardial depression.

Cardiac arrhythmias occur rarely with ether and there is no sensitization of the myocardium to circulating catecholamines.

Alimentary system

Salivary and gastric secretions are increased during light anaesthesia but decreased during deep anaesthesia. Smooth muscle of the intestine is depressed in proportion to the blood concentration of ether. Ether causes a very high incidence of postoperative nausea and vomiting by two mechanisms:

1. Solution in saliva which is swallowed and causes irritation to the stomach.
2. Stimulation of the vomiting centre.

Skeletal muscle

Ether relaxes skeletal muscle by two mechanisms:

1. Depression of spinal reflexes.
2. Blockade of the motor end-plates by a postjunctional mechanism similar, but not identical, to that of d-tubocurarine. Thus, ether potentiates the effects of non-depolarizing muscle relaxants.

Uterus and placenta

The pregnant uterus is not affected during light anaesthesia but relaxation occurs during deep anaesthesia. Placental transmission causes depression of the fetus.

Matabolism

At least 15% of ether is metabolized to carbon dioxide and water; approximately 4% is metabolized in the liver to acetaldehyde and ethanol.

Ether stimulates gluconeogenesis and therefore causes hyperglycaemia.

Clinical use of ether

Ether has a much higher therapeutic ratio than halothane, enflurane or isoflurane and is therefore safer for administration in the hands of unskilled individuals or from an uncalibrated vaporizer. Because of its high blood/gas solubility coefficient and irritant properties to the respiratory tract, induction of anaesthesia is very slow.

Administration of ether is undertaken usually using an anaesthetic breathing system with a non-calibrated vaporizer (Boyle's bottle) or calibrated vaporizer (the EMO, which may be used as a drawover or as a plenum vaporizer). It may be used safely in a closed circuit with soda lime absorption. Occasionally, ether is administered using a Schimmelbusch mask.

Vapour strengths of up to 20% are required for induction; light anaesthesia can be maintained with 3–5% and deep anaesthesia with 5–6% inspired concentrations.

The latent heat of vaporization of ether is 374 J.g^{-1} (cf. halothane, 147 J.g^{-1}) and it is necessary to avoid significant cooling, which diminishes the rate of vaporization. Thus, ether vaporizers are designed to reduce cooling (e.g. the use of a large water jacket as in the EMO apparatus).

Ether should not be used in patients with diabetes mellitus or severe liver disease. Its use is inadvisable in patients with fever, particularly in children, as such patients may develop convulsions.

AGENTS IN COMMON CLINICAL USE

In Western countries, it is customary to use one of the three modern volatile anaesthetic agents, halothane, enflurane or isoflurane, vaporized in a mixture of nitrous oxide in oxygen. In recent years, the use of halothane has declined, particularly in North America, because of medicolegal pressure relating to the very rare occurrence of hepatotoxicity. Whilst this concern is less acute in Europe there is a clear trend to avoidance of repeated halothane anaesthesia. Apart from this problem, the selection of one of these three agents is based frequently upon relatively small differences in physical and pharmacological properties.

The following account of these agents, with a comparison of their pharmacological properties,

may tend to exaggerate the differences between them. However, an equally satisfactory anaesthetic may be administered in the majority of patients with any of the three agents.

Halothane

Halothane (2-bromo-2-chloro-1,1,1-trifluoroethane) was synthesized in 1951 and introduced into clinical practice in the UK in 1956. It is a colourless liquid with a relatively pleasant smell. It is decomposed by light. The addition of 0.01% thymol and storage in amber-coloured bottles renders it stable. Although it is decomposed by soda lime, it may be used safely with this mixture. It corrodes metals in vaporizers and breathing systems. In the presence of moisture it corrodes aluminium, tin, lead, magnesium and alloys. It should be stored in a closed container away from light and heat.

Uptake and distribution

Halothane has a relatively low blood/gas solubility coefficient of 2.5 and thus induction of anaesthesia is relatively rapid. However, it may take at least 30 min for the alveolar inspired concentration to reach 50% of the inspired concentration (Fig. 8.2); this is slower than for enflurane or

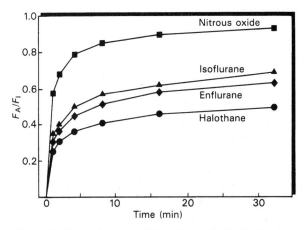

Fig. 8.2 Ratio of alveolar (F_A) to inspired (F_I) fractional concentrations of nitrous oxide, isoflurane, enflurane and halothane in the first 10 min of anaesthesia. The plot of F_A/F_I expresses the rapidity with which alveolar concentration equilibrates with inspired concentration. It is most rapid for agents with a low blood/gas partition coefficient.

isoflurane. As with all the volatile agents, it is customary to use the technique of 'over-pressure' and induce halothane anaesthesia with concentrations 2–3 times higher than the MAC value (0.75%); the inspired concentration is reduced when a stable level of anaesthesia has been achieved.

Metabolism

Approximately 20% of halothane is metabolized in the liver, usually by oxidative pathways. The end products are excreted in the urine. The major metabolites are bromine, chlorine, trifluoroacetic acid and trifluoroacetylethanol amide.

A small proportion of halothane may undergo reductive metabolism, particularly in the presence of hypoxaemia and when the hepatic microsomal enzymes have been stimulated by enzyme-inducing agents such as phenobarbitone. Reductive metabolism may result in the formation of reactive metabolites and fluoride, although normally serum fluoride ion concentrations are considerably lower than those likely to induce renal dysfunction.

Respiratory system

Halothane is non-irritant and pleasant to breathe during induction of anaesthesia. There is rapid loss of pharyngeal and laryngeal reflexes and inhibition of salivary and bronchial secretions. In the unpremedicated subject, halothane anaesthesia is associated with an increase in ventilatory rate and reduction in tidal volume. Pa_{CO_2} increases as the depth of halothane anaesthesia increases.

Halothane causes a dose-dependent decrease in mucociliary function which may persist for several hours after anaesthesia. This may contribute to postoperative sputum retention.

Halothane antagonizes bronchospasm and reduces airway resistance in patients with bronchoconstriction, possibly by central inhibition of reflex bronchoconstriction and relaxation of bronchial smooth muscle. It has been suggested that halothane exerts a β-mimetic effect on bronchial muscle.

Cardiovascular system

Halothane is a potent depressant of myocardial contractility and myocardial metabolic activity as a result of inhibition of glucose uptake by myocardial cells. During controlled ventilation, halothane anaesthesia is associated with dose-related depression of cardiac output (by decrease in myocardial contractility) with little effect on peripheral resistance. Thus, there is a reduction in arterial pressure and an increase in right atrial pressure. In spontaneously breathing patients, some of these effects may be offset by a small increase in Pa_{CO_2} which leads to a reduction in systemic vascular resistance and a shift in cardiac output back towards baseline values as a result of indirect sympathoadrenal stimulation.

The hypotensive effect of halothane is augmented by a reduction in heart rate, which commonly accompanies halothane anaesthesia. Antagonism of the bradycardia by administration of atropine frequently leads to an increase in arterial pressure.

The reduction in myocardial contractility is associated with reductions in myocardial oxygen demand and coronary blood flow. Provided that undue elevations in left ventricular diastolic pressure and undue hypotension do not occur, halothane may be advantageous in patients with coronary artery disease because of the reduced oxygen demand caused by a low heart rate and decreased contractility.

The depressant effects of halothane on cardiac output are augmented in the presence of β-blockade.

Arrhythmias are very common during halothane anaesthesia and far more frequent than with either enflurane or isoflurane. Arrhythmias are produced by:

1. Increased myocardial excitability augmented by the presence of hypercapnia, hypoxaemia or increased circulating catecholamines.

2. Bradycardia caused by central vagal stimulation.

During local infiltration with adrenaline-containing local anaesthetic solutions, multifocal ventricular extrasystoles and sinus tachycardia have been observed and cardiac arrest has been reported. Thus, caution should be exercised when these solutions are used. The following recommendations have been made:

1. Avoid hypoxaemia and hypercapnia.

2. Avoid concentrations of adrenaline greater than 1 in 100 000.

3. Avoid a dosage in adults exceeding 10 ml of 1 in 100 000 adrenaline in 10 min or 30 ml.h^{-1}.

Gastrointestinal tract

Gastrointestinal motility is inhibited. Postoperative nausea and vomiting are seldom severe.

Uterus

Halothane relaxes uterine muscle and may cause postpartum haemorrhage. It is said that a concentration of less than 0.5% is not associated with increased blood loss during anaesthesia for Caesarean section, but this concentration causes increased blood loss during therapeutic abortion.

Skeletal muscle

Halothane causes skeletal muscle relaxation and potentiates non-depolarizing relaxants. Postoperatively, shivering is common; this increases oxygen requirements and results in hypoxaemia unless oxygen is administered.

Halothane-associated hepatic dysfunction

There are two types of dysfunction which may take place after halothane anaesthesia. The first is mild and is associated with derangement in liver function tests. These changes are transient and generally resolve within a few days. Similar changes in liver function tests have also been reported after enflurane anaesthesia and, to a lesser extent, isoflurane anaesthesia.

This subclinical type of hepatic function, evidenced by an increase in glutathione-transferase (GST) concentrations, probably occurs as a result of metabolism of halothane in the liver where it reacts with hepatic macromolecules resulting in tissue necrosis which is worsened by hypoxia.

The second type of hepatic dysfunction is extremely uncommon and takes the form of severe jaundice, progressing to fulminating hepatic necrosis. The mortality of this condition is quite high and varies between 30–70%. The likelihood of this type of hepatic dysfunction is increased by repeated exposure to the drug. The mechanism

of these changes is probably the formation of a hapten–protein complex. The hapten is probably one of the metabolites of halothane, notably trifluoroacetyl (TFA)-halide as antibodies to TFA proteins have now been detected in patients who develop jaundice after halothane anaesthesia.

The incidence of type 2 liver dysfunction after halothane anaesthesia is extremely low – so low that it is extremely difficult to mount well controlled studies of the condition and consequently, this whole subject has been an area of great controversy over the last 10–15 years. Nonetheless, as a result of this concern, the Committee on Safety of Medicines has made the following recommendations in respect of halothane anaesthesia:

1. A careful anaesthetic history should be taken to determine previous exposure and any previous reaction to halothane.
2. Repeated exposure to halothane within a period of 3 months should be avoided unless there are overriding clinical circumstances.
3. A history of unexplained jaundice or pyrexia after previous exposure to halothane is an absolute contraindication to its future use in that patient.

The incidence of halothane hepatotoxicity in paediatric practice is extremely low, although there have been case reports in children. Nevertheless, halothane remains the drug of choice for paediatric anaesthesia, in preference to enflurane or isoflurane.

In summary, halothane is a very useful inhalational anaesthetic agent. Its main advantages are:

1. Rapid, smooth induction.
2. Minimal stimulation of salivary and bronchial secretions; prior administration of atropine is unnecessary.
3. Bronchodilatation.
4. Muscle relaxation.
5. Relatively rapid recovery.

The disadvantages are:

1. Poor analgesia.
2. Arrhythmias.
3. Postoperative shivering.
4. Possibility of liver toxicity, especially with repeated administrations.

Enflurane

Enflurane (2-chloro-1,1,2-trifluoroethyl difluoromethyl ether) was synthesized in 1963 and first evaluated clinically in 1966. It was introduced into clinical practice in the USA in 1971.

Physical properties

Enflurane is a clear, colourless, volatile anaesthetic agent with a pleasant ethereal smell. It is non-flammable in clinical concentrations, stable with soda lime and metals and does not require preservatives.

Uptake and distribution

Enflurane has a low blood/gas solubility coefficient of 1.9, resulting in rapid equilibration between alveolar and inspired partial pressures. Thus, induction of anaesthesia and recovery from anaesthesia are rapid (Fig. 8.2).

Metabolism

Approximately 2.5% of the absorbed dose is metabolized, predominantly to fluoride. In common with other ether anaesthetic agents (diethyl ether and isoflurane), the presence of the ether bond imparts stability to the molecule.

Defluorination of enflurane is increased in patients treated with isoniazid, but not with a classic enzyme-inducing agent such as phenobarbitone. Serum fluoride ion concentrations are greater after administration of enflurane to obese patients. To date, extensive studies have failed to demonstrate that the serum concentrations of fluoride ion reach toxic levels after enflurane anaesthesia.

Respiratory system

Enflurane is non-irritant and does not increase salivary or bronchial secretions; thus inhalational induction is relatively pleasant and rapid.

In common with all other volatile anaesthetic agents, enflurane causes a dose-dependent depression of alveolar ventilation with a reduction in tidal volume and an increase in ventilatory rate in the unpremedicated subject.

Cardiovascular system

Enflurane causes dose-dependent depression of myocardial contractility, leading to a reduction in cardiac output. In association with a small reduction in systemic vascular resistance, this leads to a dose-dependent reduction in arterial pressure. Because enflurane (unlike halothane) has no central vagal effects, hypotension leads to reflex tachycardia.

Enflurane anaesthesia is associated with a much smaller incidence of arrhythmias than halothane and much less sensitization of the myocardium to catecholamines, either endogenous or exogenous.

Uterus

Enflurane relaxes uterine muscle in a dose-related manner.

Central nervous system

Enflurane produces a dose-dependent depression of EEG activity, but at moderate to high concentrations (more than 3%) it produces epileptiform paroxysmal spike activity and burst suppression. These are accentuated by hypocapnia. Twitching of the face and arm muscles may be seen occasionally. Enflurane should be avoided in the epileptic patient.

Muscle relaxation

Enflurane produces dose-dependent muscle relaxation with potentiation of non-depolarizing neuromuscular blocking drugs to a greater extent than that produced by halothane.

Hepatotoxicity

There have been several case reports of jaundice attributable to the use of enflurane and derangement of liver enzymes also occurs after enflurane anaesthesia, although to a lesser extent than that after halothane.

Cross-sensitization has been reported between halothane and enflurane and therefore multiple administrations of halothane and enflurane should be avoided within short periods.

In summary, enflurane is a useful alternative agent to halothane. Its main advantages are:

1. Rapid induction and recovery.
2. Little biotransformation and therefore little risk of hepatic dysfunction.
3. Muscle relaxation.
4. Low incidence of arrhythmias, even in the presence of high circulating catecholamine concentrations.

Its disadvantage is:

1. Seizure activity on EEG.

Isoflurane

Isoflurane (1-chloro-2,2,2-trifluoroethyl difluoromethyl ether) is an isomer of enflurane and was synthesized in 1965. Clinical studies were undertaken in 1970, but because of early laboratory reports of carcinogenesis (which were not confirmed subsequently) it was not approved by the Food and Drug Administration in the United States until 1980.

Physical properties

Isoflurane is a colourless, volatile liquid with a slightly pungent odour. It is stable and does not react with metal or other substances and does not require preservatives. It is non-flammable in clinical concentrations.

Uptake and distribution

Isoflurane is the least (with the exception of desflurane) soluble of the modern inhalational agents and thus alveolar concentrations equilibrate more rapidly with inspired concentrations. The alveolar (or arterial) partial pressure of isoflurane increases to 50% of the inspired partial pressure within 4–8 min and to 60% by 15 min (Fig. 8.2). However, the rate of induction is limited by the pungency of the vapour and clinically may be no faster than that which can be achieved with halothane. The incidence of coughing or breath-holding on induction is significantly greater with isoflurane than with halothane.

Metabolism

Approximately 0.17% of the absorbed dose is metabolized. Metabolism takes place predominantly in the form of oxidation to produce difluromethanol and trifluoroacetic acid; the former breaks down to formic acid and fluoride. Because of the minimal metabolism, only very small concentrations of serum fluoride ions are found, even after prolonged administration. The minimal metabolism renders hepatic and renal toxicity most unlikely.

Respiratory system

In common with halothane and enflurane, isoflurane causes dose-dependent depression of ventilation; there is a decrease in tidal volume but an increase in ventilatory rate in the absence of opioid drugs.

Cardiovascular system

In vitro, isoflurane is a myocardial depressant but in clinical use there is less depression of cardiac output than with halothane or enflurane. Systemic hypotension occurs predominantly as a result of reduction in systemic vascular resistance. Arrhythmias are uncommon and there is little sensitization of the myocardium to catecholamines.

In addition to dilating systemic arterioles, isoflurane causes coronary vasodilatation. There has been some controversy recently regarding the safety of isoflurane in patients with coronary artery disease because of the possibility that the coronary steal syndrome may be induced; dilatation in normal coronary arteries offers a low resistance to flow and may reduce perfusion through stenosed vessels. It has been shown that isoflurane affects small arterioles (which makes steal a theoretical possibility), but the effect seems to occur only in end-tidal concentrations in excess of 0.5%. Production of myocardial ischaemia in clinical practice may be produced by a large number of factors in addition to coronary vasodilatation, including tachycardia, hypotension, increase in left ventricular end-diastolic pressure and reduced ventricular compliance. Attention should be directed to these factors before a diagnosis of isoflurane-induced coronary steal is considered.

Uterus

Isoflurane has an effect on the pregnant uterus similar to that of halothane and enflurane.

Central nervous system

Low concentrations of isoflurane do not cause any change in cerebral blood flow at normocapnia. In this respect, the drug is superior to enflurane and halothane, both of which cause cerebral vasodilatation. However, higher inspired concentrations of isoflurane cause vasodilatation and increase cerebral blood flow. It does not cause seizure activity on the EEG.

Muscle relaxation

Isoflurane causes dose-dependent depression of neuromuscular transmission with potentiation of non-depolarizing neuromuscular blocking drugs.

The advantages of isoflurane are:

1. Rapid induction and recovery.
2. Minimal biotransformation with little risk of hepatic or renal toxicity.
3. Cardiovascular stability.
4. Muscle relaxation.

Its disadvantages are:

1. A pungent odour which makes inhalational induction relatively unpleasant, particularly in children, and which inhibits the rate of induction of anaesthesia.
2. Coronary vasodilatation with the possibility of coronary steal syndrome at high inspired concentrations.

Comparison of halothane, enflurane and isoflurane

Pharmacokinetics

The rate of equilibration of alveolar with inspired concentrations is related to blood/gas solubility. The rate of uptake of isoflurane is faster than that of enflurane and considerably faster than that of halothane, although much slower than that of nitrous oxide (Fig. 8.2). However, rate of induction of anaesthesia with isoflurane may be reduced

because of the pungent odour compared with the more pleasant odours of halothane and enflurane.

On recovery from anaesthesia, the rate of elimination of isoflurane is faster than that of halothane or enflurane. Although it is possible using sensitive tests of psychomotor performance to demonstrate that recovery from isoflurane anaesthesia is faster than from enflurane anaesthesia (which in turn is faster than from halothane anaesthesia), tests of 'street fitness' reveal that there are no significant differences in recovery among the three agents. Recovery from these three agents to a state at which it is possible to respond to questions is in the range of 10–15 min after discontinuing administration of the volatile agent after 1–2 h of anaesthesia. More prolonged anaesthetic time prolongs the rate of recovery because of greater saturation of tissues.

Respiratory system

In unstimulated volunteers, enflurane causes greater ventilatory depression than isoflurane, which in turn causes greater depression of ventilation than halothane (Fig. 8.3). Nitrous oxide does not cause hypercapnia. Thus a reduction in inspired volatile anaesthetic concentration permitted by addition of nitrous oxide is associated with less ventilatory depression. In addition, surgical stimulation is

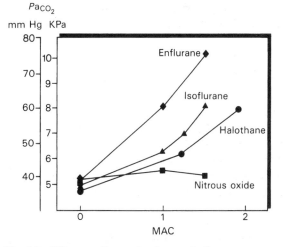

Fig. 8.3   Effects on Pa_{CO_2} of enflurane, isoflurane, halothane or nitrous oxide at equivalent MAC during spontaneous ventilation by healthy volunteers. (Nitrous oxide was administered in a hyperbaric chamber.)

responsible for considerable antagonism of ventilatory depression during anaesthesia and Pa_{CO_2} does not reach the values shown in Figure 8.3 during surgery.

With all three agents, depression of ventilation is associated with depression of whole body oxygen consumption and carbon dioxide production.

During surgery, an anaesthetic technique comprising spontaneous breathing of nitrous oxide/oxygen supplemented with halothane or isoflurane (inspired concentrations approximating to 1–1.5 MAC in total) results often in a Pa_{CO_2} value in the range 5.3–6.7 kPa (40–50 mmHg).

Cardiovascular system

In vitro studies have revealed that all three agents cause depression of contractility of isolated cardiac muscle. The effects of isoflurane and halothane are similar and greater than that of enflurane.

However, isoflurane causes relatively little depression of cardiac output in vivo whilst enflurane causes the most (Fig. 8.4); the reduction in cardiac output is produced predominantly by a decrease in stroke volume. At normocapnia, halothane has no effect on peripheral resistance, whilst isoflurane causes the greatest degree of peripheral vasodilatation (Fig. 8.5). Consequently, all three agents cause hypotension in the order enflurane > isoflurane > halothane (Fig. 8.6).

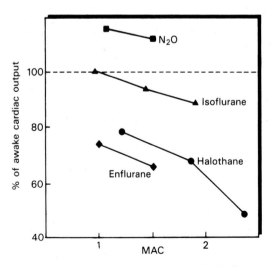

Fig. 8.4 Comparative effects of nitrous oxide, isoflurane, halothane and enflurane in healthy volunteers.

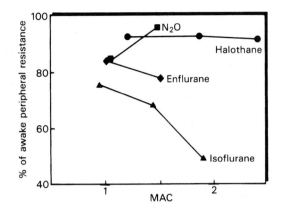

Fig. 8.5 Comparative effects of nitrous oxide, halothane, enflurane and isoflurane on peripheral vascular resistance in healthy volunteers.

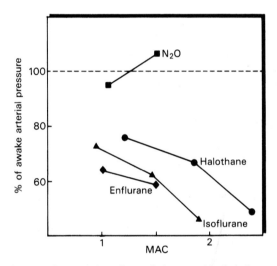

Fig. 8.6 Comparative effects of nitrous oxide, halothane, isoflurane and enflurane on arterial pressure in healthy volunteers.

With the former two agents, there is a tendency for reflex compensatory tachycardia, but this is not manifest with halothane because of its direct vagal stimulatory properties. Halothane and enflurane cause a greater increase in right atrial pressure than does isoflurane.

The data in Figures 8.4–8.6 were derived from studies in volunteers, who were not subjected to surgical stimulation and in whom artificial ventilation was used to achieve normocapnia.

Some of the cardiovascular effects of these volatile agents are antagonized by the addition of nitrous oxide. In addition, during spontaneous ventilation, the modest hypercapnia which occurs with all three agents also offsets some of the changes. With enflurane and isoflurane, for example, cardiac output may be increased compared with pre-anaesthesia levels, although there is little effect on systemic arterial pressure. The effects of enflurane and isoflurane on right atrial pressure are reduced considerably during spontaneous ventilation; indeed, there may be little change. In contrast, the right atrial pressure remains elevated in the presence of hypercapnia during halothane anaesthesia.

Arrhythmias

Arrhythmias are common during halothane, but not during enflurane or isoflurane anaesthesia.

After exogenous administration of adrenaline, stability of heart rhythm is greatest in patients anaesthetized with isoflurane, less with enflurane and least with halothane (Fig. 8.7).

Neuromuscular junction

All three agents cause relaxation sufficient to perform lower abdominal surgery in thin subjects. In addition, however, there is potentiation of non-depolarizing muscle relaxants. In this respect, isoflurane and enflurane are similar and cause markedly greater potentiation than that produced by halothane.

A comparison of other characteristics of the three agents is shown in Table 8.1, together,

for completeness, with those of the new drugs desflurane and sevoflurane.

The North American multicentre study of general anaesthetics

In a large multicentre study conducted in 15 hospitals in North America, a prospective randomized controlled comparison was made of anaesthesia with halothane, enflurane, isoflurane or fentanyl based anaesthetics.

The most significant finding was that there was no difference in major outcomes between all

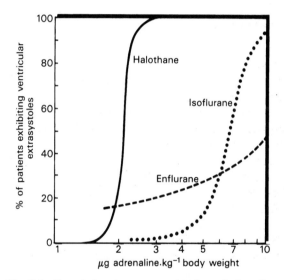

Fig. 8.7 Cumulative plots representing dose of adrenaline required to induce ventricular extrasystoles in normocapnic patients receiving 1.25 MAC of halothane, isoflurane or enflurane.

Table 8.1 Comparison of modern volatile anaesthetic agents

	Halothane	Enflurane	Isoflurane	Desflurane	Sevoflurane
Molecular weight	197.4	184.5	184.5	168	200.1
Boiling point (°C)	50	56	49	23.9	58.9
Blood/gas partition coefficient	2.5	1.9	1.4	0.42	0.6
Oil/gas partition coefficient	220	98	97	18.7	55
MAC (in O_2)	0.75	1.68	1.15	6–9	approx 2
Preservative	0.01% thymol	none	none	none	none
Percentage metabolized	20	2.4	0.17	0.02	3
Effect on EEG	depression	seizure activity	depression	depression	depression
Neuromuscular relaxation	moderate	strong	strong	strong	strong

four anaesthetics. A finding of potential clinical importance was that there was a significantly higher incidence of ventricular arrhythmias during halothane anaesthesia than with enflurane, isoflurane or fentanyl.

NEW VOLATILE ANAESTHETIC AGENTS

Sevoflurane

Sevoflurane is a methyl propyl ether which was isolated in the early 1970s and first used in 1981. The drug has been available for some time for general clinical use in Japan but only recently in the United Kingdom.

Physical properties

It is non-flammable and has a pleasant smell, a blood/gas partition coefficient of 0.6, an oil partition coefficient of 55 and a MAC value of approximately 2%. It is stable and is stored in amber-coloured bottles. In the presence of water, it undergoes some hydrolysis and this reaction also occurs with soda lime. It is therefore arguable that this agent should not be used in closed-circuit or low flow systems containing soda lime.

Uptake and distribution

It has a low blood/gas partition coefficient and therefore the rate of equilibration between alveolar and inspired concentrations is faster than that for halothane or enflurane. It is non-irritant to the upper respiratory tract and therefore the rate of induction of anaesthesia should be faster than that with either of the other agents.

Because of its higher partition coefficients in vessel-rich tissues, muscle and fat than corresponding values for desflurane, the rate of recovery is slower than that after desflurane anaesthesia.

Metabolism

Approximately 3% of the absorbed dose is metabolized by defluorination in the liver. The mean peak fluoride ion concentration after 60 min of anaesthesia at 1 MAC is 22 mmol.litre^{-1} which is significantly higher than that after an equivalent dose of isoflurane.

Because of its relatively limited clinical use to date, the safety record of sevoflurane anaesthesia has yet to be established.

Respiratory system

The drug is non-irritant to the upper respiratory tract and whilst it causes respiratory depression (in common with all volatile anaesthetic agents) there is a suggestion that it has the least effect on ventilation of all the volatile agents in current use.

Cardiovascular system

The properties of sevoflurane are similar to those of isoflurane with slightly smaller effects on heart rate and less coronary vasodilatation.

Central nervous system

Its effects are similar to those of halothane and isoflurane. There is no suggestion that it causes excitatory effects on the EEG.

Muscle relaxation

In common with isoflurane, the drug potentiates non-depolarizing muscle relaxants to a similar extent.

Desflurane

This drug was first used in humans in 1988 and it became available for general clinical use in the United Kingdom in 1993. The structure of the compound differs from that of isoflurane only in the substitution of fluorine for chlorine.

Physical properties

It is a colourless agent which is stored in amber-coloured bottles without preservative. It is not broken down by soda lime, light or metals. It is non-flammable.

Desflurane has a boiling point of 23.5°C and a vapour pressure of 664 mmHg at 20°C and it cannot be used in a standard vaporizer. Thus a special vaporizer (the TEC 6) has been developed which requires a source of electric power as it is heated and pressurized.

It has an ethereal but much less pungent odour than isoflurane but is still slightly irritant to the upper respiratory tract.

Uptake and distribution

Desflurane has a blood/gas partition coefficient of 0.42, almost the same as that of nitrous oxide. Induction of anaesthesia is therefore extremely rapid but limited somewhat by a slightly pungent nature. However, it is possible to alter the depth of anaesthesia very rapidly and the rate of recovery of anaesthesia is faster than that following any other volatile anaesthetic agent.

The rate of equilibration of alveolar with inspired concentrations of desflurane is virtually identical with that for nitrous oxide (Fig. 8.2).

Metabolism

There is very little defluorination of desflurane and after prolonged anaesthesia, there is only a very small increase in serum and urine trifluoracetic acid levels.

Respiratory system

Desflurane causes respiratory depression to a degree similar to that of isoflurane and enflurane. Because it is irritant to the upper respiratory tract it is not recommended for gaseous induction of anaesthesia.

Cardiovascular effects

The drug has effects on the cardiovascular system similar to those of isoflurane but preliminary experimental studies in animals have not detected a coronary steal phenomenon similar to that produced by isoflurane.

Central nervous system

The effects of desflurane are very similar to those of isoflurane. Further studies are required to compare its effects on cerebral blood flow and cerebral oxygen consumption to see if its effects differ from isoflurane which is currently the drug of choice for neurosurgical purposes.

ANAESTHETIC GASES

Nitrous oxide (N_2O)

Manufacture

Nitrous oxide is prepared commercially by heating ammonium nitrate to a temperature of 245–270°C. Various impurities are produced in this process, including ammonia, nitric acid, nitrogen, nitric oxide and nitrogen dioxide.

After cooling, ammonia and nitric acid are reconstituted to ammonium nitrate, which is returned to the beginning of the process. The remaining gases then pass through a series of scrubbers. The purified gases are compressed and dried in an aluminium dryer. The resultant gases are expanded in a liquefier, with the nitrogen escaping as gas. Nitrous oxide is then evaporated, compressed and passed through another aluminium dryer before being stored in cylinders.

The higher oxides of nitrogen dissolve in water to form nitrous and nitric acids. These substances are toxic and produce methaemoglobinaemia and pulmonary oedema if inhaled. In the past, there have been several reports of death occurring during anaesthesia as a result of the inhalation of nitrous oxide contaminated with higher oxides of nitrogen.

Storage

Nitrous oxide is stored in compressed form as a liquid in cylinders at a pressure of 50 bar (5000 kPa; 750 lb.in^{-2}). In the UK, the cylinders are painted blue.

Because the cylinder contains liquid and vapour, the total quantity of nitrous oxide contained in a cylinder can be ascertained only by weighing. Thus, the cylinder weights, full and empty, are stamped on the shoulder. Nitrous oxide cylinders should be kept in a vertical position during use so that the liquid phase remains at the bottom of the cylinder. During continuous use, the cylinder may cool as a result of the latent heat of vaporization of liquid anaesthetic and ice may form on the lower part of the cylinder.

Physical properties

Nitrous oxide is a sweet-smelling, non-irritant colourless gas, with a molecular weight of 44, boiling point –88°C, critical temperature 36.5°C and critical pressure 72.6 bar.

Nitrous oxide is not flammable but it supports combustion of fuels in the absence of oxygen.

Pharmacology

Nitrous oxide is frequently said to be a good analgesic but a weak anaesthetic. The latter refers to the fact that its MAC value is 105%. This value was calculated theoretically from its low oil/water solubility coefficient of 3.2 and has been confirmed experimentally in volunteers anaesthetized in a pressure chamber compressed to 2 atmospheres absolute (ata), where the MAC value was found to be 52.5% N_2O.

As it is essential to administer a minimum $F_{I_{O_2}}$ of 0.3, nitrous oxide alone is insufficient to produce an adequate depth of anaesthesia in all but the most seriously ill patient; therefore, nitrous oxide is used usually in combination with other agents. When using nitrous oxide in a relaxant technique, the inspired gas mixture should be supplemented with a low concentration of a volatile agent to minimize the possibility of awareness which may occur if nitrous oxide anaesthesia is supplemented only by the administration of opioids.

Of the anaesthetic agents in current clinical use, nitrous oxide has the lowest blood/gas solubility coefficient (0.47 at 37°C) and therefore the rate of equilibration of alveolar with inspired concentrations is very fast (Fig. 8.2).

Because of the low solubility, a change in alveolar ventilation has less effect on the rate of uptake than occurs with the more soluble agents such as halothane and ether (Fig. 8.8). Similarly, changes in cardiac output have less effect with nitrous oxide (Fig. 8.9). Nitrous oxide does not undergo metabolism in the body and is excreted unchanged.

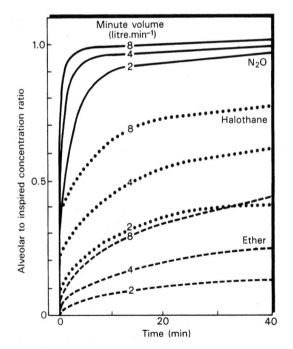

Fig. 8.8 Influence of minute volume on the rate of equilibration between alveolar and inspired concentrations of nitrous oxide, halothane and ether. The effects of ventilation are more marked on the agents with higher blood/gas solubility coefficients.

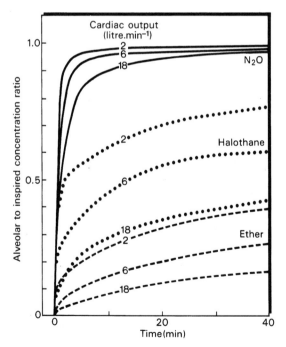

Fig. 8.9 Influence of cardiac output on the rate of equilibration between alveolar and inspired concentrations of nitrous oxide, halothane and ether. The effects of cardiac output are more marked on the agents with higher blood/gas solubility coefficients.

The concentration effect

The inspired concentration of nitrous oxide affects its rate of equilibration; the higher the inspired concentration the faster is the rate of equilibration between alveolar and inspired concentrations. Nitrous oxide is more soluble in blood than nitrogen. Thus, the volume of nitrous oxide entering pulmonary capillary blood from the alveolus is greater than the volume of nitrogen moving in the opposite direction. As a result, the total volume of gas in the alveolus diminishes and the fractional concentrations of the remaining gases increase. This has two consequences:

1. The higher the inspired concentration of nitrous oxide, the greater is the concentrating effect on the nitrous oxide remaining in the alveolus.

2. At high inspired concentrations of nitrous oxide, the reduction in alveolar gas volume causes an increase in Pa_{CO_2}. Equilibration with pulmonary capillary blood results in an increase in Pa_{CO_2}.

The result of the concentration effect on equilibration of nitrous oxide is illustrated in Figure 8.10.

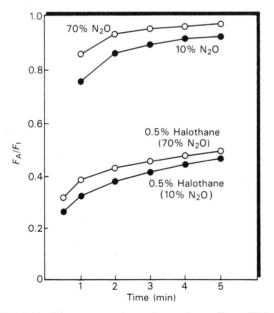

Fig. 8.10 The concentration and second gas effects. High concentrations of nitrous oxide increase the rate of increase of F_A/F_I ratio for nitrous oxide (the concentration effect) and for a volatile agent administered with nitrous oxide (the second gas effect). See text for details.

The second gas effect

When nitrous oxide is administered in a high concentration with a second anaesthetic agent, e.g. halothane, the reduction in gas volume in the alveoli caused by absorption of nitrous oxide increases the alveolar concentration of halothane, thereby augmenting the rate of equilibration with inspired gas. This is illustrated in the lower part of Figure 8.10. The second gas effect results also in small increases in Pa_{O_2} and Pa_{CO_2}.

Side effects of nitrous oxide

1. *Diffusion hypoxia.* At the end of an anaesthetic, when the inspired gas mixture is changed from nitrous oxide/oxygen to nitrogen/oxygen, hypoxaemia may occur as the volume of nitrous oxide diffusing from mixed venous blood into the alveolus is greater than the volume of nitrogen taken up from the alveolus into pulmonary capillary blood (the opposite of the concentration effect). Thus, the concentration of gases in the alveolus is diluted by nitrous oxide, leading to a reduction in Pa_{O_2} and Pa_{CO_2}. In the healthy individual, diffusion hypoxia is relatively transient, but may last for up to 10 min at the end of anaesthesia; the extent of reduction in Pa_{O_2} may be of the order of 0.5–1.5 kPa. Administration of oxygen during this period is advisable.

2. *Effect on closed gas spaces.* When blood containing nitrous oxide equilibrates with closed air-containing spaces inside the body, the volume of nitrous oxide that diffuses into the cavity exceeds the volume of nitrogen diffusing out. Thus, in compliant spaces such as the bowel lumen or the pleural or peritoneal cavities, there is an increase in volume of the space. If the space cannot expand (e.g. sinuses, middle ear) there is an increase in pressure. In the middle ear, this may cause problems with surgery on the tympanic membrane. When nitrous oxide is administered in a concentration of 75%, the volume of a cavity may increase to as much as 3–4 times the original volume within 30 min. If an air embolus occurs in a patient who is breathing nitrous oxide, equilibration with the gas bubble leads to expansion of the embolus within seconds; the volume of the embolus may double within a very short period of time.

3. *Cardiovascular depression*. Nitrous oxide is a direct myocardial depressant but in the normal individual this effect is antagonized by indirectly mediated sympathoadrenal stimulation (effects similar to those produced by carbon dioxide). Thus, healthy patients exhibit little change in the cardiovascular system during nitrous oxide anaesthesia. However, in patients with pre-existing high levels of sympathoadrenal activity and poor myocardial contractility, the administration of nitrous oxide may cause a reduction in cardiac output and arterial pressure. For this reason (in addition to avoidance of the risk of doubling the size of air emboli) nitrous oxide is avoided in some centres during anaesthesia for cardiac surgery.

4. *Toxicity*. Nitrous oxide affects vitamin B_{12} synthesis by inhibiting the enzyme methionine synthetase. This effect is of importance if the duration of nitrous oxide anaesthesia exceeds 8 h. Nitrous oxide interferes also with folic acid metabolism and impairs synthesis of DNA; prolonged exposure may cause agranulocytosis and bone marrow aplasia. Exposure of patients to nitrous oxide for 6 h or longer may result in megaloblastic anaemia. Occupational exposure to nitrous oxide may result in myeloneuropathy. This condition is similar to subacute combined degeneration of the spinal cord and has been reported in some dentists and also in individuals addicted to inhalation of nitrous oxide.

5. *Teratogenic changes*. Teratogenic changes have been observed in pregnant rats exposed to nitrous oxide for prolonged periods. There is no evidence that similar effects occur in man, but it has been suggested that nitrous oxide should be avoided in early pregnancy; however, this is not a generally held view at the present time.

OTHER GASES USED DURING ANAESTHESIA

Oxygen

Manufacture

Oxygen is manufactured commercially by fractional distillation of liquid air. Before liquefaction of air, carbon dioxide is removed and liquid oxygen and nitrogen separated by means of their different boiling points (oxygen $-183°C$, nitrogen $-195°C$).

Oxygen is supplied in cylinders at a pressure of 137 bar (approximately 2000 lb.in^{-2}) at 15°C. The cylinders are painted black with a white shoulder.

Many institutions use piped oxygen and this is supplied either by a bank of oxygen cylinders, ensuring a continuous supply, or as liquid oxygen. Premises using in excess of 150 000 litres of oxygen per week find the latter more economical. The pressure of oxygen in a hospital pipeline is approximately 4 bar (60 lb.in^{-2}), which is the same as the pressure distal to the reducing valves of gas cylinders attached to anaesthetic machines.

Oxygen is tasteless, colourless and odourless, with a specific gravity of 1.105 and a molecular weight of 32. At atmospheric pressure it liquefies at $-183°C$ but at 50 atmospheres the liquefaction temperature increases to $-119°C$.

Oxygen supports combustion, although the gas itself is not flammable.

Oxygen concentrators

Oxygen concentrators produce oxygen from ambient air by absorption of nitrogen onto some types of alumina silicates. Oxygen concentrators are useful both in hospitals and in long-term domestic use in remote areas, in developing countries and in military surgery. The gas produced by oxygen concentrators contains small quantities of inert gases (e.g. argon) which are harmless.

Physiological effects

The physiological aspects of oxygen are discussed in Chapter 1 and the clinical uses in Chapter 23.

Adverse effects of oxygen

1. *Fire*. Oxygen supports combustion of fuels. An increase in the concentration of oxygen from 21% up to 100% causes a progressive increase in the rate of combustion with the production of either conflagrations or explosions with appropriate fuels (see Ch. 15).

2. *Cardiovascular depression*. An increase in Pa_{O_2} leads to direct vasoconstriction, which occurs in peripheral vasculature and also in the cerebral,

coronary, hepatic and renal circulations. This effect is not manifest at a Pa_{O_2} of less than 30 kPa and assumes clinical importance only at hyperbaric pressures of oxygen. Hyperbaric pressures of oxygen also cause direct myocardial depression. In patients with severe cardiovascular disease, elevation of Pa_{O_2} from the normal physiological range to 80 kPa may produce clinically evident cardiovascular depression.

3. *Absorption atelectasis.* Because oxygen is highly soluble in blood, the use of 100% oxygen as the inspired gas may lead to absorption atelectasis in lung units distal to the site of airway closure. Absorption collapse may occur in as short a time as 6 min with 100% oxygen and 60 min with 85% oxygen. Thus, even small concentrations of nitrogen exert an important splinting effect and this accounts for current avoidance of 100% oxygen in estimation of pulmonary shunt ratio (Q_S/Q_T) in patients with lung pathology, in whom a greater degree of airway closure would result in greater areas of alveolar atelectasis. Absorption atelectasis has been demonstrated in volunteers breathing 100% oxygen at FRC; atelectasis is evident on chest radiography for a period of at least 24 h after exposure.

4. *CO_2 narcosis.* In patients with chronic bronchitis and chronic CO_2 retention, there may be loss of sensitivity of the central chemoreceptors and some dependence of ventilation on drive from the peripheral chemoreceptors that respond to oxygen. Administration of a high $F_{I_{O_2}}$ to such a patient may cause loss of peripheral chemoreceptor drive with the subsequent development of ventilatory failure.

5. *Pulmonary oxygen toxicity.* Chronic inhalation of a high inspired concentration of oxygen may result in the condition termed pulmonary oxygen toxicity (Lorrain–Smith effect), which is manifest by hyaline membranes, thickening of the interlobular and alveolar septa by oedema and fibroplastic proliferation. The clinical and radiological appearance of these changes is almost identical to that of the adult respiratory distress syndrome. The biochemical mechanisms underlying pulmonary oxygen toxicity probably include:

a. Oxidation of SH groups on essential enzymes such as co-enzyme A.

b. Peroxidation of lipids; the resulting lipid peroxides inhibit the function of the cell.
c. Inhibition of the pathway of reversed electron transport, possibly by inhibition of iron and SH-containing flavoproteins.

These changes lead to loss of synthesis of pulmonary surfactant, encouraging the development of absorption collapse and alveolar oedema. The onset of oxygen-induced lung pathology occurs after approximately 30 h exposure to a $P_{I_{O_2}}$ of 100 kPa.

6. *Central nervous system oxygen toxicity.* Convulsions, similar to those of grand mal epilepsy, occur during exposure to hyperbaric pressures of oxygen.

7. *Retrolental fibroplasia.* Retrolental fibroplasia (RLF) is the result of oxygen-induced retinal vasoconstriction, with obliteration of the most immature retinal vessels and subsequent new vessel formation at the site of damage in the form of a proliferative retinopathy. Leakage of intravascular fluid leads to vitreoretinal adhesions and even retinal detachment. Retrolental fibroplasia occurs in infants exposed to hyperoxia in the paediatric intensive care unit and is related not to the $F_{I_{O_2}}$ per se, but to an elevated retinal artery P_{O_2}. It is not known what the threshold of Pa_{O_2} is for the development of retinal damage, but an umbilical arterial P_{O_2} of 8–12 kPa (60–90 mmHg) is associated with a very low incidence of RLF and no signs of systemic hypoxia. It should be stressed, however, that there are many factors involved in the development of RLF in addition to arterial hyperoxia.

8. *Depressed haemopoiesis.* Long-term exposure to elevated $F_{I_{O_2}}$ leads to depression of haemopoiesis and anaemia.

Carbon dioxide

Carbon dioxide is a colourless gas with a pungent odour. It has a molecular weight of 44, a critical temperature of $-31°C$ and a critical pressure of 73.8 bar.

Carbon dioxide is obtained commercially from four sources:

1. As a byproduct of fermentation in brewing of beer.

2. As a byproduct of the manufacture of hydrogen.

3. By heating magnesium and calcium carbonate in the presence of their oxides.

4. As a combustion gas from burning fuel.

Carbon dioxide is supplied in a liquid state in grey cylinders at a pressure of 50 bar. The filling ratio (see p. 242) is 0.75 and the liquid phase occupies approximately 90–95% of the cylinder capacity.

Physiological data

The physiological aspects of CO_2 are dealt with predominantly in Chapter 1. Variations in cardiovascular state induced by alterations in Pa_{CO_2} may be similar to those induced by pain or lightness of anaesthesia and the differential diagnosis is described in Table 23.2. The cardiovascular effects of CO_2 are summarized in Table 8.2.

Uses of carbon dioxide in anaesthesia

1. During inhalational induction of anaesthesia, carbon dioxide may be used to stimulate ventilation after a heavy opioid premedication. Care should be taken to avoid undue hypercapnia.

2. To produce hyperventilation in order to facilitate blind nasal intubation.

Table 8.2 Cardiovascular effects of CO_2

Arterial pressure Cardiac output Heart rate	Biphasic response. Progressive increase in these variables with increase in Pa_{CO_2} up to approximately 10 kPa as a result of indirect sympathetic stimulation. At very high Pa_{CO_2}, these variables decrease as a result of myocardial depression
Skin Coronary circulation Cerebral circulation Gastrointestinal circulation	Dilatation with hypercapnia Constriction with hypocapnia

3. To increase cerebral blood flow during carotid artery surgery. This is an area of some controversy, as hypercapnia may induce 'stealing' of blood away from an ischaemic area of brain. Many anaesthetists prefer to maintain normocapnia during this surgical procedure.

4. To assist in reinstitution of spontaneous ventilation after a period of artificial hyperventilation.

The use of carbon dioxide in anaesthetic practice has declined as appreciation of its disadvantages has increased and as a result of the introduction of i.v. induction agents and relaxant anaesthetic techniques. Because of reports of accidental administration of high concentrations of CO_2, it is not available on some modern anaesthetic machines.

FURTHER READING

Jones R M 1994 Volatile anaesthetic agents. In: Nimmo W S, Rowbotham D J, Smith G (eds) Anaesthesia, 2nd edn. Blackwell Scientific Publications, Oxford, pp 43–74

9. Intravenous anaesthetic agents

General anaesthesia may be produced by many drugs which depress the central nervous system, including sedatives, tranquillizers and hypnotic agents. However, for some drugs the doses required to produce surgical anaesthesia are so large that cardiovascular and respiratory depression may occur commonly, and recovery is delayed for hours or even days. Only a few drugs are suitable for use routinely to produce anaesthesia after intravenous (i.v.) injection.

I.v. anaesthetic agents are commonly used to induce anaesthesia, as induction is usually more rapid and smoother than that associated with inhalational agents. I.v. anaesthetics may also be used for maintenance, either alone or in combination with nitrous oxide; they may be administered as repeated bolus doses or by continuous i.v. infusion. Other uses include sedation during regional anaesthesia, sedation in the intensive therapy unit (ITU) and treatment of status epilepticus.

Properties of the ideal intravenous anaesthetic agent

1. Rapid onset. This is achieved by an agent which is mainly un-ionized at blood pH and which is highly soluble in lipid; these properties permit penetration of the blood–brain barrier.

2. Rapid recovery. Early recovery of consciousness is usually produced by rapid redistribution of the drug from the brain into other well-perfused tissues, particularly muscle. The plasma concentration of the drug decreases, and the drug diffuses out of the brain along a concentration gradient. The quality of the later recovery period is related more to the rate of metabolism of the drug; drugs with slow metabolism are associated with a more

prolonged 'hangover' effect and accumulate if used in repeated doses or by infusion for maintenance of anaesthesia.

3. Analgesia at subanaesthetic concentrations.

4. Minimal cardiovascular and respiratory depression.

5. No emetic effects.

6. No excitatory phenomena (e.g. coughing, hiccup, involuntary movement) on induction.

7. No emergence phenomena (e.g. nightmares).

8. No interaction with neuromuscular blocking drugs.

9. No pain on injection.

10. No venous sequelae.

11. Safe if injected inadvertently into an artery.

12. No toxic effects on other organs.

13. No release of histamine.

14. No hypersensitivity reactions.

15. Water-soluble formulation.

16. Long shelf-life.

17. No stimulation of porphyria.

None of the agents available at present meets all these requirements. Features of the commonly used i.v. anaesthetic agents are compared in Table 9.1.

A classification of i.v. anaesthetic drugs is shown in Table 9.2.

Pharmacokinetics of i.v. anaesthetic drugs

After i.v. administration of a drug, there is an immediate rapid increase in plasma concentration followed by a slower decline. Anaesthesia is produced by diffusion of drug from arterial blood across the blood–brain barrier into brain. The rate of transfer into brain, and therefore the anaesthetic effect, is regulated by the following factors:

139

Table 9.1   Main properties of intravenous anaesthetics

	Thiopentone	Methohexitone	Propofol	Ketamine	Etomidate
Physical properties					
Water-soluble	+	+	−	+	+*
Stable in solution	−	−	+	+	+
Long shelf-life	−	−	+	+	+
Pain on i.v. injection	−	+	++	−	++
Non-irritant on s.c. injection	−	±	+	+	
Painful on arterial injection	+	+	−		
No sequelae from intra-arterial injection	−	±	+		
Low incidence of venous thrombosis	+	+	−	+	−
Effects on body					
Rapid onset	+	+	+	−	+
Recovery due to:					
Redistribution	+	+	+	+	
Detoxification		+	+		
Cumulation	++	+	−	−	−
Induction:					
Excitatory effects	−	++	+	+	+++
Respiratory complications	−	+	+	−	−
Cardiovascular:					
Hypotension	+	+	++	−	+
Analgesic	−	−	−	++	−
Antanalgesic	+	+	−	−	?
Interaction with relaxants	−	−	−	−	−
Postoperative vomiting	−	−	−	++	+
Emergence delirium	−	−	−	++	−
Safe in porphyria	−	−	+	+	−

*Aqueous solution not commercially available.
i.v. = Intravenous; s.c. = subcutaneous.

Table 9.2   Classification of intravenous anaesthetics

Rapidly acting (primary induction) agents
Barbiturates:
  Methohexitone
  Thiobarbiturates: thiopentone, thiamylal
Imidazole compounds: etomidate*
Sterically hindered alkyl phenols: propofol
Steroids: eltanolone
  (W: Althesin, minaxolone)
W (Eugenols: propanidid)

Slower-acting (basal narcotic) agents
Ketamine
Benzodiazepines: diazepam, flunitrazepam, midazolam
Large-dose opioids: fentanyl, alfentanil, sufentanil
Neurolept combination: opioid + neuroleptic

*Limited use as infusion.
W = Withdrawn from market.

1. Protein binding. Only unbound drug is free to cross the blood–brain barrier. Protein binding may be reduced by low plasma protein concentrations or displacement by other drugs, resulting in higher concentrations of free drug and an exaggerated anaesthetic effect. Protein binding is also affected by changes in blood pH. Thus, hyperventilation decreases protein binding and increases the anaesthetic effect.

2. Blood flow to brain. Reduced cerebral blood flow (CBF), e.g. carotid artery stenosis, results in reduced delivery of drug to brain. However, if CBF is reduced because of low cardiac output, initial blood concentrations are higher than nor-

mal after i.v. administration, and the anaesthetic effect may be delayed but enhanced.

3. Extracellular pH and pK_a of the drug. Only the non-ionized fraction of the drug penetrates the lipid blood–brain barrier; thus, the potency of the drug depends on the degree of ionization at the pH of extracellular fluid and the pK_a of the drug.

4. The relative solubilities of the drug in lipid and water. High lipid-solubility enhances transfer into the brain.

5. Speed of injection. Rapid i.v. administration results in high initial concentrations of drug. This increases speed of induction, but also the extent of cardiovascular and respiratory side-effects.

In general, any factor which increases the blood concentration of free drug, e.g. reduced protein binding or low cardiac output, also increases the intensity of side-effects.

Distribution to other tissues

The anaesthetic effect of all i.v. anaesthetic drugs in current use is terminated predominantly by distribution to other tissues. Figure 9.1 shows this distribution for thiopentone. The percentage of the injected dose in each of four body compartments as time elapses is shown after i.v. injection. A large proportion of the drug is distributed initially into the well-perfused organs (termed the vessel-rich group, or viscera — predominantly brain, liver and kidneys). Distribution into muscle (lean) is slower because of its low lipid content,

Table 9.3 Factors influencing the distribution of thiopentone in the body

	Viscera	Muscle	Fat	Others
Relative blood flow	Rich	Good	Poor	Very poor
Blood flow (litre.min⁻¹)	4.5	1.1	0.32	0.08
Tissue volume (litre; A)	6	33	15	13
Tissue/blood partition coefficient (B)	1.5	1.5	11.0	1.5
Potential capacity (litre; $A \times B$)	9	50	160	20
Time constant (capacity/flow; min)	2	45	500	250

but is quantitatively important because of its relatively good blood supply and large mass. Despite their high lipid-solubility, i.v. anaesthetic drugs distribute slowly to adipose tissue (fat) because of its poor blood supply. Fat contributes little to the initial redistribution or termination of action of i.v. anaesthetic agents, but fat depots contain a large proportion of the injected dose of thiopentone at 90 min, and 65–75% of the total remaining in the body at 24 h. There is also a small amount of redistribution to areas with a very poor blood supply, e.g. bone. Table 9.3 indicates some of the properties of the body compartments in respect of the distribution of i.v. anaesthetic agents.

After a single i.v. dose, the concentration of drug in blood decreases as distribution occurs into viscera, and particularly muscle. Drug diffuses from the brain into blood along the changing concentration gradient, and recovery of consciousness occurs. Metabolism of most i.v. anaesthetic drugs occurs predominantly in the liver; if metabolism is rapid (indicated by a short elimination half-life), it may contribute to some extent to the recovery of consciousness. However, because of the large distribution volume of i.v. anaesthetic drugs, total elimination takes many hours, or in some instances, days. A small proportion of drug may be excreted unchanged in the urine; the amount depends on the degree of ionization and the pH of urine.

BARBITURATES

Amylobarbitone and pentobarbitone were used i.v. to induce anaesthesia in the late 1920s, but their actions were unpredictable and recovery

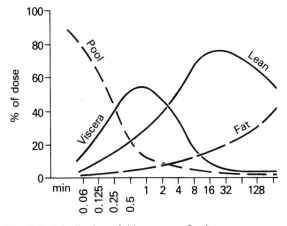

Fig. 9.1 Distribution of thiopentone after intravenous bolus administration.

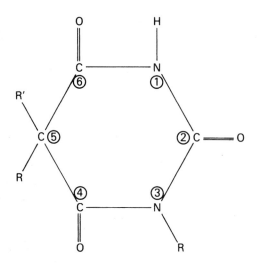

Fig. 9.2   Structure of barbiturate ring.

was prolonged. Manipulation of the barbituric acid ring (Fig. 9.2) enabled a short duration of action to be achieved by:

1. Substitution of a sulphur atom for oxygen at position 2.
2. Substitution of a methyl group at position 1; this also confers potential convulsive activity and increases the incidence of excitatory phenomena.

An increased number of carbon atoms in the side chains at position 5 increases the potency of the agent. The presence of an aromatic nucleus in an alkyl group at position 5 produces compounds with convulsant properties; direct substitution with a phenyl group confers anticonvulsant activity.

The anaesthetically active barbiturates are classified chemically into four groups (Table 9.4). The methylated oxybarbiturate hexobarbitone was moderately successful as an i.v. anaesthetic agent, but was superseded by the development in 1932 of thiopentone. Thiopentone remains probably the most commonly used i.v. anaesthetic agent throughout the world. Its pharmacology is therefore described fully in this chapter. Many of its effects are shared by other i.v. anaesthetic agents and consequently the pharmacology of these drugs is described more briefly.

Thiopentone sodium

Chemical structure

Sodium 5-ethyl-5-(1-methylbutyl)-2-thiobarbiturate.

Physical properties and presentation

Thiopentone sodium, the sulphur analogue of pentobarbitone, is a yellowish powder with a bitter taste and a faint smell of garlic. It is stored in nitrogen to prevent chemical reaction with atmospheric carbon dioxide, and mixed with 6% anhydrous sodium carbonate to increase its solubility in water. It is available in single-dose ampoules of 500 mg or multidose bottles which contain 2.5 g, and is dissolved in distilled water to produce a 2.5% (25 mg.ml^{-1}) solution with a pH of 10.8; this solution is slightly hypotonic. Freshly prepared solution may be kept for 24 h. The oil/water partition coefficient of thiopentone is 4.7, and the pK_a 7.6.

Table 9.4   Relation of chemical grouping to clinical action of barbiturates

Group	Substituents		Group characteristics when given intravenously
	Position 1	Position 2	
Oxybarbiturates	H	O	Delay in onset of action depending on 5 and 5′ side chain. Useful as basal hypnotics. Prolonged action
Methyl barbiturates	CH$_3$	O	Usually rapidly acting with fairly rapid recovery. High incidence of excitatory phenomena
Thiobarbiturates	H	S	Rapidly acting, usually smooth onset of sleep and fairly prompt recovery
Methyl thiobarbiturates	CH$_3$	S	Rapid onset of action and very rapid recovery but with so high an incidence of excitatory phenomena as to preclude use in clinical practice

Pharmacology

Central nervous system (CNS). Thiopentone produces anaesthesia usually in less than 30 s after i.v. injection, although there may be some delay in patients with a low cardiac output. There is progressive depression of the CNS, including spinal cord reflexes. The hypnotic action of thiopentone is potent, but its analgesic effect is poor, and surgical anaesthesia is difficult to achieve unless large doses are used; these are associated with cardiorespiratory depression. The cerebral metabolic rate is reduced, and there are secondary decreases in CBF, cerebral blood volume and intracranial pressure. Recovery of consciousness occurs at a higher blood concentration if a large dose is given, or if the drug is injected rapidly; this has been attributed to acute tolerance, but may represent only altered redistribution. Consciousness is usually regained in 5–10 min. At subanaesthetic blood concentrations (i.e. at low doses, or during recovery), thiopentone has an antanalgesic effect, and reduces the pain threshold; this may result in restlessness in the postoperative period. Thiopentone is a very potent anticonvulsant.

Sympathetic nervous system activity is depressed to a greater extent than parasympathetic; this may occasionally result in bradycardia. However, it is more usual for tachycardia to develop after induction of anaesthesia partly because of baroreceptor inhibition caused by modest hypotension and partly because of loss of vagal tone which may predominate normally in young healthy adults.

Cardiovascular system. Myocardial contractility is depressed and peripheral vasodilatation occurs, particularly when large doses are administered or if injection is rapid. Arterial pressure decreases, and profound hypotension may occur in the patient with hypovolaemia or cardiac disease. Heart rate may decrease, but there is often a reflex tachycardia (see above).

Respiratory system. Ventilatory drive is decreased by thiopentone as a result of reduced sensitivity of the respiratory centre to carbon dioxide. A short period of apnoea is common, frequently preceded by a few deep breaths. Respiratory depression is influenced by premedication, and is more pronounced if opioids have been administered; assisted or controlled ventilation may be required. When spontaneous ventilation is resumed, ventilatory rate and tidal volume are usually lower than normal, but they increase in response to surgical stimulation. There is an increase in bronchial muscle tone, although frank bronchospasm is uncommon.

Laryngeal spasm may be precipitated by surgical stimulation or the presence of secretions, blood or foreign bodies (e.g. an oropharyngeal or laryngeal mask airway) in the region of the pharynx or larynx. Thiopentone is less satisfactory in this respect than most other anaesthetic agents, and appears to depress the parasympathetic laryngeal reflex arc to a lesser extent than other areas of the CNS.

Skeletal muscle. Skeletal muscle tone is reduced at high blood concentrations, partly as a result of suppression of spinal cord reflexes. There is no significant direct effect on the neuromuscular junction. When thiopentone is used as the sole anaesthetic agent, there is poor muscle relaxation and movement in response to surgical stimulation is common.

Uterus and placenta. There is little effect on resting uterine tone, but uterine contractions are suppressed at high doses. Thiopentone crosses the placenta readily, although fetal blood concentrations do not reach the same levels as those observed in the mother.

Eye. Intraocular pressure is reduced by approximately 40%. The pupil dilates first, and then constricts; the light reflex remains present until surgical anaesthesia has been attained. The corneal, conjunctival, eyelash and eyelid reflexes are abolished.

Hepatorenal function. The functions of the liver and kidneys are impaired transiently after administration of thiopentone. Hepatic microsomal enzymes are induced and this may increase the metabolism and elimination of other drugs.

Pharmacokinetics

Blood concentrations of thiopentone increase rapidly after i.v. administration. Between 75 and 85% of the drug is bound to protein, mostly albumin; thus, more free drug is available if plasma protein concentrations are reduced by malnutrition or disease. Protein binding is affected by pH, and is decreased by alkalaemia; thus the concentration of free drug is increased during hyperventilation. Some drugs, e.g. phenylbutazone, occupy the same binding sites, and protein binding of thiopentone may be reduced in their presence.

Thiopentone diffuses readily into the CNS because of its lipid-solubility and predominantly un-ionized state (61%) at body pH. Consciousness returns when the brain concentration decreases to a threshold value, dependent on the individual patient, the dose of drug and its rate of administration, but at this time nearly all of the injected dose is still present in the body.

Metabolism of thiopentone occurs predominantly in the liver, and the metabolites are excreted by the kidneys; a small proportion is excreted unchanged in the urine. The terminal elimination half-life is approximately 11.5 h. Metabolism is a zero-order process; 10–15% of the remaining drug is metabolized each hour. Thus, up to 30% of the original dose may remain in the body at 24 h. Consequently, a 'hangover' effect is common; in addition, further doses of thiopentone administered within 1–2 days may result in cumulation. Elimination is impaired in the elderly. In obese patients, dosage should be based on an estimate of lean body mass, as distribution to fat is slow. However, elimination may be delayed in obese patients because of increased retention of the drug by adipose tissue.

Dosage and administration

Thiopentone is administered i.v. as a 2.5% solution; although a few anaesthetists use a 5% solution, this increases the likelihood of serious complications and is *not* recommended. A small volume, e.g. 2 ml in adults, should be administered initially; the patient should be asked if any pain is experienced in case of inadvertent intra-arterial injection (see below) before the remainder of the induction dose is given.

The dose required to produce anaesthesia varies, and the response of each patient must be assessed carefully; cardiovascular depression is exaggerated if excessive doses are given. In healthy adults, an initial dose of 4 mg.kg^{-1} should be administered over 15–20 s; if loss of the eyelash

reflex does not occur within 30 s, supplementary doses of 50–100 mg should be given slowly until consciousness is lost. In young children, a dose of 6 mg.kg^{-1} is usually necessary. Elderly patients often require smaller doses (e.g. 2.5–3 mg.kg^{-1}) than young adults.

Induction is usually smooth, and may be preceded by a taste of garlic. Side-effects are related to peak blood concentrations, and in patients in whom cardiovascular depression may occur the drug should be administered more slowly; in very frail patients, as little as 50 mg may be sufficient to induce sleep.

No other drug should be mixed with thiopentone. Muscle relaxants should *not* be given until it is certain that anaesthesia has been induced. The i.v. cannula should be flushed with saline before vecuronium or atracurium is administered, to obviate precipitation.

Supplementary doses of 25–100 mg may be given to augment nitrous oxide/oxygen anaesthesia during short surgical procedures. However, recovery may be prolonged considerably if large total doses are used (> 10 mg.kg^{-1}).

Thiopentone in a 5 or 10% solution may be administered rectally to induce basal narcosis in children. A dose of 44 mg.kg^{-1} induces sleep in 10–15 min. This technique may be used to sedate unco-operative children before anaesthesia. However, there may be loss of airway control, and the child must be supervised by skilled staff.

Adverse effects

1. *Hypotension.* The risk is increased if excessive doses are used, or if thiopentone is administered to hypovolaemic, shocked or previously hypertensive patients. Hypotension is minimized by administering the drug slowly. Thiopentone should not be administered to patients in the sitting position.

2. *Respiratory depression.* The risk is increased if excessive doses are used, or if opioid drugs have been administered. Facilities must be available to provide artificial ventilation.

3. *Tissue necrosis.* Local necrosis may follow perivenous injection. Median nerve damage may occur after extravasation in the antecubital fossa, and this site is not recommended. If perivenous injection occurs, the needle should be left in

place, and hyaluronidase injected. Tissue damage is worse if the 5% solution is used.

4. *Intra-arterial injection.* This is usually the result of inadvertent injection into the brachial artery or an aberrant ulnar artery in the antecubital fossa. The patient usually complains of intense, burning pain, and this is an indication to stop injecting the drug immediately. The forearm and hand may become blanched and blisters may appear distally. Intra-arterial thiopentone causes profound constriction of the artery accompanied by local release of noradrenaline. In addition, crystals of thiopentone form in arterioles. In combination with thrombosis caused by endarteritis, adenosine triphosphate release from damaged red cells and aggregation of platelets, these result in emboli and may cause ischaemia or gangrene in parts of the forearm, hand or fingers.

The needle should be left in the artery and a vasodilator (e.g. papaverine 20 mg) administered. Stellate ganglion or brachial plexus block may reduce arterial spasm. Heparin should be given i.v. and oral anticoagulants should be prescribed after operation.

The risk of ischaemic damage after intra-arterial injection is much greater if a 5% solution of thiopentone is used.

5. *Laryngeal spasm.* The causes have been discussed above.

6. *Bronchospasm.* This is unusual, but may be precipitated in asthmatic patients.

7. *Allergic reactions.* These range from cutaneous rashes to severe or fatal anaphylactic or anaphylactoid reactions with cardiovascular collapse. Severe reactions are rare (approximately 1 in 14–20 000). Hypersensitivity reactions to drugs administered during anaesthesia are discussed on pages 156 and 397.

8. *Thrombophlebitis.* This is relatively uncommon (Table 9.5) unless the 5% solution is used.

Indications

1. Induction of anaesthesia.
2. Maintenance of anaesthesia. Thiopentone is only suitable for short procedures because cumulation occurs with repeated doses.
3. Basal narcosis by rectal administration.
4. Treatment of status epilepticus.

Table 9.5 Percentage incidences of pain on injection and thrombophlebitis after intravenous administration of anaesthetic drugs into a large vein in the antecubital fossa or a small vein in the dorsum of the hand or wrist

Agent	Pain		Thrombophlebitis	
	Large	Small	Large	Small
Saline 0.9%	0	0	0	0
Thiopentone 2.5%	0	12	1	0
Methohexitone 1%	8	21	0	0
Propofol	10	40	0	0
Etomidate	8	80	15	20

5. Reduction of intracranial pressure (see Chapter 37).

Absolute contraindications

1. *Airway obstruction.* Intravenous anaesthesia should not be employed if there is anticipated difficulty in maintaining an adequate airway, e.g. epiglottitis, oral or pharyngeal tumours.
2. *Porphyria.* Barbiturates may precipitate lower motor neurone paralysis or severe cardiovascular collapse in patients with porphyria.
3. *Previous hypersensitivity reaction.*

Precautions

Special care is needed when thiopentone is administered in the following circumstances:

1. *Cardiovascular disease.* Patients with hypovolaemia, myocardial disease, cardiac valvular stenosis or constrictive pericarditis are particularly sensitive to the hypotensive effects of thiopentone. However, if the drug is administered with extreme caution, it is probably no more hazardous than other i.v. anaesthetic agents. Myocardial depression may be severe in patients with right-to-left intracardiac shunt because of high coronary artery concentrations of thiopentone.

2. *Severe hepatic disease.* Reduced protein binding results in higher concentrations of free drug. Metabolism may be impaired, but this has little effect on early recovery. A normal dose may be administered, but very slowly.

3. *Renal disease.* In chronic renal failure, protein

binding is reduced, but elimination is unaltered. A normal dose may be administered, but very slowly.

4. *Muscle disease.* Respiratory depression is exaggerated in patients with myasthenia gravis or dystrophia myotonica.

5. *Reduced metabolic rate.* Patients with myxoedema are exquisitely sensitive to the effects of thiopentone.

6. *Obstetrics.* An adequate dose must be given to ensure that the mother is anaesthetized. However, excessive doses may result in respiratory or cardiovascular depression in the fetus, particularly if the interval between induction and delivery is short.

7. *Outpatient anaesthesia.* Early recovery is slow in comparison with other agents. This is seldom important unless rapid return of airway reflexes is essential, e.g. after oral or dental surgery. However, slow elimination of thiopentone may result in persistent drowsiness for 24–36 h, and this impairs the ability to drive or use machinery. There is also potentiation of the effect of alcohol or sedative drugs ingested during that period. It is preferable to use a drug with more rapid elimination for patients who are ambulant within a few hours.

8. *Adrenocortical insufficiency.*

9. *Extremes of age.*

10. *Asthma.*

Methohexitone sodium

Chemical structure

Sodium   α-*dl*-5-allyl-1-methyl-5-(1-methyl-2-pentynyl) barbiturate.

Physical properties and presentation

Methohexitone has two asymmetrical carbon atoms, and therefore four isomers. The α-*dl* isomers are clinically useful. The drug is presented as a white powder mixed with 6% anhydrous sodium carbonate, and is readily soluble in distilled water. The resulting 1% (10 mg.ml^{-1}) solution has a pH of 11.1 and pK_a of 7.9. Single-dose vials of 100 mg and multidose bottles containing 500 mg or 2.5 g are available. Although the solution is

chemically stable for up to 6 weeks, the manufacturers recommend that it should not be stored for longer than 24 h because it contains no antibacterial preservative.

Pharmacology

Central nervous system. Unconsciousness is usually induced in 15–30 s. Recovery is more rapid with methohexitone than thiopentone, and occurs after 2–3 min; it is caused predominantly by redistribution. Drowsiness may persist for several hours until blood concentrations are decreased further by metabolism. Epileptiform activity has been demonstrated by electroencephalogram (EEG) in epileptic patients. However, in sufficient doses, methohexitone acts as an anticonvulsant.

Cardiovascular system. In general, there is less hypotension in otherwise healthy patients than occurs after thiopentone; the decrease in arterial pressure is predominantly mediated by vasodilatation. Heart rate may increase slightly because of a decrease in baroreceptor activity. The cardiovascular effects are more pronounced in patients with cardiac disease or hypovolaemia.

Respiratory system. Moderate hypoventilation occurs. There may be a short period of apnoea after i.v. injection.

Pharmacokinetics

A greater proportion of methohexitone than thiopentone is in the non-ionized state at body pH (approximately 75%), although the drug is less lipid-soluble than the thiobarbiturate. Binding to plasma protein occurs to a similar degree. Clearance from plasma is higher than that of thiopentone, and the elimination half-life is considerably shorter (approximately 4 h). Thus, cumulation is less likely to occur after repeated doses.

Dosage and administration

Methohexitone is administered i.v. in a dose of 1–1.5 mg.kg^{-1} to induce anaesthesia in healthy young adult patients; smaller doses are required in the elderly and infirm.

Methohexitone has been used by the intramuscular (i.m.) route in a dose of 6.6 mg.kg^{-1}, or rectally (20–25 mg.kg^{-1}) to provide heavy pre-operative sedation in children. Administration by these routes may result in unconsciousness and loss of airway reflexes, and patients must be closely supervised by trained staff.

Adverse effects

1. *Cardiovascular and respiratory depression.* This is probably less than that associated with thiopentone.
2. *Excitatory phenomena during induction,* including dyskinetic muscle movements, coughing and hiccups. Muscle movements are reduced by administration of an opioid; the incidence of cough and hiccups is reduced by premedication with an anticholinergic agent. The incidence of excitatory effects is dose-related.
3. *Epileptiform activity* on EEG in epileptic subjects.
4. *Pain on injection* (Table 9.5).
5. *Tissue damage* after perivenous injection is rare with 1% solution.
6. *Intra-arterial injection* can cause gangrene, but the risk with 1% solution is considerably less than with 2.5% thiopentone.
7. *Allergic reactions* occur, but are uncommon.
8. *Thrombophlebitis* is a rare complication.

Indications

Induction of anaesthesia, particularly when a rapid recovery is desirable. Methohexitone is used commonly as the anaesthetic agent for electro-convulsive therapy (ECT), and for induction of anaesthesia for outpatient dental and other minor procedures.

Absolute contraindications

These are the same as for thiopentone.

Precautions

These are similar to the precautions listed for thiopentone. However, methohexitone is a suitable agent for outpatients. It should not be used to induce anaesthesia in patients who are known to be epileptic.

Thiamylal sodium

This is the sulphur analogue of quinalbarbitone. It is slightly more potent than thiopentone, but otherwise almost identical in its properties. It is not available in the UK, but is used in some other countries.

NON-BARBITURATE INTRAVENOUS ANAESTHETIC AGENTS

Propofol

This phenol derivative was identified as a potentially useful intravenous anaesthetic agent in 1980, and became available commercially in 1986. It is more expensive than thiopentone or metho-hexitone, but has achieved great popularity because of its favourable recovery characteristics and its antiemetic effect.

Chemical structure

2,6-Di-isopropylphenol (Fig. 9.3).

Physical properties and presentation

Propofol is extremely lipid-soluble, but almost insoluble in water. The drug was formulated initially in Cremophor EL. However, a number of other drugs formulated in this solubilizing agent were associated with release of histamine and an unacceptably high incidence of anaphylactoid reactions, and similar reactions occurred with this

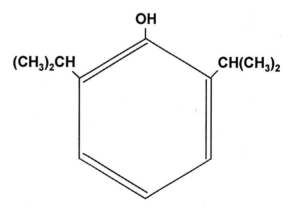

Fig. 9.3 Chemical structure of propofol (2,6-di-isopropylphenol).

formulation of propofol. Consequently, the drug was reformulated in a white, aqueous emulsion containing soyabean oil and purified egg phosphatide. Ampoules of the drug contain 200 mg of propofol in 20 ml (10 mg.ml^{-1}), and 50 and 100 ml bottles containing 1% (10 mg.ml^{-1}) or 2% (20 mg.ml^{-1}) solution are available for infusion.

Pharmacology

Central nervous system. Anaesthesia is induced within 20–40 s after i.v. administration in otherwise healthy young adults. Transfer from blood to the sites of action in the brain is slower than with thiopentone, and there is a delay in disappearance of the eyelash reflex, normally used as a sign of unconsciousness after administration of barbiturate anaesthetic agents. Overdosage of propofol, with exaggerated side-effects, may result if this clinical sign is used; loss of verbal contact is a better end-point. EEG frequency decreases, and amplitude increases. Propofol reduces the duration of seizures induced by ECT in humans. However, there have been reports of convulsions following the use of propofol and it is recommended that caution should be exercised in administration of propofol to epileptic patients. Normally cerebral metabolic rate, CBF and intracranial pressure are reduced.

Recovery of consciousness is rapid, and there is a minimal 'hangover' effect even in the immediate postanaesthetic period.

Cardiovascular system. In healthy patients, arterial pressure decreases to a greater degree after induction of anaesthesia with propofol than with thiopentone; the reduction results predominantly from vasodilatation although there is a slight negative inotropic effect. In some patients, large decreases (>40%) occur. The degree of hypotension is substantially reduced by decreasing the rate of administration of the drug and by appreciation of the kinetics of transfer from blood to brain (see above). The pressor response to tracheal intubation is attenuated to a greater degree by propofol than thiopentone. Heart rate increases slightly after induction of anaesthesia with propofol.

Respiratory system. After induction, apnoea occurs more commonly, and for a longer duration, than after thiopentone. During infusion of propofol, tidal volume is lower and respiratory rate higher than in the conscious state. There is decreased ventilatory response to carbon dioxide. As with other agents, ventilatory depression is more marked if opioids are administered.

Propofol has no effect on bronchial muscle tone and laryngospasm is particularly uncommon. The suppression of laryngeal reflexes results in a low incidence of coughing or laryngospasm when a laryngeal mask airway (LMA) is introduced, and propofol is regarded by most anaesthetists as the drug of choice when the LMA is to be used.

Skeletal muscle. Tone is reduced, but movements may occur in response to surgical stimulation.

Gastrointestinal system. Propofol has no effect on gastrointestinal motility in animals.

Uterus and placenta. Little is known of the effects of propofol on uterine tone or of its placental transfer.

Hepatorenal. There is a transient decrease in renal function, but the impairment is less than that associated with thiopentone. Hepatic blood flow is decreased by the reductions in arterial pressure and cardiac output. Liver function tests are not deranged after infusion of propofol for 24 h.

Endocrine. Plasma concentrations of cortisol are decreased after administration of propofol, but a normal response occurs to administration of Synacthen.

Pharmacokinetics

In common with other i.v. anaesthetic drugs, propofol is distributed rapidly, and blood concentrations decline exponentially. Clearance of the drug from plasma is greater than would be expected if the drug was metabolized only in the liver, and it is believed that extrahepatic sites of metabolism exist. The kidneys excrete the metabolites of propofol (mainly glucuronides); only 0.3% of the administered dose of propofol is excreted unchanged. The terminal elimination half-life of propofol is 3–4.8 h, although its effective half-life is much shorter (30–60 min). The distribution and clearance of propofol are altered by the concomitant administration of fentanyl.

Elimination of propofol remains relatively constant even after infusions lasting for several days.

Dosage and administration

In healthy, unpremedicated adults, a dose of 1.5–2.5 mg.kg^{-1} is required to induce anaesthesia. The dose should be reduced in the elderly; an initial dose of 1.25 mg.kg^{-1} is appropriate, with subsequent additional doses of 10 mg until consciousness is lost. In children, a dose of 3–3.5 mg.kg^{-1} is usually required; the drug is not recommended for use in children less than 3 years of age. Cardiovascular side-effects are reduced if the drug is injected slowly. Lower doses are required for induction in premedicated patients. Sedation during regional analgesia or endoscopy can be achieved with doses of 1.5–4.5 mg.kg^{-1}.h^{-1}. Doses of up to 15 mg.kg^{-1}.h^{-1} are required to supplement nitrous oxide/oxygen for surgical anaesthesia, although these may be reduced substantially if an opioid drug is administered. The average infusion rate is approximately 2 mg.kg^{-1}.h^{-1} in conjunction with a slow infusion of morphine (2 mg.h^{-1}) for sedation of patients in ITU.

Adverse effects

1. *Cardiovascular depression.* Unless the drug is given very slowly, cardiovascular depression following a bolus dose of propofol is greater than that associated with a bolus dose of a barbiturate, and is likely to cause profound hypotension in hypovolaemic or previously hypertensive patients and in those with cardiac disease. Cardiovascular depression is modest if the drug is administered slowly or by infusion.

2. *Respiratory depression.* Apnoea is more common and of longer duration than after barbiturate administration.

3. *Excitatory phenomena.* These are more frequent than with thiopentone, but less than with methohexitone.

4. *Pain on injection.* This occurs in up to 40% of patients (Table 9.5). The incidence is reduced if a large vein is used, if a small dose (10 mg) of lignocaine is injected shortly before propofol, or if lignocaine is mixed with propofol in the syringe

(up to 1 ml of 0.5% or 1% lignocaine per 20 ml of propofol).

5. *Allergic reactions.* Skin rashes occur occasionally. Anaphylactic reactions have also been reported, but appear to be no more common than with thiopentone.

Indications

1. *Induction of anaesthesia.* Propofol is indicated particularly when rapid early recovery of consciousness is required. Two hours after anaesthesia there is no difference in psychomotor function between patients who have received propofol and those given thiopentone or methohexitone, but the former complain of less drowsiness in the ensuing 12 h. The rapid recovery characteristics are lost if induction is followed by maintenance with inhalational agents for longer than 10–15 min. The nature of recovery from propofol may increase the risks of awareness during tracheal intubation after the administration of non-depolarizing muscle relaxants unless the lungs are ventilated with an appropriate mixture of inhaled anaesthetics (or additional doses or an infusion of propofol, administered i.v.) between induction and intubation.

2. *Sedation during surgery.* Propofol has been used successfully for sedation during regional analgesic techniques, and during endoscopy. Control of the airway may be lost at any time, and patients must be supervised continuously by an anaesthetist.

3. *Total i.v. anaesthesia* (see below). Propofol is the most suitable of the agents currently available. Recovery time is increased after infusion of propofol compared with that after a single bolus dose, but cumulation is significantly less than with the barbiturates.

4. *Sedation in ITU.* Propofol has been used successfully to sedate adult patients for several days in ITU. The level of sedation is controlled easily, and recovery is rapid (usually < 30 min).

Absolute contraindications

Airway obstruction and known hypersensitivity to the drug are probably the only contraindications. Propofol appears to be safe in porphyric patients. At present, propofol should not be used for long-term sedation of children in ITU because of a number of reports of adverse outcome.

Precautions

These are similar to those listed for thiopentone. The side-effects of propofol make it less suitable than thiopentone or methohexitone for patients with existing cardiovascular compromise unless it is administered with great care. Propofol may be more suitable than thiopentone for outpatient anaesthesia, but its use does not obviate the need for an adequate period of recovery before discharge.

Etomidate

This carboxylated imidazole compound was introduced in 1972.

Chemical structure

D-Ethyl-1-(α-methylbenzyl)-imidazole-5-carboxylate.

Physical characteristics and presentation

Etomidate is soluble but unstable in water. It is presented as a clear aqueous solution containing 35% propylene glycol. Ampoules contain 20 mg of etomidate in 10 ml (2 mg.ml^{-1}). The pH of the solution is 8.1.

Pharmacology

Etomidate is a rapidly acting general anaesthetic agent with a short duration of action (2–3 min) resulting predominantly from redistribution, although it is eliminated rapidly from the body. In healthy patients, it produces less cardiovascular depression than thiopentone; however, there is little evidence that this benefit is retained if the cardiovascular system is compromised. Large doses may produce tachycardia. Respiratory depression is less than with other agents.

Etomidate depresses the synthesis of cortisol by the adrenal gland, and impairs the response to adrenocorticotrophic hormone. Long-term infusions of the drug in ITU have been associated with increased infection and mortality, probably related to reduced immunological competence. Its effects on the adrenal gland occur also after a single bolus dose, and last for several hours.

Pharmacokinetics

Etomidate redistributes rapidly in the body. Approximately 76% is bound to protein. It is metabolized in the plasma and liver, mainly by esterase hydrolysis, and the metabolites are excreted in the urine; 2% is excreted unchanged. The terminal elimination half-life is approximately 75 min. There is little cumulation when repeated doses are given. The distribution and clearance of etomidate may be altered by the concomitant administration of fentanyl.

Dosage and administration

An average dose of 0.3 mg.kg^{-1} i.v. induces anaesthesia. The drug should be administered into a large vein to reduce the incidence of pain on injection.

Adverse effects

1. *Suppression of synthesis of cortisol.* See above.
2. *Excitatory phenomena.* Moderate or severe involuntary movements occur in up to 40% of patients during induction of anaesthesia. This incidence is reduced in patients premedicated with an opioid. Cough and hiccups occur in up to 10% of patients.
3. *Pain on injection.* This occurs in up to 80% of patients if a small vein is used, but in less than 10% when the drug is injected into a large vein in the antecubital fossa (Table 9.5). The incidence is reduced by prior injection of lignocaine 10 mg.
4. *Nausea and vomiting.* The incidence of nausea and vomiting is approximately 30%. This is very much higher than after propofol.
5. *Emergence phenomena.* The incidence of severe restlessness and delirium during recovery is greater with etomidate than barbiturates or propofol.
6. *Venous thrombosis* is more common than with other agents.

Indications

There are few positive indications for etomidate, although it is used by many anaesthetists in patients with a compromised cardiovascular system. It is suitable for outpatient anaesthesia, but has been superseded by propofol.

Absolute contraindications

1. Airway obstruction.
2. Porphyria.
3. Adrenal insufficiency.
4. Long-term infusion.

Precautions

These are similar to the precautions listed for thiopentone. Etomidate is suitable for outpatient anaesthesia. However, the incidence of excitatory phenomena is unacceptably high unless an opioid is administered; this delays recovery and is unsuitable for most outpatients.

Eltanolone

Eltanolone (3α-hydroxy-5β-pregnan-20-one; also known as 5β-pregnanolone) has undergone clinical trials as an i.v. induction agent. Like propofol, eltanolone is poorly soluble in water, and it is formulated in an emulsion with 10% Intralipid. The solution is isotonic, with a pH of 7.5. Preliminary studies have suggested that many of its clinical characteristics are similar to those of propofol, but it causes less pain on injection and less respiratory depression.

Induction of anaesthesia is slower with eltanolone than with propofol. The elimination half-life is 1–2 h, and the clearance 1–3 litre.kg^{-1}.h^{-1}. Metabolism takes place predominantly in the liver, and a proportion of unchanged drug is believed to be excreted in the bile. Recovery is prompt, with little hangover. There is a very low incidence of excitatory activity or involuntary movements.

Administration of eltanolone is associated with a significant increase in heart rate but little or no decrease in arterial pressure in volunteers and healthy patients. However, the drug does reduce cardiac output to a greater extent than does propofol; there is little change in afterload.

The dose of eltanolone which induces anaesthesia is 0.5–1.0 mg.kg^{-1}.

Ketamine hydrochloride

This is a phencyclidine derivative and was introduced in 1965. It differs from other i.v. anaesthetic agents in many respects, and produces dissociative anaesthesia rather than generalized depression of the CNS.

Chemical structure

2-(o-Chlorophenyl)-2-(methylamino)-cyclohexanone hydrochloride.

Physical characteristics and presentation

Ketamine is soluble in water and is presented as solutions of 10 mg.ml^{-1} containing sodium chloride to produce isotonicity, and 50 or 100 mg.ml^{-1} in multidose vials which contain benzethonium chloride 0.1 mg.ml^{-1} as preservative. The pH of the solutions is 3.5–5.5. The pK_a of ketamine is 7.5.

Pharmacology

Central nervous system. Ketamine is extremely lipid-soluble. After i.v. injection, it induces anaesthesia in 30–60 s. A single i.v. dose produces unconsciousness for 10–15 min. Ketamine is also effective within 3–4 min after i.m. injection, and has a duration of action of 15–25 min. It is a potent somatic analgesic at subanaesthetic blood concentrations. Amnesia often persists for up to 1 h after recovery of consciousness. Induction of anaesthesia is smooth, but emergence delirium may occur, with restlessness, disorientation and agitation. Vivid and often unpleasant nightmares or hallucinations may occur during recovery and for up to 24 h. The incidences of emergence delirium and hallucinations are reduced by avoidance of verbal and tactile stimulation during the recovery period, or by concomitant administration of opioids, butyrophenones, benzodiazepines or physostigmine; however, unpleasant dreams may persist. Nightmares are reported less commonly by children and elderly patients.

The EEG changes associated with ketamine are unlike those seen with other i.v. anaesthetics, and consist of loss of alpha rhythm and predominant theta activity. Cerebral metabolic rate is increased in several regions of the brain, and CBF, cerebral blood volume and intracranial pressure increase.

Cardiovascular system. Arterial pressure increases by up to 25%, and heart rate by approximately 20%. Cardiac output may rise, and myocardial oxygen consumption increases; the positive inotropic effect may be related to increased calcium influx by cyclic adenosine monophosphate. There is increased myocardial sensitivity to adrenaline. Sympathetic stimulation of the peripheral circulation is decreased, resulting in vasodilatation in tissues innervated predominantly by α-adrenergic receptors, and vasoconstriction in those with β-receptors.

Respiratory system. Transient apnoea may occur after i.v. injection, but ventilation is well-maintained thereafter, and may increase slightly, unless high doses are given. Pharyngeal and laryngeal reflexes and a patent airway are maintained well in comparison with other i.v. agents; however, their presence cannot be guaranteed, and normal precautions must be taken to protect the airway and prevent aspiration. Bronchial muscle is dilated.

Skeletal muscle. Muscle tone is usually increased. Spontaneous movements may occur, but reflex movement in response to surgery is uncommon.

Gastrointestinal system. Salivation is increased.

Uterus and placenta. Ketamine crosses the placenta readily. Fetal concentrations are approximately equal to those in the mother.

The eye. Intraocular pressure increases, although this effect is often transient. Eye movements often persist during surgical anaesthesia.

Pharmacokinetics

Only approximately 12% of ketamine is bound to protein. The initial peak concentration after i.v. injection decreases as the drug is distributed, but this occurs more slowly than with other i.v. anaesthetic agents. Metabolism occurs predominantly in the liver by demethylation and hydroxylation of the cyclohexanone ring; among the metabolites is norketamine, which is pharmacologically active. Approximately 80% of the injected dose is excreted renally as glucuronides; only 2.5% is excreted unchanged. The elimination half-life is approximately 2.5 h. Distribution and elimination are slower if halothane, benzodiazepines or barbiturates are administered concurrently.

After i.m. injection, peak concentrations are achieved after approximately 20 min.

Dosage and administration

Induction of anaesthesia is achieved with an average dose of 2 mg.kg^{-1} i.v.; larger doses may be required in some patients, and smaller doses in the elderly or shocked patient. In all cases, the drug should be administered slowly. Additional doses of 1–1.5 mg.kg^{-1} are required every 5–10 min. Between 8 and 10 mg.kg^{-1} is used i.m. A dose of 0.25–0.5 mg.kg^{-1} or an infusion of 50 μg.kg^{-1}.min^{-1} may be used to produce analgesia without loss of consciousness.

Adverse effects

1. *Emergence delirium, nightmares and hallucinations.*
2. *Hypertension and tachycardia.* This may be harmful in previously hypertensive patients and in those with ischaemic heart disease.
3. *Prolonged recovery.*
4. *Salivation.* Anticholinergic premedication is essential.
5. *Increased intracranial pressure.*
6. *Allergic reactions.* Skin rashes have been reported.

Indications

1. *The high-risk patient.* Ketamine is useful in the shocked patient. Arterial pressure may decrease if hypovolaemia is present, and the drug must be given cautiously. These patients are usually heavily sedated in the postoperative period, and the risk of nightmares is therefore minimized.

2. *Paediatric anaesthesia.* Children undergoing minor surgery, investigations (e.g. cardiac catheter-

ization), ophthalmic examinations or radiotherapy may be managed successfully with ketamine administered either i.m. or i.v.

3. *Difficult locations.* Ketamine has been used successfully at the site of accidents, and for analgesia and anaesthesia in casualties of war.

4. *Analgesia and sedation.* The analgesic action of ketamine may be employed when wound dressings are changed, or while positioning patients with pain before performing regional anaesthesia (e.g. fractured neck of femur). Ketamine has been used to sedate asthmatic patients in ITU.

5. *Developing countries.* Ketamine is used extensively in countries where anaesthetic equipment and trained staff are in short supply.

Absolute contraindications

1. *Airway obstruction.* Although the airway is maintained better with ketamine than other agents, its patency cannot be guaranteed. Inhalational agents should be used for induction of anaesthesia if airway obstruction is anticipated.

2. *Raised intracranial pressure.*

Precautions

1. *Cardiovascular disease.* Ketamine is unsuitable for patients with pre-existing hypertension, ischaemic heart disease or severe cardiac decompensation.

2. *Repeated administration.* Because of the prolonged recovery period, ketamine is not the most suitable drug for frequent procedures, e.g. prolonged courses of radiotherapy, as it disrupts sleep and eating patterns.

3. *Visceral stimulation.* Ketamine suppresses poorly the response to visceral stimulation; supplementation, e.g. with an opioid, is indicated if visceral stimulation is anticipated.

4. *Outpatient anaesthesia.* The prolonged recovery period and emergence phenomena make ketamine unsuitable for adult outpatients.

Other drugs

Benzodiazepines and opioids may also be used to induce general anaesthesia. However, very large doses are required, and recovery is prolonged. Their use is confined to specialist areas, e.g. cardiac anaesthesia. The pharmacology of these drugs is described in Chapter 10.

INTRAVENOUS MAINTENANCE OF ANAESTHESIA

Indications for intravenous maintenance of anaesthesia

There are a number of situations in which i.v. anaesthesia (IVA; the use of an i.v. anaesthetic to supplement nitrous oxide) or total i.v. anaesthesia (TIVA) may offer advantages over the traditional inhalational techniques. In the doses required to maintain clinical anaesthesia, i.v. agents cause minimal cardiovascular depression. In comparison with the most commonly used volatile anaesthetic agents, IVA with propofol (the only currently available i.v. anaesthetic with an appropriate pharmacokinetic profile) offers rapid recovery of consciousness and good recovery of psychomotor function, although the newer volatile anaesthetics desflurane and sevoflurane are also associated with rapid recovery and minimal hangover effects.

The use of TIVA allows a high inspired oxygen concentration in situations where hypoxaemia may otherwise occur, such as one-lung anaesthesia or in the severely ill or traumatized patient, and has obvious advantages in procedures such as laryngoscopy or bronchoscopy, when delivery of inhaled anaesthetic agents to the lungs may be difficult. TIVA can also be used to provide anaesthesia in circumstances where there are clinical reasons to avoid nitrous oxide, such as middle-ear surgery, prolonged bowel surgery and in patients with raised intracranial pressure (see Chapter 8). There are few contraindications to the use of IVA, provided that the anaesthetist is aware of the wide variability in response (see below). For surgical anaesthesia, it is desirable either to use nitrous oxide supplemented by IVA, or to infuse an opioid as well as the i.v. anaesthetic.

Principles of IVA

The calibrated vaporizer allows the anaesthetist

to establish stable conditions, usually with relatively few changes in delivered concentration of volatile anaesthetic agents during an operation. This is largely because the patient tends to come into equilibrium with the delivered concentration, irrespective of body size or physiological variations; the total dose of drug taken up by the body is variable, but is relatively unimportant, and is determined by the characteristics of the patient and the drug rather than by the anaesthetist. The task of achieving equilibrium with i.v. anaesthetic agents is more complex, as delivery must be matched to the size of the patient as well as to the expected rates of distribution and metabolism of the drug. Conventional methods of delivering i.v. agents result in the total dose of drug being determined by the anaesthetist, and the concentration achieved in the brain depends on the volume and rate of distribution, the relative solubility of the agent in various tissues, and the rate of elimination of the drug in the individual patient. Consequently, there is considerably more variability between patients in the infusion rate of an i.v. anaesthetic required to produce satisfactory anaesthesia than there is in the inspired concentration of an inhaled agent. There is concern among some anaesthetists that the difficulty in predicting the correct infusion rate for an individual patient may result in a higher risk of awareness in the paralysed patient.

Techniques of administration

Intermittent injection

Although some anaesthetists are skilled in the delivery of i.v. anaesthetic agents by intermittent bolus injection, the plasma concentrations of drug, and the anaesthetic effect, vary widely, and the technique is acceptable only for procedures of short duration in unparalysed patients.

Manual infusion techniques

The infusion rate required to achieve a predetermined plasma concentration of an i.v. drug can be calculated if the clearance of the drug from plasma is known [infusion rate ($\mu g.min^{-1}$) = steady-state plasma concentration ($\mu g.ml^{-1}$) × clearance ($ml.min^{-1}$)]. One of the difficulties is

that clearance is variable, and it is possible only to estimate the value by using population kinetics; depending on the patient's clearance in relation to the average, the actual plasma concentration achieved may be higher or lower than the intended concentration.

A fixed-rate infusion is inappropriate because the serum concentration of the drug increases only slowly, taking four to five times the elimination half-life of the drug to reach steady state (Fig. 9.4). A bolus injection followed by a continuous infusion results in achievement of an excessive concentration (with an increased incidence of side-effects) initially, and this is followed by a prolonged dip below the intended plasma concentration (Fig. 9.5). In order to achieve a reasonably constant plasma concentration (other than in very long procedures), it is necessary to use a multistep infusion regimen, a concept similar to that of over-pressure for inhaled agents. A commonly used scheme for propofol is injection of a bolus dose of 1 $mg.kg^{-1}$ followed by infusion initially at a rate of 10 $mg.kg^{-1}.h^{-1}$ for 10 min, then 8 $mg.kg^{-1}.h^{-1}$ for the next 10 min, and a maintenance infusion rate of 6 $mg.kg^{-1}.h^{-1}$ thereafter. This achieves, on average, a plasma concentration of propofol of 3 $\mu g.ml^{-1}$, and this is effective in achieving satisfactory anaesthesia in unparalysed patients who *also* receive nitrous oxide and fentanyl; higher infusion rates are required if nitrous oxide and fentanyl are not administered. These infusion rates must be regarded only as a guide,

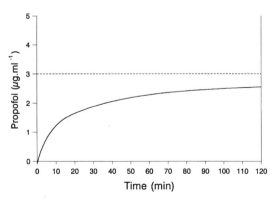

Fig. 9.4 Average blood concentration during the first 2 h of a continuous infusion of propofol at a rate of 6 $mg.kg^{-1}.h^{-1}$. Note that, even after 2 h, the equilibrium concentration of 3 $\mu g.ml^{-1}$ has not been achieved.

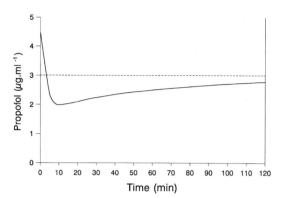

Fig. 9.5 Average blood propofol concentration following a bolus dose of propofol followed by a continuous infusion of 6 mg.kg⁻¹.h⁻¹. Note that the target concentration is initially exceeded, but that the blood concentration then falls below the target concentration, which is not achieved within 2 h.

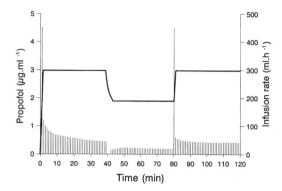

Fig. 9.6 Average blood concentrations of propofol achieved using a target-controlled infusion system. The narrow vertical lines represent the infusion rate calculated by the computer to achieve, and then to maintain, the target concentration in blood. A target concentration of 3 $\mu g.ml^{-1}$ was programmed initially. When the target concentration is reset to 2 $\mu g.ml^{-1}$, the infusion is stopped, and then restarted at a rate calculated to maintain that concentration. The target concentration is then increased to 3 $\mu g.ml^{-1}$; the infusion pump delivers a rapid infusion rate to achieve the target concentration, and then gradually decreases the infusion rate to maintain a constant blood concentration.

and must be adjusted as necessary according to clinical signs of anaesthesia.

Computer-driven infusion techniques

By programming a computer with appropriate pharmacokinetic data and equations, it is possible at frequent intervals (several times a minute) to calculate the appropriate infusion rate required to produce a preset target plasma concentration of drug. The drug is infused by a syringe driver. To produce a step increase in plasma concentration, the syringe driver infuses drug very rapidly (a slow bolus), and then delivers drug at a progressively decreasing infusion rate (Fig. 9.6). To decrease the plasma concentration, the syringe driver stops infusing until the computer calculates that the target concentration has been achieved, and then infuses drug at an appropriate rate to maintain a constant level. The anaesthetist is required only to enter the desired target concentration, and to change it when clinically indicated, in the same way as a vaporizer might be manipulated according to clinical signs of anaesthesia.

The potential advantages of such a system are its simplicity, the rapidity with which plasma concentration can be changed (particularly upwards) and avoidance of the need for the anaesthetist to undertake any calculations (resulting in less potential for error). However, the actual concentration achieved may be >50% greater than or

less than the predicted concentration, although this may not be a major practical disadvantage provided that the anaesthetist adjusts the target concentration according to clinical signs relating to adequacy of anaesthesia, rather than assuming that a specific target concentration will always result in the desired effect.

Using a target-controlled infusion system in female patients, the target concentration of propofol required to prevent movement in response to surgical incision in 50% of subjects (the equivalent of minimum alveolar concentration; MAC) was 6 $\mu g.ml^{-1}$ when patients breathed oxygen, and 4.5 $\mu g.ml^{-1}$ when 67% nitrous oxide was administered simultaneously.

Closed-loop systems

Target-controlled infusion systems may be used as part of a closed-loop system to control depth of anaesthesia. Because there is no method of measuring blood concentrations of i.v. anaesthetics on-line, it is necessary to use some form of monitor of depth of anaesthesia (such as the auditory evoked response; see Chapter 20) on the input side of the system.

DRUGS OF HISTORICAL INTEREST

Propanidid

This agent was derived from eugenol (oil of cloves), and was first used in 1964. Its duration of action was exceedingly short, as it was metabolized very rapidly by plasma cholinesterase. There were high incidences of nausea, vomiting and muscle movements. It was solubilized in Cremophor EL (polyoxylated castor oil), and was associated with an unacceptable incidence of severe anaphylactoid reactions.

γ-Hydroxybutyric acid

Anaesthesia of slow onset and recovery was produced by this agent, which is related chemically to the neurotransmitter γ-aminobutyric acid. It was introduced in 1962. It is still used for basal sedation in some European countries.

Althesin

This drug, a mixture of two steroids (alphaxalone and alphadolone), was very similar to propofol in its anaesthetic profile, but was metabolized even more rapidly. It was introduced in 1972. In common with propanidid, it was solubilized in Cremophor EL, and an unacceptable number of adverse reactions were reported.

ADVERSE REACTIONS TO INTRAVENOUS ANAESTHETIC AGENTS

These may take the form of pain on injection, venous thrombosis, involuntary muscle movement, hiccup, hypotension and postoperative delirium. All of these reactions may be modified by the anaesthetic technique.

Hypersensitivity reactions, which resemble the effects of histamine release, are more rare and less predictable. Other vasoactive agents may be released also. Reactions to i.v. anaesthetic agents are usually caused by one of the following mechanisms:

1. *Type I hypersensitivity response.* The drug interacts with specific immunoglobulin E (IgE) antibodies, which are often bound to the surface of mast cells; these become granulated and release histamine and other vasoactive amines.

2. *Classical complement-mediated reaction.* The classical complement pathway may be activated by type II (cell surface antigen) *or* type III (immune complex formation) hypersensitivity reactions. IgG or IgM antibodies are involved.

3. *Alternate complement pathway activation.* Preformed antibodies to an antigen are not necessary for activation of this pathway; thus, these reactions may occur without prior exposure to the drug.

4. *Direct pharmacological effects of the drug.* These anaphylactoid reactions result from a direct effect on mast cells and basophils. There may be local cutaneous signs only. In more severe reactions there are signs of systemic release of histamine.

Clinical features

In a severe hypersensitivity reaction, a flush may develop over the upper part of the body. There is usually hypotension, which may be profound. Cutaneous and glottic oedema may develop, and may result in hypovolaemia because of loss of fluid from the circulation. Very severe bronchospasm may also occur, although it is a feature in less than 50% of reactions. Diarrhoea often occurs some hours after the initial reaction.

Predisposing factors

1. *Age.* In general, adverse reactions are less common in children than in adults.

2. *Pregnancy.* There is an increased incidence of adverse reactions in pregnancy.

3. *Gender.* Anaphylactic reactions are more common in women.

4. *Atopy.* There may be an increased incidence of type IV (delayed hypersensitivity) reactions in non-atopic individuals, and a higher incidence of type I reactions in those with a history of extrinsic asthma, hayfever or penicillin allergy.

5. *Previous exposure.* Previous exposure to the drug, or to a drug with similar constituents, exerts a much greater influence on the incidence of reactions than does a history of atopy.

6. *Solvents.* Cremophor EL, which was used as

Table 9.6 Incidences of adverse reactions to intravenous anaesthetic agents

Drug	Incidence
Thiopentone	1:14 000–1:20 000
Methohexitone	1:1600–1:7000
Althesin	1:400–1:11 000
Propanidid	1:500–1:17 000
Etomidate	1:450 000
Propofol	1:50 000–100 000 (estimated)

a solvent for a number of i.v. anaesthetic agents, was associated with a high incidence of hypersensitivity reactions.

Incidence

The incidences of hypersensitivity reactions associated with i.v. anaesthetic agents are shown in Table 9.6.

Treatment

This is summarized in Table 9.7.

Table 9.7 Management of allergic reactions

AIMS
Correct arterial hypoxaemia
Restore intravascular fluid volume
Inhibit further release of chemical mediators

ROUTINE
Airway

Added inspired oxygen

Adrenaline (either intravenous or intramuscular, depending on the severity of the reaction) 0.5 ml of 1:1000

Fluids: both crystalloids (normal saline or Hartman's solution) and colloids. The former may be ineffective in some cases

Bronchodilators if there is bronchospasm (e.g. aminophylline, 250–500 mg i.v.). If adverse reaction occurs during anaesthesia, consider use of halothane, ether or ketamine for the relief of bronchoconstriction

Intermittent positive-pressure ventilation (IPPV): continue after resuscitation if there is pulmonary oedema

Use of inotropes to support the circulation, and *antiarrhythmic drugs*

No data to show a beneficial effect of steroids in acute allergic anaphylactic reactions
No agent affects the gastrointestinal symptoms
Isoprenaline may worsen arterial hypoxaemia, by increasing dead space
Antihistamines may be useful in angioneurotic oedema

Consider cerebral resuscitation if there is a prolonged period of arrest, hypotension or arterial hypoxaemia (e.g. mannitol, IPPV with mild hypocapnia)

FURTHER READING

Nimmo W S, Rowbotham D J, Smith G (eds) 1994 Anaesthesia, 2nd edn. Blackwell Scientific Publications. Oxford
Saidman L J 1974 Uptake, distribution and elimination of barbiturates. In: Eger E I (ed) Anesthetic uptake and action. Williams & Wilkins, Baltimore
Schwilden H, Stoeckel H, Schüttler J 1989 Closed-loop feedback control of propofol anaesthesia by quantitative EEG analysis in humans. British Journal of Anaesthesia 62: 290–296

Sear J W 1983 General kinetic and dynamic principles and their application to continuous infusion anaesthesia. Anaesthesia 38 (suppl): 10–25
Sear J W 1994 Adverse effects of drugs given by injection. In: Taylor T H, Major E (eds) Hazards and complications of anaesthesia, 2nd edn. Churchill Livingstone, Edinburgh, pp. 273–306

10. Drugs used to supplement anaesthesia

ANALGESICS

Opioids

The opioid analgesics are drugs which act on a variety of specific receptors both centrally in the CNS and peripherally. They are sometimes termed 'narcotics' but this is a US legal definition implying physical dependence and is best avoided. The term 'opiate' suggests that the drug is derived from opium but since many compounds used in anaesthetic practice are synthetic or semisynthetic, this term should also usually be avoided.

Drugs such as morphine, which bind to opioid receptors and produce dose-dependent agonist effects, are termed 'opioid agonists'. Naloxone binds to opioid receptors also, antagonizing the effects of morphine, and is termed an opioid antagonist. The term 'opioid agonist-antagonist' is applied to drugs such as nalbuphine which possess agonist effects at one receptor type and antagonist effects at another. As the dose–response relationships differ at each receptor type, biphasic clinical effects may be observed, e.g. antagonism of opioid-induced analgesia at low doses and analgesia at high doses. The partial opioid agonists, e.g. buprenorphine, have a morphine-like action in low concentrations, but the agonist effect reaches a plateau and increased doses have no further effect. Table 10.1 contains a classification of some commonly used opioids.

Endogenous opioids

These are a series of endogenous polypeptides (the endorphins and enkephalins) possessing analgesic properties similar to those of exogenous opioids. The enkephalins are found in high concentrations

Table 10.1 Classification of commonly used opioids

Opioid agonists
1. Natural opium alkaloids:
   Morphine
   Codeine
2. Semisynthetic opium alkaloid:
   Diamorphine
3. Synthetic opioids:
   Pethidine
   Fentanyl
   Alfentanil
   Sufentanil
   Remifentanil

Partial opioid agonists
Buprenorphine

Opioid agonist/antagonists
Pentazocine
Nalbuphine

Opioid antagonists
Naloxone
Naltrexone

in the central grey matter of the brain stem and the substantia gelatinosa of the spinal cord, a distribution corresponding with areas of high opioid receptor density. Enkephalins modulate pain perception both at higher centres and in the spinal cord, in the latter through a mechanism involving substance P. It is thought that whereas both enkephalins and β-endorphin have a central role, only the enkephalins act at the spinal level. β-Endorphin is structurally a much larger molecule with a longer duration of action, although only present at one-tenth the proportion of the enkephalins. It is present in high concentrations in the hypothalamic–pituitary axis and regulates endocrine function.

The enkephalins have little analgesic activity

since they are rapidly inactivated by peptidases; they are principally inhibitory neurotransmitters. In contrast, the larger β-endorphin molecule resists inactivation and has powerful, generalized analgesic properties. There is evidence that endogenous opioids are an important element in the immune system.

Opioid receptors

Opioids act on specific receptors which are distributed throughout the CNS and are the site of action of all opioids. There are three classes of receptor: μ (mu), κ (kappa) and δ (delta). The σ (sigma) receptor is associated with dysphoria and is not a true opioid receptor because its effects are not reversed by high concentrations of naloxone. Drugs which bind to σ receptors include pentazocine, nalbuphine and ketamine. Recently, the μ receptors have been subdivided into two types: high affinity μ_1 (mediating analgesia) and lower affinity μ_2 (mediating ventilatory depression). Table 10.2 lists the effects produced by pharmacological stimulation of the various receptors. Opioid receptors are also present outside the CNS at the distal ends of some C-fibres. This offers the possibility of a novel approach to pain management.

The effects of some opioid drugs on the three main receptor types are shown in Table 10.3. In theory, opioids with partial agonist effects at the μ receptor, or those with mixed agonist and antagonist actions, might produce analgesia equivalent to that of morphine but with less depression of ventilation. However, none of the drugs developed to date has achieved this goal.

Table 10.2 Effects of pharmacological stimulation of the opioid receptors

	μ_1	μ_2	δ	κ
Central analgesic effect	Yes	–	High doses only	–
Spinal analgesic effect	Yes	–	Yes	Yes
Behaviour	Euphoria	–	–	Sedation Dysphoria
Ventilation	–	Depression	–	?Depression
Pupil	Miosis	–	–	Miosis
Dependence	Yes	–	Yes	–
Gut	–	Inhibition	Endotoxic shock	–

Table 10.3 Effects of some opioid drugs on the three types of opioid receptor

Drug	μ	δ	κ
Morphine	Agonist	–	–
Pethidine	Agonist	–	–
Fentanyl	Agonist	–	–
Buprenorphine	Partial agonist	–	–
Nalbuphine	Antagonist	–	Partial agonist
Naloxone	Antagonist	Antagonist	Antagonist
Naltrexone	Antagonist	–	–
Pentazocine	Antagonist	–	Agonist
DADL (D-Ala^2-D-Leu^5-enkephalin)	–	Agonist	–

Pharmacokinetics and pharmacodynamics

Although the pattern of receptor occupancy determines the clinical effect of some opioids, the differences between the actions of the μ agonists result largely from pharmacokinetic and pharmacodynamic factors. The principles of drug distribution are described in Chapter 7. The initial distribution of opioids into CNS is related to the degree of ionization of the drug in blood and to the lipid solubility of the unionized portion. Drugs which are less soluble in lipid, e.g. morphine, reach the receptors more slowly than highly lipid-soluble agents, e.g. fentanyl. Thus, a drug of low lipid solubility has a slow onset of action; CNS concentrations decay slowly as drug is eliminated from the body by metabolism and excretion. In contrast, a lipid-soluble opioid with a short distribution half-life acts rapidly, because the drug transfers readily into CNS along a high initial blood–brain concentration gradient. The duration of action is short because brain and blood concentrations decrease after redistribution of the drug to other vessel-rich tissues. However, if a large dose is given, the effect of the drug declines only when blood concentrations decrease as a result of elimination; the duration of action is related usually to the elimination half-life of the drug. Hepatic extraction of opioids is reduced during general anaesthesia, because of reduced hepatic blood flow and impaired hepatic clearance.

Another factor which influences clinical action is the presence of active metabolites. The most significant of these is morphine-6-glucuronide, which is a more potent μ agonist than morphine itself. Although the water-soluble metabolites of morphine are normally excreted fairly rapidly, they are known to accumulate in patients with renal insufficiency and may result in a prolonged duration of action. Opioid metabolites are present in high concentrations after oral administration as a result of first-pass metabolism.

The following factors must be considered in order to minimize the risk of postoperative ventilatory depression when determining the appropriate dose of an opioid for intraoperative use.

1. *Age.* There is increased sensitivity to opioids in the elderly.

2. *Duration of surgery.* The anticipated duration of analgesic action of the chosen opioid should match the duration of surgery.

3. *Other depressant drugs.* Anaesthetic and sedative agents which depress ventilation may have additive effects with opioids.

4. *Pulmonary disease.* The respiratory depressant actions of opioids may precipitate ventilatory failure; special care is required in patients with chronic obstructive airways disease. The antitussive action of opioids may impair postoperative clearance of pulmonary or bronchial secretions. Obese patients or those with other conditions which restrict pulmonary expansion, e.g. severe kyphosis, may develop ventilatory insufficiency when given opioids. The effects of morphine on bronchial smooth muscle may aggravate bronchospasm in patients with asthma, and pethidine, although shorter-acting, may be preferable.

5. *Endocrine abnormalities.* There is increased opioid sensitivity in hypothyroidism and Addison's disease.

6. *Hepatic disease.* There may be increased sensitivity to some opioids, particularly in cirrhosis and infective hepatitis, because of reduced drug metabolism.

7. *Intracranial pathology.* Administration of opioids interferes with assessment of conscious level. Intracranial pressure may increase due to hypercapnia secondary to depression of ventilation.

8. *Miscellaneous.* There is increased sensitivity in patients who are debilitated or who have chronic infection. Patients with advanced malignancy may develop resistance and require very large doses.

Contrary to popular opinion, dose–response relationships for opioids are not related to body weight in adults.

Interaction with monoamine oxidase inhibitors (MAOI)

Life-threatening complications may follow the administration of pethidine to patients receiving MAOI therapy. Convulsions, coma, hypertensive crises and hyperpyrexia have all been reported. This situation is less clear with the other opioids but if at all possible they should be avoided in these patients.

Morphine

Although it is possible to synthesize morphine, it is produced commercially from the dried juices of the seed capsules of the poppy *Papaver somniferum*. Morphine is a tertiary amine and a weak base. It is more water-soluble than most other opioids used in anaesthetic practice. Although morphine has a number of undesirable side-effects, it is an excellent analgesic and represents the 'gold standard' against which all other opioids are judged. The drug is presented usually as morphine sulphate; 10 mg morphine sulphate contains approximately 8.5 mg anhydrous morphine.

Actions

The actions of morphine may be classified as central and peripheral (Table 10.4); it has both depressant and stimulant effects on the CNS.

Analgesia

Somatic and visceral types of pain are relieved. However, morphine is more effective against dull and continuous than sharp and intermittent pain.

Table 10.4 Summary of actions and side-effects of morphine

Central
Depressant
  Analgesia
  Sedation
  Depression of cough reflex
  Depression of respiratory centre
  Depression of metabolic rate (hypothermia)
  Depression of vasomotor centre
Excitatory
  Euphoria, hallucinations
  Convulsions (in very high dosage)
  Miosis (stimulation of oculomotor centre)
  Vomiting }
  Nausea   } (stimulation of chemoreceptor trigger zone)
  Bradycardia (vagal stimulation)
  Release of ADH and other pituitary hormones

Peripheral
Antinociceptive
Increase in smooth muscle tone
Histamine release
  Bronchospasm
  Hypotension
  Erythema
  Sensation of warmth, flushing

The pain threshold is elevated and the psychological and emotional components of pain (see Chapter 24) diminished. These effects are augmented by a sensation of euphoria and drowsiness which, as the dose is increased, progresses to sleep and eventually to an anaesthetic state characterized by decreased reflex irritability and profound ventilatory depression.

Respiratory system

Depression of ventilation occurs as a result of direct depression of the medullary respiratory centre. The carbon dioxide response curve is shifted to the right and the slope is reduced (Fig. 10.1). Both ventilatory rate and tidal volume decrease within 2–5 min after i.v. injection and more slowly after i.m. administration.

Depression of the cough reflex occurs after administration of morphine and its derivatives.

Cardiovascular system

There is little effect on arterial blood pressure in normal supine individuals. However, hypotension may occur in patients who are hypovolaemic or to whom drugs with vasodilator properties (e.g. phenothiazines) have been administered, as morphine may cause peripheral arteriolar and venous dilatation as a result of central depression of the vasomotor centre, reduction in vasoconstrictor tone and release of histamine.

Bradycardia occurs occasionally as a result of stimulation of the vagal centre.

Gastrointestinal system

Nausea and vomiting. These symptoms are distressing and unpleasant and represent one of the most common complaints after operation. Morphine stimulates the chemoreceptor trigger zone in the floor of the fourth ventricle; it may cause nausea with or without vomiting some hours after administration, persisting for 6–8 h. This side-effect appears to be a dopamine-like effect; drugs with dopamine-blocking actions, e.g. butyrophenones and phenothiazines, are effective antiemetics in opioid-induced vomiting. However, there is also a vestibular component to morphine-

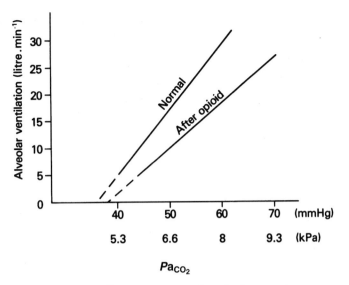

Fig. 10.1 The ventilatory response to Pa_{CO_2} in the normal individual and after administration of morphine. Note that the response curve is not only shifted to the right but that its slope is decreased also.

induced vomiting and ambulant patients are more likely to suffer from this side-effect. The emetic effects of morphine are similar to those of other opioids administered in equianalgesic doses.

Gastrointestinal motility. Morphine causes reduced peristalsis, but increased non-peristaltic contractility, in the gastrointestinal system. Gastric emptying is delayed and this may contribute to vomiting. Absorption of orally administered drugs is impaired and constipation is common with prolonged use. Increased non-peristaltic bowel contractility may contribute to dehiscence of large bowel anastomoses. Smooth muscle contraction is increased in the sphincter of Oddi, the ureter and the bladder sphincter. Morphine should be avoided in biliary and renal colic. Occasionally it may produce biliary pain if given as a premedicant in patients scheduled to undergo cholecystectomy.

Eye

Miosis (pupillary constriction) results from stimulation of the Edinger–Westphal nucleus of the oculomotor centre and may interfere with assessment of depth of anaesthesia.

Other actions

Histamine release. This is responsible for the flush and sensation of warmth which follow i.v. injection and for erythema at or near the site of injection. Bronchospasm occurs occasionally and morphine should be administered to asthmatic patients with caution.

Endocrine effects. These include release of ADH from the anterior pituitary and inhibition of release of ACTH, FSH and LH. These actions resemble those of endogenous opioids.

Metabolic. Large doses of morphine may contribute to hypothermia by decreasing muscle activity and basal metabolic rate and by increasing heat loss through vasodilatation.

Distribution and elimination

After i.v. injection, 35% of morphine is bound to protein. The remainder is distributed with a half-life of 20–25 min (Table 10.5). Plasma concentrations depend subsequently on metabolism, redistribution back into the vascular compartment, excretion and possibly enterohepatic recirculation. Metabolism occurs predominantly in the liver; the drug is inactivated by dealkylation,

Table 10.5 Physical and pharmacokinetic data related to some common opioid drugs. V_{ss} – volume of distribution at steady state; $T_{\frac{1}{2}\alpha}$ – distribution half-life; $T_{\frac{1}{2}\beta}$ – elimination half-life; Cl, clearance. Lipid solubility is expressed as octanol:water partition coefficient. Pharmacokinetic values are averages in adults; there is wide interindividual variability

Drug	V_{ss} (litre)	$T_{\frac{1}{2}\alpha}$ (min)	$T_{\frac{1}{2}\beta}$ (h)	Cl (litre.min^{-1})	Lipid solubility
Morphine	200	25	3.5	1.2	1.4
Methadone	420	10	36	0.15	116
Pethidine	250	8	3.5	0.8	40
Fentanyl	375	3	4	1.0	810
Alfentanil	36	2	1.5	0.3	130
Sufentanil	98	1	2.5	0.75	1800

oxidation and conjugation with glucuronide. The elimination half-life of morphine is 2–4 h. However, one of the two major metabolites, morphine-6-glucuronide, is active and is present in high concentrations. Consequently, the clinical effect of morphine may exceed that expected from the elimination half-life, particularly in patients who have impaired renal function and who are unable to excrete the water-soluble metabolites normally.

Morphine crosses the placental barrier and may depress neonatal ventilation profoundly.

Dosage and administration

After i.v. administration, analgesia reaches a peak after 15–20 min. Failure to appreciate this delay in onset of action may result in overdosage if incremental doses are given frequently. The dose of morphine selected for intraoperative use depends on the type of premedication, anticipated duration of surgery and general health of the patient. In a healthy adult, a single bolus dose of 10–15 mg i.v. or administration of incremental doses of 2–5 mg at 20 min intervals is appropriate.

In the postoperative period, morphine was traditionally administered by the i.m. route, in a dose of 5–20 mg; the peak effect occurs 60–90 min after administration but there is great variation between individual patients. The duration of action after either i.v. or i.m. injection is 3–4 h.

Patient-controlled analgesia (PCA) is becoming standard therapy after major operations (see below).

Oral morphine is used in the treatment of chronic pain in the form of morphine sulphate tablets (MST). The bioavailability of oral morphine is only 20–30% because of first-pass metabolism in the gut wall and liver and thus higher doses are required. However, the concentration of morphine-6-glucuronide is also higher than after i.v. or i.m. administration. Thus, oral morphine is effective in a dose of 20–40 mg. Morphine should not be administered orally in the early postoperative period, as gastric emptying is impaired.

Diamorphine

Diamorphine (diacetylmorphine) is a semisynthetic morphine derivative with similar actions and side-effects. It is approximately twice as potent as morphine and has a more rapid onset of action because of greater lipid solubility. Diamorphine undergoes rapid deacetylation, first to mono-acetylmorphine (an active opioid) and then very rapidly to morphine. It is said to produce more euphoric and antitussive actions and to cause less respiratory depression, nausea and vomiting than morphine; these claims have not been substantiated in clinical trials. Diamorphine may be regarded as a pro-drug for the active metabolites monoacetylmorphine and morphine. It is administered usually in a dose of 5–10 mg i.v. or i.m. (reduced by 50% in elderly patients).

Papaveretum

This is a partially purified extract of opium and contains 50% anhydrous morphine. The remainder comprises other alkaloids (principally codeine, noscapine, narcotine and papaverine) with a mixture of analgesic and smooth muscle effects. Consequently, papaveretum causes less spasm of smooth muscle than morphine alone. The Committee on Safety of Medicines proscribed its use in women of childbearing age because of its noscapine content but a new formulation without noscapine is now available. Papaveretum 20 mg is equipotent with morphine 12.5 mg in respect of analgesia, but there is a greater degree of sedation and possibly of ventilatory depression. The average dose for a healthy adult is 15–20 mg i.m.

Pethidine

Pethidine is a synthetic opioid with an analgesic potency approximately one-tenth that of morphine. It has mild cholinergic effects and relaxes smooth muscle. It produces sedation but little euphoria. Ventilatory depression is similar in degree to that produced by morphine in equipotent doses, but pethidine has no specific action on the cough reflex.

Unlike morphine, pethidine possesses mild quinidine-like actions which may reduce myocardial excitability and the incidence of ventricular arrhythmias. This may be related to the local anaesthetic action of pethidine. Arterial blood pressure is normally unaffected, but hypotension may occur in the hypovolaemic patient as a result of venous and arterial dilatation.

Pethidine tends to relax the tone of smooth muscle in the gastrointestinal and renal tracts. It is useful for renal colic but also reduces motility. The incidence of nausea and vomiting is similar to or slightly greater than that associated with morphine. It produces less release of histamine than morphine and is preferable for asthmatic patients.

Pethidine may be used in a dose of 25–50 mg i.v. or 100–150 mg i.m. in the healthy adult. Its duration of action is 2–3 h. It crosses the placenta and may cause ventilatory depression in the fetus; however, this is of shorter duration than that resulting from morphine. One of its metabolites, norpethidine, causes hyperexcitability and convulsions; norpethidine may accumulate if large doses of pethidine are given to patients with renal insufficiency.

Pethidine should not be given to patients taking monoamine oxidase inhibitors (see above).

Buprenorphine

This is a synthetic analgesic derived from the opium alkaloid thebaine and is closely related structurally to morphine. It is a partial agonist at the μ receptor; thus, there is a 'ceiling' to its analgesic action. Buprenorphine has a low potential for physical dependence and is not subject at present to controlled drug regulations. It has a delayed onset of action and, although its elimi-

nation half-life is 2–4.5 h, its duration of action is prolonged (6–8 h) because of slow dissociation from the μ receptor. It is a potent agent; buprenorphine 0.4 mg is equianalgesic with morphine 10 mg.

Euphoria and dysphoria occur infrequently, but marked sedation and drowsiness are common in the elderly and have limited the usefulness of the drug. Ventilatory depression may be of slow onset but prolonged duration and although in theory there is a 'ceiling', the point at which this is reached is usually not obvious. Ventilatory depression may be difficult to reverse even with large doses of naloxone; it is probably preferable to use a nonspecific ventilatory stimulant, e.g. doxapram.

A dose of 0.3–0.6 mg i.v. or i.m. is appropriate for an adult. A sublingual tablet is available in a dose of 0.2 mg which is effective after major surgery, although parenteral buprenorphine may be required initially because of the slow onset of analgesia. Buprenorphine undergoes a high degree of first-pass metabolism and has a low bioavailability if administered orally. In the event of the sublingual tablet being inadvertently swallowed, the risk of overdose is small if the dose is repeated.

Buprenorphine displaces other opioid agonists from the μ receptor and may antagonize analgesia induced previously by, for example, morphine. Consequently, if buprenorphine is to be used for provision of postoperative analgesia, it should also be employed during anaesthesia if an intraoperative analgesic is required.

Fentanyl

Fentanyl is a synthetic opioid related structurally to pethidine. Its analgesic potency is approximately 100 times that of morphine. It is very lipid-soluble and reaches opioid receptors very rapidly. Thus, its onset of action occurs in 1–2 min. After a single dose, its duration of action is limited to 20–30 min by redistribution but in high doses or after infusion its effects may last for 2–5 h and are terminated by elimination of the drug; in the elderly, its actions may last for up to 9 h.

Respiratory system

Doses in excess of 50 μg in combination with

anaesthetic drugs may result in depression of ventilation for several minutes. Large doses or an infusion of fentanyl should be used only if IPPV is planned.

Delayed ventilatory depression may occur after a bolus i.v. dose. This may be related to sequestration in gastric juice and subsequent absorption from the small intestine; this phenomenon occurs with most opioids, but peaks in blood concentration are reflected rapidly by an increase in the CNS effects of fentanyl because of its high lipid solubility.

Cardiovascular system

Fentanyl has little effect. A small reduction in arterial blood pressure may occur and heart rate may decrease because of vagal stimulation.

Other effects

Sedation is relatively poor in comparison with that produced by morphine or pethidine. The incidences of nausea and vomiting are similar to those associated with other opioids.

Chest wall rigidity may occur after large doses of fentanyl, making artificial ventilation of the lungs difficult.

Fentanyl causes little release of histamine.

Spasm of the sphincter of Oddi has occurred after moderate doses of fentanyl, mimicking the presence of a gallstone on intraoperative cholangiography.

Dosage

Fentanyl is used most commonly as an analgesic supplement during anaesthesia. Doses of 50–100 µg may be given i.v. to the spontaneously breathing patient. Larger doses (200–800 µg i.v.) are appropriate when IPPV is used; the dose selected is determined by the anticipated duration of surgery. Fentanyl has been used in very high doses, e.g. 50 µg.kg^{-1}, for major surgery in order to avoid the use of volatile anaesthetic agents. These large doses may totally suppress the metabolic effects of anaesthesia and surgery (increased plasma concentrations of glucose, cortisol, GH, ACTH, etc). However, the duration of action

is very prolonged and patients may require IPPV for some hours after operation; even if spontaneous ventilation appears adequate, observation is required in the ITU for 24 h postoperatively.

Transdermal fentanyl has been used with some success for postoperative analgesia and the control of cancer pain. An i.v. loading dose is required to establish a therapeutic plasma concentration initially. The rate at which drug reaches the circulation is governed by the characteristics of the skin patch membrane interface with the skin, and skin blood flow. Drugs must be highly lipid-soluble and of high potency if they are to be administered successfully by this route.

Alfentanil

This synthetic derivative of fentanyl has a high lipid solubility and acts within one arm–brain circulation time after i.v. administration. It has a small volume of distribution and short elimination half-life and therefore has a short duration of action even after large doses. Consequently, it is more suitable for continuous i.v. infusion during surgery than is fentanyl, as postoperative depression of ventilation is less likely. It is less cumulative than morphine when given as a long-term infusion to patients with acute renal failure.

Alfentanil depresses the cardiovascular system to a greater extent than fentanyl, particularly in the elderly and in patients of ASA classes III or IV.

Depression of ventilation is common for some minutes after administration of alfentanil and the drug should be administered only if equipment is available for IPPV.

Doses approaching 500 µg of alfentanil may be given to patients who are breathing spontaneously; the duration of action is only 5–10 min. An initial bolus dose followed by a continuous infusion (30–60 µg.min^{-1}) is appropriate for patients receiving IPPV.

Infusion of alfentanil may be preferable to morphine for patients in the intensive care unit with renal failure.

Patient-controlled analgesia (PCA)

This method of i.v. opioid delivery is replacing

the traditional i.m. regimen and is indicated after major surgery when significant pain is anticipated. Although there are some differences between PCA delivery systems, the underlying principles and operation of all are identical. Patients request an increment of opioid by pressing a button which, in turn, triggers release of the opioid through a venous cannula either from a syringe driver or a simple balloon type reservoir under pressure. The delivery system is designed so that a maximum dose predetermined by the anaesthetist is delivered per bolus increment. A 'lock-out' interval is also selected by the anaesthetist, during which requests for additional analgesic result in non-delivery of drug. A maximum dose over a longer period can sometimes be specified and the system may operate either with or without a background infusion of the chosen opioid. These safeguards make opioid overdosage unlikely provided that appropriate doses and lock-out times are employed.

A typical regimen, widely advocated, uses morphine 1 mg increments with a lock-out period of 5 min without a background infusion. Although this is pharmacokinetically flawed, in practice it provides superior analgesia, and is probably safer, than intermittent intramuscular injections. However, to be effective, it is necessary for the anaesthetist first to gain control of any pain by administering appropriate doses of opioid intravenously. Only then can the system be transferred to patient control. It is vital to impress upon patients that from that moment they are in control of their analgesia and can titrate, within set limits, the amount of intravenous opioid they receive. Other opioids have been used successfully in PCA systems, notably fentanyl and pethidine.

The supervision of this type of pain delivery system is the responsibility of the acute pain team. Nurses and junior medical staff involved in day-to-day management should understand the principle of the method and be familar with the delivery system in use. Protocols are essential to ensure standardized and effective management of drug delivery and of complications arising, especially respiratory depression and airway obstruction. Clearly, some patients will be unable to use these devices due to mental impairment, confusion or debility. Others may choose to retain closer contact with the nursing staff and to rely on traditional regimens.

Patient-controlled analgesia may be employed also for subcutaneous administration of diamorphine or other opioids for the relief of pain in the terminally ill.

Serious degrees of ventilatory depression are an uncommon, if unpredictable, sequel of PCA and there is no doubt that, from the patient's point of view, the most troublesome side-effects are nausea and vomiting. Although a wide variety of antiemetics have been used (see above), including $5HT_3$ antagonists, there is no consensus as to which is the most useful or cost-effective.

A continuous infusion of morphine is used occasionally after operation. A dose of 1–2 mg.h^{-1} is usually appropriate, but must be adjusted according to the individual patient's response. Continuous intravenous infusions of opioid must be administered only in a high-dependency or intensive therapy unit because of the risk of cumulation and ventilatory depression.

Spinal opioids (see also p. 442)

It was demonstrated in 1976 that opioid receptors exist in the spinal cord and that analgesia results if these are blocked locally by administration of opioid drugs. Many subsequent studies have confirmed that administration of opioids by either the subarachnoid or extradural route produces analgesia without the cardiovascular side-effects that result from spinal administration of local anaesthetic drugs. Many studies attest to the superior analgesic effect of subarachnoid or extradural opioids combined with local anaesthetic, usually bupivacaine, over conventional intramuscular opioid injections. Whereas the subarachnoid route is particularly suited to orthopaedic operations on the lower limb, the extradural route has more general applicability.

Almost all opioids have been administered by one or both of the spinal routes. In general, drugs which are poorly lipid-soluble may be given in smaller doses (relative to the systemic dose) than more lipid-soluble agents (Tables 10.5 and 10.6) and thus produce fewer side-effects attributable to high circulating concentrations of drug; they also have a longer duration of action. However,

Table 10.6 Doses of intrathecal and extradural opioids

Drug	Route	Bolus	Infusion
Morphine	Intrathecal	0.1–0.5 mg	–
	Extradural	2–5 mg	0.5–2 mg.kg^{-1}.h^{-1}
Pethidine	Intrathecal	0.1 mg.kg^{-1}	–
	Extradural	0.75 mg.kg^{-1}	–
Diamorphine	Intrathecal	0.5–1.0 mg	–
	Extradural	1–5 mg	0.4–0.8 mg.kg^{-1}.h^{-1}
Fentanyl	Extradural	1–2 μg.kg^{-1}	1–2 μg.kg^{-1}.h^{-1}
Sufentanil	Extradural	0.05 mg	–
Buprenorphine	Extradural	0.3 mg	–

a higher proportion of the less lipid-soluble drugs remains in CSF and may result in a greater degree of spread of analgesia. This occurs because diffusion within the CSF, and circulation of the CSF itself, carry the drug to segments of the spinal cord away from the site of injection; this increases the risk of opioid reaching the brain stem, where it may cause ventilatory depression some hours after administration ('delayed ventilatory depression').

Spinal opioids are useful after major surgery when there are no contraindications to the use of subarachnoid or extradural techniques (see Ch. 25). Bolus administration through an extradural catheter results in analgesia for 6–12 h and continuous infusions with and without local anaesthetic have also been used to provide uninterrupted pain relief for 48 h or longer. Subarachnoid administration of opioids results in analgesia of long duration with a much smaller dose than would be required systemically. The duration of analgesia, and the incidence and magnitude of side-effects, are dose-related.

Side-effects

1. *Ventilatory depression.* The incidence is highest with lipid-insoluble drugs, e.g. morphine, but is a potential risk with *any* opioid administered by the spinal route. It may occur unpredictably up to 12 h after administration. Although serious depression is uncommon, it is more likely to occur in older patients or if systemic opioids have also been administered. Ventilatory rate is not a reliable indicator of opioid-induced ventilatory depression; patients who have received spinal opioids *must* be nursed by trained recovery staff for at least 12 h after the last dose of opioid in a high dependency area equipped with peripheral oxygen saturation and ECG monitors.

2. *Urinary retention.* This occurs in approximately 90% of men. It is commoner after subarachnoid than extradural administration.

3. *Pruritus.* Itching occurs in 70–80% of patients who receive extradural morphine, although it causes distress in only 5–10%. It is less common when other opioids are used.

4. *Nausea and vomiting.* There is no doubt that, in common with patient-controlled methods of opioid administration, these are the most troublesome side-effects of spinal opioids. Of all the antiemetics which have been tried, prochlorperazine seems to provide good control without unpleasant side-effects of its own.

At present, the use of spinal opioids cannot be considered as a routine method of providing postoperative analgesia in the majority of patients because of the high incidence of side-effects and the requirement for close nursing supervision. However, these techniques are appropriate in patients undergoing very painful procedures such as total knee replacement or anterior cruciate ligament repair where other forms of pain control are either poorly effective or associated with even more undesirable side-effects.

Other opioids

Several other opioids are used occasionally during anaesthesia.

Sufentanil

This drug is related to fentanyl and is 600–700 times more potent than morphine. It is highly lipid-soluble and has a more rapid onset of action than fentanyl; its duration of action is slightly shorter. It is a suitable alternative to fentanyl for intraoperative use, in a dose of 5–10 μg for the spontaneously breathing patient and 25–30 μg in those receiving IPPV. However, it has a very high therapeutic index and doses of 10–30 μg.kg^{-1} have been used to produce hypnosis and analgesia during surgery.

Tramadol

This agent, introduced recently to the UK but available in some other European countries for some years, has agonist activity at the μ receptor. It also inhibits noradrenaline and 5-hydroxy-tryptamine uptake and the release of serotonin.

Tramadol is thought to produce less depression of ventilation than other μ agonists and its analgesic effect may not be mediated at opioid receptors. It does not appear to produce effective analgesia by the extradural route.

Methadone

Methadone is equipotent with morphine, but has a long elimination half-life (35 h) because of the limited capacity of the liver to metabolize the drug. It is not recommended for repeated administration. Analgesia lasts for approximately 20 h.

Nalbuphine

This is a synthetic agonist-antagonist opioid related to naloxone. It possesses a 'ceiling' effect in respect of ventilatory depression, but its analgesic effects are also restricted. It has a potency 0.5–0.75 times that of morphine. Nalbuphine reduces cardiac work, but has a minimal effect on arterial pressure or heart rate.

Pentazocine

Pentazocine is a synthetic agonist-antagonist opioid. Ventilatory depression is said to reach a 'ceiling'. Its analgesic potency is one-third that of morphine. Pentazocine is non-addictive but produces marked dysphoria in some patients. It can be administered by the oral, intramuscular or intravenous routes.

Opioid antagonists

These drugs act as competitive antagonists at opioid receptor sites both in the CNS and peripheral tissues. Some of the antagonists also possess intrinsic agonist activity and have different affinities for different receptor types. Thus, they may behave as competitive antagonists at one site but agonists at another. Naloxone and naltrexone are the only drugs with pure antagonist activity at all opioid receptors.

Naloxone

This opioid antagonist is related structurally to oxymorphone. It is well tolerated and rarely causes any side-effect. It acts within 1 min of i.v. injection and has a duration of action of approximately 30 min. This relatively short duration may result in return of ventilatory depression induced by an opioid of longer action. Consequently, patients should be monitored carefully for an appropriate period after its use.

All the CNS effects of opioids administered systemically are antagonized by naloxone, including analgesia. In low doses, naloxone antagonizes opioid-induced ventilatory depression and excessive sedation without affecting pain relief. Thus, the drug should be titrated slowly against the clinical effect to avoid the emergence of excessive pain. Analgesia produced by administration of spinal opioids is antagonized only by very large doses of naloxone. Arterial pressure may increase after administration of naloxone, but this results usually from reduction in the degree of sedation or emergence of pain, rather than as a direct effect. Naloxone is effective in relieving opioid-induced spasm of the sphincter of Oddi.

Ventilatory depression caused by buprenorphine is relatively resistant to reversal by naloxone because of the very high affinity of buprenorphine for the μ receptor. Naloxone is ineffective in reversing sedation or ventilatory depression induced by non-opioid drugs, e.g. barbiturates or benzodiazepines.

Naloxone is the drug of choice in antagonizing opioid-induced ventilatory depression in the neonate.

The average dose of naloxone for adults is 200–400 μg i.v.; this should be administered in increments of 50–100 μg; supplementary doses may be required after 20–30 min.

Naltrexone

This is an analogue of naloxone with similar pharmacological properties (Table 10.3) although, unlike naloxone, it can be given by mouth. It has a long duration of action (up to 24 h) and is used mainly in the treatment of opioid addiction.

Other opioid antagonists

Nalorphine

This drug is related to morphine. It antagonizes the effects of morphine at the μ receptor, but has agonist activity at other sites.

Levallorphan

This agent is related to levorphanol and, in common with nalorphine, possesses agonist and antagonist activity at different opioid receptors.

Both of these agents have been superseded by naloxone and are no longer available in the UK.

Non-opioid analgesics

These drugs may be useful after minor surgery and are used to provide analgesia during the later recovery period after major surgery. They are employed also to supplement opioid analgesia after some types of operation. The non-steroidal anti-inflammatory drugs (NSAIDs) are generally more effective than the other non-opioid analgesics after surgery or trauma because of their anti-inflammatory properties.

Non-steroidal anti-inflammatory drugs

NSAIDs produce analgesia by a peripheral effect and are effective in pain of low to moderate intensity. By reducing the activity of the enzyme cyclo-oxygenase, they inhibit the synthesis and release of prostaglandins, prostacyclins and thromboxane, which sensitize pain receptors to mechanical stimulation or to other pain mediators. The drugs differ in their precise actions on cyclo-oxygenase and in their spectrum of activity as analgesic, antipyretic and anti-inflammatory agents.

Prostaglandins are synthesized by the gastric mucosa; their inhibition by NSAIDs may result in gastric erosions or ulceration. In addition, chronic use leads occasionally to renal papillary necrosis and chronic interstitial nephritis. Uncommonly, single doses may precipitate acute renal failure, particularly in the presence of dehydration or pre-existing renal insufficiency. NSAIDs reduce platelet adhesiveness and may increase blood loss during and after surgery. They may also contribute to gastrointestinal haemorrhage. NSAIDs may precipitate bronchospasm in asthmatics.

The principal uses of the NSAIDs are for treatment of rheumatoid conditions and chronic musculoskeletal pain. However, despite the large number of potential side-effects, some drugs of this type, notably diclofenac sodium and ketorolac, have been used very successfully to provide analgesia after surgery or in association with trauma. These drugs have also been used in combination with opioids to provide a balanced analgesic regimen with the intention of enhancing analgesia and simultaneously reducing the incidence of opioid-induced side-effects.

Although there are many different classes of NSAIDs there is a dearth of well-controlled studies comparing their efficacy and toxicity. Some believe that these drugs are best given in advance of surgery in order that they can inhibit prostaglandin synthesis effectively but this has not been substantiated.

NSAIDs are contraindicated as anaesthetic supplements in the following circumstances: renal insufficiency, peptic ulcer disease, hiatus hernia, dyspepsia, asthma, bleeding/clotting diatheses, steroid or anticoagulant therapy and during pregnancy.

Acetylsalicylic acid (aspirin)

Aspirin is occasionally used for the moderate pain which persists for 3–4 days after major surgery, but more often as an antipyretic. The relatively high incidence of gastric side-effects after oral administration is reduced by the use of soluble aspirin. The drug may also be administered by the rectal route. Unfortunately, the use of aspirin in children under 12 years of age runs the risk of precipitating Reye's syndrome of encephalopathy and liver failure.

Diclofenac

This drug may be administered orally, rectally or i.m. It has been shown to reduce the amount of opioid required after abdominal surgery. It also provides pain relief equivalent to that of fentanyl following arthroscopic meniscectomy. Its use in anaesthetic practice has been limited by the absence of an intravenous preparation.

Ketorolac

This drug is available in a preparation suitable for i.v. or i.m. use. A high incidence of renal complications following the standard i.v. dose (30 mg) has led to a recommendation from the Committee on Safety of Medicines to limit the i.v. dose to 10 mg. It is not clear if ketorolac has a worthwhile analgesic effect at the lower dose.

Indomethacin

This has been used in combination with opioids to treat pain after thoracotomy or orthopaedic surgery and in patients with fractured ribs. Because of gastrointestinal side-effects and delayed gastric emptying resulting from opioid administration, it is usually most appropriate to administer indomethacin by the rectal route.

Paracetamol

This is an analgesic and antipyretic agent which does not possess the anti-inflammatory properties of the NSAIDs. However, it is effective in treatment of mild to moderate postoperative pain and has the major advantage that it does not cause gastrointestinal side-effects. If taken in overdose, it may result in fulminant hepatic failure.

BENZODIAZEPINES

These drugs are used primarily as sedatives and hypnotics, although in large doses anaesthesia is induced. In addition, they produce mild muscle relaxation and possess anticonvulsant properties. There is great variability in the response of individual patients to a given dose and there is little justification for prescribing adult doses on a weight basis.

Site and mode of action

The benzodiazepines affect polysynaptic pathways within the spinal cord and brain, particularly in the midbrain reticular formation (affecting wakefulness) and the amygdala area of the limbic system (a relay for the expression of emotion, including anxiety).

The mechanism of action is related to stimulation of the activity of the inhibitory transmitter γ-aminobutyric acid (GABA), causing presynaptic inhibition within these areas.

Central nervous system

Sedation. There is a progressive, dose-dependent transition from sedation through hypnosis to unconsciousness. In large doses anaesthesia is induced but there is wide interindividual variability in the dose required and the onset of unconsciousness is slow. In lower doses, benzodiazepines reduce the MAC value of inhalational anaesthetics (p. 121). Diazepam may induce transient analgesia after i.v. injection, but other benzodiazepines possess no analgesic properties.

Amnesia. Dose-related anterograde amnesia occurs after administration of diazepam as a result of effects on the early consolidation phase of memory processing. Although it has been claimed that some benzodiazepines induce retrograde amnesia (i.e. for events before administration), this has never been demonstrated.

Anxiolysis. Benzodiazepines are effective in alleviating acute and chronic anxiety states and are prescribed widely for this purpose. This property makes these drugs useful as premedicants in anaesthetic practice.

Anticonvulsant effect. Most benzodiazepines possess anticonvulsant properties. They do not affect the seizure focus, but prevent subcortical spread of seizure activity. Diazepam and clonazepam are useful by i.v. injection for the management of status epilepticus; clobazam is used orally as an adjunct to chronic anticonvulsant therapy.

Respiratory system

Large i.v. doses of benzodiazepines produce depression of ventilation. There is direct depression of ventilatory drive in response to both hypoxaemia and hypercapnia and a slight decrease in ventilatory muscle activity. Severe ventilatory depression may occur in elderly or debilitated patients after i.v. administration. Airway obstruction may occur if consciousness is impaired. Clinically significant decreases in oxygen saturation occur during upper gastrointestinal endoscopy when i.v. benzodiazepines are used for sedation.

Cardiovascular system

Large doses of benzodiazepines decrease cardiac output and systemic arterial pressure, particularly if given in combination with opioids, and a reflex tachycardia occurs commonly. Hypotension is more likely in the hypovolaemic patient. Benzodiazepines potentiate the effects of ganglion-blocking agents and other drugs used to induce hypotension.

Muscle relaxation

Benzodiazepines produce relaxation of smooth muscle by depression of polysynaptic transmission in the brain and spinal cord and by mild depression of motor nerve and muscle function. This effect is useful in tetanus and in spastic conditions. The muscle relaxation produced is inadequate for surgery and there is no significant potentiation of depolarizing or non-depolarizing neuromuscular blockers at the neuromuscular junction. However, the central effects of benzodiazepines may reduce requirements for neuromuscular blocking agents.

Other effects

Transfer occurs rapidly across the placenta and this may cause neonatal depression. Chronic administration of benzodiazepines may result in physical and psychological dependence.

Indications for the use of benzodiazepines in anaesthetic practice

1. *Premedication.* Diazepam, temazepam and lorazepam are used commonly by the oral route for premedication; these drugs may be admin

istered also as hypnotics at night. Midazolam is also suitable as a premedicant agent by the i.m. route.

2. *Endoscopy.* Diazepam or midazolam administered i.v. provides satisfactory sedation and amnesia during gastrointestinal or tracheobronchial endoscopy. Patients should be fasted, as laryngeal reflexes may be lost. Airway obstruction and ventilatory depression may occur and supplemental oxygen should be administered. Monitoring should include pulse oximetry.

3. *Dentistry.* Diazepam or midazolam may be administered i.v. in small doses to produce sedation and co-operation in anxious patients during minor dental procedures undertaken using local anaesthesia. Temazepam administered orally 1 h before the procedure is a useful alternative.

4. *Cardioversion.* Diazepam or midazolam may be used to induce sedation and amnesia for this procedure, but recovery is slow.

5. *Sedation in ITU.* Diazepam, lorazepam and midazolam may be administered i.v. to induce sedation and amnesia in patients who require IPPV in the ITU. Analgesics should be administered if the patient is in pain. The major disadvantage of benzodiazepines in the critically ill is prolonged sedation resulting from accumulation of the drug or its metabolites.

6. *Supplementation of anaesthesia.* Benzodiazepines are used occasionally to induce anaesthesia in patients undergoing cardiac surgery. They are used in some centres to supplement balanced anaesthesia during other procedures. It has been claimed that their amnesic effect reduces the incidence of awareness during general anaesthesia. However, there is no evidence that this is true and the drug should *not* be used primarily for this purpose.

Adverse effects

1. Residual drowsiness, impairment of mental functions, dysarthria and ataxia.

2. Ventilatory depression after i.v. administration.

3. Muscle weakness, headache, nausea and vomiting, vertigo, joint and chest pains may occur occasionally.

The incidence of these effects is higher in

elderly or debilitated patients unless a reduced dose is given.

Diazepam

This benzodiazepine is relatively lipid-soluble and water-insoluble. Absorption is slow, erratic and incomplete after i.m. administration and the drug should only be administered orally or by the i.v. route. Diazepam is available for i.v. administration as an emulsion in soya bean oil (Diazemuls) or as a viscous solution containing organic solvents (propylene glycol, ethanol and sodium benzoate in benzoic acid); both preparations contain diazepam 5 mg.ml^{-1}. The drug is available for oral use as tablets or syrup and it can also be administered by the rectal route. Its oral bioavailability is 100%.

Diazepam is effective within 30–45 min after oral administration and has a duration of action of at least 4–6 h. It induces sedation within 1–2 min after a bolus i.v. dose. The elimination half-life is extremely long (20–90 h, Table 10.7); this results partly from enterohepatic recirculation. In addition, one of its metabolites, N-desmethyl diazepam, is pharmacologically active and has a longer half-life.

Dosage

1. *Premedication.* 10–15 mg orally (1–5 mg in children).
2. *Sedation.* 7–15 mg by slow i.v. injection. The dose should be reduced by 50% in elderly patients.
3. *Intensive care.* Bolus doses of 5–15 mg i.v. Because of its prolonged half-life, there is no indication for infusion of diazepam. In tetanus, a dose of up to 5 mg.kg^{-1} may be required daily.

Table 10.7 Elimination half-lives of four commonly used benzodiazepines

	Half-life (h)	Active metabolites	Half-life (h) of metabolites
Diazepam	36	Yes	100
Midazolam	2	No	–
Temazepam	8	No	–
Lorazepam	15	No	–

4. *Status epilepticus.* 10–20 mg i.v. over 5 min, repeated if necessary after 30–60 min.

Precautions and adverse effects

Patients should be instructed in writing concerning the dangers of taking alcohol, of driving or of operating machinery within 24 h.

Intravenous administration of diazepam in organic solvents causes a high incidence of thrombophlebitis (50–60%). This complication is obviated by the use of Diazemuls.

Midazolam

This is a water-soluble benzodiazepine which has almost replaced diazepam as an i.v. sedative. It is not recommended as an anticonvulsant. It is presented both as 2-ml ampoules containing 5 mg.ml^{-1} and 5-ml ampoules containing 2 mg.ml^{-1}. The latter, more dilute formulation is preferable for i.v. injection as the dose may be titrated more accurately.

Midazolam has a slightly more rapid onset of action than diazepam after i.v. injection and a shorter duration of action; the elimination half-life is 1.5–2.5 h. Its metabolites are inactive. Metabolism is reduced in some critically ill patients which results in prolonged elimination half-life (up to 21 h) and greatly delayed recovery of consciousness.

Dosage

1. *Sedation.* 2.5–7.5 mg i.v. in the adult, with a maximum of 2.5 mg in elderly patients. The midazolam:diazepam potency ratio is between 1.5:1 and 2:1. A number of fatalities have resulted from the use of midazolam as an i.v. sedative when given in the same dose range as that recommended for diazepam. Midazolam *must* be administered slowly; the onset of its clinical effect may be delayed and there is a danger of overdosage if the drug is given rapidly without waiting to assess its effects.
2. *Premedication.* 5 mg i.m. (2.5 mg in the elderly).
3. *Intensive care.* Bolus dose of 5–10 mg i.v. followed by i.v. infusion; requirements vary widely

from 1 to 20 mg.h^{-1}. Infusions should not be maintained in high doses, as cumulation is likely.

Advantages

Midazolam has a shorter duration of action than diazepam and residual mental impairment is less marked. It is associated with a low incidence of thrombophlebitis.

Disadvantages

In common with diazepam, it may induce ventilatory depression, especially in elderly patients. Cardiovascular depression may occur in the hypovolaemic patient. Recovery is prolonged in some critically ill patients.

Temazepam

This is a short-acting benzodiazepine which produces little hangover effect. It is a useful premedicant which induces hypnosis and anxiolysis when given in a dose of 20 mg orally 1 h before surgery. In a dose of 30 mg, it is as effective as i.v. midazolam in producing sedation and anxiolysis in patients undergoing dental procedures. It is available in tablet, capsule or oral solution forms. Its very low solubility in all types of solvents has prevented the development of a parenteral preparation.

Lorazepam

This has a long duration of action (half-life 10–20 h). Its use as a premedicant in doses of 2–5 mg is associated usually with amnesia lasting several hours.

Flumazenil

Flumazenil antagonizes the central effects of benzodiazepine agonists by competing for occupancy of benzodiazepine receptors. In very high doses it has slight agonist properties and may have mild direct inverse agonist effects at lower doses. The drug is metabolized in the liver and its elimination half-life is less than 1 h.

All the central effects of benzodiazepine agonists are antagonized by flumazenil; performance in psychometric tests is restored to normal and amnesia is attenuated. EEG studies indicate that antagonism starts within 1 min. The duration of action is dose-dependent; after small but effective doses, amnesia and sedation may return within 30 min.

Indications

Antagonism of sedation. Inadvertent overdosage or undue sensitivity to the effects of benzodiazepine agonists may be antagonized by flumazenil. However, sedation may recur and the patients must be observed carefully for several hours. The routine use of flumazenil to antagonize residual effects of i.v. sedation is not recommended. Prolonged sedation resulting from accumulation of benzodiazepines in the critically ill patient is usually reversible with flumazenil. However, sedation and ventilatory depression are likely to recur unless repeated doses of flumazenil are administered or a continuous infusion instituted. It may be more appropriate to sedate patients in the ITU using a drug with a short elimination half-life rather than antagonizing a long-acting benzodiazepine with a short-acting antagonist

Self-poisoning. Deliberate overdosage with benzodiazepines may result in prolonged unconsciousness and ventilatory depression, with subsequent development of pulmonary atelectasis and infection. Flumazenil restores consciousness but repeated doses or a continuous infusion are necessary until plasma concentrations of the agonist have diminished.

Precautions

Flumazenil may induce withdrawal symptoms in patients who have received benzodiazepines for long periods.

BUTYROPHENONES

These drugs share many properties, and some structural similarities, with the phenothiazines. Their principal use in anaesthesia is as neuroleptic agents. Neurolepsis is a drug-induced state of suppressed spontaneous movements, but intact spinal and central reflexes. There is lack of initiative, disinterest in the environment, little display of emotion and a limited range of affect. Intellectual function remains intact.

Neuroleptanalgesia is the term used to describe the combined use of a neuroleptic agent with a potent analgesic, usually fentanyl. Large doses may induce profound ventilatory depression while preserving consciousness. A state may be induced in which the patient is hypoxaemic and cyanosed, but remains conscious and responds to orders to breathe (a state that has been likened to 'Ondine's curse'). This combination of neuroleptic and opioid drugs is used in moderate dosage to provide sedation during minor surgical procedures, usually as a supplement to a local anaesthetic block, e.g. during ophthalmic surgery.

Neuroleptanaesthesia is the term employed to describe the use of larger doses to supplement nitrous oxide anaesthesia. This technique is used in some centres for neurosurgical and cardiac procedures.

In addition to their effect on behaviour, the butyrophenones are powerful antiemetics. They antagonize dopamine-mediated synaptic transmission in the CNS, probably by occupation of GABA receptors. This is thought to be the major mechanism by which their therapeutic actions are mediated. The basal ganglia are rich in dopamine-mediated synapses and the major side-effect of the butyrophenones is the production of dyskinetic involuntary (extrapyramidal) movements. The incidence of extrapyramidal movements is reduced if butyrophenones are administered in combination with an opioid.

The butyrophenones have no specific analgesic action, but may prolong the duration of action of opioids.

Droperidol

This is the most widely used butyrophenone in anaesthetic practice. When administered alone, it produces a tranquil and placid appearance in the patients. However, patients may complain subsequently of unpleasant sensations of mental restlessness and agitation; these are avoided by administering an opioid or benzodiazepine simultaneously.

The onset of action of droperidol starts within 3–10 min of i.v. injection and its duration may exceed 12 h. Most of the injected dose is metabolized in the liver and reduced doses are required in patients with hepatic disease. Approximately 10% of the drug is excreted unchanged in the urine.

Cardiovascular system

Droperidol possesses mild α-blocking actions which may cause a reduction in arterial pressure. This occurs seldom after oral or i.m. administration, but may result in significant hypotension after i.v. injection, particularly if hypovolaemia is present. Droperidol has some effect in protecting the heart against catecholamine-induced arrhythmias.

Central nervous system

Droperidol causes mild cerebral vasoconstriction and a reduction in CSF pressure. Its neuroleptic properties occur within a few minutes of i.v. administration and may persist for 6–12 h. Thus, there may be re-emergence of unpleasant subjective sensations if the drug is given in conjunction with a short-acting opioid. Extrapyramidal side-effects may occur 24 h or more after administration. If severe, these may be treated with procyclidine; promethazine (12.5 mg i.v. + 12.5 mg i.m.) is usually effective if symptoms are mild.

Although droperidol possesses little intrinsic sedative activity, it may potentiate anaesthetic or sedative drugs and result in delayed recovery of consciousness.

Other effects

Total body oxygen consumption is reduced. There is little effect on ventilation.

Dosage

1. *Premedication.* 1.25–2.5 mg orally or i.m. in conjunction with a benzodiazepine or opioid. There is some evidence that doses in excess of 2.5 mg do not produce more effective antiemesis. Doses exceeding 5 mg should not be used as the effects of the drug are prolonged but sedation is not improved.

2. *Neuroleptanalgesia/anaesthesia.* Up to 10 mg i.v. with fentanyl. A mixture of fentanyl and droperidol (Thalamonal) is available and contains fentanyl 50 μg.ml^{-1} and droperidol 2.5 mg.ml^{-1}.

Haloperidol

This drug is used less commonly in anaesthesia. Its effects are similar to those of droperidol, but it has a more prolonged duration of action (up to 24 h) and virtually no α-adrenergic activity. It causes a high incidence of extrapyramidal side-effects.

α_2-ADRENERGIC AGONISTS

Clonidine

The discovery that clonidine reduces the MAC of volatile agents and decreases analgesic requirements has awakened interest in the role of adrenoceptors in anaesthesia. Clonidine activates peripheral and central α_2-receptors, thereby inhibiting noradrenaline release from nerve terminals of both peripheral and central neurones. It does not cause significant motor block but has a marked sedative effect. The drug exerts an analgesic effect after systemic, extradural and intrathecal routes of administration but is usually combined with local anaesthetic or opioid. Given intrathecally with pethidine, clonidine provides regional anaesthesia for hip replacement indistinguishable from that obtained with bupivacaine.

Irrespective of the technique, hypotension is a common complication and is of sufficient magnitude to render clonidine unsuitable for routine use.

Clonidine has been used in the management of sympathetically maintained pain syndromes where long-term opioid administration is undesirable.

Dexmedetomidine and medetomidine

These α_2-adrenergic agonists are selective for α_2 receptors whereas clonidine is thought to possess mixed agonist–antagonist properties at α_2 receptors and α_1-agonist effects. Both of these compounds, therefore, offer the possibility of improved analgesic efficacy with fewer undesirable side-effects. Neither drug is available commercially in the UK.

PHENOTHIAZINES

These agents are less potent neuroleptic drugs than the butyrophenones. Their principal use in anaesthesia is in the prevention and treatment of nausea and vomiting. In common with the butyrophenones, the phenothiazines have a specific action on the chemoreceptor trigger zone and in large doses, exert a direct depressant effect on the vomiting centre (see p. 213). In addition, some members of the group possess sedative properties and are useful for premedication. Their major side-effects are also similar to those of the butyrophenones: extrapyramidal movements, hypotension produced by α-receptor blockade and central depression of sympathetic activity.

Chlorpromazine

This phenothiazine is used widely in psychiatric practice, but some of its actions are useful in anaesthesia. It has sedative actions and has been used for premedication and to calm manic or disturbed patients in the intensive care unit. It may be used i.v. in small doses to produce α-receptor blockade. Thermoregulation is depressed and shivering reduced; this property, together with the vasodilatation induced by α-blockade, resulted in its use as an adjuvant during active cooling to induce hypothermia for neurosurgery. It is also an antiemetic.

Jaundice occurs in 0.5% of patients who receive chlorpromazine and is independent of dose or duration of treatment.

Dosage

1. *Premedication.* 25–50 mg i.m. 1 h before operation.
2. *Vasodilatation.* Increments of 2.5 mg i.v. after dilution (25 mg in 10–20 ml).

Promethazine

This drug has more marked antihistamine (H$_1$) properties than other phenothiazines. In addition, it has an atropine-like action, producing bronchodilatation and a reduction of oral and bronchial secretions. There is a spasmolytic action on the gastrointestinal tract. Its sedative action is greater than that of chlorpromazine.

The principal use of promethazine in anaesthesia is as a premedicant, usually in combination with an opioid. The combination of promethazine 25 mg and pethidine 50–100 mg i.m. is suitable especially for asthmatic or bronchitic patients.

Phenothiazines used in the treatment of nausea and vomiting are discussed on p. 212.

VENTILATORY STIMULANTS

These drugs have a limited role in the treatment of ventilatory failure in patients with chronic obstructive airways disease or in those with residual drowsiness or sedation after anaesthesia. They act by stimulating medullary centres and by an effect on peripheral chemoreceptors. They are effective only when administered i.v. and have a short duration of action. All these drugs are non-specific CNS stimulants which may produce cerebral arousal, clonic movements and convulsions. In very high doses, cortical and medullary depression occur and result in ventilatory failure and cardiovascular collapse.

The use of ventilatory stimulants in patients with chronic obstructive airways disease is controversial. Although minute volume is increased, the stimulation of muscle activity also increases oxygen consumption and carbon dioxide production. However, clearance of secretions may be improved.

Doxapram

This drug is the most specific of the analeptic drugs in its ability to stimulate ventilation without development of other signs of CNS stimulation. Tidal volume and, to a lesser extent, ventilatory rate increase for approximately 5 min after a slow bolus dose of $1-1.5$ mg.kg^{-1} i.v. If a satisfactory effect is achieved, doxapram should be administered by infusion at a rate of $0.5-4$ mg.min^{-1} and titrated against effect. Side-effects include coughing, nausea, vomiting, restlessness, hypertension, tachycardia, cardiac arrhythmias and muscle rigidity.

It has been claimed that a single bolus dose of doxapram in the early postoperative period reduces the incidence of pulmonary complications after abdominal surgery, but this has not been substantiated.

FURTHER READING

Goodman-Gilman A, Rall T W, Nies A S, Taylor P (eds) 1990 The pharmacological basis of therapeutics, 8th edn. Macmillan, New York
Vickers M D, Morgan M, Spencer PSJ 1991 Drugs in anaesthetic practice, 7th edn. Butterworths, London

Wood M, Wood A J J (eds) 1990 Drugs and anesthesia, 2nd edn. Williams & Wilkins, Baltimore

11. Neuromuscular blockade

In the last 50 years, neuromuscular blocking drugs have become an established part of anaesthetic practice. They were first administered in 1942, when Griffith and Johnson in Montreal used Intocostrin, a biologically standardized mixture of the alkaloids of the plant *Chondrodendron tomentosum*, to facilitate relaxation during cyclopropane anaesthesia. Previously, only inhalational agents (nitrous oxide, ether, cyclopropane, and chloroform) had been used during general anaesthesia, making surgical access for some procedures difficult because of lack of muscle relaxation. To achieve significant muscle relaxation it was necessary to deepen anaesthesia, which often had adverse cardiac and respiratory effects. Local analgesia was the only alternative.

At first, muscle relaxants were used only occasionally, in small doses, as an adjuvant to aid in the management of a difficult case; they were not used routinely. A tracheal tube was not necessarily passed, artificial ventilation was not instituted nor was the residual block routinely reversed; all of these caused significant morbidity and mortality, as demonstrated in the famous retrospective study by Beecher & Todd (1954). By 1946 however, it was appreciated that using drugs such as curare in larger doses allowed the depth of anaesthesia to be lightened, and it was suggested that incremental doses should be used also during prolonged surgery, rather than deepening anaesthesia — an entirely new concept at that time. The use of routine tracheal intubation and artificial ventilation then evolved.

Gray & Halton (1946) in Liverpool reported their experience of using the pure alkaloid, tubocurarine, in over 1000 patients receiving various anaesthetic agents. Over the following 6 years, they developed a concise description of the necessary ingredients of any anaesthetic technique; narcosis, analgesia and muscle relaxation were essential — the *triad* of anaesthesia. A fourth ingredient, controlled apnoea, was added at a later stage to emphasize the need for fully controlled ventilation, reducing the amount of relaxant required. This concept is the basis of the use of neuromuscular blocking drugs in modern anaesthetic practice. In particular, it has allowed seriously ill patients undergoing complex surgery to be anaesthetized safely and to be cared for postoperatively in the Intensive Therapy Unit.

PHYSIOLOGY OF NEUROMUSCULAR TRANSMISSION

Acetylcholine, the neurotransmitter at the neuromuscular junction, is released from presynaptic nerve endings on the passage of a nerve impulse (an action potential) down the axon to the nerve terminal. The neurotransmitter is synthesized from choline and acetylcoenzyme A by the enzyme *choline acetyltransferase* and stored in vesicles in the nerve terminal. The action potential depolarizes the nerve terminal to release the neurotransmitter; entry of Ca^{2+} ions into the nerve terminal is a necessary part of the process. On the arrival of an action potential, the storage vesicles are transferred to the active zones on the edge of the axonal membrane, where they fuse with the terminal wall to release the acetylcholine (Fig. 11.1). There are about a thousand active sites at each nerve ending and any one nerve action potential leads to the release of 200–300 vesicles. In addition, small *quanta* of acetylcholine, presumably equivalent to the contents of one vesicle, are released at the

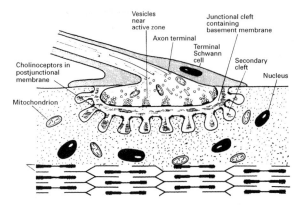

Fig. 11.1 The neuromuscular junction with an axon terminal, containing vesicles of acetylcholine. The neurotransmitter is released on arrival of an action potential and crosses the junctional cleft to stimulate the postjunctional receptors on the shoulders of the secondary clefts. (Reproduced with kind permission of Professor W. C. Bowman.)

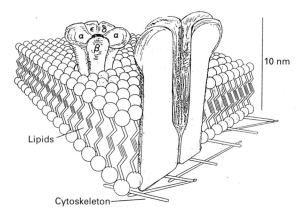

Fig. 11.2 Two postjunctional receptors, embedded in the lipid layer of the postsynaptic muscle membrane. The α, β, ε and δ subunits are demonstrated on the surface of one receptor and the ionophore is seen in cross-section on the other receptor. On stimulation of the two α subunits by two molecules of acetylcholine, the ionophore opens to allow the passage of the end-plate current. (Reproduced with kind permission of Professor W. C. Bowman.)

neuromuscular junction spontaneously, causing miniature end-plate potentials (MEPPs) on the post-synaptic membrane, but these are insufficient to generate a muscle action potential.

The active sites of release are aligned directly opposite the acetylcholine receptors on the junctional folds of the postsynaptic membrane, lying on the muscle surface. The junctional cleft, the gap between the nerve terminal and the muscle membrane, has a width of only 60 nm. It contains the enzyme *acetylcholinesterase,* which is responsible for the ultimate breakdown of acetylcholine. This enzyme is also present, in higher concentrations, in the junctional folds in the postsynaptic membrane (Fig. 11.1). The choline produced by the breakdown of acetylcholine is taken up across the nerve membrane to be re-used in the synthesis of the transmitter.

The nicotinic acetylcholine receptors on the postsynaptic membrane are organized in discrete clusters on the shoulders of the junctional folds (Fig. 11.1). Each cluster is about 0.1 µm in diameter and contains a few hundred receptors. Each receptor consists of five subunits, two of which, the alpha (α; MW = 40 000 Da), are identical. The other three, slightly larger subunits, are the beta (β), delta (δ) and epsilon (ε). In fetal muscle, the epsilon is replaced by a gamma (γ) subunit. Each subunit of the receptor is a glycosated protein — a chain of amino acids — coded by a different gene.

The receptors are arranged as a cylinder which spans the membrane, with a central, normally closed, channel — the ionophore (Fig. 11.2). Each of the α subunits carries a single acetylcholine binding region on its extracellular surface. They also bind neuromuscular blocking drugs.

Activation of the receptor requires both α sites to be occupied, producing a structural change in the receptor complex that opens the central channel running between the receptors for a very short period, about 1 ms (Fig. 11.2). This allows the movement of cations such as Na^+, K^+, Ca^{2+} and Mg^{2+} along their concentration gradients. The main change is an influx of Na^+ ions, the *end-plate current*, followed by an efflux of K^+ ions. The summation of this current through a large number of receptor channels lowers the transmembrane potential of the end-plate region sufficiently to depolarize it and generate a muscle action potential sufficient to allow muscle contraction.

At rest, the transmembrane potential is about −90 mV (inside negative). Under normal physiological conditions, a depolarization of about 40 mV occurs, lowering the potential from −90 mV to −50 mV. Once the *end-plate potential* reaches this critical threshold, it triggers an *all-or-nothing* action potential that passes around the sarcolemma to activate the muscle contractile mechanism via a mechanism involving Ca^{2+} release from the sarcoplasmic reticulum.

Each acetylcholine molecule is involved in opening one ion channel only before it is broken down rapidly by acetylcholinesterase; it does not interact with any of the other receptors. There is a large safety factor in the transmission process, in respect of both the amount of acetylcholine released and the number of postsynaptic receptors. Much more acetylcholine is released than is necessary to trigger the action potential. The end-plate region is depolarized for only a very short period (a few milliseconds) before it rapidly repolarizes and is ready to transmit another impulse.

Acetylcholine receptors are present also on the presynaptic area of the nerve terminal. It is thought that a positive feedback mechanism exists for the further release of acetylcholine, such that some of the released molecules of acetylcholine stimulate these presynaptic receptors, producing further mobilization of the neurotransmitter to the readily releasable sites, ready for the arrival of the next nerve stimulus (Fig. 11.3).

In health, postsynaptic acetylcholine receptors are restricted to the neuromuscular junction by a mechanism involving the presence of an active nerve terminal. In many disease states affecting the neuromuscular junction, this control is lost and acetylcholine receptors develop on the adjacent muscle surface. The excessive release of K^+ ions from diseased or swollen muscle on admini-

stration of suxamethonium is probably the result of stimulation of these *extrajunctional receptors*. They develop in many conditions, including polyneuropathies, severe burns and muscle disorders.

The physiology of neuromuscular transmission has been described, in detail, by Bowman (1992).

PHARMACOLOGY OF NEUROMUSCULAR TRANSMISSION

Neuromuscular blocking agents used regularly by anaesthetists are classified into *depolarizing* (or *non-competitive*) and *non-depolarizing* (or *competitive*) agents.

Depolarizing neuromuscular blocking agents

The only depolarizing relaxant now available in clinical practice is suxamethonium (known in the US as succinylcholine). Decamethonium was used clinically in Great Britain for many years, but is now available only for research purposes.

Suxamethonium chloride

This quaternary ammonium compound is comparable to two molecules of acetylcholine linked together (Fig. 11.4). The two quaternary ammonium radicals $N^+(CH_3)_3$ have the capacity to cling to each of the α units of the postsynaptic acetylcholine receptor, altering its structural conformation and opening the ion channel, but for a longer period than does a molecule of acetylcholine. Administration of suxamethonium therefore results in an initial depolarization and muscle contraction, known as *fasciculation*. As this effect persists, however, further action potentials cannot pass down the ion channels and the muscle becomes flaccid; repolarization does not occur.

The dose of suxamethonium necessary for tracheal intubation in adults is about 1.0–1.5 mg.kg^{-1}. This dose has the most rapid onset of action of any of the muscle relaxants presently available, producing profound block within 1 min. Suxamethonium is therefore of particular benefit when it is essential to achieve tracheal intubation rapidly, as in a patient with a full stomach, or an obstetric patient. It is also indicated if tracheal

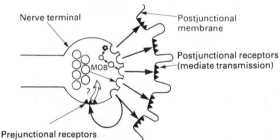

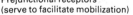

Fig. 11.3 Acetylcholine receptors are present on the shoulders of the axon terminal, as well as on the postjunctional membrane. Stimulation of the prejunctional receptors mobilizes (MOB) the vesicles of acetylcholine to move into the active zone, ready for release on arrival of another nerve impulse. The exact mechanism is unknown. (Reproduced with kind permission of Professor W. C. Bowman.)

Acetylcholine

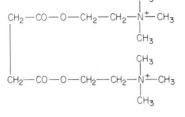

Suxamethonium

Decamethonium

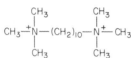

Fig. 11.4 The chemical structures of acetylcholine and suxamethonium. The similarity between the structure of suxamethonium and two molecules of acetylcholine can be seen. The structure of decamethonium is also shown. The quaternary ammonium radicals, $N^+(CH_3)_3$, cling to the α subunits of the postsynaptic receptor.

intubation is expected to be difficult for anatomical reasons, as it produces optimal intubating conditions.

The drug is metabolized predominantly in the plasma by the enzyme *plasma cholinesterase*, once known as pseudocholinesterase, at a very rapid rate. Recovery from neuromuscular block may start to occur within 3 min and is complete within 12–15 min. The use of an anticholinesterase such as neostigmine, which would inhibit such enzyme activity, is contraindicated (see below). About 10% of the drug is excreted in the urine; there is very little metabolism in the liver although some breakdown by other non-specific esterases in the plasma occurs.

If plasma cholinesterase is structurally abnormal because of inherited factors, or if its concentration is reduced by acquired factors, then the duration of action of the drug may be altered significantly.

Inherited factors. The exact structure of plasma cholinesterase is determined genetically, by autosomal genes, and has now been completely defined. Several abnormalities in the amino acid sequence of the normal enzyme, usually des-

ignated E_1^u, are recognized. The most common is produced by the atypical gene, E_1^a, which occurs in about 4% of the Caucasian population. Thus a patient who is a *heterozygote* for the atypical gene (E_1^u, E_1^a) will have a longer effect from a standard dose of suxamethonium (about 30 min). If the individual is a *homozygote* for the atypical gene (E_1^a, E_1^a), suxamethonium may have an effect for over 2 h, which can be inconvenient to the anaesthetist during an operating list. Other, rarer, abnormalities in the structure of plasma cholinesterase are also recognized, e.g. the fluoride (E_1^f) and silent (E_1^s) genes. The latter has very little capacity to metabolize suxamethonium and thus neuromuscular block in the homozygous state lasts for at least 3 h. In such patients, non-specific esterases gradually clear the drug from plasma.

It has been suggested that a source of cholinesterase, such as fresh frozen plasma, should be administered in such cases, or an anticholinesterase such as neostigmine used to reverse what has usually developed into a *dual block* (see below). However, it is wiser to:

1. Keep the patient anaesthetized and the lungs ventilated artificially.
2. Monitor neuromuscular transmission accurately until full recovery from residual neuromuscular block.

This condition is not life-threatening, but the risk of awareness is considerable, especially after the end of surgery, when the anaesthetist, who may not yet have made the diagnosis, is attempting to waken the patient. Anaesthesia must be continued until full recovery from neuromuscular block.

As plasma cholinesterase activity is reduced by the presence of suxamethonium, a plasma sample to measure the patient's cholinesterase activity should not be taken for several days after prolonged block has been experienced, by which time new enzyme will have been synthesized. A patient who is found to have reduced enzyme activity and structurally abnormal enzyme should be given a warning card or alarm bracelet, detailing their genetic status. Detailing the genetic status of the patient's immediate relatives should be considered.

Kalow & Genest (1957) first described a method

for detecting structurally abnormal cholinesterase. If plasma from a patient of normal genotype is added to a water bath containing a substrate such as benzoylcholine, a chemical reaction occurs with plasma cholinesterase, emitting light of a given wavelength, which can be detected spectrophotometrically. If dibucaine is also added to the water bath, this reaction is inhibited; no light is produced. The percentage inhibition is referred to as the *dibucaine number*. A patient with normal plasma cholinesterase has a high dibucaine number of 77–83. A heterozygote for the atypical gene has a dibucaine number of 45–68; in a homozygote, the dibucaine number is less than 30.

If fluoride is added to the solution instead of dibucaine, the fluoride gene may be detected. If there is no reaction in the presence of the substrate only, the silent gene is present.

Acquired factors. In these instances, the structure of plasma cholinesterase is normal, but its activity is reduced. Thus neuromuscular block is lengthened by only a matter of minutes, rather than hours. Causes of reduced plasma cholinesterase activity include the following:

1. *Liver disease*, because of reduced enzyme synthesis.
2. *Carcinomatosis, starvation*, for the same reason.
3. *Pregnancy*, for two reasons: an increased circulating volume (dilutional effect), and decreased enzyme synthesis.
4. *Anticholinesterases*, including those used by the anaesthetist to reverse residual neuromuscular block after a non-depolarizing muscle relaxant (e.g. *neostigmine* or *edrophonium*); these drugs inhibit plasma cholinesterase as well as acetylcholinesterase. The organophosphorus compound *ecothiopate*, used topically as a miotic in ophthalmology, is also an anticholinesterase.
5. Other drugs which are metabolized by plasma cholinesterase, and which therefore decrease its availability, include etomidate, propanidid, ester local analgesics, anticancer drugs such as methotrexate, monoamine oxidase inhibitors and esmolol (the short-acting β-blocker).
6. Hypothyroidism.
7. Cardiopulmonary bypass, plasmapheresis.
8. Renal disease.

Side-effects of suxamethonium

Although suxamethonium is a very useful drug for achieving tracheal intubation rapidly, it has several undesirable side-effects which may limit its use:

1. *Muscle pains*, especially in the patient who is ambulant soon after surgery, such as the day-case patient. The pains, thought possibly to be due to the initial fasciculations, are more common in young, fit people with a large muscle mass. They occur in unusual sites, such as the diaphragm and between the scapulae, and are not relieved easily by conventional analgesics. They may be reduced by the use of a small dose of a non-depolarizing muscle relaxant given immediately prior to the administration of the suxamethonium, e.g. gallamine 10 mg (which is thought to be most efficacious in this respect), or atracurium 2.5 mg. However, this technique, known as *pre-curarization* or *pretreatment*, reduces the potency of suxamethonium, necessitating administration of a larger dose to produce the same effect. Many other drugs have been used in an attempt to reduce the muscle pains, including lignocaine, calcium, magnesium and repeated doses of thiopentone, but none is completely reliable.

2. *Increased intraocular pressure*. This is thought to be due in part to the initial contraction of the external ocular muscles on administration of suxamethonium, but is not reduced by pre-curarization. The effect lasts for as long as the neuromuscular block and concern has been expressed that it may be sufficient to cause expulsion of the vitreal contents in the patient with an open eye injury. This is probably unlikely. Protection of the airway from gastric contents must take priority in the patient with a full stomach in addition to an eye injury, as inhalation of gastric contents can threaten life.

It is also possible that suxamethonium may increase intracranial pressure, although this is less certain.

3. *Increased intragastric pressure*. In the presence of a normal lower oesophageal sphincter, the increase in intragastric pressure produced by suxamethonium should be insufficient to produce regurgitation of gastric contents. However, in the patient with incompetence of this sphincter from, for example, a hiatus hernia, regurgitation may occur.

4. *Hyperkalaemia*. It has long been recognized that administration of suxamethonium during halothane anaesthesia increases the serum potassium concentration by 0.5 mmol.litre^{-1} (Paton, 1959). This effect is thought to be due to muscle fasciculation. It is probable that the effect is less marked with other anaesthetic techniques. A similar rise occurs in patients with renal failure, but as these patients may already have an elevated serum potassium concentration, such an increase may precipitate cardiac irregularities and even cardiac arrest.

In some conditions in which the muscle cells are swollen or damaged, or in which there is proliferation of extrajunctional receptors, this release of potassium may be exaggerated. This is most marked in the burned patient, in whom potassium levels up to 13 mmol.litre^{-1} have been reported. In such patients, pre-curarization is of no benefit. Suxamethonium is best avoided in this condition. In diseases of the muscle cell, or its nerve supply, hyperkalaemia after suxamethonium may also be exaggerated. These include the muscular dystrophies, dystrophia myotonica and paraplegia. Hyperkalaemia has been reported to cause death in such patients. Suxamethonium may also precipitate a prolonged contracture of the masseter muscles in patients with these disorders, making tracheal intubation impossible. The drug is best avoided in any patient with a neuromuscular disorder, including the patient with *malignant hyperpyrexia*, in whom the drug is a recognized trigger factor (see page 398).

Hyperkalaemia after suxamethonium has also been reported, albeit rarely, in patients with widespread intra-abdominal infection, severe trauma and closed head injury.

5. *Cardiovascular effects.* Suxamethonium has muscarinic as well as nicotinic effects, as does acetylcholine. The direct vagal effect (muscarinic) produces a sinus bradycardia, especially in patients with a high vagal tone, such as children and the physically fit. It is also more common in the patient who has not received an anticholinergic agent such as atropine, or who is given repeated increments of suxamethonium. It is advisable to use an anticholinergic routinely if more than one dose of suxamethonium is planned. Nodal or ventricular escape beats may develop in extreme circumstances.

6. *Anaphylactic reactions* to suxamethonium are rare, but may occur, especially after repeated exposure to the drug.

Characteristics of depolarizing neuromuscular block

If neuromuscular block is monitored (see below), a number of differences between depolarizing and non-depolarizing block can be defined. In the presence of a small dose of suxamethonium:

1. A decreased response to a single, low voltage (1 Hz) twitch stimulus applied to a peripheral nerve is detected. Tetanic stimulation (e.g. at 50 Hz) produces a small, but sustained, response.

2. If four twitch stimuli are applied at 2 Hz over 2 s (train-of-four stimulus), followed by a 10 s interval before the next train-of-four, no decrease in the height of successive stimuli is noted (Fig. 11.5).

3. The application of a 5 s burst of tetanic stimulation after the application of a single twitch, followed by a further twitch stimulus, produces no

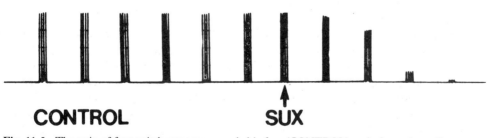

CONTROL   **SUX**

Fig. 11.5   The train-of-four twitch response recorded before (CONTROL) and after a dose of suxamethonium. Before administration of suxamethonium 1 mg.kg^{-1}, four twitches of equal height are visible. After giving the drug (SUX), the height of all four twitches decreases equally; no "fade" of the train-of-four is seen. Within a minute, the trace has been ablated.

potentiation of the twitch height; there is no *post-tetanic potentiation* (sometimes called *facilitation*).

4. Neuromuscular block is *potentiated* by the administration of an anticholinesterase such as neostigmine or edrophonium.

5. If repeated doses of suxamethonium are given, the characteristics of this depolarizing block alter; signs typical of a *non-depolarizing* block develop (see below). Initially such changes are demonstrable only at fast rates of stimulation, but with further increments of suxamethonium they can be seen at slower rates. This phenomenon is known as *dual block*.

6. Muscle fasciculation is typical of a depolarizing block.

Decamethonium

This depolarizing neuromuscular blocking agent has as rapid an onset of action as suxamethonium, but a longer duration of action (about 20 min), as it is not metabolized by plasma cholinesterase, but mainly excreted unchanged through the kidney. It is prone to produce *tachyphylaxis* — a rapid increase in the dose required incrementally to produce the same effect — which, together with its route of excretion, limit its use. It is no longer available for clinical use.

Non-depolarizing neuromuscular blocking agents

Unlike suxamethonium, these drugs do not alter the structural conformity of the postsynaptic acetylcholine receptor and therefore do not produce an initial contraction. Instead, they compete with the neurotransmitter at this site, reversibly binding to one or two of the α receptors, whenever these are not occupied by acetylcholine. The end-plate potential produced in the presence of a non-depolarizing agent is therefore smaller; it does not reach the threshold necessary to fire off a propagating action potential to activate the sarcolemma and produce an initial muscle contraction. Over 75% of the postsynaptic receptors have to be blocked in this way before there is a failure of muscle contraction: a large safety factor. However, in large doses, non-depolarizing muscle relaxants impair neuromuscular transmission sufficiently to produce profound neuromuscular block.

No metabolism of any neuromuscular blocking agent is thought to occur at the neuromuscular junction. At the end of surgery, the end-plate concentration of the relaxant is falling as the drug diffuses down a concentration gradient into the plasma, from which it is cleared. Thus more receptors are stimulated by the neurotransmitter, allowing recovery from block. An anticholinesterase given at this time increases the half-life of acetylcholine at the neuromuscular junction, facilitating recovery.

Non-depolarizing muscle relaxants are highly ionized, water-soluble drugs, which are distributed mainly in plasma and extracellular fluid. Thus they have a relatively small volume of distribution. They are of two main types of chemical structure: either *benzylisoquinolinium compounds* such as tubocurarine, alcuronium, atracurium and mivacurium, or *aminosteroid compounds* such as pancuronium, vecuronium, pipecuronium and rocuronium. All these drugs possess at least one quaternary ammonium group $N^+(CH_3)_3$, to bind to an α subunit on the postsynaptic receptor. Their structural type determines many of their chemical properties. Some benzylisoquinolinium compounds consist of quaternary ammonium groups joined by a thin chain of methyl groups. They are therefore more liable to some breakdown in the plasma than are the aminosteroids. They are also more likely to release histamine.

Non-depolarizing muscle relaxants are administered usually in multiples of the effective dose (ED) required to produce 95% neuromuscular block (ED_{95}). A dose of at least $2 \times ED_{95}$ is required to produce adequate conditions for reliable tracheal intubation in all patients.

Benzylisoquinolinium compounds

Tubocurarine chloride. This is the only naturally occurring muscle relaxant in clinical use. It is derived from the bark of the South American plant *Chondrodendron tomentosum*, and has been used for centuries by South American Indians as an arrow poison. It was the first non-depolarizing neuromuscular blocking agent to be used in humans, by Griffith and Johnson in Montreal, Canada in 1942. An intubating dose is of the order of $0.5–0.6$ mg.kg^{-1}. It is a drug with a long

Table 11.1 Time to 95% depression of the twitch response, after a dose of $2 \times ED_{95}$ of neuromuscular blocking drugs (when tracheal intubation should be possible), and time to 20–25% recovery, when an anticholinesterase can be used reliably to reverse residual block produced by a non-depolarizing drug

	95% twitch depression (s)	20–25% recovery (min)
Suxamethonium	60	10
Tubocurarine	220	80+
Alcuronium	420	70
Gallamine	300	80
Atracurium	110	43
Doxacurium	250	83
Mivacurium	170	16
Pancuronium	220	75
Vecuronium	180	33
Pipecuronium	300	95
Rocuronium	75	33
Cisatracurium	150	45

onset of action and a prolonged duration of effect (Table 11.1), and its effects are potentiated by inhalational agents and prior administration of suxamethonium. It has a marked propensity to produce histamine release and thus hypotension, with possibly a compensatory tachycardia. In large doses, it can also produce ganglion blockade, which potentiates these cardiovascular effects. It is excreted unchanged through the kidney, with some biliary excretion. Its use is declining in Great Britain.

Alcuronium chloride. This drug is a semi-synthetic derivative of toxiferin, an alkaloid of calabash curare. It has less histamine-releasing properties and therefore cardiovascular effect than tubocurarine, although it can have some vagolytic effect, producing a mild tachycardia. It also has a long onset time and nearly as long a duration of effect as tubocurarine (Table 11.1). It is almost entirely excreted unchanged through the kidney. An intubating dose is of the order of $0.2–0.25$ mg.kg^{-1}. Before the advent of atracurium and vecuronium, this cheap agent was widely used, but now its popularity is declining and it is no longer commercially available in the United Kingdom.

Gallamine triethiodide. This synthetic substance is a trisquaternary amine. It was first used in France in 1948. An intubating dose in adults is of the order of 160 mg. It has a similar onset to, but slightly shorter duration of action than,

tubocurarine, and is almost entirely excreted by the kidney. Consequently, it should not be used in patients with renal impairment. Being more lipid soluble than bisquaternary amines, it crosses the placenta to a significant degree and should not be used in obstetric practice. Gallamine has potent vagolytic properties and produces some direct sympathomimetic stimulation. Thus, it frequently increases pulse rate and blood pressure.

The only regular use of gallamine in Great Britain is as a small pretreatment dose (10 mg) prior to suxamethonium, when it seems to be more efficacious than any other non-depolarizing muscle relaxant in minimizing muscle pains.

Atracurium besylate. This drug, introduced into clinical practice in 1982, was developed by Stenlake at Strathclyde University. He recognized that quaternary ammonium compounds break down spontaneously at varying temperature and pH, a phenomenon known for over 100 years as *Hofmann degradation*. Many such substances also have neuromuscular blocking properties, and in the search for such an agent that broke down at body temperature and pH, atracurium was developed. Hofmann degradation can be considered as a 'safety net' in the sick patient with impaired liver or renal function, as atracurium will still be cleared from the body. Some renal excretion occurs in the healthy patient (10%), as does ester hydrolysis in the plasma; probably only about 45% of the drug is eliminated by Hofmann degradation in the normal patient.

Atracurium (and vecuronium) were developed in an attempt to obtain a non-depolarizing agent which had a more rapid onset, was shorter acting and had less cardiovascular effects than the older agents. Atracurium (0.5 mg.kg^{-1}) does not produce neuromuscular block as rapidly as suxamethonium; onset time is 2.0–2.5 min, depending on the dose used (Table 11.1). However, it produces more rapid recovery than the older non-depolarizing agents, and can easily be reversed 20–25 min after administration of a dose of $2 \times ED_{95}$ (0.4 mg.kg^{-1}). The drug does not have any direct cardiovascular effect, but can release histamine (about a third of that released by tubocurarine), and can therefore produce a local weal and flare around the injection site, especially if a small vein is used. This may be accompanied by a slight fall in blood pressure.

A metabolite of Hofmann degradation, *laudano-sine*, has epileptogenic properties, although this complication has never been reported in humans. The plasma levels of laudanosine required to make animals convulse are much higher than those reached during general anaesthesia, even if large doses of atracurium are given during a prolonged procedure, and there can be little concern about this metabolite in clinical practice. In patients in the ITU with multiple organ failure, who may receive atracurium for several days, laudanosine levels are higher, but as yet no reports have occurred of cerebral toxicity.

Cisatracurium. This is the most recently introduced neuromuscular blocker, and is of particular interest because it is an example of the development of specific isomers of a drug to produce a 'clean' substance with the desired clinical actions but with reduced side-effects. Cisatracurium is the R-cis R′-cis isomer of atracurium, and one of the 10 possible isomers of the parent compound. It is three to four times more potent than atracurium (ED_{95} 0.05 mg.kg^{-1}), and has a slightly longer duration of action. Its main advantage is that it does not release histamine, and therefore is associated with greater cardiovascular stability. Like atracurium, it undergoes Hofmann elimination. As a lower dose of this more potent drug is given it produces less laudanosine than an equipotent dose of atracurium.

Doxacurium chloride. This bisquaternary ammonium compound is now available in the US, but it is doubtful if it will be launched in Great Britain. It undergoes a small amount of metabolism in the plasma by cholinesterase (6%), but is excreted mainly through the kidney. It is the most potent non-depolarizing neuromuscular blocking agent available; an intubating dose is only 0.05 mg.kg^{-1}. It has a very long onset of action (Table 11.1) and a prolonged and unpredictable duration of effect. However, it has no cardiovascular effects, and may therefore be of use during long surgical procedures in which cardiovascular stability is required, e.g. cardiac surgery.

Mivacurium chloride. This drug is metabolized by plasma cholinesterase at 88% of the rate of suxamethonium. An intubating dose ($2 \times ED_{95} = 0.15$ mg.kg^{-1}) has a similar onset of action to an equipotent dose of atracurium but,

in the presence of normal plasma cholinesterase, recovery after mivacurium is much faster (Table 11.1) and administration of an anticholinesterase may not be necessary (if neuromuscular function is being monitored and good recovery can be demonstrated). Full recovery in such circumstances takes about 20–25 min, but the drug can be antagonized easily within 15 min. Mivacurium is useful particularly for surgical procedures requiring muscle relaxation in which even atracurium and vecuronium seem too long-acting, and when it is desirable to avoid the side-effects of suxamethonium, e.g. for bronchoscopy, oesophagoscopy, laparoscopy, tonsillectomy. The drug produces a similar amount of histamine release as does atracurium.

In the presence of reduced plasma cholinesterase activity, because of either inherited or acquired factors, the duration of action of mivacurium may be increased. In patients heterozygous for the atypical cholinesterase gene, the duration of action of mivacurium is comparable to that of atracurium, negating its advantages. The action of the drug may also be prolonged in patients with hepatic and renal disease.

Aminosteroid compounds

This group of non-depolarizing neuromuscular blocking agents all possess at least one quaternary ammonium group, attached to a steroid nucleus. They produce fewer adverse cardiovascular effects than do the benzylisoquinolinium compounds, and do not stimulate histamine release from mast cells to the same degree. They are excreted unchanged through the kidney and also undergo de-acetylation in the liver. The de-acetylated metabolites may possess weak neuromuscular blocking properties. The parent compound may also be excreted unchanged in the bile.

Pancuronium bromide. This bisquaternary amine, the first steroid muscle relaxant used clinically, was developed by Savege and Hewitt in the Organon laboratories and marketed in 1964. The intubating dose is 0.1 mg.kg^{-1}, which takes 3–4 min to reach its maximum effect (Table 11.1). The clinical duration of action of the drug is long, especially in the presence of potent inhalational agents or renal dysfunction, as 60% of a dose of the drug is excreted unchanged through the kidney. It is also de-acetylated in the liver; some of the metabolites have neuromuscular blocking properties.

Pancuronium does not stimulate histamine release and is therefore of use in patients with a history of allergy. However, it has direct vagolytic and sympathomimetic effects which can cause tachycardia and hypertension. It inhibits plasma cholinesterase and therefore potentiates any drug metabolized by this enzyme, e.g. suxamethonium, mivacurium.

Vecuronium bromide. This steroidal agent was developed in an attempt to reduce the cardiovascular effects of pancuronium. It is very similar in structure to the older drug, differing only in the loss of a methyl group from one quaternary ammonium radical. Thus it is a monoquaternary amine. An intubating dose of 0.1 mg.kg^{-1} produces profound neuromuscular block within 3 min, which is slightly longer than the onset time of atracurium, but shorter than tubocurarine and pancuronium. This dose produces clinical block for about 30 min. Vecuronium rarely produces histamine release, nor does it have any direct cardiovascular effects, although it allows the cardiac effects of other anaesthetic agents, such as bradycardia produced by the opioids, to go unchallenged. Vecuronium is excreted through the kidney, although to a lesser extent than pancuronium (30%), and undergoes hepatic de-acetylation; repeated doses should be used with care in patients with renal or hepatic disease.

Pipecuronium bromide. This analogue of pancuronium was developed in Hungary in 1980 and is now marketed in Eastern Europe and the US. An intubating dose is 0.07 mg.kg^{-1}. The onset time and time to recovery from block are similar to those of pancuronium (Table 11.1) and excretion of the drug through the kidney is significant (66%). In contrast to pancuronium, pipecuronium produces marked cardiovascular stability, having no vagolytic or sympathomimetic effects. It may therefore be of use during major surgery in patients with cardiac disease.

Rocuronium bromide. This monoquaternary amine is the latest aminosteroid to be introduced into clinical practice. It has the most rapid onset of any of the non-depolarizing muscle relaxants. It is six to eight times less potent than vecuronium but has approximately the same molecular weight; consequently, a greater number of drug molecules may reach the post-junctional receptors within the first few circulations, enabling faster development of neuromuscular block. In a dose of 0.6 mg.kg^{-1}, good or excellent intubating conditions are usually achieved within 60–90 s; this is only slightly slower than the onset time of suxamethonium. The clinical duration is 30–45 min.

In most other respects, rocuronium resembles vecuronium. The drug stimulates little histamine release or cardiovascular disturbance, although in high doses it has a mild vagolytic property which sometimes results in an increase in heart rate. The drug is excreted unchanged in the urine and in the bile, and thus the duration of action may be increased by severe renal or hepatic dysfunction.

Factors affecting duration of non-depolarizing neuromuscular block

The duration of action of non-depolarizing muscle relaxants is affected by a number of factors. Effects are most marked with the longer-acting agents, such as tubocurarine and pancuronium.

1. *Prior administration of suxamethonium* potentiates the effect and lengthens the duration of action of non-depolarizing drugs.

2. *Concomitant administration of a potent inhalational agent* increases the duration of block. This is most marked with the ether anaesthetic agents such as isoflurane and enflurane, but occurs to a lesser extent with halothane.

3. *pH changes.* Metabolic, and to a lesser extent, respiratory acidosis, extends the duration of block. With monoquaternary amines such as tubocurarine and vecuronium, this effect is produced probably by the ionization, under acidic conditions, of a second nitrogen atom in the molecule, making the drug more potent.

4. *Body temperature.* Hypothermia potentiates block as impairment of organ function delays metabolism and excretion of these drugs. This can be seen in patients undergoing cardiac surgery; reduced doses of muscle relaxants are required during cardiopulmonary bypass.

5. *Age*. Non-depolarizing muscle relaxants which depend on organ metabolism and excretion can be expected to have a prolonged effect in old age, as organ function deteriorates. In healthy neonates, who have a higher extracellular volume than adults, resistance may occur, but if the baby is sick or immature then, because of under-development of the neuromuscular junction and other organ function, increased sensitivity may be encountered. Children of school age tend to be relatively resistant to non-depolarizing muscle relaxants, when given on a weight basis.

6. *Electrolyte changes*. A low serum potassium concentration potentiates neuromuscular block by changing the value of the resting membrane potential of the postsynaptic membrane. A reduced ionized calcium concentration also potentiates block by impairing presynaptic acetylcholine release.

7. *Myasthenia gravis*. In this disease, the number and half-life of the postsynaptic receptors are reduced by auto-antibodies produced in the thymus gland. Thus, the patient is more sensitive to the effects of non-depolarizing muscle relaxants. Resistance to suxamethonium may be encountered.

8. *Other disease states*. Because of the altered pharmacokinetics of muscle relaxants in hepatic and renal disease, prolongation of action may be found in these conditions, especially if excretion of the drug is dependent upon these organs.

Characteristics of non-depolarizing neuromuscular block

If a small, subparalysing dose of a non-depolarizing neuromuscular blocking drug is administered, the following characteristics are recognized:

1. A decreased response to a low voltage twitch stimulus (e.g. 1 Hz) which, if repeated, decreases further in amplitude. This effect, which is in contrast to that produced by a depolarizing drug, is also seen to a greater degree when the train-of-four twitch response is applied, and with higher, tetanic rates of stimulation. It is often referred to as '*fade*', or decrement.

2. Post-tetanic potentiation (PTP) or facilitation (PTF) of the twitch response can be demonstrated (see Fig. 11.6).

3. Neuromuscular block is reversed by the administration of an anticholinesterase.

4. No muscle fasciculation is visible.

Anticholinesterases

These agents are used in clinical practice to inhibit the action of acetylcholinesterase at the neuromuscular junction, thus prolonging the half-life of acetylcholine and potentiating its effect, especially in the presence of residual amounts of non-depolarizing muscle relaxant at the end of surgery. The most commonly used anticholinesterase during anaesthesia is *neostigmine*, but *edrophonium* and *pyridostigmine* are also available. These carbamate esters are all water-soluble, quaternary ammonium compounds which are poorly absorbed from the gastrointestinal tract. The more lipid-soluble tertiary amine, *physostigmine*, has a similar effect and is more suitable for oral administration, but crosses the blood–brain barrier.

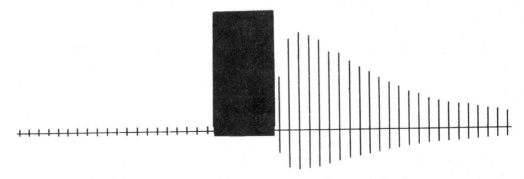

Fig. 11.6 A 5-s burst of tetanus (50 Hz), applied after a run of single twitch stimuli, causes a transient increase in the height of subsequent twitches, although they gradually decrease to their former height; this is post-tetanic potentiation (PTP) or facilitation (PTF).

Organophosphorus compounds also inhibit acetylcholinesterase, but unlike other agents, their effect is irreversible; recovery occurs only on generation of more enzyme, which takes some weeks.

Anticholinesterases are also given orally to patients with *myasthenia gravis*. In this disease, the patient possesses antibodies to the postsynaptic membrane receptor, reducing the efficacy of acetylcholine. The use of these drugs is thought to increase the amount and duration of action of acetylcholine at the neuromuscular junction, thus enhancing neuromuscular transmission.

Neostigmine. This drug combines reversibly with acetylcholinesterase by the formation of an ester linkage, which lasts about 30 min. Neostigmine is largely excreted unchanged through the kidney and has a half-life of about 45 min. It is presented in brown vials, as it breaks down on exposure to light. Neostigmine potentiates the action of acetylcholine wherever it is a neurotransmitter, including all cholinergic nerve endings; thus it produces bradycardia, salivation, sweating, bronchospasm, increased intestinal motility and blurred vision. These cholinergic effects may be reduced by the simultaneous administration of an anticholinergic agent such as atropine or glycopyrrolate. The usual dose of neostigmine is in the order of $0.035\ \text{mg.kg}^{-1}$, in combination with either atropine $0.015\ \text{mg.kg}^{-1}$ or glycopyrrolate $0.01\ \text{mg.kg}^{-1}$. Neostigmine takes at least 2 min to have an initial effect, and recovery from neuromuscular block is maximally enhanced by 5–7 min.

Edrophonium. This anticholinesterase forms an ionic bond with the enzyme but does not undergo a chemical reaction with it. The effect is therefore more short-lived than with neostigmine, of the order of only a few minutes. Edrophonium has a quicker onset of action than neostigmine, producing clinical signs of recovery within 1 min. However, its effects are more evanescent; when edrophonium is give in the presence of profound neuromuscular block, the degree of neuromuscular block may *increase* after an initial period of recovery. The dose of edrophonium is $0.5–1.0\ \text{mg.kg}^{-1}$.

Pyridostigmine. This drug has a longer onset time than neostigmine or edrophonium, and also a longer duration of action. It is used more frequently as oral therapy in patients with myasthenia gravis than in anaesthesia.

Physostigmine. This anticholinesterase, also known as *eserine*, is a tertiary amine and is more lipid-soluble than the other carbamate esters. It is therefore more easily absorbed from the gastrointestinal tract, and also crosses the blood–brain barrier.

Organophosphorus compounds. These substances are considered to be irreversible inhibitors of acetylcholinesterase, as by phosphorylation of the enzyme they produce a very stable complex which is resistant to reactivation or hydrolysis. Synthesis of new enzyme must occur before recovery. These agents, which include di-isopropyl-fluorophosphonate (DFP) and tetraethylpyrophosphate (TEPP), are used as insecticides and chemical warfare agents. They are readily absorbed through the lungs and skin. Poisoning is not uncommon among farm workers. Muscarinic effects, such as salivation, sweating and bronchospasm are combined with nicotinic effects, such as muscle weakness. Central nervous effects such as tremor and convulsions may occur, as may unconsciousness and respiratory failure. Reactivators of acetylcholinesterase are used to treat this form of poisoning; they include *pralidoxime* and *obidoxime*. Atropine, anticonvulsants and artificial ventilation may be necessary. Chronic exposure may produce a polyneuritis. Carbamates such as pyridostigmine are used prophylactically in those threatened by chemical warfare with these compounds.

Ecothiopate is an organophosphorus compound with a quaternary amine group; it was used as an eye-drop preparation in ophthalmology to produce miosis in narrow angle glaucoma. It inhibits cholinesterase by phosphorylation and will thus potentiate all esters metabolized by this enzyme. It has now been withdrawn from the British market.

A new generation of organophosphorus compounds may be beneficial in Alzheimer's disease, and clinical trials are in progress. Neuromuscular blockers must be used with great caution if these patients require anaesthesia.

NEUROMUSCULAR MONITORING

There is no clinical tool available to measure accurately neuromuscular transmission in a muscle group. Thus, neither the amount of acetylcholine released in response to a given stimulus, nor the number of postsynaptic receptors blocked by a given non-depolarizing muscle relaxant can be assessed. However, it is possible to obtain a crude estimate of muscle contraction during anaesthesia using a variety of techniques. All require the application to a peripheral nerve of a current of up to 50 mA, for a fraction of a millisecond (often 0.2 ms), necessitating a voltage of up to 300 V. Usually, a nerve which is readily accessible to the anaesthetist, such as the ulnar, facial or lateral popliteal nerve, is used. The muscle response to the nerve stimulus can then be assessed by either *visual* or *tactile* means, or it can be recorded by more sophisticated methods.

Mechanomyography. A strain-gauge transducer can be used to measure the force of contraction of, for instance, the thumb, in response to stimulation of the ulnar nerve at the wrist. This measurement can then be charted using a recording device. Accurate measurements of the twitch or tetanic response can be made, although the hand must be splinted firmly for reproducible results. This technique is primarily a research tool.

Electromyography. The electromyographic response of a muscle is measured in response to the same electrical stimulus, using recording electrodes similar to ECG pads placed over the motor point of the stimulated muscle. For instance, if the ulnar nerve is stimulated, the recording electrodes are placed over the motor point of adductor pollicis in the thumb (Fig. 11.7). A compound muscle action potential can be recorded. Although primarily a research tool, there are now several simple clinical instruments, such as the Datex Relaxograph, which give a less accurate, but similar recording. Maintaining the exact position of the hand is not as essential with electromyography as with mechanomyography.

Accelerography. With this technique, the acceleration of the thumb is measured in response to the nerve stimulus and the force of contraction can be derived (force = mass × acceleration). Clinical equipment is available (e.g. the accelerograph) which provides a quantitative assessment of, for instance, the twitch height in comparison with a control reading.

Modes of stimulation

Several different rates of stimulation can be

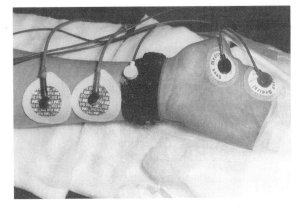

Fig. 11.7 The necessary positioning of the hand to obtain an electromyographic recording of the response of the adductor pollicis muscle to stimulation of the ulnar nerve is demonstrated. An earth electrode is placed round the wrist. Two recording electrodes are placed over the muscle on the hand; the distal one lies over the motor point.

applied to the nerve in an attempt to produce a sensitive index of neuromuscular function. It is considered essential always to apply a *supramaximal* stimulus to the nerve, i.e. the strength of the electrical stimulus (V) should be increased until the response no longer increases. It is then increased by a further 25%.

Twitch

A square-wave stimulus of short duration (0.1–0.2 ms) is applied to a peripheral nerve. In isolation, such a stimulus is of limited value, although if applied repeatedly, perhaps before and after a dose of a muscle relaxant, it may be possible to assess crudely the effects of the drug. Such rates of stimulation have the benefit of being less painful, with no untoward effects after recovery from anaesthesia.

Train-of-four twitch response

In an attempt to assess the degree of neuromuscular block clinically, Ali, Utting & Gray (1971) described a development of the twitch response which, it was hoped, would be more sensitive than repeated single twitches. Four stimuli, each of about 2 Hz, are applied over 2 s, with a 10-s gap between each train-of-four. On administration of a small dose of a non-depolarizing

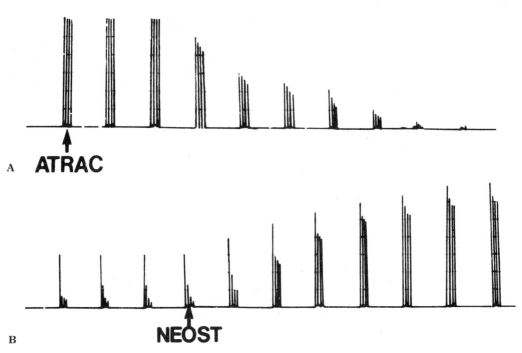

Fig. 11.8 (**A**) After the administration of a non-depolarizing muscle relaxant (in this instance atracurium 0.5 mg.kg^{-1}), the decrease in height of the fourth twitch of the train-of-four response is more marked than the decrease in height of the third twitch, which is more marked than the decrease in the second, which is greater than the decrease in the first. The effect is known as 'fade'. Within 2 min, the train-of-four response has been ablated completely. (**B**) On recovery, the first twitch response appears first, then the second, the third and finally the fourth. Marked fade is present, but on administration of an anticholinesterase, recovery of all four twitches occurs rapidly.

muscle relaxant, *fade* of the train-of-four may be visible. The ratio of the fourth to the first twitch is called the *train-of-four ratio*. In the presence of a larger dose of such a drug, the fourth twitch disappears first, then the third, followed by the second and, finally, the first twitch (Fig. 11.8A). On recovery from neuromuscular block, the first twitch appears first, then the second (when the first twitch has recovered to about 20% control), then the third, and finally the fourth (Fig. 11.8B).

It is generally thought that at least three of the four twitches must be absent to obtain adequate surgical access for upper abdominal surgery. It is also preferable to reverse residual block with an anticholinesterase only when the second twitch is visible, if good recovery is to be relied upon. After reversal, good muscle tone, as assessed clinically by the patient being able to cough, raise their head from the pillow for at least 5 s, protrude the tongue and have good grip strength, can

be anticipated when the train-of-four ratio has reached about 0.7.

It is recognized that, although the number of twitches present in the train-of-four during profound neuromuscular block can easily be assessed by visual or tactile means, it is impossible, even for the expert, to assess the value of the train-of-four *ratio* by these methods. In addition, visual or tactile evaluation fails to detect any fade of the train-of-four when the ratio is in excess of 50%. Thus, failure to detect fade with a nerve stimulator does not always guarantee adequate reversal. A recording of the response is preferable.

Tetanic stimulation

This is the most sensitive form of neuromuscular stimulation. Frequencies of 50–100 Hz are applied to a peripheral nerve to detect even minor degrees of residual neuromuscular block; thus, tetanic fade may be present when the twitch response is normal. Tetanic rates of stimulation may be applied under anaesthesia, but in the awake patient they are intolerable. Indeed, on recovery from anaesthesia in which tetanic stimulation has been applied, the patient may be aware of some discomfort in the area of application.

Post-tetanic potentiation (PTP) or facilitation (PTF)

This method of monitoring was developed in an attempt to assess more profound degrees of neuromuscular block produced by non-depolarizing neuromuscular blocking agents. If a single twitch stimulus is applied to the nerve with little or no neuromuscular response, but, after a 5 s delay, a burst of 50 Hz tetanus is given for 5 s, the effect of a further twitch stimulus 3 s later produces an enhanced effect (Fig. 11.6). In the presence of profound block, repeated single twitches applied after the tetanus until the response disappears can be counted; this is known as the *post-tetanic count*. The augmentation of the twitch is thought to be due to presynaptic mobilization of acetylcholine, as a result of the positive feedback effect of the run of tetanus.

Double burst stimulation (DBS)

In an attempt to develop a clinical tool which would allow more accurate assessment by visual or tactile means of the fade of the twitch response after administration of a non-depolarizing drug, Viby-Mogensen and his colleagues (1982) have suggested the application of two or three short bursts of 50 Hz tetanus, each comprising two or three impulses separated by a 750 ms interval.

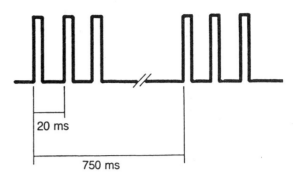

Fig. 11.9 The pattern of double-burst stimulation. Three bursts of 50 Hz tetanus, at 20 ms intervals, every 750 ms, is shown.

Each square wave impulse lasts for 0.2 ms (Fig. 11.9). If a record of the fade of the DBS and train-of-four response are compared, they are very similar, but there is evidence to suggest that visual assessment of the DBS is more accurate.

Indications for neuromuscular monitoring

It is preferable always to monitor neuromuscular function when a muscle relaxant is used during anaesthesia, but it is especially indicated in the following circumstances:

1. During prolonged anaesthesia, when repeated increments of neuromuscular blocking agents are required.
2. When infusions of muscle relaxants are given (including in the ITU).
3. In the presence of renal or hepatic dysfunction.
4. In patients with neuromuscular disorders.
5. In patients with a history of sensitivity to a muscle relaxant or poor recovery from block.
6. When poor reversal of neuromuscular block is encountered unexpectedly.

FURTHER READING

Ali H H, Utting J E, Gray T C 1971 Quantitative assessment of residual antidepolarising block (Part II). British Journal of Anaesthesia 43: 478–484

Beecher H K, Todd D P 1954 A study of the deaths associated with anaesthesia and surgery. Annals of Surgery 140: 2–34

Bevan D R, Bevan J C, Donati F 1988 Muscle relaxants in clinical anesthesia. Year Book Medical Publishers Inc, Chicago.

Bowman W C 1992 Pharmacology of neuromuscular function. John Wright and Sons, Bristol.

Gray T C, Halton J 1946 A milestone in anaesthesia? (d-tubocurarine chloride). Proceedings of the Royal Society of Medicine 39: 400–410

Kalow W, Genest K 1957 A method of detection of atypical forms of human pseudocholinesterase. Canadian Journal of Biochemistry and Physiology 35: 339–346

Paton W D M 1959 The effects of muscle relaxants other than muscle relaxation. Anesthesiology 29: 453–463

Viby-Mogensen J 1982 Clinical assessment of neuromuscular transmission. British Journal of Anaesthesia 54: 209–223

12. Drugs affecting the autonomic nervous system

THE AUTONOMIC NERVOUS SYSTEM

The term autonomic nervous system (ANS) refers to the nervous and humoral mechanisms which modify the function of the autonomous or automatic organs. These organs or functions include heart rate and force of contraction, calibre of blood vessels, contraction and relaxation of smooth muscle in gut, bladder and bronchi, visual accommodation and pupillary size, and secretion from exocrine and other glands. The ANS may be subdivided into two separate entities, the parasympathetic and sympathetic systems, on the basis of anatomical and pharmacological criteria. In order to understand the action of drugs on the ANS it is necessary initially to review these subdivisions briefly.

Parasympathetic system

The neuronal components of the parasympathetic system arise from cell bodies of the motor nuclei of the cranial nerves, III, VII, IX and X in the brain stem, and from the sacral segments of the spinal cord. The preganglionic fibres run almost to the organ innervated and synapse in ganglia within the organ, giving rise to postganglionic fibres which innervate the relevant tissues. The ganglion cells may be well-organized, as in the myenteric plexus of the intestine, or diffuse, as in the bladder or blood vessels. The chemical transmitter both at pre- and postganglionic synapses is acetylcholine (ACh). The neurotransmitter is stored in the presynaptic terminal in agranular vesicles, released by neuronal depolarization, and acts at specific receptor sites on the postsynaptic terminal. Its activity is terminated by diffusion

from the site of action and more specifically by degradation by acetylcholinesterase.

Based upon the actions of the alkaloids muscarine and nicotine, the specific receptor sites within the parasympathetic nervous system have been subdivided pharmacologically. Thus, the actions of ACh at the postganglionic neuroeffector site are mimicked by muscarine and are termed muscarinic, whereas preganglionic transmission is termed nicotinic. ACh is also the transmitter substance released from voluntary nerve endings at the neuromuscular junction. The receptor sites in this situation are also nicotinic; the pharmacology of drugs acting at this site is described in Chapter 11. Although it is possible to modify transmission at the preganglionic (nicotinic) site, drugs active at this site (ganglion-blocking drugs) are now rarely used clinically and we shall concentrate primarily in this chapter on drugs active at the postganglionic muscarinic site.

Sympathetic nervous system

The preganglionic fibres of the sympathetic nervous system arise in the cell bodies in the lateral horn of the spinal cord associated with spinal segments T1 to L2, the so-called thoracolumbar outflow. The first synapse occurs shortly after leaving the spinal cord in the sympathetic ganglionic chain, and gives rise to postganglionic fibres which innervate the effector organs. ACh is the transmitter, via a nicotinic receptor, at the preganglionic synapse (as in the parasympathetic ganglia). The adrenal medulla is innervated by preganglionic fibres from the thoracolumbar outflow, activation of which stimulates, via nicotinic ACh receptors, the release of adrenaline from this gland. At the postganglionic sympathetic endings, chemical transmission is mediated by noradrenaline, which is present in the presynaptic terminals as well as the adrenal medulla. Adrenaline is found in only insignificant amounts in the nerve endings and is released primarily as a circulating hormone from the adrenal medulla. Adrenaline and noradrenaline are composed of a basic ring structure with -OH groups in the 3 and 4 positions in relationship to a side chain ending in an amine subgroup (Fig. 12.1). Both catecholamines are synthesized from the essential amino acid phenylalanine via a number of steps including the production of dopamine, which may act as a precursor for both adrenaline and noradrenaline when administered exogenously (see below). The action of noradrenaline released from granules in the presynaptic terminals is terminated by diffusion from the site of action, reuptake back into the presynaptic nerve ending, and metabolism locally by the enzyme catechol-*o*-methyltransferase.

The actions of the catecholamines are mediated by specific postsynaptic cell surface receptors. Pharmacological subdivision of these receptors was first suggested by Ahlquist in 1948 into two groups (α and β) based upon the effects of adrenaline at peripheral sympathetic sites. These were originally termed excitatory and inhibitory receptors, respectively, because of their general tendency to produce those effects when stimulated, but as many exceptions to this general rule have been found, they are now referred to solely as α- and β-adrenoceptors. Since Ahlquist's original observations, further subdivision of both these receptor systems has been proposed on both functional and anatomical grounds. Thus, β-adrenoceptor-mediated events in the heart (β$_1$ effects; increase in force and rate of contraction) have been differentiated from those producing smooth-muscle relaxation in bronchi and blood vessels (β$_2$ effects). Similarly, α-adrenoceptor-mediated postsynaptic events (e.g. vasoconstriction) have been termed α$_1$ effects to differentiate them from the feedback inhibition by noradrenaline of its own release from the presynaptic terminals mediated via an α$_2$-adrenoceptor on the presynaptic membrane. These various subdivisions are summarized in Table 12.1.

On the basis of more recent detailed pharmacological studies, it has become apparent that this

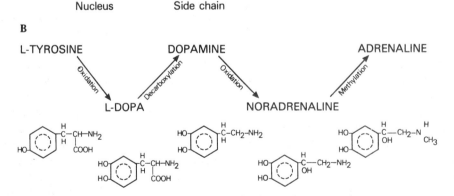

Fig. 12.1 A Standard molecular structure of catecholamines, composed of a catechol ring with –OH substitution in the 3 and 4 positions relative to the amine side chain. **B** Intermediate metabolism of naturally occurring catecholamines from the essential amino acid L-tyrosine.

Table 12.1 Responses of major effector organs to autonomic nerve impulses

Organ	Receptor subtype	Adrenergic	Cholinergic
Heart	β_1 (?β_2)	↑ Heart rate ↑ Force of contraction ↑ Automaticity and conduction velocity	↓ Heart rate ↓ Force of contraction ↓ Conduction velocity
Arteries	α_1 (?α_2) β_2	Constriction Dilatation	Dilatation
Veins	α_1 (?α_2) $\beta 2$	Constriction ++ Dilatation +	
Lung 　Bronchial muscles 　Bronchial glands	 $\beta 2$?	 Relaxation + (? Inhibition)	 Contraction ++ Stimulation +
Gastrointestinal tract 　Motility 　Sphincters	 β_2 (?α_2) α	 Decrease Contraction	 Increase +++ Relaxation
Kidney	β_2	Renin secretion	
Bladder 　Detrusor 　Sphincter	 β_2 α	 Relaxation Contraction	 Contraction +++ Relaxation ++
Liver	β_2, α	Glycogenolysis ++ Gluconeogenesis +	? Glycogen synthesis
Uterus	β_2, α	Pregnant contraction (α) Non-pregnant relaxation (β)	

anatomical subdivision of the adrenoceptor subtypes is an oversimplification. Thus, most organs and tissues contain both β_1- and β_2-adrenoceptors, which may even subserve the same function. Differentiation of β-adrenoceptor subtypes is now based more directly on the hierarchical potencies of various catecholamine agonists (isoprenaline, adrenaline and noradrenaline) and assessed on the basis of the functional or biochemical response of adrenoceptors in different tissues. Thus, at β_2-adrenoceptors, isoprenaline is more potent than adrenaline, which is more potent than noradrenaline. In contrast, adrenaline and noradrenaline are equipotent at β_1-adrenoceptors. It seems probable that postsynpatic β_1-adrenoceptors in tissues are closely associated with the noradrenergic neurone and respond to released noradrenaline, whereas β_2-adrenoceptors are at sites distant to the nerve terminals and are principally controlled by circulating adrenaline. In addition, it is now well-established that α_1- and α_2-adrenoceptors exist postsynaptically and subserve the function of vasoconstriction of resistance vessels which control arterial pressure and tissue perfusion.

However, for the purposes of general discussion of drugs acting on the sympathetic nervous system, the original anatomical subdivisions will be used and important departures from this scheme indicated where relevant. The important actions of the subdivisions of the ANS on various effector organs are summarized in Table 12.1.

Second messenger systems

Stimulation of catecholamine receptors on the extracellular surface of the cell membrane leads to activation of intracellular events by the generation of so-called second messengers. Thus, stimulation of the β-adrenoceptor leads, via coupling to the enzyme adenylate cyclase, to the generation of intracellular cyclic adenosine monophosphate (cAMP). cAMP in turn, via activation of intracellular enzyme pathways, produces the associated alteration in cell function (e.g. increased force of cardiac muscle contraction, liver glycogenolysis, bronchial smooth-muscle relaxation). The concentration of intracellular cAMP is also modulated by the enzyme phosphodiesterase, which breaks down cAMP to its inactive form. Thus, the balance between production and degradation of cAMP is an important regulatory system for cell function. This somewhat simplified scheme is illustrated in Figure 12.2. The mechanism of transduction of the signal from the β-adrenoceptors across the cell membrane to the enzyme adenylate cyclase is incompletely understood, but almost certainly involves specialized intramembranous proteins that interact with guanine nucleotides.

Since β-adrenoceptor stimulation increases production of cAMP, its association with the enzyme adenylate cyclase is termed positive coupling. The converse, receptor activation leading to reduction of intracellular cAMP, is termed negative coupling to adenylate cyclase and this results from stimulation of the α_2-adrenoceptor (Fig. 12.2). An example of this negative coupling is seen in α-adrenoceptor-mediated platelet aggregation, which is associated with a reduction in platelet cAMP content. The complex interactions between inhibitory (α_2) and stimulatory (β_1 and β_2) effects on cAMP in a single cell are still incompletely understood.

The α_1-adrenoceptor does not affect cAMP levels within the cell directly. Activation of this receptor produces changes in membrane transfer of Ca^{2+} and in intracellular calcium binding which lead, for example, to smooth-muscle contraction. The mechanism whereby the α_1-adrenoceptor alters transmembrane ionic flux is probably related to receptor-activated changes in membrane phospholipid content and the modulation of calcium channels.

DRUG EFFECTS ON THE SYMPATHETIC NERVOUS SYSTEM

Drugs which partially or completely mimic the effects of sympathetic nerve stimulation or adrenal medullary discharge are termed sympathomimetic. A wide variety of drugs has sympathomimetic activity, and they may be classified into drugs which act:

1. Directly on the adrenoceptor, e.g. the catecholamines adrenaline, noradrenaline and isoprenaline.

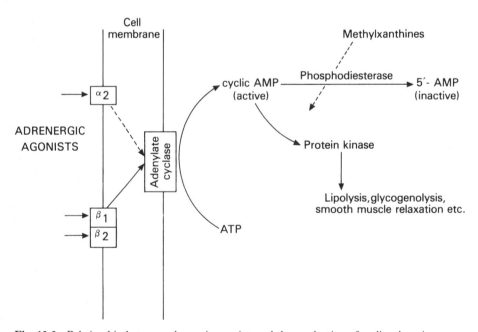

Fig. 12.2 Relationship between adrenergic agonists and the production of cyclic adenosine monophosphate (AMP). Binding of agonist to the adrenoceptors on the cell-surface membrane activates either stimulation ($\rightarrow \beta_1$, β_2) or inhibition ($--\rightarrow \alpha_2$) of the enzyme adenylate cyclase which catalyses the conversion of adenosine triphosphate (ATP) to cyclic AMP and is, in turn, inactivated by the intracellular enzyme, phosphodiesterase. Cyclic AMP interacts with cytoplasmic protein kinase to initiate various cell functions.

2. Indirectly, causing release of noradrenaline from the adrenergic nerve ending, e.g. amphetamine, ephedrine.

3. By both mechanisms, e.g. dopamine.

The major clinical effects of these drugs are produced via α- or β-adrenoceptors or both (dopamine also acts via dopamine receptors; see below), and can be classified as follows.

Cardiovascular effects

Blood-vessel calibre

Contraction and relaxation of smooth muscle in the blood vessel walls determine the calibre of the lumen and thus resistance to blood flow. Contraction of the smooth muscle produces vasoconstriction and increased peripheral resistance and is mediated via α-adrenoceptor stimulation. This comprises the normal physiological noradrenergic vasoconstrictor tone in the blood vessels. Conversely, relaxation of arterial smooth muscle produces vasodilatation via activation of β₂-adrenoceptors and is mediated physiologically by circulating adrenaline.

Cardiac contraction

Stimulation of the force and rate of cardiac contraction (inotropic and chronotropic effects respectively) is mediated via β-adrenoceptors in the heart muscle stimulated physiologically by both adrenaline and noradrenaline. Although the β₁-adrenoceptor is associated classically with this activity, recent functional and biochemical studies have indicated a role also for the β₂-adrenoceptors which are present in cardiac cells in these actions of sympathomimetic drugs.

Cardiac output

The overall effect of catecholamines on cardiac output depends on the interaction between effects on cardiac rate and contractility and changes in peripheral vascular resistance. Thus, adrenaline and isoprenaline increase cardiac output via positive inotropism coupled with peripheral vasodilatation. However, noradrenaline, particularly in high dosage, may reduce cardiac output by intense vasoconstriction despite an equally effective action on cardiac contractility.

Arterial pressure

The effects on arterial pressure depend on the balance of cardiac output and peripheral resistance and vary with the effects of different sympathomimetic agents. Drugs which increase peripheral resistance in addition to cardiac contractility are most effective in increasing arterial pressure, but this may be at the expense of intense and possibly damaging vasoconstriction.

Non-vascular smooth muscle

In general, non-vascular smooth muscle is relaxed by sympathomimetic drugs. This effect is generalized and mediated by the β₂-adrenoceptor. Thus, bladder wall smooth muscle and, more importantly, uterine smooth muscle may be relaxed by these drugs. The latter effect is more pronounced in the oestrogen-dominated uterus and sympathomimetic agents are used to reduce uterine contractility in threatened premature labour. Most important, however, is bronchodilatation; drugs specifically active at β₂-adrenoceptors (β₂-agonists) are potent bronchodilators (see Chapter 13), in addition to possessing vasodilating properties.

Metabolic effects

The metabolic effects of sympathetic nervous stimulation are related to effects on glucose and lipid metabolism. Insulin release is partially under sympathetic control and is stimulated via activation of a β₂-adrenoceptor. Likewise, adrenaline-induced glycogenolysis in both the liver and muscles is β₂-adrenoceptor-mediated. Thus, the physiological response to adrenaline release includes an increase in insulin release and provision of sufficient substrate for its action.

Stimulation of β₂-adrenoceptors on adipocytes induces mobilization and release of free fatty acids and results in increased blood concentrations.

Type 1 hypersensitivity

The release of mediators of anaphylaxis (histamine, slow-reacting substance of anaphylaxis (SRS-A)) from mast cells is inhibited by drugs which cause an increase in mast cell cAMP levels, including some sympathomimetic compounds active via the β_2-adrenoceptor on the mast cell surface. This effect may be relevant to the use of these drugs in acute asthma, and particularly anaphylaxis.

DRUGS ACTING ON THE SYMPATHETIC NERVOUS SYSTEM

We shall consider the most commonly used sympathomimetic agents in relation to this classification of actions and to their most common clinical usage in shock, hypotension and cardiac failure. The use of β-agonists as bronchodilators is discussed in Chapter 13.

Catecholamines

This group comprises naturally occurring and synthetic compounds which have a common molecular configuration based upon the catechol nucleus and amine side chain illustrated in Figure 12.1. Their effects are produced by interaction at specific catecholamine receptors (α, β and dopamine).

Adrenaline

Adrenaline has both α- and β-adrenergic effects. It is mainly used as a bronchodilator and in the treatment of acute allergic (anaphylactic) reactions. Except in emergency situations, i.v. injection is avoided because of the risk of inducing cardiac arrhythmias. Subcutaneous administration produces local vasoconstriction and a 'smoothed-out' effect by slowing absorption.

Adrenaline may be used by aerosol inhalation in bronchial asthma but its use in this context has largely been superseded by the newer β_2-agonists (see Chapter 13). Intravenous adrenaline is used in cardiac arrest to provoke ventricular fibrillation if asystole has occurred, so that electrical defibrillation can be initiated. There has been considerable interest in the administration of adrenaline by the tracheal route in emergency situations. Although apparently successful in animal models, absorption from the lungs in human cardiac arrest is limited and this route is not recommended unless direct access to the circulation is impossible.

The effects of adrenaline on arterial pressure and cardiac output are dependent on dose; although both α- and β-adrenoceptors are stimulated, β_2 vasodilatory effects are most sensitive. Thus, in large doses, direct stimulatory effects on cardiac output plus potent vasoconstriction (particularly in precapillary resistance vessels of skin, mucosa and kidney) produce a rapid increase in systolic arterial pressure. Diastolic pressure is affected less because of β_2-receptor-induced vasodilatation in muscle beds (the characteristic physiological redistribution of the circulation associated with adrenaline) and therefore pulse pressure widens. In low dosage, adrenaline may produce no overall effect on arterial pressure or a slight decrease with an increase in cardiac output.

Noradrenaline

In contrast to adrenaline, noradrenaline acts almost exclusively on α-adrenoceptors, although it is less potent at these receptor sites than adrenaline. Infusions of all doses of noradrenaline increase both systolic and diastolic arterial pressures by vasoconstriction of arteriolar and venous smooth muscle. Despite some stimulatory effects on cardiac contraction, the intense vasoconstriction leads either to no change or to a decrease in cardiac output at the cost of increased myocardial oxygen demand. In high dosage the universal vasopressor effect reduces renal blood flow and glomerular filtration rate.

The problems of induction of cardiac arrhythmias, adverse effects on renal function and intense vasoconstriction (leading to ischaemia in the periphery) have limited the clinical use of this agent in hypotension and shock.

Isoprenaline

Isoprenaline has virtually no activity at α-adrenoceptors. Its main actions are via β-adrenoceptors in the heart, smooth muscle of bronchi, skeletal muscle vasculature and the gut. Intravenous infusion reduces peripheral resistance mainly in skeletal muscle but also in renal and mesenteric vascular beds. Cardiac output is raised by an increase in venous return to the heart, combined with the positive inotropic and chronotropic actions of the drug. This may result in an increase in systolic arterial pressure.

Bronchial smooth muscle is relaxed and this effect, combined with other β_2 effects on release of mast cell mediators, has led to its widespread use in asthma, although newer specific β_2-agonists are probably preferable because of less cardiac stimulation.

Isoprenaline is absorbed unreliably by sublingual or oral routes and is usually administered by intravenous infusion or aerosol. As a direct cardiac stimulant, its most important use is in increasing the rate of cardiac contraction in heart block by direct chronotropic action on the subsidiary pacemaker; this is usually an interim measure following acute myocardial infarction before insertion of a temporary pacing wire. Its use as a positive inotropic agent in septicaemic and cardiogenic shock has been superseded by newer agents.

Dopamine

Dopamine stimulates both α- and β-adrenoceptors in addition to specific dopamine receptors in renal and mesenteric arteries. The balance of agonist properties exhibited by dopamine is closely related to dosage. It is administered only by the intravenous route.

Dopamine has a direct positive inotropic action on the myocardium via β-adrenoceptors and also by release of noradrenaline from noradrenergic nerve terminals. In low dosage (2–5 $\mu g.kg^{-1}.min^{-1}$) the major effects of dopamine are reduction of regional arterial resistance in renal and mesenteric vascular beds by an action on specific dopamine receptors. The result is an increase in renal blood flow, glomerular filtration rate and sodium excretion. Slightly higher doses (5–10 $\mu g.kg^{-1}.min^{-1}$) lead to increasing direct inotropic action with little or no peripheral vasoconstrictor effects. This combination of increased cardiac output and renal vasodilatation is particularly useful in the management of cardiogenic, traumatic, septic and hypovolaemic shock, where excessive use of direct sympathomimetics associated with a major increase in physiological sympathetic activity may lead to severe compromise of renal blood flow and peripheral circulation. At these low and intermediate doses, direct cardiac chronotropic action

is usually minimal, and tachyarrhythmias are less common than with other sympathomimetics. At these doses, dopamine increases systolic and pulse pressures, and has little effect on, or slightly increases, diastolic arterial pressure. Total peripheral resistance is usually unchanged.

In higher dosage (> 15 $\mu g.kg^{-1}.min^{-1}$), dopamine produces pronounced α-adrenoceptor activity, with direct vasoconstriction and increased cardiac stimulation (simulating infusions of noradrenaline). In general, therefore, these higher dose rates should be avoided. Occasionally the combination of a direct-acting vasodilator (e.g. sodium nitroprusside) and high-dose dopamine may be of use in cardiogenic shock, although results are generally not encouraging.

The half-life of dopamine is very short and therefore its effects are readily controlled by alteration of infusion rate.

Dobutamine

Dobutamine resembles dopamine chemically, but is primarily a β_1-agonist with little or no indirect activity. It has less β_2-agonist action than isoprenaline and no action at specific dopamine receptors. Dobutamine appears to be relatively more effective in enhancing cardiac contractile force than in increasing heart rate. Its effects on increasing sinus node automaticity, atrial and ventricular conduction velocity and enhancing atrioventricular nodal conduction are less than those of isoprenaline. Recent experimental work in both animals and humans indicates that dobutamine may exert some of its specific inotropic action via myocardial α_1-adrenoceptors. This is suggested by inhibition of the increase in cardiac output by α-adrenergic blocking agents and the relative selectivity of the active stereoisomer of dobutamine for α-agonist effects in animal models.

Infusion of dobutamine at rates ranging from 2.5 to 15 $\mu g.kg^{-1}.min^{-1}$ produces a progressive increase in cardiac output. This is associated with increased systolic arterial pressure, as peripheral resistance does not decrease initially. A decrease in pulmonary artery wedge pressure occurs also, indicating reduced diastolic filling pressure of the left ventricle. Urine output and sodium excretion are increased, presumably secondarily to the improvement in cardiovascular status, as the drug has no direct effect on renal vascular resistance.

As the effects of dobutamine on heart rate and systolic arterial pressure are minimal in comparison with other catecholamines, oxygen demands on the myocardium may be increased to a lesser degree. Thus, dobutamine appears theoretically to have some advantages over other catecholamines for improving myocardial function in heart failure when peripheral resistance and heart rate are high; in this circumstance, combination with vasodilator drugs may increase efficacy.

Non-catecholamines

This group of drugs includes a large number of synthetic amines which have a wide variety of clinical actions mimicking those of the catecholamines in different combinations. These drugs may have direct actions at adrenergic receptors or may produce effects by causing release of catecholamines after first being taken up into sympathetic nerve terminals.

Those compounds which cause release of catecholamines (e.g. amphetamine, ephedrine) have considerable effects within the central nervous system and their use has largely been superseded by newer drugs with more specific and less unpredictable actions.

Compounds with a direct action at adrenergic receptors may affect α- or β-adrenoceptors selectively. Drugs with selective α-adrenoceptor effects are potent vasoconstrictors, e.g. phenylephrine, methoxamine. Their actions on the cardiovascular system are similar to those of noradrenaline, with its associated problems (see above). Phenylephrine is now mostly used as a nasal decongestant, a mydriatic or as a local vasoconstrictor in solutions of local anaesthetics. Absorption of phenylephrine from mucous membranes may occasionally produce systemic side-effects. Drugs with a direct action at β-adrenoceptors have wider clinical use and will be considered in slightly more detail.

Selective β_2-agonists

Compounds in this group include the drugs salbutamol, terbutaline, fenoterol and rimiterol. Because of their relative specificity for β_2-adrenoceptors, these drugs relax smooth muscle of bronchi, uterus and vasculature whilst having much less stimulant effect on the heart than isoprenaline. However, these drugs are only partial agonists and their maximal stimulant activity even at β_2-adrenoceptors is less than that of isoprenaline.

The selective β_2-agonists are most widely used in the treatment of bronchospasm (see Chapter 13), thereby avoiding the direct and possibly toxic effects of isoprenaline on the heart. High dosage of these drugs by oral, intravenous or inhalational routes may still produce tachyarrhythmias and tremor.

The effects of these drugs on the cardiovascular system have recently been of interest in the treatment of cardiac failure. Intravenous administration of salbutamol decreases systemic vascular resistance and left ventricular filling pressure as a result of peripheral vasodilatation. There is a consequent increase in cardiac output in patients with cardiac decompensation. In moderate doses ($13 \, \mu g.min^{-1}$) the changes in systemic arterial pressure and heart rate are small. These indirect positive inotropic effects are supplemented by direct action of salbutamol on cardiac function probably via β_2-adrenoceptors, which are present in cardiac muscle. In high doses, salbutamol is less selective and also has some stimulant activity on cardiac β_1-adrenoceptors which may limit its use because of tachycardia. Hypotension and reflex tachycardia produced by vasodilatation may also offset the advantages of decreasing myocardial work load. For these reasons, salbutamol may be less useful in cardiogenic shock than dopamine or dobutamine.

Selective β_1-agonists

Drugs with selective β_1 effects have been developed from the group of β-adrenoceptor antagonists with intrinsic sympathomimetic (partial agonist) activity (see below). Enhancing the intrinsic activity of the β-blocking drugs produces compounds which in low dosage have stimulant activity at the β-adrenoceptor whilst at high dose they act as pure β-adrenoceptor antagonists, blocking the effects of circulating catecholamines. The degree to which the properties of agonist or antagonist are expressed depends on the compound itself as well as the status of sympathetic nervous system activation in the patient. In theory, drugs in this category would be potentially useful as positive inotropic agents in cardiac failure. Thus, at low dose, they would produce mild stimulation to contractility without the excessive chronotropic effects seen with the full agonists such as isoprenaline. At high doses, they would be expected to act more as β-blocking drugs.

The drug in this class which has been most studied in clinical practice is xamoterol, which is a β$_1$-selective partial agonist with approximately 45% of the intrinsic activity of isoprenaline in animal models and in humans. Initially, xamoterol was found to be of some benefit in patients with mild to moderate heart failure in whom activation of sympathetic drive support for the heart is low. However, in patients with more severe heart failure, in whom sympathetic drive is high, xamoterol acted more like a full antagonist and was found to cause a small but significant excess of deaths when compared to placebo.

The place of these agents in the management of heart failure is therefore uncertain and xamoterol is not presently recommended for this indication. However, it may be useful in situations where β-blockers might otherwise be indicated but are potentially problematic due to the presence of poor left ventricular function, for example in patients with angina and mild heart failure. In addition, xamoterol has been found to be a useful adjunct to standard antiarrhythmic therapy, e.g.

with amiodarone (see Chapter 13) in patients with resistant ventricular tachycardia associated with left ventricular dysfunction.

β-Adrenoceptor antagonists

In general, the β-adrenoceptor antagonists (β-blockers) are structurally similar to the β-agonists, e.g. isoprenaline. However, alteration in molecular structure (primarily in the catechol ring) has produced compounds which do not activate adenylate cyclase and the second messenger system despite binding avidly to the β-adrenoceptor. These compounds possess high affinity for the receptor but little or no intrinsic activity and therefore inhibit competitively the effects of the naturally occurring catecholamines.

There is now a wide variety of β-blockers available for clinical use and choice of the appropriate agent is made more difficult. However, the general properties of these drugs are best reviewed collectively.

Pharmacodynamic properties of β-blockers

The properties of individual drugs are summarized in Table 12.2.

The relative potency of the β-blocking drugs is less important than their relative ability to antagonize selectively effects mediated by the β-adrenoceptor subtypes. Compounds are available which block preferentially either β$_1$- or β$_2$-

Table 12.2 Pharmacological properties of β-adrenoceptor blockers

Drug	β-Blockade potency ratio; propranolol = 1	Approx. equiv. oral doses	Relative cardioselectivity	Partial agonist activity	Membrane-stabilizing effect
Acebutolol	0.3	100 mg	±	+	+
Atenolol	1	50 mg	+	0	0
Betaxolol	4	10 mg	+	–	–
Metoprolol	1	50 mg	+	0	±
Nadolol	2–4	20 mg	0	0	0
Oxprenolol	0.5–1	40–60 mg	0	++	+
Pindolol	6	5 mg	0	+++	+
Propranolol	1	40 mg	0	0	++
Sotalol	0.3	100 mg	0	0	0
Timolol	6	5 mg	0	±	0

adrenoceptors, although in clinical practice the β_1 or so-called cardioselective drugs are more important. However, β_1-selectivity is only a relative property and these drugs antagonize β_2 effects in higher doses. Practolol was the first drug to be developed with clinically useful cardioselectivity. More recent drugs are less cardioselective, e.g. atenolol, metoprolol and acebutolol. The clinical importance of cardioselectivity will be considered later.

Intrinsic sympathomimetic activity. The first drug shown to be capable of blocking β-adrenoceptors was dichloroisoprenaline. This compound has a very similar structure to isoprenaline, differing only in the substitution of two chlorine atoms for the –OH groups in the catechol ring. Because of this close similarity, it has some stimulant or agonist activity at the β-adrenoceptor, approximately equivalent to 50% of that of isoprenaline, i.e. it exhibits partial agonist or intrinsic sympathomimetic activity (ISA). This stimulant effect is apparent at low levels of sympathetic activity, but at high levels of sympathetic discharge, blockade of endogenously released catecholamines is the major clinical effect. The clinical significance of ISA is largely theoretical, but may be of some practical importance, as discussed later.

Membrane-stabilizing activity. Some β-blockers have a quinidine-like action on nerve and cardiac conducting tissue. This can be demonstrated in vivo as a stabilizing effect on the cardiac action potential, reducing the slope of phase 4 noticeably, and thus decreasing excitability and automaticity of the myocardium (see Chapter 13). The membrane-stabilizing activity is thought to have little clinical significance generally, since it occurs at drug concentrations very much higher than those achieved ordinarily in plasma after usual therapeutic doses.

Pharmacokinetic properties of β-blockers

The pharmacokinetic properties of β-blockers are summarized in Table 12.3. All β-blockers are weak bases and most are well-absorbed to produce peak plasma concentrations 1–3 h after oral administration. The effect of food is to delay the rate rather than reduce the extent of absorption. This is unlikely to have any important effect on chronic equilibrium concentrations of the drugs in plasma. An important characteristic of the highly metabolized β-blockers (e.g. propranolol) is their tendency to be affected by first pass through the liver. This reduces the bioavailability of the drugs, but this is offset by the fact that the 4-hydroxylated metabolites so formed are also active. The first-pass metabolism also tends to become saturated, so that proportionately higher plasma concentrations of the parent drug are achieved at higher oral doses. This adds an important complication to pharmacokinetic studies of these drugs, which should include measurement of pharmacological effect to be useful. The first-pass effect is also a source of wide interindividual variation in plasma

Table 12.3 Pharmacokinetic properties of β-adrenoceptor blockers

	Half-life (h)	Volume of distribution (litre.kg^{-1})	Bioavailability (%)	% Unchanged in urine	Is first-pass effect significant?	Active metabolites
Acebutolol	8	3.0	50*	35*	Yes	Yes
Atenolol	6–9	0.7	40	95	No	No
Betaxolol	12–16		90	90	No	No
Metoprolol	3–4	5.6	50	3	Yes	No
Nadolol	14–24		35	100	No	No
Oxprenolol	2	1.2	40	50	Yes	Yes
Pindolol	3–4	2.0	100	40	No	No
Propranolol	2–4	3.6	30	Under 1	Yes	Yes
Sotalol	5–13	2.4	100	75	No	No
Timolol	4	1.6	75	10	Yes	No

*Includes active metabolites.

concentrations achieved from the same dose. Other highly metabolized β-blockers, metoprolol and acebutolol, also produce active metabolites.

Atenolol, nadolol, practolol and sotalol are excreted largely unchanged in the urine and so are little affected by impairment of liver function. All β-blockers are distributed widely throughout the body and concentrations are present in the central nervous system. This is particularly true for the more lipid-soluble molecules (e.g. propranolol). Distribution is rapid over 5–30 min, so that after oral administration the β-blockers can be fitted to a one-compartment pharmacokinetic model, the distribution phase being of little clinical importance.

Most β-blockers have a half-life of 2–4 h. The less lipid-soluble drugs atenolol and practolol have longer half-lives of 6–9 and 9–12 h respectively and nadolol has the longest (24 h). Although propranolol depends less on the kidney for elimination than other β-blockers, the possible accumulation of active metabolites, which are excreted renally, should be considered when these drugs are used in patients with renal failure. The plasma concentrations of unchanged propranolol are increased in uraemia.

Interindividual variation in plasma concentrations is less with drugs excreted renally than those primarily metabolized. The plasma concentration–response relationship also shows individual variation, possibly as a result of differences in level of sympathetic tone. β-Blockers have a flat dose–response curve, so that large changes in plasma concentration may give rise to only a small change in degree of β-blockade. Differences in the formation of active metabolites amongst highly metabolized β-blockers further complicates plasma concentration–response relationships.

Cardiovascular effects of β-blockers

Antiarrhythmic activity. Although the mechanism of antiarrhythmic action of β-blockers is unknown, it appears to be a property inherent in β-blockade itself, i.e. antagonism of catecholamine effects on the cardiac action potential and muscle contractility. The result is a slowing of rate of discharge from the sinus and any ectopic pacemaker, and slowing of conduction and increased refractoriness of the atrioventricular node. β-Blockers also retard conduction in anomalous pathways of the heart. The membrane-stabilizing properties do not appear relevant to the clinical antiarrhythmic effect. Most β-blockers have comparable antiarrhythmic properties in adequate dosage; choice is based therefore on tolerance to adverse effects. Sotalol has been shown to exhibit type III antiarrhythmic activity (see Chapter 13) and may have a more specific action in treatment of cardiac arrhythmias, in particular supraventricular tachycardia.

Negative inotropism. The action of catecholamine agonists on the force of contraction of cardiac muscle is antagonized by β-blockade. The resulting negative inotropic effect is of little significance in normal hearts but may be disastrous if increased sympathetic tone is supporting the failing heart. In theory, compounds with ISA have less negative inotropism by virtue of their partial agonist activity. However, this putative benefit is of no practical use in cardiac failure when higher than normal sympathetic drive is present.

Antianginal activity. Angina pectoris occurs when oxygen demand exceeds supply. The oxygen demand of the left ventricle depends on contractility, heart rate and the pressure within the ventricle during systole. The reduction in heart rate caused by β-blockade results in a decrease in cardiac work, which reduces oxygen demand. A slower heart rate also permits longer diastolic filling time and this allows greater coronary perfusion. β-Blockade also reduces exercise-induced increases in arterial pressure, velocity of cardiac contraction and oxygen consumption at any work load.

All β-blockers, irrespective of other pharmacological properties, produce some degree of increased capacity for cardiac work in angina patients. They all limit the increase in heart rate during exercise but they differ in their effects on the heart at rest. Those with ISA have less effect on the resting heart rate; this is of benefit particularly in patients with an existing low heart rate as it reduces the risk of atrioventricular conduction disturbance. However, ISA may theoretically increase the metabolic demand of the myocardium. In practice, drugs without ISA may be more effective in patients with angina at rest or at very low levels of exercise.

Antihypertensive effect. β-Blockers are effective in controlling the arterial pressure of many hypertensive patients. The mechanism of action has not been elucidated fully but it is probable that some of the following are involved:

1. *A direct effect on the cardiovascular system.* This includes a reduction in cardiac output which correlates with a reduction in heart rate and some decrease in myocardial contractility. The significance of the reduction in heart rate is unclear, as β-blockers reduce cardiac output at rest and during exercise in paced hearts. After long-term oral treatment with β-blockers, cardiac output tends to return to pretreatment values.

2. *A reduction in sympathetic nervous activity.* This may be mediated by an action of β-blockers in the hypothalamus, altering central control of sympathetic tone. However, different drugs vary widely in their lipophilicity and consequent central nervous system penetration, but have similar effects on arterial pressure control. Thus, the significance of the central action of these drugs is uncertain.

3. *An effect on plasma renin concentrations.* β-Blockers have variable effects on resting and orthostatic release of renin. The non-selective drugs propranolol and timolol cause the greatest reduction, while drugs with ISA (oxprenolol, pindolol) or β_1-selectivity are less effective. In addition, no correlation has been found between renin-lowering effect and antihypertensive activity of these drugs or with dosage of β-blocker used.

4. *An effect on peripheral resistance.* β-Blockade does not reduce peripheral resistance directly and may even cause an increase by allowing unopposed α-stimulation. As the vasodilating effect of catecholamines on skeletal muscle is β_2-mediated, unopposed α-stimulation would be expected to be less with cardioselective drugs or with those which possess ISA. However, cardioselectivity decreases with dosage and since hypertensive patients often require a large dose of β-blocker, little real advantage is offered. Drugs with ISA may not increase peripheral resistance as much as those without.

5. *The membrane-stabilizing effect.* This was considered of possible importance when early studies indicated that the antihypertensive effect of propranolol resembled that of quinidine. However,

all β-blockers appear to reduce arterial pressure regardless of the presence of a membrane-stabilizing effect.

The full hypotensive effect of β-blockers is not achieved until about 2 weeks after the start of treatment, indicating the involvement of several mechanisms. Possibly, readjustment of cardiovascular reflexes, both central and peripheral, is an important contributory factor to the chronic antihypertensive effect. Arterial pressure reduction begins within an hour of administration of a β-blocker, but several days may elapse before the plateau is reached. During chronic administration, the hypotensive effects of β-blockers last longer than the pharmacological half-life, so that single daily dosage is adequate therapeutically.

In contrast, however, there is a more direct relationship between plasma concentration and cardiac β-blockade, so that to achieve adequate antianginal effect plasma concentrations must be maintained throughout the 24 h. To achieve this in single daily dosage, either the long-half-life drugs (e.g. atenolol, nadolol) or slow-release preparations (e.g. oxprenolol-SR, propranolol-LA, metoprolol-SR) are required. Regardless of pharmacological profile, all β-blockers are equally effective as hypotensive drugs at rest and during exercise. Patients unresponsive to one β-blocker are generally unresponsive to all.

Secondary prevention of myocardial infarction

It is now well-established that a reduction of approximately 25% in mortality during the first 2 years after myocardial infarction is possible if continuous β-blockade is provided. This is possible only in patients without contraindications to these drugs, e.g. cardiac failure, asthma. The exact mechanism of this effect is uncertain but it is probably related to antagonism of catecholamine effects on cardiac β-receptors. Most β-blockers are thought to be effective, although the best clinical trial evidence relates to timolol, propranolol and metoprolol; drugs with ISA may be less effective. β-Blocker therapy started within hours of the onset of symptoms may achieve a reduction in infarct size. However, this early intervention does not improve long-term survival beyond the improvement achieved by chronic oral treatment.

Adverse reactions to β-blocking drugs

These can be classified into:

1. *Reactions resulting from β-blockade*
   a. Induction of bronchospasm in patients who rely on sympathetically mediated bronchodilation (β_2), e.g. asthmatics, chronic bronchitics.
   b. Precipitation of heart failure in patients with compromised cardiac function. Co-administration with other drugs affecting cardiac contractility (e.g. verapamil, disopyramide, quinidine) is potentially hazardous.
   c. Production of cold extremities or worsening symptoms of Raynaud's phenomenon and peripheral vascular disease.
   d. Impairment of cardiovascular and metabolic responses to insulin-induced hypoglycaemia in diabetics; reduced cardiovascular response (tachycardia — β_1) and hepatic glycogenolysis (β_2).
   e. Increased muscle fatigue, possibly resulting from blockade of β_2-mediated vasodilatation in muscles during exercise.
   f. A withdrawal phenomenon may occur after abrupt cessation of long-term β-blocker antianginal therapy. This may take the form of rebound tachycardia, worsening angina or precipitation of myocardial infarction.
2. *Idiosyncratic reactions*
   a. Central nervous system effects occur with some β-blockers, including nightmares, hallucinations, insomnia and depression. These effects are more common with the lipophilic drugs which cross the blood–brain barrier most readily (e.g. propranolol, acebutolol, oxprenolol and metoprolol).
   b. Oculomucocutaneous syndrome was recognized in association with practolol therapy. It affects the eye, mucous and serous membranes. There is no firm evidence that any other β-blockers may provoke a similar reaction. Practolol is no longer available.

Theoretically, cardioselective (β_1-selective) drugs are less likely to aggravate bronchospasm in asthmatics, but as their selectivity is only relative, high doses still interact with bronchial β_2-adrenoceptors and therefore should not be considered safe. Similarly, β-blockers with ISA are promoted wrongly as safer in patients with mild cardiac failure, since at the higher levels of sympathetic activity seen in these patients the presence of small amounts of partial agonist activity is of no significance.

α-Adrenoceptor antagonists

α-Adrenoceptor antagonists (α-blockers) are used mainly as vasodilators and as urethral smooth-muscle relaxants. Their use has been limited because of the widespread effects of α-adrenoceptor blockade on the sympathetic nervous system; these may produce a number of undesirable effects (e.g. postural hypotension, nasal stuffiness, diarrhoea, constipation, abdominal discomfort and inhibition of ejaculation). α-Adrenoceptor blocking drugs still have a role in the preoperative management of phaeochromocytoma, although their use in other acute hypertensive situations has been replaced by directly acting vasodilators, e.g. sodium nitroprusside (see Chapters 13, 36). The α-blockers bind selectively to the α subclass of adrenoceptor and inhibit catecholamine action at these sites. Drugs in this group may bind covalently (i.e. irreversibly) to the receptor (e.g. phenoxybenzamine) or, as with the β-blockers, in a competitive reversible manner (e.g. phentolamine).

Differences in the relative abilities of the α-blockers to antagonize effects at the two subtypes of α-adrenoceptor have led to the following classification:

1. Non-selective agents (block equally α_1 and α_2), e.g. phentolamine, tolazoline.
2. α_1-Selective, e.g. prazosin, indoramin, phenoxybenzamine.
3. α_2-Selective, e.g. yohimbine.

Only classes 1 and 2 are currently relevant in clinical practice. α-Blockers produce a decrease in peripheral vascular resistance and an increase in venous capacity resulting from blockade of noradrenergic vaso- and venoconstrictor tone.

The antihypertensive action may be combined synergistically with β-blockade in order to prevent reflex sympathetic tachycardia, consequent upon vasodilatation. Prazosin and indoramin are the most commonly used agents in this class and in comparison with direct-acting vasodilators (hydralazine) and the non-selective α-blockers (phentolamine), reflex tachycardia and postural hypotension are less common. The mechanism of these changes is not completely understood, but may involve a difference in the proportions of α_1- and postsynaptic α_2-adrenoceptors in the arterial and venous smooth muscle. Thus, prazosin and indoramin may produce a more balanced effect on venous and arterial circulations. An alternative explanation is that non-selective α-antagonists block the feedback inhibition of noradrenaline on its own release at presynaptic α_2-adrenoceptors, thus encouraging increased chronotropic action of neuronally released noradrenaline at cardiac β-adrenoceptors. Non-selective α-blockers produce more postural hypotension and more reflex tachycardia, and there is a greater tendency for tolerance to develop to their therapeutic effects.

In common with other vasodilators, α-blockers may have indirect positive inotropic actions as a result of reduction in afterload and preload. Prazosin has been used for this effect as it produces balanced vaso- and venodilatation; consequently there is less likelihood of reflex tachycardia. Unfortunately, the effects of prazosin in cardiac failure are limited by the development of tachyphylaxis after a few months, and it is being superseded by other agents.

Labetalol is an oral and parenteral antihypertensive agent with both an α_1-blocking and a β-blocking action. In acute use, it may produce a prompt reduction in arterial pressure, suggesting that its α-blocking action predominates. Its β-blocking action may be the more important property during chronic administration. It has been used successfully in the preoperative management of phaeochromocytoma.

DRUG EFFECTS ON THE PARASYMPATHETIC NERVOUS SYSTEM

Stimulation of both the cholinergic synapses in ganglia and, more importantly, the postganglionic muscarinic cholinergic receptors, chiefly affects the following systems.

Cardiovascular system

Acetylcholine has three primary effects on the cardiovascular system — vasodilatation, decrease in cardiac rate (negative chronotropic effect) and a decrease in the force of cardiac contraction (negative inotropic effect). The cardiac effects are characteristic of vagal overactivity and blocked by postganglionic muscarinic antagonists (e.g. atropine). These pure effects are often obscured in the whole organism by a number of factors, in particular the release of catecholamines by ACh from cardiac and extracardiac tissues, and the dampening of direct effects by baroreceptor and other reflexes.

Gastrointestinal system

All compounds acting on the parasympathetic nervous system are capable of producing increased tone, amplitude of contractions and peristaltic activity of the alimentary tract in addition to enhanced secretory activity. This may cause nausea, belching, vomiting, cramps and defecation.

Urinary tract

Drug effects increase ureteral peristalsis, contract the detrusor muscle of the bladder and increase maximal voiding pressure, thus encouraging micturition.

Bronchial tree

Bronchoconstriction is produced in addition to increased mucus secretion. These effects may be a problem in asthmatic and allergic subjects in whom cholinergic drugs should be used with caution. Induction of bronchospasm by reflex cholinergic (vagal) effects in some asthmatics has led to the use of anticholinergics as bronchodilators (see Chapter 13).

Eye

Miosis and spasm of the ciliary muscle occur, so that the eye is accommodated for near vision.

Intraocular pressure decreases as a result of increased reabsorption of intraocular fluids.

DRUGS ACTING ON THE PARASYMPATHETIC NERVOUS SYSTEM

The major drugs in use which act on the parasympathetic nervous system are parasympathetic agonists (e.g. bethanechol and the anticholinesterases, neostigmine and pyridostigmine) and muscarinic antagonists (e.g. atropine and propantheline).

Parasympathetic agonists

Bethanechol is used as a stimulant of the smooth muscle of the gastrointestinal tract and bladder. It is given subcutaneously or orally in postoperative abdominal distension and urinary retention. Bethanechol has mainly muscarinic activity at parasympathetic nerve terminals, an action which lasts several hours, as the drug is not hydrolysed by acetylcholinesterase. Bethanechol has also been used to prevent gastro-oesophageal reflux. Generally it has little effect on the cardiovascular system, although atrial fibrillation can be precipitated in hyperthyroid patients. Bradycardia may also aggravate ischaemic heart disease. Flushing, sweating and excessive salivation are predictable adverse effects which necessitate careful dosage selection. Bethanechol is contraindicated in patients with active peptic ulcer or obstructive airways disease.

Anticholinesterase agents (e.g. neostigmine, pyridostigmine) decrease the breakdown of released ACh and exert a parasympathomimetic effect in addition to an action on skeletal neuromuscular junctions. Their use in anaesthesia to reverse the neuromuscular blockade of nondepolarizing muscle relaxants is discussed in Chapter 11. The action on the ANS tends to appear at low doses. Anticholinesterases may be used to increase gastrointestinal and bladder smooth-muscle tone in a similar way to bethanechol. Their other uses include the symptomatic management of myasthenia gravis, where pyridostigmine is a useful, relatively long-acting agent. Topical anticholinesterases are also used in ophthalmology as miotic agents.

Physostigmine differs from neostigmine and pyridostigmine in being capable of crossing into the central nervous system, producing excitation. Physostigmine has been used to arouse patients from drug-induced coma, particularly that following poisoning with anticholinergic agents, ketamine, diazepam or tricyclic antidepressants, which have anticholinergic effects. This is potentially hazardous with the last class of drug, as physostigmine can induce convulsions and may exacerbate any cardiac bradyarrhythmias associated with direct toxicity of the tricyclic group.

Parasympathetic antagonists

Parasympathetic antagonists act by blockade of the muscarinic ACh receptor. They are either tertiary or quaternary amine compounds, which differ in their ability to cross biological membranes. Tertiary amines, e.g. atropine and hyoscine, may affect central acetylcholine receptors and may produce sedative or stimulatory effects. Similar antimuscarinic drugs, e.g. benztropine and procyclidine, are useful antiparkinsonian agents because of their predominant central action.

Many other parasympathetic antagonists which have been developed are quaternary amines, which are less likely to produce central effects but which also tend to be poorly absorbed after oral administration.

Atropine. The muscarinic-blocking action of atropine affects a wide range of parasympathetic autonomic nervous functions, depending upon dosage. Salivary secretion, micturition, heart rate and visual accommodation are impaired (in that order). Central nervous system effects (sedation or excitation) are possible, but uncommon at usual therapeutic doses in medical conditions. In anaesthesia, central effects may be more common, resulting in the central anticholinergic crisis described in Chapter 18 and on page 410. Hyoscine crosses into the brain more readily and frequently produces confusion, sedation and ataxia. Hyoscine is also used as an antiemetic.

Atropine is administered subcutaneously or intravenously to counteract bradycardia in the presence of hypotension, or to prevent bradycardia associated with vagal stimulation or the use of anticholinesterase agents. Adverse cardiac effects of atropine include an increase in cardiac work and ventricular arrhythmias. Occasionally, after subcutaneous administration, atropine may produce a transient slowing of heart rate, thought to be mediated by a central action. Atropine is also used to block salivary and respiratory secretions in anaesthetic premedication (see Chapter 18).

Glycopyrronium bromide. This is a quaternary amine which has similar anticholinergic actions to atropine. It is used for its antisecretory and gastrointestinal actions. Some other quaternary amines, e.g. propantheline and dicyclomine, have a mainly peripheral parasympathetic antagonist action and are used as gastrointestinal and urinary antispasmodics. The extent to which these two agents reduce gastric acidity is limited by their lack of effect on acid secretion and the need to avoid doses which produce undesirable effects such as dry mouth and visual disturbances. Anticholinergic agents also delay gastric emptying – a disadvantage in peptic ulcer disease. Pirenzepine is an anticholinergic which has recently been developed to be rather more selective for receptor sites in the gastric mucosa. In general, anticholinergic agents have little, if any, role in the treatment of peptic ulcer disease because of the advent of histamine H_2-antagonists (see p. 212).

Ipratropium is useful topically as an anticholinergic bronchodilator aerosol.

FURTHER READING

Breckenridge A 1983 Which beta-blocker? British Medical Journal 186: 1085

Cruickshank J M, Pritchard B N C 1988 (eds) Beta blockers in clinical practice. Churchill Livingstone, Edinburgh

Goodman L S and Gilman A (eds) The pharmacological basis of therapeutics. Macmillan, New York

Opie L H 1991 Drugs for the heart, 3rd edn. W B Saunders, Philadelphia

Szabadi E, Bradshaw C M 1991 (eds) Adrenoceptors: structure, mechanisms, function. Advances in pharmaceutical sciences. Birkhauser Verlag, Basel

13. Miscellaneous drugs of importance in anaesthesia

DRUGS AFFECTING THE GASTROINTESTINAL TRACT

Gastrointestinal bleeding

Antacid or histamine H_2-antagonist therapy is used empirically to prevent bleeding from stress ulceration. H_2-antagonists are effective as prophylaxis against bleeding after severe head injury and erosive bleeding secondary to fulminant liver failure and after renal transplantation. Cimetidine does not prevent the occurrence of mucosal lesions but affects only the incidence of haemorrhage. Intravenous H_2-antagonists (preferably by continuous infusion to achieve stable serum concentrations) and hourly oral antacids are equally effective. In general, high doses of antacids are required, with adjustment according to measurement of gastric pH (pH > 4). Cimetidine, ranitidine and famotidine appear to be similarly effective on the incidence of haemorrhage although a conclusive effect on outcome remains to be demonstrated in prophylaxis or treatment of gastrointestinal bleeding. When used to treat gastrointestinal bleeding, treatment should aim to produce intragastric pH near to 7 for 3 days.

Antacids

Antacids raise gastric pH and facilitate ulcer healing only when given in large doses equivalent to around 200 ml daily of a typical magnesium–aluminium preparation. In vitro neutralizing capacity varies according to titration technique used and does not correlate with ability to relieve ulcer pain. Antacid mixtures containing local anaesthetics, barbiturates or anticholinergic agents have no proven advantages and are potentially harmful. Calcium-containing antacids should also be avoided because they can cause rebound hyperacidity and hypercalcaemia.

Magnesium compounds can produce diarrhoea whereas aluminium antacids tend to produce constipation. Particulate antacids may cause pneumonitis if aspirated and do not mix efficiently with gastric contents. Sodium citrate is preferred when preoperative antacid therapy is indicated for patients at risk of pulmonary aspiration of gastric fluid.

The high sodium content of some antacid mixtures should be taken into account when antacids are used in patients with cardiovascular or renal disease. Antacids may affect the absorption of drugs including tetracyclines, iron, ketoconazole, diflunisal, chlorpromazine, prednisone and (in high doses) cimetidine and ranitidine. Various other drugs may also be affected, so it is advisable to separate all oral medication from high-dose antacid therapy by 1–2 h.

Antisecretory agents

These include histamine H_2-receptor antagonists (cimetidine, ranitidine, famotidine and nizatidine) and proton pump inhibitors (omeprazole). Basal and stimulated gastric acid secretion is mediated by the action of locally secreted histamine on gastric parietal cells. The receptors involved are H_2-receptors which are responsible also for the effect of histamine in increasing heart rate and counteracting uterine contraction. These actions of histamine are unaffected by traditional antihistamines which act on the other elements of the histamine receptor population (H_1-receptors) which are present in bronchi, arteries and gut.

The H_2-receptor antagonists reduce acid content and volume of gastric secretions. This effect varies with dose and correlates with plasma concentrations of the drugs. They are effective in healing gastric and duodenal ulcers when given for 4–6 weeks in a twice-daily regimen or in a single (nocturnal) daily dose. Their use in single courses of treatment does not affect the high relapse rate of peptic ulcer disease.

H_2-antagonists do not appear to produce a rebound hypersecretory state after discontinuation and early reports of acute perforation after a course of treatment probably reflect the tendency for peptic ulcers to revert to their former state of activity.

A variety of adverse effects have been observed with cimetidine. Central nervous system toxicity in elderly and seriously ill patients has led to various, quickly reversible manifestations, e.g. confusion, agitation, psychosis, seizures and decreased consciousness. Pre-existing renal or hepatic impairment have been implicated. Cardiovascular toxicity, inducing bradycardia, hypotension and asystole, has been reported after rapid i.v. injection but no ECG effects have been found during continuous infusions.

Endocrine effects of long-term use include gynaecomastia, oligospermia and impotence. A range of drug interactions is known to occur as a consequence of the ability of cimetidine to inhibit drug metabolism. Of particular importance is the need to monitor the effects of drugs including anticonvulsants, aminophylline/theophylline, warfarin and lignocaine, which carry a high risk of toxicity. Dosage of these drugs may need to be reduced by 50% or more. Other drugs which may be affected include benzodiazepines, chlormethiazole, propranolol, morphine and quinidine.

Ranitidine in therapeutic doses seems free of an inhibitory effect on drug metabolism and any endocrine actions, but is capable of producing CNS disturbances.

Omeprazole produces a profound reduction of acid secretion by inhibition of the terminal stage of acid secretion – the parietal cell proton pump ($H^+/K^+/ATPase$). The inhibition is profound and long-lasting due to the irreversible inhibition requiring to be overcome by the synthesis of enzyme. Omeprazole is used orally for refractory cases of peptic ulcer disease and severe reflux oesophagitis. Diarrhoea, headache, somnolence and various manifestations of hypersensitivity are possible adverse effects. Omeprazole inhibits metabolism of diazepam, phenytoin and warfarin.

Sucralfate

Sucralfate is an aluminium salt of a sulphated sugar which is essentially unabsorbed; unwanted effects are largely limited to abdominal discomfort and constipation. Exposure to acid forms a viscous adhesive which binds to mucoproteins. It also inhibits pepsin activity and absorbs bile salts. It is used for short-term treatment of gastric ulcer and to prevent gastric bleeding in critically ill patients in the ITU, where it has largely replaced H_2 antagonists.

Antiemetic and prokinetic agents

Antiemetics are used frequently during the postoperative period. Inhibition of nausea and vomiting may be achieved by drugs which depress the vomiting centre (antihistamine/anticholinergic agents), by drugs which depress the chemoreceptor trigger zone (e.g. phenothiazines, metoclopramide) and by drugs which increase gastrointestinal motility (e.g. metoclopramide, domperidone).

Antihistamines

These agents are most useful in vestibular disorders and are thought to act mainly through an anticholinergic action which blocks stimulation of the vomiting centre by impulses from the vestibular nuclei. Drugs which possess antihistamine properties and which are used to treat peri-operative vomiting include the phenothiazine promethazine and the piperazine derivative cyclizine. Cyclizine is the most effective and least toxic of the piperazines. In opioid-induced vomiting, it is as effective as perphenazine and extra-pyramidal effects are rare. It causes some drowsiness and a dry mouth. The adult dose is 50 mg i.m. or i.v.

Phenothiazines

These are the most useful antiemetic agents in

the postoperative period. Their action is mediated probably by blockade of dopamine receptors in the chemoreceptor trigger zone. The phenothiazines are more effective in the treatment of nausea and vomiting produced by opioids than by cytotoxic drugs or motion sickness. Sedation (antihistamine and anticholinergic actions), hypotension (α-adrenoceptor blockade) and dystonic reactions (dopamine receptor blockade) are the major adverse effects. Sedation and hypotension are most frequent with chlorpromazine. Drugs based on the piperazine ring (perphenazine, prochlorperazine, thiethylperazine and trifluoperazine) are the most potent antiemetics, but also produce the highest incidence of extrapyramidal side-effects, especially if given repeatedly. Acute dystonic reactions involving eyes, head and neck are most likely to occur in children and the elderly. Phenothiazines may lower the seizure threshold and therefore should be used with caution in epileptic patients. In common with all antiemetics, phenothiazines are more effective for prophylaxis than for treatment.

Prochlorperazine is the most effective phenothiazine antiemetic currently available in the UK. It is usually administered i.m. in the postoperative period, in a dose of 12.5 mg. The duration of risk of extrapyramidal side-effects exceeds that of its antiemetic actions. Cumulation, with an increased risk of dystonic movements, may occur if the drug is given more frequently than 6-hourly.

Metoclopramide

In common with the phenothiazines, metoclopramide is a dopamine receptor antagonist which acts directly on the chemoreceptor trigger zone and the vomiting centre. It is effective in emesis induced by radiotherapy and has been used in very high doses (10 mg.kg^{-1}) to relieve sickness caused by cancer chemotherapy. Although it counteracts opioid-induced nausea and vomiting, it is less effective than the phenothiazines in relieving postoperative emesis.

Metoclopramide increases the tone of the lower oesophageal sphincter and increases gastric and intestinal motility. The peripheral actions of metoclopramide are poorly understood but it appears to mimic the effect of acetylcholine in addition

to its dopamine receptor blockade. It has virtually no sedative activity, but may induce excitement and restlessness after i.v. administration and in large doses can cause extrapyramidal effects; these are related to dopamine receptor blockade and respond to diazepam or to an anticholinergic anti-Parkinsonian agent, e.g. benztropine. Toxic effects of metoclopramide may be mistaken occasionally for idiopathic Parkinsonism.

The normal adult dose of metoclopramide is 10 mg i.m. or i.v., but this should be reduced in the presence of moderate or severe renal impairment.

Domperidone

This is a benzimidazole derivative and is not related chemically to the phenothiazines. It acts at the chemoreceptor trigger zone and the vomiting centre and increases the tone of the lower oesophageal sphincter and gastrointestinal motility. Cardiac arrhythmias and extrapyramidal reactions have been reported after i.v. use and the parenteral formulation of the drug has been withdrawn. It may be given orally or rectally to treat emesis induced by cytotoxic drugs, but is relatively ineffective in opioid-induced or postoperative vomiting.

Cisapride

Cisapride is thought to act by facilitating acetylcholine release in the myenteric plexus. It increases lower oesophageal sphincter pressure and has no antidopaminergic activity, thus avoiding many of the unwanted effects of metoclopramide.

5HT₃ antagonists

Chemotherapeutic agents, radiotherapy and vagal stimulation are believed to cause release of serotonin (5-hydroxytryptamine; 5HT) in the area postrema located on the floor of the fourth ventricle, and this can promote emesis. A number of $5HT_3$-receptor antagonists (ondansetron, granisetron, tropisetron) have been produced, and have been used extensively to treat emesis associated with chemotherapy. They have also been found to be effective in postoperative nausea and vomiting. Their main advantage is their freedom from side-effects on the central nervous system. However, they are expensive, and are not used routinely in surgical patients, being reserved usually for those with a history of severe post-operative nausea and vomiting, and for patients resistant to conventional treatment. Ondansetron is currently the only drug of this group licensed for use in postoperative patients; it is administered usually in a dose of 8 mg orally, or 4 mg i.v. or i.m.

BRONCHODILATORS

Aminophylline is probably the most widely used bronchodilator in acute bronchospasm. However, its perioperative use is controversial since individual reports of cardiac arrhythmias during anaesthesia indicate that patients under anaesthesia may be more sensitive to its toxic effects.

Xanthine bronchodilators

Theophylline and its more water-soluble ethylene diamine salt, aminophylline, are reliable bronchodilators for acute bronchospasm. Other xanthine derivatives including acepifylline, diprophylline, etamiphylline and proxyphylline have no advantages and are either too short-acting or are poorly absorbed orally.

Xanthines relax smooth muscle producing bronchodilatation, a lowering of systemic vascular resistance and a reduction in left ventricular end-diastolic pressure. Venous pooling occurs and this is beneficial in acute pulmonary oedema associated with cardiac failure. Chronotropic and inotropic effects on the heart in addition to a direct action on renal tubules produce diuresis. The smooth muscle and cardiac effects of xanthines are produced, in part, by inhibition of phosphodiesterase, the enzyme responsible for degradation of cyclic adenosine monophosphate (cAMP) within the muscle cell. Potentiation of the effects of catecholamines and calcium is thought also to be involved. In this way, the pharmacological action of xanthines mimics β adrenoceptor stimulation. The therapeutic and toxic effects of xanthines in combination with β agonists are additive.

Xanthines also cause stimulation of the central nervous system. Stimulation of the respiratory centre is exploited in the treatment of neonatal apnoea and Cheyne–Stokes respiration. CNS stimulation in high doses also produces nausea, vomiting, restlessness, irritability and convulsions. In acute situations, aminophylline should be administered i.v., since the pH (9.4) precludes the i.m. route and rectal administration is unreliable. Caution should be exercised in the i.v. use of aminophylline because the narrow therapeutic dose range requires attention to selection of dosage and rate of administration. Rapid injection of aminophylline produces high peak blood concentrations which may exceed the therapeutic range of 10–20 mg.litre^{-1} during the first 15 min or so after administration, with the risk of convulsions, tachycardia, nausea and vomiting. Aminophylline should be given i.v. over at least 10–15 min to allow complete distribution of the drug throughout the body during this period.

Variations in dose requirements arise from variations in metabolism of theophylline, resulting from age, disease and smoking habits. In otherwise healthy adults (non-smokers) the half-life of theophylline is 7–9 h, whilst the half-life is 4–5 h amongst smokers. In premature infants and patients with severe cirrhosis, the half-life is approximately 20–30 h, whereas in children (aged 1–15 years) the half-life is approximately 3–4 h.

Because aminophylline is normally metabolized rapidly, maintenance treatment is best provided by a continuous i.v. infusion following a standard loading dose of approximately 5 mg.kg^{-1}. The initial loading dose should be halved if the patient has been taking oral aminophylline/theophylline regularly. The previous recommended adult maintenance infusion rate (0.9 mg.kg^{-1}.h^{-1}) has been associated with fatalities from seizures. The initial maintenance dosage should be approximately 0.5–0.6 mg.kg^{-1}.h^{-1} and, wherever possible, should be adjusted by measurement of plasma concentration. It is important to appreciate that seizures may not be preceded by other warning symptoms (e.g. nausea). Patients also receiving cimetidine may require up to 50% reduction in maintenance dose (see above). Therapeutic benefit can be expected at plasma concentrations of 5–15 mg.litre^{-1}, with little added benefit above this range and at the cost of greatly increased toxicity above 20 mg.litre^{-1}. Other drugs (e.g. corticosteroids) should not be added to the infusion fluid. Aminophylline should not be given via a central venous catheter because of its cardiotoxicity.

Theophylline may be given orally in the salt form (choline theophyllinate) three times daily or as a slow-release preparation twice daily. In view of the need to adjust dosage individually, oral formulations of combination products of theophylline/aminophylline (with, for example, sympathomimetics) should be avoided.

β-Adrenoceptor agonists

β-Adrenoceptor agonists are based chemically on isoprenaline and structural modification has produced relatively long-acting compounds, many of which are effective orally and most of which are selective to non-cardiac (β_2) receptors in therapeutic doses.

The pharmacological profiles of selective β_2-adrenoceptor agonists are identical, differing only in duration of action. β_2-Adrenoceptor agonists are popular when administered by self-propelled aerosol. Salbutamol and terbutaline can be given also by injection, by nebulizer and orally. Fenoterol, rimiterol and reproterol are available also for aerosol administration. The majority of β_2-agonists act for 5–7 h after inhalation, except for rimiterol which lasts for only approximately 2 h. Orciprenaline is a non-selective agent. Although these agonists produce fewer cardiac effects than isoprenaline or orciprenaline, tachycardia may occur after i.v. administration or after high-dose nebulizer therapy. The cardiac effects may result partly from reduction in systemic vascular resistance. Other signs of toxicity include tremor, headache and dizziness. These side-effects are seen also during oral administration. Measurable tolerance to the therapeutic effects of long-term systemic therapy has been demonstrated and is supported by clinical impression.

The relatively small doses used in aerosol inhaler or powder insufflation (100–500 μg per metered dose) do not usually produce systemic effects. Careful attention should be paid to dosage of β_2-agonists administered via nebulizer, because the amounts of drug delivered (2.5–10 mg) are markedly greater than those given by aerosol. Drug absorbed by the lung avoids first-pass metabolism in the liver and is therefore analogous to parenteral administration. An optimal initial dose of salbutamol or terbutaline by nebulizer is 2.5–5 mg. Apart from convenience of administration, nebulizer therapy is no more effective than aerosol inhalation.

Faulty technique of aerosol administration is a common cause of poor control of chronic obstructive airways disease. Various alternative devices including an automatically triggered aerosol (rimiterol 'Autohaler'), a powder insufflation (salbutamol 'Rotahaler') and extended aerosol mouthpieces (terbutaline 'Spacer' and 'Nebuhaler'; salbutamol 'Volumatic') are available.

Intravenous salbutamol or terbutaline are as effective as aminophylline in acute asthma. Intravenous aminophylline offers the advantage of theoretical (but unproven) synergy with inhaled β_2-agonist. Salmeterol is a long-acting inhaled β-agonist for chronic asthma prophylaxis. It should not be used for immediate relief of acute attacks nor to replace existing corticosteroid therapy.

Ipratropium bromide

Ipratropium is an anticholinergic bronchodilator which may be given either by aerosol or nebulizer. It acts by blocking bronchoconstriction via cholinergic receptors and so decreases intracellular ionic calcium and cyclic guanosine monophosphate, an intracellular mediator of bronchoconstriction. Its effects occur within 15 min and peak slowly between 1–2 h. It has been found to be less effective than β_2-adrenoceptor agonists in asthmatic subjects but seems effective in chronic bronchitis. There is no evidence of systemic toxicity with inhaled ipratropium and the drug does not impair clearance of sputum. Ipratropium may have an additive bronchodilator action in combination with β_2-agonists or aminophylline in some patients.

DRUGS ACTING ON THE CARDIOVASCULAR SYSTEM

Diuretics

The management of oedema may require a planned approach to the use of diuretics, demanding an appreciation of the limitations of individual

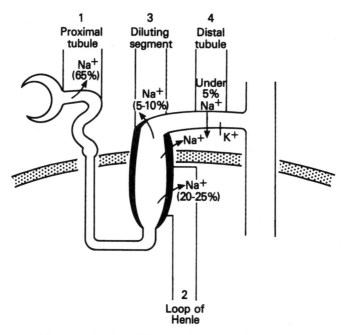

Fig. 13.1 Sites of action of diuretics. Percentages indicate the proportion of intraluminal sodium which is absorbed at different sites in the nephron.

agents and the value of combining diuretics which have different sites and mechanisms of action.

Diuretics affect sodium reabsorption at four sites in the renal tubule (Fig. 13.1).

1. The proximal tubule, where blockade of active sodium reabsorption is of limited use as a result of development of compensatory mechanisms distally.

2. The ascending loop of Henle; action at this site produces a brisk, potentially large diuresis even at low glomerular filtration rates.

3. The diluting segment; action at this site produces a moderate diuresis.

4. The distal tubule, where blockade of sodium-potassium exchange leads to a mild diuresis and conservation of potassium.

The pharmacological properties of diuretics are indicated in Table 13.1.

High-potency diuretics are useful in left ventricular failure. After i.v. administration, the immediate beneficial effect of frusemide results partly from an increase in venous capacitance and decrease in preload. Rapid diuresis may worsen electrolyte imbalance in hepatic ascites.

Spironolactone is particularly beneficial where secondary hyperaldosteronism contributes to the oedema (e.g. hepatic or cardiac failure). Potassium-retaining diuretics are potentially hazardous in the presence of declining renal function, when combined with potassium supplementation or when given with an angiotensin-converting enzyme (ACE) inhibitor. When a combination of diuretics is necessary, the objective should be to use maximum tolerable effective doses of each agent.

Cardiac glycosides

Digoxin and other cardiac glycosides improve cardiac output by an inotropic action on myocardial contractility, whilst their ability to suppress atrio-ventricular conduction is useful in controlling the ventricular rate in supraventricular arrhythmias, particularly atrial fibrillation.

The cardiovascular response to cardiac glycosides is complicated by indirect actions. In the failing heart, a slowing of heart rate occurs, brought about mainly by the reduction in sympathetic tone which results from the increase in cardiac output. In addition there is a direct

Table 13.1 Commonly used diuretics for sites of action, refer to Figure 13.1

Diuretic	Site(s) of action	Route	Onset	Duration (h)	Notes
High potency					
Frusemide	2				Effective at low GFR. Produce hyperuricaemia, hyperglycaemia, hypokalaemia and hypomagnesaemia.
Bumetanide	2	oral	30 min	4–6	Calcium excretion is increased. May cause hearing loss, tinnitus or vertigo after high doses i.v. (especially if too
		i.v.	5 min	2	rapid), very high doses orally, in uraemia, or if
Ethacrynic acid	2				combined with aminoglycosides
Medium potency					
Thiazides	1 + 3	oral	2 h	6–12 (some longer)	Ineffective at GFR less than 20 ml.min^{-1}. Maximum diuresis achieved after small increases in dose. Additive effect with high-potency diuretics. Produce
Mefruside	1 + 3	oral	2 h	12	hyperuricaemia, hyperglycaemia, hypokalaemia and hypomagnesaemia
Metolazone	1 + 3	oral	2 h	12–24	Calcium excretion is reduced. Effective at GFR less than 20 ml.min^{-1}. Synergy with high-potency diuretics. Diuresis can be profound, caution with initial dose
Low potency					
Spironolactone	4	oral	12 h	24	Acts by aldosterone inhibition. In absence of loading dose maximum effect takes 3 days
Potassium canrenoate		i.v.	12 h	24	I.v. form is the active metabolite (canrenone). Potassium retaining. Avoid in renal failure
Amiloride	4	oral	2 h	10	Independent of aldosterone. Potentially nephrotoxic. Potassium retaining. Avoid in renal failure
Triamterene	4	oral	2 h	12–16	
Actezolamide	1	oral i.v./i.m.	2 h	12	Inhibits carbonic anhydrase. Metabolic acidosis during first weeks leads to tolerance through Na$^+$–H$^+$ exchange. Synergy with high-potency diuretics

vagal stimulatory action of cardiac glycosides. Peripheral vasodilatation occurs also as sympathetic tone is diminished but there is no clinically relevant direct effect on peripheral vasculature. Although cardiac glycosides might be expected to increase cardiac work and therefore oxygen demand, the work of the failing heart is often reduced because of reduced heart rate and cardiac size.

The mechanism of action of cardiac glycosides stems from inhibition of the sodium-potassium active exchange at the myocardial cell membrane. There is an associated increase in ionic calcium within the cell because of increased influx of calcium in exchange for sodium ions. The increased availability of intracellular ionized calcium enhances excitation-contraction coupling within myofibrils.

The ability of cardiac glycosides to suppress conduction in the AV node is the basis for their use in supraventricular arrhythmias. The improve-ment in cardiac output is therefore most marked in congestive heart failure in the presence of atrial fibrillation. The use of cardiac glycosides in acute left ventricular failure has been superseded gradually by vasodilators and sympathomimetics. The glycosides are of no use in cardiogenic shock and are best avoided after acute myocardial infarction. Any long-term benefit on congestive heart failure in sinus rhythm remains to be demonstrated fully, since in many patients cardiac glycosides can be discontinued without detriment.

There is increased sensitivity to digoxin and similar cardiac glycosides in the presence of hypokalaemia, hypomagnesaemia, hypercalcaemia, renal impairment, chronic pulmonary or heart disease, myxoedema and hypoxaemia. There is decreased sensitivity in thyrotoxicosis. Quinidine and to a lesser extent amiodarone and verapamil tend to increase plasma digoxin concentrations. β-blockers and verapamil have combined effects on the AV node. Digoxin should be administered cautiously i.v. in situations where AV conduction is already suppressed.

There are various manifestations of cardiac glycoside toxicity. Ventricular arrhythmias (particularly bigeminy and trigeminy) are the commonest. Supraventricular arrhythmias may occur, often with some degree of heart block. Other symptoms are rather unpredictable and in chronic toxicity include fatigue, weakness of arms or legs, agitation, nightmares, various visual disturbances, anorexia and nausea or abdominal pain. These symptoms may not precede cardiac toxicity. Therapeutic and toxic blood concentrations overlap and plasma determinations are useful primarily to substantiate clinical impressions of digitalis toxicity. Treatment of serious arrhythmias involves careful administration of potassium chloride under ECG control (especially in the presence of heart block or renal impairment). Lignocaine or phenytoin are useful for ventricular arrhythmias, whilst β-blockade is useful in supraventricular arrhythmias. Cardioversion during cardiac glycoside therapy may produce ventricular arrhythmias.

Digoxin has a long half-life (approximately 36 h) which is sensitive to changes in renal function. In the absence of a loading dose, effective plasma concentrations (1–2 μg.litre^{-1}) occur after approximately 5–7 days if renal function is unimpaired. For an acute response, a loading (digitalizing) dose is required which should be based approximately on lean body weight. Selection of maintenance doses of digoxin should take into account the presence of renal impairment. Although the effect of an i.v. injection begins within 30–60 min, distribution into cardiac tissue takes place slowly over the first 6 h after oral or i.v. administration. The maximum response occurs 4–6 h after i.v. administration and digoxin measurements in blood samples taken before this 6 h period cannot be interpreted correctly. Intramuscular injections are painful and the drug is absorbed unreliably when given by this route.

Deslanoside has an onset of action beginning 10–30 min after i.v. administration and reaching a maximum after 1–2 h.

Digitoxin is less dependent upon renal function for its elimination. Its long half-life (4–6 days) is a disadvantage, as toxic effects are very persistent.

Vasodilators

Drugs which dilate arteries or veins are used alone or in conjunction with inotropic agents in the management of acute left ventricular failure. Arterial vasodilators are useful also in the treatment of acute hypertensive episodes and in the selective induction of controlled hypotension to reduce haemorrhage during surgery. Some vasodilators are used investigationally to reduce infarct size after myocardial infarction. The main agents are sodium nitroprusside and the nitrates (isosorbide dinitrate and glyceryl trinitrate). Hydralazine and diazoxide are also important parenteral vasodilators, whereas prazosin, minoxidil, captopril and enalapril are oral agents which have a place in the chronic management of left ventricular failure and as third-line agents in the treatment of hypertension. Calcium channel blockers also have a mainly arterial vasodilator action, including an effect on the coronary artery.

The use of vasodilators in left ventricular failure is based on their ability to reduce afterload and preload. In cardiac failure, a reflex increase in sympathetic tone creates an increase in systemic vascular resistance in the arterial bed. By lowering this resistance (afterload), the work and oxygen requirements of the heart are reduced. Those vasodilators which are capable of acting on the venous side of the circulation increase venous capacitance, reduce venous return to the heart and so decrease the left ventricular filling pressure (preload). Lowering the filling pressure in the left ventricle decreases the degree of stretch of myocardial fibres, improves myocardial contractility and cardiac output and reduces myocardial oxygen consumption for the same degree of external cardiac work performed.

Vasodilators may be classified into those which act directly on arterial smooth muscle (nitroprusside, nitrates, hydralazine, diazoxide, minoxidil, calcium channel blockers) and those which are neurohumoral antagonists (prazosin and other adrenoceptor antagonists and ACE inhibitors). This distinction is important as the drugs in the first category have a clear, often sensitive, dose–response relationship which requires haemodynamic monitoring (preferably by invasive techniques), whereas those in the second category have a relatively long duration of action and their intensity of effect is less sensitive to changes in dosage.

Another useful way of comparing vasodilators is to consider on which side of the heart they act preferentially. Hydralazine and minoxidil act mainly on afterload. Nitroprusside, the α adrenoceptor antagonists and ACE inhibitors have a balanced effect on both arteries and veins.

Sodium nitroprusside

Sodium nitroprusside has an immediate, short-lived effect (lasting only for a few minutes) which requires that it be given by continuous infusion. A smooth reduction in arterial pressure can be achieved by adjustment of the infusion rate. The nitroprusside ion is responsible for a direct action on vascular smooth muscle and it is metabolized by red cells to cyanide. Cyanide ions are detoxified by the liver and kidney to thiocyanate (requiring thiosulphate and vitamin B_{12}) which is excreted slowly in the urine.

Sodium nitroprusside produces a balanced reduction in afterload and preload. In larger doses (e.g. when used for hypotensive anaesthesia) its use leads to an increase in heart rate. There is an additive effect with other vasodilators. In medical practice, nitroprusside is well tolerated and most symptoms are non-specific (e.g. drowsiness, perspiration, nausea, dizziness) and are associated with too rapid a decrease in arterial pressure.

The accumulation of cyanide and thiocyanate, with the risk of lactic acidosis, is a possibility but is rare in the absence of impaired renal or hepatic function or if total dosage does not exceed 1.5 mg.kg^{-1}. If therapy is high-dose or prolonged, plasma bicarbonate monitoring is indicated. Plasma cyanide or thiocyanate concentrations may also be monitored if the drug is used for more than 2 days. Thiocyanate is potentially neurotoxic and can cause hypothyroidism. Thiosulphate and a specially prepared high-dose infusion of hydroxocobalamin have been used to reverse cyanide toxicity. Nitroprusside is photodegraded and infusion solutions should be protected from light.

The use of sodium nitroprusside (SNP) in hypotensive anaesthesia is considered in Chapter 36.

Nitrates

The organic nitrates, glyceryl trinitrate and isosorbide mononitrate and dinitrate, affect mainly preload and are most effective in relieving pulmonary congestion secondary to left ventricular failure. However, this selectivity of action decreases with dosage, so that a decrease in arterial pressure, tachycardia and headaches may occur. The nitrates have a short duration of action and may be given i.v. The infusion rate should be controlled carefully according to heart rate and haemodynamic effects. The action of nitrates in left ventricular failure is enhanced by agents, including hydralazine, which preferentially reduce afterload.

The nitrates are absorbed by rubber and plastics (especially PVC infusion bags), so they are best administered by syringe pump. Intravenous nitrates are used also in unstable angina. The therapeutic effects of nitrates in myocardial ischaemia result not only from preload reduction but also from counteraction of coronary vasospasm and redistribution of blood within the myocardium.

Hydralazine, diazoxide and minoxidil

These drugs are direct-acting arterial vasodilators. Their main action is to reduce afterload, with little or no effect on preload, and their main limitation is reflex tachycardia, although this is less prominent in the presence of cardiac failure.

In hypertensives, the reduction in arterial pressure is limited by reflex sympathetic discharge which tends to increase cardiac output. Their antihypertensive action is limited also by a tendency to cause sodium and water retention by a direct renal mechanism and by activation of the renin–angiotensin system. Consequently, they are often more effective if combined with a β-adrenoceptor blocker and a diuretic.

Hydralazine is the most widely used direct vasodilator drug. Its half-life is short (approximately 2.5 h) but its antihypertensive effect is relatively prolonged, permitting twice-daily dosage.

Diazoxide is of limited use because of its unpredictable duration of action, which is unrelated to its short plasma half-life. The initial i.v. dose of diazoxide must be given rapidly for maximum effect. A cumulative effect on arterial pressure may make it difficult to control the action of repeated doses. Multiple doses of diazoxide cause fluid retention and hyperglycaemia.

Minoxidil is available for oral use only and it too has a long duration of action (12–24 h) which is unrelated to its plasma half-life.

Calcium channel blockers

Calcium channel blockers, such as nifedipine and verapamil, have been used as antianginal and, more recently, as antihypertensive agents. They antagonize coronary artery spasm and relax systemic vascular smooth muscle predominantly on the arterial side of the circulation. Verapamil is also a useful drug for the treatment of supraventricular arrhythmias (see below) because it shows some preference for the AV node, through which conduction is dependent upon intracellular calcium (as opposed to sodium) influx. The antihypertensive effects of calcium channel blockers have not yet been studied widely but they appear modest and, in the case of nifedipine at least, have been inconsistent.

Intracellular calcium ion availability is important in the conduction of the cardiac action potential and in electromechanical coupling within smooth muscle cells. Drugs which affect the permeability to calcium of the extracellular or intracellular membranes can influence the size of the cytoplasmic pool of calcium ions. This action reduces cardiac contractility (producing a negative inotropic effect) and decreases vascular tone. Calcium channel blockers differ in their selectivity for myocardial or arterial tissue, verapamil being rather more selective for cardiac muscle than nifedipine. Nifedipine presents less risk of reducing contractility and has no important effect on conduction through the AV node.

Nifedipine is more potent than verapamil as a systemic and coronary arterial vasodilator, making it the more effective antianginal agent. It is effective in countering coronary artery spasm, which is thought to be an important component of all forms of angina. The antianginal effect of nifedipine is additive with that of β-adrenergic blocking drugs and nitrates. The marked negative inotropic action of verapamil presents a potential hazard when used in conjunction with β-adrenergic

blockers or other cardiodepressant drugs (including disopyramide and the volatile anaesthetic agents) in patients with limited cardiac reserve. However, the effects of these agents in individual patients are unpredictable because the failing left ventricle can benefit from reductions in afterload brought about by peripheral vasodilatation.

Side-effects of nifedipine are related to its vasodilator action and include flushing, headaches, dizziness, tiredness and palpitations. Nifedipine may also cause ankle oedema which arises from peripheral vasodilatation unrelated to any cardiodepressant action of the drug. Nifedipine is absorbed fairly rapidly from the swallowed capsule, particularly when the stomach is empty. The slow-release tablet formulation may be tolerated better as it is less likely to reduce arterial pressure acutely.

Other antianginal calcium channel blockers include nicardipine, diltiazem, amlodipine and felodipine. Nimodipine has a pronounced cerebral vasodilator effect and may be given by intravenous infusion for the prevention and treatment of cerebral ischaemia and vasospasm following subarachnoid haemorrhage.

Other interesting properties of calcium channel blockers include inhibition of platelet aggregation, protection against bronchospasm, use in Raynaud's syndrome and improvements in lower oesophageal sphincter function.

α-Adrenoceptor antagonists

The pharmacology of α adrenoceptor antagonists (e.g. phentolamine, phenoxybenzamine) has been discussed on p. 207. These agents have a balanced effect on venous capacitance and systemic arterial resistance. Oral postsynaptic (α_1) blocking agents include prazosin (also doxazosin and terazosin). Prazosin tends to produce little if any increase in heart rate. Initial administration may cause a sudden decrease in arterial pressure and so prazosin should be given as a low first dose, preferably with the patient supine. Syncope is more likely if the patient is receiving nitrates concurrently. There is concern that the short-term benefits of prazosin in left ventricular failure may not be maintained during long-term therapy.

As with many of these drugs, the duration

of vasodilator action of prazosin (approximately 12 h) does not correlate with its short half-life in plasma (3–4 h). The short-acting phentolamine and the long-acting phenoxybenzamine are other α-adrenoceptor blocking drugs which are used occasionally by the parenteral route as adjuncts in hypertension or left ventricular failure.

Angiotensin-converting enzyme (ACE) inhibitors

The orally administered ACE inhibitors such as captopril and enalapril reduce both preload and afterload. Vasodilatation and a decrease in blood volume result from blockade of the renin–angiotensin–aldosterone sequence. Captopril has a more rapid onset and shorter duration of action (plasma half-life approximately 2 h) compared with enalapril (approximately 36 h). As both drugs may produce a profound initial hypotensive response, the first dose must be small, particularly in patients already receiving diuretics.

Enalapril is de-esterified in the liver into its active form, enalaprilat. Captopril, enalapril and their active metabolites accumulate in renal failure. ACE inhibitors tend to increase plasma urea and creatinine concentrations and may produce hyperkalaemia if administered with potassium-sparing diuretics. The effects on arterial pressure and renal function are more marked in the presence of hypovolaemia or bilateral renal artery stenosis.

Other adverse effects of ACE inhibitors include disturbances of taste and a dry cough. Hypersensitivity reactions, including proteinuria, are uncommon but their incidence is increased by the use of high doses and by the presence of renal impairment or connective tissue disease. Other ACE inhibitors are now available with a similar duration of action to enalapril although some are licensed only for use in hypertension.

Antiarrhythmic agents

The aim of drug treatment of cardiac arrhythmias is either to prevent the emergence of a tachy-arrhythmia or to terminate a run of tachycardia. A continuous arrhythmia may be controlled either by slowing the primary mechanism or, in the case of supraventricular arrhythmias, by reducing the proportion of impulses transmitted through the AV node and ventricular conducting system.

The emergence of ectopic pacemaker cells may be explained by the phenomenon of re-entry. Re-entrant arrhythmias arise from retrograde conduction along a branch of tissue in which antero-grade conduction has been blocked by disease. When retrograde conduction is sufficiently slow, it can influence cells which have already discharged and repolarized, triggering a further action potential which is both premature and ectopic. A vicious circle can ensue such that these action potentials become self-sustaining (circus movements) leading to multiple ectopic beats, tachycardia or fibrillation.

The basis of treatment of specific arrhythmias has arisen largely from clinical experience. The known electrophysiological properties of anti-arrhythmics have provided explanations for observed effects and, in particular, it has become clear that any drug with an antiarrhythmic action may itself provoke arrhythmias. Consequently, antiarrhythmic agents tend to be used rather more conservatively than in the past.

Antiarrhythmic agents may be classified empirically on the basis of their effectiveness in supra-ventricular tachycardias (e.g. digoxin, β-blockers and verapamil) or in ventricular arrhythmias (lignocaine, mexiletine, tocainide, phenytoin and bretylium). Many agents (disopyramide, amiodarone, quinidine and procainamide) are effective in both supraventricular and ventricular arrhythmias.

The cardiac action potential

Antiarrhythmic agents are classified conventionally according to their effects on the cardiac action potential (Fig. 13.2) which comprises five phases, each corresponding to a changing state of depolarization of the myocardial cell.

The action potential is triggered by a low intra-cellular leak of sodium ions (and calcium ions at the AV node) until a threshold point is reached when sudden rapid influx of sodium ions generates an impulse (phase 0). The action potential starts to reverse (phase 1), but is sustained whilst there is slower inward movement of calcium ions (phase 2). Efflux of potassium ions brings about repolarization (phase 3) and the gradual

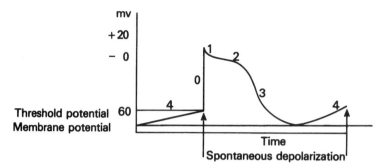

Fig. 13.2 The cardiac action potential. Phase 0 – rapid depolarization associated with fast Na^+ influx; 1 – early repolarization; 2 – maintained depolarization associated with slow Ca^{2+} influx; 3 – repolarization associated with K^+ efflux; 4 – resting membrane potential; may have upward slope representing slow spontaneous depolarization in automatic (pacemaker) tissues.

termination of the action potential. Thereafter, re-equilibration of sodium and potassium takes place and the resting membrane potential is restored (phase 4).

There are three important components of the cardiac action potential which are amenable to pharmacological intervention.

1. The *automaticity* (tendency to spontaneous discharge) of cells may be reduced. This result can be achieved by reducing the rate of leakage of sodium (reducing the slope of phase 4), by increasing the electronegativity of the resulting membrane potential or by decreasing the electronegativity of the threshold potential.

2. The speed of *conduction* of the action potential can be suppressed as indicated by a lowering of the height and slope of the phase 0 discharge. A reduction in the electronegativity of the membrane potential at the onset of phase 0 reduces both the amplitude and the slope of the phase 0 depolarization. This situation occurs if the cell discharges before it has been completely repolarized.

3. The *rate of repolarization* may be reduced, which prolongs the refractory period of the discharging cell.

On the basis of these pharmacological effects, antiarrhythmic agents can be grouped into four classes (Table 13.2). All agents in class 1 reduce automaticity by inhibiting sodium channel flux. Agents in class 1a antagonize primarily the fast influx of sodium ions and so reduce conduction

Table 13.2 Classification of antiarrhythmic agents

1. Membrane stabilization	a Quinidine, procainamide, disopyramide b Lignocaine, mexiletine, tocainide c Flecainide, propafenone
2. β-Receptor blockade	All β-blockers
3. Prolongation of action potential	Amiodarone, bretylium, sotalol (also class 2)
4. Calcium channel blockade	Verapamil

velocity, whilst prolonging the refractory period. Those in class 1b have much less effect on conduction velocity in usual therapeutic doses and they shorten the refractory period. Agents in class 1c affect conduction profoundly without altering refractoriness. β-Blockers (class 2) depress automaticity but have no other specific effect on the action potential apart from reducing the effects of catecholamines (i.e. the increases in automaticity and conduction velocity in the sinus and AV nodes). Agents in class 3 lengthen the refractory period by prolonging the action potential. Verapamil (class 4) also prolongs the action potential in addition to depressing automaticity (especially in the AV node).

An appreciation of the general class of action of different antiarrhythmic agents enables the selection of a second agent to be made from a different class in the event of failure of a primary agent or if there is need for combination therapy.

Quinidine has now been superseded largely by newer agents including disopyramide. Intravenous administration may cause severe hypotension. Toxic effects may be dose-related or arise as a result of drug idiosyncrasy. The most serious toxicity is depression of conduction and the risk of ventricular fibrillation. Visual and auditory disturbances with vertigo and gastrointestinal symptoms are signs of toxicity. Skin reactions, thrombocytopenia and agranulocytosis may occur also. Quinidine enhances digoxin toxicity by doubling plasma concentrations. It also has an additive effect with hypotensive agents and drugs with cardiodepressant properties (e.g. disopyramide, β-blockers and calcium channel blockers).

Procainamide closely resembles quinidine in its effect on the heart. It may cause hypotension after i.v. administration. Its main application is as an oral antiarrhythmic, although therapy is limited by its short half-life (3 h) which necessitates frequent administration or the use of a sustained-release oral preparation. Procainamide is restricted usually to short-term use because of the risk of drug-induced systemic lupus erythematosus. Other manifestations of hypersensitivity include fever, rash, arthralgia and agranulocytosis.

Disopyramide has properties in common with both quinidine and lignocaine. It is useful in supraventricular tachycardias and as a second-line agent to lignocaine in ventricular arrhythmias. Its half-life (8 h) is prolonged in renal impairment and after myocardial infarction, necessitating dosage reduction. Side-effects result mainly from the anticholinergic effect of the parent drug and a major metabolite, which can produce urinary retention and blurred vision. Disopyramide is markedly cardiodepressant, especially in combination with β-blockers, quinidine, procainamide or verapamil

Lignocaine remains the drug of first choice for ventricular arrhythmias. It has a short half-life of less than 2 h, although this is prolonged after myocardial infarction, in liver disease and during cimetidine treatment. The effect of a single loading dose may be brief as lignocaine distributes rapidly after an i.v. bolus, which may need to be repeated twice. A continuous infusion is used to maintain the effect, with the rate of infusion adjusted according to response. Close adjustment of the infusion rate is required to avoid toxicity (confusion, slurring of speech, numbness, dizziness and convulsions). The presence of heart failure, β blockade or liver disease should be an indication to reduce maintenance dosage by half. A reduced loading dose is necessary also in heart failure. The presence of hypokalaemia is a common reason for failure of response to lignocaine.

Mexiletine is a longer-acting, orally effective lignocaine analogue which has a half-life of 10 h. It shares lignocaine's low margin of safety, especially after i.v. administration when hypotension and bradycardia have been reported. Most frequent adverse effects involve the central nervous system and include tremors, nystagmus, confusion, speech disturbances, tinnitus, paraesthesiae and convulsions. Gastrointestinal effects are also common during oral treatment.

Tocainide is another lignocaine analogue which can be given orally or parenterally. It has a half-life of 13 h. Arrhythmias which do not respond to lignocaine are unlikely to respond to tocainide. Adverse effects resemble those of mexiletine and include blood dyscrasias.

Flecainide is another class 1 agent which may be administered orally or i.v. It differs from other drugs in this class by having little effect on the refractory period. Its half-life is 7–23 h, but this may be prolonged in renal failure.

Propafenone is a class 1 agent with complex pharmacology including weak β adrenoceptor blocking action which necessitates caution in patients with obstructive airways disease. Interaction with digoxin may increase plasma digoxin concentrations.

Phenytoin is unique in that it accelerates intraventricular conduction and is particularly effective in controlling digitalis-induced ventricular arrhythmias.

β-Blockers are used mainly in sinus and supraventricular tachycardias, especially those provoked by emotion or exercise. Their cardiodepressant effects are a disadvantage in the management of arrhythmias after acute myocardial infarction. For further discussion of the pharmacology of β-blockers see Chapter 12.

Amiodarone is a very effective agent against both supraventricular and ventricular arrhythmias. It has a long half-life (over 30 days) so that oral treatment should be started with a week of high doses to establish a therapeutic effect. Intravenous administration may cause bradycardia, hypotension (vasodilatation), heart block and thrombophlebitis. It must be diluted in an infusion of glucose. Long-term accumulation produces reversible microdeposits in the cornea which generally do not interfere with vision. Deposition in the skin produces photosensitivity and blue-grey discoloration. As amiodarone is an iodinated compound, it may disturb thyroid function tests and may produce clinical hyperthyroidism or, less commonly, hypothyroidism. Long-term treatment is associated with pulmonary fibrosis and hepatotoxicity. Amiodarone may increase blood concentrations of digoxin.

Adenosine blocks conduction in calcium-dependent tissue. It is used to treat paroxysmal supraventricular tachycardia. Unwanted effects include dyspnoea, bronchospasm and bradycardia.

Bretylium is a quaternary ammonium compound which prevents noradrenaline uptake into sympathetic nerve endings. It is used in resuscitation for resistant life-threatening ventricular arrhythmias/fibrillation. There is an initial increase in catecholamine release and it has a positive inotropic effect and disturbance of blood pressure. It may cause bradycardia or asystole and may worsen ventricular arrhythmias, particularly those due to cardiac glycosides.

Verapamil is also a coronary and peripheral vasodilator which is useful in angina and hypertension and effective both orally and i.v. It is very effective in supraventricular tachycardias, in which it acts by depressing AV conduction and blocking re-entry mechanisms. Similarly, it controls the ventricular rate in atrial fibrillation. Intravenous administration may reduce arterial pressure (by vasodilatation) and caution is necessary in low-output states and in patients treated with negative inotropic agents, e.g. β-blockers, disopyramide, quinidine and procainamide.

DRUGS AFFECTING THE IMMUNE SYSTEM

The major drugs used in acute conditions involving the activation of immunological and inflammatory mechanisms are the corticosteroids and the antihistamines.

Corticosteroids

The corticosteroids have been advocated in a variety of acute life-threatening conditions, although few recommendations are supported by firm evidence of efficacy. Included in these conditions are bacteraemic and anaphylactic shock, adult respiratory distress syndrome, status asthmaticus and cerebral oedema.

Amongst the many complex actions of pharmacological doses of corticosteroids, those affecting the cellular and microvascular components of the inflammatory response are more relevant to any therapeutic benefit achieved in critically ill patients. These pharmacological effects seem to parallel the glucocorticoid properties of individual corticosteroids which are shown in Table 13.3.

Table 13.3 Glucocorticoid corticosteroids

	Equivalent dosage (mg)	Mean dose to suppress HPA* (mg.day^{-1})	Half-life in plasma (h)	Half-life of pharmacological effect** (h)
Hydrocortisone	20	15–30	1.5	8–12
Cortisone	25	20–35	1.5	8–12
Prednisolone	5	7.5–10	3+	18–36
Prednisone	5	7.5–10	3+	18–36
Methylprednisolone	4	7.5–10	3+	18–36
Dexamethasone	0.75	1–1.5	5+	36–54
Triamcinolone	4	7.5–10	3+	18–36
Betamethasone	0.6	1–1.5	5+	36–54

* HPA = hypothalamic-pituitary-adrenal axis
** Based on duration of suppression of HPA axis

The anti-inflammatory action of corticosteroids involves reduction in the permeability of capillaries to intravascular fluid, proteins and chemical mediators of the inflammatory process. The migration and phagocytosis of polymorphonuclear leucocytes is inhibited. In high doses, corticosteroids prevent tissue damage by stabilizing lysosomal membranes; this reduces the extent of autolysis and hinders the perpetuation of the local inflammatory response. Corticosteroid administration leads to a relative lymphocytopenia which results from redistribution into the reticulo-endothelial system and a cytolytic action affecting preferentially the T lymphocyte population. The action on B lymphocytes is less marked and antibody formation is reduced only by high doses.

High doses of steroids have a cardiac inotropic effect and they also reduce systemic and pulmonary vascular resistance. Capillary flow is increased and there is mobilization of interstitial fluid and protein.

The use of corticosteroids in septic shock gained theoretical support from the knowledge that the inflammatory process includes an early phase of vasodilatation and extensive capillary leakage which leads to hypovolaemia. β-Endorphin is probably also involved in vasodilatation and it is derived from the same precursor molecule as ACTH. Early administration of high-dose corticosteroids may conceivably affect both ACTH and β-endorphin release. However, the results of clinical studies carried out to date indicate that corticosteroids are not of benefit. There is also no evidence for any beneficial effect of corticosteroids in cardiogenic shock.

An effect on pulmonary capillary leakage formed the theoretical basis for the use of corticosteroids in the adult respiratory distress syndrome. Experimentally, steroids have been demonstrated to be beneficial in animal models of ARDS. It is likely that the drugs should be given early to be effective and this may be practical when respiratory distress is provoked by a specific event such as pulmonary aspiration. However, current evidence suggests that corticosteroids are of no benefit in adult respiratory distress syndrome and there is likely to be a greater risk of infection if steroids are used routinely.

In acute allergic emergencies, including status asthmaticus, the use of corticosteroids is empirical, hydrocortisone being used most commonly. Intensive corticosteroid therapy should be for as short a period as possible (ideally limited to 48–72 h). In such instances, the dosage need not be tapered, or may be tapered quickly over the next 48–72 h, except in conditions (such as asthma) in which there may be a relapse unless dosage is reduced carefully. In asthma, a change to oral prednisolone should be undertaken when an adequate response has been obtained. Dosage can be tapered gradually over 1–2 weeks. There is no evidence that very high doses of potent steroids are more effective than conventional doses of hydrocortisone in acute allergy.

In cerebral oedema, corticosteroids (most commonly dexamethasone) have been used successfully to reduce raised intracranial pressure associated with cerebral tumours and symptomatic improvement can be obtained when oedema results from benign intracranial hypertension. In head injury or stroke, corticosteroids are of no value. In cerebral malaria, steroid treatment is detrimental.

The potential hazards of corticosteroids argue against their use in indications where their effectiveness is in doubt. The most important risk is infection, as a consequence of the suppressed inflammatory response. Glucose intolerance and gastrointestinal haemorrhage are also risks to be considered, although an accurate assessment of their clinical importance is lacking. Effective antimicrobial cover is essential whenever corticosteroids are used in the critically ill.

Antihistamines

Although there are two distinct populations of histamine receptor (H_1 and H_2) the term 'antihistamines' is used to refer to those drugs which block selectively histamine H_1-receptors found in the bronchi, arteries and gut. No compound currently in therapeutic use influences both H_1- and H_2-receptors.

Histamine is only one of many mediators which may be involved in acute allergic reactions. Some consequences of these substances (e.g. hypotension and bronchospasm) may be counteracted most effectively by adrenaline and other β-adrenoceptor agonists. Antihistamines (e.g.

chlorpheniramine, promethazine) tend to have only a secondary role in the management of acute allergy. They are most effective against symptoms such as itch, oedema and urticaria. They are less effective against hypotension and ineffective against bronchospasm, fever and arthralgia.

The most important adverse effect of anti-histamines is sedation, although occasionally they may produce central nervous system stimulation (e.g. agitation or convulsions), especially in children. A new generation of antihistamines with less sedative properties, e.g. terfenadine, has been developed.

All antihistamines have anticholinergic effects which tend to dry mucosal secretions and may cause tachycardia.

FURTHER READING

DePiro J T, Talbert R L, Hayes P E, Yee G C, Matzke G R, Posey L M (eds) 1992 Pharmacotherapy, a pathophysiologic approach, 2nd edn. Elsevier, New York

Dollery C (ed) 1991 Therapeutic drugs, vols 1, 2 and supplement 1. Churchill Livingstone, London

Goodman-Gilman A, Rall T W, Nies A S, Taylor P 1990 The pharmacological basis of therapeutics, 8th edn. Macmillan, New York

Ritter J M, Lewis L D, Mant T G K 1994 A textbook of clinical pharmacology, 3rd edn. Hodder and Stoughton, London

14. Local anaesthetic agents

Local anaesthetic drugs act by producing a reversible block to the transmission of peripheral nerve impulses. A reversible block may be produced also by physical factors including pressure and cold. Although nerve compression is of purely historical interest, cold (produced by the evaporation of ethyl chloride, the application of ice packs or use of, the cryoprobe) still has a limited use.

Many types of drug have local anaesthetic actions (e.g. β-blockers and antihistamines), but all those known and used as local anaesthetics have originated from cocaine, the alkaloid found in the leaves of the South American bush *Erythroxylum coca*. Its local anaesthetic action was demonstrated first by Koller, an ophthalmic surgeon working in Vienna. Although most of the major local anaesthetic techniques were described within a few years of that discovery, the drug was not used widely other than as a topical agent because of its systemic toxicity, central nervous stimulant and addictive properties and tendency to produce allergic reactions.

The demonstration of the physical structure of cocaine as an ester of benzoic acid permitted the production of safer agents, all with the same general structure of an aromatic group joined to an amine by an intermediate chain (Fig. 14.1). Procaine, synthesized in 1904, was the first significant advance and it allowed wider use of local anaesthetic techniques. Many other drugs were introduced, but none displaced procaine as the standard until the synthesis of lignocaine in the 1940s. The intermediate chain in lignocaine contains an amide bond and this obviated many of the problems associated with the ester group present in the older drugs. The subsequent production of other amide agents with varying clinical profiles

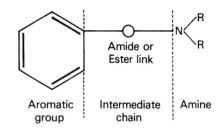

Fig. 14.1 General formula for local anaesthetic drugs.

has greatly extended the scope of modern local anaesthesia.

The mode of action of local anaesthetics is by blocking membrane depolarization in all excitable tissues. Since local anaesthetics are injected at their site of action, only peripheral nerve is usually exposed to concentrations high enough to have a significant effect. However, if sufficient drug reaches other organs via the circulation, more widespread effects occur.

MODE OF ACTION

Neural transmission (Fig. 14.2)

During the resting phase the interior of a peripheral nerve fibre has a potential difference of about −70 mV relative to the outside. When the nerve is stimulated there is a rapid increase in the membrane potential to approximately +20 mV, followed by an immediate restoration to the resting level. This depolarization/repolarization sequence lasts 1–2 ms and produces the familiar action potential associated with the passage of a nerve impulse.

The resting potential is the net result of several factors affecting the distribution of ions across

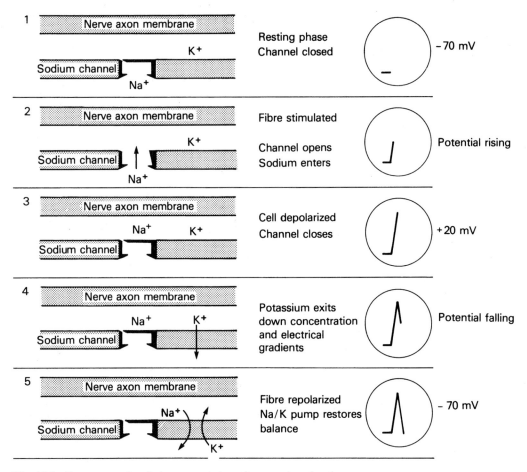

Fig. 14.2 Events occurring during transmission of a nerve impulse along an axon.

the cell membrane. Electrochemical and concentration gradients modify ionic diffusion, which is adjusted further by the semipermeable nature of the membrane and the action of the sodium/potassium pump.

Depolarization of the fibre is the result of a sudden increase in membrane permeability to sodium which can thus diffuse down both electrochemical and concentration gradients. Sodium ions enter the cell through large protein molecules in the membrane (known as channels), which are closed during the resting phase. Stimulation of the nerve changes the configuration of these protein molecules so that the channels open and allow positively charged sodium ions to enter the cell. This increases the membrane potential to approximately +20 mV, when the electrochemical and concentration gradients for sodium balance each

other and the channels close. Both concentration and electrochemical gradients then favour movement of potassium out through the membrane until the resting potential is restored. Relative to the total amounts present, only small numbers of ions take part in this exchange and the sodium/potassium pump restores their distribution during the resting phase.

At sensory nerve endings, the initial opening of sodium channels is produced by the appropriate physiological stimulus, which may be chemically mediated in some instances. The impulse is transmitted along the axon because a local current flows between the depolarized segment of nerve (which has a positive charge) and the next segment (which has a negative charge). The voltage change associated with this current causes the configurational change in the sodium channels in the next

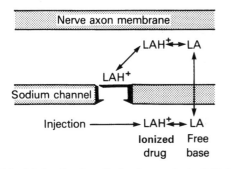

Fig. 14.3 Mode of action of a local anaesthetic (LA) drug. In order to penetrate the lipid cell membrane, the drug must be in free base form, while to effect a block reionization must occur.

segment, so that the action potential is propagated along the nerve.

Effect of local anaesthetic drugs (Fig. 14.3)

Local anaesthetics are usually injected in an acid solution as the hydrochloride salt (pH approximately 5). The tertiary amine group becomes quaternary and they are thus soluble in water and suitable for injection. Following injection, the pH increases as a result of buffering in the tissues and a proportion of the drug, determined by the pK, dissociates to release free base. As it is lipid-soluble, the free base is able to pass through the lipid cell membrane to the interior of the axon, where reionization takes place. The reionized portion enters the sodium channels, and may be thought of simply as plugging them so that sodium ions cannot enter the cell. As a result, no action potential is generated or transmitted, and conduction blockade has occurred. Because it is the ionized form of drug that is active and reionization has to take place intracellularly, individual drug pK has little effect on rate of onset of blockade.

In addition to diffusing into nerves at the site of injection, the drug also enters capillaries and is removed by the circulation. Eventually, tissue concentration decreases below that in the nerves and the drug diffuses out, so allowing restoration of normal function.

Systemic toxicity

If significant amounts of local anaesthetic drug reach the tissues of heart and brain they exert the same membrane-stabilizing effect as on peripheral nerve, resulting in a progressive depression of function. The earliest feature of systemic toxicity is numbness or tingling of the tongue and circumoral area; this is the result of a rich blood supply depositing enough drug to have an effect on the nerve endings. The patient may become light-headed, anxious, drowsy and/or complain of tinnitus. If concentrations continue to rise, consciousness is lost and this may be preceded or followed by convulsions.

Coma and apnoea may develop subsequently. Cardiovascular collapse may result from direct myocardial depression and vasodilatation, but more commonly it is a result of hypoxaemia secondary to apnoea.

Factors affecting toxicity

The most common cause of life-threatening systemic toxicity is an inadvertent intravascular injection, but it may result also from absolute overdosage. The changes in plasma concentration of drug following injection (Fig. 14.4) are dependent on the total dose administered, the rate of absorption, the pattern of distribution to other tissues and the rate of metabolism.

Absorption. Absorption from the site of injection depends on the blood flow; the higher the blood flow, the more rapid is the increase in plasma concentration, and the greater the resultant peak. Of the common sites of injection of large doses, the intercostal space has the highest blood supply, followed in turn by the extradural space, the brachial plexus and the sites of major lower limb nerve block. Absorption is slowest after infiltration anaesthesia.

Intravenous regional anaesthesia is a special case. If the tourniquet deflates immediately after drug injection, a large dose enters the circulation very rapidly. After 20 min of tourniquet application, sufficient drug has diffused out of the vessels into the tissues to result in the increase in systemic concentration being smaller than that following brachial plexus block.

Blood supply may be modified by the inherent vasoactive properties of the particular drug or by the addition of vasoconstrictors to the solution.

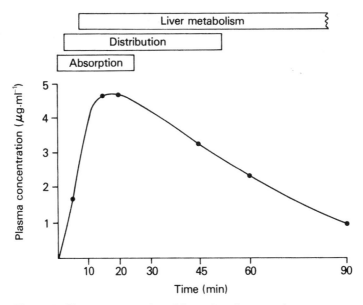

Fig. 14.4 Plasma concentration of lignocaine. Concentrations are shown after the injection into the lumbar extradural space of 400 mg of lignocaine without adrenaline. The injection was made at time zero and the phases of absorption, distribution and metabolism are indicated.

Use of the latter permits the safe dose to be increased by 50–100%.

Distribution (Fig. 14.5). After absorption, local anaesthetic drugs are distributed rapidly to, and taken up by, organs with a large blood supply and high affinity, e.g. brain, heart, liver and lungs. Muscle and fat, with low blood supplies, equilibrate more slowly, but the high affinity of fat for these drugs ensures that a large amount is taken up into adipose tissues. The lungs sequester (and possibly metabolize) local anaesthetic drugs, thereby preventing a large proportion of the injected dose from reaching the coronary and cerebral circulations.

Metabolism. In general, ester drugs are broken down so rapidly by plasma cholinesterase that systemic toxicity is unusual. Toxicity may occur with some of the slowly hydrolysed drugs or in patients with abnormal enzymes (cf. suxamethonium). The amides are metabolized by amidases

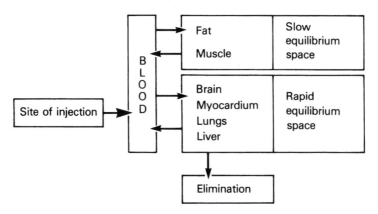

Fig. 14.5 Distribution of local anaesthetic drug after absorption from the site of injection.

located predominantly in the liver. Hepatocellular disease has to be severe before the rate of metabolism is slowed significantly, and in general the rate of disappearance of drug is dependent more upon liver blood flow. This has practical relevance to the use of lignocaine as an antiarrhythmic in cardiogenic shock, where liver blood flow is diminished.

Protein binding. Local anaesthetics are bound to plasma proteins to varying degrees. It is assumed sometimes that drugs with the greatest degrees of protein binding are less toxic because only a small fraction of the total amount in plasma is free to diffuse into the tissues and produce toxic effects. However, values for protein binding are obtained under laboratory conditions and probably bear little relationship to the dynamic situation that exists during the phase of rapid absorption. Furthermore, even if a drug is bound to protein, it is still available to diffuse into the tissues down a concentration gradient, as the bound portion is in equilibrium with that in solution in plasma. Thus, values for protein binding do not relate to acute toxicity of a drug.

Placental transfer. Much theoretical concern has been expressed about the mechanisms and effects of placental transfer of local anaesthetics administered to the mother during labour. Local anaesthetics cross the placenta as readily as other membranes, but their effects are of minimal significance when compared with those of conventional methods of analgesia and anaesthesia.

Fetal plasma protein may bind some drugs to a lesser extent than maternal protein so that *total* plasma concentration may be lower in the baby. It is claimed that such drugs are safer for the fetus. However, the concentration of *free* drug on each side of the placental membrane is the same and as a result tissue concentrations are more similar in mother and fetus than total plasma concentrations. The neonatal liver metabolizes drugs slowly, but provided that delivery does not occur immediately after a toxic reaction, there should be little concern about effects on the baby.

Prevention of toxicity

The single most important factor in the prevention of toxicity is the avoidance of accidental intra-vascular injection. Careful aspiration tests are vital and should be repeated each time the needle is moved. However, a negative test is not an absolute guarantee, especially when a catheter technique is used. The initial injection of 2–3 ml of a solution that contains adrenaline (1 : 200 000) has been advocated; an increase in heart rate during the succeeding 1–2 min should indicate intravascular injection. However, adrenaline is not the safest of drugs and this method is no guarantee against subsequent migration of needle or cannula into a vessel.

An alternative is to repeat the aspiration test after each 5–10 ml of solution, and to inject slowly. The patient should be watched for early signs of toxicity so that the injection may be stopped before there are major sequelae. Particular care should be taken when performing head and neck blocks because a very small dose may produce a major reaction if injected into a carotid or vertebral artery.

Overdosage may be avoided by consideration of the behaviour of the various drugs after injection at the particular site. Most practical manuals indicate the appropriate drug and dosage for each block, and these recommendations should be followed. Maximum safe dosages (for use in any situation) are often quoted for local anaesthetics with and without vasoconstrictor, but such recommendations are not really helpful since they ignore variations caused by factors such as the site of injection, the patient's general condition and the concomitant use of a general anaesthetic. If the same total dose is used, variations in drug concentration have no effect on toxicity. In adults, body weight correlates poorly with the risk of toxicity and it is better to modify the dose on the basis of an informed assessment of the patient's general condition.

Treatment of toxicity

No matter how careful the anaesthetist is with regard to prevention, facilities for treatment must always be available. The airway is maintained and oxygen administered by face mask, using artificial ventilation if apnoea occurs. Convulsions may be controlled with small increments of either diazepam (2.5 mg) or thiopentone (50 mg). The latter is usually more readily available and acts more rapidly. Excessive doses should not be given to control convulsions, since cardiorespiratory depression may be exacerbated. If cardiovascular collapse occurs despite adequate oxygenation (and this is *rare*), it should be treated with an adrenergic drug with α- and β-agonist properties, e.g. ephedrine in 3–5 mg increments.

Additional side-effects

Local anaesthetics are remarkably free from side-effects other than systemic toxicity which is an extension of pharmacological action. Complications of specific drugs are discussed later, but there are two general features — allergic reactions and drug interactions.

Allergic reactions

Allergy to the esters was relatively common, particularly with procaine, and was caused by *para*-aminobenzoic acid produced on hydrolysis. Most reactions were dermal in personnel handling the drugs, but fatal anaphylaxis has been recorded. Allergy to the amides is extremely rare and most reactions result from systemic toxicity, overdosage with vasoconstrictors, or are manifestations of anxiety. The occasional genuine allergic reaction is usually to a preservative in the solution rather than the drug itself.

Drug interactions

Interactions with other drugs do occur, although they rarely give rise to clinical problems. Therapy with anticholinesterases for myasthenia, or the concomitant administration of other drugs hydrolysed by plasma cholinesterase, increases the toxicity of the ester drugs, and competition for plasma protein binding sites may occur with the amides. Of more practical importance is that heavy sedation with anticonvulsants (e.g. benzodiazepines) may mask the early signs of toxicity. These drugs may even prevent convulsions, so that if a severe reaction does occur the patient may suddenly become deeply unconscious.

PHARMACOLOGY OF INDIVIDUAL DRUGS

The local anaesthetic drugs in current use vary in their clinical profile (stability, potency, duration, toxicity, etc.). These differences may be related to variations in physico-chemical properties.

Local anaesthetic drug chemistry

As indicated above (Fig. 14.1), all the local anaesthetic drugs have a three-part structure, with either an ester or amide bond at the centre. The important effects of the nature of this linkage on the route of metabolism and allergenicity have been discussed. The ester drugs also have short shelf-lives because they tend to hydrolyse spontaneously, especially on warming. The amides may be stored for long periods without loss of potency and are not heat-sensitive unless mixed with glucose to produce hyperbaric spinal solutions. As a general rule, solutions of amides in glucose and solutions of any ester may be heat-sterilized once, and should be used soon after autoclaving.

The aromatic end of the molecule determines fat-solubility and the amine affects its water-solubility. Addition of other organic groups to any part of the molecule increases lipid-solubility, and therefore potency, since ability to penetrate the lipid cell membrane is increased. The duration of action increases in proportion to the extent of protein binding, which is also a property of the aromatic group. Sodium channels are formed from large protein molecules and drugs with longer durations of action bind to these proteins for longer periods.

The effects of a local anaesthetic drug on blood vessels also modify its profile. Cocaine is a vasoconstrictor, but most of the other agents produce some degree of vasodilatation, which tends to shorten duration of action and increase toxicity.

The effects of differences in molecular structure often interact in complex ways, but a simple example of a structure–activity relationship is the addition of a butyl group to mepivacaine to produce bupivacaine, which is four times as potent and significantly longer-acting. Alterations in structure also affect the rate, and the products, of metabolism.

Differential sensory and motor blockade

It is often stated that small diameter axons, such as C fibres, are more susceptible to local anaesthetic block than are larger diameter fibres. In terms of absolute sensitivity, the reverse is actually true; large diameter fibres are more sensitive than small ones. However, large diameter fibres are usually more heavily myelinated than small fibres and the myelin sheath presents a significant barrier to drug diffusion. This means that small, unmyelinated fibres are blocked more rapidly by most local anaesthetic drugs. This difference in rate of blockade may be manipulated clinically with the aim of producing analgesia with relatively little motor blockade because skeletal muscle is innervated by larger, heavily myelinated fibres. Thus weak solutions (e.g. bupivacaine 0.125%) are employed with this aim. The newer agent, ropivacaine, appears to produce even greater separation of sensory and motor blockade, and may become the agent of choice for epidural use in obstetrics and the postoperative period.

Clinical factors affecting drug profile

Increasing the dose of a drug shortens its onset time and increases the duration of block. Dose may be increased by using either a higher concentration or a larger volume; a large volume of a dilute solution is usually more effective.

The site of injection also affects onset time and duration (in addition to potential toxicity). Onset is almost immediate after infiltration and is progressively delayed with subarachnoid, peripheral nerve and extradural blocks respectively. The slowest onset follows brachial plexus block. The dose required and the likely duration of action tend to increase in much the same order as for onset time.

Pregnancy and age are said to increase segmental spread of extradurals. For many blocks, young, fit, tall patients seem to require more drug, as do obese, alcoholic or anxious patients, the last perhaps because they react to any sensation from the operative area.

Individual drug properties

Only when all the above factors are taken into account may the properties of various drugs be compared. It is doubtful if, at *equipotent* concentrations, there are any real differences in speed of onset, but there are certainly variations in potency, duration and toxicity. The features of individual drugs are described below and in Table 14.1. Appropriate volumes and concentrations of local anaesthetic agents used commonly for specific blocks are detailed in Chapter 25.

Cocaine

Cocaine has no place in modern anaesthetic practice, although it is used in ear, nose and throat

Table 14.1 The features of individual local anaesthetic drugs

Proper name/ formula	% equivalent concentration*	Relative duration*	Toxicity	pK_a	Partition coefficient	% protein bound	Main use by anaesthetists in the UK
Cocaine	1	0.5	Very high	8.7	?	?	Nil
Benzocaine	NA	2	Low	NA	132	?	Topical
Procaine	2	0.75	Low	8.9	3.1	5.8	Nil

Table 14.1 (*cont'd*)

Proper name/ formula	% equivalent concentration*	Relative duration*	Toxicity	pK_a	Partition coefficient	% protein bound	Main use by anaesthetists in the UK
Chloroprocaine	1	0.75	Low	9.1	17	?	Not available
Amethocaine	0.25	2	High	8.4	541	76	Topical
Lignocaine	1	1	Medium	7.8	110	64	Infiltration Nerve block Epidural
Mepivacaine	1	1	Medium	7.7	42	77	Not available
Prilocaine	1	1.5	Low	7.7	50	55	Infiltration Nerve block IVRA
Cinchocaine	0.25	2	High	7.9	?	?	Not available
Ropivacaine	0.25	2–4	Medium	8.1	230	94	Not yet marketed
Bupivacaine	0.25	2–4	Medium	8.1	560	95	Extradural Spinal Nerve block
Etidocaine	0.5	2–4	Medium	7.9	1853	94	Not available

*Lignocaine = 1; NA = not applicable (not used in solution); ? = information not available. NB: published figures vary. See Strichartz et al (1990) for more details.

surgery for its vasoconstrictor action. Because of its use as a drug of addiction, it is increasingly difficult to obtain cocaine legitimately at a reasonable price.

Benzocaine

This is an excellent topical agent of low toxicity. It does not ionize and therefore its use is limited to topical application. In addition, its mode of action cannot be explained according to the theory outlined above. Instead, it is thought that benzocaine diffuses into the cell membrane, but not into the cytoplasm, and either causes the membrane to expand in the same way as is suggested for general anaesthetics (see Chapter 4) or enters the sodium channel from the lipid phase of the membrane. Whichever is the case, the mechanism may also be relevant to the action of the other agents.

Procaine

The incidence of allergic problems, short shelf-life and brief duration of action of procaine have resulted in its infrequent use at the present time.

Chloroprocaine

This is a relatively new ester which is widely used in the USA. Its profile is very similar to procaine, from which it differs only by the addition of a chlorine atom (Table 14.1). As a result, it is hydrolysed four times as quickly by cholinesterase and seems to be less allergenic. It is claimed to have a more rapid onset than any other agent but this may relate to its very low toxicity, which permits the use of relatively larger doses. There has been some concern that chloroprocaine might be neurotoxic, because of a number of reports of paraplegia after its accidental intrathecal injection. However, the evidence suggests that it was the preservative in the solution that caused the problems and not the drug itself.

Amethocaine

This drug (also known as tetracaine) is relatively toxic for an ester because it is hydrolysed very slowly by cholinesterase. It is also very potent and is the standard drug in North America for subarachnoid anaesthesia. It has a prolonged duration of action, but also a slow onset time. It can be used intrathecally in hyperbaric or isobaric solutions. Its use in the UK is restricted to topical anaesthesia.

Lignocaine

Having been used safely and effectively for every possible type of local anaesthetic procedure, lignocaine is currently the standard agent. It has no unusual features and is also a standard anti-arrhythmic. Lignocaine is used commonly for infiltration in concentrations of 0.5–1.0% and for peripheral nerve blocks if an intermediate duration is required. It can be used for intravenous regional anaesthesia, although prilocaine is preferred. Lignocaine 5% has been used for subarachnoid anaesthesia, although the degree of spread is unpredictable, and the duration of action relatively short. In a concentration of 1–2%, lignocaine produces epidural anaesthesia with a short onset time. Lignocaine 2–4% is used by many anaesthetists as a topical solution for anaesthesia of the upper airway prior to awake fibreoptic intubation.

Mepivacaine

This agent is very similar to lignocaine and seems to have neither advantages nor disadvantages in comparison.

Prilocaine

This is an underrated agent. It is equipotent to lignocaine, but has virtually no vasodilator action, is either metabolized or sequestered to a greater degree by the lungs, and is more rapidly metabolized by the liver. As a result, it is slightly longer-acting, considerably less toxic and is the drug of choice when the risk of toxicity is high. Metabolism produces o-toluidine, which reduces haemoglobin; thus, methaemoglobinaemia may occur but is rare unless the dose is considerably in excess of 600 mg. Cyanosis appears when 1.5 g.dl^{-1} of haemoglobin is converted, and treatment with methylene blue (1 mg.kg^{-1}) is effective immediately. Fetal haemoglobin is more sensitive, and prilocaine should not be used for extradural block during labour. Prilocaine is used mostly for infiltration and for intravenous regional anaesthesia.

Cinchocaine

Cinchocaine was the first amide agent to be produced (two decades before lignocaine). It is very potent and toxic. Like amethocaine, it was used mainly for subarachnoid anaesthesia, but the drug is no longer available for clinical use.

Bupivacaine

The introduction of bupivacaine represented a significant advance in anaesthesia. Relative to potency, its acute central nervous system toxicity is only slightly less than that of lignocaine, but its longer duration of action reduces the need for repeated doses, and thus the risks of cumulative toxicity.

A number of deaths have occurred after the accidental intravenous administration of large doses of bupivacaine, and some concern has been expressed that this drug might have a more toxic effect on the myocardium than other local anaesthetic agents. There is some experimental evidence that this is so, but very large doses must be given rapidly and intravenously for the effect to be clinically apparent.

Bupivacaine can be used for infiltration, although only in small doses because of its toxicity. It is used frequently for peripheral nerve blockade, and for subarachnoid and extradural anaesthesia because of its prolonged duration of action.

Bupivacaine 0.5% is the most commonly used drug for subarachnoid anaesthesia in the UK. It may be used in a plain solution, or in a hyperbaric formulation (see Chapter 25).

Etidocaine

This is an amide derived from lignocaine. It may be even longer-acting than bupivacaine and is of particular interest because it seems to produce a more profound effect on motor than sensory nerves; the reverse is probably true with other agents.

Ropivacaine

The cardiovascular toxicity of bupivacaine has stimulated interest in finding other long-acting agents which do not possess this effect. Ropivacaine is similar chemically to bupivacaine (the butyl group attached to the amine is replaced by a propyl group). It is slightly less potent than bupivacaine, and produces a block of slightly shorter duration. At equipotent concentrations, ropivacaine appears to be less likely than bupivacaine to cause cardiac collapse and arrhythmias, and cardiac resuscitation is more likely to be successful if cardiotoxicity does occur.

Additives

Many substances are added to local anaesthetics for pharmaceutical purposes. Sodium hydroxide and hydrochloric acid are used to adjust the pH, sodium chloride the tonicity, and glucose and water the baricity of solutions. Preservatives, e.g. methyl hydroxybenzoate, are added to multidose bottles and manufacturers recommend that these should not be used for subarachnoid or extradural block. Other additions are made for pharmacological reasons.

Vasoconstrictors

The addition of a vasoconstrictor to a solution of local anaesthetic drug slows the rate of absorption, reduces toxicity, prolongs duration and may result in a more profound block. These are all desirable effects, but vasoconstrictors are not used universally for several reasons. They are absolutely contraindicated for injection close to end-arteries (ring blocks of digits and penis) and in intravenous regional anaesthesia because of the risk of ischaemia.

There is also a theoretical risk that the use of vasoconstrictors may increase the risk of permanent neurological deficit by rendering nerve tissue ischaemic. While evidence is inconclusive, many anaesthetists feel that vasoconstrictors should not be used unless there is no alternative method of prolonging duration or reducing toxicity in the specific clinical situation.

Adrenaline is the most potent agent. It produces

systemic toxicity, and should be used with particular care, if at all, in patients with cardiac disease. Even in healthy patients concentrations greater than 1:200 000 should not be used, and the maximum dose administered should not exceed 0.5 mg. Interactions with other sympathomimetic drugs, including tricyclic antidepressants, may occur, especially when adrenergic drugs are used systemically to treat hypotension.

Felypressin is a safer drug, although it causes pallor and may constrict the coronary circulation. It is available usually for dental use only.

Carbon dioxide

In order to speed the onset of blockade, some local anaesthetics have been produced as the carbonated salt, with carbon dioxide dissolved under pressure in the solution. The rationale for the use of these solutions is that after injection the carbon dioxide lowers intracellular pH and favours formation of more of the ionized active form of the drug. With blocks of slower onset there is good evidence that a significant improvement is obtained.

Dextrans

There have been many attempts to prolong duration of action by mixing local anaesthetics with high-molecular-weight dextrans. The results are inconclusive, but the very large dextrans may be effective, especially in combination with adrenaline. 'Macromolecules' may be formed between dextran and local anaesthetic so that the latter is held in the tissues for longer periods.

Hyaluronidase

For many years the enzyme hyaluronidase was added to local anaesthetics to aid spread by breaking down tissue barriers. There was little evidence that it had a significant effect and this practice has been abandoned.

Mixtures

Some practitioners deliberately mix different local anaesthetics together in an attempt to obtain the advantages of both. One such combination (sometimes referred to as compounding) is lignocaine and bupivacaine; the aim is to achieve the rapid onset of the former and the long duration of the latter with a single injection. Another advantage claimed for compounding two drugs is a decrease in toxicity. However, local anaesthetic drug toxicity is additive, so that the use of 'half a dose' of each of two drugs is of no benefit. If an ester is combined with an amide, toxicity may increase because the amide slows hydrolysis of the ester by inhibiting plasma cholinesterase. It is more appropriate to use a catheter technique, to initiate the block with a dose of lignocaine and to maintain it with a dose of bupivacaine as the effect of lignocaine starts to regress.

A more effective combination is the eutectic mixture of local anaesthetics (EMLA). This is a mixture of the base (un-ionized) forms of lignocaine and prilocaine in a cream formulation. It is a local anaesthetic preparation which penetrates intact skin with some reliability. It takes up to 1 h to become effective but is very useful in paediatric practice, especially in children who need repeated venepuncture. It may also be of value for poor-risk patients undergoing skin grafting.

CHOICE OF LOCAL ANAESTHETIC AGENT

When using a local technique the anaesthetist has to decide upon the concentration, volume and nature of the agent to be used. For lignocaine (the relative potencies of other agents are shown in Table 14.1) concentrations required are:

skin infiltration } IVRA	0.5%
minor nerve block	1.0%
brachial plexus } sciatic/femoral	1.0–1.5%
extradural	1.5–2.0%
subarachnoid	2.0–5.0%

Higher concentrations than these may be used to produce more profound peripheral blocks of faster onset. The volumes required for specific techniques are described in Chapter 25 and the interrelationships that exist between patient status and the required amount of drug have been discussed above.

Ideally, several drugs of different potency, duration and toxicity should be available to permit a rational choice based upon the required dose, the particular risk of toxicity in that block and patient, and the likely duration of surgery. Often this is not possible, mainly for commercial reasons. For example, in the UK, lignocaine and bupivacaine are marketed in a full range of concentrations, but little else is available apart from the more dilute solutions of prilocaine. The availability of spinal anaesthetic solutions is particularly poor. For more peripheral blocks, lignocaine and bupivacaine may be used safely unless the risk of toxicity is relatively high (e.g. intravenous regional anaesthesia) when prilocaine is the drug of choice. When large volumes of more concentrated solutions are needed and the higher concentrations of prilocaine are not available, then one of the other agents should be used in combination with adrenaline.

FURTHER READING

Covino B G 1980 The mechanisms of local anaesthesia. In: Norman J, Whitman J G (eds) Topical reviews in anaesthesia. John Wright, Bristol

Covino B G, Vassallo H G 1976 Local anesthetics: mechanisms of action and clinical use. Grune & Stratton, New York

Henderson J J, Nimmo W S 1983 Practical regional anaesthesia. Blackwell Scientific Publications, Oxford

Stanton-Hicks M d'A (ed) 1978 Regional anesthesia: advances and selected topics. International Anesthesiology Clinics 16 (4)

Stricharz et al 1990 Fundamental properties of local anaesthetics II measured octanol: buffer partition coefficients and pKa values of clinically used drugs. Anesthesia and Analgesia 71: 158–170

Wildsmith J A W, Armitage E N 1993 Principles and practice of regional anaesthesia, 2nd edn. Churchill Livingstone, Edinburgh

15. Basic physics for the anaesthetist

The application of physics in anaesthesia

A knowledge of simple physics is required in order to understand fully the function of many items of anaesthetic apparatus. This chapter is designed to emphasize the more elementary aspects of physical principles and it is hoped that the reader will be stimulated to read some of the excellent books which are designed for anaesthetists and examine this topic in greater detail (see Further Reading). Sophisticated measurement techniques may be required for more complex types of anaesthesia, in the intensive therapy unit and during anaesthesia for severely ill patients and an understanding of the principles involved in performing such measurements is required in the later stages of the anaesthetist's training.

This chapter does not describe all the physical principles which may be encountered in the early stages of anaesthetic training (e.g. magnetism and light), but concentrates on the more common applications, including pressure and flow in gases and liquids, electricity and electrical safety. However, it is necessary first to consider some basic definitions.

BASIC DEFINITIONS

It is now customary in medical practice to employ the International System (SI) of units. Common exceptions to the use of the SI system include measurement of arterial pressure and, to a lesser extent, gas pressure measurements. Arterial pressure is frequently measured using a mercury column and so 'mmHg' is retained. Pressures in gas cylinders are also referred to frequently in terms of the 'normal' atmospheric pressure of 760 mmHg; this is equal to 1.01 bar (or approximately 1 bar). Low pressures are expressed usually in the SI units of kPa whilst higher pressures are referred to in bar (100 kPa = 1 bar). The basic and derived units of the SI system are shown in Table 15.1.

The fundamental quantities in physics are mass, length and time.

Mass (m) is defined as the amount of matter in a body. The unit of mass is the kilogram (kg), for which the standard is a block of platinum held in a Physics Reference Laboratory.

Length (l) is defined as the distance between two points. The SI unit is the metre (m), which is defined as the distance occupied by a specified number of wavelengths of light.

Time (t) is measured in seconds. The reference standard for time is based on the frequency of resonation of the caesium atom.

From these basic definitions, several units of measurement may be derived.

Velocity is defined as the distance travelled per unit time:

$$\text{velocity } (v) = \frac{\text{distance}}{\text{time}} \text{ m.s}^{-1}$$

Acceleration is defined as the rate of change of velocity:

$$\text{acceleration } (a) = \frac{\text{velocity}}{\text{time}} \text{ m.s}^{-2}$$

Force is that which is required to give a mass acceleration:

$$\text{force} = \text{mass} \times \text{acceleration}$$
$$= ma$$

The SI unit of force is the newton (N). One newton

Table 15.1 Physical quantities

Quantity	Definition	Symbol	SI Unit
Length	Unit of distance	l	metre (m)
Mass	Amount of matter	m	kilogram (kg)
Density	Mass per unit volume (m/v)	ρ	kg.m^{-3}
Time		t	second (s)
Velocity	Distance per unit time (l/t)	v	m.s^{-1}
Acceleration	Rate of change of velocity (v/t)	a	m.s^{-2}
Force	Gives acceleration to a mass (ma)	F	newton (N) (kg.m.s^{-2})
Weight	Force exerted by gravity on a mass (mg)	W	kg $\times$ 9.81 m.s^{-2}
Pressure	Force per unit area (F/A)	P	N.m^{-2}
Temperature	Tendency to gain or lose heat	T	kelvin (K) or degree Celsius (°C)
Work	Performed when a force moves an object (force $\times$ distance)	U	joule (J) (Nm)
Energy	Capacity for doing work (force $\times$ distance)	U	joule (J) (Nm)
Power	Rate of performing work (joules per second)	P	watt (W) (J.s^{-1})

is the force required to give a mass of 1 kg an acceleration of 1 m.s^{-2}:

$$1\,N = 1\,kg.m.s^{-2}$$

Weight is the force of the earth's attraction for a body. When a body falls freely under the influence of gravity, it accelerates at a rate of 9.81 m.s^{-2}:

$$\begin{aligned}\text{weight} &= \text{mass} \times g\\ &= m \times g\\ &= m \times 9.81\,m.s^{-2}\end{aligned}$$

Momentum is defined as mass multiplied by velocity:

$$\text{momentum} = m \times v$$

Work is undertaken when a force moves an object:

$$\begin{aligned}\text{work} &= \text{force} \times \text{distance}\\ &= F \times l\\ &= U\,Nm \text{ or joules (J)}\end{aligned}$$

Energy is the capacity for undertaking work. Thus it has the same units as those of work.

Power is the rate of doing work. The SI unit of power is the watt, which is equal to 1 J.s^{-1}:

$$\begin{aligned}\text{power} &= \text{work per unit time}\\ &= \text{joules per second}\\ &= \text{watt (W)}\end{aligned}$$

Pressure is defined as force per unit area:

$$\begin{aligned}\text{pressure }(P) &= \frac{\text{force}}{\text{area}}\\ &= N.m^{-2}\\ &= \text{pascal (Pa)}\end{aligned}$$

As 1 Pa is a rather small unit, it is more common in medical practice to use the kilopascal (kPa).

FLUIDS

Substances may exist in solid, liquid or gaseous form. These forms or phases differ from each other according to the random movement of their constituent atoms or molecules. In solids, molecules oscillate about a fixed point, whereas in liquids the molecules possess higher velocities and move more freely and thus do not bear a constant relationship in space to other molecules. The molecules of gases also move freely, but to an even greater extent.

Both gases and liquids are termed fluids. Liquids are incompressible and at constant temperature occupy a fixed volume, conforming to the shape of a container; gases have no fixed volume but expand to occupy the total space of a container.

Heating a liquid increases the kinetic energy of its molecules, permitting some to escape from the surface into the vapour phase. Random loss of molecules with higher kinetic energies from a liquid occurs in the process of vaporization. As these molecules possess higher kinetic states, this leads to a reduction in the energy state and cooling of the liquid.

Collision of randomly moving molecules in the gaseous phase with the walls of a container is responsible for the pressure exerted by a gas.

Gas pressures

There are three important laws which determine the behaviour of gases and which are important to anaesthetists.

Boyle's law states that, at constant temperature, the volume (V) of a given mass of gas varies inversely with its absolute pressure (P):

$$PV = k_1$$

Charles' law states that, at constant pressure, the volume of a given mass of gas varies directly with its absolute temperature (T):

$$V = k_2T$$

The third gas law states that, at constant volume, the absolute pressure of a given mass of gas varies directly with its absolute temperature:

$$P = k_3T$$

Combining these three gas laws:

$$PV = kT$$

or,

$$\frac{P_1V_1}{T_1} = \frac{P_2V_2}{T_2}$$

The behaviour of a mixture of gases in a container is described by *Dalton's law of partial pressures*. This states that, in a mixture of gases, the pressure exerted by each gas is the same as that which it would exert if it alone occupied the container.

Thus, in a cylinder of compressed air at a pressure of 100 bar, the pressure exerted by nitrogen is equal to 79 bar (as the fractional concentration of nitrogen is 0.79).

Avogadro's hypothesis

Avogadro's hypothesis states that equal volumes of gases at the same temperature and pressure contain equal numbers of molecules.

Avogadro's number is the number of molecules in 1 gram molecular weight of a substance and is equal to 6.022×10^{23}.

Under conditions of standard temperature and pressure, 1 gram molecular weight of any gas occupies a volume of 22.4 litres.

These data are useful in calculating, for example, the quantity of gas produced from liquid nitrous oxide. The molecular weight of nitrous oxide is 44. Thus, 44 g of N_2O occupy a volume of 22.4 litres at standard temperature and pressure (STP). If a full cylinder of N_2O contains 3.0 kg of liquid, then vaporization of all the liquid would yield:

$$\frac{22.4 \times 3.0 \times 1000}{44} \text{ litres}$$
$$= 1527 \text{ litres at STP}$$

Critical temperature

The critical temperature of a substance is the temperature above which that substance cannot be liquefied by pressure, irrespective of its magnitude.

The critical temperature of oxygen is $-118°C$, that of nitrogen $-147°C$ and that of air $-141°C$. Thus, at room temperature, cylinders of these substances contain gases. In contrast, the critical temperature of carbon dioxide is $31°C$ and that of nitrous oxide $36.4°C$. The critical pressures are 73.8 bar and 72.5 bar respectively; at higher pressures, cylinders of these substances contain a mixture of gas and liquid.

Clinical application of the gas laws

A 'full' cylinder of oxygen on an anaesthetic machine contains compressed gaseous oxygen at a pressure of 137 bar (2000 lb.in^{-2}). If the cylinder of oxygen empties at constant temperature, the volume of gas contained is related linearly to its pressure (by Boyle's law). In practice, linearity is not followed because temperature falls as a result of adiabatic expansion of the compressed gas; the term adiabatic implies a change in the state of a gas without exchange of heat energy with its surroundings.

In contrast, the pressure in a cylinder of nitrous

oxide remains relatively constant as the cylinder empties to the point at which liquid has totally vaporized. Subsequently, there is a linear decline in pressure proportional to the volume of gas remaining within the cylinder.

Filling ratio

The degree of filling of a nitrous oxide cylinder is expressed as the mass of nitrous oxide in the cylinder divided by the mass of water which the cylinder could hold. Normally, a cylinder of nitrous oxide is filled to a ratio of 0.67. This should not be confused with the volume of liquid nitrous oxide in a cylinder. A 'full' cylinder of nitrous oxide at room temperature is filled to the point at which approximately 90% of the interior of the cylinder is occupied by liquid, the remaining 10% being occupied by gaseous nitrous oxide. Incomplete filling of a cylinder is necessary, because thermally induced expansion of the liquid in a totally full cylinder may cause an explosion.

Entonox

Entonox is the trade name for a compressed gas mixture containing 50% oxygen and 50% nitrous oxide. The mixture is compressed into cylinders containing gas at a pressure of 137 bar (2000 lb.in^{-2}). The nitrous oxide does not liquefy because the two gases in this mixture 'dissolve' in each other at high pressure. In other words, the presence of oxygen reduces the critical temperature of nitrous oxide. The critical temperature of the mixture is $-7°C$. Cooling of a cylinder of Entonox to a temperature below $-7°C$ results in separation of liquid nitrous oxide. Use of such a cylinder results in oxygen-rich gas being emitted initially, followed by a hypoxic nitrous oxide rich gas. Consequently, it is recommended that when an Entonox cylinder may have been exposed to low temperatures, it should be stored horizontally for a period of not less than 24 h at a temperature of 5°C or above. In addition, the cylinder should be inverted several times before use.

Pressure notation in anaesthesia

Although the use of SI units of measurement is generally accepted in medicine, a variety of ways of expressing pressure is still used, reflecting custom and practice. Arterial pressure is still referred to universally in terms of mmHg because a column of mercury is one of the most common means of measurement of pressure and is used also to calibrate electronic devices.

Similarly, measurement of central venous pressure is referred to customarily in cmH$_2$O.

Atmospheric pressure (P_B) exerts a pressure sufficient to support a column of mercury of height 760 mm (Fig. 15.1).

$$
\begin{aligned}
1 \text{ atmospheric pressure} &= 760 \text{ mmHg} \\
&= 1.01325 \text{ bar} \\
&= 760 \text{ torr} \\
&= 1 \text{ atmosphere absolute (ata)} \\
&= 14.7 \text{ lb.in}^{-2} \\
&= 101.325 \text{ kPa}
\end{aligned}
$$

In considering pressure, it is necessary to indicate whether or not atmospheric pressure is taken into account. Thus, a diver working 10 m below the surface of the sea may be described as compressed to a depth of 1 atmosphere or working at a pressure of 2 atmospheres absolute (2 ata).

In order to avoid confusion when discussing compressed cylinders of gases, the term gauge pressure is used. This refers to the difference between the pressure of the contents of the cylinder and the ambient pressure. Thus, a full cylinder of oxygen has a gauge pressure of 137 bar, but the contents are at a pressure of 138 bar absolute.

Pressure relief valves

The Heidbrink valve is a common component of many anaesthesia breathing systems. In the Magill breathing system, the anaesthetist may vary the force in the spring(s), thereby controlling the pressure within the breathing system (Fig. 15.2). At equilibrium, the force exerted by the spring is equal to the force exerted by gas within the system:

Force (F) = Gas pressure (P) × Disc area (a)

Modern anaesthesia systems contain a variety of pressure relief valves, in each of which the force is fixed so as to provide a gas escape mechanism when pressure reaches a preset level. Thus, an

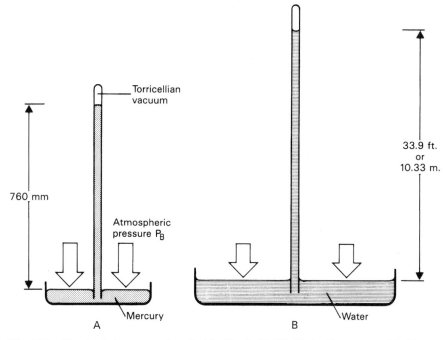

Fig. 15.1 The simple barometer described by Torricelli; (**A**) filled with mercury, (**B**) filled with water.

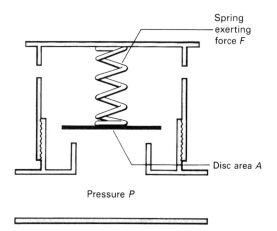

Fig. 15.2 A pressure relief valve.

anaesthetic machine may contain a pressure relief valve operating at 35 kPa, situated on the back bar of the machine between the vaporizers and the breathing system. Modern ventilators may contain a pressure relief valve set at 7 kPa. A much lower pressure is set in relief valves which form part of anaesthetic scavenging systems and these may operate at pressures of 0.2–0.3 kPa.

Pressure-reducing valves (pressure regulators)

Pressure regulators have two important functions in anaesthetic machines:

1. They reduce high pressures of compressed gases to manageable levels (acting as pressure-reducing valves).
2. They minimize fluctuations in the pressure within an anaesthetic machine which would necessitate frequent manipulations of flowmeter controls.

Modern anaesthetic machines are designed to operate with an inlet gas supply at a pressure of 3–4 bar (usually 4 bar in the UK). Hospital pipeline supplies also operate at a pressure of 4 bar and therefore pressure regulators are not required between a hospital pipeline supply and an anaesthetic machine. In contrast, the contents of cylinders of all medical gases (i.e. oxygen, nitrous oxide and carbon dioxide) are at much higher pressures. Thus, cylinders of these gases require a pressure-reducing valve between the cylinder and the flowmeter.

The principle on which the simplest type of pressure-reducing valve operates is shown in Figure 15.3. High-pressure gas enters through the valve and forces the flexible diaphragm upwards, tending to close the valve and prevent further ingress of gas from the high-pressure source.

If there is no tension in the spring, the relationship between the reduced pressure (p) and the high pressure (P) is very approximately equal to the ratio of the areas of the valve seating (a) and the diaphragm (A):

$$\frac{p}{P} = \frac{a}{A}$$

By tensing the spring, a force F is produced which offsets the closing effect of the valve. Thus, p may be increased by increasing the force in the spring.

Without the spring, the simple pressure regulator has the disadvantage that reduced pressure decreases proportionally with the decrease in cylinder pressure. The addition of a force from the spring considerably reduces but does not eliminate this problem and in order to overcome it newer pressure regulators contain an extra closing spring.

The S60 M regulator (BOC) is a modern regulator used widely in the UK and is illustrated in Figure 15.4. It should be noted that the high pressure tends to close the valve.

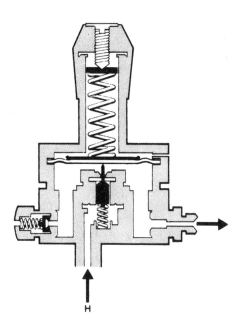

Fig. 15.4 A modern pressure-regulating valve: the S60 M regulator (BOC).

Pressure demand regulators

These are regulators in which gas flow occurs when an inspiratory effort is applied to the outlet port. The Entonox valve is a two-stage regulator and its mode of action is demonstrated in Figure 15.5.

Measurement of pressure in fluids

Gases

The simplest method of measuring pressure in gases is by the use of a manometer, illustrated in Figure 15.6. The manometer may be filled with water to measure low pressures; for measurement of larger pressures, the column is filled with mercury, which possesses a density 13.6 times greater than that of water. It is clear that liquid-filled manometers are not appropriate for measurement of either gas or liquid pressures in the majority of clinical situations.

In anaesthetic practice, pressures in gases may be measured by sensitive electrical pressure transducers similar to those used for measurement of intravascular pressures.

Pressure gauges on anaesthetic ventilators

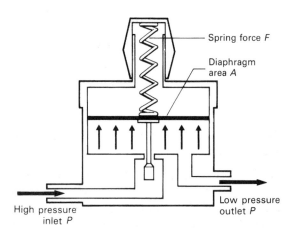

Spring force *F*

Diaphragm area *A*

Low pressure outlet *P*

High pressure inlet *P*

Fig. 15.3 A simple pressure-reducing valve.

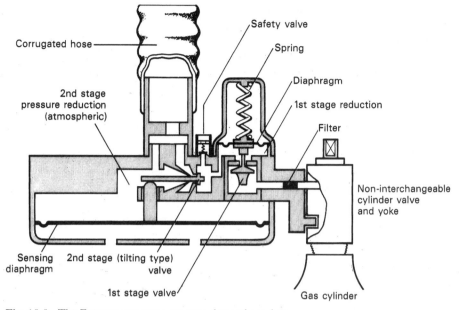

Fig. 15.5   The Entonox two-stage pressure demand regulator.

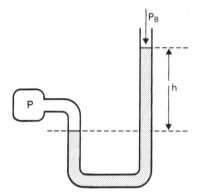

Fig. 15.6   A simple fluid-filled manometer for measurement of pressure *P*.

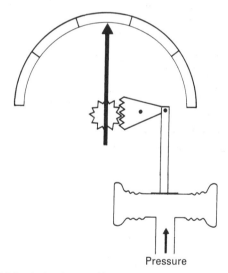

Fig. 15.7   A simple aneroid pressure gauge.

usually comprise a simple bellows type of aneroid gauge (Fig. 15.7) whilst high gas pressure (e.g. in medical gas cylinders) are measured using a type of Bourdon gauge (Fig. 15.8).

Liquids

In anaesthetic practice, measurement of pressures in liquids is required in assessment of the circulation. The simple manometer, filled with water, is used frequently for measurement of central venous pressure (see p. 343). Measurement

of arterial pressure is undertaken by a variety of different means including:

1. Sphygmomanometry. A pressure occlusion cuff is applied to the upper arm and the pressure raised until flow through the brachial artery ceases. The pressure within the cuff is measured by using either a simple mercury-filled manometer

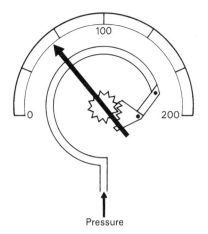

Fig. 15.8 A Bourdon type of pressure gauge. Increase in pressure tends to straighten the coiled metal tube.

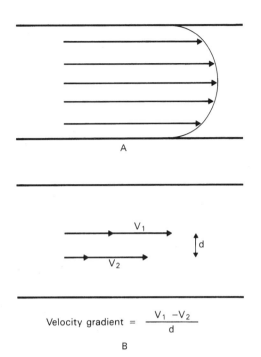

$$\text{Velocity gradient} = \frac{V_1 - V_2}{d}$$

B

Fig. 15.9 (**A**) Diagrammatic illustration of laminar flow. (**B**) Velocity gradient.

or an aneroid manometer. Flow beyond the cuff may be detected by:

a. Palpation of the radial artery.
b. Auscultation of the brachial artery.
c. Application of a Doppler flowmeter over the radial artery (a method used principally in paediatric practice).
d. By the use of finger plethysmography.
e. By means of a special double cuff which is incorporated in a device termed the oscillotonometer.

2. Direct measurement of pressure by an electronic transducer connected through a fluid-filled column to a cannula sited in the arterial system.

These clinical methods of measuring arterial blood pressure are described in detail in Chapter 20.

Flow of fluids

Viscosity is defined as that property of a fluid which causes it to resist flow. The coefficient of viscosity (η) is defined as:

$$\eta = \frac{\text{force}}{\text{area}} \times \text{velocity gradient}$$

In this context, velocity gradient is equal to the difference between velocities of different fluid molecules divided by the distance between molecules (Fig. 15.9B). The units of the coefficient of viscosity are Pascal seconds.

Fluids which obey this formula are referred to as Newtonian fluids and η is a constant for each fluid. However, some biological fluids are non-Newtonian. A prime example is blood; viscosity changes with the rate of flow of blood (as a result of change in distribution of cells) and, in stored blood, with time (blood thickens on storage).

Viscosity of liquids diminishes with increase in temperature, whereas viscosity of a gas increases with increase in temperature.

Laminar flow

Laminar flow through a tube is illustrated in Figure 15.9A. In this situation, there is a smooth orderly flow of fluid such that molecules travel with the greatest velocity in the axial stream whilst the velocity of those in contact with the wall of the tube may be virtually zero. The linear velocity of axial flow may be twice the average linear velocity of flow.

In a tube, the factors determining flow are given by the Hagen–Poiseuille formula:

$$\dot{Q} = \frac{\pi P r^4}{8\eta l}$$

where $\dot{Q}$ = flow; P = pressure gradient along the tube; r = radius of the tube; η = viscosity of fluid; and l = length of the tube.

The Hagen–Poiseuille formula applies only to Newtonian fluids. In non-Newtonian fluids such as blood, increase in velocity of flow may alter viscosity because of variation in the dispersion of cells within plasma.

Turbulent flow

In turbulent flow, fluid no longer moves in orderly planes but swirls and eddies around in a haphazard manner as illustrated in Figure 15.10. Although viscosity affects laminar flow, it should be noted that this does not apply to turbulent flow, which is affected by changes in density.

It may be seen from Figure 15.11 that the rela-

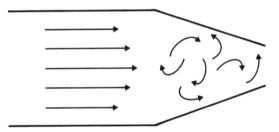

Fig. 15.10 Diagrammatic illustration of turbulent flow.

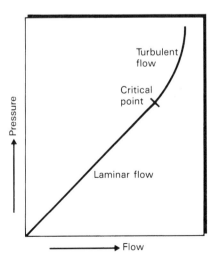

Fig. 15.11 The relationship between pressure and flow in a fluid is linear up to the critical point, above which flow becomes turbulent.

tionship between pressure and flow is linear within certain limits. However, as velocity increases, a point is reached (the critical point or critical velocity) at which the characteristics of flow change from laminar to turbulent. The critical point is dependent upon several factors which were investigated by the physicist Reynolds. The factors are related by the formula used for calculation of Reynolds' number:

$$\text{Reynolds' number} = \frac{v\rho r}{\eta}$$

where v = linear velocity; r = radius of tube; ρ = density; and η = viscosity.

Studies with cylindrical tubes have shown that if Reynolds' number exceeds 2000, flow is likely to be turbulent, whereas a Reynolds' number of less than 2000 is associated usually with laminar flow.

Flow of fluids through orifices

In an orifice, the diameter of the fluid pathway exceeds the length. The flow rate of a fluid through an orifice is dependent upon:

1. The square root of the pressure difference across the orifice.
2. The square of the diameter of the orifice.
3. The density of the fluid, as flow through an orifice inevitably involves some degree of turbulence.

Applications in anaesthetic practice

1. In upper respiratory tract obstruction of any severity, flow is inevitably turbulent; thus for the same respiratory effort, a lower tidal volume is achieved than when flow is laminar. The extent of turbulent flow may be reduced by reducing gas density; clinically it is common practice to administer oxygen-enriched helium rather than oxygen alone (the density of oxygen is 1.3 and that of helium is 0.16).

2. In anaesthetic breathing systems, a sudden change in diameter of tubing or irregularity of the wall may be responsible for a change from laminar to turbulent flow. Thus, tracheal and other breathing tubes should possess smooth

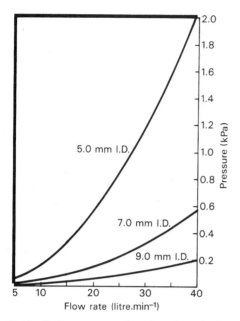

Fig. 15.12 Resistance to gas flow through tracheal tubes of different internal diameter (ID).

internal surfaces, gradual bends, no constrictions and be of as large a diameter and as short a length as possible.

3. Resistance to breathing is much greater when a tracheal tube of small diameter is used (Fig. 15.12).

MEASUREMENT OF GAS VOLUMES

Spirometers

Spirometers may be classified as dry (e.g. the 'Vitalograph') or wet (e.g. the 'Benedict Roth' spirometer). Both the Vitalograph and Benedict Roth spirometers measure volumes of gases of the order of a few litres. Larger volumes of gases may be measured by the dry gas meter, an instrument used for measuring volumes in domestic gas supplies.

In anaesthesia, the Wright respirometer (see p. 350) is a convenient method of measuring gas volumes.

MEASUREMENT OF FLOW

Flowmeters

The principles of gas flow described above are

used in the construction of anaesthetic flowmeters. There are two types of flowmeter: variable-orifice (constant-pressure) or fixed-orifice (variable-pressure).

Fixed-orifice flowmeters

The only common type of fixed-orifice meter used in anaesthetic practice comprises a Bourdon pressure gauge which measures the pressure through a small fixed orifice, beyond which the pressure varies little. Consequently, the flow rate is proportional to the pressure proximal to the fixed orifice and the pressure gauge may be calibrated in units of flow.

Variable-orifice flowmeters

These instruments may be either ball flowmeters or bobbin flowmeters, as illustrated in Figure 15.13. The commonest flowmeter used by the anaesthetist is the bobbin flowmeter, which is referred to frequently by the trade name of Rotameter. Readings are taken from the middle of the ball in a ball flowmeter, but from the top of the bobbin in a bobbin flowmeter.

In the Rotameter, the bobbin possesses small slots which cause it to rotate. Rotation reduces errors caused by friction between the walls of the tube and the bobbin. In order to reduce electrostatic charges and sticking of the bobbin, some

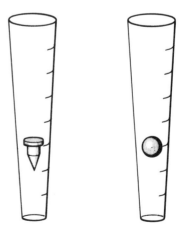

Fig. 15.13 The bobbin (left) and ball (right) flowmeters in exaggerated diagrammatic form to show tapering of tubes.

modern flowmeter tubes are coated with a thin layer of tin (stannous oxide).

The pressure across the bobbin remains relatively constant, producing a force which is equal to the force of gravity on the bobbin. As the flow rate increases, the bobbin rises higher in the tube and the size of the annulus between the bobbin and the walls of the tube increases. At low flow rates, the narrow annular space between the bobbin and the wall mimics a tube. At high flow rates, the width of the annulus is large relative to the height of the bobbin and the annular space forms an orifice. Thus at low flow rates, the viscosity of gas determines the position of the bobbin, whereas at higher rates the effect of density of the gas becomes more important. Consequently, flowmeters must be calibrated for individual gases.

The Wright peak flowmeter depends upon the variable-orifice principle.

Pneumotachograph

The pneumotachograph is an instrument for measuring flow rate by sensing the pressure drop across a laminar resistance, i.e. a resistance through which laminar flow occurs.

The Fleisch pneumotachograph (Fig. 15.14) comprises a series of parallel tubes which generate laminar flow even at variable or high flow rates; the pressure change across the tubes is determined using a differential pressure transducer. The major problem with this device is condensation of water vapour; in order to prevent this, the

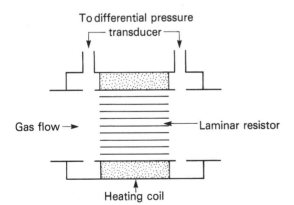

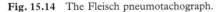

Fig. 15.14 The Fleisch pneumotachograph.

laminar resistor may be surrounded by a heated coil. In addition, heating maintains a constant temperature which prevents errors caused by variations in gas viscosity.

Measurement of flow in liquids

Several methods exist for measurement of blood flow in the circulation.

1. *Limb plethysmography*. This simple technique for measuring blood flow in the limb entails temporary occlusion of venous outflow from the limb; the consequent increase in volume of the limb corresponds to arterial inflow. The increase in volume of the limb may be calculated either from volume displacement in a water container or from the increase in girth of the limb measured by a mercury-in-rubber strain gauge.

2. *The Fick principle*. This principle may be used for measurement of blood flow through a variety of organs, including heart, brain, liver and kidney. Total cardiac output may be measured by the use of the Fick principle as applied to the lung.

In essence, the principle states that the amount of substance or tracer taken up or given off by an organ in unit time is equal to the product of blood flow through the organ and the concentration difference of the substance across the organ:

$$\frac{\text{amount}}{\text{time}} = \text{flow} \times (A - V) \text{ content difference}$$

where A = arterial and V = venous.

Cardiac output ($\dot{Q}_t$) may be calculated by measuring oxygen consumption ($\dot{V}_{O_2}$) with a spirometer, and the oxygen contents of arterial (Ca_{O_2}) and mixed venous ($C\bar{v}_{O_2}$) blood samples drawn simultaneously from the radial artery and pulmonary artery. Then:

$$\dot{Q}_t = \frac{\dot{V}_{O_2}}{(Ca_{O_2} - C\bar{v}_{O_2})}$$

Typical values are:

$$5 \text{ litre.min}^{-1} = \frac{250 \text{ ml.min}^{-1}}{(20 - 15) \text{ ml.dl}^{-1}}$$

3. *Electromagnetic flowmeter*. This instrument operates on the principle of electromagnetic in-

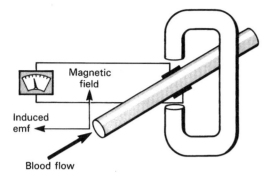

Fig. 15.15 Faraday's left-hand rule of electromagnetic induction in the principle underlying the electromagnetic flowmeter.

duction. As blood (which is a conductor of electricity) moves through a magnetic field, an electric potential is induced which is proportional to the rate of movement of the blood. The potential is induced in a plane perpendicular to both the magnetic field and the direction of blood flow according to Faraday's left-hand rule (Fig. 15.15).

4. *Ultrasonic flowmeters.* These devices provide good qualitative but not quantitative information on flow.

5. *Dye-dilution and thermal dilution techniques.* These techniques are used clinically for measurement of cardiac output (see p. 346).

THE INJECTOR

The injector is frequently termed a Venturi, although the principles governing such an apparatus were formulated by Bernoulli in 1778, some 60 years earlier than Venturi. The principle is illustrated in Figure 15.16. As fluid passes through a constriction, there is an increase in velocity of the fluid; beyond the constriction, velocity decreases to the initial value. At point A, the energy in the fluid is both potential and kinetic, but at point B the amount of kinetic energy is much greater because of the increased velocity. As the total energy state must remain constant, potential energy is reduced at point B and this is reflected by a reduction in pressure. Venturi's contribution to the injector lay in the design of the tube distal to the site of the constriction. For optimum performance, it is necessary for fluid flow to remain laminar in such a tube. In the Venturi tube, the pressure is least at the site of maximum constriction and by gradual opening of the tube beyond the constriction a subatmospheric pressure may be induced distal to the constriction (Fig. 15.17).

The injector principle may be seen in anaesthetic practice in the following situations:

1. *Oxygen therapy.* Several types of Venturi oxygen masks are available which provide oxygen-enriched air. With an appropriate flow of oxygen (usually exceeding 4 litre.min^{-1}) there is a large degree of entrainment of air. This results in a total gas flow that exceeds the patient's peak inspiratory flow rate, thus ensuring that the inspired oxygen concentration remains constant, and it prevents an increase in apparatus dead space which always accompanies the use of low-flow oxygen devices (see p. 420).

2. *Nebulizers.* These are used to entrain water from a reservoir. If the water inlet is suitably positioned, the entrained water may be broken up into a fine mist by the high gas velocity.

3. *Portable suction apparatus.*

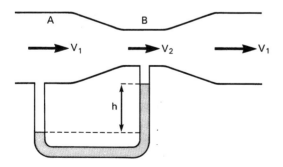

Fig. 15.16 The Bernoulli principle.

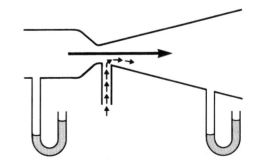

Fig. 15.17 Fluid entrainment by a Venturi injector.

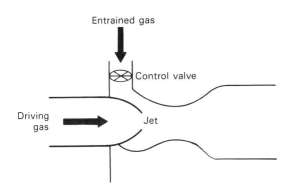

Fig. 15.18 A simple injector.

4. *Oxygen tents.*
5. *As a driving gas in a ventilator* (Fig. 15.18).

The Coanda effect

The Coanda effect describes a phenomenon whereby gas flow through a tube with two Venturis tends to cling either to one side of the tube or to the other. The principle has been used in anaesthetic ventilators (termed fluidic ventilators), as the application of a small pressure distal to the restriction may enable gas flow to be switched from one side to another (Fig. 15.19).

HEAT AND TEMPERATURE

Temperature is a measure of the tendency of an object to gain or lose heat. Heat is the energy which can be transferred from a body at a hotter temperature to one at a colder temperature.

Thermometry

In the SI system, the unit of temperature is the kelvin (K). The zero reference point on this scale is absolute zero (0 K or $-273.15°C$) and the upper point is the triple point of water (the temperature at which water exists simultaneously in solid, liquid and gaseous states); this corresponds to 273.16 K or 0.01°C.

Temperature is measured in clinical practice by one of the following techniques:

1. *Mercury in glass thermometer.*
2. *Thermistor.* This is a semiconductor which exhibits a reduction in electrical resistance with increase in temperature.
3. *Thermocouple.* This relies on the Seebeck effect. When two metal conductors are joined together to form a circuit, a potential difference is produced which is proportional to the difference in temperatures of the two junctions. In order to measure temperature, one junction has to be kept at a constant temperature.

Heat capacity

The heat capacity of a body is the amount of heat required to raise the temperature of the body by 1°C; in the SI nomenclature, heat capacity is measured in units of joules per kelvin ($J.K^{-1}$).

Specific heat capacity

The specific heat capacity of a substance is the energy required to raise the temperature of 1 kg of a substance by 1 K. Thus:

heat capacity = mass × specific heat capacity

The specific heat capacity of different substances is of interest because anaesthetists are frequently concerned with maintenance of body temperature in unconscious patients.

Heat is lost from patients by the processes of:

1. Conduction
2. Convection
3. Radiation
4. Evaporation.

The specific heat capacity of gases is up to 1000 times smaller than that of liquids. Consequently, humidification of inspired gases is a more important method of conserving heat than warming dry gases; in addition, the use of humidified gases

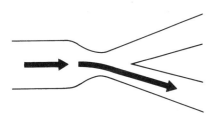

Fig. 15.19 The Coanda effect.

minimizes the very large energy loss produced by evaporation of fluid from the respiratory tract.

The skin of man acts as an almost perfect radiator; radiant losses in susceptible patients may be reduced by the use of reflective aluminium foil ('space blanket').

VAPORIZATION AND VAPORIZERS

In a liquid, molecules are in a state of continuous motion because of mutual attraction by Van der Waal's forces. Some molecules may develop velocities sufficient to escape from these forces and if they are close to the surface of a liquid these molecules may escape to enter the vapour phase. Increasing the temperature of a liquid increases its kinetic energy and a greater number of molecules escape. As the faster moving molecules escape into the vapour phase, the net velocity of the remaining molecules reduces; thus the energy state and therefore temperature of the liquid phase are reduced. The amount of heat required to convert unit mass of liquid into a vapour without a change in temperature of the liquid is termed the heat of vaporization.

In a closed vessel containing liquid and gas, a state of equilibrium is reached when the number of molecules escaping from the liquid is equal to the number of molecules re-entering the liquid phase. The vapour concentration is then said to be saturated at the specified temperature. Saturated vapour pressure of liquids is independent of the ambient pressure, but increases with increasing temperature.

The boiling point of a liquid is the temperature at which its saturated vapour pressure becomes equal to the ambient pressure. Thus, on the graph in Figure 15.20, the boiling point of each liquid at 1 atmosphere is the temperature at which its saturated vapour pressure is 101.3 kPa.

Vaporizers

Vaporizers may be classified into two types:

1. Drawover vaporizers.
2. Plenum vaporizers.

In the former type, gas is pulled through the vaporizer when the patient inspires, creating a subatmospheric pressure. In the latter type, gas is forced through the vaporizer by the pressure of the fresh gas supply. Consequently, the resistance

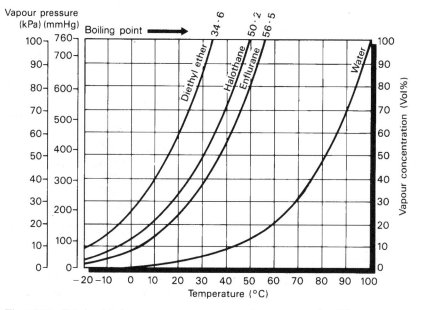

Fig. 15.20 Relationship between vapour pressure and temperature for different anaesthetic agents.

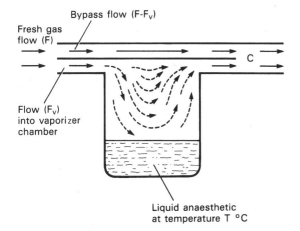

Fig. 15.21 A simple type of vaporizer.

to gas flow through a drawover vaporizer must be extremely small; the resistance of a plenum vaporizer may be high enough to prevent its use as a drawover vaporizer, although this is not necessarily so.

The principles of both devices are similar. If we consider the simplest form of vaporizer (Fig. 15.21), the concentration (*C*) of anaesthetic in the gas mixture emerging from the outlet port is dependent upon:

1. *The saturated vapour pressure* of the anaesthetic liquid in the vaporizer. Thus, a highly volatile agent such as diethyl ether is present in a much higher concentration than a less volatile agent (i.e. with a lower saturated vapour pressure) such as halothane.

2. The *temperature* of the liquid anaesthetic agent, as this determines its saturated vapour pressure.

3. The *splitting ratio*, i.e. the flow rate of gas through the vaporizing chamber (F_v) in comparison with that through the bypass ($F - F_v$). Regulation of the splitting ratio is the usual mechanism whereby the anaesthetist controls the output concentration from a vaporizer.

4. The *surface area* of the anaesthetic agent in the vaporizer. If the surface area is relatively small during use, the flow of gas through the vaporizing chamber may be too rapid to achieve complete saturation with anaesthetic molecules of the gas above the liquid.

5. *Duration of use.* As the liquid in the vaporiz-

ing chamber evaporates, its temperature, and thus its saturated vapour pressure, decreases. This leads to a reduction in concentration of anaesthetic in the mixture leaving the exit port.

6. The *flow characteristics* through the vaporizing chamber. In the simple vaporizer illustrated, gas passing through the vaporizing chamber may fail to mix completely with vapour as a result of streaming because of poor design. This lack of mixing is flow-dependent.

Modern anaesthetic vaporizers overcome many of the problems described above. Maintenance of full saturation may be achieved by making available a large surface area for vaporization. In the Tec series of vaporizers this is achieved by the use of wicks which draw up liquid anaesthetic and provide a very large surface area. Efficient vaporization and prevention of streaming of gas through the vaporizing chamber are achieved by ensuring that gas travels through a concentric helix which is bounded by the fabric wicks. Another method of ensuring full saturation is to bubble gas through liquid anaesthetic via a sintered disc. This method is used in the Halox vaporizer and in the Copper Kettle vaporizer. In both these types of vaporizer the final concentration is determined by mixing a known flow of fresh gas with a measured flow of fully saturated vapour.

Temperature compensation

Temperature-compensated vaporizers possess a mechanism which produces an increase in flow through the vaporizing chamber (i.e. an increased splitting ratio) as the temperature of liquid anaesthetic decreases. In the TEC vaporizers, a bimetallic strip controls (by bending) a valve which alters flow through the exit port of the vaporizing chamber. In the EMO and Ohio vaporizers, a bellows mechanism is used to regulate the valve (by shortening with decreased temperature) whilst in the Drager Vapor 19 vaporizers a metal rod acts in a similar fashion.

In the Copper Kettle and Halox vaporizers, the temperature in the vaporizer is measured and the flow rate adjusted according to a calibration chart. In addition, reduction in temperature is minimized in the Copper Kettle vaporizer by the method of construction; this comprises a large mass of copper which provides a large heat capacity and efficient conduction of heat from the anaesthetic machine to which the vaporizer is attached.

Back pressure (pumping effect)

Some gas-driven mechanical ventilators (e.g. Manley) produce a considerable increase in pressure in the outlet port and back bar of the anaesthetic machine. This pressure is highest during the inspiratory phase of ventilation. If the simple vaporizer shown in Figure 15.21 is attached to the back bar, the increased pressure during inspiration compresses the gas in the vaporizer; some gas in the region of the outlet port of the vaporizer is forced back into the vaporizing chamber, where more vapour is added to it. Subsequently, there is a temporary surge in anaesthetic concentration when the pressure decreases at the end of the inspiratory cycle.

This effect is minimal with efficient vaporizers (i.e. those which saturate gas fully in the vaporization chamber) because gas in the outlet port is already saturated with vapour. However, when pressure reduces at the end of inspiration, some saturated gas passes retrogradely out of the inspiratory port and mixes with the bypass gas. Thus, a temporary increase in total vapour concentration may still occur in the gas supplied to the patient. Methods of overcoming this problem include:

1. Incorporation of a one-way valve in the outlet port.
2. Construction of a bypass chamber and vaporizing chamber which are of equal volumes so that the gas in each is compressed or expanded equally.
3. Construction of a long inlet tube to the vaporizing chamber so that retrograde flow from the vaporizing chamber does not reach the bypass channel (as in the Mark 3 TEC vaporizers).

HUMIDITY AND HUMIDIFICATION

Absolute humidity is the mass of water vapour present in a given volume of gas. Relative humidity is the ratio of mass of water vapour in a given volume of gas to the mass required to saturate that volume of gas at the same temperature.

Relative humidity (RH) may be expressed as:

$$RH = \frac{\text{actual vapour pressure}}{\text{saturated vapour pressure}}$$

In normal practice, relative humidity may be measured using:

1. The *hair hygrometer*. This operates on the principle that a hair elongates if humidity increases; the hair length controls a pointer. This simple device may be mounted on a wall. It is reasonably accurate only in the range 15–85% relative humidity.
2. The *wet and dry bulb hygrometer*. The dry bulb measures the actual temperature, whereas the wet bulb measures a lower temperature as a result of the cooling effect of evaporation of water. The rate of vaporization is related to the humidity of the ambient gas and the difference between the two temperatures is a measure of ambient humidity; the relative humidity is obtained from a set of tables.
3. *Regnault's hygrometer*. This consists of a thin silver tube containing ether and a thermometer to show the temperature of the ether. Air is pumped through the ether to produce evaporation, thereby cooling the silver tube. When gas in contact with the tube is saturated with water vapour it condenses as a mist on the bright silver. The temperature at which this takes place is known as the *dew point*, from which relative humidity is obtained from tables.

Humidification in the respiratory tract

Air drawn into the respiratory tract becomes fully saturated in the trachea at a temperature of 37°C. Under these conditions, the SVP of water is 6.3 kPa (47 mmHg); this represents a fractional concentration of 6.2%. The concentration of water is 44 mg.litre^{-1}. At 21°C, saturated water vapour contains 2.4% water vapour or 18 mg.litre^{-1}. Thus, there is a considerable capacity for patients to lose both water and heat when the lungs are ventilated with dry gases.

There are three means of humidifying inspired gas:

1. Heated humidifier (water vaporizer).
2. Nebulizer.
3. Condenser humidifier (also known as heat and moisture exchanging humidifier).

The hot water bath humidifier is a simple device for heating water to 45–60°C. These devices have several potential problems, including infection if the water temperature decreases below 45°C, scalding the patient if the temperature exceeds 60°C (these high temperatures may be employed to prevent growth of bacteria) and condensation of water in the inspiratory anaesthetic tubing. These devices are approximately 80% efficient.

Some nebulizers are based upon a Venturi system; a gas supply entrains water which is broken up into a large number of droplets. The ultrasonic nebulizer operates by dropping water on to a surface which is vibrated at a frequency of 2 MHz. This breaks up the water particles into extremely small droplets. The main problem with these nebulizers is the possibility that supersaturation of inspired gas may occur and the patient may be overloaded with water.

The condenser humidifier (or artificial nose) may consist of a simple wire mesh which is inserted between the tracheal tube and anaesthetic breathing system. More recently, humidifiers constructed of rolled corrugated paper have been introduced. These devices are approximately 70% efficient.

SOLUTION OF GASES

Henry's law states that, at a given temperature, the amount of a gas which dissolves in a liquid is directly proportional to the partial pressure of the gas in equilibrium with the liquid. If a liquid is heated and its temperature rises, the partial pressure of its vapour increases. As the total ambient pressure remains constant, the partial pressure of any dissolved gas must decrease.

It is customary to confine the term 'tension' to the partial pressure of a gas exerted by gas molecules in solution.

Solubility coefficients

The Bunsen solubility coefficient is the volume of gas which dissolves in unit volume of liquid at a given temperature when the gas in equilibrium with the liquid is at a pressure of one atmosphere.

The Ostwald solubility coefficient is the volume of gas which dissolves in unit volume of liquid at a given temperature. Thus, the Ostwald solubility coefficient is independent of pressure.

The partition coefficient is the ratio of the amount of substance in one phase compared with a second phase, each phase being of equal volume and in equilibrium. As with the Ostwald coefficient, it is necessary to define the temperature, but not the pressure. The partition coefficient may be applied to two liquids, but the Ostwald coefficient applies to partition between gas and liquid.

DIFFUSION AND OSMOSIS

If two different gases or liquids are separated in a container by an impermeable partition which is then removed, gradual mixing of the two different substances occurs as a result of the kinetic activity of each molecule. This is illustrated in Figure 15.22. The principle governing this process is described by Fick's law of diffusion, which states that the rate of diffusion of a substance across unit area is proportional to the concentration gradient. Graham's law (which applies to gases only) states that the rate of diffusion of a

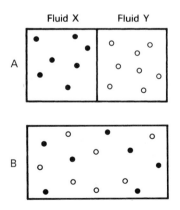

Fig. 15.22 Illustration of diffusion in fluids: (**A**) fluid X and Y separated by partition; (**B**) mixing of fluids after removal of partition.

gas is inversely proportional to the square root of its molecular weight.

In the example shown in Figure 15.22B, the interface between fluids X and Y after removal of the partition would be the surface of the fluid. In biology, however, there is normally a membrane separating gases or separating gas and liquids.

The rate of diffusion of gases may be affected by the nature of the membrane. In the lungs, the alveolar membrane is moist and may be regarded as a water film. Thus, diffusion of gases through the alveolar membrane is dependent not only on the properties of diffusion described above but also on the solubility of gas in the water film. As carbon dioxide is highly soluble compared with oxygen, it diffuses more rapidly across the alveolar membrane, despite the larger partial pressure gradient for oxygen.

Osmosis

In the examples given above, the membranes are permeable to all substances. However, in biology, membranes are frequently semipermeable, i.e. they allow the passage of some substances but are impermeable to others. This is illustrated in Figure 15.23. In Figure 15.23A, initially equal volumes of water and glucose solution are separated by a semipermeable membrane. Water molecules pass freely through the membrane to dilute the glucose solution (Fig. 15.23B). By application of a hydrostatic pressure (Fig. 15.23C), the process of transfer of water molecules can be prevented; this pressure (P) is equal to the osmotic pressure exerted by the glucose solution.

Substances in dilute solution behave in accordance with the gas laws. Thus, 1 gram molecular weight of a dissolved substance occupying 22.4 litres of solvent exerts an osmotic pressure of 1 bar at 273 K. Dalton's law applies also; the total osmotic pressure of a mixture of solutes is equal to the sum of osmotic pressures exerted independently by each substance.

The osmotic pressure of a solution depends on the number of dissolved particles per litre. Thus, a molar solution of a substance which ionizes into two particles exerts twice the osmotic pressure exerted by a molar solution of a non-ionizing substance.

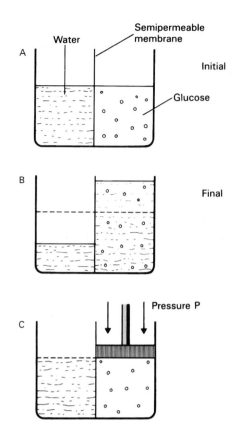

Fig. 15.23 Diagram to illustrate osmotic pressure: (**A**) water and glucose placed into two compartments separated by a semipermeable membrane; (**B**) at equilibrium, water has passed into the glucose compartment to balance osmotic pressure; (**C**) the magnitude of osmotic pressure of the glucose is denoted by a hydraulic pressure P applied to the glucose to prevent any movement of water into the glucose compartment.

The term osmolarity refers to the osmotic pressure produced by all substances in a fluid. Thus, it is the sum of the individual molarities of each particle.

The term osmolality refers to the number of osmoles per kilogram of water or other solvent (whilst molarity refers to osmoles per litre of solution). Thus, osmolarity may vary slightly from osmolality as a result of changes in density due to the effect of temperature on volume, although in biological terms the difference is extremely small.

In the circulation, water and the majority of ions are freely permeable across the endothelial membrane, but plasma protein does not traverse into the interstitial fluid. The term oncotic pressure is used to describe the osmotic pressure exerted by the plasma proteins alone. Plasma oncotic pressure is relatively small (approximately 1 mosmol.litre^{-1}) in relation to total osmotic pressure exerted by plasma (approximately 300 mosmol.litre^{-1}).

ELECTRICAL SAFETY

The anaesthetist is in daily contact with a large amount of equipment which is powered by mains supply electricity; this includes monitoring equipment, some ventilators, suction apparatus, defibrillators and diathermy equipment.

Whilst a total understanding of this equipment and its mode of action may depend upon a detailed knowledge of electronics, the equipment can usually be used safely as a type of 'black box' (i.e. the inside of the box may be a mystery, but the anaesthetist must be familiar with the operating controls and the ways in which the apparatus may malfunction or, if a recording instrument, give rise to artefacts).

It is not possible in this brief chapter to provide a synopsis of the basic principles of electricity and electronics, but it is essential to stress some elements which have a bearing on the safety of both the patient and the anaesthetist in the operating theatre.

In the UK, the mains electricity is supplied at a voltage of 240 V with a frequency of 50 Hz and in the USA at a voltage of 110 V and a frequency of 60 Hz. These voltages are potentially dangerous, although the danger is related predominantly to the current which flows through the patient:

$$\text{current } (I) = \frac{\text{voltage } (V)}{\text{resistance } (R)} \text{ (Ohm's law)}$$

When dealing with alternating current, it is necessary to use the term impedance in place of resistance, as impedance takes into account the presence of capacitors and resistors. Direct current cannot pass through capacitors; the resistance of a capacitor is inversely proportional to the frequency of an alternating current.

If an increasing electrical current at 50 Hz passes through the body, there is initially a tingling sensation at a current of 1 mA. Increase in the current produces increasing pain and muscle spasm until, at 80–100 mA, arrhythmias and ventricular fibrillation may occur.

The damage to tissue by alternating current is related also to the current density; a current passing through a small area is more dangerous than the same current passing through a much larger area. Other factors relating to the likelihood of ventricular fibrillation are the duration of passage of the current and its frequency. Radio frequencies (such as those used in diathermy) have no potential for fibrillating the heart.

It is clear from Ohm's law that the size of the current is dependent upon the size of the impedance to current flow. A common way of reducing the risk of a large current injuring the anaesthetist in the operating theatre is to wear antistatic shoes and to stand on the antistatic floor. This provides a high impedance (see below).

There are three classes of electrical insulation which are designed to minimize the risk of a patient or anaesthetist forming part of an electrical circuit between the live conductor of a piece of equipment and ground.

1. *Class I equipment.* The main supply lead has three cores (live, neutral and earth). The earth is connected to all exposed conductive parts and in the event of a fault developing which short-circuits current to the casing of the equipment, current flows from the case to earth and blows a fuse.

2. *Class II equipment.* This has no protective earth. The power cable has only live and neutral conductors and these are 'double-insulated'. The casing is normally made of non-conductive material.

3. *Class III equipment.* This relies on a power supply at a very low voltage produced from a secondary transformer situated some distance away from the device. Potentials do not exceed 24 V AC or 50 V DC. Electric heating blankets, for example, are rendered safer in this way.

Isolation circuits

All modern patient-monitoring equipment uses an isolation transformer so that the patient is connected only to the secondary circuit of the transformer, which is not earthed. Thus, even if the patient makes contact between the live circuit of the secondary transformer and ground, no current is transmitted to ground.

Microshock

Mains electricity supplies may induce currents in other circuits or on cases of instruments. The resulting induced currents are termed leakage currents and may pass through either the patient or anaesthetist to ground. Although the currents are very small, they may present problems to patients with an intracardiac pacemaker or a saline-filled intracardiac monitoring catheter.

The International Electrotechnical Commission has produced recommendations (adopted by the British Standards Institute) defining the levels of permitted leakage currents and patient currents from different types of electromedical equipment.

FIRES AND EXPLOSIONS

Although the use of inflammable anaesthetic agents has declined greatly over the last 2–3 decades, ether is still used commonly in many countries. In addition, other inflammable agents may be utilized in the operating theatre, e.g. alcohol for skin sterilization. Thus the anaesthetist should have some understanding of the problems and risks of fire occurring in the operating theatre.

Fires are produced when fuels undergo combustion. A conflagration differs from a fire in having a more rapid and more violent rate of combustion. A fire becomes an explosion if the combustion is sufficiently rapid to cause pressure waves which in turn cause sound waves. If these pressure waves possess sufficient energy to ignite adjacent fuels, the combustion is extremely violent and termed a detonation.

Fires require three ingredients:

1. Fuel.
2. Oxygen or other substance capable of supporting combustion.
3. Source of ignition, i.e. a source of heat sufficient to raise the fuel temperature to its ignition temperature. This quantity of heat is termed the activation energy.

Fuels

The modern volatile anaesthetic agents (halothane, enflurane and isoflurane) are non-flammable and non-explosive at room temperature in either air or oxygen.

Oils and greases are petroleum-based and form excellent fuels. In the presence of high pressures of oxygen, nitrous oxide or compressed air, these fuels may ignite spontaneously, an event termed dieseling (an analogy with the diesel engine). Thus oil or grease must not be used in compressed air, nitrous oxide or oxygen supplies.

Surgical spirit burns readily in air and the risk is increased in the presence of oxygen or nitrous oxide. Other non-anaesthetic inflammable substances include methane in the gut (which may be ignited by diathermy when the gut is opened), paper dressings and plastics found in the operating theatre suite.

Ether burns in air slowly with a blue flame but mixtures of nitrous oxide, oxygen and ether are always explosive. It has been suggested that if administration of ether is discontinued 5 min before exposure to a source of ignition, the patient's expired gas is unlikely to burn provided that an open circuit has been used after discontinuation of ether.

The stoichiometric concentration of a fuel and oxidizing agent is the concentration at which all combustible vapour and agent are completely utilized. Thus the most violent reactions take place in stoichiometric mixtures and as the concentration of the fuel moves away from the stoichiometric range the reaction gradually declines until a point is reached (the flammability limit) at which ignition does not occur.

The inflammability range for ether is 2–82% in oxygen, 2–36% in air and 1.5–24% in nitrous oxide. The stoichiometric concentration of ether in oxygen is 14% and there is a risk of explosion with ether concentrations of approximately 12–40% in oxygen. In air, the stoichiometric concentration of ether is 3.4% and explosions do not occur.

Support of combustion

It should always be remembered that as the concentration of oxygen increases so does the likelihood of ignition of a fuel and the conversion of the reaction from fire to explosion.

Nitrous oxide supports combustion. During laparoscopy, there is a risk of perforation of the bowel and escape of methane or hydrogen into the peritoneal cavity. Consequently, the use of nitrous oxide to produce a pneumoperitoneum for this procedure is not recommended; carbon dioxide is to be preferred, as it does not support combustion (and in addition has a much greater solubility in blood than nitrous oxide, thereby diminishing the risk of gas embolism).

Sources of ignition

The two main sources of ignition in the operating theatre are static electricity and diathermy.

Static electricity

Static charges are produced on non-conductive material, such as rubber mattresses, plastic pillow cases and sheets, woollen blankets, nylon, terylene, hosiery garments, rubber tops of stools and non-conducting parts of anaesthetic machines and breathing systems.

Diathermy

Diathermy equipment has now become an essential element of most surgical practice. However, it should not be used in the presence of inflammable agents.

Other sources of ignition

1. Faulty electrical equipment.
2. Heat from endoscopes, thermocautery, lasers, etc.
3. Electric sparks from motor switches, X-ray machines, etc.

Prevention of static charges

Where possible, antistatic conducting material should be used in place of non-conductors. The resistance of antistatic material should be between 50 kΩ.cm^{-1} and 10 MΩ.cm^{-1}.

All material should be allowed to leak static charges through the floor of the operating theatre. However, if the conductivity of the floor is too high there is a risk of electrocution if an individual forms a contact between mains voltage and ground. Consequently, the floor of the operating theatre is designed to have a resistance of 25–50 kΩ when measured between two electrodes placed 1 m apart. This allows the gradual discharge of static electricity to earth. Personnel should wear conducting shoes, each with a resistance of between 0.1 and 1 MΩ.

Moisture encourages the leakage of static charges along surfaces to the floor. The risk of sparks from accumulated static electricity charges is reduced if the relative humidity of the atmosphere is kept above 50%.

FURTHER READING

Mushin W W, Jones P L 1987 Physics for the anaesthetist, 4th edn. Blackwell Scientific Publications, Oxford
Parbrook G D, Davis P D, Parbrook E O 1985 Basic physics and measurement in anaesthesia, 2nd edn.

Heinemann, London
Sykes M K, Vickers M D, Hull C J 1981 Principles of clinical measurement, 2nd edn. Blackwell Scientific Publications, Oxford

16. Anaesthetic apparatus

In cannot be stressed too highly that anaesthetists should have a sound understanding and firm knowledge of the functioning of all anaesthetic equipment in common use. Although primary malfunction of equipment has not featured highly in surveys of anaesthetic-related morbidity and mortality, failure to understand the use of equipment features in these reports as a cause of morbidity and mortality. This is true especially of ventilators, where lack of knowledge regarding the function of equipment may result in a patient being subjected to the dangers of hypoxaemia and/or hypercapnia.

It is essential that the anaesthetist checks that all equipment is functioning correctly before he proceeds to anaesthetize patients. In some respects, the routine of testing anaesthetic equipment resembles the airline pilot's check list which is an essential preliminary to aircraft flight. Adverse events occur during anaesthesia with great rapidity and faced with an imminent disaster, the anaesthetist must be assured in advance that any equipment which he proposes to use is functioning correctly.

The purpose of this chapter is to describe briefly apparatus which is used in delivery of gases, from the sources of supply to the patient's lungs. Clearly, it is not possible to describe in detail equivalent models produced by all manufacturers. Consequently, this chapter concentrates only on principles and some equipment which is used commonly.

It is convenient to describe anaesthetic apparatus sequentially from the supply of gases to point of delivery to the patient. This sequence is shown in Table 16.1.

Table 16.1 Classification of anaesthetic equipment described in this chapter

Supply of gases
– from outside the operating theatre
– from cylinders within the operating theatre, together with the connections involved

The anaesthetic machine
– unions
– cylinders
– reducing valves
– flowmeters
– vaporizers

Safety features of the anaesthetic machine

Anaesthetic breathing systems

Ventilators

Apparatus used in scavenging waste anaesthetic gases

Apparatus used in interfacing the patient to the anaesthetic breathing system
– laryngoscopes
– anaesthetic masks and airways

Tracheal tubes

Accessory apparatus for the airway
– forceps
– laryngeal sprays
– bougies
– mouth gags
– stilletes
– catheter mounts

GAS SUPPLIES

Bulk supply of anaesthetic gases

In the majority of modern hospitals, piped medical gases and vacuum systems (PMGV) have been installed. These obviate the necessity for holding large numbers of cylinders in the operating theatre suite. Normally, only a few cylinders are kept in reserve, attached usually to the anaesthetic machine.

The advantages of the PMGV system are reductions in cost, in the necessity to transport cylinders and in accidents caused by cylinders becoming exhausted. However, there have been several well-publicized incidents in which anaesthetic morbidity or mortality has resulted from incorrect connections in piped medical gas supplies.

The PMGV services comprise five sections:

1. Bulk store.
2. Distribution pipelines in the hospital.
3. Terminal outlets, situated usually on the walls or ceilings of the operating theatre suite and other sites.
4. Flexible hoses connecting the terminal outlets to the anaesthetic machine.
5. Connections between flexible hoses and anaesthetic machines.

Responsibility for items 1–3 lies with the Engineering and Pharmacy Departments. Within the operating theatre, it is partly the anaesthetist's responsibility to check the correct functioning of items 4 and 5 (see below).

Bulk store

Oxygen

In small hospitals, oxygen may be supplied to the PMGV from a bank of several oxygen cylinders attached to a manifold. However, in larger hospitals, pipeline oxygen originates from a liquid oxygen store. Liquid oxygen is stored at a temperature of approximately –165°C at 10.5 bar in a giant Thermos flask – a vacuum insulated evaporator (VIE). Some heat passes from the environment through the insulating layer between the two shells of the flask, increasing the tendency to evaporation and elevation of pressure within the chamber. Pressure is maintained constant by transfer of gaseous oxygen into the pipeline system (via a warming device). However, if the pressure increases above 17 bar a safety valve opens and oxygen runs to waste. When the supply of oxygen resulting from the slow evaporation from the surface in the VIE is inadequate, the pressure decreases and a valve opens to allow liquid oxygen to pass into an evaporator, from which gas passes into the pipeline system.

Liquid oxygen plants are housed some distance away from hospital buildings because of the risk of fire. Even when a hospital possesses a liquid oxygen plant, it is still necessary to hold reserve banks of oxygen cylinders in case of supply failure.

Oxygen concentrators. Recently, oxygen concentrators have been used to supply hospitals and it is likely that the use of these devices will increase in future. The oxygen concentrator depends upon the ability of an artificial zeolight to entrap molecules of nitrogen. These devices cannot produce pure oxygen, but the concentration usually exceeds 90%; the remainder comprises nitrogen, argon and other inert gases. Small oxygen concentrators are provided for domiciliary use.

Nitrous oxide

Nitrous oxide and Entonox may be supplied from banks of cylinders connected to manifolds similar to those used for oxygen.

Medical compressed air

Compressed air is supplied from a bank of cylinders into the PMGV system. Air of medical quality is required, as industrial compressed air may contain fine particles of oil.

Piped medical vacuum

Piped medical vacuum is provided by large vacuum pumps which discharge via a filter and silencer to a suitable point, usually roof level, where gases are vented to atmosphere. Although concern has been expressed regarding the possibility of volatile anaesthetic agents dissolving in the lubricating oil of vacuum pumps and causing malfunction, this fear has not been substantiated.

Terminal outlets

There has been standardization of terminal outlets in the United Kingdom since 1978, but there is no universal standard.

Seven types of terminal outlet are found commonly in the operating theatre. The terminals are colour-coded and also have non-interchangeable connections specific to each gas:

1. Vacuum (coloured yellow). A vacuum of at least 53 kPa (400 mmHg) should be maintained at the outlet, which should be able to take a free flow of air of at least 40 litre.min^{-1}.

2. Compressed air (coloured white/black) at 4 bar. This is used for anaesthetic breathing systems and ventilators.

3. Air (coloured white/black) at 7 bar. This is to be used only for powering compressed air tools and is confined usually to the orthopaedic operating theatre.

4. Nitrous oxide (coloured blue) at 4 bar.

5. Oxygen (coloured white) at 4 bar.

6. Scavenging. There is a variety of scavenging outlets from the operating theatre. The passive systems are designed to accept a standard 30 mm connection.

Whenever a new pipeline system has been installed or servicing of an existing pipeline system has been undertaken, a designated member of the pharmacy staff should test the gas obtained from the sockets, using an oxygen analyser. Malfunction of an oxygen/air mixing device may result in entry of compressed air into the oxygen pipeline, rendering an anaesthetic mixture hypoxic. Because of this possibility, it has been advocated that oxygen analysers be used routinely during anaesthesia.

Gas supplies

Gas supplies to the anaesthetic machine should be checked at the beginning of each session to ensure that the gas which issues from the pipeline or cylinder is the same as that which passes through the appropriate flowmeter. This ensures that pipelines are not connected incorrectly. Both the machine in the operating theatre and that in the anaesthetic room should be checked. The following procedure has been recommended:

1. Check that the cylinders are in position, attached correctly to their yokes and switched off.

2. Open the oxygen and nitrous oxide flowmeter valves by 2–3 full turns and ensure that all others are closed. No flow should occur.

3. Turn on the oxygen cylinder. Check the oxygen gauge to ensure that sufficient oxygen is present in the cylinder. The oxygen flowmeter should be adjusted to provide a flow rate of 4 litre.min^{-1}. If there is any flow in the nitrous oxide flowmeter, the machine should be rejected.

4. Turn on the nitrous oxide cylinder and check that the flowmeter registers a low flow. If the oxygen flow changes, the machine should be rejected.

5. Set the oxygen failure device in operation, if it is not automatic.

6. Turn off the oxygen cylinder. Check that the oxygen bobbin falls completely to the bottom of the tube. Check that the oxygen failure device works. If the oxygen flowmeter registers any flow when the nitrous oxide only is turned on, the machine should be rejected.

7. Insert the probe into the wall connection for the oxygen supply. This should cancel the operation of the oxygen failure alarm. Apply a tug to ensure that it is connected correctly. Check the oxygen flowmeter, which should still show a flow rate of 4 litre.min^{-1}.

8. Turn off the nitrous oxide cylinder. If the oxygen bobbin demonstrates any fall when nitrous oxide is turned off, the machine should be rejected.

9. Insert the nitrous oxide connection into the pipeline system and apply a tug. If there is any change in the position of the oxygen bobbin, the machine should be rejected.

10. Complete the check by occluding the outlet of the machine and ensure that the pressure relief valve on the back bar operates.

CYLINDERS

Modern cylinders are constructed from molybdenum steel. They are checked at intervals by the manufacturer to ensure that they can withstand hydraulic pressures considerably in excess of those to which they are subjected in normal use. One cylinder in every 100 is cut into strips to test the metal for tensile strength, flattening impact and bend tests.

Medical gas cylinders are tested hydraulically every 5 years and the tests recorded by a mark stamped on the neck of the cylinder.

The cylinders are provided in a variety of sizes, and colour coded according to the gas supplied.

The cylinders comprise a body and a shoulder containing threads into which are fitted either a pin index valve block, a bull-nosed valve or a handwheel valve.

The pin index system was devised to prevent interchangeability of cylinders of different gases. Pin index valves are provided for the smaller cylinders of oxygen and nitrous oxide (and also carbon dioxide) which may be attached to anaesthetic machines. The pegs on the inlet connection slot into corresponding holes on the cylinder valve.

Full cylinders are supplied usually with a plastic dust cover in order to prevent contamination by dirt. This cover should not be removed until immediately before the cylinder is fitted to the anaesthetic machine. When fitting the cylinder to a machine, the yoke is positioned and tightened with the handle of the yoke spindle. After fitting, the cylinder should be opened to make sure that it is full and that there are no leaks at the gland nut or the pin index valve junction caused, for example, by absence of or damage to the washer. The washer used is normally a Bodok seal which has a metal periphery designed to keep the seal in good condition for a long period.

Cylinder valves should be opened slowly to prevent sudden surges of pressure and should be closed with no more force than is necessary, otherwise the valve seating may be damaged.

The sealing material between the valve and the neck of the cylinder may be constructed of a fusable material which melts in the event of fire and allows the contents of the cylinder to escape around the threads of the joint.

The colour codes used for medical gas cylinders are shown in Table 16.2 and the cylinder sizes and capacities are shown in Table 16.3.

THE ANAESTHETIC MACHINE

The anaesthetic machine comprises:

1. A means of supplying gases either from attached cylinders or from piped medical supplies via appropriate unions on the machine.
2. Methods of measuring flow rate of gases.
3. Apparatus for vaporizing volatile anaesthetic agents.
4. Breathing systems for delivery of gases and vapours from the machine to the patient.
5. Apparatus for scavenging anaesthetic gases in order to minimize environmental pollution.

Supply of gases

In the United Kingdom, gases are supplied at a pipeline pressure of 4 bar (400 kPa; 60 lb.in^{-2}) and this pressure is transferred directly to the bank of flowmeters and back bar of the anaesthetic machine. The gas issuing from other medical gas cylinders is at a much higher pressure, necessitating the interposition of a pressure regulator between the cylinder and the bank of flowmeters. In some older anaesthetic machines (and in some other countries), the pressure in the pipelines of the anaesthetic machine may be 3 bar (300 kPa; 45 lb.in^{-2}).

Table 16.2 Medical gas cylinders

| | Colour | | Pressure at 15°C | |
	Body	Shoulder	lb.in^{-2}	bar
Oxygen	Black	White	1987	137
Nitrous oxide	Blue	Blue	638	44
CO_2	Grey	Grey	725	50
Helium	Brown	Brown	1987	137
Air	Grey	White/black quarters	1987	137
O_2/helium	Black	White/brown quarters	1987	137
O_2/CO_2	Black	White/grey quarters	1987	137
N_2O/O_2 (Entonox)	Blue	White/blue quarters	1987	137

Table 16.3 Medical gas cylinder sizes and capacities

Cylinder size	A	B	C	D	E	F	G	J
Height (in)	10	10	14	18	31	34	49	57
Capacities (litres)								
Oxygen			170	340	680	1360	3400	6800
Nitrous oxide			450	900	1800	3600	9000	
CO_2			450	900	1800			
Helium				300		1200		
Air							3200	6400
O_2/helium					600	1200		
O_2/CO_2						1360	3400	
Entonox							3200	6400

Pressure regulators

Pressure regulators are used on anaesthetic machines for three purposes:

1. To reduce the high pressure of gas in a cylinder to a safe working level.

2. To prevent damage to equipment on the anaesthetic machine, e.g. flow control valves.

3. As the contents of the cylinder are used, the pressure within the cylinder decreases and the regulating mechanism maintains a constant reduced pressure, obviating the necessity to make continuous adjustments to the flowmeter controls.

The principles underlying the operation of flowmeters are described in detail in Chapter 15.

A modern anaesthetic reducing valve, the BOC S60M, is shown in Figure 15.4. Its mechanism of action will be clear from careful study of the diagram.

Flow restrictors

Pressure regulators are omitted usually when anaesthetic machines are supplied directly from a pipeline at a pressure of 4 bar. Changes in pipeline pressure would cause changes in flow rate, necessitating adjustment of the flow control valves. This is prevented by the use of a flow restrictor upstream of the flowmeter (flow restrictors are simply constrictions in the low-pressure circuit).

A different type of flow restrictor may be fitted also to the downstream end of the vaporizers to prevent back pressure effects (see Ch. 15). The absence of such a flow restrictor may be detected if a ventilator such as the Manley is employed, as this leads to fluctuations in the positions of the flowmeter bobbins during the respiratory cycle.

Pressure relief valves on regulators

Pressure relief valves are often fitted on the downstream side of regulators to allow escape of gas if the regulators were to fail (thereby causing a high output pressure). Relief valves are set usually at approximately 7 bar for regulators designed to give an output pressure of 4 bar.

Flowmeters

The principles of flowmeters are described in detail in Chapter 15.

Problems with flowmeters

1. *Non-vertical tube.* This causes a change in shape of the annulus and therefore variation in flow. If the bobbin touches the side of the tube, resulting friction causes an even more inaccurate reading.

2. *Static electricity.* This may cause inaccuracy (by as much as 35%) and sticking of the bobbin, especially at low flows. This may be reduced by coating the inside of the tube with a transparent film of gold or tin.

3. *Dirt.* Dirt on the bobbin may cause sticking or alteration in size of the annulus and therefore inaccuracies.

4. *Back pressure.* Changes in accuracy may be produced by back pressure. For example, the Manley ventilator may exert a back pressure and depress the bobbin; there may be as much as 10% more gas flow than that indicated on the flowmeter. Similar problems may be produced by the insertion of any equipment which restricts flow downstream, e.g. Selectatec head, vaporizer.

5. *Leakage.* This results usually from defects in the top sealing washer of a Rotameter.

It is unfortunate that in the United Kingdom the standard position of the flowmeters from left to right is oxygen, carbon dioxide, nitrous oxide (if all three gases are supplied). On several recorded occasions, patients have suffered damage from hypoxia because of leakage of a broken flowmeter tube in this type of arrangement, as oxygen, being at the upstream end, passes out to atmosphere through any leak. This problem is reduced if the oxygen flowmeter is placed downstream (i.e. on the right-hand side of the bank of flowmeters) as is standard practice in the USA. In the UK, this problem is now avoided by designing the outlet from the oxygen flowmeter to enter the back bar distal to the outlets of other flowmeters.

On modern anaesthetic machines, the emergency oxygen flush lever is situated downstream from the vaporizer. This leads to dilution of the anaesthetic mixture with excess oxygen if the emergency oxygen tap is opened partially by mistake and results in the possibility of awareness. In addition, a much higher fresh gas flow is delivered than the anaesthetist has set on the flowmeter controls.

Quantiflex

The Quantiflex mixer flowmeter (Fig. 16.1) eliminates the possibility of reducing the oxygen supply inadvertently. One dial is set to the desired percentage of oxygen and the total flow rate adjusted independently. The percentage of oxygen gas passes through a flowmeter to provide evidence of correct functioning of the linked valves. Both gases arrive via linked pressure-reducing regulators. The Quantiflex is useful in particular for varying the volume of fresh gas flow from

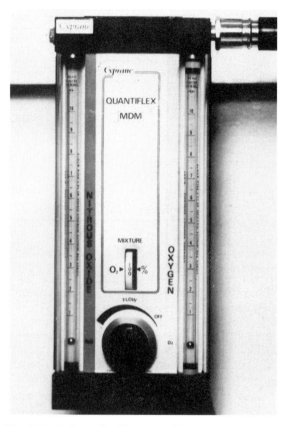

Fig. 16.1 A Quantiflex flowmeter. The required oxygen percentage is selected using the dial, and total flow of oxygen/nitrous oxide mixture adjusted using the black knob.

moment to moment whilst keeping the proportions constant. In addition, the oxygen flowmeter is situated downstream of the nitrous oxide flowmeter.

Linked flowmeters

The majority of modern anaesthetic machines such as that shown in Fig. 16.2 (a Datex Flexima with fully integrated monitoring) possess a mechanical linkage between the N_2O and O_2 flowmeters. This causes the N_2O flow to cease if the oxygen flowmeter is adjusted to give less than 30% O_2.

Vaporizers

The principles of vaporizers have been described in detail in Chapter 15.

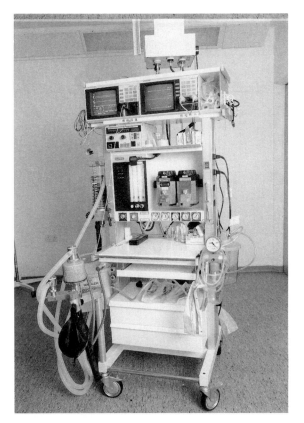

Fig. 16.2 A Datex Flexima with fully integrated monitoring.

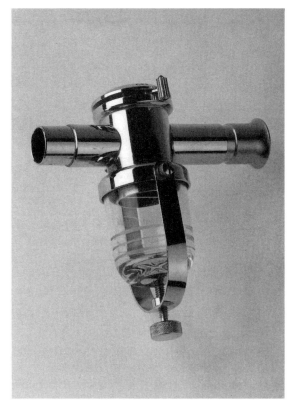

Fig. 16.3 The Goldman drawover vaporizer.

Modern vaporizers may be classified as:

1. *Plenum vaporizers*. These are intended for unidirectional gas flow, have a relatively high resistance to flow and are unsuitable for use either as drawover vaporizers or in a circle system. Examples include the 'TEC' type in which there is a variable bypass flow and the Kettle type in which measured flows are used. Commonly used types of equipment are shown in Figures 16.3 to 16.6.

2. *Drawover vaporizers*. These have a very low resistance to gas flow and may be used in a circle system (e.g. Goldman vaporizer), for emergency use in the field (e.g. Oxford miniature vaporizer) or in underdeveloped countries (e.g. EMO vaporizer).

Methods of temperature regulation include a bimetallic strip (TEC), bellows (EMO and Blease

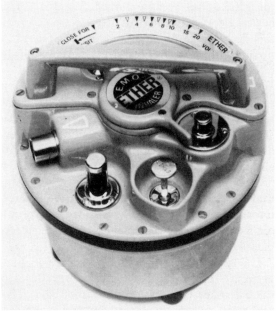

Fig. 16.4 The EMO (Epstein and Macintosh of Oxford) drawover ether vaporizer. A cutaway diagram is shown in Fig. 16.5.

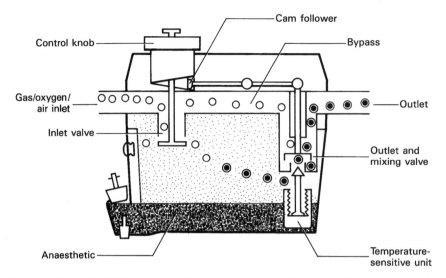

Fig. 16.5 Working principles of the EMO vaporizer. The water jacket provides a heat sink to reduce the decrease in temperature during vaporization. Temperature compensation is provided by a valve operated by bellows, filled with ether vapour. When the control lever is moved to the 'closed' position, the ether chamber is sealed to prevent spillage during transit.

Universal vaporizer) and manual compensation (Drager Vapor and Copper Kettle).

Desflurane presents a particular challenge as it possesses a boiling point of 23.5°C and above this temperature the liquid changes to gas. In order to combat this problem a new vaporizer, the TEC 6, has been developed (Fig. 16.7). It is heated electrically and possesses electronic monitors of vaporizer function and alarms. The functioning of the vaporizer is shown diagrammatically in Figure 16.8.

Anaesthetic-specific connections are available to link the supply bottle (container of liquid anaesthetic agent) to the appropriate vaporizer (Fig. 16.9). These connections reduce the extent of spillage (and thus atmospheric pollution) and also the likelihood of filling the vaporizer with an inappropriate liquid. In addition to being designed specifically for each liquid, the connections themselves may be colour-coded (e.g. purple for isoflurane, orange for enflurane and red for halothane).

Halothane contains a non-volatile stabilizing agent (0.01% thymol) to prevent breakdown of the halothane by heat and ultraviolet light. Thymol is less volatile than halothane and its concentration in the vaporizer increases as halothane is vaporized. If the vaporizer is used and refilled

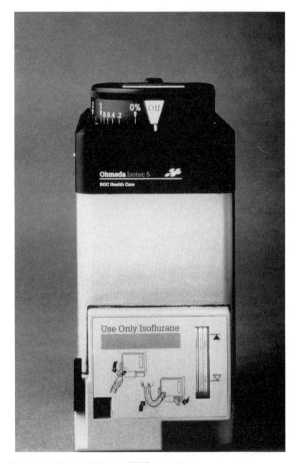

Fig. 16.6(A) A Mark 5 TEC vaporizer.

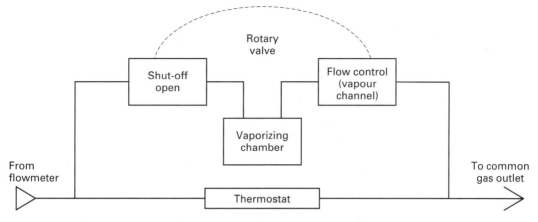

Fig. 16.6(B) Schematic diagram of the Mark 5 TEC vaporizer.

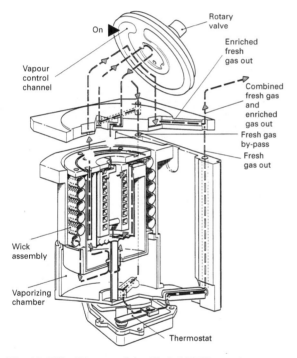

Fig. 16.6(C) Diagram of the Mark 5 TEC vaporizer.

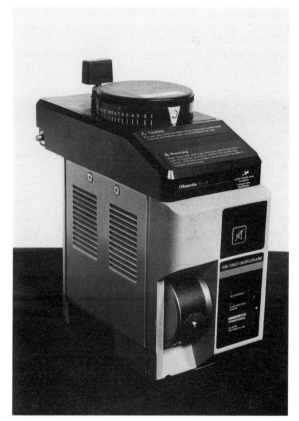

Fig. 16.7 The TEC 6 desflurane vaporizer.

regularly, the concentration of thymol may become sufficiently high to impair vaporization of halothane. In addition, very high concentrations may result in a significant degree of thymol vaporization, which may be harmful to the patient. Consequently, it is recommended that halothane

vaporizers be drained once every 2 weeks. Enflurane and isoflurane vaporizers require to be emptied at much less frequent intervals.

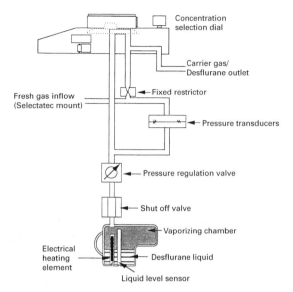

Concentration selection dial

Carrier gas/ Desflurane outlet

Fixed restrictor

Fresh gas inflow (Selectatec mount)

Pressure transducers

Pressure regulation valve

Shut off valve

Vaporizing chamber

Electrical heating element

Desflurane liquid

Liquid level sensor

Fig. 16.8 The TEC 6 desflurane vaporizer. Liquid in the vaporizing chamber is heated and mixed with fresh gas; the pressure-regulating valve balances both fresh gas pressure and anaesthetic vapour pressure.

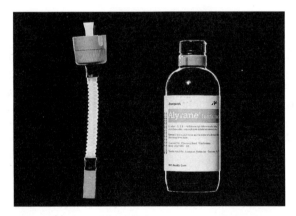

Fig. 16.9 An agent-specific connector for filling a vaporizer.

SAFETY FEATURES OF THE MODERN ANAESTHETIC MACHINE

1. Specificity of probes on flexible hoses between terminal outlets and connections with the anaesthetic machine.

2. Pin index system to prevent incorrect attachment of gas cylinders to anaesthetic machine.

3. Pressure relief valves on downstream side of regulators.

4. Flow restrictors on upstream side of flowmeters.

5. Arrangement of bank of flowmeters, such that oxygen flowmeter is on the right (i.e. downstream side).

6. Non-return valves. Sometimes a single regulator and contents meter is used both for cylinders in use and for the reserve cylinder. When one cylinder runs out, the presence of a non-return valve prevents the empty cylinder from being refilled by the reserve cylinder and also enables the empty cylinder to be removed and replaced without interrupting the supply of gas to the patient.

7. An oxygen bypass valve (emergency oxygen) delivers oxygen directly from a point upstream of the flowmeters to a point downstream of the vaporizers. When operated, the oxygen bypass should give a flow of at least 35 litre.min^{-1}.

8. Mounting of vaporizers on the back bar. Temperature-compensated vaporizers should be mounted upstream because they contain wicks which absorb a considerable amount of anaesthetic agent. If two such vaporizers are mounted in series, the downstream vaporizer could become contaminated to a dangerous degree with the agent from the upstream vaporizer. It is preferable to have only one temperature-compensated calibrated vaporizer on the back bar. The Selectatec block enables vaporizers to be changed very quickly, provides versatility and removes the necessity to have more than one vaporizer on the back bar. A development has been a back bar carrying two Selectatec vaporizers but with a control which permits only one to be in use at any one time (Fig. 16.10).

9. Pressure-linked flow controls. Some anaesthetic machines possess a device which switches off the supply of nitrous oxide automatically in the event of failure of the oxygen supply.

10. A non-return valve situated downstream of the vaporizers prevents back pressure (e.g. when using a Manley ventilator) which may cause output of high concentrations of vapour.

11. A relief valve may be situated downstream of the vaporizer, opening at 34 kPa to prevent damage to the flowmeters or vaporizers if the outlet is obstructed.

12. A pressure relief valve set to blow off at a low pressure of 5 kPa may be fitted to prevent the patient's lungs from being damaged by high

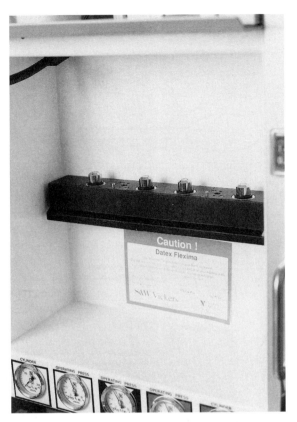

Fig. 16.10 A Selectatec block on the back bar of an anaesthetic machine. This permits the vaporizer to be changed rapidly without interrupting the flow of carrier gas to the patient.

pressure. The presence of such a valve prevents the use of the machine with minute volume divider ventilators, such as the Manley.

13. Oxygen failure warning devices. There is a variety of oxygen failure warning devices. The ideal warning device:

a. Does not depend on the pressure of any gas other than the oxygen itself.

b. Does not use a battery or mains power.

c. Gives a signal which is audible and of sufficient duration and volume and of distinctive character.

d. Should give a warning of impending failure and a further warning that failure has occurred.

e. Should interrupt the flow of all other gases when it comes into operation. The breathing system should open to atmosphere, inspired oxygen concentration should be at least equal to that of air and accumulation of carbon dioxide should not occur. In addition, it should be impossible to resume anaesthesia until the oxygen supply has been restored.

14. The rubber reservoir bag in an anaesthetic breathing system is highly distensible and seldom reaches pressures exceeding 5 kPa.

BREATHING SYSTEMS

The delivery system which conducts anaesthetic gases from the machine to the patient is termed colloquially a 'circuit' but is described more accurately as a breathing system. Terms such as 'open circuits', 'semi-open circuits' or 'semi-closed circuits' should be avoided. The 'closed circuit', or circle system, is the only true circuit, as anaesthetic gases are recycled.

Adjustable pressure-limiting valve

Most breathing systems incorporate an adjustable pressure-limiting valve (spill valve; 'pop-off' valve; expiratory valve) which is designed to vent gas when there is a positive pressure within the system. During spontaneous ventilation, the valve opens when the patient generates a positive pressure within the system during expiration; during positive pressure ventilation, the valve is adjusted to produce a controlled leak during the inspiratory phase.

Several valves of this type are available. They comprise a light-weight disc (Fig. 16.11) which rests on a 'knife-edge' seating to minimize the area of contact and reduce the risk of adhesion resulting from surface tension of condensed water. The disc has a stem which acts as a guide to position the disc correctly. A light spring is incorporated in the valve so that the pressure required to open the valve may be adjusted. During spontaneous breathing, the tension of the spring is low so that the resistance to expiration is minimized. During controlled ventilation, the valve top is screwed down to increase the tension in the spring so that gas leaves the system at a higher pressure than during spontaneous ventilation.

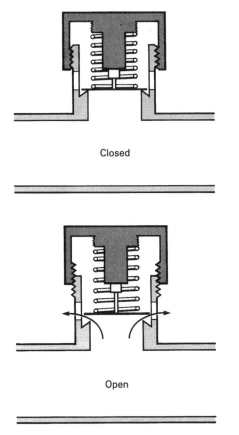

Fig. 16.11 Diagram of a spill valve. See text for details.

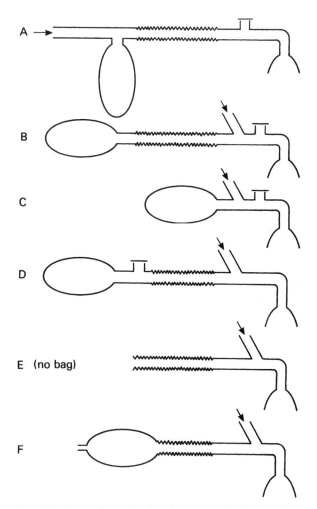

Fig. 16.12 Mapleson classification of anaesthetic breathing systems. The arrow indicates entry of fresh gas to the system.

Classification of breathing systems

In 1954, Mapleson classified anaesthetic breathing systems into five types (Fig. 16.12); the Mapleson E system was modified subsequently by Rees, but is classified as the Mapleson F system. The systems differ considerably in their 'efficiency', which is measured in terms of the fresh gas flow rate required to prevent rebreathing of alveolar gas during ventilation.

Mapleson A systems

The most commonly used version is the Magill attachment. The corrugated hose should be of adequate length (usually approximately 110 cm). It is the most efficient system during spontaneous ventilation, but one of the least efficient when ventilation is controlled.

During spontaneous ventilation, there are three phases in the ventilatory cycle: inspiratory, expiratory and the expiratory pause. Gas is inhaled from the system during inspiration (Fig. 16.13B). During the initial part of expiration, the reservoir bag is not full and thus the pressure in the system does not increase; exhaled gas (the initial portion of which is dead space gas) passes along the corrugated tubing towards the bag (Fig. 16.13C), which is filled also by fresh gas from the anaesthetic machine. During the latter part of expiration, the bag becomes full, the pressure in the system increases and the spill valve opens, venting all subsequent exhaled gas to atmosphere. During the expiratory pause, continued flow of fresh gas

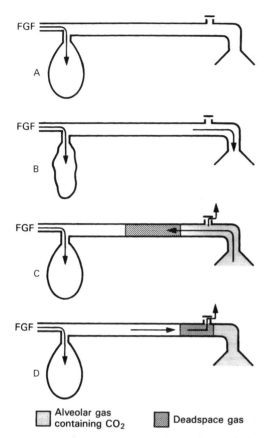

Fig. 16.13 Mode of action of Magill attachment during spontaneous ventilation. See text for details. FGF = fresh gas flow.

the extent of dead space but it remains too high to allow use of the system in infants or small children (less than 4 years of age).

The characteristics of the Mapleson A system are different during controlled ventilation (Fig. 16.14). At the end of inspiration (produced by the anaesthetist squeezing the reservoir bag), the bag is usually less than half full (see below). During expiration, dead space and alveolar gas pass along the corrugated tube and are likely to reach the reservoir bag, which therefore contains some carbon dioxide (Fig. 16.14A). During inspiration, the valve does not open initially because its opening pressure has been increased by the anaesthetist in order to generate a sufficient pressure within the system to inflate the lungs. Thus, alveolar gas re-enters the patient's lungs and is followed by a mixture of fresh, dead space and alveolar gases (Fig. 16.14B). When the valve does open, it is this mixture which is vented (Fig. 16.14C). Consequently, fresh gas flow rate must be very high (at least three times alveolar minute volume) to prevent rebreathing. The volume of gas squeezed from the reservoir bag

from the machine pushes exhaled gas distally along the corrugated tube to be vented through the spill valve (Fig. 16.13D). Provided that the fresh gas flow rate is sufficiently high to vent all *alveolar* gas before the next inspiration, no rebreathing takes place from the corrugated tube. If the system is functioning correctly and no leaks are present, a fresh gas flow (FGF) rate equal to the patient's alveolar minute ventilation is sufficient to prevent rebreathing. In practice, a higher FGF is selected in order to compensate for leaks; the rate selected is usually equal to the patient's total minute volume (approximately 6 litre.min^{-1} for a 70 kg adult).

The system increases dead space to the extent of the volume of the anaesthetic facemask and anglepiece to the spill valve. The volume of this dead space may amount to 100 ml or more for an adult facemask. Paediatric facemasks reduce

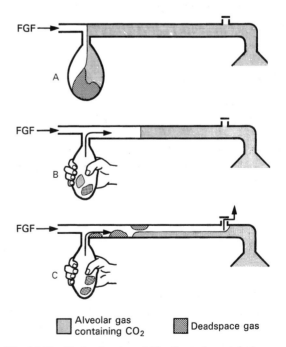

Fig. 16.14 Mode of action of Magill attachment during controlled ventilation. See text for details. FGF = fresh gas flow.

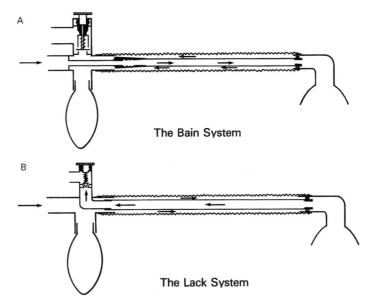

A

The Bain System

B

The Lack System

Fig. 16.15 Coaxial anaesthetic breathing systems. (**A**) Bain system (Mapleson D). (**B**) Lack system (Mapleson A).

must be sufficient both to inflate the lungs and to vent gas from the system.

The major disadvantage of the Magill attachment during surgery is that the spill valve is attached close to the mask. This makes the system heavy, particularly when a scavenging system is used, and it is inconvenient if the valve is in this position during surgery of the head or neck. The Lack system (Fig. 16.15) is a modification of the Mapleson A system with a coaxial arrangement of tubing. This permits positioning of the spill valve at the proximal end of the system. The inner tube must be of sufficiently wide bore to allow the patient to exhale with minimal resistance. The Lack system is not quite as efficient as the Magill attachment.

Mapleson B and C systems

These systems cause mixing of alveolar and fresh gas during spontaneous or controlled ventilation. Very high FGF rates are required to prevent rebreathing. There is no clinical role for the Mapleson B system. The Mapleson C system is used in some hospitals to ventilate the lungs with oxygen during transport, but a self-inflating bag with a non-rebreathing valve is preferable.

Mapleson D system

The Mapleson D arrangement is inefficient during spontaneous breathing (Fig. 16.16). During expiration, exhaled gas and fresh gas mix in the corrugated tube and travel towards the reservoir bag (Fig. 16.16B). When the reservoir bag is full, the pressure in the system increases, the spill valve opens and a mixture of fresh and exhaled gas is vented; this includes the dead space gas, which reaches the reservoir bag first (Fig. 16.16C). Although fresh gas pushes alveolar gas towards the valve during the expiratory pause, a mixture of alveolar and fresh gases is inhaled from the corrugated tube unless FGF rate is at least twice as great as the patient's minute volume (i.e. at least 12 litre.min^{-1} in the adult); in some patients, a fresh gas flow rate of 250 ml.kg^{-1}.min^{-1} is required to prevent rebreathing.

However, the Mapleson D system is more efficient than the Mapleson A during controlled ventilation (Fig. 16.17), especially if an expiratory pause is incorporated into the ventilatory cycle. During expiration, the corrugated tubing and reservoir bag fill with a mixture of fresh and alveolar gas (Fig. 16.17A). Fresh gas fills the distal part of the corrugated tube during the expiratory pause (Fig. 16.17B). When the reservoir bag is

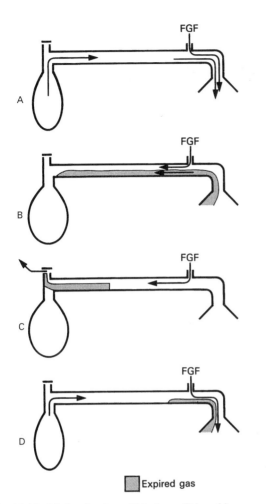

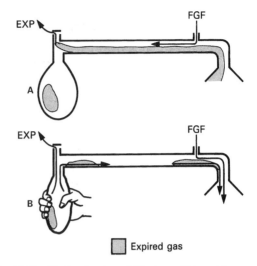

Fig. 16.17   Mode of action of Mapleson D breathing system during controlled ventilation. See text for details. FGF = fresh gas flow.

Fig. 16.16   Mode of action of Mapleson D breathing system during spontaneous ventilation. See text for details. FGF = fresh gas flow.

squeezed, this fresh gas enters the lungs and when the spill valve opens a mixture of fresh and alveolar gas is vented. The degree of rebreathing may thus be controlled by adjustment of the fresh gas flow rate, but this should always exceed the patient's minute volume.

The Bain coaxial system (Fig. 16.15) is the most commonly used version of the Mapleson D system. FGF is supplied through a narrow inner tube. This tube may become disconnected, resulting in hypoxaemia and hypercapnia. Before use, the system should be tested by occluding the distal end of the inner tube transiently with a finger or the plunger of a 2-ml syringe; there should be a reduction in the flowmeter bobbin

reading during occlusion and an audible release of pressure when occlusion is discontinued. Movement of the reservoir bag during anaesthesia does *not* indicate that fresh gas is being delivered to the patient.

The Bain system may be used to ventilate the patient's lungs with some types of automatic ventilator (e.g. Penlon Nuffield 200). A 1-m length of corrugated tubing is interposed between the patient valve of the ventilator and the reservoir bag mount (Fig. 16.18); the spill valve *must* be closed completely. An appropriate tidal volume and ventilatory rate are selected on the ventilator and anaesthetic gases are supplied to the Bain system. During inspiration, the gas from the ventilator pushes a mixture of anaesthetic and alveolar gas from the corrugated outer tube into the patient's lungs; during expiration, the ventilator gas and some of the alveolar gas are vented through the exhaust valve of the ventilator. The degree of rebreathing is regulated by the anaesthetic gas flow rate; a flow of $70–80 \text{ ml.kg}^{-1}.\text{min}^{-1}$ should result in normocapnia and a flow of $100 \text{ ml.kg}^{-1}.\text{min}^{-1}$ in moderate hypocapnia. A secure connection between the Bain system and the anaesthetic machine must be assured. If this connection is loose, a leak of fresh gas occurs; this causes rebreathing of ventilator gas and results in awareness, hypoxaemia and hypercapnia.

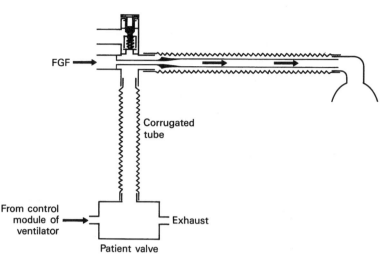

Fig. 16.18 The Bain system for controlled ventilation by a mechanical ventilator (e.g. Nuffield 200). A 1 m length of corrugated tubing with a capacity of at least 500 ml is required to prevent gas from the ventilator reaching the patient's lungs. Pa_{CO_2} is controlled by varying the fresh gas flow rate (FGF).

Mapleson E and F systems

The Mapleson E system, or Ayre's T-piece, has virtually no resistance to expiration and was used extensively in paediatric anaesthesia before the advantages of continuous positive airways pressure (CPAP) were recognized. It functions in a manner similar to the Mapleson D system in that the corrugated tube fills with a mixture of exhaled and fresh gas during expiration and with fresh gas during the expiratory pause. Rebreathing is prevented if the FGF rate is 2.5–3 times the patient's minute volume. If the volume of the corrugated tube is less than the patient's tidal volume, some air may be inhaled at the end of inspiration; consequently, a fresh gas flow rate of at least 4 litre.min^{-1} is recommended with a paediatric Mapleson E system.

During spontaneous ventilation, there is no indication of the presence, or the adequacy, of ventilation. It is possible to attach a visual indicator, such as a piece of tissue paper or a feather, at the end of the corrugated tube, but this is not very satisfactory.

IPPV may be applied by occluding the end of the corrugated tube with a finger; however, there is no way of assessing the pressure in the system and there is a possibility of exposing the patient's lungs to excessive volumes and pressures.

The Mapleson F system, or Rees' modification of the Ayre's T-piece, includes an open-ended bag attached to the end of the corrugated tube. This confers several advantages:

1. It provides visual evidence of breathing during spontaneous ventilation.

2. By occluding the open end of the bag temporarily, it is possible to confirm that fresh gas is entering the system.

3. It provides a degree of CPAP during spontaneous ventilation and PEEP during IPPV.

4. It provides a convenient method of assisting or controlling ventilation. The open end of the reservoir bag is occluded between the fourth and fifth fingers and the bag squeezed between the thumb and index finger; the fourth and fifth fingers are relaxed during expiration to allow gas to escape from the bag. It is possible with experience to assess (approximately) the inflation pressure and to detect changes in lung and chest wall compliance.

Drawover systems

Occasionally, it is necessary to administer anaesthesia at the scene of a major accident. If inhalational anaesthesia is required, it is necessary to use simple, portable equipment. The Triservice

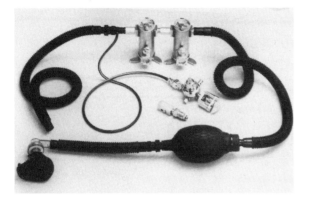

Fig. 16.19 The Triservice apparatus. See text for details.

Table 16.4 Composition of soda lime

$Ca(OH)_2$	94%
NaOH	5%
KOH	1%
Silica	0.2%
Moisture content	14–19%

apparatus (Fig. 16.19) has been designed by the British armed forces for use in battle conditions. It comprises a self-inflating bag, a non-rebreathing valve (e.g. Ambu E, Rubens) which vents all expired gases to atmosphere, one or two Oxford miniature vaporizers (which have a low internal resistance), an oxygen supply and a length of corrugated tubing which serves as an oxygen reservoir. Either spontaneous or controlled ventilation may be employed using this apparatus.

Rebreathing systems

Anaesthetic breathing systems in which the same gases are rebreathed by the patient were designed originally to economize in the use of cyclopropane. In addition, they reduce the risk of atmospheric pollution and increase the humidity of inspired gases, thereby reducing heat loss from the patient. Rebreathing systems may be used as 'closed' systems, in which fresh gas is introduced only to replace oxygen and anaesthetic agents absorbed by the patient. More commonly, the system is used with a small leak through a spill valve and a fresh gas supply which exceeds basal oxygen requirements. Because rebreathing occurs, these systems must incorporate a means of absorbing carbon dioxide from exhaled alveolar gas.

Soda lime

Soda lime is the substance used most commonly for absorption of carbon dioxide in rebreathing systems. The composition of soda lime is shown

in Table 16.4. The major constituent is calcium hydroxide, but sodium and potassium hydroxides are present also. Absorption of carbon dioxide occurs by the following chemical reactions:

$$CO_2 + 2NaOH \rightarrow Na_2CO_3 + H_2O + heat$$
$$Na_2CO_3 + Ca(OH)_2 \rightarrow 2NaOH + CaCO_3$$

Water is required for efficient absorption. There is some water in soda lime and more is added from the patient's expired gas and from the chemical reaction. The reaction generates heat and the temperature in the centre of a soda lime canister may exceed 60°C. Trichloroethylene degenerates at high temperatures, forming toxic substances including the neurotoxin dichloroacetylene; consequently, trichloroethylene must never be used in rebreathing systems which contain soda lime.

The size of soda lime granule is important. If granules are too large, the surface area for absorption is insufficient; if they are too small, the narrow space between granules results in a high resistance to breathing. Silica is added to soda lime to reduce the tendency of the granules to disintegrate into powder. In addition, soda lime contains an indicator which changes colour as the active constituents become exhausted. The rate at which soda lime becomes exhausted depends on the capacity of the canister, the fresh gas flow rate and the rate of carbon dioxide production. In a completely closed system, a standard 450-g canister becomes inefficient after approximately 2 h.

'To-and-fro' (Waters') system

This breathing system comprises a Mapleson C breathing system with a canister of soda lime interposed between the spill valve and reservoir bag (Fig. 16.20). The soda lime granules nearest the patient become exhausted first, increasing the

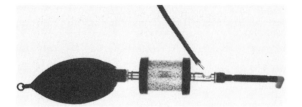

Fig. 16.20 Waters' anaesthetic breathing system, incorporating a canister of soda lime.

dead space of the system; in addition, the canister is positioned horizontally and gas may be channelled above the soda lime unless the canister is packed tightly. The system is cumbersome and there is a risk that patients may inhale soda lime dust from the canister.

Circle system

This system has replaced the 'to-and-fro' system in most centres. The soda lime canister is mounted usually on the anaesthetic machine and inspiratory and expiratory corrugated tubing conduct gas to and from the patient (Fig. 16.21). The system incorporates a reservoir bag and spill valve and two low-resistance one-way valves to ensure unidirectional movement of gas. These valves are mounted normally in glass domes so that they may be observed to be functioning correctly. The spill valve may be mounted close to the patient or beside the absorber; during surgery to the head or neck, it is more convenient to use a valve near the absorber. Fresh gas enters the system between the absorber and the inspiratory tubing.

The soda lime canister is mounted vertically and thus channelling of gas through unfilled areas is not possible. The canister cannot contribute to dead space; consequently, a large canister may be used and the soda lime needs to be changed less often.

The major disadvantage of the circle system arises from its volume. If the system is filled with air initially, low flow rates of anaesthetic gases are diluted substantially and adequate concentrations cannot be achieved. Even if the system is primed with a mixture of anaesthetic gases, the initial rapid uptake by the patient results in a marked decrease in concentrations of anaesthetic

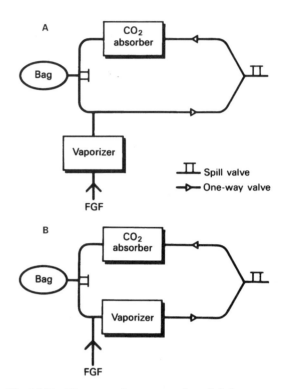

Fig. 16.21 Diagrammatic representation of circle system. (**A**) Vaporizer outside the circle (VOC). (**B**) Vaporizer inside the circle (VIC).

agents in the system, resulting in light anaesthesia. Consequently, it is necessary usually to provide a total fresh gas flow rate of 3–4 litre.min^{-1} to the system initially. This flow rate may be reduced subsequently, but it must be remembered that dilution of fresh gas continues at low flow rates and that rapid changes in depth of anaesthesia cannot be achieved.

Volatile anaesthetic agents may be delivered to a circle system in two ways:

1. *Vaporizer outside the circle (VOC)*. If a standard vaporizer (e.g. TEC series) is used, it must be placed on the back bar of the anaesthetic machine because of its high internal resistance. If low FGF rates (< 1 litre.min^{-1}) are used, the change in concentration of volatile anaesthetic agent achieved in the circle system is very small because of dilution, even if the vaporizer is set to deliver a high concentration (Fig. 16.22A), and it may be necessary to change FGF rate rather than the vaporizer setting to achieve a rapid change in depth of anaesthesia. The concentration of volatile

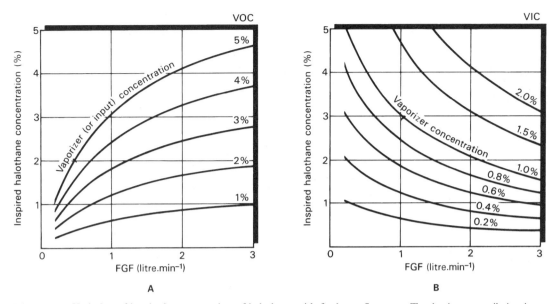

Fig. 16.22 Variation of inspired concentration of halothane with fresh gas flow rate. Total minute ventilation is 5 litre.min^{-1}. (**A**) Vaporizer outside the circle (VOC); note that dilution of the fresh gas results in much lower concentrations in the circle system than the concentration set on the vaporizer unless fresh gas flow rate approaches 3 litre.min^{-1}. (**B**) Vaporizer inside the circle (VIC); at low flow rates, lack of dilution of expired halothane concentrations, with additional halothane vaporized during each inspiration, results in inspired concentrations much higher than those set on the vaporizer. Even at a fresh gas flow rate of 3 litre.min^{-1}, inspired concentration is approximately 50% higher than the vaporizer setting.

agent in the system depends on the patient's expired concentration (which is recycled), the rate of uptake by the patient (which decreases with time and is slower with agents of low blood/gas solubility coefficient), the concentration of agent supplied and the fresh gas slow rate.

2. *Vaporizer inside the circle (VIC)*. Drawover vaporizers with a low internal resistance (e.g. Goldman) may be placed within the circle system. During each inspiration, vapour is added to the inspired gas mixture. In contrast to a VOC system, the inspired concentration is higher at low FGF rates because the expired concentration is diluted to a lesser extent (Fig. 16.22B) and the vaporizer *adds* to the concentration present in the expired gas. Very high concentrations of volatile agent may be inspired if minute volume is large; this risk is greatest if IPPV is employed.

If FGF rate is low, the use of the circle system by the inexperienced anaesthetist may result either in inadequate anaesthesia or in severe cardiovascular and respiratory depression. In addition, a hypoxic gas mixture may be delivered if low

flow rates of a nitrous oxide/oxygen mixture are supplied, because after 10–15 min oxygen is taken up in larger volumes than nitrous oxide. These difficulties may be overcome by monitoring the inspired concentrations of oxygen and volatile anaesthetic agent continuously (see Ch. 20). The trainee anaesthetist *must* be aware that:

1. It is inadvisable to use a VIC system unless inspired concentrations of anaesthetic agents are monitored continuously.

2. IPPV must *never* be used with a VIC system unless inspired concentrations of anaesthetic agents are monitored continuously, because of the risk of generating very high concentrations of volatile agent.

3. Nitrous oxide must *not* be used in any circle system if the total fresh gas flow rate is less than 1000 ml.min^{-1}, unless inspired oxygen concentration is measured continuously.

VENTILATORS

Mechanical ventilation of the lung may be achieved

by several mechanisms, including the generation of a negative pressure around the whole of the patient's body except the head and neck (cabinet ventilator or 'iron lung'), a negative pressure over the thorax and abdomen (cuirass ventilators) or a positive pressure over the thorax and abdomen (inflatable cuirass ventilators). However, during anaesthesia, and in the majority of patients who require mechanical ventilation in the intensive therapy unit, ventilation is achieved by the application of positive pressure to the lungs through a tracheal tube. Only this mode of ventilation is described here.

An enormous selection of ventilators exists and it is possible in this section to discuss only the principles involved in their use. Before using any ventilator, it is *essential* that the trainee understands its functions fully; failure to do so may result in the delivery of a hypoxic gas mixture, rebreathing of carbon dioxide and/or delivery of a mixture that contains no anaesthetic gases. If an unfamiliar ventilator is encountered, it may be helpful to use a 'dummy lung' (a small reservoir bag on the patient connection) and to discuss the capabilities and limitations of the machine with a senior colleague. In addition, the manufacturer's 'user handbook' may be consulted or details may be obtained from a specialist book.

With simple ventilators, observation of the patient is the only means of assessing the adequacy of ventilation. Continuous clinical monitoring is essential when any ventilator is used, even those which incorporate sophisticated monitoring and warning devices. In addition to standard clinical monitoring systems attached to the patient (see Ch. 20), the minimum acceptable monitoring of ventilator function includes measurement of expired tidal volume, airway pressure and inspired oxygen concentration; in addition, a ventilator disconnection alarm should be incorporated in the system. Continuous monitoring of end-tidal carbon dioxide and inspired anaesthetic gas concentrations is essential. Pulse oximetry is necessary.

The incorporation of a humidifier in the inspiratory limb, or of a condenser humidifier at the connection with the tracheal tube, is essential in long-term ventilation in ITU. Bacterial filters may be desirable in patients with infected pulmonary secretions.

The principles of operation of ventilators are described best by considering each phase of the ventilatory cycle.

Inspiration

The pattern of volume change in the lung is determined by the characteristics of the ventilator. Ventilators may deliver a predetermined flow of gas (*flow generators*) or exert a predetermined pressure (*pressure generators*), although some machines produce a pattern which does not conform to either category. Most flow generators produce a constant flow of gas during inspiration, although a few generate a sinusoidal flow pattern if the ventilator bellows is driven via a crank, e.g. Cape–Waine ventilator. The characteristics of constant flow and constant pressure generators are shown in Figure 16.23.

Constant pressure generator. The East–Radcliffe ventilator is the only true pressure generator in common use. This machine contains a bellows with a capacity that greatly exceeds the normal tidal volume. The inspiratory pressure is generated by weights on top of the bellows. The bellows cease to empty when the pressure generated by the weights equals the pressure in the patient's alveoli. To a certain extent, the machine can compensate for leaks, as the bellows are large and continue to empty until a predetermined pressure has been achieved in the lungs. However, that pressure may be achieved after delivery to the lungs of different volumes of gas if the lung/chest wall compliance changes (Fig. 16.24). For example, if the patient is tipped head-down, compliance decreases and a smaller tidal volume is delivered (compliance = volume/pressure). If airways resistance increases, the flow rate of gas is decreased and the pressure in the lungs may not reach bellows pressure before the end of the inspiratory cycle; consequently, tidal volume decreases. Tidal volume is decreased also if a large leak develops.

Constant flow generator. Changes in resistance or compliance make little difference to the volume delivered (unless the ventilator is pressure-cycled; see below), although airway and alveolar pressures may change (Fig. 16.25). For example, decreased compliance results in delivery of a normal tidal volume; however, the rate of increase

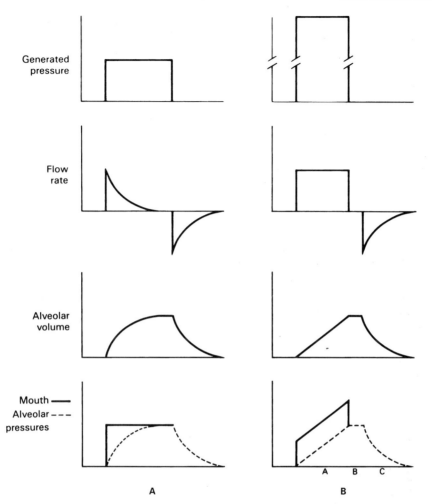

Fig. 16.23 Graphs of generated pressure, mouth (or tracheal tube) and alveolar pressures, flow rate and alveolar volume changes during inspiration and subsequent expiration produced by (**A**) a constant pressure generator and (**B**) a constant flow generator. A constant pressure generator exerts a low (e.g. 1.5 kPa; 15 cmH$_2$O) pressure. At the start of inspiration, the pressure in the alveoli is zero. Gas flows rapidly into the alveoli at a rate determined by airways resistance resulting in rapid increases in alveolar volume and pressure. The mouth–alveolar pressure gradient decreases and flow rate, and consequently the rate of increase of alveolar volume and pressure, decrease also. When the alveolar pressure equals ventilator pressure, flow ceases.

A constant flow generator generates a very high internal pressure (e.g. 400 kPa) but has a high internal resistance to limit flow rate. The pressure gradient between machine and alveoli remains virtually constant throughout inspiration and thus flow rate is constant. The increases in alveolar volume and (assuming constant compliance) pressure are linear. Because flow rate is constant, the pressure gradient between mouth and alveoli is constant throughout inspiration (A). Mouth pressure decreases to equal alveolar pressure during the inspiratory pause when flow ceases (B).

Gas flow out of the lung during expiration (C) is passive.

of alveolar pressure is greater than normal (i.e. the slope is greater) and airway pressure is correspondingly higher to maintain a gradient between the tracheal tube and the alveoli. If airway resistance increases, the pressure at the tracheal tube (and the gradient between tracheal tube and alveolar pressures) is higher than normal throughout inspiration, but alveolar pressure and the slopes of both pressure curves are normal. Constant flow generators do not compensate for leaks; the tidal volume delivered to the lungs decreases.

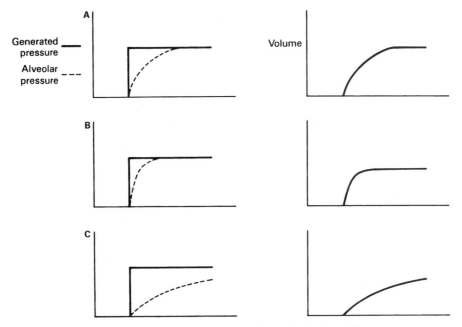

Fig. 16.24 Generated and alveolar pressures, and alveolar volume, during inspiration with a constant pressure generator. (**A**) Normal. (**B**) Decreased compliance. (**C**) Increased airway resistance. Note that both abnormalities reduce alveolar volume.

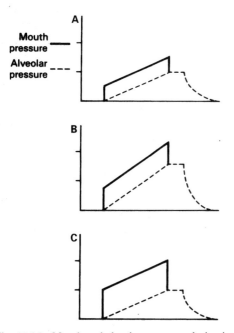

Fig. 16.25 Mouth and alveolar pressures during inspiration with a constant flow generator. (**A**) Normal. (**B**) Decreased compliance. (**C**) Increased airway resistance. Alveolar volume remains constant because flow rate is constant. Decreased compliance results in an increased rate of increase of alveolar pressure; mouth pressure also increases more steeply, but the gradient between mouth and alveolar pressures remains normal. Increased airway resistance increases the mouth–alveolar pressure gradient.

Some ventilators, e.g. Blease Brompton, generate a pressure rather higher than that required to inflate the lungs but not high enough to maintain constant flow throughout inspiration. The flow, volume and pressure changes within the lung are shown in Figure 16.26.

Change from inspiration to expiration

This is termed 'cycling', and may be achieved in one of three ways:

1. *Volume-cycling.* The ventilator cycles into expiration whenever a predetermined tidal volume has been delivered. The duration of inspiration is determined by the inspiratory flow rate.

2. *Pressure-cycling.* The ventilator cycles into expiration when a preset *airway* pressure is achieved. This allows compensation for small leaks but, in common with a constant pressure generator, a pressure-cycled ventilator delivers a different tidal volume if compliance or resistance changes. In addition, inspiratory time varies with changes in compliance and resistance.

3. *Time-cycling.* This is the method used most commonly by modern ventilators. The duration of inspiration is predetermined. With a constant

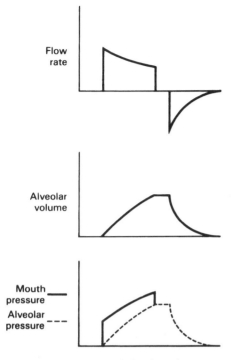

Fig. 16.26 Pressure, flow and alveolar volume characteristics during inspiration with a ventilator with a moderately high internal pressure (e.g. Blease Brompton). At higher bellows pressures, and in a patient with normal compliance and airway resistance, the characteristics approximate to those of a constant flow generator (Fig. 16.23). At low bellows pressures, if compliance decreases or if airway resistance increases, the pattern is similar to that of a constant pressure generator.

flow generator, it may be desirable to preset a tidal volume; when this has been delivered, there is a short inspiratory pause (which improves gas distribution within the lung) before the inspiratory cycle ends. The use of this *'volume-preset'* mechanism must be differentiated from volume-cycling. When a constant pressure generator is time-cycled, the tidal volume delivered depends on the compliance and resistance of the lungs and on the pressure within the bellows.

Expiration

Usually, the patient is allowed to exhale to atmospheric pressure; flow rate decreases exponentially. Subatmospheric pressure should not be used during expiration as it induces small airways closure and air trapping. Positive end-expiratory

pressure (PEEP) may be applied in some circumstances (see Ch. 41).

Change from expiration to inspiration

On most ventilators, this is achieved by time-cycling. However, it may be desirable occasionally to use pressure-cycling in response to a sub-atmospheric pressure generated by the patient's inspiratory effort.

Delivery of anaesthetic gas

Some ventilators deliver a minute volume determined by a preset tidal volume and rate. When used in anaesthesia, these machines must be supplied with a flow rate of anaesthetic gases which equals or exceeds the minute volume delivered or else air, or gas used to drive the ventilator, is entrained and delivered to the patient. A number of ventilators which are driven by the anaesthetic gas supply can deliver only that gas and divide it into predetermined tidal volumes (*minute volume dividers*). Ventilators may be used to compress bellows in a separate system which contains anaesthetic gases ('bag-in-a-bottle'); it is possible to provide IPPV in a circle system in this way. Some devices may be used also to ventilate the patient through a Bain system (see below).

The characteristics of several common ventilators are summarized in Table 16.5.

High-frequency ventilation

High-frequency jet ventilation is used during some operations on the larynx, trachea or lung and in a small number of patients in ITU. Gas exchange may be unpredictable and the technique should not be used by the trainee without supervision.

SCAVENGING

The possible adverse effects of pollution on staff in the operating theatre environment are discussed in Chapter 17. The principal sources of pollution by anaesthetic gases and vapours include:

1. Gas discharge from ventilators.
2. Expired gas vented from the spill valve of an anaesthetic breathing system.

Table 16.5   Classification of some common ventilators used during anaesthesia

Ventilator	Driven by	Cycling to expiration	Cycling to inspiration	Pressure/flow generator	Minute volume divider	Volume preset
Manley MP2, MN2, NO3	Anaesthetic gases	Time	Time	Pressure	Yes	Yes
Manley Pulmovent	Anaesthetic gases	Volume	Time	Flow	Yes	Yes
Blease Brompton	Anaesthetic gases	Volume or time	Time	Mixed	Yes	Yes
Philips AV1	Anaesthetic gases	Time (electrically operated valves)	Time (electrically operated valves)	Flow	Yes	No
Cape–Waine	Electric motor	Time	Time	Flow (sine wave)	Yes	No
East–Radcliffe	Electric motor	Time	Time	Pressure	No	No
Manley Servovent	Compressed air or oxygen	Volume	Time	Flow	No	Yes
Oxford	Compressed air or oxygen	Time	Time	Flow	No	Yes
Nuffield 200	Compressed air or oxygen	Time	Time	Flow	No	No
Servo 900	Anaesthetic gases	Time (electrically operated valves)	Time (electrically operated valves)	Flow (usually)	No	Yes

3. Leaks from equipment, e.g. from an ill-fitting facemask.

4. Gas exhaled by the patient after anaesthesia. This may occur in the operating theatre, corridors and recovery room.

5. Spillage during filling of vaporizers.

Although most attention has centred on removing gas from expiratory ports of breathing systems and ventilators, other methods of reducing pollution should be considered also:

1. *Reduced use of anaesthetic gases and vapours.* The use of the circle system reduces the potential for atmospheric pollution. The use of inhalational anaesthetics may be obviated totally by employing total intravenous anaesthesia or local anaesthetic techniques.

2. *Air conditioning.* Air conditioning units which produce a rapid change of air in the operating theatre reduce pollution substantially. However, some systems recycle air and older operating theatres, dental surgeries and obstetric delivery suites may not be equipped with air conditioning.

3. *Care in filling vaporizers.* Great care should be taken not to spill volatile anaesthetic agents when vaporizers are filled. The use of agent-specific connections (see Fig. 16.9) reduces the risk of spillage. In some countries, vaporizers may be filled only in a portable fume cupboard.

Scavenging apparatus

Anaesthetic gases vented from the breathing system are removed by a collecting system. A variety of purpose-built scavenging spill valves is available; an example is shown in Figure 16.27. Waste gases from ventilators are collected by attaching

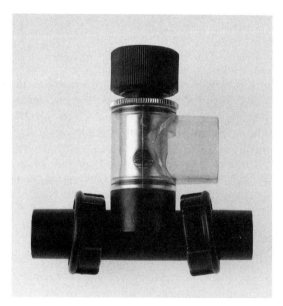

Fig. 16.27   An expiratory spill valve with scavenging attachment.

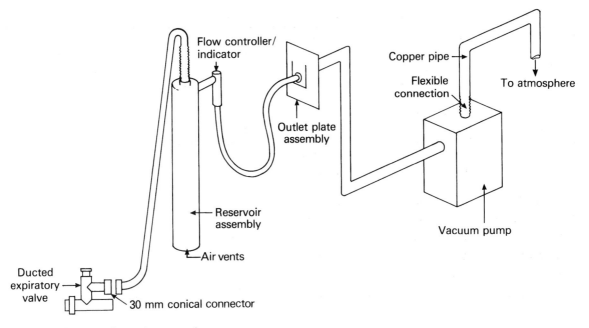

Fig. 16.28 Diagram of an active scavenging system.

the scavenging system to the expiratory port of the ventilator. Connectors on scavenging systems have a diameter of 30 mm to ensure that inappropriate connections with anaesthetic apparatus cannot be made.

Disposal systems may be active, semi-active or passive.

Active systems

These employ apparatus to generate a negative pressure within the scavenging system which propels waste gases to the outside atmosphere. The system may be powered by a vacuum pump (Fig. 16.28) or a Venturi system (Fig. 16.29). The exhaust should be capable of accommodating 75 litre.min^{-1} continuous flow with a peak of 130 litre.min^{-1}. Usually, a reservoir system is used to permit high peak flow rates to be accommodated. In addition, there must be a pressure-limiting device within the system to prevent the application of negative pressure to the patient's lungs.

Semi-active systems

The waste gases may be conducted to the extrac-

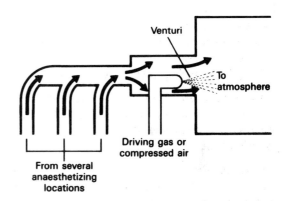

Fig. 16.29 Diagram of a Venturi system for active scavenging of anaesthetic gases.

tion side of the air-conditioning system, which generates a small negative pressure within the scavenging tubing. These systems have variable performance and efficiency.

Passive systems

These systems vent the expired gas to the outside atmosphere (Fig. 16.30). Gas movement is generated by the patient. Consequently, the total length of tubing must not be excessive or resistance to expiration is high. The pressure within

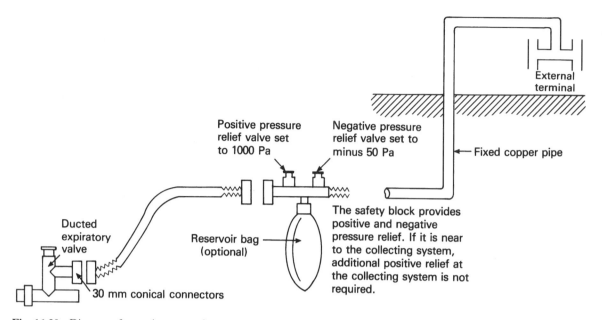

Fig. 16.30 Diagram of a passive scavenging system.

the system may be altered by wind conditions at the external terminal; on occasions, these may generate a negative pressure, but may also generate high positive pressures. Each scavenging location should have a separate external terminal to prevent gases being vented into adjacent locations. Relief valves must be incorporated to prevent negative or high positive pressures within the system.

Irrespective of the type of disposal system, tubing used for scavenging must not be allowed to lie on the floor of the operating theatre as compression (e.g. by feet or by items of equipment) results in increased resistance to expiration and may generate dangerously high pressure within the patient's lungs.

LARYNGOSCOPES

Curved blade

The most commonly used adult laryngoscope blade is the Macintosh curved blade, which is manufactured in several sizes (Figs 16.31 and 16.32).

The tip of the laryngoscope blade is advanced carefully over the surface of the tongue until it

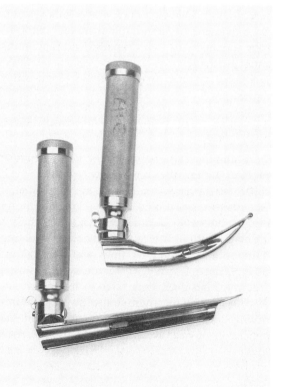

Fig. 16.31 Two laryngoscopes with Magill adult blade (below) and Macintosh adult blade (above).

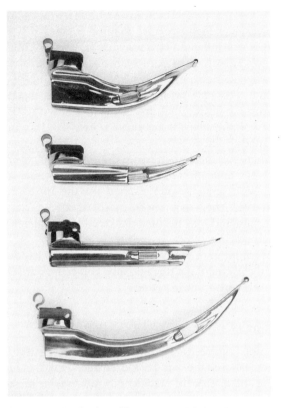

Fig. 16.32   A selection of laryngoscope blades. From above downwards: Macintosh infant blade, Robertshaw blade, Magill infant blade and large adult Macintosh blade.

reaches the vallecula (see Fig. 19.3). The tip of the blade is rotated upwards and the laryngoscope lifted along the axis of the handle to lift the larynx; the incisor teeth must not be used as a fulcrum to lever the tip of the blade upwards. When the arytenoids and posterior part of the cords are seen, gentle pressure on the larynx using the right thumb, or provided by an assistant, may help to improve the view.

Straight blade

The technique of laryngoscopy is slightly different when a straight blade (e.g. Magill) is used (see Fig. 19.3). Instead of placing the tip of the blade in the vallecula, it is advanced over the posterior border of the epiglottis, which is then lifted directly by the blade to provide a view of the larynx. This technique is useful particularly in babies, in whom the epiglottis is rather floppy

and may obscure the view of the larynx if a curved blade is used. However, bruising of the epiglottis is more likely with a straight blade.

Most laryngoscopes are powered by batteries contained within the handle; these must be replaced regularly to prevent failure during laryngoscopy. On many laryngoscopes, the light source is a bulb which screws into a socket on the blade; a tight connection should be ensured before laryngoscopy is attempted. It is usual for the electrical circuit between the batteries and the bulb to be closed by a switch which operates automatically when the blade is opened. However, the electrical contacts of the switch may become corroded, causing a reduction in power or total failure. Because of these potential problems, it is important that the function of the laryngoscope is checked carefully before use. It is also wise to have a spare functioning laryngoscope and a variety of blades available.

TRACHEAL TUBES

Most tracheal tubes are constructed either of red rubber or plastic. Red rubber tubes are reusable, although they may start to show signs of deterioration after 2–3 years. Disposable plastic tubes are preferred in most centres as they eliminate the need to collect, clean, sterilize and check tubes after use. Plastic tubes are presented in a sterile pack and should be cut to an appropriate length before use.

Tube size

In adults, there is little to be gained in the way of reduced resistance to breathing by selecting a tube larger than 8.0 mm internal diameter. However, it is common to use a tube of 9.0–9.5 mm internal diameter for male adults and 8.0–8.5 mm for females. Tubes of wide diameter may exert pressure on the laryngeal cords after insertion. Appropriate sizes of tracheal tubes for children are shown in Appendix IXa, p. 757.

Plain tubes

Uncuffed tubes are used in children. A cuff is unnecessary to secure an airtight fit if the correct diameter of tube is selected, because the narrowest part of the airway is in the trachea at the level of the cricoid cartilage. However, the larynx is the narrowest part of the airway in the adult and a leak occurs if an uncuffed tube is used; in addition, there is a risk of aspiration of fluid from the pharynx into the trachea. However, nasotracheal intubation is less traumatic if an uncuffed tube is used. The incidence of sore throat is not influenced by the presence of a cuff on the tracheal tube.

Cuffed tubes

It is usual to use a cuffed tube whenever tracheal intubation is required in the adult. It is almost mandatory if IPPV is to be employed and is essential if there is a risk of blood, pus or gastric fluid entering the pharynx. Tracheal tubes with a streamlined cuff are available and are suitable for nasotracheal intubation.

Cuff volume

A tube with a low-volume cuff (Fig. 16.33) may require inflation to a high pressure to effect a seal within the trachea. The pressure within a low-volume cuff does not necessarily relate to the pres-

sure exerted by the cuff on the tracheal mucosa. However, a high pressure may be exerted if the cuff is overinflated. This may occur inadvertently during anaesthesia because nitrous oxide diffuses through some types of plastic. Some anaesthetists inflate the cuff with an oxygen/nitrous oxide mixture to obviate this problem. Alternatively, the cuff volume may be readjusted after 10–15 min of anaesthesia.

High-volume, low-pressure ('floppy') cuffs cover a larger area of tracheal wall and may effect a seal with less pressure exerted on the mucosa. However, they may cause more trauma during insertion and may become puckered in a relatively small trachea.

Herniation of an overinflated cuff may occlude the distal end of the tracheal tube and cause partial or total airway obstruction.

Shape of tube

In most centres, a curved tracheal tube is used. These should be cut to the correct length and there is a risk of accidental intubation of a bronchus (usually the right main bronchus) if the tip is inserted too far. The Oxford tube is L-shaped and the angle of the tube lies in the pharynx; the distal end is of a fixed length. It is claimed that the use of an Oxford tube reduces the risk of bronchial intubation. There may be less risk of an Oxford tube kinking if the head is flexed during surgery. However, an introducer is required to pass an Oxford tube through the larynx.

Some plastic tracheal tubes are preformed in shapes which either fit the pharyngeal contour or carry the proximal end of the tube away from the mouth (Fig. 16.34); the latter design is useful when surgery on the face or head is planned.

Specialized tubes

An armoured latex tube (Fig. 16.35) is useful if there is a danger of the tube kinking during surgery; a nylon spiral is incorporated in the wall of the tube and prevents obliteration of the lumen. Alternatively, a flexometallic tube, with a metal spiral in the wall, may be used. These tubes are very floppy and a wire stilette is required for their insertion.

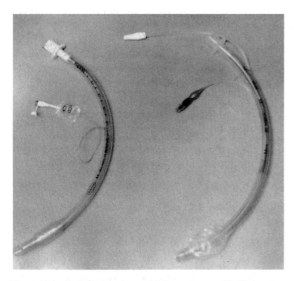

Fig. 16.33 Left: low-volume, high-pressure cuff. Right: high-volume, low-pressure ('floppy') cuff on tracheal tubes.

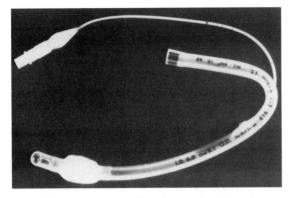

Fig. 16.34 A pre-formed disposable plastic tracheal tube.

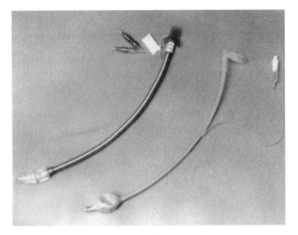

Fig. 16.36 Flexible metal tube and a metal-coated plastic tube suitable for use during laser surgery to the airway.

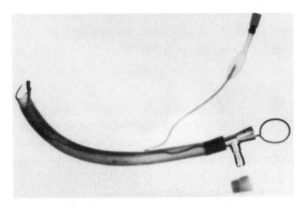

Fig. 16.35 Armoured latex cuffed tracheal tube, with stilette for introduction.

A flexible mental tube (Fig. 16.36) may be employed during procedures that require the use of lasers in the airway; plastic tubes may ignite if struck by the laser beam.

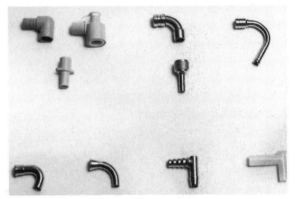

Fig. 16.37 A variety of tracheal tube connectors. From top left in clockwise rotation: Portex and Portex swivel with 15-mm tracheal tube connector, Nosworthy, Worcester, Cobbs, Rowbotham, Magill oral, Magill nasal.

Connections

British standard connections with a 22-mm diameter taper are used in breathing systems. All modern adult tracheal tube connectors have a 15-mm diameter taper.

Tracheal tube connectors

Disposable 15-mm diameter connectors are provided with plastic disposable tubes; the diameter of the distal end is of an appropriate size to fit the internal diameter of the tube. A number of other connections (Fig. 16.37) may be used with plastic or rubber tracheal tubes. The Nosworthy connector is less bulky than the 15-mm disposable connector and is used often in paediatric practice. The Magill connectors are useful, particularly during surgery of the head or neck.

THE LARYNGEAL MASK

This device consists of a shortened conventional silicone tracheal tube with an elliptical cuff, inflated through a pilot tube, attached to the distal end (Fig. 16.38). The cuff, which resembles a miniature face mask, has been designed to form

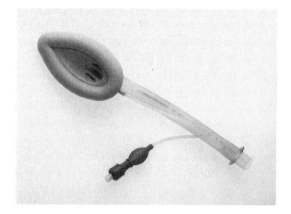

Fig. 16.38 Laryngeal mask.

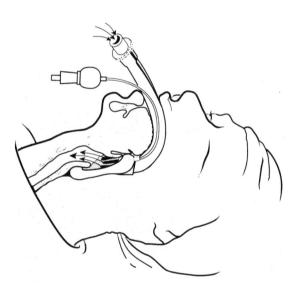

Fig. 16.39 Diagram of a laryngeal mask in situ.

a (relatively) airtight seal around the posterior perimeter of the larynx (Fig. 16.39). A variety of sizes of cuff is available. The mask is inserted and the cuff inflated until no air leak is present; an introducer may be required to ensure that the epiglottis is in the correct position in relation to the proximal end of the cuff. The device is very effective in maintaining a patent airway in the spontaneously breathing patient. Positive pressure ventilation can be applied if necessary. The mask is not suitable for patients who are at risk from regurgitation of gastric contents or in whom pharyngeal soiling is anticipated.

OTHER APPARATUS

Face masks

These are designed to fit the face perfectly so that no leak of gas occurs, but without applying excessive pressure to the skin. An appropriate size of face mask must be selected to ensure a proper fit, but the smallest size possible should be used to minimize dead space. Adult face masks have a 22 mm taper connection and a 90° angle-piece is inserted usually between the mask and the anaesthetic breathing system.

A harness system (e.g. Clausen harness) is used by some anaesthetists to hold the mask on the face during surgery. However, airway obstruction may occur at any time and the excursion of the reservoir bag must be observed constantly.

Intubating forceps

The most commonly used intubating forceps is that designed by Magill (Fig. 16.40). The instrument is employed to manipulate a nasotracheal or nasogastric tube through the oropharynx and into the correct position. A laryngoscope is used to obtain a view of the oropharynx.

Laryngeal spray

This is used to deposit a fine mist of local anaesthetic solution (usually lignocaine 4%) on the mucosa of the larynx and upper trachea. An

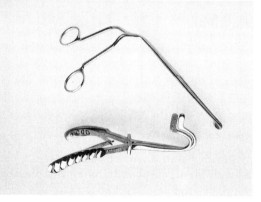

Fig. 16.40 (Above) Magill intubating forceps. (Below) The Ferguson mouth gag.

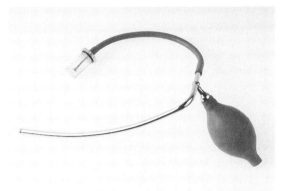

Fig. 16.41   Forrester laryngeal spray.

example of a laryngeal spray is shown in Figure 16.41.

Mouth gag

A mouth gag (Fig. 16.40) may be employed during dental anaesthesia and is required occasionally to open the mouth in patients with trismus or if masseter spasm is present. It is positioned between the molar teeth and must be used with great care to avoid dental trauma.

Gum elastic bougie

If the larynx cannot be seen adequately during laryngoscopy, or if the tracheal tube cannot be manoeuvred into the laryngeal inlet, a gum elastic bougie may be used as an aid to tracheal intubation. The lubricated bougie is inserted into the trachea to act as a guide for the tracheal tube. The tube should be rotated so that the bevel does not become lodged against the aryepiglottic fold.

Stilettes

A malleable metal stilette may be used to adjust the degree of curvature of a tracheal tube as an aid to its insertion. The stilette must not protrude from the distal end of the tube.

Airways

An *oropharyngeal* airway (Guedel airway; Fig. 16.42) may be required to prevent obstruction caused by the tongue or collapse of the pharynx in the unintubated patient. A *nasopharyngeal* airway (Fig. 16.42) is tolerated better during light anaesthesia and may be used also if it is difficult to insert an oropharyngeal airway, e.g. trismus.

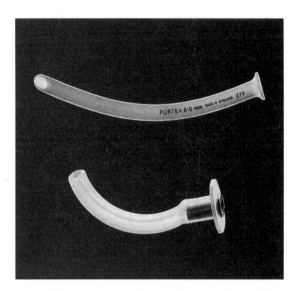

Fig. 16.42   Nasopharyngeal airway (above) and Guedel airway (below).

FURTHER READING

Davey A, Moyle J T B, Ward C S 1992 Anaesthetic equipment, 3rd edn. W B Saunders, London
Nimmo W S, Rowbotham D J, Smith G 1994 Anaesthesia, 2nd edn. Blackwell Scientific Publications, Oxford
Scurr C, Feldman S, Soni N 1990 Scientific foundations of anaesthesia, 4th edn. Butterworth Heinemann, London

17. The operating theatre environment

Until the middle of the 19th century, surgery was carried out in any convenient room, frequently one which was used for other purposes. Although the introduction of antisepsis resulted in the washing of instruments and operating table, the operating room itself was ignored as a source of infection. Operating rooms were designed with tiers of wooden benches around the operating table for spectators; thus the term operating theatre was introduced. During the early part of the 20th century, large windows were incorporated, as artificial light was relatively ineffective, and high ceilings were introduced to improve ventilation. Additional facilities became necessary for preparing and anaesthetizing the patient, for sterilization of instruments and for the surgeon and other theatre staff to change clothes and scrub up. In addition, the design of operating theatres changed, and smaller theatres were introduced to facilitate frequent cleaning.

A modern operating theatre incorporates the following design features:

1. Environmental controls of varying degrees of complexity, to reduce the risk of air-borne infection.
2. Services for surgical and anaesthetic equipment.
3. An operating table on which the patient may be placed in the position required for surgery.
4. Artificial lighting appropriate for the requirements of both surgeon and anaesthetist.
5. Measures to ensure the safety of patient and staff.

In addition, provision should be made immediately adjacent to the operating theatre for anaesthetizing the patient, preparing instruments, cleaning dirty instruments and for the surgeon to scrub up. There should also be separate areas for reception and recovery of patients. It is now common practice for each hospital to have a suite of theatres, rather than operating theatres close to each of the surgical wards. The use of theatre suites permits more flexible and efficient use of staff and resources.

THE OPERATING THEATRE SUITE

The number of operating theatres required is difficult to calculate, but approximates in most British cities to one for every 40 000 of the population served. Ideally, the operating theatre suite should be close to the surgical wards, and adjacent to, and on the same floor as, the accident and emergency department, intensive care unit, X-ray department, day-case ward and sterile supplies unit. It is logical for the anaesthetic department to be immediately adjacent to, or an integral part of, the operating theatre suite, although this seldom occurs in practice.

The main purpose of the operating theatre environment is to minimize the risk of transmission of infection to the patient from the air, the building or the staff. The operating theatre suite contains four zones of increasing degree of cleanliness (Table 17.1).

Transfer of patient

There is some evidence that anxiety in the surgical patient peaks as transfer from the ward to the operating theatre begins, and it is important that

293

Table 17.1   Zones of cleanliness in the operating theatre suite

Outer zone
Hospital areas up to and including the reception area

Clean zone
The circulation area used by staff after they have changed, and the route taken by patients from the transfer bay to the anaesthetic room

Aseptic zone
Scrub-up and gowning area, anaesthetic room, theatre preparation room, operating room, exit bay

Disposal zone
Disposal area for waste products and soiled or used equipment and supplies

---

facilities for transfer minimize stress. A nurse from the ward usually accompanies the patient, but it is customary for the ward nurse to leave adult patients before anaesthesia has been induced. In paediatric practice, it is now the normal routine that a ward nurse and parent remain with the child during induction of anaesthesia.

On arrival at the reception area, the patient's identity and surgical procedure are checked. In a theatre suite, it may be necessary for patients to wait for some time in the reception area to prevent delays in the operating schedules. Consequently, adequate space should be provided for a number of beds, and there should be screens for patients who wish privacy. The staff in the reception area should include nurses. The décor should be cheerful, and the lighting subdued.

Transport should involve the minimum number of changes of trolley. A trolley is used commonly to transfer the patient to the operating theatre suite, but changes of trolley may be required to enter the clean area and also for transfer to the operating table after anaesthesia has been induced. Alternatively, the patient's own bed may be taken to the operating theatre suite. If the patient is infirm or in severe pain, the bed may be taken to the anaesthetic room, and transfer delayed until after induction of anaesthesia, but this is appropriate only if the bed has the facility to be tipped head-down if necessary. In some hospitals, a single transfer is effected by transporting the patient to the theatre suite in bed, where the patient is moved on to the operating theatre table-top, which is mounted on a wheeled frame. After induction of anaesthesia, the table-top is wheeled into the theatre and the top attached to a fixed base, which allows it to be positioned for surgery.

There is no universal method of transferring patients from one trolley to another. This may be achieved by the use of canvas and poles, rollers or lifting the patient bodily. There is increasing awareness of the risk of injury to operating theatre personnel as a result of lifting patients, and thus an increasing tendency to install transfer systems which do not require great physical effort.

All trolleys in the operating theatre suite should be equipped with oxygen, and this should be administered routinely to patients during transfer from theatre to the recovery room at the end of the procedure if general anaesthesia has been used.

Anaesthetic room

In a number of countries, the anaesthetic room has developed from a small annexe to the theatre to an integral part of the operating theatre suite. However, this is not universal, and in many parts of the world anaesthesia is induced in the operating theatre after the patient has been transferred on to the operating table. The main advantages of the anaesthetic room are:

1. The patient's anxiety may be reduced by avoiding the sights and sounds of the operating theatre. This is of special importance in children.
2. The equipment which may be necessary during induction of anaesthesia may be stored in a readily accessible form.
3. Time is saved by inducing anaesthesia while surgery is being completed on another patient. This is useful particularly if preparation is prolonged, e.g. performance of local anaesthetic blocks or establishment of invasive cardiovascular monitoring.

However, there are a number of disadvantages:

1. Anaesthetic and monitoring equipment must be duplicated, or moved to the operating theatre with the patient; this usually necessitates temporary disconnection from electrical or gas supplies.
2. Hazards are involved in transferring an

unconscious patient from a trolley to the operating table.

3. Construction and maintenance of anaesthetic rooms are expensive.

Even in countries where anaesthetic rooms are used, it is customary to induce anaesthesia in the high-risk patient on the operating table, as the delay between onset of unconsciousness and the start of surgery must be kept to a minimum, e.g. for emergency Caesarean section or severe haemorrhage.

The design of the anaesthetic room should allow easy access all round the patient's trolley, and should provide space for anaesthetic and monitoring equipment, and storage cupboards and shelves. The minimum floor area recommended by the Department of Health in the UK is 17 m^2, but this is inadequate. A floor area of 21 m^2 is more appropriate. Piped gases and suction and electrical sockets are required near the head of the trolley. An anaesthetic machine, mechanical ventilator and monitoring system are also necessary. Cupboards must be available to store equipment and drugs, and work tops must be of sufficient size to allow syringes, needles, cannulae and drugs to be prepared. There should be a clock with a second hand.

Operating room

The operating room is designed around its centrally situated operating table with overhead lighting and ventilation systems. The ideal shape for the operating room is circular, but this is inefficient and most operating rooms are square or nearly square. In 1980, the Royal College of Surgeons of England suggested that the floor should be 625 ft^2 (approximately 58 m^2) in area, and no smaller than 484 ft^2 (approximately 45 m^2). Theatres for specialized surgery may require a larger area to accommodate bulky equipment.

Outlets for piped gases and electrical sockets must be positioned close to the head of the operating table; they are provided most conveniently by a boom or stalactite system. Electrical cables should not lie across the floor. The operating room should be of sufficient size to allow all types of surgery without moving the position of

the head of the table; this location should be reached easily and without complex manoeuvres as the patient enters the theatre from the anaesthetic room.

Temperature, humidity and ventilation

The temperature in the operating theatre and anaesthetic room should be sufficiently high to minimize the risk of inducing hypothermia in the patient, but must be comfortable for theatre staff. The patient may develop hypothermia at an ambient temperature of less than 21°C. Temperatures of 22–24°C are usually acceptable in the operating room, with a relative humidity of 50–60%; a higher environmental temperature is required during surgery in the neonate or infant. Slightly lower temperature and humidity are acceptable in other parts of the theatre suite. Controls for temperature and humidity should be located within the operating theatre.

Heating and humidity are controlled usually by an air-conditioning and ventilation system, which provides an ambient pressure inside the operating room slightly higher than atmospheric. In general, air is introduced directly over the operating table, and leaves at the periphery through ducts positioned near floor level. In the area of the table, 400 air changes per hour are required to minimize the risk of air-borne transmission of infection. More effective systems of ventilation, involving radial exponential air flow away from the operating table, or laminar flow, are used in some centres for some types of surgery, e.g. total hip replacement, in which infection is especially undesirable. High-flow systems may accelerate cooling of the patient.

Light

Daylight is not necessary in the operating theatre, although it is more pleasant for staff if there are windows in the theatre suite, e.g. in corridors and common rooms. A high level of illumination is required over the operating table, and ceiling-mounted lamps are standard; it is preferable if they can be positioned directly by the surgeon.

The intensity and colour temperature of general lighting are very important to the anaesthetist, as appreciation of skin colour is affected by the spectrum of the source of illumination. The spectrum provided by lighting tubes should be similar to that of daylight, with an emission temperature of 4000–5000 K. The colour of the décor should be neutral and uniform. The intensity of general illumination should be up to 325 lm.m^{-2} in the operating theatre, and it should be diffuse to avoid glare. In the anaesthetic room and recovery area, a light intensity of approximately 220 lm.m^{-2} is acceptable, but a spotlight should be available if increased illumination is required for specific procedures.

Safety in the operating theatre

Electrocution and gas explosions are the two main hazards to staff and patients in the operating theatre. In addition, there may be a risk to staff from pollution of the atmosphere with anaesthetic gases and vapours, and of contracting infection, particularly human immunodeficiency virus (HIV) or hepatitis, from infected patients.

Electrical safety

Although some mention is made of electrical hazards in the operating theatre in Chapter 15, a detailed description is beyond the scope of this book, and the reader is referred to the article by Hull (1978). The electrical supply to the operating theatre and all electrical equipment connected to the patient incorporate design features which minimize the risk of electrical currents being transmitted through the patient to earth.

Explosions

The use of explosive anaesthetic gases and vapours has diminished greatly in recent years. However, diethyl ether is still used occasionally. Ether burns in air, but forms an explosive mixture with oxygen. An explosion may be initiated by a spark of very low energy ($< 1 \mu J$) or by contact with a temperature of 300°C or higher. The risk of explosion is highest within and close to the anaesthetic breathing system because of the presence of a high oxygen concentration. Beyond a distance of 10 cm from the breathing system,

the oxygen concentration diminishes, and the risk is reduced.

The construction of anaesthetic apparatus is designed to minimize explosion hazards from generation of sparks caused by cumulation of static electricity. All rubber is conductive, so that electrical charges leak to earth, and non-conductive substances are treated with antistatic material. In most existing theatres, the operating theatre floor has a high but finite resistance, so that static charges leak to earth but electrocution risks are minimized. Theatre footwear is designed also to earth static charges. Sparks may be generated by clothing made of synthetic materials such as nylon. The risk of accumulation of static electricity on walls and equipment is reduced if the environmental humidity exceeds 70%. Diathermy must not be used if explosive anaesthetics are employed. However, the use of these agents has virtually ceased in the UK and most other First-World countries, and many of the precautions, particularly the use of expensive antistatic flooring, are becoming unnecessary. In addition, modern monitoring apparatus is unsuitable for use with flammable or explosive anaesthetics. Most new operating theatres are built without antistatic precautions, but this must be indicated clearly by labels so that explosive agents are not employed.

Atmospheric pollution

There has been considerable controversy regarding the risk to theatre staff from atmospheric pollution by anaesthetic gases and vapours. Earlier investigations suggested that theatre staff are more likely than other hospital personnel to suffer from hepatic and renal disease, to have non-specific neurological symptoms and for their children to have an increased risk of congenital abnormality. However, none of these problems has been substantiated.

There was more convincing evidence from the early studies that female staff who worked in the operating theatre during the early months of pregnancy suffered an increased incidence of spontaneous abortion, and there is experimental evidence to suggest that constant exposure of rats to a concentration of more than 1000 p.p.m.

of nitrous oxide produces adverse results on their reproduction. However, the most recent, comprehensive and only randomized prospective investigation of operating theatre staff failed to demonstrate any increased health risk.

Trace concentrations of anaesthetic gases have been implicated in another area of concern — impairment of professional performance. Motor and intellectual performance were shown in an early laboratory study in volunteers to deteriorate in the presence of concentrations of nitrous oxide of 500 p.p.m., with or without halothane 15 p.p.m. However, subsequent studies failed to confirm these findings, and the consensus of several studies is that concentrations of 8–12% nitrous oxide are required before significant impairment of performance occurs. Such concentrations might be inhaled if the anaesthetist is close to an unscavenged expiratory valve, or during inhalational induction of anaesthesia, but exceed those present in other areas of an adequately ventilated operating theatre.

Nevertheless, it is sensible to minimize atmospheric pollution in the operating theatre, and hospital regulations in both western Europe and North America require the installation of anaesthetic gas-scavenging systems in all areas where anaesthesia is administered. In the USA, the National Institute of Occupational Safety and Hygiene (a Federal regulatory body) dictates that environmental concentrations of anaesthetic gases should not exceed a value of 25 p.p.m. of nitrous oxide and 2 p.p.m. of volatile agent. In the UK, the Health and Safety Executive introduced maximum limits of exposure to anaesthetic agents in January 1996; these are shown in Table 17.2, and may necessitate major alterations in anaesthetic techniques. Scavenging systems are described in Chapter 16.

Anaesthetic gases are not the only source of environmental pollution in the operating theatre; volatile skin-cleaning fluids and aerosol sprays, e.g. iodine or plastic skin dressing, should be used sensibly, and inhalation of vapours should be avoided. Ethyl chloride is used by some anaesthetists to produce local anaesthesia of the skin before venepuncture; ethyl chloride is both explosive and an atmospheric pollutant, and should not be used for this purpose.

Table 17.2 Maximum levels of exposure to anaesthetic agents in the operating theatre suite over an 8-h time-weighted average reference period, as laid down in the UK by the Health and Safety Executive

Agent	Maximum concentration (p.p.m.)
Nitrous oxide	100
Halothane	10
Enflurane	50
Isoflurane	50

Infection

The most serious types of acquired infection in operating theatre staff are HIV and hepatitis, which may be contracted by contact with blood or body fluids from an infected patient. A number of health care workers have been infected in this way, either by a needlestick injury, or through cuts and abrasions. The risk of percutaneous transmission of HIV is believed to be extremely low; the incidence of seroconversion after occupational exposure to HIV is 0.39%. However, the risk is 5–30% after an occupational inoculation injury.

Two thousand cases of hepatitis B are reported each year in the UK, although the true incidence is probably very much higher. Hepatitis B surface antigen persists for at least 6 months in 5–10% of infected individuals. The virus is highly infectious, and minute amounts of blood may transmit the disease. The Association of Anaesthetists of Great Britain and Ireland recommends that all anaesthetists should receive active immunization against hepatitis B. A single dose of hepatitis B immunoglobulin combined with active immunization is required immediately if an unprotected individual is inoculated with infected material.

Hepatitis C and D viruses are also blood-borne. Up to 50% of people infected with the hepatitis C virus develop chronic liver disease. Occupational transmission of this virus has been reported.

The incidence of acquired immunodeficiency syndrome (AIDS) continues to increase, and is not confined to homosexuals and drug abusers. For every patient with fully developed AIDS, there are estimated to be five with a less severe form of the disease, and up to 50 asymptomatic carriers. At present, it is unclear what proportion of these will develop AIDS, but probably it may approach 100%. Thus, anaesthetists are likely to be exposed to an increasing number of patients who may transmit HIV. At present, compulsory screening of hospital patients for HIV is regarded as unacceptable. Consequently, precautions must be taken in patients who are believed to be at high risk of being HIV-positive; these include homosexual or bisexual men, haemophiliacs and sexual partners of high-risk patients. In some locations, it has been recommended that precautions should be taken with all patients.

Human T-cell leukaemia virus (HTLV-I) is another virus which is of potential importance.

The following precautions are recommended to reduce the risks of transmission of HIV; these are also applicable when patients infected with other blood-borne viruses are anaesthetized.

1. Gloves must be worn during induction of anaesthesia, performance of venepuncture or insertion of any intravascular cannula, and during insertion or removal of airways and tracheal tubes. A plastic apron, mask and eye protection should be worn if substantial spillage of blood is anticipated, e.g. during insertion of an arterial cannula. Gloves should normally be discarded on taking the patient into the operating theatre and a fresh pair donned when any of these procedures are carried out during or at the end of anaesthesia. Equipment, notes and other articles must not be handled with contaminated gloves.

2. Needles which have been in contact with the patient must not be resheathed, or handed from one person to another.

3. All needles and other sharp objects should be disposed of in an appropriate tough disposal bin; cardboard bins are unsatisfactory.

4. Cuts or abrasions on the anaesthetist's hands should be covered with a waterproof dressing. An anaesthetist with considerable skin lesions such as eczema, chapping or several scratches is particularly at risk of being infected.

5. If a needlestick injury or contamination of a cut or abrasion occurs, bleeding should be encouraged and the skin washed thoroughly with soap and water.

6. Advice should be obtained immediately from the hospital's occupational health department if there is reason to believe that contamination has occurred.

7. Disposable equipment should be used where possible. Non-disposable equipment should be decontaminated with 2% glutaraldehyde, washed with soap and water and left in glutaraldehyde for a further 3 h. Contaminated floors and surfaces should be washed with 1% hypochlorite solution. Gloves must be worn.

It has been recommended that a bacterial filter should be placed between the tracheal tube or airway and the anaesthetic breathing system in all patients to prevent cross-infection from a patient with undiagnosed infection.

Recovery room

A recovery room or ward is an essential requirement in the operating theatre environment. All patients require close surveillance in the immediate postoperative period, and for up to 24 h after major surgery.

The recovery room should be an integral part of the operating theatre suite, and should be located within the clean area. Department of Health guidelines suggest that there should be 1.5 places in the recovery area for each operating theatre, although a greater number may be required if surgery with a high turnover, e.g. gynaecology or day-case surgery, is common. Each place requires a minimum floor area of approximately 10 m², and there must be sufficient space to move a patient without disturbing the remainder.

It is appropriate for most patients to lie on a trolley in the recovery room, but beds should be available for those who are likely to stay for more than 30–45 min, e.g. patients who have undergone major surgery, or American Society of Anesthesiology grade III or IV patients who may require prolonged observation even after minor surgery. Each place should have piped oxygen and suction outlets on the wall, with an oxygen flowmeter and suction apparatus attached to a wall rail. Lighting should conform to the same standards as apply to the operating theatre, and additional spotlights should be provided. It is not common practice in the UK to monitor the electrocardiogram in all patients in the recovery ward, but oxygen saturation and blood pressure should be monitored routinely. Most large recovery areas have two or three places which are fully equipped with piped nitrous oxide, a mechanical ventilator and complete cardiovascular monitoring facilities.

An anaesthetic machine, defibrillator and equipment and drugs for resuscitation should be available in the recovery room. Oxygen is usually administered by disposable face mask, but each place should have a self-inflating resuscitation bag and anaesthetic mask.

Drug cupboards and storage space for equipment should be provided and, in a large recovery area, several telephones are required. Nursing staff spend most of their time with the patient, but require a nursing station at which notes may be written and theatres and wards contacted by telephone. At least one nurse is required for each three bed spaces. At present, there is no specific training course in the UK for recovery room nurses. Student nurses receive only 1 week of training in this area.

In many hospitals, it is possible to provide supervision of patients in the recovery ward for up to 24 h after major surgery. This is highly desirable in the absence of a separate high-dependency unit, as intensive care facilities are often overwhelmed in large hospitals.

Clinical aspects of recovery room care are discussed in Chapter 23.

High-dependency unit

A high-dependency unit is an area for patients who require more invasive observation, treatment and nursing care than can be provided on a general ward. It would not normally accept patients requiring mechanical ventilation, but could manage those receiving invasive monitoring. A survey conducted by the Association of Anaesthetists of Great Britain and Ireland (1991) indicated that many intensive care units admitted patients who could have been managed appropriately in a high-dependency unit. An unknown number of patients return from the recovery area to a general ward requiring monitoring or an intensity of nursing or medical care which cannot be provided safely in that location.

The facilities required to provide high-dependency care vary. Essential features are a high nurse-to-patient ratio, provision of piped oxygen and suction at every bed, and appropriate monitoring equipment. Protocols must be in place for admission and discharge criteria, and medical staffing must be clearly defined. In large hospitals, several units may be desirable, each dedicated to the care of specific groups of patients; in smaller hospitals, a single, multi-user unit may be more appropriate.

Other accommodation

Storage space is required for large items of equipment. In most modern operating theatre suites, instruments are sterilized in a separate department, which should be situated in close proximity. Access to blood gas analysis and measurement of serum electrolyte concentrations are essential, especially if major surgery is to be undertaken, and large operating theatre suites usually contain a small laboratory.

Staff accommodation includes changing rooms and rest rooms. There should be facilities for beverages and snacks. Offices are provided for the theatre supervisor and senior operating department assistants, and there should be a tutorial or seminar room for staff training. Some theatre suites incorporate an office for the anaesthetic department.

Other anaesthetizing locations

The anaesthetist is often required to work in areas outside the operating theatre suite. Many hospitals have peripheral theatres for some types of surgery, e.g. a self-contained day-case unit. In addition, patients may require anaesthesia in the accident and emergency unit, the radiology and radiotherapy departments or, in some instances (e.g. paediatric oncology), the side room of a ward. In these circumstances, where conditions are frequently not ideal, it is essential that the same precautions are taken as in the operating theatre suite to ensure that the identity of the patient is checked, that equipment is functioning correctly, that skilled help for the anaesthetist is available and that recovery facilities and staff are satisfactory.

Ancillary staff

Skilled and dedicated help should be available to the anaesthetist at all times. In the majority of hospitals in the UK, this is provided by operating department practitioners (ODPs), who undergo a 2-year training programme in recognized institutions and are required to sit examinations. In some hospitals, anaesthetic nurses assist the anaesthetist. It is important to differentiate between anaesthetic nurses and the nurse anaesthetists who are trained to deliver anaesthesia in some countries (e.g. CRNAs in the USA). The anaesthetic nurse performs essentially the same functions as the ODP. These include:

1. Preparation and preliminary checking of equipment. It should be stressed that this does not absolve the anaesthetist from the responsibility of checking the equipment fully before an operating list is started.

2. Alleviation of anxiety by reassurance and constant communication with the patient while awaiting anaesthesia.

3. The ODP or anaesthetic nurse is involved in checking the correct identity of the patient. However, it is the joint responsibility of the surgeon and anaesthetist to ensure that the appropriate procedure is undertaken on the correct patient, and this is one of the many reasons why the anaesthetist must see every patient preoperatively.

4. Preparation of intravenous infusions, cardiovascular monitoring transducers, etc.

5. Assistance during anaesthesia, particularly during induction, when special manoeuvres such as cricoid pressure may be required, and after transfer to the operating theatre to assist in re-establishment of monitoring.

6. Assistance in positioning the patient for local or regional blocks.

7. Assistance in obtaining drugs or equipment if complications arise during anaesthesia.

8. Assistance in the immediate postoperative period before the patient is transferred to the recovery room.

The ODP or anaesthetic nurse should *never* be left alone with an anaesthetized patient unless a dire emergency requires the anaesthetist's presence elsewhere.

THE MEDICOLEGAL ENVIRONMENT

The increasing volume of litigation instituted by patients in respect of alleged or actual injury arising from treatment is causing great concern within the medical profession. Insurance premiums for medical practice have escalated rapidly. Anaesthesia represents a high insurance risk, because anaesthetists manipulate the physiology of the cardiovascular and respiratory systems to administer potentially lethal drugs for reasons which are not primarily therapeutic; consequently, when a serious accident occurs, it may result in death or permanent neurological damage. In addition, even minor morbidity caused by anaesthesia or the anaesthetist may be regarded by the patient as unacceptable when it does not appear to be related to the primary illness.

Mortality associated with anaesthesia

The overwhelming majority of anaesthetics are uneventful. However, both surgery and anaesthesia carry a finite risk. Mortality is usually related to the extent of surgery and the preoperative condition of the patient (see Table 18.3). However, avoidable deaths occur. In 1982, Lunn & Mushin estimated that the risk of death attributable to anaesthesia alone was approximately 1 in 10 000. In a subsequent study of more than half a million operations (Confidential Enquiry into Perioperative Deaths; CEPOD), the overall death rate after anaesthesia and surgery was 0.7% (Buck et al 1987). Anaesthesia alone was responsible for death in approximately 1 in 180 000 operations, but *contributed* to 14% of all deaths; in almost one-fifth of these deaths, avoidable errors occurred. Factors which contributed to death in these instances are listed in Table 17.3.

Morbidity associated with anaesthesia

The incidence of major morbidity (causing perma-

Table 17.3 Factors involved in deaths attributable in part to anaesthesia, in decreasing order of frequency (CEPOD report)

Failure to apply knowledge
Lack of care
Failure of organization
Lack of experience
Lack of knowledge
Drug effect
Failure of equipment
Fatigue

Table 17.4 Causes of anaesthetic-related death or cerebral damage reported to the Medical Defence Union between 1970 and 1982

Mainly misadventure		Mainly error	
Coexisting disease	14%	Faulty technique	43%
Unknown	6%	Failure of postoperative care	9%
Drug sensitivity	5%		
Hypotension/blood loss	4%	Drug overdosage	5%
Halothane-associated hepatic failure	3%	Inadequate preoperative assessment	3%
Hyperpyrexia	2%		
Embolism	2%	Drug error	1%
		Anaesthetist's failure	1%

nent disability) related to anaesthesia is difficult to assess. Its causes are often similar to those associated with mortality. Table 17.4 lists the causes of death or cerebral damage reported to the Medical Defence Union between 1970 and 1982; Table 17.5 shows the detailed causes of the incidents resulting from errors in technique. Permanent disability may result also from spinal cord damage.

Other, albeit less serious incidents may result in distress or physical injury to patients. Table 17.6 lists untoward events, other than death and cerebral damage, reported to the Medical Defence Union.

Table 17.5 Causes of anaesthetic-related death or cerebral damage reported to the Medical Defence Union and thought to be the result of errors in technique

Cause	% of total
Errors associated with tracheal intubation	31
Misuse of apparatus	23
Inhalation of gastric contents	14
Errors associated with induced hypotension	8
Hypoxia	4
Obstructed airway	4
Accidental pneumothorax/haemopericardium	4
Errors associated with extradural analgesia	3
Use of nitrous oxide instead of oxygen	2
Use of carbon dioxide instead of oxygen	2
Errors associated with Bier's block	2
Underventilation	1
Use of halothane with adrenaline	1
Mismatched blood transfusion	<1
Vasovagal attack	<1

Table 17.6 Untoward anaesthetic-related events (other than death or cerebral damage) reported to the Medical Defence Union between 1970 and 1982

Event	% of total
Damage to teeth	52
Peripheral nerve damage	9
Extradural foreign bodies (needles, catheter tips)	7
Superficial thrombophlebitis and minor injuries (e.g. abrasions)	7
Awareness	7
Spinal cord damage	4
Pneumothoraces	3
Extravasation of injected drugs	2
Lacerations, falls from table	2
Impaired renal function (mismatched blood)	1
Burns	1
Other	5

Critical incidents

These are incidents that could or do lead to death, permanent disability or prolongation of hospital stay. Most critical incidents in anaesthesia are detected before damage occurs; their incidence is 4–500 times greater than that of death or serious injury attributable to anaesthesia. It has been estimated that a critical incident occurs on average once in every 80 anaesthetics. Analysis of the causes of critical incidents is valuable in indicating the potential causes of anaesthetic-related mortality and major morbidity. Human error is responsible for approximately 70% of critical incidents in anaesthesia; the commonest errors are shown in Table 17.7. Factors associated with critical incidents are shown in Table 17.8.

Table 17.7 Types of human error contributing to critical incidents during anaesthesia

Type of error	% of total
Wrong drug administered	24
Misuse of anaesthetic machine	22
Problem with airway management	16
Problem with breathing system	11
Fluid therapy mismanagement	5
Intravenous infusion disconnection	6
Failure of monitoring	4
Others	12

Table 17.8 Associated factors producing critical incidents during anaesthesia, in decreasing order of frequency

Failure to check
First experience of procedure
Inadequate experience
Inattention/carelessness
Haste
Unfamiliarity
Visual restriction
Fatigue

Minimizing the risk

The most effective means of reducing the risk of an anaesthetic accident is to ensure that every aspect of anaesthetic management is conducted competently (Table 17.9). Preoperative assessment (see Chapter 18) is essential. In the anaesthetic room, the anaesthetist must check the identity of the patient before proceeding. The information contained in Tables 17.4–17.8 indicates areas of particular concern regarding intraoperative management. All anaesthetic equipment must be checked before use. The anaesthetist must understand the principles of all the equipment used, especially mechanical ventilators. Drug doses must be calculated carefully and syringes labelled. After induction of anaesthesia, the correct placement of the tracheal tube must be confirmed on every occasion.

Studies of critical incidents indicate that the time of highest risk is during maintenance of anaesthesia. For this reason, appropriate clinical and instrumental monitoring (see Chapter 20) must be used throughout anaesthesia. After operation, the anaesthetist is responsible for the patient until consciousness has returned and until the cardiovascular and respiratory systems are stable. He or she may be required to defend a decision to delegate the care of the patient to a nurse in the recovery room.

The following factors should be considered also:

1. *Awareness*. Patients may recall intraoperative events, and may experience pain and discomfort, if the doses or concentrations of anaesthetic drugs are insufficient (see p. 403). In high-risk groups, it may be advisable to warn the patient of the possibility of awareness.

2. *Anaesthetic record*. A legible and comprehensive record must be made of every anaesthetic. The record should include details of preoperative findings, the doses and timing of all drugs administered during anaesthesia, frequent and regular recordings of cardiovascular and respiratory measurements and notes regarding any untoward intraoperative event. This is an important document because it provides information which may assist other anaesthetists in the future and because a comprehensive record is *essential* in the event of medicolegal proceedings.

3. *Communication*. If a mishap occurs, failure

Table 17.9 Summary of important factors which should minimize the risk of accidents during anaesthesia and the risk of litigation against the anaesthetist

Careful preoperative assessment should be undertaken to identify risk factors such as concurrent disease, chronic medication, history of allergy or other untoward reactions to anaesthesia, and potential difficulties in tracheal intubation

Anaesthetic equipment must be maintained according to the manufacturers' recommendations, and checked thoroughly before every operating theatre session, or when the equipment is changed during an operating session

The anaesthetic technique should be recognized as appropriate for the individual patient and for the proposed type of surgery

The anaesthetist must be present at all times during anaesthesia

Appropriate monitoring, in accordance with national recommendations, should be employed at all times during anaesthesia and in the immediate recovery period. Alarms should be set at appropriate levels, and must not be disabled

At the end of anaesthesia, the anaesthetist should transfer the care of the patient only to an appropriately qualified recovery room nurse

All anaesthetists should be taught how to manage uncommon emergencies, such as failed intubation, anaphylaxis or malignant hyperthermia. It is advisable to have protocols available in every anaesthetizing location to act as an *aide-memoire* for uncommon emergencies, and anaesthetists and operating room staff should rehearse emergency management on a regular basis

The anaesthetist should keep careful records

on the part of the anaesthetist to communicate with the patient or relatives may arouse feelings of anger and suspicion. While no admission (or accusations) of liability should be made, an explanation should be offered. An interview with a patient or relatives in these circumstances requires skill and tact; the trainee should discuss the event with a consultant, and if possible, the consultant should be present at the interview. Any untoward event, or any complaint by a patient, should be reported promptly to the anaesthetist's defence society.

Each anaesthetic department should ensure that the channels of communication between trainees and consultants are clear, especially with regard to emergency procedures.

4. *Audit*. Standards of anaesthetic practice may be improved by identifying areas in which patient care has been suboptimal. Although case reports published in anaesthetic journals form a useful source of information, local meetings to discuss morbidity and mortality related to anaesthesia and surgery, together with critical incident analysis, should be convened regularly.

FURTHER READING

Association of Anaesthetists of Great Britain and Ireland 1991 The high dependency unit: acute care in the future. Association of Anaesthetists of Great Britain and Ireland, London

Association of Anaesthetists of Great Britain and Ireland 1992 HIV and other blood borne viruses: guidance for anaesthetists. Association of Anaesthetists of Great Britain and Ireland, London

Aitkenhead A R 1994 The pattern of litigation against anaesthetists. British Journal of Anaesthesia 73: 10

Buck N, Devlin H B, Lunn J N 1987 The report of a confidential enquiry into perioperative deaths. Nuffield Provincial Hospitals Trust, London

Drain C B, Christoph S S 1987 The recovery room, 2nd edn. W B Saunders, Philadelphia

Johnston I D A, Hunter A R (eds) 1984 The design and utilisation of operating theatres. Edward Arnold, London

Hull C J 1978 Electrical hazards in the operating theatre. British Journal of Anaesthesia 50: 647

Lunn J N, Mushin W W 1982 Mortality associated with anaesthesia. Nuffield Provincial Hospitals Trust, London

Runciman W B, Sellen A, Webb R K, Williamson J A, Currie M, Morgan C A, Russell W J 1993 Errors, incidents and accidents in anaesthetic practice. Anaesthesia and Intensive Care 21: 506

Spence A A 1987 Environmental pollution by inhalation of anaesthetics. British Journal of Anaesthesia 59: 96

Taylor T H, Major E (eds) 1994 Hazards and complications of anaesthesia, 2nd edn. Churchill Livingstone, Edinburgh

18. Preoperative assessment and premedication

Several of the large-scale epidemiological studies (e.g. the CEPOD study) have indicated that inadequate preoperative preparation of the patient may be a major contributory factor to the primary anaesthetic causes of perioperative mortality. It is therefore essential that the anaesthetist visits every patient in the ward before surgery to assess 'fitness for anaesthesia', as this function cannot be undertaken by surgical staff. Unfortunately, the anaesthetist is frequently under pressure to proceed with the planned operating theatre lists as he usually sees the patient on the ward only 1 day before the scheduled date for surgery and cancellation would lead to inefficient use of operating theatre time and inconvenience for the patient. This problem may be obviated by the provision of anaesthetic outpatient assessment clinics, to which a patient is referred before an admission date is given. This allows the anaesthetist to plan optimum preparation of the patient for anaesthesia and surgery. Unfortunately, such anaesthetic assessment clinics are uncommon. Nevertheless, failure by the anaesthetist to perform a preoperative visit and assessment may be regarded as negligent if anaesthetic morbidity or mortality occur subsequently and therefore the anaesthetist *must* undertake a preoperative visit.

The purposes of the preoperative visit are to:

1. Establish rapport with the patient.
2. Obtain a history and perform a physical examination.
3. Order special investigations.
4. Assess the risks of anaesthesia and surgery and if necessary postpone or cancel the date of surgery.
5. Institute preoperative management.

6. Prescribe premedication and plan the anaesthetic management.

ESTABLISHMENT OF RAPPORT

The preoperative visit enables the patient to meet the doctor and discuss possible causes of anxiety regarding the anaesthetic or surgical management. The anaesthetist may explain in simple terms how the patient will be cared for during and after anaesthesia and the measures that will be taken to provide postoperative pain relief. The anaesthetist can also assure himself that the patient understands the proposed scope of surgery and that informed consent has been given for the proposed procedure.

HISTORY AND PHYSICAL EXAMINATION

Normally the patient has been clerked and examined by a house physician or house surgeon and the anaesthetist may concentrate on physiological systems of greatest relevance, e.g. the cardiovascular and respiratory systems.

Systematic evaluation of each system should be undertaken as described in most standard textbooks of medicine.

History

Direct questions should be asked about the following items of particular anaesthetic relevance:

1. A family history of hereditary conditions associated with anaesthetic problems, e.g. porphyria, malignant hyperpyrexia, hypercholesterol-

305

aemia, haemophilia, cholinesterase abnormalities, dystrophia myotonica.

2. Diseases of the cardiovascular and respiratory systems are the most relevant in respect of fitness for anaesthesia. Specific questions should be addressed regarding exertional dyspnoea, paroxysmal nocturnal dyspnoea, orthopnoea, angina of effort, etc. It may be difficult to elicit a history of exertional dyspnoea if exercise is limited by arthritis, intermittent claudication, etc.

3. If relevant, enquiries should be made regarding possible pregnancy. The presence of pregnancy is a contraindication to elective surgery. In the early stages of pregnancy, anaesthetics are teratogenic (at least theoretically), but a more likely problem is the induction of spontaneous abortion. In late pregnancy, the patient presents risks of regurgitation and acid aspiration syndrome (see p. 560).

4. A history of previous anaesthesia should be sought and specific questions asked concerning drug allergy, postoperative nausea and vomiting, deep vein thrombosis or respiratory problems. If previous anaesthetic records are available, they should be inspected carefully; problems with tracheal intubation should be documented and the type of anaesthetic technique employed should be described in detail. The current recommendation of the Committee of Safety of Medicines is that halothane anaesthesia should not be repeated within 6 months of a previous halothane anaesthetic.

5. A history of allergies to drugs, plaster, rubber, etc. should be sought.

6. A history of HIV infection or jaundice, particularly viral hepatitis, has important implications for the patient and medical personnel (see p. 297).

Smoking

Deleterious effects of smoking include vascular disease of the peripheral, coronary and cerebral circulations, carcinoma of the lung and chronic bronchitis. It has been suggested recently that there are good theoretical reasons for advising all patients to cease cigarette smoking for at least 12 h prior to surgery.

The cardiovascular effects of smoking are caused by the action of nicotine on the sympathetic nervous system, producing tachycardia and hypertension. Furthermore, smoking causes an increase in coronary vascular resistance; cessation of smoking improves the symptoms of angina.

Cigarette smoke contains carbon monoxide, which converts haemoglobin to carboxyhaemoglobin. In heavy smokers, this may result in a reduction in available oxygen by as much as 25%. The half-life of carboxyhaemoglobin is short and therefore abstinence for 12 h leads to an increase in arterial oxygen content.

The effect of smoking on the respiratory tract leads to a sixfold increase in postoperative respiratory morbidity. It has been suggested that abstinence for 6 weeks results in reduced bronchoconstriction and mucus secretion in the tracheobronchial tree.

Alcohol

Regular alcohol intake leads to induction of liver enzymes and tolerance to anaesthetic drugs. Excessive alcohol intake causes both hepatic and cardiac damage. Delirium tremens may occur in alcoholics during the postoperative recovery phase as a result of withdrawal of the drug.

Drug history

It is essential that a complete history is obtained regarding concurrent medication. Many drugs interact with agents employed by the anaesthetist; the most important interactions are listed in Table 18.1.

In general terms, administration of most drugs should be continued up to and including the morning of operation, although some adjustment in dosage may be required (e.g. antihypertensives, insulin). Knowledge of the pharmacology of drug therapy is essential to permit the anaesthetist to adjust the dosage of anaesthetic agents appropriately and to avoid possibly dangerous interactions.

Some drugs should be discontinued preoperatively. The monoamine oxidase inhibitors (MAOI) should be withdrawn 2–3 weeks before surgery because of the risk of interactions with drugs used during anaesthesia; psychiatric advice may be required for the prescription of alternative antidepressant therapy. This standard teaching has

Table 18.1 Drug interactions in anaesthesia

Drug	Problems and interactions	Recommendations
Alcohol	*Acute intoxication* Effects of sedatives, opioids and anaesthetics enhanced	Continue with reduced dosage anaesthetic drugs
	Chronic alcoholism Tolerance to effect of these drugs as a result of enzyme induction	Increased dosage usually required
Adrenaline	Arrhythmias with volatile anaesthetic agents halothane > enflurane > isoflurane	Do not exceed 1 µg.kg^{-1} of adrenaline in the presence of halothane
Antibiotics (streptomycin, kanamycin, neomycin, polymyxin, bacitracin, colistin)	Some of these agents may produce neuromuscular block alone and prolong the block produced by muscle relaxant	Caution using relaxant drugs. Monitor neuromuscular transmission May be antagonized with Ca^{2+}
Anticoagulants	Bleeding from nasotracheal intubation, i.m. injections and local anaesthetic injections Surgical haemorrhage	Avoid i.m. injections Control anticoagulant therapy as described on page 99 Avoid subarachnoid/extradural blocks
Anticholinesterases (ecothiopate eye drops, organophosphorus insecticides)	Inhibition of plasma cholinesterase causes potentiation of suxamethonium and antagonism of curare	Avoid suxamethonium
Anticonvulsants phenytoin phenobarbitone carbamazepine	All these drugs induce liver enzymes	May increase requirements for sedative/anaesthetic agents Avoid enflurane
Antihypertensives reserpine methyldopa guanethidine clonidine	Reserpine depletes noradrenaline stores	Hypotension with all anaesthetic agents, so reduce dosage. Clonidine may allow reduction in dosage of anaesthetics. Action of sympathomimetics increased by guanethidine
Antimitotic drugs cyclophosphamide thiotepa	Inhibit plasma cholinesterase	Caution with suxamethonium
β-Blockers propranolol oxprenolol metoprolol atenolol, etc. timolol eyedrops — may be absorbed systemically	Negative inotropic effects additive with anaesthetic agents to cause exaggerated hypotension. Mask compensatory tachycardia	Monitor β-blockade therapy in perioperative period. Caution with dosage of all CVS-depressant drugs
Barbiturates	Long-term dosage induces liver enzymes and increases metabolism of many drugs	May need to increase dosage of induction agent and opioids
Benzodiazepines	Additive effect with many CNS-depressant drugs Additive effect with competitive muscle relaxants	Caution with induction agents and opioids. Curare potentiated. Suxamethonium antagonized
Ca^{2+} channel blockers verapamil	Depresses AV conduction and excitability. Interacts with volatile anaesthetic agents — bradyarrhythmias and decreased cardiac output	Caution with dosage of volatile anaesthetic agents
nifedipine diltiazem	Vasodilators and negative inotropes interact with volatile agents to produce hypotension. May augment action of competitive muscle relaxants	
Contraceptive pill	Increased incidence of DVT. This risk does not exist with progesterone-only tablets	Discontinue o.c. for at least 6 weeks and cover with alternative contraceptive methods. Use low-dose heparin therapy if surgery is urgent and o.c. cannot be stopped.

Table 18.1 (Cont'd)

Drug	Problems and interactions	Recommendations
Digoxin	Arrhythmias enhanced by calcium. Toxicity enhanced by hypokalaemia. Suxamethonium enhances toxicity. Danger of bradycardia	Avoid calcium. Check serum K^+. Caution in use of suxamethonium
Diuretics	May cause hypokalaemia which prolongs competitive neuromuscular block	Check K^+
Insulins	Hypoglycaemia augmented by subarachnoid and extradural anaesthesia and β-blocking drugs	Further recommendations given on page 676
Monoamine oxidase inhibitors (MAOI) phenelzine iproniazid tranylcypromine isocarboxazide	React with opioids — coma, twitching, CNS excitement → trauma. Severe hypertensive response to pressor agents	Adverse effects do not occur in all patients. Probably safest to withdraw drugs (takes 2–3 weeks) and utilize alternative antidepressants
Lithium	Potentiates non-depolarizing relaxants	Discontinue 48–72 h before anaesthesia
L-Dopa	Risks of tachycardia and arrhythmias with halothane. Actions antagonized by droperidol. Augments hyperglycaemia in diabetes	Discontinue on day of operation
Magnesium	Potentiation of muscle relaxants	Caution with dosage
Phenothiazines	Interact with other hypotensive agents	Caution with dosage of all agents affecting CVS
Quinidine	I.v. quinidine may cause neuromuscular block, especially after suxamethonium	Caution with muscle relaxants
Steroids	Possible hypotension unless increased steroid cover is given	Avoid sympathomimetic amines because of danger of pressor responses
Sulphonamides	Potentiation of thiopentone	
Tricyclic antidepressants	Inhibit the metabolism of catecholamines → arrhythmias. Imipramine potentiates the CVS effects of adrenaline	

been questioned recently in a review of patients taking MAOI who had undergone surgery. However, care must be taken to avoid the well known interactions of MAOI with pethidine and sympathomimetic agents. If opioids are required, morphine is the best drug to use, but in reduced dosage.

The oral contraceptive pill should be discontinued at least 6 weeks before elective surgery because of the increased risk of venous thrombosis.

Physical examination

A full physical examination should be undertaken *and documented in the case records*. The examination should include all systems, even if not directly relevant to the operation. Even in an otherwise healthy individual presenting for relatively minor surgery, it is important to document the findings of full physical examination in case unexpected morbidity arises postoperatively, e.g. foot drop as a result of incorrect positioning on the operating theatre table, prolonged sensory anaesthesia following local anaesthetic techniques, etc.

In addition, the anaesthetist pays particular attention to assessment of the ease of tracheal intubation. The teeth should be inspected closely for the presence of caries, caps, loose teeth and particularly protruding upper incisors. The extent of mouth opening is assessed together with the degree of flexion of the cervical spine and extension of the atlanto-occipital joint. Features associated with difficulty in performing tracheal intubation are described on page 391.

SPECIAL INVESTIGATIONS

It is generally accepted that the clinical history and physical examination represent the best method of screening for the presence of disease. Routine laboratory tests in patients who are apparently healthy on clinical examination and history are invariably of little use and a waste of resources. Before ordering extensive investigations, the anaesthetist should ask himself the following questions:

1. Will this investigation yield information not revealed by physical examination?
2. Will the results of the investigation alter the management of the patient?

In order to reduce the volume of routine preoperative investigations, the following suggestions are made. It should be noted that these are guidelines only and should be modified according to the assessment obtained from the history and clinical examination.

Urine analysis

This should be performed on every patient. It is normally very inexpensive and may occasionally reveal an undiagnosed diabetic or the presence of urinary tract infection.

Haemoglobin concentration

Haemoglobin concentration should be measured in the following situations:

1. Males over 50 years of age.
2. All females.
3. Before major surgery.
4. When clinically indicated, e.g. history of blood loss, pallor, etc.
5. All Asian patients.

Urea and electrolyte concentrations

Serum urea and electrolyte concentrations are not required routinely in patients less than 50 years of age, but should be obtained in the following situations:

1. If there is a history of diarrhoea, vomiting or metabolic disease.
2. In the presence of renal or hepatic disease, diabetes or an abnormal nutritional state.
3. In patients receiving medication with diuretics, digoxin, antihypertensives, steroids or hypoglycaemic agents.

It is important to appreciate that patient who receive preoperative bowel preparation for colonic or rectal surgery may become dehydrated; intravenous fluid replacement may be required and electrolyte status should be monitored carefully.

Liver function tests

Liver function tests are required only in patients with:

1. Hepatic disease.
2. Abnormal nutritional state or metabolic disease.
3. A history of large intake of alcohol (> 80 g.day^{-1}).

Chest X-ray

A chest X-ray is not required routinely in patients below 60 years of age but should be obtained in the following situations:

1. If there is a history or physical signs of cardiac or respiratory disease.
2. If there may be metastases from carcinoma.
3. Before thoracic surgery.
4. In recent immigrants (who have not had a chest X-ray within the previous 12 months) from countries where tuberculosis is endemic.

Other X-rays

Cervical spine X-rays are required in all patients in whom there is anticipated difficulty with tracheal intubation, e.g. in the presence of rheumatoid arthritis. Thoracic inlet X-rays are required in patients with thyroid enlargement.

ECG

A 12-lead electrocardiogram should be obtained in the following situations:

1. If there is a history or physical signs of cardiac disease.

2. In the presence of hypertension.

3. In all patients over the age of 50 years.

Blood sugar concentration

Blood sugar measurement is required in patients receiving corticosteroid drugs and in those who have diabetes or vascular disease.

Sickle status

Patients whose ethnic origin or family history suggests that a haemoglobinopathy may be present should have haemoglobin concentration measured and haemoglobin electrophoresis undertaken. If such patients are scheduled for emergency surgery, a Sickledex test should be performed; if this is positive, haemoglobin electrophoresis should be undertaken as soon as possible but should not delay emergency surgery.

Pulmonary function tests

Peak expiratory flow rate, forced vital capacity and FEV_1 should be measured in all patients with severe dyspnoea on mild to moderate exertion.

Blood gas analysis

Arterial blood gas analysis is required in all patients with dyspnoea at rest and in patients scheduled for elective thoracotomy.

Coagulation tests

Coagulation tests (PTTK and INR) are required in patients who give a history of bleeding disorders, in patients receiving anticoagulant therapy and in those with liver disease.

RISK ASSESSMENT

Preoperative assessment of risk should embrace two broad questions:

1. Is the patient in optimum physical condition for anaesthesia?

2. Are the anticipated benefits of surgery greater than the anaesthetic and surgical risks produced by concurrent medical disease?

In principle, if there is any medical condition which may be improved, (e.g. pulmonary disease, hypertension, cardiac failure, chronic bronchitis, renal disease), surgery should be postponed and appropriate therapy instituted.

There has been great interest recently in quantifying factors preoperatively which correlate with the development of postoperative morbidity and mortality. Some accuracy is possible for populations of patients, but precision does not extend to accurate prediction of risk for an individual patient. Frequently, the decision to proceed can be made only by discussion between surgeon and anaesthetist.

Over a broad range of surgery and patient age, the overall mortality rate from surgery is of the order of 0.6%. This is many times greater than the overall mortality rate attributable to anaesthesia *per se* (approximately 1 in 10 000).

In many large-scale studies of mortality, common factors which have emerged as contributing to anaesthetic mortality include inadequate assessment of patients in the preoperative period, inadequate supervision and monitoring in the intraoperative period and inadequate postoperative supervision and management.

ASA grading

The ASA grading system (Table 18.2) was introduced originally as a simple description of the physical state of a patient. Despite its apparent simplicity, it remains one of the few prospective

Table 18.2 The ASA Physical Status Scale

Class I	A normally healthy individual
Class II	A patient with mild systemic disease
Class III	A patient with severe systemic disease that is not incapacitating
Class IV	A patient with incapacitating systemic disease that is a constant threat to life
Class V	A moribund patient who is not expected to survive 24 h with or without operation
Class E	Added as a suffix for emergency operation.

Table 18.3 Mortality rates after anaesthesia and surgery for each ASA physical status — emergency and elective cases

ASA rating	Mortality rate (%)
I	0.1
II	0.2
III	1.8
IV	7.8
V	9.4

descriptions of the patient which correlate with the risk of anaesthesia and surgery (Table 18.3). However, it does not embrace all aspects of anaesthetic risk, as there is no allowance for inclusion of many criteria such as age or difficulty in intubation. Nevertheless, it is extremely useful and should be applied to all patients who present for surgery.

Cardiovascular disease

Myocardial infarction

A large number of studies undertaken retrospectively in the 1970s demonstrated that the incidence of perioperative myocardial infarction (MI) was 0.1–0.4% in previously healthy patients, but 3.2–7.7% in patients who had suffered a previous MI. The majority of perioperative infarctions occur on the third day after surgery and 50% are silent. The mortality associated with perioperative MI is 40–60%.

It is accepted generally that the development of perioperative reinfarction is related closely to the time interval between the first MI and surgery and that an interval of 6 months or less is associated with the highest incidence of reinfarction. However, two studies suggested that the rate of reinfarction and also cardiac death in patients with recent MI may be reduced greatly if patients are subjected to intensive invasive monitoring (radial artery cannulation and pulmonary artery catheterization) and if heart rate and systemic arterial pressure are not allowed to fluctuate by more than 20% from preoperative values. In these studies, arrhythmias and tachycardia were treated immediately and monitoring and treatment were continued in the ITU for 3–4 days after surgery. Unfortunately, it is not possible to

monitor all patients for such a prolonged period of time in ITU and there are no data to identify which subgroup of patients requires more extensive monitoring or treatment than others. Consequently, it is still recommended that a myocardial infarction within 6 months of proposed surgery is a contraindication to elective anaesthesia and surgery, unless the risks of postponing surgery outweigh the likelihood of perioperative infarction.

Hypertension

There is some dispute as to whether or not arterial hypertension increases the risk of morbidity after anaesthesia and surgery. Arterial pressure increases with age and on admission to the ward there is often some degree of hypertension associated with anxiety. The arterial pressure should therefore be measured at regular intervals in the preoperative period in order to assess the resting baseline level. The question then arises as to what constitutes hypertension. It is difficult to be precise on this point, but several authorities have formed the view that a diastolic pressure in excess of 110 mmHg is associated with an increased risk of myocardial ischaemia.

Gross hypertensive responses, with ECG evidence of ischaemia on some occasions, are likely to occur in response to noxious stimuli during anaesthesia in hypertensive patients, whether treated or not, if the preoperative diastolic pressure exceeds 110 mmHg. Episodes of marked hypertension, ischaemic ST changes on ECG and the combination of hypotension and tachycardia are associated with an increased incidence of postoperative myocardial infarction. It follows that patients should be prepared for surgery in such a way that these changes are less likely to occur. Thus, patients who present preoperatively with a diastolic arterial pressure in excess of 110 mmHg should receive antihypertensive treatment. As several days or weeks may be required to stabilize the cardiovascular system, surgery should be postponed for 2–3 weeks.

Multifactorial assessment of risk

Goldman and his colleagues have examined by multivariate analysis a number of risk factors

Table 18.4 Goldman's index of cardiac risk in non-cardiac procedures (modified)

Risk factor	Points
3rd heart sound or jugular venous distension	11
MI in preceding 6 months	10
Rhythm other than sinus or premature atrial contractions	7
More than 5 ventricular ectopic beats per min	7
Abdominal, thoracic, or aortic operation	3
Age > 70 years	5
Important aortic stenosis	3
Emergency operation	4
Poor condition as defined by any one of:	3
$PaO_2 < 8\,kPa$ $PaCO_2 > 6.5\,kPa$ $K^+ < 3.0\,mmol.litre^{-1}$ $HCO_3^- < 20\,mmol.litre^{-1}$ urea $> 7.5\,mmol.litre^{-1}$ creatinine $> 270\,\mu mol.litre^{-1}$ SGOT abnormal chronic liver disease	
Total	53

0–5 points — major cardiac complications 0.3–3%
6–12 points — major cardiac complications 1–10%
13–25 points — major cardiac complications 3–30%
26–53 points — major cardiac complications 19–75%

in patients undergoing non-cardiac surgery and produced a risk index (Table 18.4) for the development of life-threatening cardiovascular complications in the perioperative period. The 'Goldman Cardiac Risk Index' has been shown in several studies to provide a reasonable prognostic indication of the risk of developing cardiac complications postoperatively.

Pulmonary disease

Patients at risk of developing postoperative pulmonary complications include smokers, those with pre-existing lung disease, the obese and those undergoing thoracic and abdominal surgery.

Unfortunately, sophisticated tests of pulmonary function (e.g. FRC, closing capacity, pulmonary diffusing capacity, etc.) are no more valuable in assessment of lung disease than simple spirometric tests, particularly vital capacity, forced vital capacity and FEV_1. Blood gas analysis is the most sensitive method of predicting the need for IPPV in the postoperative period.

Age

It is generally agreed that the elderly are subject to increased risks of anaesthesia and surgery. This is largely because of the association between many diseases of the cardiovascular or respiratory systems and age and also because routine clinical evaluation often fails to detect cardiorespiratory dysfunction in geriatric patients.

Prediction of risk factors in general

Factors which are of greatest importance in predicting the development of postoperative morbidity and mortality include, in decreasing order of importance:

1. Clinical assessment – ASA greater than 3.
2. Cardiac failure.
3. Cardiac risk index.
4. Pulmonary disease.
5. Pulmonary abnormalities confirmed by X-ray.
6. ECG abnormalities.

Common causes for postponing surgery

1. *Acute upper respiratory tract infection* (common cold). Although many patients may admit to the presence of a cold, clarification of such an admission should be made. In general, the presence of nasal secretions, pyrexia or the unexpected presence of physical signs on clinical examination of the chest suggest that surgery should be postponed for a few weeks until the patient has recovered.

2. *Existing medical disease* (cardiac, respiratory, endocrine, etc.), which is not under optimum control (see Ch. 40).

3. *Emergency surgery for which the patient has not been resuscitated adequately.* Postponement may be necessary for only 1–2 h to permit restoration of circulating blood volume. This important principle may be breached if haemorrhage is extensive and continuous.

4. *Recent ingestion of food.* In general, anaesthesia for elective surgery should not be undertaken within 4–6 h of ingestion of food. Recently, it has been suggested that it may be safe for patients to take clear fluids up to 3 h before surgery.

5. *Failure to obtain informed consent.* Informed consent for surgery should be obtained from all patients. Consent is invalid if obtained after the patient has received premedicant drugs. Consent from a parent or guardian is required if the patient is under 16 years of age in England or Wales or under 14 years of age in Scotland. If parents or guardians cannot be contacted, consent may be obtained from a court of law or, in the case of emergency surgery, from a District Medical Officer.

6. *Drug therapy.* It is unwise to proceed to anaesthesia if the patient is receiving drug therapy which is not under optimum control.

PREOPERATIVE THERAPY

Having taken a full clinical history and performed a physical examination, reviewed the special investigations and decided that it is reasonable to proceed to anaesthesia and surgery, the anaesthetist should decide if further measures are required to prepare the patient satisfactorily. Some common problems are detailed below.

Respiratory disease

In patients with respiratory disease who are regarded as fit for surgery, chest physiotherapy should be started preoperatively. In addition, sputum should be obtained for bacteriological examination and culture to determine optimum antibiotic therapy in the event of postoperative chest infection.

Asthma

Chest physiotherapy should be started preoperatively. If severe asthma is present, instruction may be required in the use of appropriate bronchodilators, e.g. salbutamol by inhaler.

Cardiovascular disease

Subacute bacterial endocarditis

For those at risk of developing subacute bacterial endocarditis, prophylactic antibiotics are required, as described in Appendix IIIc (p. 738).

Hypertension

In patients who are found to be hypertensive on admission, regular measurement of arterial pressure should be undertaken. Frequently, pressure declines as the initial anxiety of admission becomes attenuated. If the diastolic pressure decreases below 110 mmHg, it is reasonable to proceed with surgery. If diastolic pressure remains above 110 mmHg, surgery should be postponed and the patient referred to a physician. If the patient is a known hypertensive receiving therapy, adjustment of the dosage of antihypertensives may be required.

It is essential that antihypertensive therapy be continued throughout the postoperative period. Many β-blocking drugs have a relatively short half-life and if a patient is receiving such therapy it may be preferable to change to a drug with a long duration of action, such as atenolol or nadolol. If bowel function is likely to remain disturbed for several days postoperatively, it may be necessary to use an i.v. infusion of atenolol $2-6$ mg.h^{-1} or labetalol $2.5-10$ mg.h^{-1}.

Diabetic management

See page 677.

Obstructive jaundice

This is associated with the hepatorenal syndrome and bleeding problems. To minimize the risk of renal failure, an i.v. infusion should be started on the night before surgery. Glucose 5% should be infused at a rate of 100 ml.h^{-1}. In addition, mannitol 20 g should be given just before or at induction of anaesthesia. Vitamin K may be prescribed in a dose of 10 mg i.m. daily preoperatively and postoperatively for 3 days.

Blood transfusion requests

Blood is an expensive commodity and blood transfusion carries very small but finite risks of incompatibility reactions and transmission of infection. Blood should therefore be used only if absolutely necessary. The object of transfusion is to ensure that the postoperative haemoglobin concentration does not decline to less than 10 g.dl^{-1}.

Thus the amount of blood ordered from the blood transfusion service depends upon both the patient's preoperative haemoglobin concentration and the extent of surgery.

Guidelines on the quantity of blood to request from the blood transfusion service are shown in Table 18.5.

PREMEDICATION

Premedication refers to the administration of drugs in the period 1–2 h before induction of anaesthesia. The objectives of premedication are to:

1. Allay anxiety and fear.
2. Reduce secretions.
3. Enhance the hypnotic effect of general anaesthetic agents.
4. Reduce postoperative nausea and vomiting.
5. Produce amnesia.
6. Reduce the volume and increase the pH of gastric contents.
7. Attenuate vagal reflexes.
8. Attenuate sympathoadrenal responses.

Table 18.5 Guidelines for ordering blood for routine surgery

Group and screen only
Amputation
Bladder tumour: transurethral resection
Cervical rib and thoracic inlet exploration
Cholecystectomy and exploration of bile duct
Colostomy, gastrostomy: closure or formation of
Cone biopsy of cervix
Embolectomy
Femoral nail: removal of
Glossectomy
Hysterectomy
Laminectomy
Laparoscopy
Laparotomy: planned exploratory
Mastectomy: simple
Mastoidectomy
Mediastinoscopy
Osteotomy: bone biopsy
Ovary: wedge resection
Pacemaker: insertion of
Palate: resection of
Parathyroidectomy
Pinning of long bone (planned)
Prostatectomy: transurethral
Salivary gland: dissection of
Splenectomy
Sympathectomy: abdominal
Tonsillectomy
Tracheostomy
Tubal (Fallopian) surgery
Ureters: reimplantation
Vagotomy and pyloroplasty

Group, screen and crossmatch one unit of blood
Carotid or femoral endarterectomy
Ovarian cystectomy
Pinning fractured neck of femur

Group, screen and crossmatch two units of blood
Abdominoperineal resection
Arthroplasty knee/shoulder
Atrioventricular septal defect
Brachial plexus repair
Fallot's tetralogy (depends on age)
Laryngectomy

Mastectomy: radical
Maxillectomy
Myomectomy
Nephrectomy or graft nephrectomy
Ovarian carcinoma
Patent ductus arteriosus
Prostatectomy: suprapubic
Pyelolithotomy: 1st operation
Renal transplantation
Spinal fusion
Thoracotomy: pneumonectomy
                wedge resection
Total or hemicolectomy or anterior resection of rectum

Group, screen and crossmatch three units of blood
Adrenalectomy
Femoropopliteal bypass
Gastrectomy: partial
Hip: arthroplasty
Hysterectomy: Wertheim
Pulmonary valvulotomy

Group, screen and crossmatch four units of blood
Aortoiliac or aortofemoral bypass
Commando operation
Coronary vein graft
Gastrectomy: total
Hip prosthesis: change of
Mitral commissurotomy
Pancreatectomy: partial
Pyelolithotomy: repeat operations

Group, screen and crossmatch six units of blood
Coronary vein grafts: repeat operations
Oesophagectomy
Pancreatectomy: total
Partial hepatectomy
Radical cystectomy
Valve replacement: single
Ventricular aneurysm

Group, screen and crossmatch eight units of blood
Aortic aneurysm: abdominal
Aortic aneurysm: thoracic
Valve replacement: double
Vein graft and valve replacement

Relief from anxiety

Surgical patients have a high incidence of anxiety and there is a significant inverse relationship between anxiety and smoothness of induction of anaesthesia. Relief from anxiety is accomplished most effectively by non-pharmacological means, which may be termed psychotherapy. This is effected at the preoperative visit by establishment of rapport, explanation of events which occur in the perioperative period and reassurance regarding the patient's expressed anxieties and fears. There is good evidence that psychotherapy has a significant calming effect.

In some patients, reassurance and explanation may be insufficient to allay anxiety. Thus it is customary and traditional to prescribe anxiolytic medication; the benzodiazepine drugs are the most effective for this purpose.

Reduction in secretions

The older anaesthetic agents, ether and cyclopropane, stimulate the production of secretions from pharyngeal and bronchial glands. This effect occurs only to a minor degree with modern anaesthetic agents and so anticholinergic premedication is not essential. However, many anaesthetists continue to prescribe anticholinergic drugs to reduce the secretions produced by the presence of an airway or tracheal tube in the mouth and larynx.

Ketamine tends to promote secretions and an anticholinergic premedication should be prescribed before using this agent.

Sedation

Sedation is not synonymous with anxiolysis. Some drugs, e.g. the barbiturates and to a lesser extent the opioids, possess sedative but no anxiolytic properties. In general, it is unnecessary to use a sedative preoperatively unless the patient expresses a preference for this. An exception to this may be in paediatric practice.

Postoperative antiemesis

Nausea and vomiting are extremely common after anaesthesia. Opioid drugs administered during and after operation are often responsible. Occasionally, antiemetics may be given with the premedication, but they are more effective if administered intravenously during anaesthesia.

Amnesia

Under some circumstances it may be desirable for patients, especially children, to be amnesic for the immediate perioperative period in case unpleasant memories cause difficulties if subsequent operations are required. However, some anaesthetists believe that amnesia should not be induced in children, otherwise they may associate natural sleep with awakening to find a surgical incision.

Although claims have been made for retrograde amnesia, it is unlikely that this is ever achieved. However, anterograde amnesia (after administration of a drug) is produced commonly by the benzodiazepines; in this respect, lorazepam is two to five times more potent than diazepam. It is totally inappropriate to prescribe an amnesic drug with the object of reducing the risks of awareness during anaesthesia.

Reduction in gastric volume and elevation of gastric pH

In patients who are at risk of vomiting or regurgitation (e.g. emergency patients with a full stomach or elective patients with hiatus hernia or pharyngeal pouch), it may be desirable to promote gastric emptying and elevate the pH of residual gastric contents. Gastric emptying may be enhanced by the administration of metoclopramide, which also possesses some antiemetic properties, whilst elevation of the pH of gastric contents may be produced by administration of sodium citrate. This topic is described in greater detail in Chapter 13.

Reduction in vagal reflexes

Vagal bradycardia, which may be severe, may occur in several situations:

1. Traction on the eye muscles, particularly the rectus medialis during squint surgery, leads to bradycardia and/or arrhythmias (the oculocardiac

reflex). Premedication with atropine protects against this, but it is not as effective as the i.v. administration of atropine at induction of anaesthesia or in anticipation of traction on the muscles.

2. Repeated administration of suxamethonium commonly gives rise to bradycardia, which may proceed to asystole. Administration of atropine should always precede the administration of a second dose of suxamethonium.

3. Induction of anaesthesia with halothane, particularly in children, may be associated with bradycardia.

4. Surgical stimulation during an opioid/relaxant technique employing one of the newer muscle relaxants (atracurium or vecuronium) may be associated with bradycardia.

Limitation of sympathoadrenal responses

Induction of anaesthesia and tracheal intubation may be associated with marked sympathoadrenal activity, manifest by tachycardia, hypertension and elevation of plasma catecholamine concentrations. These responses are undesirable in the healthy individual and may be harmful in patients with hypertension or ischaemic heart disease. β-blockings drugs are sometimes given with the premedication in order to attenuate these responses.

Some of the objectives listed above may be achieved by administration of drugs at induction or during maintenance of anaesthesia. The only essential requirement of premedication in the period before anaesthesia is anxiolysis. The ability to achieve all objectives by administration of a variety of drugs either preoperatively or at induction is responsible for the wide variation in prescribing habits amongst anaesthetists. The commonest regimens used for premedication are shown in Table 18.6.

Drugs used for premedication

Benzodiazepines

The benzodiazepines possess several properties which are useful for premedication, including anxiolysis, sedation and amnesia. The extent of each of these effects differs among individual drugs. Lorazepam produces a greater degree of amnesia than diazepam. In addition, diazepam and lorazepam may produce anxiolysis in doses that do not produce excessive sedation. The drugs are thought to increase brain receptor sensitivity to γ-aminobutyric acid (GABA).

Absorption of diazepam after i.m. administration is relatively poor; absorption from the gastrointestinal tract is more reliable. This accounts for the popularity of the oral route for administration of diazepam. In contrast, lorazepam is absorbed equally well after i.m. or oral administration. Standard preparations of diazepam should not be given by the i.v. route because of the high incidence of thrombophlebitis; the incidence is reduced substantially if diazepam is administered in a lipid emulsion (Diazemuls).

In patients who are particularly anxious, it is common practice to prescribe a benzodiazepine as a hypnotic on the night before operation and to employ the same drug for premedication the following morning.

Table 18.6 Common premedication regimens (doses are suitable only for healthy adult male)

Drug (combination)	Dose (mg)	Route of administration	Comments
Papaveretum Hyoscine	20 0.4	i.m. i.m. }	Profound sedation. 'Omnopon & scopolamine' still very commonly used combination
Diazepam	10–15	oral	Good anxiolysis but effect variable
Lorazepam	2–3	oral	Marked anterograde amnesia. Prolonged action
Diazepam Metoclopramide	10 10	oral oral }	Metoclopramide increases the tone of the lower oesophageal sphincter and possesses antiemetic effect
Morphine Atrophine	10 0.6	i.m. i.m. }	Frequently used when less profound sedation is required than 'Omnopon & scopolamine'
Promethazine Atropine	50 0.6	i.m. i.m. }	Frequently prescribed for asthmatic patients

Cimetidine delays the plasma clearance of diazepam but not lorazepam.

Unfortunately, there is a very wide variation in response to benzodiazepines and effects may be unpredictable. Although physostigmine has been used in the past to reverse excessive sedation produced by benzodiazepines, a specific antagonist (flumazenil) is now available.

Opioid analgesics

It is necessary to prescribe opioid analgesic drugs for premedication only when patients are in pain preoperatively. This is uncommon except in the emergency situation; nevertheless, opioid drugs are employed commonly for premedication.

The opioids cause sedation, but are not good anxiolytic agents. Although they produce euphoria in the presence of pain, they tend to cause dysphoria in its absence. Because of their long duration of action, they contribute to a smoother intraoperative course and provide some analgesia in the early postoperative period. Tachypnoea, which occurs during spontaneous breathing of volatile agents, is reduced and a lower concentration of anaesthetic agent is required for maintenance of anaesthesia. However, it is more logical in many respects to administer opioids intravenously at or after induction of anaesthesia rather than intramuscularly for premedication.

There are several important side-effects of the opioids:

1. Depression of ventilation and delayed resumption of spontaneous ventilation at the end of N_2O/O_2 relaxant techniques.

2. Nausea and vomiting produced by stimulation of the chemoreceptor trigger zone in the medulla are extremely common. Opioids should always be used in combination with an antiemetic agent, such as hyoscine, a phenothiazine or a butyrophenone.

3. Morphine causes spasm of the sphincter of Oddi and this may result in right upper quadrant pain, particularly in patients presenting for surgery on the biliary tract.

4. Morphine causes histamine release and is generally regarded as contraindicated in asthmatics.

Butyrophenones

Of the two butyrophenones, haloperidol and droperidol, only the latter enjoys current popularity in anaesthetic practice. This drug possesses neuroleptic effects (which may be manifest as withdrawal and seclusion), α-blocking actions and antiemetic effects. Occasionally, droperidol may produce dose-dependent dysphoric reactions and extrapyramidal side-effects.

Butyrophenones possess a very long duration of action and this may delay recovery from anaesthesia, particularly in elderly patients. The commonest use for droperidol in anaesthetic practice is as an antiemetic agent, administered either with the premedication in a dose of 2.5 mg or intravenously during anaesthesia in a dose of 1.25 mg.

Phenothiazines

These are useful agents for premedication because they produce the following effects:

1. Central antiemetic action.
2. Sedation.
3. Anxiolysis.
4. H_2-receptor antagonism.
5. α-adrenergic antagonism.
6. Anticholinergic properties.
7. Potentiation of opioid analgesia.

Disadvantages include extrapyramidal side-effects, synergism with opioids which may delay postoperative recovery and potentiation of the hypotensive effects of anaesthetic agents. Postoperatively (particularly in children given trimeprazine) the patient may exhibit pallor with mild tachycardia and hypotension, mimicking the signs of hypovolaemia.

Anticholinergic agents

The three anticholinergic agents used commonly in anaesthesia are atropine, hyoscine and glycopyrronium. Atropine and hyoscine are tertiary amines that cross the blood–brain barrier; glycopyrronium is a quarternary amine, does not cross the blood–brain barrier and is not absorbed from the gastrointestinal tract. Although atropine is absorbed from the gastrointestinal tract, this occurs in an unpredictable manner and is dependent upon gastric content, pH and motility.

These three drugs differ with respect to their dose–response effects at various cholinergic receptors. In standard clinical doses, hyoscine 0.4 mg differs from atropine 0.6 mg in that there is greater antisialagogue effect and little action on cardiac vagal receptors. Hyoscine possesses sedative and amnesic actions and, in contrast to atropine, does not cause stimulation of higher centres. Hyoscine should be avoided in the elderly (over 60 years) as it produces dysphoria and restlessness. Glycopyrronium has no central effects, a much longer duration of action and in a standard clinical dose of 0.4 mg causes less change in heart rate than atropine 0.6 mg.

Anticholinergic drugs are used clinically to produce:

1. *Antisialagogue effects.* Glycopyrronium and hyoscine are more potent in this respect than atropine. These drugs block secretions when irritant anaesthetic gases are used and reduce excessive secretions and bradycardia associated with suxamethonium when it is given either repeatedly or as an infusion.

2. *Sedative and amnesic effects.* In combination with morphine, hyoscine produces powerful sedative and amnesic effects.

3. *Prevention of reflex bradycardia.* Anticholinergics are given for both prophylaxis and treatment of bradycardia. Atropine is used very commonly as premedication in ophthalmic surgery to block the oculocardiac reflex in patients undergoing squint surgery and is used also in small children to reduce the bradycardia which may occur in association with halothane anaesthesia.

Side effects of anticholinergic drugs include:

1. *CNS toxicity.* The *central anticholinergic syndrome* is produced by stimulation of the CNS (usually by atropine). Symptoms include restlessness, agitation and somnolence and, in extreme cases, convulsions and coma. With hyoscine there is more commonly prolonged somnolence. Physostigmine 1–2 mg i.v. has been recommended to reverse the central anticholinergic syndrome and should be given in combination with glycopyrronium to prevent profound muscarinic effects produced by physostigmine.

2. *Reduction in lower oesophageal sphincter tone.* Theoretically, a reduction in tone may lead to increased risk of gastro-oesophageal reflux, although in clinical practice there is no suggestion that the use of anticholinergics for premedication is associated with an increased incidence of preoperative aspiration.

3. *Tachycardia,* which should be avoided in cardiac conditions (e.g. obstructive cardiomyopathy, valvular stenosis and ischaemic heart disease) or when a hypotensive anaesthetic technique is planned.

4. *Mydriasis and cycloplegia,* which lead to visual impairment. This may be troublesome, but is not a serious side-effect. Theoretically, mydriasis may be associated with reduced drainage of aqueous from the anterior chamber of the eye, thereby increasing intraocular pressure in patients with glaucoma. However, this effect is not important in practice and atropine may be prescribed safely to patients with glaucoma provided that appropriate therapy is maintained.

5. *Pyrexia.* By suppressing secretion of sweat, anticholinergics predispose to elevation in body temperature. These drugs should therefore be avoided in the presence of pyrexia, particularly in children.

6. *Excessive drying.* Although anticholinergics are given for the specific purpose of producing antisialagogue effects, this may be most unpleasant for the patient.

7. *Increased physiological dead space.* Atropine and hyoscine increase physiological dead space by 20–25% but this is compensated for by an increase in ventilation.

FURTHER READING

Fee J P H, McCaughey W 1994 Preoperative preparation, premedication and concurrent drug therapy. In: Nimmo W S, Rowbotham D J, Smith G (eds) Anaesthesia. Blackwell Scientific Publications, London, p 677–703

Mason R A 1994 Anaesthesia databook, 2nd edn. A clinical practice compendium. Churchill Livingstone, Edinburgh

Strunin L 1993 How long should patients fast before surgery? Time for new guidelines. British Journal of Anaesthesia 70: 1–3

19. The practical conduct of anaesthesia

Planning the conduct of anaesthesia starts normally after details concerning the surgical procedure and the medical condition of the patient have been ascertained at the preoperative visit. Preoperative assessment and selection of appropriate premedication are discussed in Chapter 18.

PREPARATION FOR ANAESTHESIA

Before embarking on the anaesthetic, consideration should be given to the induction and maintenance of anaesthesia, the position of the patient on the operating table, equipment necessary for monitoring, the use of intravenous fluids or blood for infusion and the postoperative care and recovery facilities which will be required.

Table 19.1 Equipment required for tracheal intubation

Correct size of laryngoscope and spare (in case of light failure)

Tracheal tube of correct size + an alternative smaller size

Tracheal tube connector

Wire stilette

Gum elastic bougies

Magill forceps

Cuff-inflating syringe

Artery forceps

Securing tape or bandage

Catheter mount(s)

Local anaesthetic spray – 4% lignocaine

Cocaine spray/gel for nasal intubation

Tracheal tube lubricant

Throat packs

Anaesthetic breathing system and face masks – tested with O_2 to ensure no leaks present

The anaesthetic machine to be used must be tested for leaks, misconnections and proper function. A check list, for example that published by the Association of Anaesthetists of Great Britain and Ireland, is recommended.

The availability and function of all anaesthetic equipment should be checked before starting (see Table 19.1). After the patient's arrival in the anaesthetic room, the anaesthetist should be satisfied that the correct operation is being performed upon the correct patient and that consent has been given. The patient must be on a tilting bed or trolley and the anaesthetist should have a competent assistant.

INDUCTION OF ANAESTHESIA

Anaesthesia is induced using one of the following techniques.

Inhalational induction

The most common indications for induction of anaesthesia by an inhalational technique are listed in Table 19.2.

The proposed procedure should be explained to the patient before starting. A 'no-mask' technique using a cupped hand around the fresh gas

Table 19.2 Indications for inhalational induction

Young children

Upper airway obstruction, e.g. epiglottitis

Lower airway obstruction with foreign body

Bronchopleural fistula or empyema

No accessible veins

delivery tube may be preferred for young children; some anaesthetists favour allowing the child to play with the mask before connecting the anaesthetic tubing. The mask or hand is introduced *gradually* to the face from the side as the sight of a black mask descending on to the face may be disturbing. While talking to the patient and encouraging him to breathe normally, the anaesthetist adjusts the mixture of the fresh gas flow and observes the patient's reactions. Initially, nitrous oxide 70% in oxygen is used and anaesthesia is deepened by the gradual introduction of increments of a volatile agent, e.g. halothane 1–3%. Maintenance concentrations of halothane (1–2%), enflurane (1.5–2.5%) or isoflurane (1–2%) are used when anaesthesia has been established.

A single-breath technique of inhalational induction has been advocated for patients who are able to cooperate. One vital capacity breath from a prefilled 4-litre reservoir bag containing a high concentration of volatile agent (e.g. halothane 5%) in oxygen (or nitrous oxide 50% in oxygen) results in smooth induction of anaesthesia within 20–30 s.

Observation of the colour of the patient's skin and pattern of ventilation, palpation of the peripheral pulse, ECG and Sp_{O_2} monitoring and measurement of arterial pressure are important accompaniments to the technique of inhalational induction.

If spontaneous ventilation is to be maintained throughout the procedure, the mask is applied more firmly as consciousness is lost and the airway is supported manually. Insertion of an oropharyngeal airway, a laryngeal mask airway or a tracheal tube may be considered when anaesthesia has been established.

Difficulties and complications

1. Slow induction of anaesthesia.
2. Problems particularly during stage 2 (see below).
3. Airway obstruction, bronchospasm.
4. Laryngeal spasm, hiccups.
5. Environmental pollution.

Intravenous induction

Induction of anaesthesia with an i.v. agent is suitable for most routine purposes and avoids many of the complications associated with the inhalational technique. It is the most appropriate method of rapid induction for the patient undergoing emergency surgery, in whom there is a risk of regurgitation of gastric contents during induction. All drugs which may be required at induction should be prepared and a cannula inserted into a suitable vein before starting.

If an existing i.v. cannula is to be used, its function must be checked. 'Butterfly' type needles or cannulae with a side injection port ('Venflon' type) are useful; large cannulae (e.g. 16G, 14G) are necessary for transfusion of fluids or blood. A vein in the forearm or back of the hand is preferable; veins in the antecubital fossa are best avoided because of the risks of intra-arterial injection. After selection of a suitable vein, skin preparation is performed using iodine or alcohol. Subcutaneous local anaesthetic should be used where a large cannula is to be employed. Alternatively, 'EMLA' local anaesthetic cream may have been applied preoperatively. Intravenous entry is confirmed with blood aspiration and the device secured firmly with tape. 'Opsite' dressing may be used when long-term use is anticipated.

Monitoring should be commenced before induction of anaesthesia, including Sp_{O_2}, ECG and arterial pressure measurement. Preoxygenation may be started, using a close-fitting facemask and 100% oxygen delivered, for example, by a Magill breathing system for 5 min. Alternatively 3–4 large (vital capacity) breaths may be used.

Doses of the common i.v. agents are shown in Table 19.3. The induction dose varies with the patient's weight, age, state of nutrition, circulatory status, premedication and any concurrent medication. A small test dose is administered commonly and its effects are observed. Slow injection is

Table 19.3 Intravenous induction agents

Agent	Induction dose (mg.kg^{-1})
Thiopentone	3–5
Methohexitone	1–1.5
Etomidate	0.3
Propofol	1.5–2.5
Ketamine	2

recommended in the aged and in those with a slow circulation time (e.g. shock, hypovolaemia, cardiovascular disease) while the effects of the drug on the cardiovascular and respiratory systems are monitored.

A rapid-sequence induction technique is indicated for patients undergoing emergency surgery and for those in whom vomiting or regurgitation is a potential problem. After i.v. induction, a rapid transition to stage 3 anaesthesia (see below) is achieved; this is maintained by the introduction of an inhalational agent or by repeated bolus injections or a continuous infusion of an i.v. anaesthetic agent. Emergency anaesthesia is discussed fully in Chapter 31.

Complications and difficulties

1. *Regurgitation and vomiting.* If regurgitation occurs, the patient should be placed immediately into the Trendelenburg position and material aspirated with suction apparatus. Should inhalation of gastric contents occur, treatment with 100% oxygen, bronchodilators, tracheal suction and toilet, steroids and antibiotics should be started immediately. Continued IPPV may be required if the resultant pneumonitis is severe.

2. *Intra-arterial injection of thiopentone.* This causes pain and blanching in hand and fingers as a result of crystal formation in the capillaries. The needle should be left in the artery and 5 ml 0.5% procaine and 40 mg papaverine injected. Further treatment includes stellate ganglion block, brachial plexus block or sympathetic block with i.v. guanethidine.

3. *Perivenous injection.* This causes blanching and pain and may result in a small degree of tissue necrosis. Methohexitone and propofol produce less tissue damage than thiopentone. Hyaluronidase may be used to speed dispersal of the drug.

4. *Cardiovascular depression.* This is likely to occur particularly in the elderly, the hypovolaemic or the untreated hypertensive patient. Reducing the dose and speed of injection is recommended in these patients. Infusion of i.v. fluid (e.g. 500 ml colloid or 1000 ml crystalloid solution) is usually successful in restoring arterial pressure.

5. *Respiratory depression.* Slow injection of an induction agent may reduce the extent of respiratory depression. Respiratory adequacy must be assessed carefully and the anaesthetist should be ready to assist ventilation of the lungs if necessary.

6. *Histamine release.* Thiopentone or methohexitone may cause release of histamine with subsequent formation of typical weals. Severe reactions may occur to individual agents and appropriate drugs and fluids should be available in the anaesthetic room for treatment. Guidelines for emergency management of acute major anaphylaxis are available (Association of Anaesthetists of Great Britain and Ireland) and may be displayed in the anaesthetic room.

7. *Porphyria.* An acute porphyric episode may be precipitated by barbiturates in susceptible individuals.

8. *Other complications.* Pain on injection (especially with methohexitone, etomidate or propofol), hiccup or muscular movements may occur.

POSITION OF PATIENT FOR SURGERY

After induction of anaesthesia, the patient is placed on the operating table in a position appropriate for the proposed surgery. When positioning the patient, the anaesthetist should take into account surgical access, patient safety, anaesthetic technique, monitoring and position of i.v. lines, etc.

Some commonly used positions are shown in Figure 19.1. Each may have adverse effects in terms of skeletal, neurological, ventilatory and circulatory effects.

1. The *lithotomy* position may result in nerve damage on the medial or lateral side of the leg from pressure exerted by the stirrups, which must be well padded. Care must be taken to elevate both legs simultaneously so that pelvic asymmetry and resultant backache are avoided. The sacrum should be supported on the operating table and not allowed to slip off the end.

2. The *lateral* position may result in asymmetrical lung ventilation (see Ch. 38). Care is required with arm position and i.v. infusions. The pelvis and shoulders must be supported to prevent the patient from rolling either backwards (with a risk of falling from the table) or forwards into the recovery position.

3. The *prone* position may cause abdominal

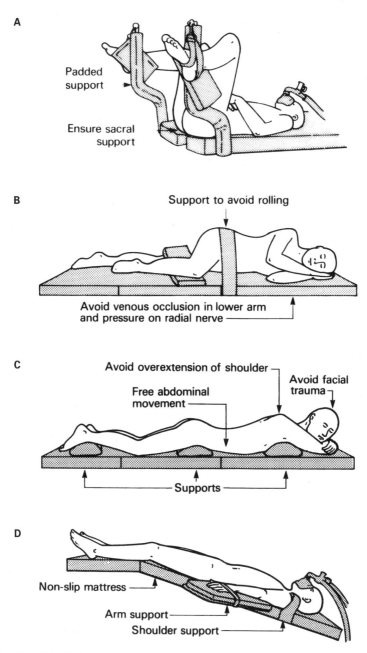

Fig. 19.1 Positions on the operating table; (**A**) lithotomy; (**B**) lateral; (**C**) prone; (**D**) Trendelenburg.

compression which may result in ventilatory and circulatory embarrassment. To prevent this, support must be provided beneath the shoulders and iliac crests. Excessive extension of the shoulders should be avoided. The face, and particularly the eyes, must be protected from trauma. The

tracheal tube must be secured firmly in place as it is almost impossible to reinsert it with the patient in this position.

4. The *Trendelenburg* position may produce upward pressure on the diaphragm because of the weight of the abdominal contents. Damage to the

brachial plexus may occur as a result of pressure from shoulder supports, especially if the arms are abducted.

5. The *sitting* position requires careful support of the head. In addition, venous pooling and resultant cardiovascular instability may occur.

6. The *supine* position carries the risk of the supine hypotensive syndrome during pregnancy (see Ch. 32) or in patients with a large abdominal mass.

MAINTENANCE OF ANAESTHESIA

Anaesthesia may be continued using inhalational agents, i.v. anaesthetic agents or i.v. opioids either alone or in combination. Tracheal intubation with or without muscle relaxants may be employed. Regional anaesthesia may be used to supplement any of these techniques.

Inhalational anaesthesia with spontaneous ventilation

This is an appropriate form of maintenance for superficial operations, minor procedures which produce little reflex or painful stimulation and operations for which profound muscle relaxation is not required.

Conduct

After induction of anaesthesia, inhalational and/or volatile agents may be used in the spontaneously breathing patient. Depending on the nature of surgery, the provision of analgesia in the premedication and the patient's response (assessed by observation of ventilation, circulation and heart rate and rhythm), halothane 1–2% inspired concentration may be employed in a mixture with nitrous oxide 70% in oxygen; enflurane 1.5–2.5% or isoflurane 1–2% are alternatives to halothane.

Minimum alveolar concentration (MAC)

MAC is the minimum alveolar concentration of an inhaled anaesthetic agent which prevents reflex movement in response to surgical incision in 50% of subjects. MAC values of commonly used inhalational agents are shown in Appendix II (p. 733). MAC varies little with metabolic factors but is reduced by opioid premedication and in the presence of hypothermia. MAC is higher in neonates and is reduced in the elderly (see Ch. 8).

The effects of inhalational anaesthetics are additive; thus 1 MAC-equivalent could be achieved by producing an alveolar concentration of 70% nitrous oxide (0.67 MAC) and 0.25% halothane (0.33 MAC).

The rate at which MAC is attained may be increased by raising the inspired concentration and by avoidance of airway obstruction. Increasing ventilation at a constant inspired concentration produces more rapid equilibration between inspired and alveolar concentrations. The time taken for equilibration increases with the blood/gas solubility coefficient of the agent; those with a high blood/gas solubility coefficient do not reach equilibrium for several hours (see Ch. 8). It follows therefore that the inspired concentration must be considerably higher than MAC to produce an adequate alveolar concentration when such agents are used.

Control of depth of anaesthesia by varying the inspired concentration of volatile agent requires constant assessment of the patient's reaction to anaesthesia and surgery to produce adequate anaesthesia while avoiding overdosage and excessively 'deep' anaesthesia. This rapid control is one of the main advantages of inhalational anaesthesia. The signs of inadequate depth of anaesthesia include tachypnoea, tachycardia, hypertension and sweating.

Signs of anaesthesia (Fig. 19.2)

Guedel's classic signs of anaesthesia are those seen in patients premedicated with morphine and atropine and breathing ether in air. The clinical signs associated with anaesthesia produced by other inhalational agents follow a similar course, but the divisions between the stages and planes are less precise.

Stage 1: the stage of analgesia. This is the stage attained when using nitrous oxide 50% in oxygen, as employed in the technique of relative analgesia (see Ch. 34).

Stage 2: stage of excitement. This is seen with inhalational induction, but rapidly passed during

STAGE	RESPIRATION	PUPILS	EYE REFLEXES	URT & RESPIRATORY REFLEXES
1 Analgesia	Regular Small volume	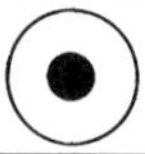 ⬤		
2 Excitement	Irregular	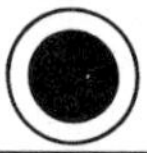 ⬤	Eyelash absent	
3 Anaesthesia Plane I	Regular Large volume	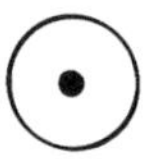 ⊙	Eyelid absent Conjunctival depressed	Pharyngeal & vomiting depressed
Plane II	Regular Large volume	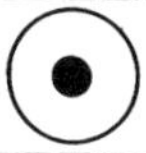 ⊙	Corneal depressed	
Plane III	Regular Becoming diaphragmatic Small volume	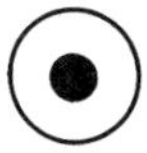 ⊙		Laryngeal depressed
Plane IV	Irregular Diaphragmatic Small volume	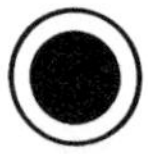 ⬤		Carinal depressed
4 Overdose	Apnoea	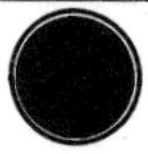 ⬤		

Fig. 19.2 Stages of anaesthesia (modified from Guedel).

i.v. induction. Respiration is erratic, breath-holding may occur, laryngeal and pharyngeal reflexes are active and stimulation of pharynx or larynx, e.g. by insertion of a Guedel or laryngeal mask airway, can produce laryngeal spasm. The eyelash reflex (used as a sign of unconsciousness with i.v. induction) is abolished in stage 2, but the eyelid reflex (resistance to elevation of eyelid) remains present.

Stage 3: surgical anaesthesia. This deepens through 4 planes (in practice, 3 – light, medium, deep) with increasing concentration of anaesthetic drug. Respiration assumes a rhythmic pattern and the thoracic component diminishes with depth of anaesthesia. Respiratory reflexes become suppressed but the carinal reflex is abolished only at plane IV (therefore a tracheal tube which is too long may produce carinal stimulation at an otherwise adequate depth). The pupils are central and gradually enlarge with depth of anaesthesia. Lacrimation is active in light planes but absent

in planes III and IV – a useful sign in a patient not premedicated with an anticholinergic.

Stage 4: stage of impending respiratory and circulatory failure. Brainstem reflexes are depressed by the high anaesthetic concentration. Pupils are enlarged and unreactive. The patient should not be permitted to reach this stage. Withdrawal of the anaesthetic agents and administration of 100% oxygen lightens anaesthesia.

Observation of other reflexes provides a guide to depth of anaesthesia. Swallowing occurs in the light plane of stage 3. The gag reflex is abolished in upper stage 3. Stretching of the anal sphincter produces reflex laryngospasm even at plane III of stage 3.

Complications and difficulties

Airway obstruction. Relieved by appropriate positioning and equipment (see below).

Laryngeal spasm. This may occur as a result

of stimulation above light-medium stage 3. Treatment is to stop the stimulation and gently deepen anaesthesia. If spasm is severe, 100% oxygen is applied with the face mask held tightly, while the airway is maintained by hand and pressure is applied to the reservoir bag. Attempts to ventilate the patient's lungs usually result only in gastric inflation. However, as the larynx partially opens, 100% oxygen flows through under pressure. Further gentle deepening of anaesthesia may then take place. In severe laryngeal spasm, i.v. suxamethonium may be required and after the lungs have been inflated with oxygen it is advisable to intubate the trachea.

Bronchospasm. This may occur if volatile anaesthetic agents are introduced rapidly, particularly in smokers with excessive bronchial secretions. Humidification and warming of gases may minimize the problem. Bronchospasm may accompany laryngospasm. Administration of bronchodilators may be required. These respiratory reflexes are induced more readily in the presence of an upper respiratory tract infection.

Malignant hyperthermia. Volatile agents, suxamethonium or amide-type local anaesthetic agents may trigger this syndrome in susceptible individuals (see Ch. 22).

Raised intracranial pressure (ICP). All volatile agents may produce an increase in ICP and this is accentuated by retention of CO_2 which accompanies the use of volatile agents in the spontaneously breathing patient. A spontaneous ventilation technique is therefore contraindicated in patients with an intracranial space-occupying lesion or cerebral oedema.

Atmospheric pollution. The use of the appropriate scavenging apparatus helps to reduce levels of theatre pollution by volatile and gaseous agents (see Ch. 16).

Delivery of inhalational agents – airway maintenance

Maintenance of the airway is one of the most important of the anaesthetist's tasks. Inhalational agents may be delivered via a face mask, a laryngeal mask airway (LMA) or a tracheal tube. Insufflation techniques, although once popular, are used rarely now.

Use of the face mask. Inhalational anaesthesia usually involves the use of a face mask which is applied after loss of consciousness at anaesthetic induction. The face mask has many variants of type and size and selection of the correct fit is important to provide a gas-tight seal.

For children, a mask with excessive dead space should be avoided. Nasal masks are required during dental anaesthesia. The patient's head position during mask anaesthesia is important; the mandible is held 'into' the mask by the anaesthetist, with his fingers holding the mandible itself rather than pressing into the soft tissues, which may result in airway obstruction (especially in children). The mandible is held forward, helping to prevent posterior movement of the tongue and obstruction of the airway.

The importance of observation of the airway during mask anaesthesia cannot be overemphasized. Soft tissue indrawing in the suprasternal and supraclavicular areas is evidence of obstruction of the upper airway. Noisy ventilation or inspiratory stridor provides further evidence that airway obstruction requires correction. Maintenance of the airway may be assisted further by the use of an oropharyngeal (Guedel) airway. An appropriate stage of anaesthesia must be reached before insertion of the airway as stimulation of the pharynx at stage 2 or at light stage 3 will produce coughing, laryngospasm or breath-holding. The use of local anaesthetic spray or jelly to coat the airway may permit its insertion at an earlier stage. A nasopharyngeal airway may be tolerated better.

When the airway has been established and the patient's ventilatory pattern is regular, a Clausen harness may be used to support the mask. The straps should be applied carefully and symmetrically for success. Support for the mandible may be achieved with a well-padded tongue spatula or an oropharyngeal airway inserted between the straps.

Use of the laryngeal mask airway (LMA)

Indications

1. To provide a clear airway without the need for the anaesthetist's hands to support a mask.

2. To avoid the use of tracheal intubation during spontaneous ventilation.

3. In a case of difficult intubation, to facilitate subsequent insertion of a tracheal tube either via the LMA or after use of a gum elastic bougie (see Ch. 16).

Contraindications

1. A patient with a 'full stomach' or with any condition leading to delayed gastric emptying.

2. A patient in whom regurgitation of gastric contents into the oesophagus is possible (e.g. hiatus hernia).

3. Where surgical access (e.g. to the pharynx) is impeded by the cuff of the LMA.

Conduct of LMA insertion. An appropriate depth of anaesthesia is required for successful insertion of the LMA. Fewer difficulties are encountered after i.v. induction of anaesthesia with propofol than with thiopentone because of the greater tendency of the former to suppress pharyngeal reflexes. The patient's head is extended, the mouth is opened and, if necessary, the mandible can be held down by an assistant. The LMA cuff is evacuated and the LMA is inserted into the pharynx in a direction along the axis of the hard palate so that the cuff encounters the posterior pharyngeal wall and is swept distally into the laryngopharynx. The cuff then lies posterior to the larynx. Air is then injected into the cuff and the breathing system is attached via a catheter mount to the 22 mm proximal connector. The LMA is secured in place with tape or a bandage after confirmation of correct placement by observation of movement of the reservoir bag or the chest after a gentle manual inflation of the lungs.

Tracheal intubation

Indications

1. Provision of a clear airway, e.g. anticipated difficulty in using mask anaesthesia in the edentulous patient.

2. An 'unusual' position, e.g. prone or sitting. A reinforced non-kinking tube may be necessary.

3. Operations on the head and neck, e.g. ENT, dental. A nasotracheal tube may be required.

4. Protection of the respiratory tract, e.g. from blood during upper respiratory tract or oral surgery and from inhalation of gastric contents in emergency surgery or patients with oesophageal obstruction. The use of a cuffed tube for adults is mandatory in these circumstances.

5. During anaesthesia using IPPV and muscle relaxants.

6. To facilitate suction of the respiratory tract.

7. During thoracic operations.

Contraindications. There are few contraindications. In emergency situations, hypoxaemia must be relieved if at all possible before insertion of a tracheal tube.

Preparation

Before starting, the anaesthetist must check the availability and function of the necessary equipment. He should have a 'dedicated' and experienced assistant. Laryngoscopes of the correct size are chosen and the function of bulb and batteries checked, the patency of the tracheal tube is checked and the integrity of the cuff ensured. Various aids to intubation must also be present (see Table 19.1).

Choice of equipment

Laryngoscopes. Laryngoscopes are manufactured in many shapes and sizes. There are two basic types of blade – straight or curved. Straight-blade laryngoscopes (e.g. Magill) are favoured for children, in whom the epiglottis is floppy, and are designed to pass posterior to the epiglottis and to lift it anteriorly, exposing the larynx. The curved blade (e.g. Macintosh) is designed so that the tip lies anterior to the epiglottis in the vallecula, pressing on the hyoepiglottic ligament and moving it anteriorly to expose the larynx and vocal cords (Fig. 19.3).

Tracheal tubes. Most tracheal tubes are made of either rubber or PVC. The latter are disposable and less irritant to the tracheal mucosa. In some circumstances, e.g. head and neck or throat surgery, the tracheal tube may be subject to direct or indirect pressure and standard tubes may kink or become compressed. It may be appropriate to use a tube which is reinforced with a nylon or steel spiral in such cases. Tracheal

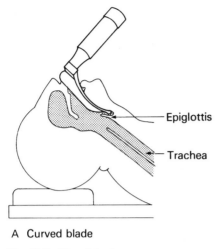

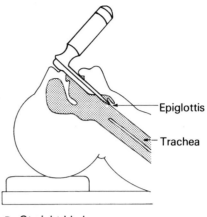

A Curved blade   B Straight blade

Fig. 19.3 Use of the laryngoscope.

tubes are introduced usually through the mouth, although it may be preferable to pass the tube through the nose, particularly for oral surgery. The length of disposable tubes exceeds that required normally for oral intubation and the tube should be cut to the appropriate length before use. During thoracic surgery, it may be necessary to ventilate the lungs independently and a bronchial or double-lumen tube is required (see Ch. 38).

In order to seal the airway, most tracheal tubes are manufactured with an inflatable cuff at the distal end. The cuff may be of low or high volume; low-volume cuffs produce a seal over a smaller area of tracheal mucosa and tend to exert a high pressure on the mucosal cells, reducing the capillary blood supply and rendering the cells potentially ischaemic. High-volume cuffs cover a wide area of mucosa; the pressure exerted varies during the respiratory cycle, but on average is lower than that produced by a low-volume cuff.

Tracheal tubes of different sizes are required. The size quoted usually is the internal diameter (ID). Adult males require normally a tube of 9–9.5 mm ID and females 8–8.5 mm. For oral intubation, the tube should be 20–23 cm in length. The appropriate internal diameter of tube for paediatric use can be calculated from the formula (age/4) + 4 mm. This is an approximation and a tube 0.5 mm smaller and 0.5 mm larger should also be prepared. The length of tube required for oral intubation in children is approxi-

mately equal to (age/2) + 12 cm. A tube of slightly smaller internal diameter may be required for nasal intubation and its length may be calculated from the formula (age/2) + 15 cm.

An appropriate connector is required between the tracheal tube and the anaesthetic breathing system, e.g. curved connector for nasal tube, lightweight plastic with low dead space for children or a connector with a suction port for thoracic surgery.

Anaesthesia for tracheal intubation

Tracheal intubation may be performed under local anaesthesia (using topical spray, transtracheal spray and superior laryngeal nerve block) or under general anaesthesia (either i.v. or inhalational, with or without the use of muscle relaxation). The usual approach is to provide general anaesthesia and muscle relaxation, to perform laryngoscopy and direct vision intubation and then to maintain anaesthesia via the tracheal tube with spontaneous or controlled ventilation. Adequate anaesthesia and muscle relaxation must be provided for laryngoscopy.

Inhalational technique for intubation. Adequate depth of anaesthesia is necessary to depress the laryngeal reflexes and provide a degree of relaxation of the laryngeal and pharyngeal muscles. Halothane in concentrations up to 4% may provide rapid attainment of the necessary depth, which can be judged from the pattern of respiration with predominance of diaphragmatic breathing (a useful sign in children is the 'dissociation' of the thoracic and abdominal excursion). The mask is removed and laryngoscopy and intubation performed. The anaesthetic circuit is then connected to the tracheal tube and anaesthesia maintained at a depth appropriate for surgery.

Relaxant anaesthesia for intubation. After i.v. or inhalational induction of anaesthesia, the short-acting depolarizing muscle relaxant suxamethonium may be used to provide relaxation for tracheal intubation. After loss of consciousness, the patient breathes 100% oxygen or 50% nitrous oxide in oxygen and suxamethonium is administered in a dose of 1–1.5 mg.kg^{-1}. Assisted ventilation is maintained via the face mask until muscle relaxation occurs (except in emergency patients and those likely to regurgitate) and laryngoscopy and intubation are performed. Inhalational anaesthesia may be continued with manual ventilation until the effects of the relaxant have ceased, whereupon spontaneous ventilation is resumed. Alternatively, non-depolarizing neuromuscular blockade is instituted and ventilation controlled.

Conduct of laryngoscopy

The position of the patient's head and neck is important. The neck should be flexed and the head extended with support of a pillow; thus the oral, pharyngeal and tracheal axes are brought into alignment (Fig. 19.4). The laryngoscope is designed for left hand use and is introduced into

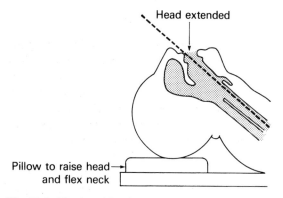

Head extended

Pillow to raise head and flex neck

Fig. 19.4 Head position for laryngoscopy.

the right side of the mouth while the right hand opens the mouth, parting the lips to avoid interposing them between laryngoscope and teeth. The teeth may be protected from blade trauma with the fingers or the use of a plastic 'guard'. The laryngoscope blade deflects the tongue to the left and the length of the blade is passed over the contour of the tongue. The laryngoscope is lifted upwards and forwards, avoiding a levering movement which can damage the upper teeth. Using a straight blade, the tip is passed posterior to the epiglottis, which is lifted anteriorly and the vocal cords visualized. With a curved blade, the tip is inserted into the vallecula and pressure on the hyoepiglottic ligament moves the epiglottis to expose the vocal cords. External pressure on the thyroid cartilage by an assistant may aid laryngeal visualization at this stage.

Conduct of intubation

After laryngeal visualization, the supraglottic area and cords may be sprayed, if required, with local anaesthetic solution (lignocaine 4%). The tracheal tube is passed from the right side of the mouth (which may be held open by the assistant's finger if necessary, permitting a clear view of the midline) and between the vocal cords into the trachea until the cuff is below the vocal cords. A semirigid stilette may be used during intubation to provide the correct degree of curvature of the tracheal tube to facilitate intubation.

The tube cuff is inflated sufficiently to abolish audible gas leaks on inflation of the lungs. The correct position of the tube must now be confirmed. If the tube has been seen clearly at laryngoscopy to pass through the vocal cords into the trachea, then equal movement of both sides of the chest during ventilation should be confirmed and auscultation in each axilla for breath sounds should be performed to ensure that the tip of the tracheal tube has not passed too far distally to enter, or occlude, one of the main bronchi (see p. 390); if there is unilateral air entry, the tube should be withdrawn slowly and carefully until air entry is equal in both lungs. If the tube has not been seen clearly to enter the trachea, or if there is *any* reason to suspect that its distal end is not in the trachea, then the steps outlined in Chapter 22 (p. 390) must be undertaken immediately to identify possible oesophageal intubation.

After its correct position has been determined, the tube is secured with cotton tape, bandage or sticking plaster strips. Correct fixation of the tube is important, particularly if the head is inaccessible during surgery, e.g. when the patient is in the prone position.

Nasal intubation

Nasal intubation may be employed for dental operations, ENT operations, etc. and may be preferred for long-term intubation by providing easier tube fixation, easier oral toilet and greater patient comfort.

A slightly smaller tube is used and is introduced preferentially to the right nostril since the left-facing bevel of the tube favours this approach. The tube is passed along the floor of the nose and advanced *gently* into the pharynx, avoiding excessive force. Laryngoscopy takes place and the tube is advanced into the trachea by manipulation of the proximal end or by grasping the tip with Magill's intubating forceps to pass it between the cords.

Packing of the throat may be employed after intubation especially for oropharyngeal operations. The moist gauze pack is introduced using the laryngoscope and Magill forceps. The pharynx should be packed on each side of the tracheal tube. The pack should be applied gently to avoid abrasion of the mucosa. A 'tail' of the pack is left protruding from the mouth and the anaesthetist must accept responsibility for removal of the pack before extubation. A latex 'foam' pack may be used as an alternative to cotton gauze.

Difficult intubation

Difficult intubation may be anticipated or unanticipated. Difficulty may be anticipated from evidence sought at the preoperative visit. The unexpected case should be acknowledged as such at the time of intubation and the anaesthetist should have contingency plans to overcome the situation. This subject is discussed in Chapter 22.

Complications of tracheal intubation

Complications may be mechanical, respiratory or cardiovascular and may occur early or late.

Early complications. Trauma may occur to lips and teeth or dental crowns. Jaw dislocation and dislocation of arytenoids may be produced. Trauma during intubation may result in damage to larynx and vocal cords. Nasal intubation may produce epistaxis, trauma to the pharyngeal wall or dislodgement of adenoid tissue. Obstruction or kinking of the tube can occur and carinal stimulation or bronchial intubation may take place if the tube is too long. Laryngeal trauma may produce postoperative croup, bronchospasm or laryngospasm, especially in children. Mechanical complications may be avoided with a careful technique. Broken teeth must be retrieved and the event documented. Immediate postoperative respiratory complications may be minimized by humidification of inspired gases. Cardiovascular complications of intubation include arrhythmias and hypertension, especially in untreated hypertensive patients.

Late complications. These are more common after long-term intubation. Tracheal stenosis is rare, but damage to tracheal mucosa from a cuffed tube may be related to its design; high-volume low-pressure cuffs may be preferred for long-term intubation. Trauma to vocal cords may result in ulceration or granulomata which may require surgical removal. Cord trauma may be more common in the presence of an upper respiratory tract infection.

Relaxant anaesthesia

Indications for relaxant anaesthesia

As an alternative to deep anaesthesia with spontaneous ventilation and volatile agents leading to multisystem depression, the triad of sleep, suppression of reflexes and muscle relaxation may be provided separately with specific agents. Relaxation anaesthesia provides muscle relaxation, permitting lighter anaesthesia with less risk of cardiovascular depression. Thus the technique is appropriate for major abdominal, intraperitoneal, thoracic or intracranial operations, prolonged operations in which spontaneous ventilation would lead to respiratory depression and operations in a position in which ventilation is impaired mechanically.

Conduct of relaxant anaesthesia

Induction of anaesthesia is followed by tracheal intubation after administration of a depolarizing muscle relaxant. When its action has subsided relaxation is provided by a longer-acting non-depolarizing relaxant (Table 11.1). The choice of agent depends upon operative indications (e.g. tubocurarine has been employed traditionally during induced hypotension) or the patient's condition (e.g. vecuronium and atracurium produce little cardiovascular depression).

Controlled ventilation is instituted, first manually by compression of the reservoir bag and then by a mechanical ventilator delivering the appropriate tidal and minute volume (see Appendix X, p. 760). Anaesthesia and analgesia are provided usually by nitrous oxide/oxygen, together with a volatile agent and/or i.v. analgesic. When ventilation is controlled volatile agents are used in an inspired concentration less than MAC. Intravenous opioids, e.g. morphine or fentanyl, are employed in small bolus doses. Analgesia may also be supplemented by opioid premedication or by use of regional or local anaesthetic techniques.

Assessment of relaxant anaesthesia

Light anaesthesia with preservation of reflexes permits the use of physical signs for the continued assessment of the adequacy of anaesthesia.

Adequacy of anaesthesia. Autonomic reflex activity with lacrimation, sweating, tachycardia, hypertension or reflex movement in response to surgery indicate 'light' anaesthesia and response to surgical stimulation and warn that the depth of anaesthesia should be increased or further increments of i.v. analgesic given.

Awareness during anaesthesia. The possibility of conscious or unconscious awareness exists in a patient who is under the influence of a neuromuscular blocking drug if nitrous oxide/oxygen anaesthesia is unsupplemented or is supplemented by an opioid with little or no volatile agent. The anaesthetist should ensure that this possibility is avoided by constant observation of the patient for clinical signs of light anaesthesia and by use of small concentrations of a volatile agent. Up to 1% of patients may recall intra-operative events spontaneously if a mixture of nitrous oxide 67% in oxygen is administered, even with an i.v. opioid, and a proportion of these patients experience pain. Awareness during anaesthesia is now a common source of litigation. An appropriate concentration of volatile anaesthetic agent should be used routinely during elective surgery.

Adequacy of muscle relaxation. Clinical signs of return of muscle tone include retraction of the wound edges during abdominal operations and abdominal muscle, diaphragmatic or facial movement. An increase in airway pressure (with a time- or volume-cycled ventilator) may indicate a return of muscle tone. Quantitative estimation of neuromuscular status may be obtained with a peripheral nerve stimulator (see Ch. 11). Small increments (e.g. 25–35% of the original dose of muscle relaxant) may be given to maintain relaxation; alternatively, an infusion of vecuronium or atracurium may be a more convenient method of administration, but the use of a peripheral nerve stimulator is mandatory with this technique.

Adequacy of ventilation. Clinical signs of inadequate ventilation and an increase in Pa_{CO_2} include venous dilatation, wound oozing, tachycardia, hypertension and attempts at spontaneous ventilation by the patient.

Measurement of airway pressure and end-expired P_{CO_2} with a capnograph are strongly recommended during relaxant anaesthesia and controlled ventilation. Monitoring expired gas volume provides useful information to adjust the degree of mechanical ventilation and occasionally arterial P_{CO_2} measurement may be employed.

Reversal of relaxation

At the end of operation, residual neuromuscular blockade is antagonized and spontaneous ventilation established before the tracheal tube is removed and the patient awakened. Residual neuromuscular block is antagonized with neostigmine 2.5–5 mg (0.05–0.08 mg.kg^{-1} in children). Atropine 1.2 mg or glycopyrronium 0.5 mg counteracts the muscarinic side effects of the anticholinesterase and may be given before, or with, neostigmine. Care should be exercised in the use of an anticholinergic agent in the presence of existing tachycardia, pyrexia, carbon dioxide retention or ischaemic heart disease.

Resumption of spontaneous ventilation should occur if normocapnic ventilation has been employed and assured by monitoring the end expired P_{CO_2}. Tracheobronchial suction (see below) has the beneficial side-effect of stimulating respiration if used at this stage.

Conduct of extubation

This may take place with the patient supine if the anaesthetist is satisfied that airway patency can be maintained by the patient in this position and there is no risk of regurgitation. In patients at risk of regurgitation and potential aspiration, the lateral position is preferred. However, it is safer to employ the lateral recovery position after extubation (Fig. 19.5). Return of respiratory reflexes is signified by coughing and resistance to the presence of the tracheal tube.

Tracheobronchial suction via the tracheal tube is carried out using a soft sterile suction catheter with an external diameter less than half the internal diameter of the tube. Preoxygenation precedes suctioning as the oxygen stores may be depleted by tracheal suction. The catheter is occluded during insertion and suction applied during withdrawal.

Pharyngeal suction is performed best under direct vision, avoiding trauma to the pharyngeal mucosa, uvula or epiglottis.

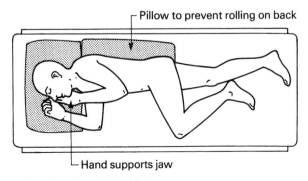

Fig. 19.5   Recovery position.

Oxygen 100% replaces the anaesthetic gas mixture before extubation to avoid the potential effects of diffusion hypoxia (p. 415) and to provide a pulmonary reservoir of oxygen in case breath-holding or coughing occurs.

Extubation is performed preferably during an inspiration when the larynx dilates; the cuff is deflated and the tube withdrawn along its curved axis since careless withdrawal in a straight line may damage laryngeal structures. Some anaesthetists generate a positive pressure in the trachea during this manoeuvre by 'squeezing the bag' in order to propel secretions into the pharynx.

After extubation, the patient's ability to maintain the airway is ensured, the ability to cough and clear secretions is assessed and an oropharyngeal airway employed if required. Administration of oxygen is continued by face mask. Preparations are made for recovery.

Complications of tracheal extubation

Laryngeal spasm. This may follow stimulation during extubation. Extubation during deep anaesthesia and subsequent maintenance with a mask may be used. Local anaesthetic spray to the larynx may block the reflex and pharyngeal suction before extubation removes secretions which may cause stimulation.

Regurgitation/inhalation. Aspiration via the nasogastric tube (if present) should be performed before tracheal extubation to remove gastric liquid. In emergency patients, extubation should be performed with the patient awake so that airway control is continuous. Partial incompetence of laryngeal reflexes may occur in the immediate post-extubation period, especially if local anaesthetic spray has been employed. In this event, recovery should take place with the patient in the lateral head-down position, with facilities at hand for suction, oxygenation and reintubation.

EMERGENCE AND RECOVERY

After tracheal extubation or at the end of mask anaesthesia, anaesthetic agents are withdrawn and oxygen 100% is delivered via the face mask. The patient's airway is supported until respiratory reflexes are intact. The patient's muscle power and coordination are assessed by testing hand grip, tongue protrusion or lifting the head from the pillow in response to command. Return of adequate muscle power must be ensured before the patient leaves theatre.

The patient is then ready for transfer from the operating table to a bed or trolley and further recovery takes place in a recovery area of theatre or in the recovery ward (Ch. 23).

The lateral recovery position (Fig. 19.5) is adopted unless the anaesthetist is satisfied that this is unnecessary. The patient is turned on one side, upper leg flexed and lower extended; the head is on one side and the tongue falls forward under gravity, thus avoiding airway obstruction.

FURTHER READING

Association of Anaesthetists of Great Britain and Ireland 1990 Checklist for anaesthetic machines. AAGBI, London
Association of Anaesthetists of Great Britain and Ireland 1990 Anaphylactic reactions associated with anaesthesia. AAGBI, London
Birmingham P K, Cheney F W, Ward R J 1986 Esophageal intubation: a review of detection techniques. Anesthesia and Analgesia 65: 886

Brain A I J The Intavent laryngeal mask instruction manual, 2nd edn. Intavent, Pangbourne
Jones R M 1994 Volatile anaesthetic agents. In: Nimmo W S, Rowbotham D J, Smith G (eds) Anaesthesia, 2nd edn. Blackwell Scientific Publications, Oxford
Stenquist O, Nilsson K 1982 Postoperative sore throat related to tracheal cuff design. Canadian Anaesthetists Society Journal 29: 384

20. Monitoring during anaesthesia

The word monitor is derived from the Latin verb *monere* – to warn. The purpose of a monitoring device is to measure a physiological variable and to indicate trends of change, thus enabling appropriate therapeutic action to be taken.

As the derivation suggests, a monitor can only warn. No mechanical or electrical device can replace conscientious observations of the patient by the anaesthetist. Information from monitoring equipment requires clinical interpretation.

It is essential to ensure that all monitoring equipment is maintained correctly and that it functions accurately, so that the information which it provides is reliable. The user should understand the basic principles on which monitoring equipment is based and be able to interpret the information provided.

The anaesthetic record

Varying levels of complexity of monitoring are appropriate during anaesthesia in different clinical situations; for instance, major cardiovascular surgery and dilatation and curettage represent opposite ends of the monitoring spectrum.

The importance of meticulous record-keeping for all patients undergoing anaesthesia cannot be stressed too highly. Detailed, accurate charts provide not only a valuable record of trends occurring during anaesthesia, but are also useful for reference purposes, if further administration of anaesthesia is necessary. In addition, they may be required for medicolegal purposes. Litigation may arise many years after the event and claims are almost impossible to defend in the absence of comprehensive records. A suitable chart is shown in Figure 20.1. The basic requirements of a chart are that it should provide space to record the following:

1. Details of preoperative assessment, including drug history.
2. Cardiovascular variables, including heart rate, arterial pressure, central venous pressure (CVP) and urine output.
3. Respiratory variables, including ventilator settings, airway pressure, arterial oxygen saturation, end-tidal carbon dioxide concentration and fractional inspired concentration of oxygen (F_{IO_2}).
4. Details of apparatus employed.
5. Dosages of all drugs, including the concentrations of nitrous oxide and volatile agent employed.
6. Details of all intravenous (i.v.) fluids.
7. Volume of blood lost.
8. Any problems or difficulties encountered.
9. Postoperative instructions.

Automated anaesthetic records

It is estimated that up to 20% of anaesthetic time is taken up with documentation. Inevitably, update from the anaesthetist's memory occurs following intense periods of activity such as anaesthetic induction, or the management of critical incidents and mishaps and this may lead to inaccuracies. Automated documentation could fill this gap.

Such a system should produce a standardized and legible document providing a continuous record of information, ideally recording data both from the monitoring apparatus and the anaesthetic machine. The facility for recording other

333

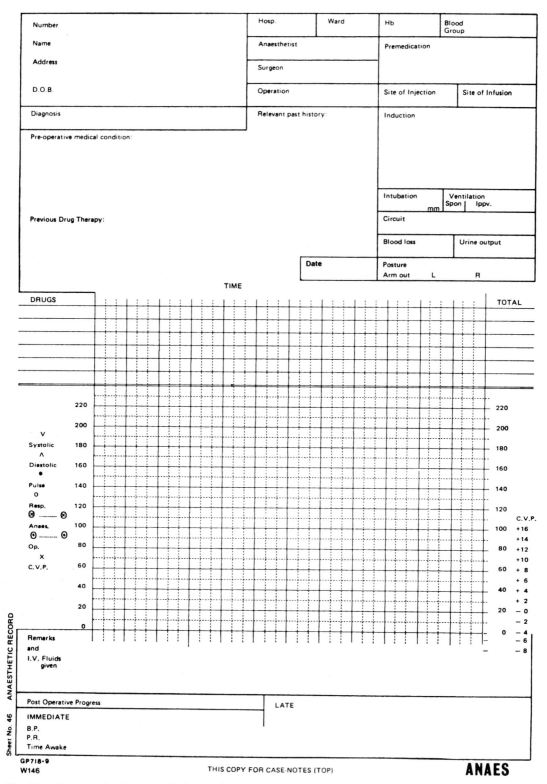

Fig. 20.1   An example of an anaesthetic record.

administrative data should also be possible. Data should be displayed graphically where appropriate. For the ideal system, a personal computer at every work station would be necessary and the vast amount of data generated would need to be stored safely and to satisfy the requirements of the Data Protection Act.

Systems currently available show a lack of standardization with regard to interfaces for the hardware as well as for the design of the chart.

Advantages of automated systems are the high quality of documentation produced and a possible reduction in workload for the anaesthetist. However, these advantages must be set against the considerable disadvantages of recording artefactual data and bypassing the interface in the anaesthetist's mind which constantly records and evaluates the information presented. These issues must be evaluated fully. An example of a computer-generated record is shown in Figure 20.2.

THE CARDIOVASCULAR SYSTEM

Electrocardiography

Valuable information concerning cardiac rhythm may be obtained by monitoring the electrocardiogram (ECG). Most ECG machines calculate ventricular rate. This should not distract the anaesthetist from monitoring peripheral pulse rate.

ECG monitors have become increasingly reliable and less subject to interference. As the technique is non-invasive, simple and accurate, it is now regarded as mandatory in the UK that the ECG should be monitored in all patients undergoing anaesthesia, no matter how minor the surgical procedure.

Standard lead II monitoring is used widely. However, the CM5 lead configuration (Fig. 20.3) has been advocated for routine intraoperative monitoring because it reveals more readily ST segment changes produced by left ventricular ischaemia.

It is important to appreciate that the ECG is an index only of electrical activity. It is possible for a normal electrical waveform to exist in the presence of a negligible cardiac output. Consequently, information from the ECG should be used in conjunction with data acquired from monitoring of perfusion.

Monitoring the circulation

Maintenance of perfusion of vital organs is one of the principal tasks of the anaesthetist during surgery. Adequate perfusion is dependent on adequate venous return to the heart, cardiac performance and arterial pressure.

Direct measurements of cardiac output and blood volume are difficult during anaesthesia and require invasive procedures which are inappropriate in many situations. However, adequacy of cardiac output and circulating blood volume may be inferred indirectly from observation of the following variables:

1. Peripheral pulse.
2. Arterial oxygen saturation.
3. Peripheral perfusion.
4. Urine production.
5. Arterial pressure.

The peripheral pulse

Regular palpation of the peripheral pulse is one of the simplest and most useful methods of monitoring during anaesthesia and is mandatory for even the most minor surgery. Information may be obtained by observation of the rate, volume and rhythm.

Pulse plethysmography

Automated devices are available for monitoring peripheral pulsation. They are based on the principle of photoplethysmography. The skin of a suitable digit, or of the pinna of the ear, is illuminated by a weak source of light. The intensity of light transmitted through, or reflected by, the digit waxes and wanes with each capillary pulsation, and this is detected by a photoelectric cell, the signal of which is transduced to display a waveform on an oscilloscope. When a finger is used, inflation of an arterial pressure-recording cuff causes the waveform from the pulse meter to flatten. Oscillations reappear when the cuff is deflated below systolic arterial pressure.

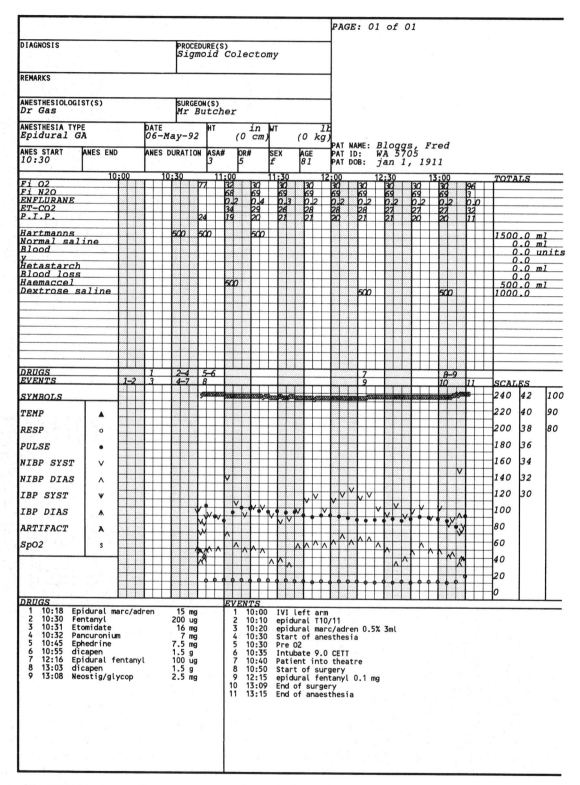

Fig. 20.2   An example of a computer-generated anaesthetic record.

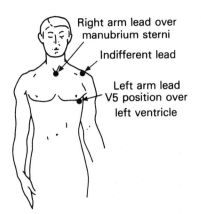

Fig. 20.3 CM5 lead configuration for electrocardiogram monitoring.

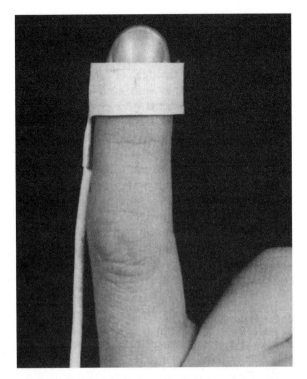

Fig. 20.5 Disposable finger probe for pulse oximeter.

The pulse monitor provides a guide to the pulse pressure. Thus an increased signal may be seen in peripheral vasodilatation or increased cardiac output, and a low pulse pressure is seen during vasoconstriction or low cardiac output states.

Pulse oximetry

Pulse oximeters measure the arterial oxygen saturation and the pulse rate non-invasively and accurately to within ±2%. A simple probe is attached to a finger (Fig. 20.4), an ear lobe, flexed across the nasal bridge, or wrapped around a child's digit (Fig. 20.5) and connected to the oximeter (Fig. 20.6). The probe contains two light-emitting diodes, one for red and one for infrared light,

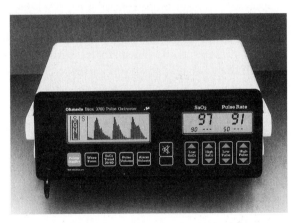

Fig. 20.6 Pulse oximeter control and display module.

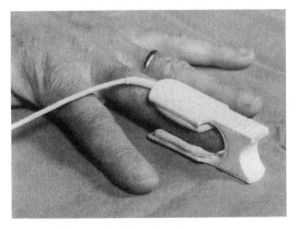

Fig. 20.4 Finger probe for pulse oximeter.

and a single detector positioned on the opposite side of the digit or ear lobe.

The function of the instrument is based on the following principle. The proportion of light absorbed by blood depends on two factors: the wavelength of the light, and the ratio of oxy-haemoglobin to deoxyhaemoglobin (Fig. 20.7). At the isobestic point, absorption is identical; at other

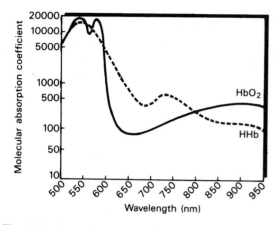

Fig. 20.7   Absorption spectra of reduced (HHb) and oxygenated (HbO$_2$) haemoglobin.

wavelengths, the absorption is different but the ratio of absorptions is known. As both forms of haemoglobin are present within a sample of blood the saturation of haemoglobin may be calculated by measuring the absorption at two different wavelengths. Developments in electronics have made it possible to separate the incident light absorbed by the tissues from that absorbed by the pulsatile arterial component (Fig. 20.8). Thus, the pulse oximeter records only the saturation of arterial blood.

The software is designed to recognize the shape of the pulse waveform so that the saturation of arterial blood only is assessed and in order

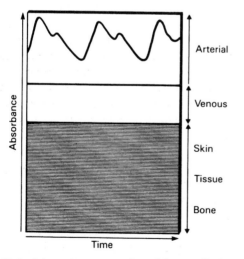

Fig. 20.8   Schematic representation of the contribution of various body components to absorbance of light.

to minimize errors caused by movement artefact. Pulse oximeters linked to an ECG signal have been introduced in an attempt to increase the accuracy of pulse detection.

Advantages. Pulse oximeters are simple to use, non-invasive and require no warm-up time. They provide an overall assessment of the integrity of all the systems involved in delivering oxygen to the tissues:

1. Oxygen supply to the patient.
2. Oxygen uptake by the lungs.
3. Oxygen delivery to the tissues via the circulatory system.

Their function is unaffected by pigmented skin. This is a significant advantage in patients of African or Asian origin, in whom hypoxaemia is more difficult to detect clinically.

Disadvantages. Because of the sigmoid shape of the oxyhaemoglobin dissociation curve, there may be a substantial decrease in arterial oxygen tension (Pa_{O_2}) before saturation begins to decrease; a large change in Pa_{O_2} above 10 kPa (75 mmHg) produces a small change in saturation, but if Pa_{O_2} is less than 10 kPa a small change produces a large change in saturation. A saturation of 94% corresponds to a Pa_{O_2} of 10 kPa. Therefore, the lower alarm limit should be set at this point.

Pulse oximeters read inaccurately in the presence of other forms of haemoglobin, e.g. carboxyhaemoglobin, methaemoglobin or other pigments, e.g. bilirubin. Some models are inaccurate in the presence of poor tissue perfusion or excessive vasoconstriction because of attenuation of the light signal, and also in the presence of excessive incident light.

Pulse oximeters are particularly useful in the following circumstances:

1. Anaesthesia in infants and children.
2. Situations in which rapid fluctuations in oxygen saturation may occur, e.g. during recovery from anaesthesia.
3. One-lung anaesthesia.
4. Conditions of reduced lighting, e.g. in the X-ray department or during ear, nose and throat procedures.
5. During regional anaesthesia with accompanying sedation.
6. Endoscopic examination.

7. Transport of the critically ill patient.
8. Exacerbations of chronic respiratory disease.
9. Sleep studies.

It is now accepted that pulse oximetry should be used routinely throughout anaesthesia because of the ability of the technique to detect abnormalities of cardiorespiratory function at an early stage.

Peripheral perfusion

Peripheral perfusion is assessed most usefully by observation of the patient's extremities. Warm, dry, pink skin indicates adequate peripheral perfusion; cold white peripheries imply the converse. This is particularly true in children, in whom cool peripheries usually indicate a degree of hypovolaemia. Other methods exist for estimating peripheral blood flow, including ultrasound and venous occlusion plethysmography, but these are not useful for routine monitoring.

The core–peripheral temperature gradient is a useful index of adequacy of peripheral perfusion. One temperature probe is placed centrally (e.g. in the nasopharynx) and the other peripherally (e.g. on the great toe). The temperature gradient increases with vasoconstriction and low cardiac output, and decreases gradually as vasodilatation occurs with increasing limb blood flow consequent upon increasing cardiac output.

Urine output

Adequacy of renal perfusion may be inferred from the volume of urine produced. The kidney is the only organ whose function may be monitored directly in this way. Adequate production of urine implies that perfusion of other vital organs is likely to be adequate. Accurate measurement of urine volumes with, for example, a urimeter, is particularly indicated in the following situations:

1. Major vascular surgery.
2. Massive fluid or blood loss.
3. Major trauma.
4. Critically ill/shocked patients.
5. Cardiac surgery.
6. Surgery in the jaundiced patient.

The aim is to achieve a urine production of $0.5–1 \text{ ml.kg}^{-1}.\text{h}^{-1}$.

Table 20.1 Classification of methods of arterial pressure measurement

Indirect	Direct
Palpation	Intra-arterial manometry
Auscultation	
Oscillotonometry	
Oscillometry	
Doppler ultrasound	

Systemic arterial pressure

Measurement of arterial pressure may be classified into indirect or direct methods (Table 20.1).

Measurement of arterial pressure is mandatory during anaesthesia in all patients. It is an indirect method of estimating adequacy of cardiac output, because:

$$\text{Blood pressure} = \text{cardiac output} \times \text{peripheral resistance}$$

In conjunction with estimation of peripheral perfusion, it is an invaluable measurement. Indirect, non-invasive methods of measurement are appropriate for most types of surgery.

Palpation. Palpation of the radial pulse as the sphygmomanometer cuff is deflated is a simple method of measuring systolic pressure, but is inaccurate at low pressures or when vasoconstriction is present.

Auscultation. Auscultation of the Korotkoff sounds is too cumbersome for routine use during anaesthesia.

Oscillometry. The indirect measurement of arterial pressure using automated oscillometry has become popular, although the accuracy of the various machines now available is no better, and in some cases is worse, than conventional methods. However, these devices may free the anaesthetist to perform other tasks.

An example of an automated oscillometer is shown in Figure 20.9. These devices incorporate a microprocessor which controls the inflation and deflation sequence. An air pump inflates the cuff; a bleed-valve then deflates it in discrete decrements of pressure. A pressure transducer records the pressure signals, which in turn are interpreted by the microprocessor.

The single-bladder cuff usually possesses two

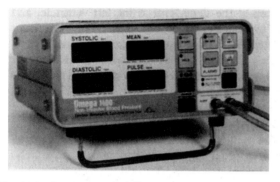

Fig. 20.9 An automated oscillometer.

tubular connections. Inflation of the cuff occurs through one, and pressure fluctuations are sensed through the other, which is connected to the pressure transducer. An example of the signal generated is shown in Figure 20.10. Systolic, diastolic and mean pressures can be estimated, mean pressure being the minimum pressure at which maximal arterial wall expansion occurs. Heart rate is determined as the median rate calculated from an analysis of all the pressure pulses received during a single determination sequence. Measurements may be automatically instituted at preset intervals.

A recent review showed that all models tested were inaccurate at a systolic pressure of less than 60 mmHg. In addition, under-reading occurred at high systolic pressures. Invasive methods of measurement are preferable in the shocked patient. Determinations may be impossible during episodes of arrhythmia, and the oscillometer is unable to follow rapid swings in arterial pressure.

Frequent repeated cuff inflations have resulted in ulnar nerve palsy, and may cause petechial haemorrhages of the skin immediately beneath the cuff. Clearly, it is imprudent to apply the cuff to an arm with an i.v. infusion in progress.

Continuous non-invasive blood pressure monitoring

Finapres. This instrument produces a calibrated arterial waveform based on the arterial volume clamp method. A cuff is placed around a finger (Fig. 20.11) and inflated to a pressure just less than that which causes the digital artery to collapse. This pressure is called the zero transmural pressure. As the pressure changes, the volume of the blood in the artery changes. This is sensed by infrared photoelectric receivers in the cuff, which operate a pump which then adjusts the cuff inflation to maintain zero transmural pressure.

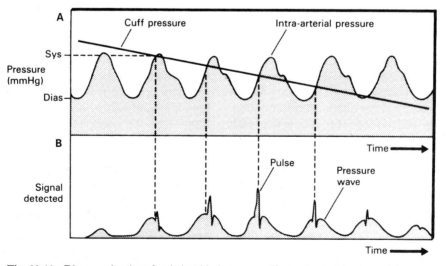

Fig. 20.10 Diagram showing: **A** relationship between cuff pressure and intra-arterial pressure as cuff pressure decreases during oscillometry; **B** the signal created by the relative pressure changes in **A**. The sharp spikes of pressure in **B** are created by the walls of the artery opening and closing. These spikes are detected by a transducer first when the cuff pressure is just below systolic arterial pressure; their amplitude reaches a peak at mean arterial pressure and they cease when the cuff pressure is below diastolic arterial pressure.

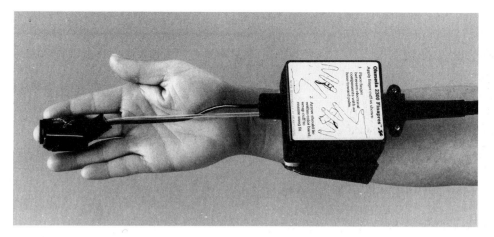

Fig. 20.11   Finapres cuff and pneumatic transducer strapped to the forearm.

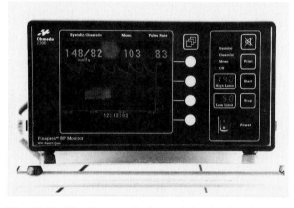

Fig. 20.12   The Finapres display module, showing the arterial pressure waveform.

Thus, cuff pressure reflects intra-arterial pressure at all times. The resultant pressure signal is transduced and a waveform is displayed on a screen which gives a continuous display of heart rate, systolic, mean and diastolic pressures (Fig. 20.12).

The method is said to be at least as accurate as oscillometry but less so than readings from an intra-arterial device. However, the cuff *must* be properly sited. The pneumatic transducer is cumbersome and must be placed at the level of the right atrium.

Accuracy of measurement deteriorates with long-term use, probably due to vasoconstriction. Agreement with intra-arterial pressures is good for systolic readings, but less well-correlated with diastolic and mean pressures. The device performs better in the vasodilated than in the vasoconstricted patient.

Doppler ultrasound. The Doppler principle is utilized in the Arteriosonde. An ultrasound emitter and receiver are placed over the brachial artery and surrounded by an inflatable cuff. As the cuff deflates from just above systolic pressure, the vessel walls begin to move apart during systole. Each movement generates a signal detected by the machine. As the pressure in the cuff decreases further, the vessel walls remain open for longer during each pulsation, and when the cuff pressure equals diastolic pressure, they do not move. Two mercury columns display systolic and diastolic pressures. The main advantages of the method are that it is accurate at low pressures, and that it is suitable for use in children. Disadvantages include its expense and size.

Direct measurement of arterial pressure

This is achieved by attaching a transducer to an intra-arterial cannula inserted percutaneously into a peripheral artery. This is an invasive procedure which carries potential morbidity. Thus, the method is only justified when rapid changes in arterial pressure are anticipated during anaesthesia. Some indications for arterial cannulation are shown in Table 20.2.

The radial or dorsalis pedis arteries are selected most frequently for cannulation. When using the radial artery, the non-dominant hand should be

Table 20.2 Common indications for arterial cannulation

Major vascular surgery

Cardiothoracic surgery

Induced hypotension

Critically ill and shocked patients

Surgery for phaeochromocytoma

Neurosurgery

Necessity for frequent blood gas analysis

Table 20.3 Morbidity associated with long-term arterial cannulation

Arterial wall damage and thrombosis

Embolization

Disconnection and haemorrhage

Sepsis

Tissue necrosis

used if possible. Complications of short-term cannulation (up to 48 h) are relatively minor and infrequent. Long-term cannulation carries risks of morbidity (Table 20.3). Most of these may be minimized by meticulous attention to antisepsis, continuous slow flushing of the cannula with heparinized saline, the use of a Teflon, parallel-sided cannula of small diameter (20- or 22-gauge), and the use of Luer-Lok connections.

The availability of accurate, low-volume displacement miniature strain-gauge transducers has helped simplify recording of arterial pressure. The transducer should be zeroed, i.e. placed at the same level as the left ventricle, and the system should be calibrated. The transducer is connected to the arterial cannula via a short piece of stiff-walled, saline-filled manometer tubing. The pressure signal is usually displayed as a waveform on an oscilloscope screen (Fig. 20.13) and systolic, diastolic and mean arterial pressures displayed digitally.

Damping of the system should be carefully adjusted in order to reproduce pressures accurately. The commonest causes of a damped trace are:

1. Air bubbles/blood in the system.
2. Kinking of the cannula.
3. Arterial spasm.

Central venous pressure

A central venous catheter positioned with its tip in the superior vena cava provides valuable information concerning the volume status of the circulation during anaesthesia. Measurement of CVP is useful in situations similar to those warranting direct measurement of arterial pressure.

Catheters are usually inserted percutaneously via one of the following routes:

1. *Peripheral arm vein.* This route is the least likely to provide correct placement of the catheter (approximately 40%). However, it avoids most of the serious complications of other routes of insertion. Thrombophlebitis and sepsis are common when a peripheral arm vein is used, particularly if the catheter is left in place for more than 48 h.

2. *Internal jugular vein.* This route is associated with the highest incidence of correct catheter placement (approximately 90%). Numerous techniques have been described for insertion of a catheter into the internal jugular vein. Common complications are listed in Table 20.4. Secure fixation of an internal jugular catheter is difficult.

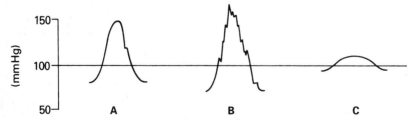

Fig. 20.13 Arterial pressure waveform. **A** Correct, optimally damped waveform. **B** Underdamped waveform, resulting in overestimation of systolic and underestimation of diastolic pressure. **C** Overdamped waveform, resulting in underestimation of systolic and overestimation of diastolic pressure.

Table 20.4 Complications of internal jugular cannulation

Air embolism

Carotid artery puncture

Brachial plexus/phrenic nerve damage

Ectopic placement (numerous sites)

Sepsis

Pneumothorax

Table 20.5 Complications of subclavian vein cannulation

Pneumothorax

Subclavian artery puncture

Air embolism

Damage to thoracic duct (left side)

3. *Subclavian vein.* This approach is more hazardous than the internal jugular, and less likely to provide correct catheter placement. However, it is the most suitable route if long-term cannulation is contemplated, e.g. to facilitate parenteral feeding. The main complications of insertion at this site are shown in Table 20.5.

Whichever route is chosen, meticulous attention to antisepsis is necessary. Free back-flow of blood should always be confirmed before starting infusion of fluid. Numerous complications have been documented, particularly associated with routes of entry in the neck, and these approaches are unsuitable for the unskilled unless properly supervised.

Oscillations of pressure should be observed with ventilation. Large oscillations in time with heart rate may indicate insertion into the right ventricle, and the catheter should be withdrawn accordingly.

The position of every central venous catheter should be confirmed by chest X-ray as soon as possible after insertion. The tip of the catheter should lie above the level of the pericardium to minimize the risk of erosion through the wall of the right atrium.

Measurement of CVP. The catheter is connected to a fluid-filled water manometer column via a three-way stopcock (Fig. 20.14). Alternatively, the catheter may be connected to a transducer, as with arterial pressure monitoring, and the waveform displayed on a screen. The surface markings of the right atrium, the true zero

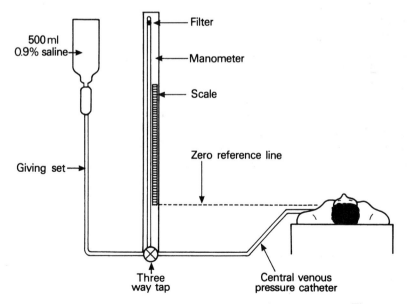

Fig. 20.14 Measurement of central venous pressure using a manometer. The manometer tubing is filled from the infusion bag and the tap turned to connect the manometer to the central venous catheter. The fluid level in the manometer falls until the height of the fluid column above the zero reference point is equal to the central venous pressure.

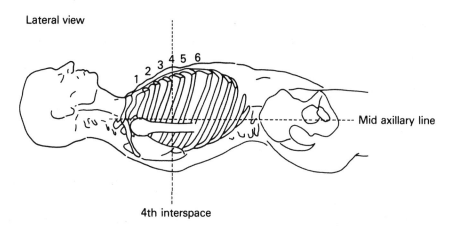

Lateral view

Mid axillary line

4th interspace

Fig. 20.15 Surface markings used to identify the position of the right atrium.

reference point, are shown in Figure 20.15. The normal range of values is 0–6 cmH₂O in the spontaneously breathing patient. It is sometimes simpler to use the manubriosternal junction as the reference point, in which case the value obtained for CVP is 5 cmH₂O lower than the true right atrial measurement at the mid axillary line. In patients receiving intermittent positive-pressure ventilation (IPPV), values of CVP are approximately 5 cmH₂O higher because of the increased mean intrathoracic pressure.

Trends in measured observations are more valuable than absolute values. For example, in a patient undergoing major arterial surgery, a decrease in CVP from +5 to +1 cmH₂O indicates considerable fluid loss which warrants therapeutic intervention, even though the lower value is still within the normal range.

Measurement of CVP is a valuable aid to blood and fluid replacement. If CVP increases above normal and remains high with no improvement in arterial pressure, it is likely that myocardial failure has occurred and inotropic support may be required.

Pulmonary artery pressure monitoring

In the normal individual, CVP measurement provides a reasonably accurate estimate of the filling pressures of both right and left atria. In some clinical situations, however, the central venous or right atrial pressure does not correlate with pressure in the left atrium, and infusion of fluids

or inotropic agents titrated against CVP may not result in optimum cardiac function. Dissociation between left atrial and central venous (right atrial) pressures occurs particularly in the following situations:

1. Left ventricular failure with pulmonary oedema.
2. Interstitial pulmonary oedema of any aetiology.
3. Chronic pulmonary disease.
4. Valvular heart disease.

If such patients are about to undergo major surgery, it may be desirable to monitor pressures in the pulmonary circulation and left side of the heart. This is achieved by the use of a balloon-tipped flow-directed pulmonary artery catheter (Figs 20.16 and 20.17).

The simplest form of catheter has two channels, one for inflation of the balloon and one for measurement of pressure at the tip. It is marked at 10-cm intervals in order to facilitate insertion. More sophisticated versions of this device have four lumina.

1. *The proximal lumen.* This is situated approximately 25 cm from the tip and should lie in the right atrium after final placement of the catheter. CVP may be measured using this lumen.

2. *The distal lumen.* Situated at the tip of the catheter, this lumen lies in a major branch of the pulmonary artery when the catheter is placed correctly and is used to measure pulmonary artery pressure by connecting it to a suitable transducer.

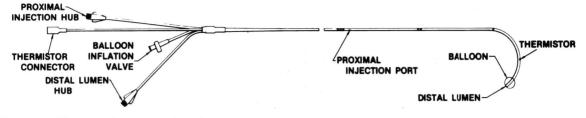

Fig. 20.16 Diagrammatic representation of a pulmonary artery catheter.

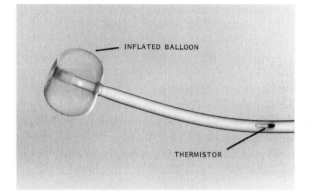

Fig. 20.17 Distal end of pulmonary artery catheter showing inflated balloon and thermistor.

3. *The balloon lumen*. This lumen permits the introduction of approximately 1.5 ml of air into the balloon which surrounds the distal tip of the catheter.

4. *Thermistor lumen*. A bead thermistor is situated 4 cm from the tip of the catheter and measures the temperature of blood at this site.

This is used in measurement of cardiac output (see below).

The pulmonary artery catheter is inserted via a central vein, usually the internal jugular or subclavian. A vein dilator is necessary to facilitate its introduction. The port of the distal lumen is connected to a pressure transducer and the pressure signal displayed on an oscilloscope screen. When the catheter reaches the right atrium (indicated by a venous pressure waveform on the screen; Fig. 20.18) the balloon is inflated and the catheter advanced slowly and gently. The balloon helps to 'float' the catheter through the right ventricle, where the typical ventricular waveform replaces that of the atrium. The catheter then passes into the pulmonary artery, when the waveform again alters. Further advancement of the catheter into a branch of the pulmonary artery should show typical 'wedging' of the waveform. At this stage, a continuous column of fluid connects the left atrium via the pulmonary veins and capillaries to the catheter. Thus, the pressure measured

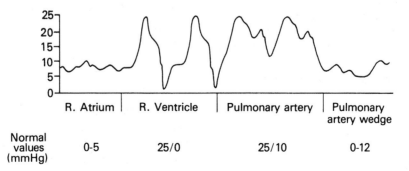

Fig. 20.18 Diagrammatic representation of pressure waveforms seen on an oscilloscope as the tip of a pulmonary artery catheter is advanced through the right atrium and right ventricle to lie in the pulmonary artery. The pulmonary artery wedge waveform is seen when the balloon is inflated with the tip of the catheter in a branch of the pulmonary artery. Normal values shown represent pressures in a spontaneously breathing patient.

reflects left atrial pressure. As soon as this pressure is obtained, the balloon is deflated. Constant inflation may cause pulmonary infarction.

Occasionally, arrhythmias may be encountered during insertion, and suitable therapeutic agents should be available.

Use of the pulmonary artery catheter includes the following:

1. The assessment of the volume status of the patient in conditions where CVP is unreliable (see above).
2. Sampling of mixed venous blood in order to calculate shunt fraction (see Chapter 1).
3. Measurement of cardiac output using the thermodilution method.
4. Derivation of other cardiovascular indices, such as the peripheral vascular resistance.

Measurement of cardiac output. The thermistor lead is connected to a cardiac output computer. Cold glucose 5% (10 ml) is injected as quickly as possible through the proximal lumen. The temperature of the blood arriving at the thermistor near the tip of the catheter is measured. The computer calculates the degree of dilution of the relatively cold injectate, and from this extrapolates the cardiac output. This method has been shown to correlate well with the Fick method of measuring cardiac output.

Complications of pulmonary artery catheterization are not negligible and include the following:

1. Arrhythmias on insertion.
2. Knotting of the catheter in the right ventricle.
3. Balloon rupture.
4. Pulmonary infarction.
5. Infection.

The device should be used for as short a period of time as necessary, and only in exceptional circumstances for longer than 48 h.

Non-invasive measurement of cardiac output

Thoracic impedance cardiography. If a high-frequency alternating current is applied across the chest, cyclical changes occur in transthoracic impedance during the cardiac cycle because of ejection of blood, which possesses a relatively high conductance, into the thoracic cavity. These changes are related to stroke volume. Two electrodes are used to apply the alternating current, and the voltage changes are detected by a second pair of electrodes. Impedance cardiography is less accurate than thermodilution in measuring absolute cardiac output, but provides a reliable indication of trends.

Doppler systems. Doppler ultrasound provides a non-invasive and virtually continuous method of measuring cardiac output. Two values must be determined: the blood velocity and the aortic diameter. The first may be measured, but the second must be calculated (albeit from known measurements), and this results in the major inaccuracy of the technique. The probe may be placed either over the suprasternal notch, which may not be easily accessible during anaesthesia, or behind the descending aorta.

Transoesophageal Doppler echocardiography. Transoesophageal Doppler ultrasound of descending aortic blood flow is now increasingly used for continuous haemodynamic monitoring both in the operating theatre and on the intensive care unit. A continuous visual display of velocity–time waveforms is obtained, from which several variables can be derived (Fig. 20.19). The area under each waveform allows stroke volume to be derived when the patient's age, weight and height are entered. Flow time correlates with the time of systolic flow in the aorta. Corrected flow time, that is, flow time divided by the square root of cycle time, gives a guide to left ventricular filling and thus volume status. Peak velocity relates to left ventricular contractility and function. In addition to its use for making haemodynamic measurements, transoesophageal echocardiography is used to assess cardiac anatomy and also to observe myocardial contractility directly (Fig. 20.20). Reported complications of this technique are few.

Recently an ultrasound probe mounted at the end of an endotracheal tube has been described. The reliability of this device remains to be assessed.

Measurement of blood loss

Losses of up to 10% of blood volume (i.e. approxi-

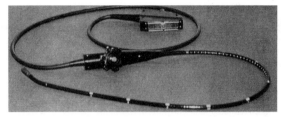

A

VELOCITY

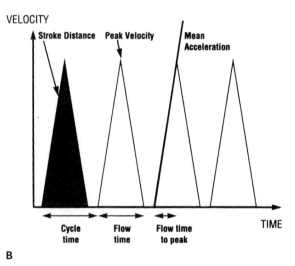

B

Fig. 20.19 **A** Adult transoesophageal echocardiography probe. The ultrasound transducer is mounted on the end of a flexible endoscope. **B** Velocity–time waveforms and derived variables.

mately 7 ml.kg^{-1} in the adult) are tolerated well and may be replaced by an appropriate volume of crystalloid solution. Blood loss in excess of 15% of blood volume during surgery should be replaced by blood.

It is prudent to weigh surgical swabs when losses appear to be mounting and then subtract the weight of an equivalent number of dry swabs in order to obtain an estimate of blood loss. This is particularly important in children. However, the method is notoriously inaccurate; it ignores blood lost on drapes, gowns, etc., and unless weighing is carried out promptly, weight is lost because of evaporation of water. A more accurate method is that which employs colorimetry; swabs, gowns and drapes are washed with a known volume of fluid, and the haemoglobin content measured colorimetrically. Clearly, this can be performed only at the end of the procedure.

THE RESPIRATORY SYSTEM

Clinical monitoring of ventilation

Continuous observation should be made of the following: the patient's colour, respiratory rate, adequacy of chest movement and the movement of the reservoir bag or ventilator bellows. Auscultation of both lung fields should also be performed frequently in order to detect equality of air entry, intubation of a bronchus, presence of secretions or the occurrence of a pneumothorax. In addition, the anaesthetist must check regularly for signs of respiratory obstruction as evidenced by tracheal tug, paradoxical abdominal movement and absence of bag deflation. Some ventilators make a regular noise during part of the ventilating cycle and this is a valuable audible monitor.

Oesophageal stethoscope

This method of monitoring the cardiovascular and respiratory systems (Fig. 20.21) is in common use in the USA, but is not frequently employed in the UK. It permits the anaesthetist to monitor heart and breath sounds continuously. A moulded ear piece renders the device more comfortable. Alterations in heart sounds, air entry to the tracheobronchial tree and the development of abnormal breath sounds, e.g. crepitations or rhonchi, may be detected readily. In procedures subject to the risk of air embolism, e.g. hip joint replacement and some neurosurgical operations, air is audible if it enters the great veins or cardiac chambers.

The oesophageal stethoscope is simple, cheap, safe, non-invasive and free from electrical interference. Its routine use is recommended for intraoperative monitoring.

Measurement of airway pressure

A simple manometer which measures the pressure of the gases delivered to the airway is incorporated into most mechanical ventilators. Observation of changes in this pressure is vital. Airway pressure may reflect changes in lung and chest wall compliance if the ventilator is of the volume-cycled or time-cycled volume-preset variety (see Chapter 16). Chest wall compliance may be influenced by the degree of muscle paralysis, surgical manipulation

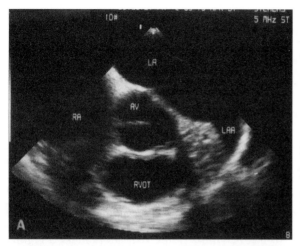

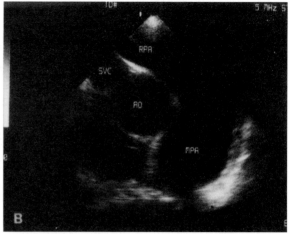

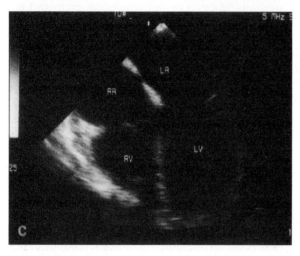

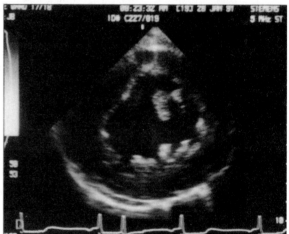

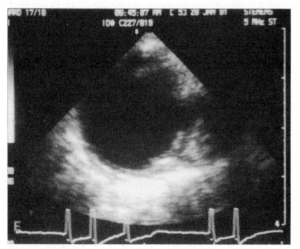

Fig. 20.20 Five different views of the cardiac chambers obtained by transoesophageal echocardiography. LA = Left atrium; LAA = left atrial appendage; RA = right atrium; RVOT = right ventricular outflow tract; AV = aortic valve; MPA = main pulmonary artery; RPA = right pulmonary artery; SVC = superior vena cava. **A** Good view of aortic valve; **B** good view of aortic route; **C** four-chamber view; **D** view of left ventricle; **E** descending aorta and arch of aorta.

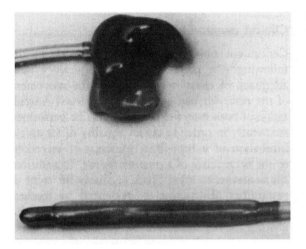

Fig. 20.21   An oesophageal stethoscope.

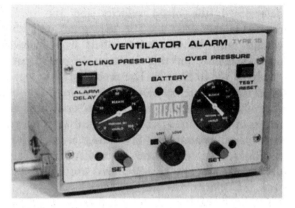

Fig. 20.22   A ventilator disconnection alarm.

and the position of the patient, and lung compliance by accumulation of secretions, or the development of a pneumothorax. Increased resistance to air flow caused by bronchospasm or obstruction of the tracheal tube is reflected by an increased peak airway pressure.

Causes of excessive elevation of airway pressure

1. Kinking of ventilator tubing or tracheal tube.
2. Overinflation of the tracheal tube cuff with consequent obstruction of the lumen of the tube.
3. Increased secretions.
4. Pneumothorax.
5. Bronchospasm.
6. Inadequate muscle relaxation.

Disconnection alarm

When the lungs are ventilated mechanically, the continuity of the anaesthetic breathing system, and thus of gas delivery to the patient, should be monitored using a disconnection alarm (Fig. 20.22). The alarm is activated if the airway pressure decreases below a preset minimum for a preset time interval. A large leak, or total disconnection, is indicated if the alarm is triggered. In addition, most of these devices sound an alarm if excessive airway pressures are generated. A disconnection alarm does not obviate the need for visual surveillance of the continuity of the breathing system.

Measurement of inspired and expired volumes

A device for measuring inspired and expired lung volumes should always be incorporated into the breathing system when a patient receives IPPV. A Wright respirometer (Fig. 20.23) is commonly used and is usually mounted in the expiratory limb of the breathing system, so that leaks which occur in the inspiratory limb are eliminated from the evaluation of expired minute volume. It should be sited as near to the tracheal tube as possible to minimize the effects of system compliance on its function.

The Wright respirometer is a vane anemometer. The vane rotates within a small cylinder, the walls of which are perforated with a number of tangential slits, so that the air stream causes the vane to rotate. Rotation of the vane drives the pointer around the dial and gas volume is recorded. It tends to over-read at high tidal volumes and under-read at low volumes as a result of its inertia. Its function is affected by moisture, which causes the pointer to stick; thus, it should be switched off when not in use. In the electronic version, rotation of the vane is detected electronically; this reduces the inaccuracies caused by water condensation.

Spirometry

It is now possible to obtain real-time displays of flow–volume and pressure–volume loops to calculate compliance and to measure other respi-

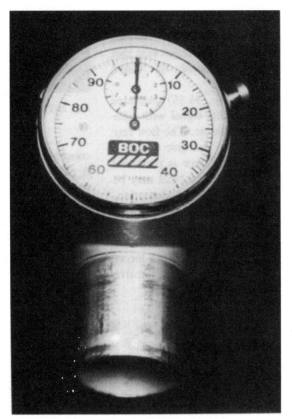

A

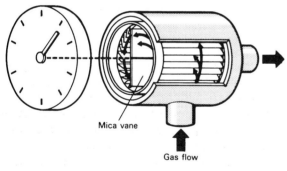

Mica vane

Gas flow

B

Fig. 20.23 A Wright respirometer. **B** Diagrammatic representation of mechanism (see text for details).

ratory pressures and volumes using side-stream spirometry.

The Datex 'Ultima' uses a single airway adaptor (the D lite adaptor; Fig. 20.24) which is inserted into the breathing system close to the tracheal tube. This adaptor is a bi-directional, pressure-based flow sensor. A gas sampling tube is attached to a separate connection on the adaptor.

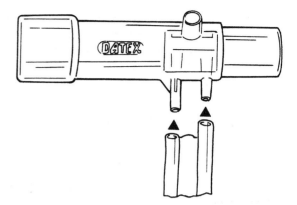

Fig. 20.24 Diagrammatic representation of the D lite adaptor showing the separate connecting ports for gas sampling and spirometry tubing.

Continuous measurement of gas flow and volume are based on the measurement of kinetic gas pressures using the pitot effect. In this way, numerical values of inspired and expired tidal volumes, minute volume and the pressures P_{peak}, $P_{plateau}$ and positive end-expiratory pressure (PEEP) are continuously displayed on the screen. Inspiratory:expiratory ratio, compliance and forced expiratory volume in 1 s (FEV_1) are also shown (Fig. 20.25). Pressure–volume and flow–volume loops can also be displayed.

This device has many applications in anaesthesia and is indicated during operations, or patient conditions in which respiratory mechanics are likely to vary, for example in asthmatic patients or during one-lung anaesthesia. It can also indi-

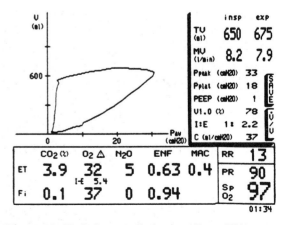

Fig. 20.25 Typical screen display from Datex Ultima monitoring system.

cate obstruction of the tracheal tube or endo-bronchial intubation. Because of the smaller volumes generated it is a less useful monitor in patients who are breathing spontaneously than in those receiving IPPV.

MONITORING GAS DELIVERY AND EXCRETION

Oxygen delivery to the patient

Before using an anaesthetic machine, the anaesthetist must assess whether it is functioning correctly, particularly with regard to delivery of oxygen. All anaesthetic machines should be fitted with an oxygen failure alarm which provides an audible and/or visual warning if the oxygen pressure decreases. A full spare cylinder of oxygen should always be available on the anaesthetic machine when piped gases are in use.

Inspired oxygen concentration

An oxygen analyser should be used in every anaesthetic breathing system to ensure that the required concentration of oxygen is delivered to the patient. A galvanic (fuel cell) oxygen analyser (Fig. 20.26) generates a current proportional to the partial pressure of oxygen; this is achieved by reduction of oxygen at a silver cathode connected through a thin film of electrolyte solution to a lead anode. These instruments may be placed in the inspira-

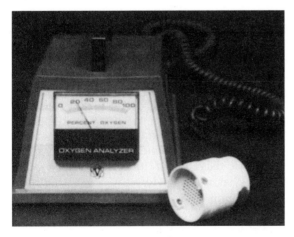

Fig. 20.26 A fuel cell oxygen analyser.

tory limb of the breathing system, and have a 90% response time of approximately 20 s. They are accurate to within ±3%, are calibrated simply using air, are not affected by humidity and are powered by battery.

It is important to appreciate that oxygen analysers measure partial pressure, although the display is calibrated in percentage of oxygen. If these devices are positioned between the gas outlet port of an anaesthetic machine and a gas-driven ventilator (e.g. Manley), the total gas pressure to which the detector is subjected increases by as much as 25–30%. The partial pressure of oxygen increases by the same percentage, and the display indicates an erroneously high oxygen concentration. The analyser should be positioned in the inspiratory limb of the breathing system to overcome this problem.

Oxygen delivery to the tissues

Pulse oximetry

This has become the standard method of measuring oxygen delivery to the tissues. It is described fully on pages 337–339.

Transcutaneous partial pressure of oxygen (Ptc_{O_2}) measurement

The instrument used to measure this parameter is a modified Clark electrode (Fig. 20.27) applied to the skin surface. However, to ensure that Ptc_{O_2} approximates to Pa_{O_2} the skin must be rendered hyperaemic by heating to 45°C. The transcutaneous Po_2 electrode provides a continuous, non-invasive estimate of arterial oxygen tension.

The instrument requires a warm-up period of 15 min, calibration and subsequently a 5-min equilibration period. There is good correlation — at least in infants — between Ptc_{O_2} and Pa_{O_2}. The response time is 10–15 s when the skin is thin, and the device is reliable in following trends. However, the equipment is cumbersome and expensive. In adults with a thicker skin, correlation is not as good and decreases with increasing age.

Carbon dioxide excretion in expired gas

It is important to ensure adequate carbon dioxide

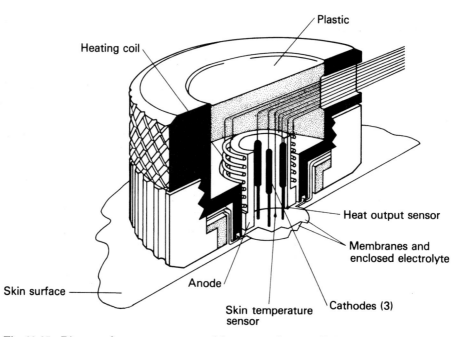

Plastic

Heating coil

Heat output sensor

Membranes and enclosed electrolyte

Skin surface

Anode

Cathodes (3)

Skin temperature sensor

Fig. 20.27 Diagram of a transcutaneous partial pressure of oxygen (Po_2) electrode.

elimination during anaesthesia because of the deleterious effects of a high arterial carbon dioxide tension (Pa_{CO_2}).

End-tidal carbon dioxide tension (PE'_{CO_2})

PE'_{CO_2} correlates well with Pa_{CO_2} in patients who have no significant pulmonary disease. The normal Pa_{CO_2}–PE'_{CO_2} gradient is approximately 0.7 kPa (5 mmHg). End-tidal carbon dioxide concentration may be measured using the principle of infrared absorption spectrophotometry. Infrared rays are passed through two identical channels; one contains the sampled gas and the other acts as a reference. Carbon dioxide absorbs infrared light and the extent of absorption is measured as a reduction in heat generated at a detector. Infrared light is absorbed by many gases, including nitrous oxide and anaesthetic vapours, and appropriate measures are taken to minimize errors caused by their presence in the sample.

A number of machines are marketed which measure carbon dioxide concentration breath-by-breath. Many also measure the inspired and expired concentrations of oxygen, nitrous oxide and anaesthetic vapour, and also display respiratory rate. The sampling probe is placed as near as possible to the patient's mouth. Tracheal tubes are available which incorporate a pilot tube to sample gas near the tip; these ensure a more representative end-tidal sample. A digital or analogue signal of end-tidal carbon dioxide is displayed by the capnograph.

A printer may be used to provide a permanent record of expired carbon dioxide concentrations, permitting trended information to be obtained. Information regarding ventilation/perfusion ($\dot{V}/\dot{Q}$) inequalities and rebreathing may be gleaned from the printed capnogram (Fig. 20.28).

Capnography is useful particularly in the following circumstances.

1. To provide evidence of correct placement of the tracheal tube. Capnography is the only method available which provides rapid and reliable diagnosis of intubation of the oesophagus.
2. For routine monitoring of the adequacy of ventilation and the effects of IPPV.
3. To detect rebreathing.
4. To detect air, fat or pulmonary embolism; a

%CO₂

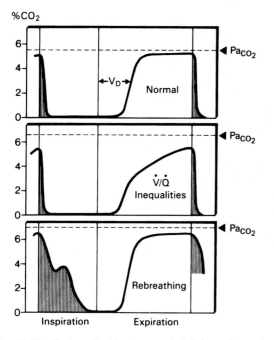

Fig. 20.28 Carbon dioxide traces recorded from the proximal end of the tracheal tube to illustrate the altered pattern of alveolar plateau in a patient with ventilation/perfusion ($\dot{V}/\dot{Q}$) inequalities. The bottom trace shows the presence of carbon dioxide in inspired gas during spontaneous ventilation with a Bain breathing system supplied with an inadequate flow rate of fresh gas. Pa_{CO_2} = Arterial carbon dioxide tension.

sudden decrease in PE'_{CO_2} occurs as a result of increased dead space.

5. To detect malignant hyperthermia; a progressive increase in PE'_{CO_2} results from increased muscle metabolism.

6. To ensure normocapnia in elderly patients in an attempt to maintain adequate cerebral perfusion.

7. To maintain normal PE'_{CO_2} during carotid artery surgery in order to maintain cerebral perfusion.

The technique may provide inaccurate estimation of Pa_{CO_2} in the presence of the following:

1. Rapid respiratory frequencies.
2. Chronic respiratory disease ($\dot{V}/\dot{Q}$ abnormalities).
3. Hypotension and blood loss ($\dot{V}/\dot{Q}$ abnormalities).
4. High inspired oxygen concentrations.

Carbon dioxide excretion in tissues

Transcutaneous partial pressure of carbon dioxide (Ptc_{CO_2}) monitoring

Devices for measurement of Ptc_{CO_2} have proved useful in the management of acutely ill neonates. In adults, there are numerous technical problems.

Ptc_{CO_2} changes much less rapidly than Pa_{CO_2} after apnoea, making Ptc_{CO_2} less useful as an emergency warning device. In addition, the instrument has a slow response time: 5 min to 90% response.

Ptc_{CO_2} consistently reads higher than arterial Pco_2, but there is a good correlation over a wide range of values up to 8 kPa. The skin must be heated to increase blood flow and reduce the arterial–capillary Pco_2 gradient.

Anaesthetic vapour delivery

Inspired and expired concentrations of halothane, enflurane and isoflurane may be measured on a breath-by-breath basis. Devices may be classified into two categories, based on the physical principle employed. Infrared analysers are employed most commonly.

Infrared analysers

Gas is sampled from the breathing system into a measuring chamber, where the concentration of vapour is measured using infrared absorption spectrophotometry (see above). Volatile vapours absorb infrared light to varying degrees depending on their concentration and composition. The resulting transmitted radiation is converted into an electrical signal. Sample flow is approximately 200 ml.min⁻¹ but this gas can be returned to the breathing system; thus, these instruments are suitable for use during closed-circuit anaesthesia. Readings are unaffected by the presence of nitrous oxide or carbon dioxide. Water vapour has a negligible effect. The response time of this instrument may be inadequate to give accurate breath-by-breath monitoring at high respiratory frequencies.

Quartz crystal oscillators

The EMMA multigas analyser is an example of

this type of machine. The resonant frequency of a highly stable quartz crystal oscillator changes as a result of interaction between the coating of the crystal and its surrounding gas. This oscillation produces an electrical signal proportional to the vapour concentration. The crystal is mounted in a compact measuring head which is positioned in the anaesthetic breathing system. Water vapour produces some artefact, and this, together with the weight of the measuring head, makes the device less suitable for use with the closed circuit.

Both types of instrument may be used to check the calibration of vaporizers.

Mass spectrometer

At present, this versatile but bulky and expensive instrument is mainly used as a research tool. It provides extremely rapid and accurate measurements of a number of gases simultaneously. Smaller, cheaper devices will be available in the near future for use in the operating theatre.

THE NERVOUS SYSTEM

Central nervous system

Monitoring of the central nervous system during anaesthesia is primarily concerned with estimation of depth of unconsciousness, in order to avoid awareness or vivid unpleasant dreams.

Clinical monitoring

Observations of the signs of sympathetic over-activity (lacrimation, sweating, increase in pupil size, increase in heart rate or arterial pressure) and reflex movements indicate that anaesthesia is too light. However, numerous investigations have shown that these signs are unreliable indicators of inadequate narcosis.

A more sophisticated attempt to detect the occurrence of awareness comprises isolation of one arm from the remainder of the circulation by inflation of a tourniquet on the upper arm before injection of relaxant into the systemic circulation. It is suggested that in this way contact may be maintained with the patient, who indicates when he or she is aware by responding to the anaesthetist's questions with a squeeze of the isolated hand. However, many anaesthetists regard this technique as unsatisfactory.

Cerebral function monitor

The conventional electroencephalograph (EEG) is too cumbersome for routine theatre use. The cerebral function monitor (CFM) is a device which integrates the total electrical activity in the brain.

Two parietal needle electrodes record the electrical signal for display on an $X–Y$ plotter. The height of the signal against the axis is proportional to the amplitude of cerebral electrical rhythms. Changes in the height and width of the trace correspond to changes in cerebral electrical function (Fig. 20.29). This device appears to be capable of detecting changes in depth of total i.v. anaesthesia, but is unreliable when volatile agents are used. It is principally employed in situations where cerebral ischaemia may occur, e.g. carotid artery or cardiac surgery.

The cerebral function analysing monitor (CFAM) provides the facility to display both the amplitude and frequency of cerebral electrical activity separately, again indicating trends in cerebral activity. Separate electrodes enable the function of each hemisphere to be monitored. The data provided are amenable to statistical analysis by computer. This device is also capable of computing evoked potentials (see Chapter 4) and of measuring the spontaneous scalp electromyogram (EMG). Increasing amplitude of the EMG reflects an increase in patient activity. Facial and scalp muscles are less sensitive to muscle relaxants than peripheral muscles and this may be a promising way of detecting pain and awareness during relaxant anaesthesia.

The CFM may be useful in the following situations:

1. Cardiac surgery.
2. Carotid artery surgery.
3. Neurosurgery
4. Total i.v. anaesthesia.
5. Status epilepticus – if neuromuscular blockers are used.
6. Hypotensive anaesthesia.
7. Drug overdose.

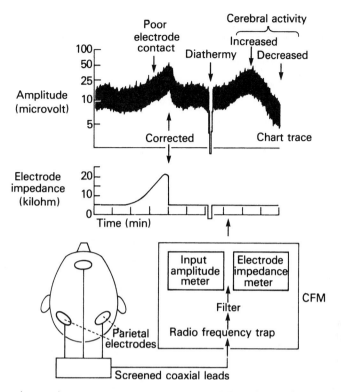

Fig. 20.29 The cerebral function monitor (CFM). Screened electrical signals displayed on the upper trace depict cerebral activity. Allowance must be made for alterations in electrode impedance and interference from extraneous electrical sources.

Evoked potentials

This technique shows promise as a monitor of the depth of anaesthesia. The auditory evoked response (AER) is the response in the EEG to a noise stimulus. By repeating the stimulus and employing computer averaging techniques, a series of waves are produced on the monitor screen which represent the passage of the electrical activity along the auditory pathway from cochlea to cortex (Fig. 20.30).

The EEG is recorded from scalp electrodes and the average response to a repeated sound stimulus is derived. The response is divided into three phases — the brain stem response, the early cortical response and the late cortical response.

Increasing concentrations of the anaesthetic agents increase brain stem wave latencies III and V and also increase interpeak intervals I–III, I–V and III–V. Increased latency of the Pa and Nb components of the early cortical response have also been noted with inhalational agents.

Intravenous agents have little effect on the brain stem response but produce similar changes to those associated with inhalational agents in the early cortical response. Because of this, the early cortical response shows promise as a general indicator of the depth of anaesthesia as it shows dose-related changes in latencies which are similar with different general anaesthetic agents.

Cerebral blood flow

The measurement of cerebral blood flow using a gamma camera and radioactive isotope injection provides the most accurate measurement of cerebral perfusion. However, this method is too cumbersome and complicated for routine application.

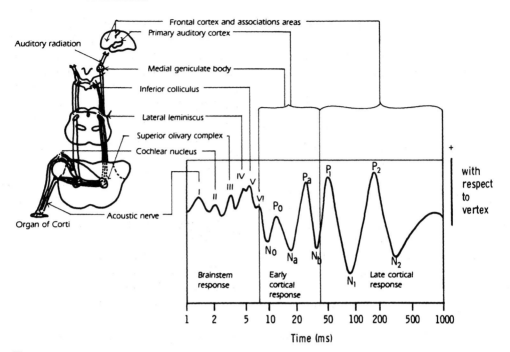

Fig. 20.30 The auditory evoked response consists of a series of waves generated from specific anatomical sites in the auditory pathway as indicated. Activity passes from the cochlea through the brain stem to the cortex.

MONITORING THE NEUROMUSCULAR JUNCTION

See Chapter 11.

MONITORING OF METABOLISM

Homeostasis of the main metabolic processes of the body must be assured during anaesthesia. Monitoring of the following functions should be considered for all but minor surgery.

Temperature regulation

General anaesthesia inhibits the patient's ability to maintain body temperature by depressing the thermoregulatory centre in the hypothalamus. Heat loss during anaesthesia is potentiated by surgery of long duration and exposure of large surface areas of tissue, e.g. the abdominal contents during gastrointestinal operations. The use of wet packs and dry inspired gases compounds the problem. These sources of heat loss assume even more importance in children, especially small babies, whose surface area is much larger in proportion to body weight than in the adult.

During operations where these factors are important, core temperature must be monitored and efforts made to minimize heat loss. Measures to minimize heat loss include the following:

1. The operating room temperature should be as high as is comfortable for the theatre staff.
2. A warming mattress should be placed beneath the patient.
3. Exposed surfaces should be swaddled with warm gauze or foil, especially in neonates.
4. All i.v. infusion fluids should be warmed.
5. Inspired gases should be warmed and humidified.

The thermistor probe is the most commonly used type of temperature-measuring device. It consists of a bead of a mixture of non-metal oxides which is thermally sensitive and the resistance of which varies non-linearly with temperature.

The probe may be placed in the following positions in order to measure core temperature:

1. The nasopharynx (approximates to brain temperature).

2. The oesophagus (approximates to cardiac temperature).
3. The tympanic membrane (best for core temperature, but the membrane is delicate and easily damaged).
4. The rectum.

It is useful also to measure the temperature of the inspired gases when an efficient humidifier is employed in order to avoid thermal burns to the respiratory tract.

If core temperature decreases during anaesthesia, this may result in intense shivering during recovery. This in turn results in increased oxygen consumption (5–10 times normal), disturbances of blood gas homeostasis, increased demands on the cardiovascular system and discomfort to the patient.

Rarely, a rapid increase in temperature occurs during anaesthesia. This is usually associated with the rare inherited disorder of malignant hyperthermia. The rapid increases in muscle metabolism and temperature result in profound metabolic acidosis, hypercapnia and hyperkalaemia. Prompt therapeutic action is required to prevent a fatal outcome (see p. 400).

Fluid and electrolyte status

Blood and fluid losses may be considerable during surgery and empirical calculations of electrolyte losses may be erroneous. Estimation of fluid losses includes measurement of blood loss on swabs and drapes (see above), fluid collection in suction jars and an allowance for evaporative loss. Fluid input and output must be measured as accurately as possible in babies and young children.

Measurement of serum sodium and potassium concentrations in the laboratory is relatively simple and this provides guidance on replacement with appropriate i.v. fluids. However, there may be some delay in obtaining laboratory results. Flame photometers and ion-specific electrodes are now available for measurement of serum and urine electrolytes in the operating theatre suite or intensive therapy unit.

Blood gas and acid–base status

Monitoring of oxygen and carbon dioxide contents in blood is achieved most accurately by the measurement of arterial blood gases. This is facilitated by the presence of an arterial cannula and the availability of an automated blood gas analyser. Modern blood gas analysers use microelectrode systems and require very small quantities (approximately 0.2 ml) of heparinized blood. These machines provide results within 2–3 min and have helped to improve the management of patients undergoing major surgery.

Measurement of blood gases or acid–base status is indicated in the following situations:

1. Major vascular surgery, including cardiac surgery.
2. One-lung anaesthesia.
3. Hypotensive anaesthesia.
4. Critically ill patients.
5. Neurosurgical anaesthesia.

Monitoring of hormonal status

The metabolic response to anaesthesia and surgery consists of an elevation of the plasma concentrations of all the catabolic hormones (cortisol, catecholamines, growth hormone) and depression of the secretion of insulin. The magnitude of this response is proportional to the extent and duration of surgery.

The resulting elevation of blood sugar concentrations may be detrimental, particularly to the diabetic patient and to patients who are critically ill and already in a catabolic phase. In such patients, blood sugar concentration should be monitored at appropriate intervals and an insulin infusion administered as appropriate. Blood sugar concentration may be estimated rapidly and accurately if a sample of blood from a thumb prick is applied to a test strip, e.g. Dextrostix or BM test.

Assessment of clotting status

Assessment of the adequacy of blood coagulation is of obvious importance during surgery. However, in specific situations, e.g. patients with inherent disorders of clotting, those given a massive blood transfusion, those receiving anticoagulant therapy or those suspected of developing disseminated intravascular coagulation (DIC), it is mandatory to monitor clotting status.

Massive transfusion

Storage of blood induces the following changes:

1. Decrease in platelet count.
2. Decrease in concentrations of labile clotting factors (mainly V and VIII).
3. Decrease in 2,3-diphosphoglycerate concentrations.
4. Increase in extracellular potassium ion concentration.
5. Decrease in ionized calcium concentration.
6. Decrease in pH (6.6–7.1).

When large quantities of stored blood are transfused, coagulation may be affected adversely. The following tests may be helpful in assessing the necessity for platelet transfusion, transfusion of fresh frozen plasma or calcium therapy:

1. Platelet count (normal range 150–300×10^9 litre^{-1}).
2. Prothrombin time (normal range 12–15 s) or international normalized ratio (INR; normal range 1.0–1.2) — tests extrinsic system.
3. Partial thromboplastin time (PTT; normal range 35–45 s) — tests intrinsic system.

If PTT is prolonged to more than twice normal, infusion of fresh frozen plasma is indicated. Spontaneous bleeding may not occur until the platelet count is less than 10×10^9 litre^{-1} but platelet transfusion should be considered if the platelet count is less than 50×10^9 litre^{-1} and the patient is bleeding actively. If DIC is suspected the fibrinogen level (normally 1.5 g.litre^{-1}) and fibrin degradation product titre (normally < 10 mg.litre^{-1}) should also be measured.

Table 20.6 Summary of recommendations for standards of monitoring during anaesthesia and recovery (Association of Anaesthetists of Great Britain and Ireland, 1994)

The Association of Anaesthetists of Great Britain and Ireland strongly recommends that the standard of monitoring used during general anaesthesia should be uniform in all circumstances, irrespective of the duration of anaesthesia or the location of administration

An anaesthetist must be present throughout the conduct of general anaesthesia

Monitoring should be commenced before induction and continued until the patient has recovered from the effects of anaesthesia

These recommendations also apply to the administration of local anaesthesia, regional analgesia or sedation where there is a risk of unconsciousness or cardiovascular or respiratory complications

The anaesthetist should check all equipment before use. Monitoring of anaesthetic machine function during the administration of anaesthesia should include an oxygen analyser with alarms. During spontaneous ventilation, clinical observation and a capnometer should be used to detect leaks, disconnections, rebreathing and high pressure in the breathing system. Measurement of airway pressure, expired volume and carbon dioxide concentration is strongly recommended when mechanical ventilation is employed

A pulse oximeter and capnometer must be available for every patient

It is strongly recommended that clinical observation of the patient should be supplemented by continuous monitoring devices displaying heart rate, pulse volume or arterial pressure, oxygen saturation, the electrocardiogram and expired carbon dioxide concentration. Devices for measuring intravascular pressures, body temperature and other parameters should be used when appropriate. It is useful to have both waveform and numerical display

Intermittent non-invasive arterial pressure measurement must be recorded regularly if invasive monitoring is not indicated. If neuromuscular blocking drugs are used, a means of assessing neuromuscular function should be available

Additional monitoring may be required in certain situations. These recommendations may be extended at any time on the judgement of the anaesthetist

A printed record of monitoring measurements provides a contemporaneous record during emergency situations and allows the anaesthetist to concentrate on managing the patient

When handing over to recovery staff, anaesthetists should issue clear instructions concerning monitoring during postoperative care. Monitoring of oxygen saturation is strongly recommended for all patients and temperature monitoring is recommended for patients at risk of hypothermia

Standards of monitoring during transfer of sedated, anaesthetized or unconscious patients should be as high as during the administration of anaesthesia. All patients should have oxygen saturation, electrocardiogram and arterial pressure monitored. Other monitors may be appropriate in certain circumstances

For interhospital transfers, a specialist retrieval team based at the receiving hospital can have advantages

---

Anticoagulant therapy

Patients receiving oral anticoagulants should not be considered for surgery until the INR is less than twice normal. If emergency surgery is necessary, fresh frozen plasma should be available.

Peroperative heparin therapy may be monitored by measuring the activated clotting time. A commercially available kit (Haemochron) may be used in the operating theatre. It consists of a test tube which contains a magnet and some diatomaceous earth. The blood sample is injected into the test tube, which is placed in the machine. The test tube is slowly rotated and when a clot forms it enmeshes the magnet which then rotates along with the tube and activates a detector. The activated clotting time is kept at two to three times normal (normal range 80–135 s) for adequate heparin anticoagulation.

ESSENTIAL MONITORING

The question of what constitutes generally applicable minimum standards for monitoring has generated much debate worldwide. This debate has arisen because of an increasingly litigious climate over the past decade which has resulted in an escalation of awards for damages, and consequently of indemnity premiums. Adequate monitoring appears to be one of the more critical factors in preventing injury to patients during anaesthesia in that analysis of anaesthetic mishaps often identifies events which might have been prevented by the use of an appropriate monitor. In addition, contemporaneous recordings of data acquired from monitoring apparatus are invaluable in assessing the validity of a claim that injury has occurred during anaesthesia.

The recommended standards for minimal monitoring published by the Association of Anaesthetists of Great Britain and Ireland are reprinted in Table 20.6. Such standards have been widely published and embraced by the specialty in many countries. Table 20.7 shows a scheme for essential and desirable monitoring in various types of surgery.

Table 20.7 Essential and desirable patient monitoring in addition to that incorporated in the breathing system and ventilator

Operation category	Monitoring	

Minor
Less than 30 min
	Essential
	Pulse
	   Palpation
	   Stethoscope { oesophageal / precordial
	   Finger plethysmograph
	ECG
	Indirect arterial pressure
	Pulse oximeter
		Desirable

Standard Less than 3 h Relatively healthy patient Endotracheal anaesthesia Blood loss < 10% of blood volume	As for minor Expired volume (if IPPV is employed)	End-tidal CO_2 Neuromuscular blockade Temperature

Major
Longer than 3 h
Blood loss > 10% of blood volume
Operations on:
   chest
   central nervous system
   cardiovascular system
	ECG
	Pulse oximeter
	Direct arterial pressure
	Central venous pressure
	Blood loss measurement
	Urine output
	Temperature
	   patient
	   blood warmer, mattress
	   inspired gas
	Blood gas analysis
	Serum potassium concentration
	Coagulation status
		Neuromuscular blockade

GA = general anaesthetic; ECG = electrocardiogram; CO_2 = carbon dioxide; IPPV = intermittent positive-pressure ventilation.

In the last few years a reduction in the number and severity of medical malpractice insurance claims in the USA has resulted in decreased insurance premiums for anaesthetists.

There is also strong evidence that the number and severity of intraoperative critical incidents has decreased over the last few years. It is likely that this is a reflection not only of the publication of, and adherence to, accepted monitoring standards but also of other factors such as improved quality of personnel entering anaesthesia, improved continuing education, better training, better equipment, risk management initiatives and possibly additional factors.

Clearly, modification — and possibly extension — of these recommendations may be dictated by preoperative assessment of the patient's condition, and the physiological changes caused by specific operations.

The adoption of these standards demands enormous expenditure on the part of hospital authorities, and not all are likely to acquiesce to the requests of anaesthetists for purchase of new equipment. However, it is likely that if any mishap occurs during an anaesthetic in which monitoring does not meet the published standards, the anaesthetist may be judged to have been negligent.

FURTHER READING

Blith C D 1990 Monitoring in anaesthesia and critical care medicine. Churchill Livingstone, Edinburgh

Desmonts J M 1992 Outcome after anaesthesia and surgery. Baillières Clinical Anaesthesiology: International Practice and Research 6(3): 463–690

Jones J G 1989 Depth of anaesthesia. Baillière's Clinical Anaesthesiology: International Practice and Research 3(3): 451–668

Lake C 1994 Clinical monitoring. W B Saunders, London

Sykes M K, Vickers M D, Hull C J 1991 Principles of measurement and monitoring in anaesthesia and intensive care. Blackwell Scientific Publications, Oxford

21. Fluid, electrolyte and acid–base balance

The realization that the enzyme systems and metabolic processes responsible for the maintenance of cellular function are dependent on an environment with stable electrolyte and hydrogen ion concentrations led Claude Bernard over 100 years ago to describe the 'milieu interieur'. Complex homoeostatic mechanisms have evolved to maintain the constancy of this internal environment and thus prevent cellular dysfunction.

Basic definitions

Osmosis refers to the movement of *solvent* molecules across a membrane into a region in which there is a higher concentration of *solute*. This movement may be prevented by applying a pressure to the more concentrated solution – the effective osmotic pressure. This is a colligative property; the magnitude of effective osmotic pressure exerted by a solution depends on the *number* rather than the type of particles present.

The amounts of osmotically active particles present in solution are expressed in *osmoles*. One osmole of a substance is equal to its molecular weight in grams (one mole) divided by the number of freely moving particles which each molecule liberates in solution. Thus, 180 g of glucose in 1 litre of water represents a solution with a molar concentration of 1 mol.litre^{-1} and an *osmolarity* of 1 osmol.litre^{-1}. Sodium chloride ionizes in solution and each ion represents an osmotically active particle. Assuming complete dissociation into Na^+ and Cl^-, 58.5 g of NaCl dissolved in 1 litre of water has a molar concentration of 1 mol.litre^{-1} and an osmolarity of 2 osmol.litre^{-1}. In body fluids, solute concentrations are much lower (mmol.litre^{-1}) and dissociation is incomplete. Consequently, a solution of NaCl containing 1 mmol.litre^{-1} contributes slightly less than 2 mosmol.litre^{-1}.

The term *osmolality* refers to the number of osmoles per unit of total weight of solvent and, unlike osmolarity, is not affected by the volume of various solutes in solution. Confusion regarding the apparently interchangeable use of the terms osmolarity (measured in osmol.litre^{-1}) and osmolality (measured in osmol.kg^{-1}) is caused by their numerical equivalence in body fluids; plasma osmolarity is 280–310 mosmol.litre^{-1} and plasma osmolality is 280–310 mosmol.kg^{-1}. This equivalence is explained by the almost negligible solute volume contained in biological fluids and the fact that most osmotically active particles are dissolved in water, which has a density of one, i.e. osmol.litre^{-1} = osmol.kg^{-1}). As the number of osmoles in plasma is estimated by measurement of the magnitude of freezing point depression, the more accurate term in clinical practice is osmolality.

Cations (principally Na^+) and anions (Cl^- and HCO_3^-) are the major osmotically active particles in plasma. Glucose and urea make a smaller contribution. Plasma osmolality (P_{osm}) may be estimated from the formula:

$$P_{osm} = 2\,[Na^+] \quad + Blood \quad + Blood$$
$$\text{(mmol.litre}^{-1}) \quad \text{glucose} \quad \text{urea}$$
$$\text{(mmol.litre}^{-1}) \text{ (mmol.litre}^{-1})$$
$$= 290 \text{ mosmol.kg}^{-1}$$

Osmolality is a chemical term and may be confused with the physiological term of *tonicity*. This term is used to describe the effective osmotic pressure of a solution relative to that of plasma. The critical difference between osmolality and tonicity is that *all* solutes contribute to osmolality but only solutes that do not cross the cell membrane contribute to tonicity. Thus, tonicity expresses the osmolal activity of solutes restricted to the extracellular compartment, i.e. those which exert an osmotic force affecting the distribution of water between ICF and ECF. As urea diffuses freely across cell membranes, it does not alter the distribution of water between these two body fluid compartments and does not contribute to tonicity. Other solutes that contribute to plasma osmolality but not tonicity include ethanol and methanol, both of which distribute rapidly throughout the total body water. In contrast, mannitol and sorbitol are restricted to the ECF and contribute to both osmolality and tonicity. The tonicity of plasma may be estimated from the formula:

$$\begin{array}{rl} \text{Plasma} & = 2 \, [\text{Na}^+] + \text{Blood glucose} \\ \text{tonicity} & \quad (\text{mmol.litre}^{-1}) \quad (\text{mmol.litre}^{-1}) \\ & = 285 \text{ mosmol.kg}^{-1} \end{array}$$

Compartmental distribution of total body water

The volume of total body water (TBW) may be measured using radioactive dilution techniques involving either deuterium or tritium, both of which cross all membranes freely and equilibrate rapidly with hydrogen atoms in body water. Such measurements show that approximately 60% of lean body mass (LBM) is water in the average

70 kg male adult. As fat contains little water, females have proportionately less TBW (55%) relative to LBM. TBW decreases with age, falling to 45–50% in later life.

The distribution of TBW between the main body compartments is illustrated in Fig. 21.1. One-third of TBW is contained in the extracellular fluid volume (ECFV) and two-thirds in the intracellular fluid volume (ICFV). The ECFV is subdivided further into the interstitial and intravascular compartments. In addition to the absolute volumes of each compartment, Fig. 21.1 shows the relative size of each compartment compared with body weight.

Solute composition of body fluid compartments

Extracellular fluid (ECF)

The capillary endothelium behaves as a freely permeable membrane to water, cations, anions and many soluble substances such as glucose and urea (but *not* protein). As a result, the solute compositions of interstitial fluid and plasma are similar. Each contains sodium as the principal cation and chloride as the principal anion. Protein behaves as a non-diffusible anion and is present in a higher concentration in plasma. The concentration of Cl$^-$ is slightly higher in interstitial fluid in order to maintain electrical neutrality (Donnan equilibrium).

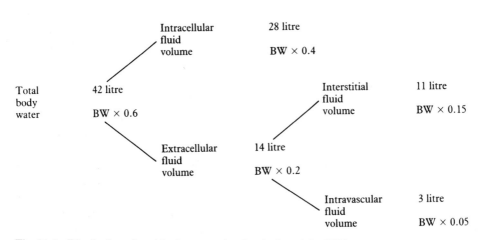

Fig. 21.1 Distribution of total body water related to body weight (BW).

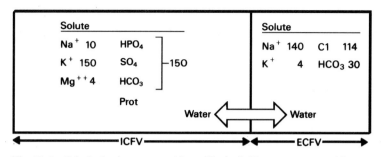

Fig. 21.2 Principal solute composition of body fluid compartments. All concentrations are expressed in mmol.litre^{-1}.

Intracellular fluid (ICF)

This differs from ECF in that the principal cation is potassium and the principal anion is phosphate. In addition, there is a high protein content. In contrast to the capillary endothelium, the cell membrane is permeable *selectively* to different ions and freely permeable to water. Thus, equalization of osmotic forces occurs continuously and is achieved by the movement of water across the cell membrane. The osmolalities of ICF and ECF at equilibrium must be equal. Water moves rapidly between ICF and ECF to eliminate any induced osmolal gradient. This principle is fundamental to an understanding of fluid and electrolyte physiology.

Figure 21.2 shows the solute composition of the main body fluid compartments. Although the total concentration of intracellular ions exceeds that of extracellular ions the numbers of osmotically active particles (and thus the osmolalities) are the same on each side of the cell membrane (290 mosmol.kg^{-1} of solution).

Water homoeostasis

Normal day-to-day fluctuations in TBW are small (< 0.2%) because of a fine balance between input, controlled by the thirst mechanisms, and output, controlled mainly by the renal–ADH system.

The principal sources of body water are ingested fluid, water present in solid food and water produced as an end product of metabolism. Intravenous fluids are another common source in hospital patients. Actual and potential outlets for water are classified conventionally as sensible and insensible losses. Insensible losses emanate

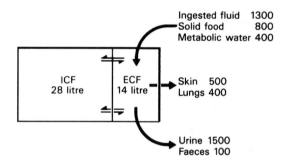

Fig. 21.3 Daily water balance. Input and output in ml.

from the skin and lungs; sensible losses occur mainly from the kidneys and gastrointestinal tract. Figure 21.3 depicts the daily water balance in a 70 kg adult in whom input and output balance. It should be noted that sources of potential loss are not evident in this diagram. For example, over 5 litres of fluid are secreted daily into the gut in the form of saliva, bile, gastric juices and succus entericus, yet only 100 ml of fluid is present in faeces. This illustrates the potential that exists for significant fluid loss in the presence of disease.

PRACTICAL FLUID BALANCE

Calculation of the daily prescription of fluid is an arithmetic exercise to balance the input and output of water and electrolytes.

Table 21.1 shows the electrolyte contents of five intravenous solutions used commonly in the United Kingdom. These solutions are adequate for most clinical situations. Two self-evident but important generalizations may be made regarding solutions for intravenous infusion.

Table 21.1 Electrolyte contents of commonly used intravenous fluids

Solution	Electrolyte content (mmol.litre^{-1})		Osmolality (mosmol.kg^{-1})
Saline 0.9% ('normal saline')	Na$^+$ 154	Cl$^-$ 154	308
Saline 0.45% ('half-normal saline')	Na$^+$ 77	Cl$^-$ 77	154
Glucose 4%/saline 0.18% (glucose–saline)	Na$^+$ 31	Cl$^-$ 31	284
Glucose 5%	nil		278
Compound sodium lactate (Hartmann's solution)	Na$^+$ 131 K$^+$ 5 Ca^{2+} 4	Cl$^-$ 112 HCO$_3^-$ 29 (as lactate)	281

Rule 1

All infused Na$^+$ remains in the ECF; Na$^+$ cannot gain access to the ICF because of the sodium pump. Thus, if saline 0.9% is infused, all Na$^+$ remains in the ECF. As this is an isotonic solution, there is no change in ECF osmolality and therefore no water exchange occurs across the cell membrane. Thus, saline 0.9% expands ECFV only. However, if saline 0.45% is given, ECF osmolality decreases; this causes a shift of water from ECF to ICF. If saline 1.8% is administered, all Na$^+$ remains in the ECF, its osmolality increases and water moves from ICF to ECF to maintain osmotic equality.

Rule 2

Water without sodium expands the TBW. After infusion of a solution of glucose 5%, the glucose enters cells and is metabolized. The infused water enters both ICF and ECF in proportion to their initial volumes.

Table 21.2 illustrates the results of infusion of

Table 21.2 Compartmental expansion resulting from infusion of 1 litre of saline 0.9%, saline 0.45% or glucose 5%

Intravenous infusion of 1000 ml	Change in volume (ml)		Remarks
	ECF	ICF	
Saline 0.9%	+1000	0	Na$^+$ remains in ECF
Glucose 5%	+333	+666	66% of TBW is ICF
Saline 0.45%	+666	+333	33% of TBW is ECF

1 litre of saline 0.9%, saline 0.45% or glucose 5% in a 70 kg adult.

Assessment of daily fluid requirements may be allocated usefully into three processes:

1. Normal maintenance needs.
2. Abnormal losses resulting from the underlying pathology.
3. Correction of pre-existing deficits.

Normal maintenance needs

Water

Regardless of the disease process, water and electrolyte losses occur in urine and as evaporative losses from skin and lungs. It is evident from Figure 21.3 that a normothermic 70 kg patient with a normal metabolic rate may lose 2500 ml of water per day. Allowing for a gain of 400 ml from water of metabolism, this hypothetical patient needs 2000 mlH$_2$O.day^{-1}. As a rule of thumb, a volume of 30–35 mlH$_2$O.kg^{-1}.day^{-1} is a useful estimate for daily maintenance needs.

Sodium

The normal requirement is 1 mmol.kg^{-1}.day^{-1} (50–80 mmol.day^{-1}) for adults.

Potassium

The normal requirement is 1 mmol.kg^{-1}.day^{-1} (50–80 mmol.day^{-1}) for adults.

Thus, a 70 kg patient requires daily provision of 2000–2500 ml of water and approximately 70 mmol each of Na$^+$ and K$^+$. This could be administered as:

1. 2000 ml of glucose 5% + 500 ml of saline 0.9%; or
2. 2500 ml of glucose 4%/saline 0.18%;

plus potassium as KCl, 1 g (13 mmol) added to each 500 ml of fluid.

Abnormal losses

These are common in surgical patients. They may be sensible or insensible and either overt or covert.

Losses from the gut are common, e.g. naso-gastric suction, diarrhoea and vomiting or seques-tration of fluid within the gut lumen (e.g. intestinal obstruction). Although the composition of gastro-intestinal secretions is variable, replacement should be with saline 0.9% with 13–26 mmol.litre^{-1} of potassium as KCl. If losses are considerable (> 1000 ml.day^{-1}), a sample of the appropriate fluid should be sent for biochemical analysis so that electrolyte replacement may be rationalized.

Increased insensible losses from the skin and lungs occur in the presence of fever or hyper-ventilation. The usual insensible loss of 0.5 ml.kg^{-1}.h^{-1} increases by 12% for each degree Celsius rise in temperature.

Sequestration of fluid at the site of operative trauma is a form of fluid loss which is common in surgical patients. Plasma-like fluid is seques-tered in any area of tissue injury; its volume is proportional to the extent of trauma. This fluid is frequently referred to as 'third-space' loss because it ceases to take part in normal metabolic processes. However, it is not contained in an anatomically separate compartment; it represents an expansion of ECFV. Third-space losses are not measured easily. Sequestered fluid is reabsorbed after 48–72 h.

Existing deficits

These occur preoperatively and arise primarily from the gut. The difficulty in correcting these deficits relates to an inability to quantify their magnitude accurately. Fluid and electrolyte defi-cits occur directly from the ECF. If the fluid lost is isotonic, only ECFV is reduced; however, if water alone or hypotonic fluid is lost, redistri-bution of the remaining TBW occurs from ICF to ECF to equalize osmotic forces.

Dehydration with accompanying salt loss is a common disorder in the acute surgical patient.

Assessment of dehydration

This is a clinical assessment based upon:

1. *History.* How long has the patient had abnor-mal loss of fluid? How much has occurred, e.g. frequency of vomiting?

2. *Examination.* Specific features are thirst, dry-ness of mucous membranes, loss of skin turgor, orthostatic hypotension or tachycardia, reduced JVP or CVP and decreased urine output. In the presence of normal renal function, dehydration is associated usually with a urine output of less than 0.5 ml.kg^{-1}.h^{-1}. The severity of dehydration may be described clinically as mild, moderate or severe and each category is associated with the following water loss relative to body weight.

Mild. Loss of 4% body weight (approximately 3 litres in a 70 kg patient); reduced skin turgor, sunken eyes, dry mucous membranes.

Moderate. Loss of 5–8% body weight (approximately 4–6 litres in a 70 kg patient); oliguria, orthostatic hypotension and tachycardia in addition to the above.

Severe. Loss of 8–10% body weight (approxi-mately 7 litres in a 70 kg patient); profound oliguria and compromised cardiovascular function.

Laboratory assessment

The degree of haemoconcentration and increase in albumin concentration may be helpful in the absence of anaemia and hypoproteinaemia. Increased blood urea concentration and urine osmolality (> 650 mosmol.kg^{-1}) confirms the clinical diagnosis.

Perioperative fluid therapy

In addition to normal maintenance requirements of water and electrolytes, patients may require fluid in the perioperative period to restore TBW after a period of fasting and to replace small blood losses, loss of ECF into the 'third space' and losses of water from the skin, gut and lungs.

Blood losses in excess of 15% of blood volume in the adult are replaced usually by infusion of stored blood. Smaller blood losses may be re-placed by a crystalloid electrolyte solution such as compound sodium lactate; however, because these solutions are distributed throughout ECF, blood volume is maintained only if at least three times the volume of blood loss is infused. Alterna-tively, a colloid solution (human albumin solution or a synthetic substitute) may be infused in a volume equal to that of the estimated loss.

'Third-space' losses are replaced usually as compound sodium lactate. In abdominal surgery (e.g. cholecystectomy), a volume of 5 ml.kg^{-1}.h^{-1} during operation, in addition to normal maintenance requirements (approximately 1.5 ml.kg^{-1}.h^{-1}) and blood loss replacement, is usually sufficient. Larger volumes may be required in more major procedures, but should be guided by measurement of CVP.

In the postoperative period, normal maintenance fluids should be administered (see above). Additional fluid (given as saline 0.9% or compound sodium lactate) may be required in the following circumstances:

1. If blood or serum is lost from drains (colloid solutions should be used if losses exceed 500 ml).
2. If gastrointestinal losses continue, e.g. from a nasogastric tube or a fistula.
3. After major surgery (e.g. total gastrectomy, repair of aortic aneurysm), when additional water and electrolytes may be required for 24–48 h to replace continuing 'third-space' losses.
4. During rewarming if the patient has become hypothermic during surgery.

Normally, potassium is not administered in the first 24 h after surgery as endogenous release of potassium from tissue trauma and catabolism warrants restriction. The postoperative patient differs from the 'normal' patient in that the stress reaction modifies homoeostatic mechanisms; stress-induced release of ADH, aldosterone and cortisol causes retention of Na$^+$ and water and increased renal excretion of potassium. However, restriction of fluid and sodium in the postoperative period is inappropriate despite a low urine output because of increased losses by evaporation and into the 'third space'. The stress response lasts for 24–72 h and recovery is heralded usually by a diuresis.

After major surgery, assessment of fluid and electrolyte requirements is achieved best by measurement of CVP and serum electrolyte concentrations.

Fluid and electrolyte requirements in infants and small children differ from those in the adult (see Ch. 33).

Patients with renal failure require fluid replacement for abnormal losses, although the total volume of fluid infused should be reduced to a degree determined by the urine output.

SODIUM AND POTASSIUM

Sodium balance

Daily ingestion amounts to 50–300 mmol. Losses in sweat and faeces are minimal (approximately 10 mmol.day^{-1}) and final adjustments are made by the kidney. Urine sodium excretion may be as little as 2 mmol.day^{-1} during salt restriction or may exceed 700 mmol.day^{-1} after salt loading. Sodium balance is related intimately to ECFV and water balance.

Disorders of sodium/water balance

Hypernatraemia

Hypernatraemia is defined as a plasma sodium concentration of more than 150 mmol.litre^{-1} and may result from pure water loss, hypotonic fluid loss or salt gain. In the first two conditions, ECFV is reduced, whereas salt gain is associated with an expanded ECFV. For this reason, the clinical assessment of volaemic status is important in the diagnosis and management of hypernatraemic states. The common causes of hypernatraemia are summarized in Table 21.3. The abnormality common to all hypernatraemic states is intracellular dehydration secondary to ECF hyperosmolality.

Table 21.3 Causes of hypernatraemia

Pure water depletion	
Extrarenal loss	Failure of water intake (coma, elderly, postoperative)
	Mucocutaneous loss
	Fever, hyperventilation, thyrotoxicosis
Renal loss	Diabetes insipidus (cranial, nephrogenic)
	Chronic renal failure
Hypotonic fluid loss	
Extrarenal loss	Gastrointestinal (vomiting, diarrhoea)
	Skin (excessive sweating)
Renal loss	Osmotic diuresis (glucose, urea, mannitol)
Salt gain	Iatrogenic (NaHCO$_3$, hypertonic saline)
	Salt ingestion
	Steroid excess

Primary water loss resulting in hypernatraemia may occur during prolonged fever, hyperventilation or during severe exercise in hot, dry climates. However, a more common cause is the renal water loss that occurs when there is a defect in either the production or release of ADH (cranial diabetes insipidus) or an abnormality in response to ADH (nephrogenic diabetes insipidus).

The administration of osmotic diuretics results temporarily in plasma hyperosmolality. An osmotic diuresis may occur also in hyperglycaemia. During an osmotic diuresis, the solute causing the diuresis (e.g. glucose, mannitol) constitutes a significant fraction of urine solute and the sodium content of the urine becomes hypotonic relative to plasma sodium. Thus, osmotic diuretics cause hypotonic urine losses which may result in hypernatraemic dehydration.

Hypertonic dehydration may occur also in paediatric practice. Diarrhoea, vomiting and anorexia lead to loss of water in excess of solute (hypotonic loss). Concomitant fever, hyperventilation and the use of high-solute feeds may combine to exaggerate the problem. ECFV is maintained by movement of water from ICF to ECF to equalize osmolality and clinical evidence of dehydration may not be apparent until 10–15% of body weight has been lost. Rehydration must be undertaken gradually to prevent the development of cerebral oedema.

Measurement of urine and plasma osmolalities and assessment of urine output help in the diagnosis of hypernatraemic, volume-depleted states. If urine output is low and urine osmolality exceeds 800 mosmol.kg^{-1}, then both ADH secretion and the renal response to ADH are present. The most likely causes are extrarenal water loss (e.g. diarrhoea, vomiting or evaporation) or insufficient intake. High urine output and high urine osmolality suggest an osmotic diuresis. If urine osmolality is less than plasma osmolality, reduced ADH secretion or impairment of the renal response to ADH should be suspected; in both cases, urine output is high.

Usually, hypernatraemia caused by salt gain is iatrogenic in origin. It occurs when excessive amounts of hypertonic sodium bicarbonate are administered during resuscitation or when isotonic fluids are given to patients who have only

insensible losses. Treatment comprises induction of a diuresis with a loop diuretic if renal function is normal; urine output is replaced in part with glucose 5%. Dialysis or haemofiltration is necessary in patients with renal dysfunction.

Consequences of hypernatraemia. The major clinical manifestations of hypernatraemia involve the central nervous system. Severity depends on the rapidity with which hyperosmolality develops. Acute hypernatraemia is associated with a prompt osmotic shift of water from the intracellular compartment causing a reduction in cell volume and water content of the brain. This results in increased permeability and even rupture of the capillaries in the brain and subarachnoid space. The patient may present with pyrexia (a manifestation of impaired thermoregulation), nausea, vomiting, convulsions, coma and virtually any type of focal neurological syndrome. The mortality and long-term morbidity of sustained hypernatraemia (Na$^+$ > 160 mmol.litre^{-1} for over 48 h) is high irrespective of the underlying aetiology. In many cases the development of hypernatraemia can be anticipated and prevented, e.g. cranial diabetes insipidus associated with head injury, but in situations where preventative strategies have failed treatment should be instituted without hesitation.

Treatment of hypernatraemia. The magnitude of the water deficit can be estimated from the measured plasma sodium concentration and calculated total body water:

$$\text{Water deficit} = (\text{measured } [\text{Na}^+]/140 \times \text{TBW}) - \text{TBW}$$

Thus in a 75 kg patient with a serum sodium of 170 mmol.litre^{-1}:

$$\begin{aligned}
\text{Water deficit} &= (170/140 \times 0.6 \times 75) - (0.6 \times 75) \\
&= 54.6 - 45 \\
&= 9.6 \text{ litres}
\end{aligned}$$

For hypernatraemic patients *without* volume depletion 5% glucose is sufficient to correct the water deficit. However, the majority of hypernatraemic patients are frankly hypovolaemic and intravenous fluids should be prescribed to repair both the sodium and the water deficit. Regardless of the severity of the condition, isotonic saline is the initial treatment of choice in the volume-depleted, hypernatraemic patient as even this fluid is *relatively* hypotonic in patients with severe hypernatraemia. Once volume depletion has been corrected then further repair of any water deficit can be accomplished with hypotonic fluids. Fluid therapy should be prescribed with the intention of correcting hypernatraemia over a period of 48–72 h to prevent the onset of cerebral oedema.

Hyponatraemia

This is defined as a plasma sodium concentration of less than 135 mmol.litre⁻¹. Hyponatraemia is a common finding in hospital patients. It may occur as a result of water retention, sodium loss or both; consequently, it may be associated with an expanded, normal or contracted ECFV. As in hypernatraemia, the state of ECFV is impor-

tant in determining the cause of the electrolyte imbalance.

As plasma osmolality decreases, an osmolal gradient is created across the cell membrane and results in movement of water into the ICF. The resulting expansion of brain cells is responsible for the symptomatology of hyponatraemia or 'water intoxication': nausea, vomiting, lethargy, weakness and obtundation. In severe cases (plasma Na⁺ < 115 mmol.litre⁻¹), seizures and coma may result.

A scheme depicting the causes of hyponatraemia is shown in Fig. 21.4. True hyponatraemia must be distinguished from pseudohyponatraemia. Sodium ions are present only in plasma water, which constitutes 93% of normal plasma. In the laboratory the concentration of sodium in plasma is measured in an aliquot of whole plasma and

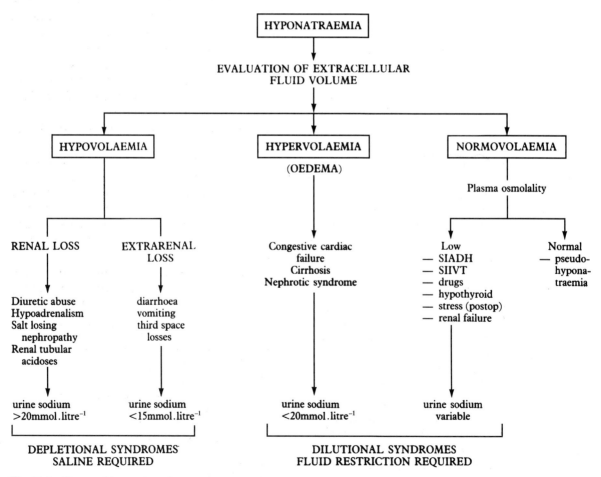

Fig. 21.4 Causes of hyponatraemia.

the concentration is expressed in terms of plasma volume (mmol.litre^{-1} of whole plasma). If the percentage of water present in plasma is decreased, as in hyperlipidaemia or hyperproteinaemia, the amount of Na$^+$ in each aliquot of plasma is decreased also, even if its concentration in plasma water is normal. A clue to this cause of hyponatraemia is the finding of a normal plasma osmolality. Pseudohyponatraemia is not encountered when plasma sodium concentration is measured by increasingly employed ion-specific electrodes, because this method assesses directly the sodium concentration in the aqueous phase of plasma.

True hyponatraemic states may be classified conveniently into *depletional* and *dilutional* types. Depletional hyponatraemia occurs when a deficit in TBW is associated with an even greater deficit of total body sodium. Assessment of volaemic status reveals hypovolaemia. Losses may be *renal* or *extrarenal*. Excessive renal loss of sodium occurs in Addison's disease, diuretic administration, renal tubular acidosis and salt-losing nephropathies; usually, urine sodium concentration exceeds 20 mmol.litre^{-1}. Extrarenal losses occur usually from the gastrointestinal tract (e.g. diarrhoea, vomiting) or from sequestration into the 'third space' (e.g. peritonitis, surgery). Normal kidneys respond by conserving sodium and water to produce a urine that is hyperosmolal and low in sodium. In both situations, treatment should be directed at expanding the ECFV with saline 0.9%.

Dilutional hyponatraemic states may be associated with hypervolaemia and oedema or with normovolaemia. Again, assessment of volaemic status is important. If oedema is present, there is an excess of total body sodium with a proportionately greater excess of TBW. This is seen in congestive heart failure, cirrhosis and the nephrotic syndrome and is caused by secondary hyperaldosteronism. Treatment comprises salt and water restriction and spironolactone.

In normovolaemic hyponatraemia there is a modest excess of TBW and a modest increase in ECFV associated with a normal total body sodium. Pseudohyponatraemia is excluded by finding high protein or lipid levels and a normal plasma osmolality. True normovolaemic hyponatraemia is commonly iatrogenic in origin. The syndrome of inappropriate intravenous therapy (SIIVT) is caused usually by administration of intravenous fluids with a low sodium content to patients with isotonic losses.

A more chronic water overload may occur in patients with hypothyroidism and in conditions associated with an inappropriately elevated level of ADH. The syndrome of inappropriate ADH secretion (SIADH) is characterized by hyponatraemia, low plasma osmolality and an inappropriate antidiuresis, i.e. a urine osmolality higher than anticipated for the degree of hyponatraemia. It occurs in the presence of malignant tumours which produce ADH-like substances (e.g. lung, prostate, pancreas), in neurological disorders (e.g. head injury, tumours, infections) and in some severe pneumonias. A number of drugs are associated with increased ADH secretion or potentiate the effects of ADH (Table 21.4). In patients with SIADH, the urine is concentrated in spite of hyponatraemia. Management comprises restriction of fluid intake to encourage a negative fluid balance. In severe or refractory cases, demeclocycline or lithium may result in improvement. Both drugs induce a state of functional diabetes insipidus and have been used effectively in SIADH if the primary disease cannot be treated.

Consequences of hyponatraemia. Symptoms vary with the underlying aetiology, the magnitude of the reduction of plasma sodium and the rapidity with which the plasma sodium concentration falls. Serious consequences involve the central nervous system and result from intracellular overhydration, cerebral oedema and raised intracranial pressure. Nausea, vomiting, delirium, convulsions and coma result.

Treatment of hyponatraemia. Acute symptomatic hyponatraemia is a medical emergency

Table 21.4 Drugs associated with antidiuresis and hyponatraemia

---

Increased ADH secretion
  Hypnotics — barbiturates
  Analgesics — opioids
  Hypoglycaemics — chlorpropamide, tolbutamide
  Anticonvulsants — carbamazepine
  Miscellaneous — phenothiazines, tricyclics

Potentiation of ADH at distal tubule
  Paracetamol
  Indomethacin
  Chlorpropamide

and requires prompt intervention using hypertonic saline. The rapidity with which hyponatraemia should be corrected is the subject of controversy because of observations that rapid correction may cause central pontine myelinolysis, a disorder characterized by paralysis, coma and death. As a causal relationship between this syndrome and the rate of rise of plasma sodium has not been established and it is clear that there is a prohibitive mortality associated with inadequately treated water intoxication, rapid correction of the symptomatic hyponatraemic state is warranted. Sufficient sodium should be given to return the plasma concentration to 125 mmol.litre^{-1} only and this should be administered over a period of no less than 12 h. The amount of sodium needed to cause the desired correction in the plasma sodium can be calculated as follows:

$$Na^+ \text{ required (mmol)} = TBW \times (\text{desired } [Na^+] - \text{measured } [Na^+])$$

Hypertonic saline (3%) contains 514 mmol.litre^{-1} of Na^+ and administration poses the risk of pulmonary oedema, especially in oedematous patients in whom renal dialysis is preferable.

Potassium balance

The normal daily intake of potassium is 50–200 mmol. Minimal amounts are lost via the skin and faeces; the kidney is the primary regulator. However, the mechanisms for the retention of potassium are less efficient than those for sodium. In periods of K^+ depletion, daily urinary excretion cannot decrease to less than 5–10 mmol. A considerable deficit of total body potassium occurs if intake is not restored. Hypokalaemia is a more common abnormality than hyperkalaemia.

Hypokalaemia. This is defined as a plasma potassium concentration of less than 3.5 mmol.litre^{-1}. Non-specific symptoms of hypokalaemia include anorexia and nausea, effects on skeletal and smooth muscle (muscle weakness, paralytic ileus) and cardiac conduction (delayed repolarization with ST segment depression, reduced height of the T wave, increased height of the U wave and a widened QRS complex).

The causes of hypokalaemia are summarized in Table 21.5. Management includes diagnosis

Table 21.5 Causes of hypokalaemia

Cause	Comments
Reduced intake	Usually only contributory
Tissue redistribution	Insulin therapy, alkalaemia, β_2-adrenergic agonists, familial periodic paralysis, vitamin B_{12} therapy
Increased loss	
Gastrointestinal (urine K^+ < 20 mmol.litre^{-1})	Diarrhoea, vomiting, fistulae, nasogastric suction, colonic villous adenoma
Renal	Diuretic therapy, primary or secondary hyperaldosteronism, malignant hypertension, renal artery stenosis (high renin), renal tubular acidosis, hypomagnesaemia, renal failure (diuretic phase)

and treatment of the underlying disorder in addition to repletion of total body potassium stores. As a general rule, a reduction in plasma K^+ concentration by 1 mmol.litre^{-1} reflects a total body K^+ deficit of approximately 100 mmol. Potassium supplements may be given orally or i.v. The maximum infusion rate should not exceed 0.5 mmol.kg^{-1}.h^{-1} to allow equilibration with the intracellular compartment; much slower rates are employed usually.

The potassium salt used for replacement therapy is important. In most situations, and especially in the presence of alkalosis, potassium should be replaced as the chloride salt. Supplements are available also as the bicarbonate and phosphate salts.

Hyperkalaemia. This is defined as a plasma potassium concentration exceeding 5 mmol.litre^{-1}. Vague muscle weakness progressing to flaccid paralysis may occur. However, the major clinical feature of an increasing plasma potassium concentration is the characteristic sequence of ECG abnormalities. The earliest change is the development of tall, peaked T waves and a shortened QT interval, reflecting more rapid repolarization (6–7 mmol.litre^{-1}). As plasma K^+ increases (8–10 mmol.litre^{-1}), abnormalities in depolarization become manifest as widened QRS complexes and widening, and eventually loss, of the P wave; the widened QRS complexes merge finally into the T waves (*sine wave pattern*). Plasma concentrations

Table 21.6 Causes of hyperkalaemia

Factitious (pseudohyperkalaemia)	– in vitro haemolysis – thrombocytosis – leucocytosis – tourniquet – exercise
Impaired excretion	– renal failure – acute or chronic hyperaldosteronism – Addison's disease – K^+-sparing diuretics – indomethacin
Tissue redistribution	– tissue damage (burns, trauma) – rhabdomyolysis – tumour necrosis – hyperkalaemic periodic paralysis – massive intravascular haemolysis – suxamethonium
Excessive intake	– blood transfusion – excessive i.v. administration

in excess of 10 mmol.litre^{-1} are associated with ventricular fibrillation. The cardiac toxicity of K^+ is enhanced by hypocalcaemia, hyponatraemia or acidaemia. The causes of hyperkalaemia are summarized in Table 21.6.

Immediate treatment is necessary if the plasma potassium concentration exceeds 7 mmol.litre^{-1} or if there are any serious ECG abnormalities. Specific treatment may be achieved by four mechanisms:

1. Chemical antagonism of the membrane effects.
2. Enhanced cellular uptake of K^+.
3. Dilution of ECF.
4. Removal of K^+ from the body.

Methods by which the plasma potassium concentration may be reduced are summarized in Table 21.7.

Table 21.7 Treatment of hyperkalaemia

Calcium gluconate 10% i.v. (0.5 ml.kg^{-1} to maximum of 20 ml) given over 5 min. No change in plasma $[K^+]$. Effect immediate but transient

Glucose 50 g (0.5–1.0 g.kg^{-1}) plus insulin 20 units (0.3 unit.kg^{-1}) as single i.v. bolus dose. Then infusion of glucose 20%, plus insulin 6–20 units.h^{-1} (depending on blood glucose)

Sodium bicarbonate 1.5–2.0 mmol.kg^{-1} i.v. over 5–10 min

Calcium resonium 15 g p.o. or 30 g p.r. 8-hourly

Peritoneal or haemodialysis

ACID–BASE BALANCE

The concentration of hydrogen ions (H^+) in body fluids is extremely small and the pH notation was adopted for the sake of practicality. This system expresses H^+ concentration $[H^+]$ on a logarithmic scale:

$$pH = -\log_{10}[H^+]$$

A more logical arithmetic convention which expresses $[H^+]$ in nmol.litre^{-1} is gaining popularity. Table 21.8 compares values of $[H^+]$ expressed as pH and nmol.litre^{-1} and reveals a number of disadvantages of the pH notation. The most obvious disadvantage is that it moves in the opposite direction to $[H^+]$; a decrease in pH is associated with increased $[H^+]$ and vice versa. It is also apparent that the logarithmic scale distorts the quantitative estimate of change in $[H^+]$; for example, twice as many hydrogen ions are required to reduce pH from 7.1 to 7.0 as are needed to reduce it from 7.4 to 7.3. The pH scale gives the false impression that there is relatively little difference in the sensitivity of biological systems to an equivalent increase or decrease in $[H^+]$. However, when $[H^+]$ is expressed in nmol.litre^{-1}, it becomes apparent that tolerance is limited to a reduction in $[H^+]$ of only 24 nmol.litre^{-1} from normal, but to an increase of up to 120 nmol.litre^{-1}. Nevertheless, the pH notation remains the most widely used system and is employed in the remainder of this chapter.

Table 21.8 Comparison of logarithmic and arithmetic methods of expressing hydrogen ion concentration in the range of blood $[H^+]$ compatible with life

pH	$[H^+]$ (nmol.litre^{-1})	
7.8	16	
7.7	20	
7.6	25	*Alkalaemia*
7.5	32	
7.4	**40**	*Normal*
7.3	50	
7.2	63	
7.1	80	
7.0	100	*Acidaemia*
6.9	125	
6.8	160	

Basic definitions

An *acid* is a substance that dissociates in water to produce H^+; a *base* is a substance that can accept H^+. Strong acids dissociate completely in aqueous solution, whereas weak acids (e.g. carbonic acid, H_2CO_3) dissociate only partially. The *conjugate base* of an acid is its dissociated anionic product. For example, bicarbonate ion (HCO_3^-) is the conjugate base of carbonic acid:

$$H_2CO_3 \rightleftharpoons H^+ + HCO_3^-$$

A *buffer* is a combination of a weak acid and its conjugate base (usually as a salt) which acts to minimize any change in $[H^+]$ that would occur if a strong acid or base was added to it. Buffers in body fluids represent an important defence against $[H^+]$ change. The carbonic acid/bicarbonate system is an important buffer in blood. The pH of a buffer system may be determined from the Henderson–Hasselbalch equation which, for the carbonic acid/bicarbonate system, relates pH, $[H_2CO_3]$ and $[HCO_3^-]$:

$$pH = pK + \log_{10} \frac{[HCO_3^-]}{[H_2CO_3]}$$

where K = dissociation constant and $pK = -\log_{10}K$.

This equation shows that $[H^+]$ in body fluids is a function of the *ratio* of base to acid. For the bicarbonate buffer system, pK is 6.1. As most of the carbonic acid pool exists as dissolved CO_2, the equation may be rewritten:

$$pH = 6.1 + \log_{10} \frac{[HCO_3^-]}{0.225 \times PCO_2}$$

The value 0.225 represents the solubility coefficient of CO_2 in blood ($ml.kPa^{-1}$). Normally, $[HCO_3^-]$ is 24 $mmol.litre^{-1}$ and Pa_{CO_2} is 5.3 kPa. Thus:

$$pH = 6.1 + \log_{10} \frac{24}{0.225 \times 5.3} = 7.4$$

Most acid–base disorders may be formulated in terms of the Henderson–Hasselbalch equation. The pH of plasma is kept remarkably constant at 7.36–7.44, i.e. a hydrogen ion concentration of 40 ± 5 $nmol.litre^{-1}$. This is achieved by:

1. Regulation of H^+ excretion and bicarbonate regeneration by the kidney.

2. Regulation of CO_2 by the alveolar ventilation of the lungs.

Cellular metabolism poses a constant threat to buffer systems by the production of 'volatile acid', i.e. CO_2, from cellular respiration and the formation of 'fixed' or 'non-volatile' acids by intermediary metabolism. Thus, the acid–base status of body fluids reflects the metabolism of both H^+ and CO_2.

Acid–base disorders

The normal pH of body fluids is 7.36–7.44. Conventional acid–base nomenclature involves the following definitions:

1. An *acidosis* is a process that causes acid to accumulate.
2. An *acidaemia* is present if pH < 7.36.
3. An *alkalosis* is a process that causes base to accumulate.
4. An *alkalaemia* is present if pH > 7.44.

Simple acid–base disorders are common in clinical practice and their successful management requires logical analysis of pH, $[HCO_3^-]$ and Pa_{CO_2}. The first step involves diagnosis of the primary disorder; this is followed by an assessment of the extent and appropriateness of any compensation.

Primary acid–base disorders are either *respiratory* or *metabolic*. The disorder is respiratory if the primary disturbance involves CO_2 and metabolic if it involves HCO_3^-. Thus, four potential primary disturbances exist (Table 21.9) and each may be identified by analysis of pH, $[HCO_3^-]$ and Pa_{CO_2}. Both pH and Pa_{CO_2} are measured directly by the blood gas machine. $[HCO_3^-]$ is measured directly on the electrolyte profile but is derived in most blood gas machines. Other derived parameters include *standard bicarbonate* and *base excess*. The standard bicarbonate is not the actual bicarbonate of the sample but an estimate of bicarbonate concentration after elimination of any abnormal respiratory contribution to $[HCO_3^-]$, i.e. an estimate of $[HCO_3^-]$ at a Pa_{CO_2} of 5.3 kPa. The base excess (in alkalosis) or base deficit (in acidosis) is the amount of acid or base (in mmol) required to return the pH of 1 litre of blood to normal at a

Table 21.9 Compensatory mechanisms in acid–base disturbances. ↓↓ or ↑↑ denotes the primary abnormality. The final pH depends on the degree of compensation. Respiratory compensation for metabolic disorders is rapid; renal compensation for respiratory disorders is slow

Primary disorder		pH	HCO_3^-	Pa_{CO_2}	Compensation
Metabolic	acidosis	↓	↓↓		Hyperventilation ↓ Pa_{CO_2}
	alkalosis	↑	↑↑		Hypoventilation ↑ Pa_{CO_2}
Respiratory	acidosis	↓		↑↑	Renal retention of HCO_3^-
	alkalosis	↑		↓↓	Renal elimination of HCO_3^-

Pa_{CO_2} of 5.3 kPa; it is a measure of the magnitude of the metabolic component of the acid–base disorder.

After the primary disorder has been identified, it is necessary to consider if it is acute or chronic and if any compensation has occurred. The body defends itself against changes in pH by compensatory mechanisms which *tend* to return pH towards normal. Primary respiratory disorders are compensated by a metabolic mechanism and vice versa. For example, a primary respiratory acidosis is compensated for by renal retention of HCO_3^-, whereas a primary metabolic acidosis is compensated for by hyperventilation and a decrease in Pa_{CO_2}. Thus, in each case the *acidaemia* produced by the primary acidosis is reduced by a compensatory alkalosis. The response to a respiratory alkalosis is increased renal elimination of HCO_3^- and a metabolic alkalosis results in hypoventilation and increased Pa_{CO_2}. pH is restored towards normal by the compensatory respiratory acidosis. In each case, the efficiency of compensatory mechanisms is limited; compensation is usually only partial and rarely complete. Overcompensation does not occur.

Metabolic acidosis

This is characterized by decreased $[HCO_3^-]$ and a variable degree of acidaemia. The extent of the acidaemia depends upon the nature, severity and duration of the initiating pathology in addition to the efficiency of compensatory mechanisms.

An important clue to the nature of the abnormality is given by the measurement of the *anion gap* in plasma:

$$anion\ gap = ([Na^+] + [K^+]) - ([Cl^-] + [HCO_3^-])$$

In reality, the numbers of cations and anions in plasma are the same and an anion gap exists because negatively charged proteins, together with phosphate, lactate and organic anions (which maintain electrical neutrality) are not measured. The normal anion gap is 12–18 mmol.litre^{-1}.

Clinically, it is useful to divide the metabolic acidoses into those associated with a normal anion gap and those with an increased anion gap. The former are caused by loss of HCO_3^- from the body and replacement with chloride. In acidoses associated with an increased anion gap, HCO_3^- has been titrated by either endogenous, e.g. lactic, or exogenous acids, thus increasing the number of unmeasured plasma anions without altering the plasma chloride concentration (Table 21.10).

Clinical effects and treatment. Metabolic acidosis results in widespread physiological disturbances, including reduced cardiac output, pulmonary hypertension, arrhythmias, Kussmaul respiration and hyperkalaemia; the severity of the disturbances are related to the extent of the *acidaemia*. Treatment should be directed initially at identifying and reversing the cause. If acidaemia

Table 21.10 Types and causes of metabolic acidosis

High anion gap	
Overproduction of acid	– diabetic ketoacidosis
	– lactic acidosis type A (hypoxia, shock) or type B (biguanides)
	– starvation
Exogenous acid	– salicylates
	– methanol
	– ethylene glycol
Reduced excretion	– renal failure
Normal anion gap	
Bicarbonate loss	– *Extrarenal* diarrhoea biliary/pancreatic fistula ileostomy ureterosigmoidostomy
	– *Renal* renal tubular acidosis carbonic anhydrase inhibitors
Addition of acid (with chloride)	– HCl, NH_4Cl, arginine or lysine hydrochloride

is considered to be life-threatening (pH < 7.2, $[HCO_3^-] < 10$ mmol.litre^{-1}), measures may be required to restore blood pH to normal. Overzealous use of sodium bicarbonate may lead to rapid correction of blood pH, with the risks of tetany and convulsions in the short term and volume overload and hypernatraemia in the longer term. The required quantity of bicarbonate should be calculated:

bicarbonate requirement (mmol) = body weight (kg) × base deficit (mmol.litre^{-1}) × 0.3

Administration of sodium bicarbonate should be followed by repeated measurements of plasma $[HCO_3^-]$ and pH. Sodium bicarbonate is available as isotonic (1.4%; 163 mmol.litre^{-1}) and hypertonic 8.4%; 1000 mmol.litre^{-1}) solutions. Slow infusion of the hypertonic solution is advisable to minimize adverse effects.

When considering the use of sodium bicarbonate in the context of metabolic acidaemia it is important to distinguish those acidoses associated with tissue hypoxia (e.g. cardiac arrest, septic shock) as it appears that therapy with sodium bicarbonate often exacerbates the acidosis in the presence of tissue hypoxia. In patients with cardiac arrest, $NaHCO_3$ increases mixed venous and arterial P_{CO_2}, resulting in either an unchanged or a reduced arterial pH in addition to hypernatraemia and hyperosmolality. Current guidelines for the management of cardiopulmonary arrest no longer recommend the routine use of sodium bicarbonate. However, if the acidosis is not associated with tissue hypoxia (e.g. uraemic acidosis) then the use of sodium bicarbonate will result in a potentially beneficial increase in arterial pH.

Metabolic alkalosis

This is characterized by a primary increase in plasma $[HCO_3^-]$ and a variable degree of alkalaemia. The compensatory response of hypoventilation is limited and not very effective. For diagnostic and therapeutic reasons it is usual to subdivide metabolic alkalosis into the chloride-responsive and chloride-resistant varieties (Table 21.11). The differential diagnosis of metabolic alkalosis, and in particular the separation of patients on the basis of the urinary chloride concentration, is

Table 21.11 Types and causes of metabolic alkalosis

Chloride-responsive (urine chloride < 20 mmol.litre^{-1})	
Loss of acid	– vomiting – nasogastric suction – gastrocolic fistula
Chloride depletion	– diarrhoea – diuretic abuse
Excessive alkali	– $NaHCO_3$ administration – antacid abuse
Chloride-resistant (urine chloride > 20 mmol.litre^{-1}) Primary or secondary hyperaldosteronism	
Cushing's syndrome	
Severe hypokalaemia	
Carbenoxolone	

important because of the differences in treatment of the two groups. In chloride-responsive alkalosis, the administration of saline causes volume expansion and results in the excretion of excess bicarbonate; if potassium is required, it should be given as the chloride salt. In patients in whom volume administration is contraindicated, the use of acetazolamide results in renal loss of HCO_3^- and an improvement in pH. H_2-receptor antagonists may be helpful if nasogastric suction is contributing to hydrogen ion loss.

Severe alkalaemia with compensatory hypoventilation may result in seizures or CNS depression. In life-threatening metabolic alkalosis, rapid correction is necessary and may be achieved by administration of hydrogen ions in the form of dilute hydrochloric acid. Acid administration requires central vein cannulation as peripheral infusion causes sclerosis of veins. Acid is given as 0.1 normal HCl in glucose 5% at a rate no greater than 0.2 mmol.kg^{-1}.h^{-1}.

Respiratory acidosis

This abnormality is characterized by a primary increase in Pa_{CO_2} which results in acidaemia to an extent proportional to the degree of hypercapnia. Buffering processes are activated rapidly in acute hypercapnia and may remove enough H^+ from the extracellular fluid to result in a secondary increase in plasma HCO_3^-. The compensation is less efficient than in metabolic alkalosis and pH is seldom more than 7.35.

Usually, hypoxaemia and the manifestations of the underlying disease dominate the clinical picture but hypercapnia *per se* may result in coma, raised intracranial pressure and a hyperdynamic cardiovascular system (tachycardia, vasodilatation, ventricular arrhythmias) resulting from release of catecholamines.

There are many causes of respiratory acidosis; the most important are classified in Table 21.12. Treatment consists of reversing the underlying pathology if possible and mechanical ventilatory support if required.

Respiratory alkalosis

This is characterized by a primary decrease in Pa_{CO_2} (alveolar ventilation in excess of metabolic needs) which increases pH above 7.44. Usually, hypocapnia indicates a disturbances of ventilatory control (in patients not receiving mechanical ventilation). As in respiratory acidosis, the manifestations of the underlying disease usually dominate the clinical picture. Acute hypocapnia results in cerebral vasoconstriction and reduced cerebral blood flow and may cause lightheadedness, confusion and, in severe cases, seizures. Circumoral paraesthesia, hyperreflexia and tetany are common. Cardiovascular manifestations include tachycardia and ventricular arrhythmias secondary to the alkalaemia.

The causes of respiratory alkalosis are summarized in Table 21.13. Treatment comprises correction of the underlying cause and thus differential diagnosis is important.

Table 21.12   Causes of respiratory acidosis

Central nervous system
Drug overdose
Trauma
Tumour
Degeneration or infection
Cerebrovascular accident
Cervical cord trauma

Peripheral nervous system
Polyneuropathy
Myasthenia gravis
Poliomyelitis
Botulism
Tetanus
Organophosphorus poisoning

Primary pulmonary disease

Airway obstruction	– asthma
	– laryngospasm
	– chronic obstructive airways disease
Parenchymal disease	– ARDS
	– pneumonia
	– severe pulmonary oedema
	– chronic obstructive airways disease
Loss of mechanical integrity	– flail chest

Table 21.13   Causes of respiratory alkalosis

Supratentorial
Voluntary/hysterical hyperventilation
Pain, anxiety

Specific conditions

CNS disease	– meningitis/encephalitis
	– cerebrovascular accident
	– tumour
	– trauma
Respiratory disease	– pneumonia
	– pulmonary embolism
	– early pulmonary oedema or ARDS
	– high altitude
Shock	– cardiogenic
	– hypovolaemic
	– septic
Miscellaneous	– cirrhosis
	– Gram-negative septicaemia
	– pregnancy
	– IPPV
Drugs/hormones	– salicylates
	– aminophylline
	– progesterone

FURTHER READING

Arieff A I 1991 Indications for the use of bicarbonate in patients with metabolic acidosis. British Journal of Anaesthesia 67: 165–178
Askanazi J, Starker P M, Weissman C (eds) 1986 Fluid and electrolyte balance in critical care. Butterworths, Boston
Swales J D 1991 Management of hyponatraemia. British Journal of Anaesthesia 67: 146–154
Walmsley R N, Guerin M D 1984 Disorders of fluid and electrolyte balance. Wright, Bristol
Willatts S M 1987 Lecture notes on fluid and electrolyte balance, 2nd edn. Blackwell, Oxford

22. Complications during anaesthesia

Most intraoperative complications involve the patient, although staff are also at risk (see Chapter 17). Information about the type, incidence and outcome of complications is provided by studies of anaesthetic morbidity, mortality and critical incidents. At least one intraoperative complication occurs in 9% of all patients undergoing surgery. The risk increases with the duration of surgery and is higher in the morbidly obese, patients at the extremes of age and those undergoing emergency or obstetric anaesthesia.

The most frequent complications during anaesthesia are arrhythmia, hypotension, adverse drug effects and inadequate ventilation of the lungs. Inadequate ventilation is commonly caused by unrecognized oesophageal intubation, poorly managed or difficult tracheal intubation, pulmonary aspiration of gastric contents, breathing system disconnections and gas supply failure. These complications are also the major causes of anaesthetic mortality, preventable intraoperative cardiac arrest and permanent neurological damage. In particular, hypotension and hypoxaemia are implicated consistently in poor patient outcome from anaesthesia. The source of most anaesthetic complications is human error, often in association with poor monitoring, equipment malfunction and organizational failure.

There are important implications for the anaesthetist. As most complications are preventable, meticulous preparation of both the patient and anaesthetic equipment is essential to reduce the risk of an adverse event. Should an intraoperative complication occur, the anaesthetist must be able to rapidly recognize and effectively manage the problem. This demands constant vigilance, the use of appropriate monitoring and a well-rehearsed and effective plan of action. The use of specific protocols for managing critical incidents is recommended.

ARRHYTHMIAS (and disorders of rate)

Aetiology (Table 22.1)

Arrhythmias are the most frequently reported critical incident. During anaesthesia, bradycardia and tachycardia may be defined as any cardiac rhythm with a rate less than 60 or greater than 100 beat.min^{-1} respectively. Most intraoperative arrhythmias are caused by pharmacological or physiological alterations in autonomic tone and are therefore potentially avoidable or easily treated by correcting the precipitating factor.

Bradycardia

Sinus bradycardia originates from the sinoatrial node. It is common during anaesthesia in healthy patients and is associated with the use of opioids or deep levels of anaesthesia. Surgical manipulations such as eyeball traction, cervical dilatation and peritoneal traction can increase vagal tone, producing bradycardia and occasionally sinus arrest. Suxamethonium is a well-known cause of bradycardia, especially following repeat doses. Drugs without sympathomimetic activity, such as atracurium and vecuronium, can be associated with bradycardia if used concurrently with opioids or β-blocking agents. Halothane, and to a lesser extent enflurane, cause a dose-dependent depression of sinus node automaticity. This may produce bradycardia and emergence of an ectopic pacemaker, often as a wandering atrial pacemaker or junctional escape rhythm. Both halothane

Table 22.1 Causes of arrhythmia during anaesthesia

Cardiorespiratory	Hypoxaemia Hypotension Hypo/hypercapnia Myocardial ischaemia		
Metabolic	Catecholamines	Endogenous	Inadequate analgesia Inadequate anaesthesia Airway manipulation Hyperthyroidism
		Exogenous	Sympathomimetics
	Hypo/hyperkalaemia Malignant hyperthermia		
Surgical	Increased vagal tone (eye surgery, anal stretch, mesenteric traction) Direct cardiac stimulation (chest surgery, CVP cannulae) Dental surgery		
Drugs	Vagolytics (atropine, pancuronium) Sympathomimetics (adrenaline, ephedrine) Halothane, enflurane Digoxin		

and enflurane also depress atrioventricular conduction. Calcium channel blockers, β-blockers and digoxin potentiate this effect. Bradycardia is clinically significant if associated with an escape rhythm or a decrease in cardiac output.

Tachycardia

Sinus tachycardia with sympathetic nervous stimulation is a normal physiological response. It is observed in most patients at some time during the perioperative period. Sympathetic tone is most commonly increased by hypoxaemia, inadequate anaesthesia and/or analgesia, hypovolaemia, hypotension and airway manipulations such as laryngoscopy and extubation. Other signs of sympathetic nervous activity may be present, including hypertension and ventricular ectopy. Tachycardia is also associated with an increase in metabolic rate (sepsis, burns, hyperthyroidism), the use of vagolytic drugs (atropine, pancuronium) and sympathomimetic drugs (ephedrine, adrenaline). Tachycardia reduces the duration of diastolic coronary artery filling and simultaneously increases myocardial work. This may precipitate myocardial ischaemia in patients with coronary artery or hypertensive heart disease.

Extracellular potassium concentration

Extracellular potassium concentration has a pro-

found effect on myocardial electrical activity. Intraoperative abnormalities are most likely to occur in patients with preoperative potassium, fluid or acid–base imbalance, especially if inadequately treated prior to anaesthesia. Hypokalaemia increases ventricular irritability and the risk of ventricular ectopy and ventricular tachycardia/fibrillation. This effect is potentiated in patients with ischaemic heart disease and in those receiving digoxin. Hyperventilation alters acid–base balance with acute transmembrane redistribution of potassium. Serum potassium concentration can decrease by 0.5 mmol.litre^{-1} for every 1.3 kPa decrease in CO_2 tension. Life-threatening hyperkalaemia with atrioventricular conduction block or ventricular fibrillation can occur if suxamethonium is used in patients with burns or denervating injuries. Electrolyte disorders are further discussed in Chapter 21.

Management

Preoperative correction of fluid, electrolyte and acid–base imbalance is essential. Continuous intraoperative ECG monitoring is mandatory as arrhythmias are extremely common. Lead II best demonstrates atrial activity and its use is recommended for routine ECG monitoring. As the ECG gives no indication of cardiac output or tissue perfusion, the detection of an abnormal cardiac rhythm should be followed by rapid assessment of the circulation. An absent pulse, severe hypotension or ventricular tachycardia or fibrillation should be treated as a cardiac arrest.

The anaesthetist should always exclude hypoxaemia, hypotension, inadequate analgesia and light anaesthesia. Correcting the precipitating factor is often the only treatment required. If the arrhythmia persists, intervention with a specific antiarrhythmic agent or cardioversion is indicated if the arrhythmia predisposes to ventricular tachycardia or fibrillation, causes a significant decrease in cardiac output or is associated with myocardial ischaemia.

Bradycardia can be treated with an anticholinergic agent such as glycopyrrolate or atropine, with the choice and dose depending on the clinical urgency. If the bradycardia is refractory to treatment, intravenous isoprenaline or cardiac pacing may be indicated. An anticholinergic drug may be given prophylactically where surgical stimulation increases the risk of bradycardia (e.g. ophthalmic surgery) or with a second dose of suxamethonium. If sinus tachycardia is associated with myocardial ischaemia, it may be controlled by careful intravenous administration of a β-blocker such as propranolol or esmolol. Serum potassium concentration should be measured if ventricular arrhythmias occur, especially if the patient is receiving digoxin.

Atrial arrhythmias

These can reduce the atrial contribution to left ventricular filling, with a decrease in cardiac output.

Junctional rhythm. This bradycardia is associated usually with the use of halothane. A reduction in concentration and/or a change of volatile agent is indicated. An anticholinergic drug may be required to restore sinus rhythm.

Accelerated nodal rhythm. This may be precipitated by an increase in sympathetic tone in the presence of sensitizing volatile agents. Adjusting the depth of anaesthesia and/or changing the anaesthetic agent is appropriate treatment.

Supraventricular tachycardia (SVT). SVT can occur at any time during the perioperative period in susceptible patients, such as those with Wolff–Parkinson–White or other 'pre-excitation' syndromes. If attempts to increase vagal tone and

terminate the SVT by carotid sinus massage are unsuccessful, the treatment of choice is adenosine by fast intravenous injection. This is safe and effective during haemodynamic instability as adenosine has a duration of action of less than 60 s and blocks atrioventricular conduction without compromising ventricular function. Adenosine should not be given to patients with asthma or atrioventricular conduction block. If adenosine is unavailable and the patient is normotensive, intravenous verapamil can be given in 1–2 mg increments up to 10 mg. However, verapamil can cause prolonged hypotension and depression of ventricular function, especially in the presence of anaesthetic agents causing myocardial depression. Cardioversion is indicated if the SVT is associated with hypotension and adenosine is unavailable.

Atrial flutter/fibrillation. During anaesthesia, these arrhythmias are most commonly observed as a paroxysmal increase in ventricular rate in patients with pre-existing atrial flutter/fibrillation. After correcting any precipitating factors, digoxin by slow intravenous injection is the treatment of choice. Alternative therapy with amiodarone or a β-blocker may be necessary to control the ventricular rate in patients receiving digoxin preoperatively. Immediate cardioversion should be considered if the ventricular fate is fast with a clinically significant reduction in cardiac output.

Ventricular arrhythmias

Premature ventricular contractions (PVCs). PVCs are common in healthy patients and may be present preoperatively. If associated with a slow atrial rate (escape beats), increasing the sinus rate with an anticholinergic drug will abolish them. In other situations, an underlying cause should be sought before antiarrhythmic agents are considered, as PVCs rarely progress to more serious arrhythmias unless there is underlying myocardial ischaemia or hypoxaemia. Halothane lowers the threshold for catecholamine-induced ventricular arrhythmias. This is exacerbated by hypercapnia. Halothane should be used with care in patients receiving sympathomimetic drugs (including those undergoing tissue infiltration with local anaesthetics containing adrenaline) and in patients taking aminophylline or drugs which block noradrenaline reuptake, such as tricyclic antidepressants. The maximum recommended dose of adrenaline for infiltration in the presence of halothane is 100 μg (10 ml of 1 in 100 000 concentration) during any 10 min period, although the rate of absorption depends on the site of injection. The use of enflurane or isoflurane reduces the risk. Isoflurane is associated with a low incidence of intraoperative arrhythmias.

Although uncommon, other ventricular arrhythmias such as ventricular tachycardia and fibrillation should be treated as a cardiac arrest.

Heart block

This is discussed in Chapter 40.

HYPOTENSION

In healthy patients, hypotension during anaesthesia may be defined as a mean arterial pressure less than 60 mmHg. A systolic blood pressure 25% less than the patient's preoperative level also indicates hypotension, especially in patients with pre-existing hypertension. Hypotension is clinically significant if vital organ perfusion is compromised (e.g. myocardial ischaemia or oliguria). As left ventricular coronary blood flow occurs predominantly in diastole, diastolic blood pressure is important in patients with coronary artery disease.

Aetiology

Hypotension is caused by a decrease in cardiac output and/or systemic vascular resistance (vasodilatation). Table 22.2 classifies the causes of hypotension during anaesthesia. During anaesthesia, hypotension is usually multifactorial, with hypovolaemia a common underlying factor (see below). As most anaesthetic agents reduce both systemic vascular resistance and myocardial contractility, relative overdosing can cause significant hypotension, especially in hypovolaemic or elderly patients. The hypotensive effects of anaesthetic agents are potentiated by calcium channel blockers, β-blockers and other antihypertensive drugs. Drug-induced vasodilatation can result from a direct action on vasculature or indirectly by histamine release or chemical sympathectomy (central neural blockade with local anaesthetic).

Management

Preoperative correction of hypovolaemia is essential. The anaesthetist should anticipate the cardiovascular effects of anaesthetic agents; appropriate doses of drugs should be used and intravenous fluid preloading should be con-

Table 22.2 Causes of hypotension during anaesthesia

Decreased cardiac output		
Decreased venous return	Hypovolaemia	Inadequate preoperative resuscitation
		Gastrointestinal fluid loss
		Haemorrhage
	Obstruction	Pulmonary embolus
		Aorta/caval compression (surgery, pregnancy, tumour)
	Increased ITP	IPPV/PEEP
		Pneumothorax
	Head-up position	
Myocardial	Reduced contractility	Drugs (most anaesthetic agents, β-blockers, calcium antagonists, acidosis)
		Ischaemia/infarction
	Arrhythmias	
	Pericardial tamponade	
Vasodilatation		
Drugs	Relative/absolute overdose (most anaesthetic agents, antihypertensives)	
	Central regional blockade (local anaesthetics)	
	Hypersensitivity (drugs, colloids, blood)	
	Direct histamine release (morphine, tubocurarine)	
Septicaemia		

ITP, intrathoracic pressure; IPPV, intermittent positive pressure ventilation; PEEP, positive end-expiratory pressure

sidered. If intraoperative hypotension occurs and the measurement is validated, ensure adequate oxygenation, increase venous return by raising the legs or using head-down tilt, decrease the concentration or infusion rate of anaesthetic agents and give intravenous fluid as necessary. This will be effective in most patients. If hypotension persists and the cause is not obvious, consider drug hypersensitivity and exclude factors that decrease venous return, especially concealed haemorrhage and pneumothorax. Examine the ECG to exclude arrhythmias and myocardial ischaemia. Hypotension from profound vasodilatation requires further fluid administration and the use of a vasoconstrictor such as ephedrine or phenylephrine. If cardiac output remains low, careful fluid loading is indicated using central venous pressure as a guide. Pulmonary arterial catheter insertion and inotropic support with dobutamine should also be considered.

Hypovolaemia

Hypovolaemia refers to a fluid deficit with reduced intravascular volume (Table 22.3).

Clinical features. Hypovolaemia most often occurs in the emergency patient. The clinical picture depends on the rate, volume and type of fluid loss and may include thirst, dryness of mucous membranes, reduced tissue turgor, tachycardia and postural or absolute hypotension. β-blocking drugs can prevent compensatory tachycardia. Vasoconstriction reduces peripheral tissue perfusion causing cool limbs and an increase in the skin–core temperature difference. Oliguria (urine output less than 0.5 ml.kg^{-1}.h^{-1}) and evidence of haemoconcentration or anaemia may be present. Hypokalaemia and other electrolyte abnormalities are often associated with fluid deficits, in particular gastrointestinal losses.

Management. It is essential to assess intravascular fluid volume and fluid balance preoperatively in all patients undergoing non-elective surgery. Fluid deficit and replacement are easily underestimated, especially in patients with intestinal obstruction or concealed haemorrhage. Unless immediately life-saving, surgery should be delayed to allow adequate fluid resuscitation. The response of the CVP to fluid challenge is a useful guide when assessing and treating patients with significant hypovolaemia.

As most anaesthetic agents abolish compensatory vasoconstriction and cause myocardial depression, relative overdosing will reveal hypovolaemia and inadequate fluid resuscitation, resulting in hypotension and sometimes cardiovascular collapse. These effects are exaggerated in the elderly and in patients with decreased cardiac reserve or pre-existing hypertension. The risk of hypotension at induction can be reduced by giving a fluid preload and carefully titrating induction agents to effect. Etomidate produces less cardiovascular depression than other induction agents. Ketamine can be used for induction in patients with severe hypovolaemia where immediate operation may be life-saving.

The anaesthetist must monitor fluid balance closely during surgery. Adequate intraoperative fluid replacement must account for maintenance requirements, evaporative loss, 'third space' tissue sequestration and blood loss. For example, during abdominal operations, up to 5 ml.kg^{-1}.h^{-1} may be required to replace evaporative and third space losses in addition to maintenance requirements.

Haemorrhage

Adults who have lost 15% of circulating blood volume require red blood cell transfusion to maintain oxygen carrying capacity. Blood loss can be estimated by weighing swabs, measuring the

Table 22.3 Causes of hypovolaemia and fluid loss

Preoperative	
Haemorrhage	Trauma
	Obstetric
	Gastrointestinal
	Major vessel rupture (aortic aneurysm)
Gastrointestinal	Vomiting
	Obstruction
	Fistulae
	Diarrhoea
Other	Fasting
	Diuretics
	Fever
	Burns
Intraoperative	Haemorrhage
	Insensible loss (evaporation)
	Drainage of stomach, bowel or ascites
	'Third space' loss – tissue sequestration

volume of blood in suction bottles and assessing the clinical response to fluid therapy. Estimation is often difficult where large volumes of irrigation fluid have been used, for example during transurethral resection of the prostate. With severe or ongoing haemorrhage, maintenance of intravascular volume is essential. An effective fluid warming device should be used when giving any cold fluid and is advisable when giving any infusion rapidly. The problems of massive transfusion are discussed on page 531.

HYPERTENSION

Intraoperative hypertension may be defined as a systolic blood pressure 25% greater than the patient's preoperative level. Hypertension increases myocardial work by increasing afterload and left ventricular wall tension. It is often associated with tachycardia. This is particularly undesirable in patients with ischaemic heart disease or left ventricular hypertrophy as the myocardial oxygen supply/demand balance is easily compromised. The subendocardium is most susceptible to ischaemia in these situations. Hypertension also increases the risk of ischaemia, infarction and haemorrhage in other organs such as the brain.

Aetiology

Table 22.4 shows the common causes of hypertension during anaesthesia. Hypertension is most often caused by an increase in sympathetic tone and systemic vascular resistance. This can be a physiological response to light anaesthesia, pain or airway manipulation or a pharmacological response (e.g. sympathomimetic drug overdose). Tachycardia and arrhythmias are associated signs of sympathetic nervous stimulation. The anaesthetist should be aware of the less common causes of hypertension such as phaeochromocytoma and malignant hyperthermia.

Management

Preoperative control of hypertension is essential. Patients with poorly controlled hypertension exhibit exaggerated vascular responses during anaesthesia and suffer greater intraoperative and postoperative morbidity and mortality. Where

Table 22.4   Causes of hypertension during anaesthesia

Pre-existing	Undiagnosed or poorly controlled Pregnancy-induced
Increased sympathetic tone	Inadequate analgesia Inadequate anaesthesia Hypoxaemia Airway manipulation (laryngoscopy, extubation) Hypercapnia
Drug overdose	Adrenaline Ephedrine Ketamine Ergometrine
Other	Hypervolaemia Aortic cross-clamping Phaeochromocytoma Malignant hyperthermia

possible, surgery should be postponed until adequate control is achieved (e.g. arterial pressure less than 180/100 mmHg) and target organ function (e.g. heart and kidney) assessed. Premedication may be indicated to reduce anxiety. The anaesthetist should anticipate the anaesthetic and surgical events that increase sympathetic tone. The pressor response to laryngoscopy can be obtunded by the use of an adequate dose of short-acting opioid such as alfentanil. In patients in whom the sympathetic response to extubation is undesirable, extubation can be performed during deep anaesthesia or after giving intravenous lignocaine $1–1.5$ mg.kg^{-1}. The response to aortic cross-clamping can be controlled by careful use of volatile agents and/or nitrate infusion. The use of ketamine should be avoided in hypertensive patients.

If hypertension occurs in other clinical situations, ensure adequate oxygenation, depth of anaesthesia and analgesia. The use of an antihypertensive agent such as labetalol or hydralazine may then be indicated for persistent hypertension. As the effect of these drugs is potentiated by anaesthetic agents, careful titration is advisable.

HYPERVOLAEMIA

Hypervolaemia is fluid excess with an overfilled intravascular compartment.

Clinical features

Hypervolaemia is usually caused by excessive

transfusion with blood or other intravenous fluids. Significant fluid overload produces tachycardia, elevated JVP/CVP, added heart sounds and lung crepitations. Severe overloading may cause pulmonary oedema with raised lung inflation pressures, hypoxaemia, hypotension or oedema fluid in the airway.

Fluid absorption occurs during operations in which continuous irrigation is used. The volume absorbed is proportional to the duration of irrigation and can be rapid. If the fluid is hypotonic, dilutional hyponatraemia can develop. Classically, this occurs during transurethral resection of the prostate. Reduced serum osmolality promotes extravascular fluid shifts and increases the risk of pulmonary and cerebral oedema. Elderly patients and those with cardiac disease, renal disease or hypoproteinaemia are most susceptible. Hyponatraemia is associated with arrhythmias and QRS widening on the ECG. In the past, the use of irrigation fluid containing citrate was associated with metabolic alkalosis, sometimes severe and life-threatening.

Management

Careful monitoring of preoperative and intraoperative fluid balance is essential. Should hypervolaemia occur, intravenous infusions and surgical irrigation should be stopped, the inspired oxygen concentration increased and the operation terminated as soon as possible. Serum biochemistry and arterial blood gas analysis will identify associated electrolyte or acid–base disorders. Fluid restriction and a loop diuretic are indicated in mild cases, with postoperative monitoring of serum electrolytes and cardiorespiratory function. In severe cases with evidence of pulmonary or cerebral oedema, tracheal intubation and ventilation may be necessary to protect the airway and enable control of arterial blood gas tensions. Inotropic support with dobutamine, invasive cardiovascular monitoring and haemofiltration should be considered.

MYOCARDIAL ISCHAEMIA

Aetiology

Myocardial ischaemia occurs when myocardial oxygen demand exceeds supply. The subendocardium is particularly vulnerable. Hypertension increases myocardial afterload and therefore oxygen demand. Hypotension can reduce oxygen supply by reducing coronary blood flow. However, tachycardia is the most important determinant of the myocardial oxygen supply/demand ratio as the duration of diastolic coronary filling is reduced simultaneously with an increase in myocardial work. Furthermore, it is the heart rate that determines the level of hypotension or hypertension at the ischaemic threshold. Intraoperative ischaemia can also occur without significant haemodynamic changes. Stimulating procedures such as laryngoscopy and surgical incision may produce coronary vasospasm and ischaemia in some patients.

Clinical features

Patients with coronary artery disease are most at risk. Intraoperative myocardial ischaemia manifests clinically as arrhythmias, hypotension or pulmonary oedema. It is diagnosed by ECG ST segment changes although these are not always detected reliably without computer assisted analysis. The use of the V5 electrode is recommended for ECG monitoring in susceptible patients (e.g. the CM5 configuration) as it is the most sensitive ECG lead for the detection of left ventricular ischaemia. A rise in left ventricular end-diastolic pressure often precedes ECG changes and is detected by an increase in the pulmonary capillary wedge pressure if a pulmonary arterial catheter is in situ. Transoesophageal echocardiography can detect abnormal myocardial wall motion, a sensitive indicator of ischaemia. Regional wall dysfunction often persists into the postoperative period without clinical signs. Increased myocardial work during this period can precipitate further ischaemia or infarction in susceptible patients although the risk of infarction in the general surgical population is low.

Management

The aims of management are prevention of ischaemia by the use of an appropriate anaesthetic technique and early detection in susceptible patients by the use of appropriate monitoring. If ischaemia is detected, ensure adequate arterial oxygenation, normocapnia, analgesia and depth of anaesthesia. Significant hypertension, hypotension and tachycardia can then be controlled pharmacologically. If signs of myocardial ischaemia persist, the use of a coronary vasodilator such as glyceryl trinitrate by intravenous infusion should be considered.

CARDIAC ARREST (see Chapter 43)

EMBOLISM

Gas

Aetiology

Gas embolism describes the entry of gas bubbles into the circulation, usually via the venous route. Embolism of room air is possible if atmospheric pressure is greater than intravenous pressure at the site of an open vein. This is most likely with surgical sites above the level of the right atrium, for example during head and neck operations in the head-up position. Vascular catheters are another potential route for air entry. Gas embolism, usually carbon dioxide, can also occur during insufflation procedures such as laparoscopy. Table 22.5 lists the procedures associated with gas embolism.

Clinical features

The clinical presentation varies with the volume and rate of gas entry into the circulation. An entry rate of $0.5\ ml.kg^{-1}.min^{-1}$ or greater has been reported to produce clinical signs. If a significant volume of gas enters the right side of the heart,

blood flow is obstructed, reducing cardiac output and arterial pressure. A 'millwheel' murmur may be auscultated via the praecordial or oesophageal stethoscope. A fall in cardiac output with gas in the pulmonary circulation increases pulmonary dead space. This is detected by a rapid decrease in end-tidal carbon dioxide concentration. Hypoxaemia, tachycardia, arrhythmias and an increase in pulmonary artery pressure follow. In extreme cases, cardiac pumping is ineffective with severe hypotension and asphyxia. Praecordial or oesophageal Doppler ultrasound is a highly sensitive monitor of gas entry into the circulation. As the foramen ovale is potentially patent in more than 25% of the population, an increase in right heart pressure can open the foramen in these patients. Paradoxical gas embolism via this route or across the pulmonary capillary bed to the coronary or cerebral circulations can cause myocardial ischaemia or convulsions.

Management

If air embolism is detected, further air entry should be prevented by flooding the operative site with saline and covering it with wet gauze. During head and neck procedures, the venous pressure at the surgical site should be elevated by compressing the jugular veins, lowering the operative site where possible and applying continuous positive airway pressure. The lungs should be ventilated with 100% oxygen (nitrous oxide should be discontinued to avoid gas bubble expansion). Gas can sometimes be aspirated from the right heart if a right atrial cannula is present, otherwise cannula insertion is usually impractical and time-consuming. Expansion of the intravascular fluid

Table 22.5 Procedures associated with gas embolism

Head and neck surgery	ENT surgery (sinus, mastoid) Neurosurgery (posterior fossa, sitting position)
Insufflation techniques	Laparoscopy Hysteroscopy Arthroscopy
Orthopaedic surgery	Arthrography Hip and spinal surgery
Chest surgery	Breast and open cardiac operations
Other	Intravascular cannulae (venous, arterial) Extradural injection

volume, inotropic support of the circulation and external cardiac massage may be necessary.

Thrombus

Aetiology

Risk factors for venous thromboembolism include immobility, malignancy, smoking, pelvic and limb surgery, medication with the contraceptive pill and a past history of venous thromboembolism. Thrombosis is usually sited in the deep venous system of the lower limbs or in the pelvis. There is a high risk of thrombus formation in susceptible patients during the intraoperative period. Venous stasis in the lower limbs is produced by direct venous compression, hypovolaemia, hypotension, hypothermia and the use of tourniquets and head-up positioning. Veins can sustain trauma during positioning and surgery. Increased blood coagulability is a consequence of the stress response to surgery.

Management

Although venous embolism during surgery is uncommon, thromboprophylaxis must begin pre-operatively for maximum benefit. This includes correction of risk factors where possible, adequate hydration and the use of subcutaneous heparin and leg compression stockings. During the intra-operative period, venous stasis in the lower limb can be reduced by raising the legs, avoiding leg trauma and using apparatus for pneumatic leg compression or electrical calf muscle stimulation. A good anaesthetic and surgical technique ensures adequate fluid therapy and minimizes heat loss and tourniquet times. The use of subarachnoid or epidural anaesthesia is associated with a lower incidence of early postoperative venous thrombo-embolism.

Pulmonary embolism during anaesthesia is uncommon but may present with tachycardia, hypoxaemia, arrhythmia, difficulty with ventila-tion, an acute decrease in the end-tidal carbon dioxide concentration or cardiovascular collapse. Other causes should be excluded before making this diagnosis. If pulmonary embolism is diag-nosed, ventilate the lungs with 100% oxygen and consider bronchodilator therapy, fluid loading

and inotropic support of the circulation. After management of the initial haemodynamic dis-turbance, thrombolytic therapy, anticoagulation and in extreme cases surgical removal of the embolus may be indicated.

Other

Air or clot may embolize via arterial cannulae and produce distal ischaemia. Fat embolism to the lungs can occur in patients with fractures. Although an acute presentation during anaes-thesia is unusual, fat emboli can cause severe hypoxaemia. Tumour fragments can embolize during cancer surgery. Amniotic fluid embolus can occur in obstetric patients.

HYPOXAEMIA

Hypoxaemia refers to arterial haemoglobin desaturation or reduced arterial oxygen tension; hypoxia is oxygen deficiency at the tissue level.

Aetiology

A practical classification of the causes of hypoxaemia is given in Table 22.6. Equipment problems such as leaks and disconnections are common. $\dot{V}/\dot{Q}$ mis-match can result from either inadequate ven-tilation or reduced pulmonary perfusion. Unless hypoxaemia is promptly recognized and treated, the consequences can be disastrous.

Clinical features

Hypoxaemia is a common perioperative event. Cyanosis is an unreliable sign of hypoxaemia, especially in the operating theatre environment. Hypoxaemia produces tachycardia, sweating, hyper-tension and arrhythmias, although bradycardia is the usual response to hypoxaemia in children. Tachypnoea occurs in spontaneously breathing patients. There may be clinical signs associated with the cause. As arterial desaturation progresses, bradycardia, hypotension and cardiac arrest follow.

Management

The complications of hypoxaemia are preventable. Cyanosis should seldom be witnessed by the

Table 22.6   Causes of hypoxaemia during anaesthesia

Hypoxic inspired gas mixture		
Equipment	Oxygen supply (cylinder/pipeline failure, misconnection)	
	Flowmeters (inaccurate settings, leak)	
	Breathing system (obstruction, leak)	
Hypoventilation		
Equipment	Ventilator failure	
	Breathing system (obstruction, leak, disconnection)	
	Tracheal tube (obstruction, oesophageal intubation)	
Patient	Respiratory depression in spontaneously breathing patients	
	Obstruction (see Table 22.7)	
$\dot{V}/\dot{Q}$ *mismatch*		
Patient	Inadequate ventilation	Endobronchial intubation
		Secretions
		Atelectasis
		Pneumothorax
		Bronchospasm
		Pulmonary aspiration
		Pulmonary oedema
	Inadequate perfusion	Embolus (gas, thrombus, amniotic fluid)
		Low cardiac output (see Table 22.2)
Other	Methaemoglobinaemia, malignant hyperthermia	

vigilant anaesthetist as the routine use of pulse oximetry allows early detection and treatment of hypoxaemia. If hypoxaemia is detected, the following plan should be instituted.

1. Palpate the carotid pulse. Simultaneously assess the ECG and cardiac rhythm. Treat as for cardiac arrest if there is inadequate cardiac output or ventricular tachycardia/fibrillation.

2. Exclude delivery of a hypoxic gas mixture using an oxygen analyser. Increase the inspired oxygen concentration to 100%.

3. Test the integrity of the breathing system by manual ventilation of the lungs and confirm bilateral chest movement and breath sounds. Blow down the tracheal tube if necessary. Confirm the position and patency of the tracheal tube by assessing the capnograph, passing a suction catheter through the tracheal tube and auscultating the chest.

4. Search for clinical evidence of the causes of V/Q mismatch with early exclusion of pneumothorax. If atelectasis is likely, gentle hyperinflation of the lungs should improve oxygenation. Lung volumes can be maintained by applying CPAP or PEEP.

5. If the diagnosis is difficult, measure core temperature and consider arterial blood gas analysis and chest X-ray examination.

HYPERCAPNIA

Hypercapnia refers to carbon dioxide accumulation in the blood. During anaesthesia, this is indicated by an arterial carbon dioxide tension (kPa) or end-tidal carbon dioxide concentration (%) greater than 6.0.

Aetiology

Intraoperative hypercapnia is caused by inadequate carbon dioxide removal or excessive carbon dioxide production. Inadequate carbon dioxide removal is most commonly caused by hypoventilation (Table 22.6), but may result also from inadequate fresh gas flow and exhausted soda lime. Carbon dioxide production rises with the metabolic rate during fever, sepsis, malignant hyperthermia, drug reactions and hyperthyroidism. Inadvertent or excessive carbon dioxide delivery from the anaesthetic machine and the use of carbon dioxide during laparoscopic procedures are other causes of hypercapnia.

Clinical features

Progressive hypercapnia stimulates sympathetic nervous activity with tachycardia, sweating and arrhythmias. Increased cerebral blood flow and alterations in blood pressure may occur. As anaesthesia suppresses autonomic responses, these signs may not occur until carbon dioxide tension is markedly increased. Acute respiratory acidosis produces an increase in serum potassium. Increased carbon dioxide production in the spontaneously breathing patient stimulates tachypnoea.

Management

This is directed at the underlying cause. Mild degrees of hypercapnia are usually well tolerated in spontaneously breathing patients unless there is a contraindication such as head injury. If signs of hypercapnia occur, the anaesthetist should control ventilation.

HYPOCAPNIA

Hypocapnia refers to a carbon dioxide deficit in the blood. During anaesthesia, this is indicated by an arterial carbon dioxide tension (kPa) or end-tidal carbon dioxide concentration (%) less than 4.0. Unintentional hyperventilation in association with decreased carbon dioxide production is the usual cause during anaesthesia. Hypocapnia produces respiratory alkalosis with a decrease

in serum potassium concentration. There are reductions in cerebral blood flow, cardiac output and tissue oxygen delivery. There may also be a delay in onset of spontaneous ventilation at the conclusion of anaesthesia. Decreasing the ventilatory minute volume or increasing the breathing system dead space reduce carbon dioxide removal.

RESPIRATORY OBSTRUCTION

Aetiology

Table 22.7 shows the causes of respiratory obstruction. It is a common and potentially hazardous anaesthetic complication. The tracheal tube is a frequent site of obstruction, although problems can occur at any point in the breathing system or airway. Inadequate ventilation can lead to hypercapnia, hypoxaemia and reduced uptake of volatile agent. Total obstruction rapidly produces hypoxaemia.

Clinical features

Spontaneously breathing patients

Partial obstruction is indicated by noisy breathing or stridor, whereas complete obstruction is silent.

Table 22.7 Causes of respiratory obstruction during anaesthesia

Equipment	
Breathing system	Valve malfunction, kinking
Tracheal tube	External compression (surgical gag/manipulation, kinking)
	Occlusion of lumen (secretions, blood)
	Cuff (overinflation, herniation)
	Oesophageal or endobronchial intubation
Patient	
Oropharynx	Soft tissue (oedema from trauma/infection, reduced muscle tone)
	Secretions (blood, surgical packs)
	Tumour
Larynx	Laryngospasm
	Recurrent laryngeal nerve palsy
	Oedema (drug hypersensitivity, pre-eclampsia, infection)
	Tumour
Trachea	Laryngotracheobronchitis
	External compression (surgical manipulation, haemorrhage, thyroid tumour)
	Stricture (radiotherapy)
Bronchi	Secretions
	Pneumothorax
	Bronchospasm
	Tumour
	Surgical manipulation

Tracheal tug, paradoxical chest and abdominal movement ('see-saw' respiration) and inadequate reservoir bag movement are other signs. The generation of large negative intrathoracic pressures can precipitate pulmonary oedema in some patients.

Artificially ventilated patients

Respiratory obstruction can be associated with increased inflation pressures, prolonged expiratory phase, hypercapnia and alteration of the end-tidal carbon dioxide waveform. Hypoxaemia may be the first sign.

Management

Early detection and prevention of hypoxaemia is essential.

Spontaneously breathing patients

Reduced muscle tone with apposition of the tongue and pharyngeal soft tissue is a common cause of upper airway obstruction. This is usually overcome by jaw lift and use of an oral or nasopharyngeal airway. Suction will remove accumulated secretions, but care is required as laryngospasm may be precipitated during light anaesthesia. If obstruction persists, ventilate the lungs manually with 100% oxygen and exclude the breathing system as the site of obstruction. Confirm the presence of bilateral chest movement and breath sounds and exclude other causes of obstruction such as laryngospasm, bronchospasm, aspiration and pneumothorax. If airway maintenance is difficult, insertion of a laryngeal mask or tracheal intubation should be considered.

Artificially ventilated patients (including patients with an artificial airway)

Systematically exclude causes of obstruction in the breathing system and patient. Complete obstruction suggests an equipment problem. The easy passage of a suction catheter throughout the length of the tracheal tube confirms its patency. The distal orifice of the tracheal tube can be obstructed by the tracheal wall or a herniated cuff. This is unlikely if the tracheal tube has a

Murphy Eye. Surgical manipulations during neck and thoracic surgery easily distort tracheal and bronchial anatomy and can displace the tracheal tube, especially endobronchial tubes. If obstruction persists and no obvious cause is identified, assume that the tracheal tube or laryngeal mask is the site of obstruction. Immediately replace it using manual ventilation with 100% oxygen by mask to prevent hypoxaemia.

The management of specific lower airway problems is discussed below.

Laryngospasm

Aetiology

Laryngospasm is a reflex, prolonged closure of the vocal cords in response to a trigger, usually airway stimulation during light anaesthesia. Therefore, laryngospasm is most common during induction and emergence, often precipitated by premature insertion of an oral airway, the presence of pharyngeal secretions or blood, or airway irritation by volatile agents. Laryngospasm can also be produced by surgical and visceral stimuli such as incision, peritoneal traction, anal stretch and cervical dilatation. Children are particularly prone to laryngospasm. The use of intravenous barbiturates disinhibits laryngeal reflexes and increases the risk of laryngospasm in comparison to propofol. Poor management of laryngospasm can lead to inadequate ventilation with hypoxaemia, hypercapnia and reduced depth of anaesthesia. Crowing inspiratory noises with signs of respiratory obstruction suggest partial laryngospasm. Complete laryngospasm is silent.

Management

Where possible, avoid airway and surgical stimulation during light anaesthesia and use the lateral position for control of secretions during extubation and transfer. Surgical stimuli should be anticipated with appropriate adjustment of anaesthetic depth. If laryngospasm occurs, hypoxaemia must be prevented. The anaesthetist should remove the offending stimulus, give 100% oxygen and provide a clear airway using an oral or pharyngeal airway and gentle pharyngeal suction. Unnecessary airway manipulation can exacerbate laryngospasm. Where appropriate, anaesthetic depth can be increased with an intravenous agent and the lungs ventilated manually with care, applying continuous positive airway pressure to prevent hypoxaemia. Most episodes of laryngospasm respond to this treatment. If laryngospasm persists and hypoxaemia ensues, a small dose of suxamethonium (e.g. 25 mg in adults) relaxes the vocal cords and allows manual ventilation and oxygenation. A full dose of suxamethonium can be given if tracheal intubation is indicated. Doxapram has also been used successfully in the treatment of laryngospasm.

Bronchospasm

Aetiology

General anaesthesia can alter airway resistance by influencing bronchomotor tone, lung volumes and bronchial secretions. Patients with increased airway reactivity from recent respiratory infection, asthma, atopy or smoking are more susceptible to bronchospasm during anaesthesia. Bronchospasm may be precipitated by insertion of an artificial airway during light anaesthesia, carinal or bronchial stimulation by the tracheal tube and by drugs causing β-blockade or histamine release. Drug hypersensitivity, pulmonary aspiration and foreign bodies in the lower airway can also present with bronchospasm.

Clinical features

Bronchospasm can cause expiratory wheeze, a prolonged expiratory phase, increased inflation pressures and an upwardly sloping end-tidal carbon dioxide plateau. Wheezing may occur with other causes of respiratory obstruction and these should be excluded. If bronchospasm is severe, ventilation may be quiet, with signs of hypoxaemia.

Management

Management must prevent hypoxaemia and resolve the bronchospasm. Initially give 100% oxygen, deepen anaesthesia if appropriate and remove any precipitating factors (e.g. reposition the tracheal tube, stop the operation). If further treatment is necessary, give a bronchodilator in increments according to the response. Recommended drugs include intravenous aminophylline (up to 6 mg.kg^{-1}) or salbutamol (up to 3 μg.kg^{-1}). Volatile agents and ketamine are also effective bronchodilators. Adrenaline is indicated in life-threatening situations. Consider tracheal intubation and ventilation if hypoxaemia develops in the spontaneously breathing patient. In patients receiving IPPV, ventilation should be adjusted to minimize peak airway pressure and allow sufficient expiratory time. Steroids and H$_1$ receptor antagonists have no immediate effect but may be indicated in the later management of severe cases.

Anaesthesia for asthmatic patients. Elective surgery should proceed only if symptoms are optimally controlled. Premedication with the patient's usual bronchodilator therapy or an inhaled β$_2$-agonist is recommended and the use of an anxiolytic should be considered. If regional anaesthesia is contraindicated, use a general anaesthetic technique with minimal airway stimulation. Avoid using drugs which release histamine where possible and give all drugs slowly and after dilution. If tracheal intubation is necessary, ensure an adequate depth of anaesthesia. The provision of postoperative oxygen and maintenance bronchodilator therapy is essential.

Pneumothorax

Aetiology

The causes of pneumothorax during anaesthesia are listed in Table 22.8. Patients with recent chest trauma, asthma and chronic lung disease with bullae are most at risk, especially during IPPV. Air in the pleural space reduces ipsilateral lung ventilation. Nitrous oxide diffuses into air-filled spaces and causes a pneumothorax to expand. IPPV forces gas into the pleural space, with a rapid increase in the size of the pneumothorax. Increasing $\dot{V}/\dot{Q}$ mismatch and hypoxaemia follow. If the pneumothorax is under tension, hypoxaemia, mediastinal shift, reduced venous return and impairment of cardiac output can be life-threatening.

Clinical features

A pneumothorax should be excluded if un-

Table 22.8 Causes of pneumothorax during anaesthesia

Traumatic	Chest injury (rib fracture, flail, penetrating injury)
Iatrogenic	Subclavian/internal jugular venous cannulae Brachial plexus block Cervical/thoracic surgery Barotrauma
Spontaneous	Bullae, emphysema, asthma Marfan's syndrome Rapid decompression of divers

explained tachycardia, hypotension, hypoxaemia, cyanosis, difficulty with ventilation or high inflation pressures occur intraoperatively. Examination may demonstrate unequal air entry and/or chest movement, bronchospasm, surgical emphysema or mediastinal shift. Chest X-ray examination provides a definitive diagnosis (caution below).

Management

Prior to anaesthesia, it is desirable to exclude a pneumothorax by X-ray examination in all patients with recent chest trauma or central venous cannula insertion. However, this does not preclude later development of a pneumothorax during the perioperative period and a high index of suspicion is advisable in these patients. In patients with recent chest trauma, including rib fractures, regional analgesia or a technique using spontaneous ventilation is advised where possible. If tracheal intubation and IPPV are indicated, a chest drain should be inserted prior to anaesthesia.

If a pneumothorax is suspected intraoperatively, *treatment should not be delayed to confirm the diagnosis by chest X-ray examination.* Nitrous oxide should be discontinued and the lungs ventilated with 100% oxygen. The presence of air in the pleural space can be confirmed by careful needle aspiration on the suspected side via the second intercostal space in the midclavicular line and/or the fifth space in the midaxillary line. If the pneumothorax is under tension, there may be a gush of air. Temporary decompression using one or more large-bore intravenous cannulae may be life-saving prior to insertion of a chest drain. The presence of a bronchopleural fistula with substantial air leak can make ventilation ineffective.

In this situation, the affected lung can be isolated by insertion of a double lumen tube or gas exchange improved by the use of high frequency ventilation.

INTUBATION PROBLEMS

Unintentional endobronchial intubation

Unintentional endobronchial intubation produces one lung ventilation with a large shunt, hypoxaemia, decreased uptake of volatile agents and collapse of the contralateral lung. Intubation of the right main bronchus is more common. The likelihood of this complication is reduced by cutting the tracheal tube to an appropriate length prior to intubation and confirmation of its position by auscultation after intubation and changes in position.

Oesophageal intubation

Unrecognized oesophageal intubation is an important and preventable cause of anaesthetic mortality. Direct visual confirmation of the tracheal tube passing into the larynx anterior to the arytenoid cartilages confirms correct placement, although the tracheal tube may subsequently be displaced. Where direct vision is not possible, evidence of tracheal placement must be sought actively. Auscultation of breath sounds and chest or abdominal movement with ventilation are misleading indicators of tracheal tube placement. Furthermore, preoxygenation delays the onset of arterial oxygen desaturation after oesophageal intubation; therefore neither clinical signs nor the use of pulse oximetry can be relied upon to confirm correct tracheal tube placement. A persistent and normal expired carbon dioxide waveform confirms placement of the tracheal tube and therefore the early use of capnography after intubation is recommended strongly.

Mechanical devices such as the Wee oesophageal detector can also be used reliably to confirm the correct position of the tracheal tube. These devices use a large syringe or rubber evacuator bulb to aspirate air from the tracheal tube after intubation and prior to ventilation. Free aspiration of air indicates tracheal placement as the cartilaginous tracheal rings maintain patency, unlike the oesophageal walls which collapse and cause a resistance to aspiration. Disposable chemical indicators that detect expired carbon dioxide and transtracheal illumination via the tracheal tube with a special lighted stilette are alternative methods to confirm tracheal intubation. The use of fibreoptic bronchoscopy to visualize the trachea and bronchi directly via the tracheal tube gives a certain diagnosis, but is impractical in most clinical situations. If there is doubt regarding the position of the tracheal tube or if hypoxaemia occurs, removal of the tracheal tube and ventilation by mask may be life-saving.

Difficult intubation

The reported incidence of difficult intubation is one in every 65 patients. In practice, most cases represent difficulty with laryngoscopy. Poor management of difficult intubation is a significant cause of anaesthetic morbidity and mortality. Sequelae include dental and airway trauma, pulmonary aspiration and hypoxaemia.

Aetiology

Table 22.9 shows the common causes of difficult intubation. The single most important cause is an inexperienced or inadequately prepared anaesthetist, often complicated by equipment malfunction. There are numerous causes of difficult laryngoscopy related to patients. The anatomical features associated with difficult laryngoscopy are listed in Table 22.10. Of these, the atlanto-occipital distance is the best predictor of difficulty but requires an X-ray examination. Many of these factors are normal anatomical variations, but they may also be congenital or acquired.

Congenital. Many syndromes are associated with multiple anatomical abnormalities such as a small mouth, large tongue and cleft palate. Patients with encephalocoele, cystic hygroma and hydrocephalus may have restricted head or jaw movement. Morquio and Down syndromes are associated with cervical spine instability.

Acquired. Acquired factors can affect jaw opening, neck movement or the airway itself. Reduced jaw movement is a common cause of difficult laryngoscopy. Trauma and infection can cause reflex spasm of the masseter and medial pterygoid muscles (trismus). This typically occurs with dental abscess and fractures of the mandible and is usually relaxed by anaesthetic agents. In contrast, the reduced jaw movement associated

Table 22.9 Causes of difficult intubation

Anaesthetist		
Inadequate preoperative assessment		
Inadequate equipment preparation		
Inexperience, poor technique		
Equipment		
Malfunction		
Unavailability		
No trained assistance		
Patient		
Congenital	Syndromes (Down's, Pierre Robin, Treacher Collins, Marfan's)	
	Achondroplasia, cystic hygroma, encephalocoele	
Acquired	Reduced jaw movement	Trismus (abscess/infection, fracture, tetanus)
		Fibrosis (postinfection/radiotherapy/trauma)
		Rheumatoid arthritis, ankylosing spondylitis
		Tumours, jaw-wiring
	Reduced neck movement	Rheumatoid/osteoarthritis, ankylosing spondylitis
		Cervical fracture/instability/fusion
	Airway	Oedema (abscess/infection, trauma, angioedema, burns)
		Compression (goitre, surgical haemorrhage)
		Scarring (radiotherapy, infection, burns)
		Tumours/polyps, foreign body, nerve palsy
	Morbid obesity, pregnancy, acromegaly	

Table 22.10 Anatomical factors associated with difficult laryngoscopy

Short, muscular neck
Protruding incisors (buck teeth)
Long, high arched palate
Receding lower jaw
Poor mobility of the mandible
Increased anterior depth of mandible
Increased posterior depth of mandible (reduces jaw opening, requires X-ray)
Decreased atlanto-occipital distance (reduces neck extension, requires X-ray)

Table 22.11 Preoperative assessment of the airway.

1. General appearance of the neck, face, maxilla, and mandible
2. Jaw movement
3. Head extension and neck movement
4. The teeth and oropharynx
5. The soft tissues of the neck
6. Recent chest and cervical spine X-rays
7. Previous anaesthetic records

Management

Preoperative assessment. Preoperative examination of the airway (Table 22.11) is essential. Identifying patients with a potentially difficult airway (Tables 22.9 and 22.10) will allow time for planning an appropriate anaesthetic technique. Previous anaesthetic records should always be consulted. However, a past record of normal tracheal intubation is no guarantee for future anaesthesia as airway anatomy can be altered. Pregnancy is a common example. The presence of stridor or hoarse voice are warning signs for the anaesthetist. As it is impossible to identify all patients with a difficult airway during preoperative assessment, the anaesthetist must be prepared to manage the unexpected difficult laryngoscopy.

Many additional clinical tests to predict difficult laryngoscopy have been described. None of these tests is totally reliable, but their use may complement routine examination of the airway. The 'Mallampati' test is a widely used and simple classification of the pharyngeal view obtained during maximal mouth opening and tongue protrusion (Fig. 22.1). In practice, this test suggests a higher incidence of difficult laryngoscopy if the posterior pharyngeal wall is not visualized. The predictive value of this test may be strengthened if the thyromental distance (thyroid cartilage prominence to the bony point of the chin during full head extension) is less than 6.5 cm. The Mallampati classification correlates with the view obtained at laryngoscopy (Fig. 22.2). The difficulty associated with a 'grade 3' laryngoscopy can usually be overcome by posterior laryngeal displacement and/or the use of a gum elastic bougie. A patient whose epiglottis is not visible at laryngoscopy ('grade 4') usually has obvious preoperative anatomical abnormalities. Management of these patients requires the use of special techniques such as fibreoptic laryngoscopy.

with temporomandibular joint fibrosis is usually fixed. This can complicate chronic infection, rheumatoid arthritis, ankylosing spondylitis and radiotherapy. Any local soft tissue swelling or mass can also reduce jaw movement.

Reduced head movement is another important cause of difficult laryngoscopy as optimal positioning for laryngoscopy requires extension of the head at the atlanto-occipital joint. This joint may be damaged in patients with rheumatoid arthritis, osteoarthritis and ankylosing spondylitis. Cervical spine movement can also be reduced by surgical fusion, fibrosis and soft tissue swellings of the head and neck. Cervical spine instability (e.g. fractures, tumours, rheumatoid arthritis) makes neck movement undesirable.

Disorders of the airway itself may pose a serious threat to ventilation as well as preventing normal laryngoscopy. Soft tissue oedema of the face/upper airway from dental abscess, other infections, drug hypersensitivity, burns and trauma can cause considerable anatomical distortion with life-threatening airway obstruction. Foreign bodies, tumours and scarring after infection, burns and radiotherapy can also cause difficult laryngoscopy. Vocal cord apposition from recurrent laryngeal nerve palsy can hinder passage of the tracheal tube through the larynx. Positioning of the tracheal tube in the trachea can be difficult if there is compression or deviation caused by thyroid tumours, haematoma (traumatic, surgical) and thymic or lymph node tumours. Other rare disorders include vascular rings and laryngotracheomalacia. In clinical practice, the cause of difficult laryngoscopy is often multifactorial, for example in patients with morbid obesity, pregnancy and rheumatoid arthritis.

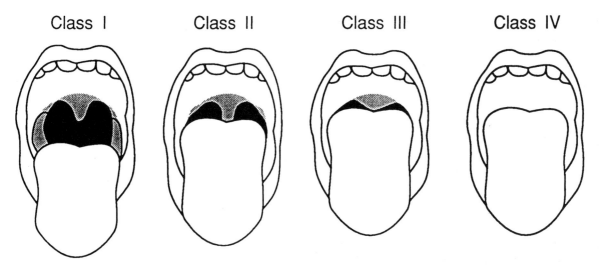

Fig. 22.1 Classification of the pharyngeal view when performing the Mallampati test. The patient must fully extend the tongue during maximal mouth opening. Class I: Pharyngeal pillars, soft palate, uvula visible. Class II: Only soft palate, uvula visible. Class III: Only soft palate visible. Class IV: Soft palate not visible.

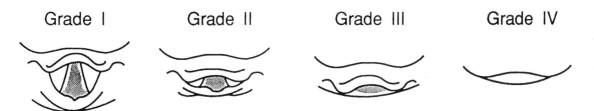

Fig. 22.2 Grading of the laryngoscopic view. Grade I: Vocal cords visible. Grade II: Arytenoid cartilages and posterior part of vocal cords visible. Grade III: Epiglottis visible. Grade IV: Epiglottis not visible. Note: the pharyngeal view (Fig. 22.1) is a clinical guide to the likely laryngoscopic view.

Preoperative preparation. Premedication with an antisialagogue reduces airway secretions. This is advantageous prior to inhalational induction and essential for awake fibreoptic laryngoscopy to maximize the effectiveness of topical local anaesthesia. An anxiolytic can also be given but is contraindicated in patients with airway obstruction. The presence of a trained assistant is essential and the availability of an experienced anaesthetist and a special 'difficult intubation' trolley with a range of equipment such as gum elastic bougies, laryngoscopes and tracheal tubes is desirable.

Regional anaesthesia. This should be used wherever possible in patients with a difficult airway, although the patient, anaesthetist and equipment must be prepared for general anaesthesia should a complication arise.

General anaesthesia. Unless tracheal intubation is essential for airway protection or to enable muscle relaxation and ventilation, the use of an artificial airway such as the laryngeal mask with spontaneous ventilation is a safe technique. If intubation is essential, the appropriate anaesthetic technique depends on the anticipated degree of difficulty, the presence of airway obstruction and the risk of regurgitation and aspiration. There is no place for the use of a long-acting muscle relaxant to facilitate intubation where difficulty is anticipated. Correct positioning of the head and neck is essential and the lungs should be preoxygenated after establishing intravenous access and appropriate monitoring. The safest anaesthetic technique can usually be chosen from the following clinical examples.

1. Patients with an increased risk of regurgitation and aspiration (e.g. full stomach, intra-abdominal pathology, pregnancy). An inhalational induction is inappropriate in these patients. Regional anaesthesia is preferable in the parturient (see Chapter 32). Preoxygenation and a rapid sequence induction with suxamethonium can be used if there is little anticipated difficulty. If intubation is unsuccessful, no further doses of muscle relaxant should be used, the patient allowed to wake and further assistance sought. If there is a high degree of anticipated difficulty, an awake technique is recommended (see below).

2. Patients with little anticipated difficulty and no airway obstruction (e.g. mild reduction of jaw or neck movement). After a sleep dose of intravenous induction agent and confirmation of the ability to ventilate the lungs manually by mask, suxamethonium can be given to provide the best conditions for tracheal intubation. If difficulty is encountered, the patient is allowed to wake up and the procedure replanned. Where appropriate, anaesthesia can be deepened by spontaneous ventilation using a volatile agent and alternative techniques to facilitate tracheal intubation used (see below).

3. Patients with severe anticipated difficulty and no airway obstruction (e.g. severe reduction of jaw or neck movement). Appropriate techniques include inhalational induction with halothane or the use of fibreoptic laryngoscopy either in the awake patient or after inhalational induction. A muscle relaxant must not be used until the ability to ventilate the lungs manually and view the vocal cords is confirmed.

4. Patients with airway obstruction (e.g. burns, infection, trauma). An inhalational induction may be used, otherwise an awake technique should be considered. Muscle relaxants should not be used until tracheal intubation is confirmed.

5. Extreme clinical situations. Tracheostomy performed under local anaesthesia may be the safest technique.

Inhalational induction. Premedication with an antisialagogue is desirable. Depth of anaesthesia is increased carefully by spontaneous ventilation of increasing concentrations of a volatile agent in 100% oxygen until laryngoscopy can be per- formed safely. Sevoflurane gives the best conditions for this purpose. If the larynx is viewed easily, intubation can be performed with or without suxamethonium. If the view is limited, the use of a gum elastic bougie will assist passage of the tracheal tube through the larynx. This is confirmed by detecting tracheal rings or resistance when the smaller bronchi are encountered. The tracheal tube is then 'railroaded' over the bougie into the trachea, often made easier by rotating the tracheal tube through 90° in an anticlockwise direction to align the bevel as it passes through the larynx. If this is unsuccessful, anaesthesia can be maintained and the use of fibreoptic laryngoscopy, blind nasal intubation or a retrograde technique considered. The last technique involves passage of an epidural catheter via a Tuohy needle through the cricothyroid membrane into the mouth and 'railroading' of the tracheal tube over the catheter into the trachea. The position of the tracheal tube should be confirmed using the methods described earlier. Trauma and bleeding can complicate this procedure, therefore other methods are probably safer in inexperienced hands.

Awake intubation. Fibreoptic laryngoscopy and intubation requires special equipment, skill and time. It can be performed by the nasal or oral route after topical anaesthesia is achieved by spraying the nasal and oropharyngeal mucosa and/or gargling viscous preparations. The injection of 3–5 ml of lignocaine 2% through the cricothyroid membrane induces coughing and anaesthetizes the tracheal and laryngeal mucosa. Conventional laryngoscopy can also be performed in awake patients. After cricothyroid injection of lignocaine, laryngoscopy is performed in stages. The oropharynx is progressively anaesthetized with lignocaine spray until the patient tolerates deep insertion of the laryngoscope, enabling the larynx to be viewed.

Failed intubation

The incidence of failed tracheal intubation is approximately one in 2000 in general surgical patients but one in 300 in obstetric patients. Poor management of failed intubation is a significant cause of anaesthetic morbidity and mortality. The aims of management are to maintain oxygenation and prevent aspiration of gastric contents. The 'failed intubation drill' is now established as an important skill for safe anaesthetic practice. An early decision to use a failed intubation protocol and call for assistance is essential, as continued attempts at intubation may result in airway trauma, pulmonary aspiration and hypoxaemia. Figure 22.3 suggests a protocol for managing failed intubation. The obstetric patient is a special case and is considered in Chapter 32.

If the airway is obstructed and ventilation inadequate during management of a failed intubation, there are several useful and potentially life-saving pieces of anaesthetic equipment available for use. The laryngeal mask is an essential piece of emergency airway equipment. It has been used successfully to provide an airway and allow ventilation when attempts to intubate and ventilate by other means have failed. It is also possible to pass a small diameter tracheal tube or a bougie through the laryngeal mask into the trachea. However, the laryngeal mask should not be regarded as protection against pulmonary aspiration. The oesophageal obturator airway and similar devices are alternatives in an emergency, but there are doubts about their efficacy and reports of misplacement and oesophageal rupture associated with their use.

In extreme situations, transtracheal ventilation can be life-saving. The cricothyroid membrane (CTM) is punctured using a large-bore needle or intravenous cannula. Aspiration of air confirms tracheal placement. High pressure 'jet' ventilation from a Sanders injector or the high pressure oxygen outlet on the anaesthetic machine is delivered via the cannula. This should allow oxygenation until the patient wakes. The laryngeal inlet must be patent to allow expiration, otherwise additional cannulae must be sited in the CTM. Seldinger-type tracheostomy devices or surgical cricothyroidotomy can also be used to gain access to the tracheal lumen during emergency situations. These techniques can produce tissue injury and barotrauma.

If surgery is essential, the decision to continue anaesthesia should be made by an experienced anaesthetist. It is safe practice to maintain oxygenation, protect the airway and allow the patient to awaken.

ASPIRATION OF GASTRIC CONTENTS

Aetiology

Regurgitation and pulmonary aspiration of gastric contents is more likely to occur in patients with intra-abdominal pathology, delayed gastric emptying (pain, trauma, alcohol) or inadequate gastro-oesophageal sphincter function (hiatus hernia, raised intra-abdominal pressure). Patients with reduced laryngeal reflexes, such as the elderly or sedated, are also at risk. Aspiration is more common during difficult intubation and therefore in emergency, obese and obstetric patients. Bronchospasm may be the first sign of pulmonary aspiration. If significant, respiratory obstruction, ventilation–perfusion mismatch and intrapulmonary shunting can produce severe hypoxaemia, with chemical pneumonitis and subsequent infection.

Management

The aims of preoperative management in at-risk patients are to reduce the volume and acidity of gastric contents (see Chapter 13). If general anaesthesia is essential, the airway must be protected using a rapid sequence induction with cricoid pressure and tracheal intubation. During emergence, extubation should not be performed until protective airway reflexes are regained. If aspiration occurs during anaesthesia, further regurgitation should be prevented by immediate application or maintenance of cricoid pressure. In all but mild cases, the trachea should be intubated to facilitate removal of the aspirate by suction prior to the use of positive pressure ventilation. However, ventilation should not be delayed if hypoxaemia is imminent. Bronchodilator therapy may be required and the inspired oxygen concentration can be increased with the addition of PEEP if hypoxaemia ensues. Surgery should be postponed or abandoned as soon as possible. Bronchoscopy will allow removal of solid matter and a chest X-ray and arterial blood gas measurement will help assess the severity of injury. The patient should be transferred to the intensive care unit for further monitoring and respiratory care.

HICCUPS

Unco-ordinated, spasmodic diaphragmatic move-

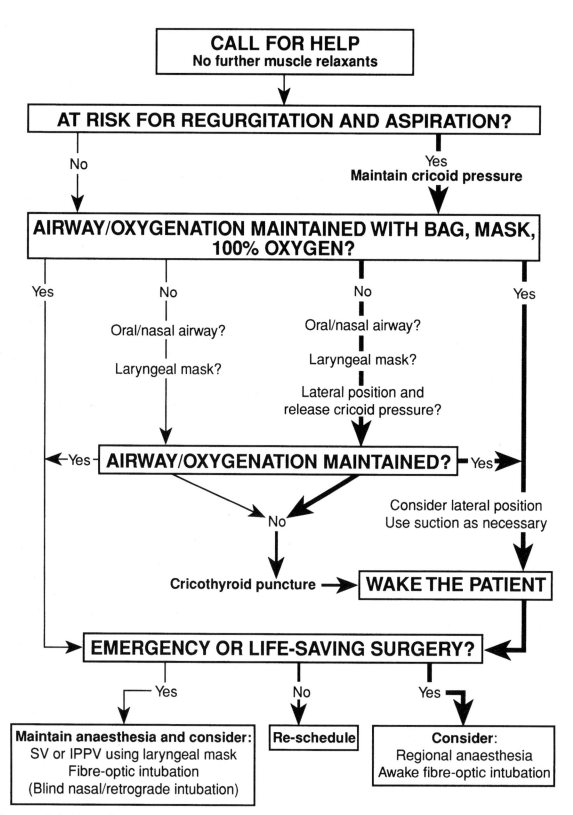

Fig. 22.3 Failed intubation protocol. Make an early decision to enter the protocol. Basic monitoring, optimal head positioning, use of bougie/stilette assumed. NOT APPLICABLE TO OBSTETRIC PATIENTS.

ments can occur during induction with intravenous agents such as etomidate and methohexitone or with vagal stimulation during light anaesthesia. Anticholinergic premedication reduces the incidence of hiccups. Although difficult to treat, hiccups are of little consequence unless surgery, or rarely oxygenation, is compromised. Persistent hiccups may be abolished by deepening anaesthesia, stimulating the nasopharynx with a suction catheter or administering metoclopramide or droperidol. Profound muscle relaxation may be justified to stop all diaphragmatic movement if hiccups are causing surgical difficulty.

ADVERSE DRUG EFFECTS

Table 22.12 shows a classification of drug-related complications. Although uncommon, hypersensitivity (allergy) and idiosyncratic reactions are potentially disastrous without early recognition and effective management. In contrast, drug interactions and the incorrect use of drugs are common problems. These are usually predictable, preventable and the result of human error. The risk of an adverse reaction increases in a non-linear fashion with the number of drugs given to a patient. Therefore, as polypharmacy is usual during anaesthesia, there is a substantial risk of a drug reaction.

Hypersensitivity

Aetiology

True hypersensitivity describes an enhanced immunological reaction. The incidence of perioperative drug hypersensitivity in anaesthetic practice is about one in 11 000. Most reactions during general anaesthesia follow intravenous drug administration. Hypersensitivity reactions may be either anaphylactic or anaphylactoid. These reactions differ from direct, drug-induced histamine release which does not have an immunological basis.

Anaphylaxis (immediate hypersensitivity or Gell and Coombs type 1 reaction). This is an antibody-mediated reaction to an antigen, characterized by a sudden, life-threatening, generalized pathophysiological response involving the cutaneous, respiratory and cardiovascular systems. Primary antigen exposure stimulates the production of specific IgE antibodies which bind to mast cells. Re-exposure with antigen bridging of these IgE antibodies stimulates mast cell degranulation and systemic release of the mediators of anaphylaxis. Mediators include histamine, prostaglandins, platelet activating factor and leukotrienes. Anaphylaxis has been reported in patients without apparent previous exposure to the specific antigen, probably due to immunological cross-reactivity.

Anaphylactoid reactions. These are not IgE-mediated although the clinical presentation resembles anaphylaxis. The precise immunological mechanism is not always evident, although many reactions involve complement, kinin and coagulation pathway activation.

Non-immunological histamine release. This is caused by the direct action of a drug on mast cells. The clinical response depends on both the drug dose and rate of delivery but is usually benign and confined to the skin. Anaesthetic drugs which release histamine directly include *d*-tubocurarine, atracurium, doxacurium, mivacurium (all of similar chemical derivation), morphine and pethidine. Clinical evidence of histamine release, usually cutaneous, occurs in up to 30% of patients during anaesthesia.

Table 22.12 Drug complications

Hypersensitivity	Allergic	Mostly unpredictable, uncommon
Idiosyncratic	Genetic	
Interactions	Pharmacokinetic Pharmacodynamic	Predictable, preventable, common
Other	Incorrect choice, dose, route Other unwanted effects	

Important agents in anaesthetic practice

Most drugs are capable of precipitating a hypersensitivity reaction.

Intravenous induction agents. The incidence of severe reactions to thiopentone has been reported as about one in 14 000. Methohexitone is associated with a higher reported incidence of hypersensitivity and there is cross-reactivity among barbiturates. Barbiturates can also cause direct histamine release. Propofol has caused anaphylaxis. Drugs solubilized in Cremophor EL are associated with a high incidence of anaphylactoid reactions. For this reason, Althesin and propanidid are no longer available for use in human anaesthetic practice. Hypersensitivity to benzodiazepines and etomidate is rare and these drugs do not cause direct histamine release.

Muscle relaxants. These are the most common cause of hypersensitivity in anaesthetic practice with an overall incidence of about one in 5000. Suxamethonium is the most immunogenic, although reactions to vecuronium, atracurium, alcuronium, gallamine and *d*-tubocurarine are well documented. The majority of reactions are IgE-mediated. There is significant cross-reactivity between muscle relaxants and with other drugs having quaternary ammonium molecules.

Opioids. Anaphylaxis has been reported with most opioids. Fentanyl is a rare cause of anaphylaxis and does not lead to significant direct histamine release. Morphine, codeine and pethidine can cause dose-dependent, non-immunological, cutaneous histamine release.

Local anaesthetics. Hypersensitivity to local anaesthetics is rare. Reactions are more likely to be dose-related toxicity, sensitivity to the effects of added vasoconstrictor or a reaction to preservatives such as paraben and benzoates. Amide local anaesthetic agents are considered safer than esters in patients with a previous history of sensitivity.

Colloid solutions. The overall reported incidence of hypersensitivity is 0.033%, with plasma protein and gelatin solutions presenting the lowest and highest risks respectively. The mechanism of reaction is often uncertain although gelatin solutions can cause both direct histamine release and anaphylaxis. All hyperosmolar solutions can release histamine directly. These solutions, for example mannitol, should be infused slowly.

Antibiotics. The anaesthetist is often asked to give antibiotics prior to induction for prophylaxis of wound infection. Penicillins are frequently prescribed and are most often implicated in hypersensitivity reactions. There is some cross-reactivity with cephalosporin antibiotics.

Radiocontrast media. Hypersensitivity reactions have been reported in up to 3% of patients although vasomotor symptoms such as flushing, warmth, nausea and cutaneous phenomena are more common. Reactions can be severe and most occur within minutes of administration. The risk of a reaction is markedly increased if the patient has suffered a previous reaction. Newer agents are associated with a lower risk.

Blood products. See Chapter 6.

Others. Protamine, streptokinase, aprotinin, atropine, bone cement and latex-containing products are just a few of the many substances that can cause severe reactions during the perioperative period.

Clinical features (Table 22.13)

As the patient is unable to volunteer symptoms during general anaesthesia, drug hypersensitivity should be considered with priority in the differential diagnosis of any major cardiorespiratory problem. Reactions are more common in females, with a history of allergy, atopy or previous exposure to anaesthetic agents, and over 90% of reactions occur immediately after induction of anaesthesia. There is a clinical spectrum of severity related to the degree of mast cell degranulation and host response.

Coughing, skin erythema, difficulty with ventilation or loss of a palpable pulse are often the first signs of a reaction. Erythema of the skin may be shortlived or absent as cyanosis from poor tissue perfusion and hypoxaemia may be profound. The awake patient may experience a sense of impending doom, dyspnoea, nausea and vomiting. The differential diagnosis should include anaesthetic drug overdose and other causes of bronchospasm, hypotension and hypoxaemia.

Management

Emergency management. Early recognition and effective action are essential as mortality in-

Table 22.13   Clinical features of drug hypersensitivity. Any one, or any combination, may occur

Skin	
Symptoms	Pruritus, burning
Signs	Erythema, urticaria, oedema (head/neck/airway/generalized)
Respiratory	
Symptoms	Shortness of breath, wheeze
Signs	Cough, laryngospasm, bronchospasm, increased inflation pressure, pulmonary oedema
Cardiovascular	
Symptoms	Feeling faint
Signs	Syncope, tachycardia, hypotension, absent peripheral pulses, arrhythmia, cyanosis, cardiovascular collapse/arrest
Gastrointestinal	
Symptoms	Abdominal cramps, nausea, vomiting, diarrhoea

creases with the delay in treatment. Deaths result from inadequate cardiorespiratory function. The aims of management are to prevent or correct hypoxaemia, maintain cerebral and tissue perfusion and to stop mediator release. Table 22.14 shows a protocol for the emergency management of anaphylaxis during general anaesthesia. *The use of intravenous adrenaline is essential treatment in the management of anaphylaxis.* It is life-saving if given early as it produces peripheral vasoconstriction, mast cell stabilization and bronchodilatation. Corticosteroids and H_1 receptor antagonists have a delayed onset of action and therefore have a role only in later management.

Later management. After stabilization, the patient should be transferred to the intensive care unit. Progressive oedema involving the airway often develops rapidly. Tracheal intubation and mechanical ventilation are recommended until the patient is clinically stable and airway patency can be guaranteed after a period of observation. Sequential blood sampling over a 24 h period for subsequent analysis of plasma histamine, tryptase, complement and IgE may enable identification of the causative agent and mechanism of the reaction. Blood coagulation should also be monitored. The patient should be reviewed after discharge by an appropriate clinician. Further investigations such as intradermal or skin prick tests and radioallergosorbent (RAST) tests for specific IgE antibodies should be performed. A Medicalert bracelet or other form of hazard alert should be carried by the patient. The details of the reaction must be recorded in the medical records and reported to the appropriate adverse drug reactions body. The patient's general practitioner must be informed.

Anaesthesia in the susceptible patient. Regional anaesthesia should be used where possible. In patients requiring general anaesthesia, the preoperative use of sodium cromoglycate, nebulized bronchodilators, corticosteroids and H_1- and H_2-receptor antagonists should be considered. A safe technique will avoid re-exposure to implicated agents and use drugs with a low potential for hypersensitivity and direct histamine release. These include volatile agents, etomidate, fentanyl and benzodiazepines. All drugs should be given slowly in dilution. Full resuscitation facilities must be immediately available.

Idiosyncratic reactions

An idiosyncratic drug reaction is a qualitatively abnormal and harmful drug effect occurring in a small number of individuals and precipitated usually by small drug doses. There is often an associated genetic defect and the reaction may be fatal. Suxamethonium sensitivity (see Chapter 11), malignant hyperthermia and acute intermittent porphyria are important examples of drug idiosyncrasy in anaesthetic practice.

Malignant hyperthermia (MH)

MH is an inherited myopathic disorder characterized by a marked increase in metabolic rate. The reported incidence varies considerably but is approximately one in 50 000. Rapid and effective treatment can reduce mortality from greater than 60% to less than 20%.

Table 22.14 Emergency management of acute major anaphylaxis under general anaesthesia

All doses for 70 kg patient – adjust as necessary.
Basic monitoring assumed.
Exercise caution if the diagnosis is not certain.

Immediate therapy
1. Discontinue administration of the suspect drug.
2. SUMMON HELP.
3. Discontinue surgery and anaesthesia if feasible.
4. Maintain airway with 100% oxygen (consider tracheal intubation and IPPV).
5. Give intravenous ADRENALINE especially if bronchospasm present, 50–100 µg (0.5–1.0 ml 1 : 10 000).
   Further 1 ml aliquots as necessary for hypotension and bronchospasm. Prolonged therapy may be
   necessary occasionally. (5–8 µg.kg^{-1} is the usual dose range.)
6. Start intravascular volume expansion, preferably colloid. 10 ml.kg^{-1} rapidly.
7. Consider external chest compression.

Secondary management
1. Adrenaline-resistant bronchospasm:
   Consider: SALBUTAMOL 250 µg i.v. loading dose. 5–20 µg.min^{-1} i.v. maintenance
   or TERBUTALINE 250–500 µg i.v. loading dose. 1.5 µg.min^{-1} i.v. maintenance
   or AMINOPHYLLINE 6 mg.kg^{-1} i.v. over 20 min.
2. Bronchospasm and/or cardiovascular collapse:
   Steroids: HYDROCORTISONE 500 mg i.v. or METHYL PREDNISOLONE 2 g i.v.
3. Antihistamines: CHLORPHENIRAMINE 20 mg i.v. diluted given slowly.
4. SODIUM BICARBONATE if acidosis severe after 20 min treatment.
5. Catecholamine infusions:
   Adrenaline: 5 mg in 500 ml (10 µg.ml^{-1}). Start at 10 ml.h^{-1} – up to 85 ml.h^{-1}
   Noradrenaline: 4 mg in 500 ml (8 µg.ml^{-1}). Start at 25 ml.h^{-1} – up to 100 ml.h^{-1}
6. Consider possibility of coagulopathy: clotting screen.
7. Measure arterial blood gas tensions for oxygenation and acid–base status.

From 1990 Anaphylactic reactions associated with anaesthesia. Association of Anaesthetists of Great Britain
and Ireland, London.

Aetiology. Inheritance of the MH gene (located on chromosome 19) gives rise to a defect in calcium binding within the sarcoplasmic reticulum of skeletal and possibly cardiac muscle. Contact with specific agents can trigger abnormal calcium release into the cytoplasm causing myofibrillar contraction, depletion of high energy muscle phosphate stores, accelerated metabolic rate, increased carbon dioxide and heat production, increased oxygen consumption and metabolic acidosis. The usual triggering agents are suxamethonium and any volatile agent. There is an uncertain clinical relationship between MH, other myopathies and musculoskeletal disorders such as squint.

Clinical features. The MH syndrome may present at any time during the perioperative period. The clinical features and their severity vary considerably. The most consistent early sign is unexplained and progressive tachycardia. Spontaneously breathing patients may present with tachypnoea and an increase in end-tidal carbon dioxide concentration. MH should always be considered if the patient's body temperature increases during anaesthesia. Classically the temperature rises by more than 2°C per hour and may exceed 40°C in some patients, although this is not a universal feature. Muscle rigidity is common and often involves the limbs. Without treatment, the full MH syndrome can develop with progressive deterioration and cardiovascular collapse. The syndrome is characterized by sweating, cyanosis, mottled skin, hypoxaemia, ventricular arrhythmias and severe metabolic and respiratory acidosis. Muscle injury can cause significant potassium release with ECG signs of hyperkalaemia. Coagulopathy, hypocalcaemia, elevated creatine kinase, oliguria, myoglobinuria and acute renal failure are other sequelae.

An alternative presentation of MH is masseter spasm shortly after the use of suxamethonium for tracheal intubation. Less than 10% of patients with this presentation progress to the full MH syndrome.

Management. Administration of volatile agents should be discontinued immediately and the lungs hyperventilated with 100% oxygen. If end-tidal carbon dioxide monitoring is unavailable, use at least twice the predicted minute volume. The trachea should be intubated at the earliest opportunity if a tracheal tube is not already in place. Experienced help in both theatre and the laboratory should be obtained and the operation abandoned as soon as possible. Intravenous dantrolene is indicated specifically and should be given in 1–2 mg.kg^{-1} doses every 5 min until the rise in arterial carbon dioxide tension is controlled and decreasing. The mean and maximum doses used are 2.5 and 10 mg.kg^{-1} respectively. Dantrolene is packaged as a powder that requires several minutes to reconstitute, forming an alkaline solution. It is a skeletal muscle relaxant and will cause muscle weakness if a sufficient dose is given. MH is associated with severe, life-threatening acidosis which can develop rapidly. Therefore the early use of intravenous sodium bicarbonate should be considered and large amounts may be necessary.

The patient should be cooled actively with ice packs to the axillae and groins and chilled intravenous saline infused. If necessary, gastric and rectal lavage with iced saline can be performed. Peritoneal dialysis and cardiopulmonary bypass have also been used to cool patients with MH. If possible, substitute the anaesthetic breathing system for an unused system. Monitor core temperature, central venous pressure, direct arterial pressure and urine output. Early and serial blood samples should be collected for analysis of acid–base status, arterial blood gas tensions, coagulation and serum electrolyte concentrations, especially potassium and glucose. Hyperkalaemia should be treated with intravenous insulin and dextrose. Arrhythmias usually resolve after treatment of hyperkalaemia and acidosis, otherwise specific antiarrhythmic drugs may be indicated. A urine output greater than 1 ml.kg^{-1}.h^{-1} should be encouraged by ensuring an adequate circulating blood volume, giving a renal vasodilator such as dopamine and using intravenous mannitol where necessary. Haemofiltration may be indicated in the management of biochemical abnormalities and/or renal dysfunction. The patient must be managed in an intensive care unit for at least 48 h as the syndrome can recur during this time. Treatment with oral dantrolene is recommended for 48 h.

Any patient who experiences a clinical episode resembling MH, as well as the first-degree relatives of patients with confirmed MH, should be referred to a specialist centre for further assessment. The tests used to identify individuals with MH susceptibility vary between centres. The most common test is halothane and caffeine-induced contracture of a muscle specimen. Less invasive genetic tests are being developed.

Anaesthesia in the susceptible patient. This should be a planned inpatient procedure with the facility for extended postoperative monitoring. The aim of management is to prevent contact with volatile agents and suxamethonium. A 'clean' anaesthetic machine can be prepared by flushing the machine overnight with 100% oxygen and using a new breathing system. The use of anticholinergic premedication is not advisable as it interferes with thermoregulation. Full resuscitation facilities and dantrolene should be immediately available. Regional anaesthesia should be used where possible. Safe drugs for use in susceptible patients include barbiturates, propofol, etomidate, benzodiazepines, non-depolarizing muscle relaxants, opioids and local anaesthetic agents. Total intravenous anaesthesia with propofol is one recommended technique. Monitoring of end-tidal carbon dioxide concentration, ECG, arterial pressure, oxygen saturation and continuous core temperature is mandatory.

Acute intermittent porphyria (AIP)

AIP is a rare but serious metabolic disorder caused by an inherited deficiency of an enzyme required for haem synthesis. This allows potential accumulation of porphyrin precursors in the pathway. The hepatic synthesis of these porphyrin precursors is controlled by the enzyme delta-amino laevulinic acid synthetase. Induction of this enzyme by barbiturates and many other drugs causes precursor accumulation and manifests clinically with acute neuropathy, abdominal pain and delirium. On occasions, the abdominal pain can mimic an acute abdomen, leading to surgical intervention. If an at-risk patient is identified, porphyrinogenic drugs including barbiturates must be avoided as AIP can be fatal. Drugs considered safe for use in patients with AIP include propofol, midazolam, suxamethonium, vecuronium, nitrous oxide, morphine, fentanyl, neostigmine and atropine.

Interactions

Pharmacokinetic

This describes modification of the absorption, distribution, metabolism or excretion of one drug by another. Examples include the reduction in clearance of warfarin and lignocaine by cimetidine and the effect of opioids on the absorption of orally administered drugs by increasing gastric emptying time.

Pharmacodynamic

This describes interactions in which the pharmacological response to a drug is changed by the presence of another. Examples include potentiation of the myocardial depressant effect of volatile agents and intravenous induction agents in patients receiving β-blockers or calcium antagonists and the enhancement of neuromuscular blockade by aminoglycoside antibiotics.

Other drug complications

The incorrect choices of a drug, its dose or route of administration are common, preventable complications. Errors involving ampoule and syringe identification can be prevented by a sound anaesthetic technique including the use of labels. Inappropriate mixing of incompatible drugs can cause precipitation due to a change in pH, most often caused by mixing acidic and alkaline drugs. Absolute or relative overdosage is a frequent event and can be disastrous. Excessively rapid drug administration can also cause complications such as histamine release (e.g. muscle relaxants).

Most drugs have undesirable side-effects. For example, etomidate inhibits cortisol synthesis and can increase mortality in critically ill patients when used continuously for sedation. Nitrous oxide interferes with methionine synthesis and haemopoiesis as well as diffusing into gas-filled spaces. For example, the use of 70% nitrous oxide for 2 h doubles the volume of bowel gas and may compromise gut blood supply, reduce surgical access and increase the incidence of postoperative nausea and vomiting. Nitrous oxide also increases the size and/or pressure in gas-filled spaces such as a pneumothorax.

HYPOTHERMIA

Hypothermia during anaesthesia may be defined as a core body temperature less than 36.0°C.

Aetiology

Heat loss exceeds production in anaesthetized patients. Heat production falls as anaesthetic agents alter hypothalamic function, reduce metabolic rate, abolish the behavioural response to heat loss and reduce the ability to shiver. Many factors increase heat loss. During the first hour of anaesthesia, vasodilatation redistributes body heat to the periphery causing a rapid fall in core temperature followed by a slower but steady decrease. Over 50% of heat loss is from radiation. This is exacerbated when the ambient temperature is less than 24°C, during surgery with open body cavities and during transfer with inadequate covering. Evaporative heat loss is increased by ventilation of the lungs with dry, cold anaesthetic gases, the use of wet packs, sweating and operations with open body cavities. High theatre air flow rates promote convective heat loss. Irrigation or intravenous infusion with cold fluids and long duration of surgery are associated with increased heat loss. The risk of hypothermia is greater in neonates, patients with a low metabolic rate such as the elderly and patients with burns.

The effects of hypothermia are proportional to the change in temperature. Metabolic rate is reduced by up to 10% for every 1°C fall in body temperature. There is a decrease in cardiac output and an increase in haemoglobin oxygen affinity. This leads to a reduction in tissue oxygen delivery. Significant hypothermia is associated with metabolic acidosis, oliguria, altered platelet and clotting function and reduced hepatic blood flow with slower drug metabolism. The MAC for volatile agents is reduced and muscle relaxants have a longer duration of effect. Postoperative shivering increases oxygen consumption and myocardial work.

Management

Measures to minimize heat loss should begin when the patient leaves the ward for theatre (Table 22.15). Patients are particularly vulnerable during transfers and the first hour of anaesthesia. Induced hypothermia is occasionally used in some centres for highly specialized paediatric neurological and cardiac operations where circulatory arrest provides optimal operating conditions. Lowering the metabolic rate reduces tissue oxygen consumption and allows a short time of deliberate circulatory arrest. Hypothermia reduces intracranial pressure and is occasionally induced in the management of paediatric head injuries.

HYPERTHERMIA

Hyperthermia during anaesthesia may be defined as a core body temperature greater than 37.5°C or an increase in temperature of greater than 2°C per hour.

Aetiology

Hyperthermia is usually caused by an increase in heat production. Causes include sepsis, drug reactions, excessive catecholamine secretion (phaeochromocytoma, thyroid storm) and malignant hyperthermia. Elevated metabolic rate and oxygen consumption increase cardiac output and minute ventilation and can lead to acidosis. Without treatment, sweating and vasodilatation will produce hypovolaemia. Extreme hyperthermia results in seizures and central nervous system damage.

Management

General measures include exposure of the body surface, application of ice packs, the use of fans and administration of cooled intravenous fluids. Specific measures depend on the cause.

AWARENESS

Aetiology

Awareness during anaesthesia refers to a patient experiencing an intraoperative event. As the brain is capable of processing information and memory function during anaesthesia, there is probably a spectrum of awareness that correlates with depth of anaesthesia. Of clinical importance is the patient who recalls the event postoperatively. Although awareness is most likely to occur in obstetric patients undergoing emergency Caesarean section under general anaesthesia, all patients undergoing general anaesthesia are at risk. The reported incidence in non-obstetric anaesthesia is about two per 1000. Awareness is associated with a poor anaesthetic technique, the use of low concentrations of volatile agents (either inappropriately or during a hypotensive episode) and equipment problems such as breathing system disconnections and leaks.

Management

Assessment of the depth of anaesthesia is difficult. It has been based traditionally on activity of the autonomic nervous system (e.g. tachycardia, sweating), although these signs are not always a reliable indication of anaesthetic depth. The use of muscle relaxants with a balanced anaesthetic technique further obscures some of the signs of light anaesthesia. The isolated forearm technique and monitoring of lower oesophageal motility are other unreliable techniques for assessing the depth of anaesthesia. However, changes in the auditory evoked potential with anaesthesia appear

Table 22.15   Measures to reduce heat loss

Environment	Increase the ambient temperature and humidity
Patient	Cover patient during transfers and induction of anaesthesia
	Warm all irrigation, intravenous fluids and blood
	Insulate patient with plastic wrap, swaddling (limbs, head)
	Warming blanket (more effective on top of patient)
	Enclose exposed viscera in plastic bags
	Warm and humidify inspired gases

to correlate with anaesthetic depth and this technique has potential for clinical application.

If a patient enquires about awareness at the preoperative visit, the risks and causes of awareness should be discussed to allay anxiety. It may also be appropriate electively to discuss the topic with patients planning Caesarean section under general anaesthesia. Reducing the risk of awareness by meticulous preparation of equipment and the use of an appropriate anaesthetic technique is essential. If a patient complains of recall, the anaesthetist should be informed and should visit the patient forthwith, preferably with a senior colleague. The anaesthetist should establish the perioperative timing of the episode and distinguish between dreaming and awareness. If there is genuine awareness and a clear anaesthetic error, then honest admission and apology are advisable. All details should be recorded in the case notes. Although the majority of recalled events are not painful (up to 90% of patients with awareness have not experienced pain), awareness is a traumatic experience for the patient. This can lead to psychological sequelae including insomnia, depression and fear of death. The situation is exacerbated if staff disbelieve or ignore the patient. It is essential to offer follow-up counselling for the patient.

INJURY

Most intraoperative injuries are sustained as a result of poor positioning or tracheal intubation. Neural, dental and ophthalmic injuries are common causes of litigation, although most are preventable. Thermal and electrical injuries are less common but potentially disastrous.

Neural

Although neurological deficits present during the postoperative period, they are usually sustained intraoperatively.

Peripheral

The reported incidence of peripheral nerve injury is about one in every 1000 anaesthetics. Poor positioning is a common underlying factor. The brachial plexus and superficial nerves of the limbs (ulnar, radial and common peroneal) are the most frequently affected nerves. The usual mechanism of injury to superficial nerves is ischaemia from compression of the vasa vasorum by surgical retractors, leg stirrups and contact with other equipment. This is more likely to occur during periods of poor peripheral perfusion from hypotension and hypothermia. The mechanism of brachial plexus injury is usually traction by excessive shoulder abduction. Needle-stick or chemical injury can occur during regional anaesthesia.

Meticulous care is necessary when positioning the patient. Padding should be used beneath tourniquets and to protect pressure points. Extreme joint positions should be avoided. Close surveillance of tourniquet ischaemia times is essential. Although most injuries recover within several months, all patients with a peripheral nerve injury must be referred to a neurologist for continuing care. Many ulnar nerve palsies occur in patients with an anatomical predisposition, which can usually be deduced from a history of numbness after sleep or as a result of posture at work. In these patients, the elbows should not be flexed during surgery.

Central

Central nervous system injury ranges from minimal dysfunction to stroke or death. The mechanism is usually hypoxaemia and/or hypotension and the causes have been outlined previously. The cervical cord can be damaged during tracheal intubation and positioning in patients with cervical spine instability from fractures, rheumatoid arthritis and some congenital conditions such as Klippel–Feil, Morquio and Down syndromes. Extreme positions of the head and neck can occasionally cause cerebral ischaemia in patients with vertebrobasilar insufficiency. Ischaemic injury to the cord can occur during major vascular and spinal surgery.

Dental

Dental damage is the most frequently reported anaesthetic injury and is usually sustained during careless or difficult laryngoscopy. The injury varies from chipping and scratches to fracture and avulsion, most often involving the upper incisors. Preoperative assessment and documentation of dentition is essential. If a tooth is accidentally avulsed it should be reimplanted in its socket with minimal interference and a dental surgeon consulted at the earliest opportunity.

Ophthalmic

Corneal abrasions are associated with inadequate eye protection, especially during transfer or use of the prone position. The use of adhesive tape to close the eyelids is also a risk factor. Lubricated dressings such as sterile paraffin gauze may be a preferable method of securing the eyelids. Mechanical pressure to the globes should be avoided at all times. Retinal detachment has been reported with extreme Trendelenburg positioning and as a result of pressure exerted on the eye in patients placed in the prone position.

Thermal and electrical

The high density electrical current used with surgical diathermy is a potential source of injury. If the return current path is interrupted by incorrect application of the diathermy pad, then the ECG electrodes or points of skin–metal contact can provide an alternative electrical path, producing serious burns. Failure of thermostatic control of warming devices is also a source of thermal injury.

EQUIPMENT PROBLEMS

About a third of all critical incidents are related to equipment failure and most are preventable. Most equipment problems have implications for the patient and these have previously been described where clinically relevant (e.g. leaks and disconnections involving the anaesthetic machine and gas delivery system). Additional important problems can involve monitoring equipment and the use of limb tourniquets.

Monitoring

The equipment used for monitoring can provide inaccurate data and mislead the inexperienced anaesthetist. For example, non-invasive blood pressure equipment can be unreliable at low and high blood pressures and pulse oximeters can fail to provide data in patients with poor peripheral perfusion. Ultimately, the anaesthetist must rely on clinical skills during the conduct of anaesthesia. Invasive monitoring is a further source of complications. Central venous and pulmonary arterial catheterization are associated with numerous problems including thrombosis, sepsis, pneumothorax and damage to deep structures. The use of arterial and peripheral venous cannulae can lead to thrombophlebitis, sepsis, air embolism and tissue damage from extravasation of fluids and drugs.

Tourniquets

The incorrect use of tourniquets and bandages can traumatize skin, dislodge deep venous thrombi and produce nerve and muscle ischaemia. Deflation of a tourniquet after a period of limb ischaemia is associated with translocation of acidotic blood to the circulation. Hypercapnia, acidosis and depression of cardiac function may be clinically significant in patients with poor cardiorespiratory function. Limb tourniquets are contraindicated in patients with sickle cell disease, peripheral neuropathy, limb infections and peripheral vascular disease including deep venous thrombosis. Tourniquets should be applied with adequate padding to the proximal limb avoiding bony prominences. The correct pressure for arm and leg tourniquet inflation is 50 mmHg and 100 mmHg respectively above systolic blood pressure. The duration of limb ischaemia in healthy patients should not exceed 2 h without a reperfusion time of at least 20 min.

FURTHER READING

Brown D L (ed) 1992 Risk and outcome in anesthesia, 2nd edn. JB Lippincott, Philadelphia
Buck N, Devlin H B, Lunn J N 1987 The report of a confidential enquiry into perioperative deaths. The Nuffield Provincial Hospitals Trust, London

Cooper J B, Newbower R S, Kitz R J 1984 An analysis of major errors and equipment failures in anesthesia management: considerations for prevention and detection. Anesthesiology 60, 34
Harrison G G, Meissner P N, Hift R J 1993 Anaesthesia

for the porphyric patient. Anaesthesia 48, 417

Hunter J M 1993 Editorial: histamine release and neuromuscular blocking drugs. Anaesthesia 48, 561

King T A, Adams A P 1990 Failed tracheal intubation. British Journal of Anaesthesia 65, 400

Latto I P, Rosen M (eds) 1985 Difficulties in tracheal intubation. Baillière Tindall, London

Levy J H 1992 Anaphylactic reactions in anesthesia and intensive care, 2nd edn. Butterworth Heinemann, Boston

Taylor T H 1992 Editorial: avoiding iatrogenic injuries in theatre. British Medical Journal 305, 595

Taylor T H, Major E (eds) 1993 Hazards and complications of anaesthesia, 2nd edn. Churchill Livingstone, London

Tunstall M E 1976 Failed intubation drill. Anaesthesia 31, 850

23. Postoperative care

In modern anaesthetic practice, the patient is monitored and supervised closely and continuously during induction and throughout the operative procedure. However, many problems associated with anaesthesia and surgery may occur in the immediate postoperative period, and it is essential that supervision by adequately trained and experienced personnel is continued during the recovery period. In addition, some major and minor complications of anaesthesia and surgery may occur at any time in the first few days after operation.

THE EARLY RECOVERY PERIOD

Most hospitals have a recovery ward in close proximity to the operating theatre suite (see Chapter 17). Many recovery areas are closed at night and at weekends; at these times, and in hospitals with no recovery ward, the patient is supervised usually in a corridor close to the operating theatre and often by inadequately trained staff. This section describes common problems which occur in the immediate postoperative period and refers specifically to their management in a recovery ward; however, the same principles are applicable to recovery in other locations.

The recovery period starts as soon as the patient leaves the operating table and the direct supervision of the anaesthetist. All the complications listed below may occur at any time, including the period of transfer from operating theatre to recovery ward; in some operating theatre suites, the transfer to the recovery ward may last for several minutes, and it is essential that the standard of observation does not diminish during the journey. The patient must be supervised and monitored closely *at all times*.

Systems affected

Central nervous system

Consciousness may not return for several minutes after the end of general anaesthesia, and may be impaired for a longer period of time. During this period, a patent airway must be maintained. There is a risk of aspiration into the lungs of any material, e.g. gastric content or blood, which is present in the pharynx. Consciousness may also be depressed in patients who have received sedation to facilitate endoscopy or regional anaesthesia.

Excitement and confusion may occur during recovery and may result in injury. Pain may be severe if long-acting analgesics have not been given during surgery.

Cardiovascular system

Peripheral resistance and cardiac output may be reduced because of residual effects of anaesthetic drugs in the absence of surgical stimulation. Hypovolaemia may be present because of inadequate fluid replacement during surgery, continued bleeding postoperatively or expansion of capacitance of the vascular system as a result of rewarming. Cardiac output may also be reduced as a result of arrhythmias or pre-existing disease. Hypertension may occur as a result of increased sympathoadrenal activity after restoration of consciousness, especially if analgesia is inadequate.

Respiratory system

Hypoventilation occurs commonly, usually as a result of residual effects of anaesthetic drugs or incomplete antagonism of neuromuscular blocking drugs. Hypoxaemia may result from hypoventilation, ventilation/perfusion imbalance or increased oxygen consumption produced by restlessness or shivering.

Gastrointestinal

Nausea and vomiting are common in the immediate postoperative period.

Staff, equipment and monitoring

The recovery ward should be staffed by trained and experienced nurses; one nurse must remain with each unconscious patient at all times. The responsibility for the patient's welfare remains with the anaesthetist. In many hospitals, an anaesthetist is designated to be available immediately to treat complications detected by the nursing staff.

The patient is nursed in a bed if a prolonged stay is anticipated, but more commonly on a trolley (Fig. 23.1). All beds and trolleys must have the facility to be tipped head-down. Suction apparatus, including catheters, an oxygen supply with appropriate face mask, a self-inflating resuscitation bag and anaesthetic mask, a pulse oximeter and an oscillometer (or at least a sphygmomano-

meter) must be available for each patient. In addition, there should be a complete range of resuscitation equipment within the recovery area; this includes an anaesthetic machine, a range of laryngoscopes, tracheal tubes, bougies, intravenous (i.v.) cannulae, fluids, emergency drugs, electrocardiogram (ECG) monitor and defibrillator. Facilities for cricothyroid cannulation, e.g. minitracheotomy set, or for formal tracheostomy should also be available.

A wide range of drugs should be stored in the recovery area for the treatment of common complications and also emergency events (Table 23.1).

All patients should be monitored by measurement of pulse rate, arterial pressure, arterial oxygen saturation and respiratory rate and by assessment of level of consciousness, peripheral circulation and adequacy of ventilation; in some circumstances, minute volume may be measured using a respirometer (e.g. Wright's). Depending on the nature of work undertaken in the theatre suite, a proportion of bed stations should have the facility for monitoring ECG, systemic and pulmonary arterial pressures and central venous pressure (CVP) continuously; this may be required in high-risk patients or those who have undergone major surgery. At least one mechanical ventilator should

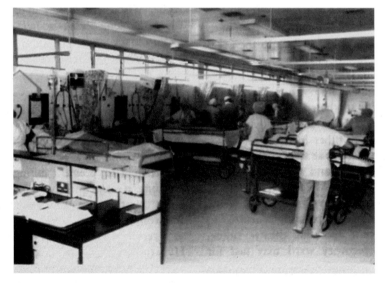

Fig. 23.1 A recovery ward. Most patients are nursed on a trolley, but a bed is used for those who need to stay for several hours.

Table 23.1 Drugs which should be available in the recovery room

Adenosine	Insulin
Adrenaline	Isoprenaline
Alfentanil	Ketamine
Aminophylline	Ketorolac
Antibiotics	Labetalol
Aprotinin	Lignocaine
Aspirin	Metaraminol
Atracurium	Methoxamine
Atropine	Methylprednisolone
Bupivacaine	Metoclopramide
Calcium chloride	Midazolam
Calcium gluconate	Morphine
Calcium heparin	Naloxone
Chlorpheniramine	Neostigmine
Co-proxamol	Nifedipine
Cyclizine	Noradrenaline
Dexamethasone	Ondansetron
Diazepam	Papaverine
Diclofenac	Paracetamol
Digoxin	Pethidine
Dobutamine	Phentolamine
Dopamine	Phenytoin
Doxapram	Phytomenadione
Edrophonium	Potassium chloride
Ephedrine	Procainamide
Fentanyl	Prochlorperazine
Flumazenil	Propranolol
Frusemide	Protamine
Glucose	Ranitidine
Glyceryl trinitrate	Salbutamol
Glycopyrronium	Sodium citrate
Hyaluronidase	Sodium nitroprusside
Hydralazine	Suxamethonium
Hydrocortisone	Tranexamic acid
Hyoscine	Verapamil

be available. Urine output should be measured routinely in patients who have undergone major surgery.

Wounds and surgical drains should be inspected regularly for signs of bleeding.

The patient should not be discharged to the surgical ward until:

1. Consciousness has returned fully, and a patent airway can be maintained.
2. Ventilation is adequate and stable.
3. The cardiovascular system is stable.
4. Excessive surgical blood loss has stopped.

A record should be made of pulse rate, blood pressure and arterial oxygen saturation, together with any other relevant physiological observations, while the patient is in the recovery area. In most units, these recordings are made every 5 min,

at least until consciousness has returned. Records should also be made of any complications which occur, and of all drugs administered.

High-risk patients, or those who have undergone major surgery, should stay in the recovery ward for up to 24 h. If this is not feasible, or if instability persists for longer than 24 h, the patient should be transferred to a high-dependency or intensive therapy unit.

Although the recovery room nurse undertakes the direct care of the patient, the responsibility for the patient remains with the anaesthetist. Patients must only be discharged to the ward with the anaesthetist's consent.

The remainder of this chapter is devoted to the diagnosis and management of common problems which occur in the postoperative period. Some of these occur most frequently in the immediate recovery period, while others may occur at any time during the patient's convalescence from surgery. Some surgical procedures are associated with specific complications.

CENTRAL NERVOUS SYSTEM

Conscious level

Many patients are unconscious on arrival in the recovery ward because of residual effects of anaesthetic drugs. The duration of impaired consciousness depends on:

1. *The drugs used.* Recovery of consciousness may be delayed if the following agents have been used:
   a. Volatile anaesthetics with high blood/gas solubility coefficient.
   b. Barbiturates, particularly if large total doses have been given.
   c. Benzodiazepines.
   d. Opioids with a long duration of action, including large doses of fentanyl.
2. *The timing of drug use.* Delayed recovery may occur if a long-acting i.v. anaesthetic or analgesic drug has been given towards the end of the procedure, or if the more soluble volatile agents have been continued until the end of surgery.
3. *Pain.* The presence of pain speeds recovery of consciousness. Recovery may be delayed after minor procedures or if potent analgesia has

been provided by administration of opioids or by regional anaesthesia.

Undue prolongation of consciousness should not be attributed to these factors alone. Other causes should be considered, as their early recognition may prevent serious sequelae.

Hypoglycaemia

This occurs most commonly in diabetic patients treated with oral hypoglycaemic agents or insulin, and an inadequate intake of glucose. The perioperative management of the diabetic patient is discussed in Chapter 40.

Hyperglycaemia

Hyperglycaemia in known diabetics may occur as a result of inadequate provision of insulin or injudicious infusion of glucose. However, coma is unusual in acute hyperglycaemia. Undiagnosed diabetics with hyperglycaemia and ketosis may present for surgery because of abdominal pain, and prolonged postoperative coma may occur unless the metabolic defect is diagnosed and treated.

Cerebral pathology

Consciousness may be impaired by functional or structural cerebral damage. Possible causes include:

1. Episodes of cerebral ischaemia (e.g. carotid artery surgery, profound hypotension) or hypoxia during anaesthesia.
2. Intracranial haemorrhage, thrombosis or infarction. These may occur fortuitously, or may have been associated with intraoperative hypertension, hypotension or arrhythmias.
3. Pre-existing cerebral lesions, e.g. tumour, trauma. Anaesthetic techniques which increase intracranial pressure are likely to impair cerebral function.
4. Epilepsy. Convulsions may have been masked by anaesthesia or neuromuscular blocking drugs.
5. Air embolism.
6. Intracranial spread of local anaesthetic solution after subarachnoid injection. Introduction

into the subarachnoid space may be accidental, e.g. during extradural block or, rarely, interscalene brachial plexus block. Unconsciousness is almost always accompanied by apnoea.

Other causes

1. *Hypoxaemia.* In the presence of an adequate circulation, coma occurs only if profound hypoxaemia is present.
2. *Hypercapnia.* Unconsciousness may occur if arterial carbon dioxide tension (Pa_{CO_2}) exceeds 9–10 kPa.
3. *Hypotension.*
4. *Hypothermia.*
5. *Hypo-osmolar or TURP syndrome.* This results most commonly from absorption of water from the bladder during transurethral resection of the prostate (TURP). The investigation and management of this condition are described on p. 476.
6. *Hypothyroidism.*
7. *Hepatic or renal failure.*

Confusion and agitation

These occasionally occur during emergence from an otherwise uncomplicated anaesthetic. They are more common in elderly patients, particularly if hyoscine has been given as a premedicant. Atropine also crosses the blood–brain barrier and may result in the central anticholinergic syndrome, characterized by restlessness and confusion, together with obvious antimuscarinic effects. Glycopyrronium does not cross the blood–brain barrier, and is preferable to atropine for antagonism of the muscarinic effects of neostigmine in elderly patients; in addition to its lack of central effects, it produces less tachycardia and antagonizes the effects of neostigmine for a longer period.

All the factors listed above as causes of prolonged coma may also result in confusion and agitation. Pain may also contribute, although it is seldom responsible alone. Emergence delirium is particularly associated with the use of ketamine, and may occur after the administration of etomidate. Septicaemia may result in confusion, as may distension of the stomach or bladder.

A lightly sedated, conscious patient with inadequate antagonism of neuromuscular blocking drugs may appear to the inexperienced observer to be agitated and confused. Movements are unco-ordinated. The condition is distressing to the patient and is an indication of a poor anaesthetic technique. It should never be allowed to develop.

Pain

This subject is discussed fully in Chapter 24. The effects of pain should be differentiated from those of hypercapnia and hypovolaemia (Table 23.2).

RESPIRATORY SYSTEM

Hypoventilation

Common causes of hypoventilation in the immediate postoperative period are listed in Table 23.3. Hypoventilation results in an increase in Pa_{CO_2} (Fig. 23.2), and a decrease in alveolar oxygen tension (PA_{O_2}), and thus hypoxaemia, which may be corrected by increasing the inspired concentration of oxygen.

Airway obstruction

Airway obstruction caused by the tongue, by indrawing of the pharyngeal muscles or by blood or secretions in the pharynx, is ameliorated by placing the patient in the lateral or recovery position (see Fig. 19.5). This position should be used for all unconscious patients who have undergone oral or ear, nose and throat surgery, and for patients at risk of gastric aspiration.

Partial obstruction of the airway is characterized by noisy ventilation. As the obstruction increases, tracheal tug and indrawing of the supraclavicular area occur during inspiration. Total obstruction is signalled by absent sounds of breathing and paradoxical movement of the chest wall and abdomen.

In many patients, a clear airway is only maintained by displacing the mandible anteriorly and

Table 23.2 Common problems in the recovery room: symptoms and signs

	Pain	Hypercapnia	Hypovolaemia
Conscious level	May be restless May be quiescent if severe pain	Comatose	Restless or quiescent depending on extent of analgesia and residual anaesthesia
Periphery	Vasoconstriction, pallor ± sweating	Warm, flushed with bounding pulse (if normovolaemic)	Vasoconstriction, pallor ± sweating
Heart rate	Tachycardia	Tachycardia	Tachycardia
Arterial pressure	Systolic ↑ Diastolic ↑ Pulse pressure normal	Systolic ↑ Diastolic ↑ ↓ Pulse pressure ↑	Systolic and diastolic may be normal until marked reduction in stroke volume then ↓ Pulse pressure ↓

Table 23.3 Causes of postoperative hypoventilation

Factors affecting airway	Factors affecting ventilatory drive	Peripheral factors
Upper airway obstruction: Tongue Laryngospasm Oedema Foreign body Tumour Bronchospasm	Respiratory depressant drugs Preoperative CNS pathology Intra- or postoperative cerebrovascular accident Hypothermia Recent hyperventilation (Pa_{CO_2} low)	Muscle weakness: Residual neuromuscular block Preoperative neuromuscular disease Electrolyte abnormalities Pain Abdominal distension Obesity Tight dressings Pneumo-/haemothorax

CNS = Central nervous system; Pa_{CO_2} = arterial carbon dioxide tension.

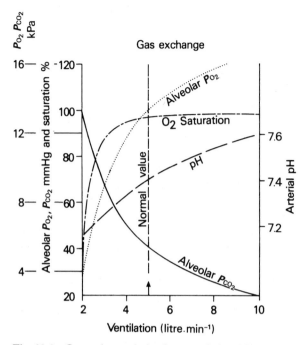

Fig. 23.2 Gas exchange during hypoventilation. Note the relatively rapid increase in alveolar partial pressure of carbon dioxide (P_{CO_2}) compared with the slow decrease in arterial oxygen saturation. P_{O_2} = Partial pressure of oxygen.

extending the head. In some, it is necessary also to insert an oropharyngeal airway, although this may stimulate coughing, gagging and laryngospasm during recovery of consciousness. A nasopharyngeal airway is often tolerated better, but there is a risk of causing haemorrhage from the nasopharyngeal mucosa. Very occasionally, tracheal intubation is necessary to maintain the airway until consciousness has returned fully.

Blood, oral secretions or regurgitated gastric fluid which have accumulated in the pharynx should be aspirated and the patient placed in the recovery position to allow any further fluid to drain anteriorly.

Foreign bodies, such as dentures (particularly partial dentures) or throat packs may cause airway obstruction. It may be difficult to maintain a patent airway in unconscious patients with an oral, pharyngeal or laryngeal tumour.

Obstruction of the upper airway occurs intermittently after recovery from anaesthesia. Obstructive sleep apnoea is common in the postoperative period, and may result in decreases of arterial oxyhaemoglobin saturation (Sa_{O_2}) to less than 75%. Episodes occur with the greatest frequency in the first 4 h after anaesthesia, and are more common and severe in patients who receive opioids for postoperative analgesia than those in whom analgesia is provided by a regional technique.

Airway obstruction may result from haemorrhage after surgery to the neck, including thyroid surgery; the wound should be opened urgently, and the haematoma drained. Occasionally, tracheal collapse occurs after thyroidectomy in patients who have developed chondromalacia of the cartilaginous rings of the trachea caused by pressure from a large goitre. Inspiratory stridor may be present or there may be total obstruction during inspiration; the trachea must be reintubated immediately.

Laryngeal spasm

This complication is relatively common after general anaesthesia. It may be partial or complete, and is usually caused by direct stimulation of the cords by secretions or blood, or of the epiglottis by an oropharyngeal airway. It may follow extubation of the trachea in the semiconscious patient. It may be difficult to differentiate this condition from airway obstruction caused by the pharyngeal wall; if airway obstruction persists despite implementation of the measures described above, laryngoscopy should be undertaken.

Any obvious foreign material causing laryngospasm should be removed by aspiration, and oxygen 100% administered. If obstruction is complete, positive-pressure ventilation by mask may force some oxygen through the cords to maintain arterial oxygenation until the spasm has subsided; there is a significant risk of inflating the stomach with oxygen during this procedure. If attempts to oxygenate the lungs fail, suxamethonium should be administered, and the lungs ventilated with oxygen. When oxygenation has been achieved, it may be advisable to intubate the trachea to reduce the risk of regurgitation of gastric contents, as the stomach may have been inflated with oxygen, and to administer 60–65% nitrous oxide in oxygen to minimize the risk of awareness if the patient regains consciousness before muscle power returns. When the effects of suxamethonium have terminated, oxygen 100% is administered, and the trachea extubated when the patient regains consciousness.

Rarely, laryngeal obstruction occurs after thyroid surgery if both recurrent laryngeal nerves have been traumatized.

Laryngeal oedema

This occasionally occurs after tracheal intubation and may result in severe obstruction, particularly in a child. Treatment depends on the severity of the obstruction; immediate reintubation may be required if obstruction is complete, but partial obstruction may subside if the patient is treated with heated humidified gases. Dexamethasone may hasten resolution of the oedema.

Bronchospasm

This may result from stimulation of the airway by inhaled material. It is commoner in asthmatic or bronchitic patients, and in smokers. It may result directly from intrinsic asthma, or may be part of an anaphylactic reaction. Several drugs used in anaesthetic practice may precipitate bronchospasm either by a direct effect on bronchial muscle or by releasing histamine; these include barbiturates, d-tubocararine, morphine and atracurium. Treatment comprises the removal of any predisposing factor and the administration of oxygen and bronchodilators.

Ventilatory drive

There are several possible causes of reduced ventilatory drive during recovery from anaesthesia (Table 23.3). The presence of intracranial pathology, e.g. tumour, trauma or haemorrhage, may affect ventilatory drive in the postoperative period. Ventilation is reduced in the presence of hypothermia, although it is usually appropriate for the metabolic needs of the body. Hypoventilation occurs in the hypocapnic patient, e.g. after a period of hyperventilation, until Pa_{CO_2} is restored to normal, and in the presence of primary metabolic alkalosis.

The most important cause of reduced ventilatory drive during recovery is the effect of drugs administered by the anaesthetist in the perioperative period. All the volatile and i.v. anaesthetic agents — with the exception of ketamine — depress the respiratory centre; significant concentrations of these drugs remain in the brain stem during the early postoperative period.

All opioid analgesics depress ventilation. With most opioids the effect is dose-dependent, although the agonist–antagonist agents are claimed to have a ceiling effect. In the majority of patients opioids do not produce apnoea, but result in decreased ventilatory drive and an increase in Pa_{CO_2} which plateaus at an elevated value. The elderly are particularly sensitive to drug-induced ventilatory depression. The treatment of postoperative pain begins in the recovery area, often by administration of i.v. opioids by the medical or nursing staff, and ventilation must be carefully monitored after each dose.

Spinal opioids, particularly lipid-insoluble agents such as morphine, may produce ventilatory depression some hours after administration. Patients who have received subarachnoid or extradural opioids should remain in the recovery ward or in a high-dependency unit for at least 12 h after administration of the last dose of spinal morphine, or at least 4 h after fentanyl.

Reduced ventilatory drive is easy to diagnose if the ventilatory rate or tidal volume is clearly reduced. However, lesser degrees of hypoventilation may be difficult to detect, and the signs of moderate hypercapnia, e.g. hypertension and tachycardia, may be masked by the residual effects of anaesthetic agents, or misdiagnosed as pain-induced (Table 23.2).

Mild hypoventilation is acceptable provided that oxygenation remains adequate; this can easily be achieved by a modest increase in fractional concentration of oxygen (F_{IO_2}; see below). If ventilatory drive is reduced excessively by opioids, with an increasing Pa_{CO_2} or delayed recovery of consciousness, naloxone in increments of 1.5–3 $\mu g.kg^{-1}$ should be administered every 2–3 min until improvement occurs. Administration of excessive doses of naloxone reverses the analgesia induced by systemic, but not spinal, opioids; large doses may cause severe hypertension and have been associated with cardiac arrest on rare occasions. The effects of i.v. naloxone only last for

20–30 min; in order to prevent the recurrence of reduced ventilation after long-acting opioids, an additional dose (50% of the effective i.v. dose) may be administered intramuscularly, or an i.v. infusion instituted.

Peripheral factors

The commonest peripheral factor associated with hypoventilation is residual neuromuscular blockade. This may be exaggerated by disease of the neuromuscular junction, e.g. myasthenia gravis, or by electrolyte disturbances. Inadequate reversal of neuromuscular blockade is usually associated with unco-ordinated, jerky movements, although these may occur occasionally during recovery of consciousness in patients with normal neuromuscular function. Measurement of tidal volume is not a reliable guide to adequacy of reversal of neuromuscular blockade; a normal tidal volume may be achieved with only 20% return of diaphragmatic power, but the ability to cough remains severely impaired. If the patient is able to lift the head from the trolley for 5 s or can maintain a good hand-grip, it is likely that there is sufficient return of neuromuscular function for adequate ventilation and maintenance of the airway. Some more objective means of assessment are listed in Table 23.4, but these require the co-operation of the patient. In the unconscious or unco-operative patient, nerve stimulation (see Chapter 11) provides the best means of assessing neuromuscular function, although there are differences among the non-depolarizing relaxants in the relationship between their actions in the forearm and diaphragm.

If residual non-depolarizing blockade is confirmed, further doses of neostigmine may be administered (with atropine or glycopyrronium) up to a total of 5 mg; in higher doses, neostigmine can worsen neuromuscular function. If the block

Table 23.4 Clinical assessment of the adequacy of antagonism of neuromuscular block

Subjective
Grip strength
Adequate cough

Objective
Ability to sustain head lift for at least 5 s
Ability to produce vital capacity of at least 10 ml.kg^{-1}

persists, artificial ventilation must be maintained while the cause is sought.

Factors responsible most commonly for difficulty in antagonism of neuromuscular block include overdosage with muscle relaxant, too short an interval between administration of the drug and the antagonist, hypokalaemia, respiratory or metabolic acidosis, administration of aminoglycoside antibiotics, local anaesthetic agents, diseases affecting neuromuscular transmission and muscle disease.

Delayed elimination of all of the non-depolarizing muscle relaxants (except atracurium) has been reported, and causes prolonged neuromuscular block. Delayed elimination occurs most frequently in the presence of renal or hepatic insufficiency, or in dehydrated patients with low urine output. Muscle paralysis may recur 30–60 min after administration of neostigmine if elimination of the relaxant is inadequate, even if antagonism appears to be satisfactory initially. A similar phenomenon may occur if acidosis develops, or when patients who have been hypothermic are rewarmed.

Prolonged neuromuscular block after suxamethonium or mivacurium occurs in the presence of atypical plasma cholinesterase, or a low concentration of normal plasma cholinesterase. Paralysis after suxamethonium may persist for up to 8 h, although in most instances recovery occurs within 20–120 min. Neostigmine should not be administered if prolonged neuromuscular block occurs after administration of suxamethonium.

Artificial ventilation of the lungs must be maintained or resumed in any patient who has inadequate neuromuscular function. Anaesthesia should be provided to prevent awareness; this is achieved most easily with nitrous oxide and a low concentration of a volatile anaesthetic agent.

Hypoventilation may be caused also by restriction of diaphragmatic movement resulting from abdominal distension, obesity, tight dressings or abdominal binders. Pain, particularly from thoracic or upper abdominal wounds, may cause reduced ventilation.

The presence of air or fluid in the pleural cavity may result in hypoventilation. Pneumothorax may occur during intermittent positive-pressure ventilation (IPPV). It is an occasional complication in healthy patients, but is a particular risk in those with chronic obstructive airways disease, especially if bullae are present, and after chest trauma. It may complicate brachial plexus nerve block, central venous cannulation or surgery of the kidney or neck. Haemothorax may result from chest trauma or central venous cannulation. Hydrothorax may be caused by pleural effusions or inadvertent infusion of fluids through a misplaced central venous catheter. These rapidly remediable causes of hypoventilation are often overlooked.

Treatment

This consists primarily of treatment of the cause. Mild or moderate hypoventilation resulting from residual effects of anaesthetic drugs may respond to a bolus dose or infusion of doxapram. Artificial ventilation should be reinstituted if severe hypercapnia is present or Pa_{CO_2} continues to rise, or if the clinical condition of the patient is deteriorating.

Hypoxaemia

A functional classification of causes of hypoxaemia in the early recovery period is shown in Table 23.5. An inspired oxygen concentration of less than 21% should never occur, although Pa_{O_2} is decreased when air is breathed at high altitudes.

Ventilation–perfusion abnormalities

These are the commonest cause of hypoxaemia in the recovery room. Cardiac output and pulmonary arterial pressure may be reduced after general or regional anaesthesia, causing impaired perfusion of some areas of the lungs. Functional residual capacity (FRC) is reduced during and immediately after anaesthesia, and closing capacity

Table 23.5 Functional classification of the causes of hypoxaemia in the postoperative period

Reduced inspired oxygen concentration

Ventilation–perfusion abnormalities

Shunting

Hypoventilation

Diffusion deficits

Diffusion hypoxia after nitrous oxide anaesthesia

(see p. 13) may encroach on the tidal breathing range, resulting in reduced ventilation of some lung units, particularly those in dependent alveoli. Thus the scatter of ventilation/perfusion ($\dot{V}/\dot{Q}$) ratios is increased. Areas of lung with increased $\dot{V}/\dot{Q}$ ratios constitute physiological dead space; unless there is central depression of ventilation, an increase in dead space is usually followed by an increase in minute volume. Areas of lung with low $\dot{V}/\dot{Q}$ ratios increase venous admixture, which results in hypoxaemia.

Shunt

Physiological shunt may be increased in the immediate postoperative period if small airways closure has been extreme. Shunting may be present also in patients with pulmonary oedema of any aetiology, or if there is consolidation in the lung. More commonly, shunt is increased in the later postoperative period secondary to retention of secretions and underventilation of the lung bases because of pain; these changes lead to alveolar consolidation and collapse.

Hypoventilation

This has been discussed in detail above. Moderate hyperventilation, with some elevation of Pa_{CO_2}, leads to a modest reduction in Pa_{O_2} (Fig. 23.3). Obstructive sleep apnoea may produce profound transient but repeated decreases in arterial oxygenation. Sa_{O_2} may decrease to less than 75%, corresponding to a Pa_{O_2} of less than 5 kPa (40 mmHg). These repeated episodes of hypoxaemia cause temporary, and possibly permanent, defects in cognitive function in elderly patients, and may contribute to perioperative myocardial infarction.

Diffusion defects

Interstitial oedema produced by overtransfusion of fluids or by left ventricular dysfunction may cause hypoxaemia by impairment of oxygen transfer across the alveolar–capillary membrane.

Diffusion hypoxia

Nitrous oxide is 40 times more soluble in blood

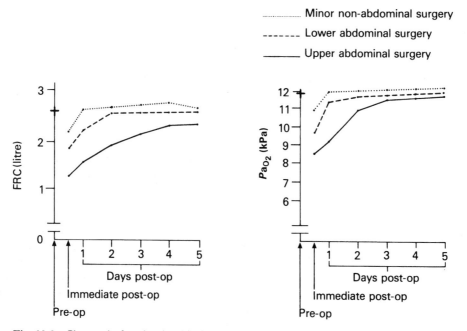

Fig. 23.3   Changes in functional residual capacity (FRC) and arterial oxygen tension (Pa_{O_2}) postoperatively.

than nitrogen. When administration of nitrous oxide is discontinued at the end of anaesthesia, nitrous oxide diffuses out of blood into the alveoli in larger volumes than nitrogen diffuses in the opposite direction. Consequently, the alveolar concentrations of other gases are diluted. Pa_{O_2} is reduced and arterial oxygenation impaired if the patient breathes air; Pa_{O_2} is also reduced, causing hypoventilation. Sa_{O_2} is reduced to values as low as 90% for several minutes in normal individuals after breathing 50% nitrous oxide in oxygen. Arterial desaturation is greater in elderly patients, if higher concentrations of nitrous oxide have been used, or if Pa_{O_2} is initially low because of hyperventilation.

Diffusion hypoxia is avoided by the administration of oxygen for 10 min after discontinuation of nitrous oxide anaesthesia.

Reduced venous oxygen content

Assuming that oxygen consumption remains unchanged, anaemia or reduced cardiac output result in increased oxygen extraction from circulating arterial blood, and consequently a reduction

in mixed venous oxygen content. In the presence of increased ventilation/perfusion scatter or intrapulmonary shunt, this causes a variable degree of arterial hypoxaemia. Similarly, if cardiac output remains constant, increased oxygen utilization by the tissues (as may occur during shivering, restlessness or malignant hyperpyrexia) causes a reduction in mixed venous oxygen content and a worsening of arterial hypoxaemia if any shunt is present.

Tissue hypoxia

Oxygenation of the tissues is a function of arterial oxygenation, oxygen carriage in blood, delivery of blood to the tissues and transfer of oxygen from the blood. It may be impaired by respiratory or cardiovascular dysfunction, by severe anaemia or by a leftward shift of the oxyhaemoglobin dissociation curve (reduced P_{50}).

Pulmonary changes after abdominal surgery

Patients with previously normal lungs suffer impairment of oxygenation for at least 48 h after abdominal surgery. The extent of this impairment is related to the site of operation. It is less marked after lower abdominal surgery and worse after thoraoabdominal procedures, or midline or paramedian incisions in the upper abdomen. In these circumstances, the differences between pre- and postoperative Pa_{O_2} may be as much as 4 kPa.

Impairment of oxygenation in the postoperative period is related to a reduction in FRC. After induction of anaesthesia there is an abrupt decrease in FRC. The magnitude of the decrease is similar for anaesthetic techniques in which the patient breathes spontaneously and those in which IPPV is employed. Postoperatively, this decrease is maintained by wound pain, which causes spasm of the expiratory muscles, and abdominal distension leading to diaphragmatic splinting. This is also influenced by the site of surgical incision; the greatest reduction follows thoracic or upper abdominal surgery. The supine position also reduces FRC.

The reduction in FRC may lead to closing capacity impinging upon the tidal breathing range. This results in small airways closure during normal tidal ventilation. Gas trapping occurs in the affected airways and subsequent absorption of air may lead to the development of small, discrete areas of atelectasis which are not visible radiologically. This occurs mainly in the dependent parts of the lung, and can be demonstrated very soon after induction of anaesthesia. The end-result is an increase in the number of areas of low $\dot{V}/\dot{Q}$ ratio within the lungs. The relationship between changes in FRC and Pa_{O_2} postoperatively is shown in Figure 23.3.

In most patients, these abnormalities return towards normal by the fifth or sixth postoperative day. However, if the changes have been marked, the areas of low $\dot{V}/\dot{Q}$ ratio may become a focus for infection, particularly in the presence of retained secretions. Factors which contribute to the retention of secretions after surgery are:

1. *Inability to cough.* This results mostly from wound pain. However, excessive sedation may contribute also. Postoperative electrolyte imbalance, especially hypokalaemia or hypophosphataemia, may compound the situation by interfering with muscle function.

2. *Suppression of bronchial mucosal ciliary activity.* This results from the use of unhumidified anaesthetic gases.

3. *Antisialagogue drugs.* When antisialagogue premedicants have been used the secretions become more viscid. The dry mucosa itself is more prone to inflammatory reaction. If this occurs, the exudate produced increases the problem still further.

4. *Infection.* If pulmonary infection supervenes, impairment of oxygenation may contribute to a lack of co-operation in clearing secretions.

A combination of these factors may result in retention of secretions, leading to areas of radiologically visible pulmonary collapse, and an increase in the work of breathing. Ultimately, oxygenation of the blood may become inadequate despite oxygen therapy, or carbon dioxide retention may occur. The sequence of events that culminate in ventilatory failure is shown in Figure 23.4.

Predisposing factors

1. *Site of surgery.* Pulmonary complications occur more commonly after upper abdominal or thoracic surgery than after lower abdominal operations.
2. *Pre-existing respiratory disease* increases the complication rate. This is particularly so in the presence of concurrent infection or excessive secretions.
3. *Smokers* have an increased incidence of pulmonary complications compared with non-smokers.
4. *Obesity* is associated with a high incidence of pulmonary complications. Obese patients have a low FRC and increased work of breathing postoperatively.

The anaesthetic technique has little effect on the incidence of postoperative pulmonary complications.

Clinical findings

Collapse of lung units. In patients who develop clinical symptoms, the first signs of atelectasis are usually seen within 24 h of opera-

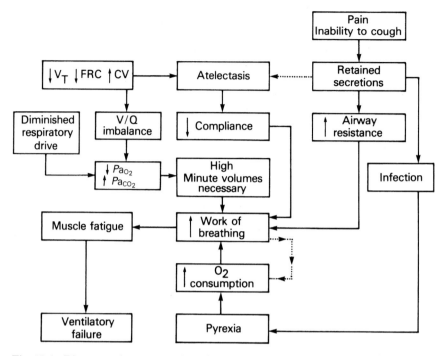

Fig. 23.4 Diagrammatic representation of events that result in postoperative ventilatory failure. V_T = Tidal volume; FRC = functional residual capacity; CV = closing volume; V/Q = ventilation/perfusion; Pa_{O_2} = arterial oxygen tension; Pa_{CO_2} = arterial carbon dioxide tension.

tion. The triad of pyrexia, tachycardia and tachypnoea is often present. Temperature is usually in the range of 38–39°C. There is often a productive cough. If atelectasis is extensive, the patient is cyanosed. On physical examination, localizing signs are uncommon unless the area of involvement is large. Chest X-ray reveals patchy areas of atelectasis.

Pneumonia. Lobar pneumonia is rarely seen postoperatively. Bronchopneumonia is more common, especially in the elderly. The onset of symptoms is not as rapid as in atelectasis. There is usually fever and associated tachycardia with an increase in the ventilatory rate. Physical examination usually reveals areas of consolidation, predominantly at the lung bases, which are evident radiologically.

Treatment

If a pulmonary complication is suspected, a sputum sample should be sent to the laboratory for bacteriological analysis. Appropriate antibiotic

therapy may then be started. Intensive physiotherapy should be prescribed in an attempt to remove secretions and re-expand atelectatic areas of the lung.

Patients with pulmonary collapse are usually hypoxaemic, but Pa_{CO_2} remains normal or may be low as a result of tachypnoea, at least in the early stages. Usually, oxygen in moderate concentrations (30–40%) is sufficient to correct hypoxaemia, but this should be confirmed by blood gas analysis. If the patient fails to respond to these measures, signs of respiratory distress develop. The patient becomes drowsy and ventilation is laboured, with rapid shallow breathing involving the accessory muscles. Pa_{CO_2} increases and arterial oxygenation deteriorates despite oxygen therapy. The presence of continued deterioration in blood gases is an indication for ventilatory support.

Reducing pulmonary complications

Preoperative

Measures to reduce pulmonary complications

should begin preoperatively. Upper and lower respiratory tract infections should be treated before surgery. Dental sepsis and sinus infections should be eradicated. Pre-existing chronic respiratory disorders should be treated so that the patient is in optimal condition before surgery. Spirometry is useful to monitor such treatment, but arterial blood gas analysis is the only assessment which has been demonstrated to correlate well with the need for postoperative ventilatory support. Smoking should be discouraged and weight loss encouraged where indicated. In patients with increased risk factors, heavy premedication should be avoided to ensure minimal ventilatory depression at the end of the procedure.

Intraoperative

At induction, care should be taken not to introduce infection by contaminated equipment. During prolonged procedures, the anaesthetic gases should be humidified. If neuromuscular blocking agents are used, particular care should be taken to ensure that antagonism is adequate.

Postoperative

Analgesia should be optimal to ensure adequate coughing and co-operation during physiotherapy, which should be started as soon as possible after operation.

Oxygen therapy

Hypoxaemia may occur to some degree in *any* patient during the early recovery period as a result of one or more of the mechanisms described above. Consequently, *all* patients should receive additional oxygen for the first 10 min after general anaesthesia has been discontinued. Oxygen therapy should be continued for a longer period in the presence of any of the conditions listed in Table 23.6.

Oxygen therapy is particularly beneficial in treating hypoxaemia caused by hypoventilation; Pa_{O_2} is substantially increased by a modest increase in FI_{O_2}. In contrast, higher concentrations are required in the presence of a shunt fraction in excess of 0.1–0.15 (Fig. 23.5). Known concentra-

Table 23.6 Conditions in which prolonged oxygen therapy is required after operation

Hypotension
Ischaemic heart disease
Reduced cardiac output
Anaemia
Obesity
Shivering
Hypothermia
Hyperthermia
Pulmonary oedema
Airway obstruction
After major surgery

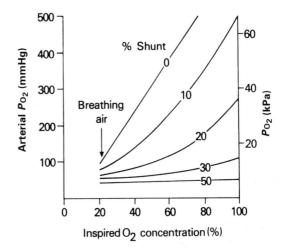

Fig. 23.5 Response of arterial partial pressure of oxygen (Po_2) to increased inspired oxygen concentrations in the presence of various degrees of shunt. Note that arterial Po_2 remains well below the normal value when 100% oxygen is breathed. Nevertheless, useful increases in arterial oxygenation occur with a shunt of up to 30%.

tions of oxygen may be administered by a tightly fitting mask supplied with metered flows of air and oxygen via either an anaesthetic breathing system or a continuous positive airways pressure (CPAP) system (see Chapter 41). In small children, an oxygen tent or headbox may be used. However, oxygen is usually administered by less cumbersome disposable equipment.

Oxygen therapy devices

The characteristics of oxygen face masks depend

predominantly on their volume, the flow rate of gas supplied and the presence of holes in the side of the mask. If no gas is supplied, face masks act as increased dead space and result in hypercapnia unless minute volume is increased; the increase in dead space is proportional to the volume of the mask. If the mask contains holes, air is entrained readily during inspiration.

When oxygen is supplied, the inspired oxygen concentration increases, but to an extent which depends upon the relationship between the oxygen flow rate and the ventilatory pattern. If there is a pause between expiration and inspiration, the mask fills with oxygen and a high concentration is available at the start of inspiration; during inspiration, the inspired oxygen is diluted by air drawn in through the holes when the inspiratory flow rate exceeds the flow rate of oxygen. During normal tidal ventilation, the peak inspiratory flow rate (PIFR) is 20–30 litre.min^{-1}, but is considerably higher during deep inspiration or in the hyperventilating patient. If there is no expiratory pause, alveolar gas may be rebreathed from the mask at the start of inspiration; this occurs especially when the oxygen flow rate is low, or no holes are present in the mask. A predictable and constant inspired oxygen concentration may be achieved only if the total gas flow to the mask exceeds the patient's PIFR.

Fixed-performance devices. These masks, termed also high air flow oxygen enrichment (HAFOE) devices, provide a constant and predictable inspired oxygen concentration irrespective of the patient's ventilatory pattern. This is achieved by supplying the mask with oxygen and air at a high total flow rate. Oxygen is passed through a jet which entrains air (Fig. 23.6). The mask is designed in such a way that the total flow rate of gas to the mask exceeds the expected PIFR of most patients who require oxygen therapy. For example, if a jet designed to supply 28% oxygen is supplied with an oxygen flow rate of 4 litre.min^{-1}, approximately 41 litre.min^{-1} of air is entrained and a total flow of 45 litre.min^{-1} passes to the patient's face.

Various types of HAFOE device are available; some examples are shown in Figure 23.7. Ventimasks are the most accurate, but a different mask is required for each of the range of oxygen concentrations available. Some manufacturers produce masks in which the jet device can be changed by the user, so that the oxygen concentration may be adjusted as appropriate.

The air-entraining jets of HAFOE devices provide a relatively constant oxygen concentration irrespective of the flow rate of oxygen. The recommended oxygen flow rates are larger when jets providing a high concentration are used (e.g. 8 litre.min^{-1} for 40%, 15 litre.min^{-1} for 60%) so that the total flow rate supplied to the mask remains adequate despite the smaller proportion of air entrained. The total flow rates through masks which deliver more than 28% oxygen are between 20 and 30 litre.min^{-1} when the recom-

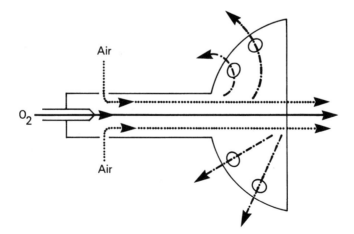

Fig. 23.6 Diagram of high air flow oxygen enrichment (HAFOE) mask (see text for details).

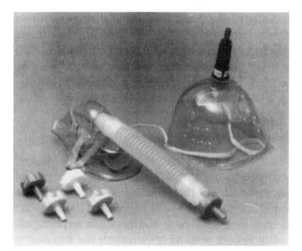

Fig. 23.7 High air flow oxygen enrichment (HAFOE) masks.

Table 23.7 Oxygen masks, flow rates and approximate oxygen concentrations delivered

Type of mask	Oxygen flow (litre.min⁻¹)	Oxygen concentration (%)
Edinburgh	1	24–29
	2	29–36
	4	33–39
Nasal cannulae	1	25–29
	2	29–35
	4	32–39
Hudson	2	24–38
	4	35–45
	6	51–61
	8	57–67
	10	61–73
MC	2	28–50
	4	41–70
	6	53–74
	8	60–77
	10	67–81

mended oxygen flow rates are provided; higher flow rates of oxygen may be used in patients who are thought to have an increased PIFR.

Because of the high fresh gas flow rate, expired gas is rapidly flushed from the mask. Thus, re-breathing does not occur, i.e. fixed-performance devices do not act as an additional dead space.

Variable-performance devices. All other disposable oxygen masks, and nasal cannulae, provide an oxygen concentration which varies with the oxygen flow rate and the patient's ventilatory pattern. Although there is no increase in dead space when nasal cannulae are used, all variable-performance disposable face masks add dead space, the magnitude of which depends on the patient's pattern of ventilation. Table 23.7 gives an indication of the range of oxygen concentrations achieved with a number of commonly used variable-performance devices; some examples are shown in Figure 23.8.

Oxygen therapy in the recovery ward

The large majority of patients recovering after anaesthesia require only a modest increase in $F_{I_{O_2}}$ to overcome the combined effects of mild hypoventilation, diffusion hypoxia and some degree of increased $\dot{V}/\dot{Q}$ scatter. Usually, an inspired concentration of 30% is adequate and this may be achieved in most instances by supplying an oxygen flow rate of 4 litre.min⁻¹ to any of the variable-

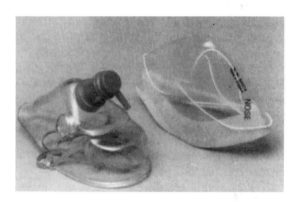

Fig. 23.8 Variable-performance masks.

performance devices (Table 23.7). However, in a small proportion of patients, it is necessary to control the $F_{I_{O_2}}$ more strictly.

Controlled oxygen therapy. This is required in two categories of patient:

1. Some patients with chronic bronchitis develop chronic hypercapnia, and ventilatory drive is largely produced by hypoxaemia. If Pa_{O_2} increases above the level which stimulates breathing, ventilatory depression may occur. However, these patients may become dangerously hypoxaemic after anaesthesia, and oxygen therapy is required so that adequate oxygenation of the tissues is maintained. The aim of oxygen therapy in these

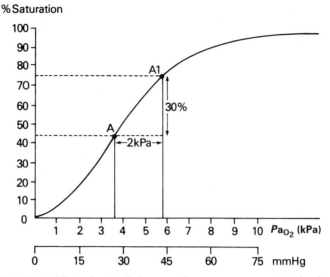

Fig. 23.9   Effect of controlled oxygen therapy on oxygen saturation in a hypoxaemic chronic bronchitic patient. A small increase in inspired oxygen concentration produces a modest increase in arterial oxygen tension (Pa_{O_2}) but a substantial increase in arterial oxygen saturation.

circumstances is to increase arterial oxygen content without an excessive increase in Pa_{O_2}. This is achieved by a modest increase in F_{IO_2}. In the hypoxaemic patient, the relationship between arterial oxygen tension and saturation (and therefore oxygen content) is represented by the steep portion of the oxyhaemoglobin dissociation curve, and a small increase in oxygen tension results in significant increased in saturation and oxygen content (Fig. 23.9).

The use of a variable-performance device in these patients is unsatisfactory, as an unacceptably high F_{IO_2} may be delivered. A fixed-performance device delivering 24% oxygen should be used initially, and the response assessed. If the patient remains clinically well, and the Pa_{CO_2} does not increase by more than 1–1.5 kPa, 28% oxygen, and subsequently higher concentrations, may be administered if further increases in Pa_{O_2} are desirable.

Most patients with chronic bronchitis do not depend on hypoxaemia for respiratory drive, and should not be denied adequate concentrations of oxygen. Patients at risk may usually be detected preoperatively by the presence of central cyanosis; hypoxaemia and hypercapnia are confirmed by blood gas analysis.

2. Patients with increased shunt, e.g. those with acute respiratory distress syndrome (ARDS), pulmonary oedema or pulmonary consolidation, may require a high inspired oxygen concentration (Fig. 23.5), which cannot be guaranteed if a variable-performance device is used. In addition, serial blood gas analysis is used normally to assess improvement or deterioration in their condition. Changes in Pa_{O_2} and the degree of shunt may be interpreted accurately only if the F_{IO_2} is known. Thus, controlled oxygen therapy should be employed, using a fixed-performance device which delivers 40% oxygen or more.

CARDIOVASCULAR SYSTEM

Hypotension

Residual effects of anaesthetic drugs

Hypotension may result from the residual vasodilator effect of i.v. or inhalational anaesthetic drugs, particularly in patients who are experiencing little pain. Subarachnoid or extradural nerve block may also cause hypotension which persists into the postoperative period. Heart rate is seldom elevated, and the peripheries are warm if anaesthetic drugs or regional anaesthesia are the cause of hypotension. A systolic arterial pressure of 80–90 mmHg is tolerated well except by the elderly or patients with myocardial disease. No treatment is required in most patients. Elevation of the legs often increases arterial pressure by increasing venous return. Intravenous infusion of 7–10 ml.kg^{-1} of colloid solution is usually effective in restoring normotension if there is concern; infusion should be undertaken cautiously in elderly patients and in those with cardiovascular disease.

Other causes of hypotension in the recovery period are more sinister, and must be excluded before it may be assumed that residual anaesthesia is responsible.

Hypovolaemia

This may result from inadequate or inappropriate replacement of preoperative or intraoperative fluid and blood losses, or from postoperative haemorrhage. Surgical bleeding may be obvious from inspection of wounds and drains, but may be concealed, particularly in the abdomen, retroperitoneal space or thorax, even when drains are present.

Inadequate surgical haemostasis is the usual cause of postoperative bleeding but coagulation disorders may be present in the following circumstances:

1. After massive blood transfusion, which results in decreased concentrations of clotting factors and reduced platelet numbers.
2. Pre-existing bleeding tendency, e.g. haemophilia.
3. Disseminated intravascular coagulation produced by sepsis, amniotic fluid embolism, etc.
4. If anticoagulant drugs have been administered.

A coagulation disorder is frequently associated with prolonged bleeding after venepuncture, oozing from the wound and the development of petechiae or bruises. The investigation and management of coagulation disorders are discussed in Chapter 6.

Hypotension caused by hypovolaemia is accompanied by signs of poor peripheral perfusion, e.g.

cold, clammy extremities and pallor. Tachycardia may be present but is masked not infrequently by the effects of drugs (e.g. anticholinesterases, β-blockers). CVP may be low or normal. Urine output is reduced (< 30 ml.h^{-1}). The effects of hypovolaemia on arterial pressure are more pronounced in the presence of vasodilatation or reduced myocardial contractility resulting from the effects of residual anaesthetic drugs, or antihypertensive, calcium-channel or β-blocker therapy. In patients who have undergone prolonged surgery, and particularly if the core temperature is below normal, vasoconstriction may be profound and hypovolaemia may be unmasked at a relatively late stage, as normal vasomotor tone returns with rewarming.

Treatment comprises elevation of the legs and administration of appropriate crystalloid or colloid solutions; in elderly or high-risk patients, or if hypovolaemia is profound, administration of fluids should be monitored by measurement of CVP. Clotting factors or platelets should be administered if appropriate, and surgical bleeding treated by reoperation if necessary.

Arrhythmias

These are discussed below.

Ventricular failure

Left or right ventricular failure may cause hypotension. Right ventricular failure is uncommon, and is secondary usually to acute pulmonary disease, e.g. ARDS.

Left ventricular failure in the postoperative period is associated most commonly with perioperative myocardial infarction or overtransfusion. The peripheral circulation is poor. Usually, tachycardia is present, and there is clinical and radiological evidence of pulmonary oedema. Jugular venous pulse and CVP are usually elevated, but they may remain normal despite a substantial increase in left atrial pressure, particularly if right ventricular hypertrophy is present. Thus, left ventricular failure may be misdiagnosed as hypovolaemia in some patients, and in some instances the two conditions coexist. If there is doubt about the diagnosis, a small fluid load may be administered (no more than 200 ml), and the response of arterial pressure and CVP monitored; if the diagnosis remains uncertain, a pulmonary artery catheter should be inserted to measure pulmonary artery and left atrial pressures.

Treatment comprises administration of oxygen, fluid restriction, diuretics and, if necessary, inotropic support or vasodilator therapy. ECG, arterial pressure and CVP should be monitored. The possibility of myocardial infarction should be investigated.

Septic shock

In this condition, hypotension is accompanied by raised cardiac output and peripheral vasodilatation in the early stages, followed by vasoconstriction and reduced cardiac output caused partly by loss of fluid from the circulation. CVP monitoring is essential and a pulmonary artery catheter desirable. Treatment includes infusion of appropriate volumes of colloid, inotropic support, antibiotic therapy and, if necessary, surgical treatment of the source.

Hypertension

Arterial hypertension is a common complication in the early postoperative period. The causes include:

1. Pain.
2. Pre-existing hypertension, particularly if controlled inadequately.
3. Hypoxaemia.
4. Hypercapnia.
5. Administration of vasopressor drugs.
6. After aortic surgery, as a result partly of increased plasma concentration of renin.

A combination of these causes may be present. Hypertension results in increased cardiac work and myocardial oxygen consumption, and may result in myocardial ischaemia or infarction, left ventricular failure or cerebral haemorrhage. The cause should be elicited rapidly and treated if possible. Oxygen should be administered. If no remediable cause is found, vasodilatation with hydralazine, sodium nitroprusside or glyceryl trinitrate should be started. Alternatively, labetalol

may be used, particularly if there is a degree of tachycardia. Such treatment may unmask hypovolaemia (see above) and additional i.v. fluids may be required.

Arrhythmias (see also pp. 657–658)

These are common during and immediately after anaesthesia. The majority are benign and require no treatment. However, the cause should be sought and their effect on the circulation assessed. Common causes include:

1. Residual anaesthetic agents, especially halothane.
2. Hypercapnia.
3. Hypoxaemia.
4. Electrolyte or acid–base disturbance.
5. Vagal stimulation, e.g. by tracheal tube or suction catheters.
6. Myocardial ischaemia or infarction.
7. Pain.

Sinus tachycardia is common, and may be a reflex response to hypovolaemia or hypotension. It also occurs in the presence of hypercapnia, anaemia or hypoxaemia, and if the metabolic rate is elevated by fever, shivering, restlessness or malignant hyperpyrexia. The commonest cause is pain. Tachycardia increases myocardial oxygen consumption, and decreases coronary artery perfusion by reducing diastolic time. The combination of arterial hypertension and tachycardia is dangerous in the presence of ischaemic heart disease and should *not* be allowed to persist as it may result in myocardial infarction. Sinus tachycardia should be treated specifically only if it persists after therapy for underlying causes has been given; a small i.v. dose of a cardioselective β-blocker (e.g. metoprolol 1–2 mg) should be administered slowly. The ECG must be monitored.

Sinus bradycardia may result from inadequate antagonism by atropine of vagal stimulation by neostigmine, pharyngeal stimulation during suction or the residual effects of volatile anaesthetic agents. Other causes include hypoxaemia (especially in neonates and infants), raised intracranial pressure, myocardial infarction and some cardiac drugs, e.g. β-blockers, digoxin. Oxygen should be administered. Intravenous atropine is usually effective, and should be given in a dose of 0.4–0.6 mg in adults if the heart rate is less than 45 beat.min^{-1}, or if there is associated hypotension. In the presence of severe bradycardia, external cardiac massage is necessary to increase cardiac output.

Bradycardia may also occur as a result of complete heart block.

Supraventricular arrhythmias, including atrial fibrillation, flutter or supraventricular tachycardia, are treated as in other circumstances. Rapid arrhythmias are best treated by cardioversion, but may require pharmacological therapy to prevent recurrence. Nodal rhythm with a normal heart rate is common in the perioperative period, particularly when volatile anaesthetic agents have been used. Supraventricular arrhythmias may cause moderate hypotension because of the loss of synchronization between atrial and ventricular contractions.

Ventricular arrhythmias. Premature ventricular contractions (PVCs) may require treatment with i.v. lignocaine 1–1.5 mg.kg^{-1} if they are frequent (< 5 min^{-1}), multifocal or occur close to the preceding T wave; however, most cardiologists regard PVCs as benign if cardiac output is adequate. Ventricular tachycardia requires immediate treatment with lignocaine or cardioversion. The management of ventricular fibrillation and asystole are discussed in Chapter 43.

Conduction defects

In the perioperative period these usually occur in patients with pre-existing heart disease (see pp. 658–659). Heart rate and cardiac output in complete heart block may increase in response to isoprenaline, but electrical pacing should be started as soon as possible. Patients who develop second-degree heart block during anaesthesia or in the recovery ward should be transferred to a coronary care or intensive therapy unit for an appropriate period of observation.

Myocardial ischaemia

This occurs most commonly in patients with pre-existing coronary artery disease, and most often in the presence of hypoxaemia, hypotension,

hypertension or tachycardia. The ECG should be monitored throughout the recovery period in patients known to be at risk, and precipitating factors should be avoided. Angina occurring during the recovery period should be treated by elimination of any predisposing factor and administration of glyceryl trinitrate sublingually or intravenously.

Myocardial infarction

The average incidence of myocardial infarction (MI) is 1–2% in unselected patients over 40 years of age undergoing major non-cardiac surgery. Pre-existing coronary artery disease, and in particular, evidence of a previous MI, result in a higher risk. Mortality in patients who suffer a perioperative MI may be as high as 60%. Perioperative MI occurs most commonly on the third postoperative day, but may happen at any time during or after surgery.

A number of factors which may be detected during preoperative assessment are known to increase the likelihood of perioperative MI. The most important of these is the time interval between surgery and a previous MI. One extensive study of risk factors which might predict major cardiac complications (including, but not exclusively, MI) showed that preoperative evidence of cardiac failure, arrhythmias (of any type) or aortic stenosis, and age were also associated with a high risk. In addition, there is evidence that pre-existing uncontrolled hypertension is associated with increased risk, and that in elderly patients haemodynamic abnormalities detected only by pulmonary artery catheterization (e.g. elevated left atrial pressure) may affect the incidence of MI in the perioperative period. These problems are discussed more fully in Chapter 18.

The incidence of perioperative MI is also related to intraoperative and postoperative factors. The magnitude of surgery is an important determinant; in patients with a history of previous MI, the incidence of perioperative reinfarction associated with major vascular surgery is considerably higher than when surgery is performed outside the thorax and abdomen. In patients with ischaemic heart disease, postoperative MI is more likely if there is evidence of ischaemic changes on ECG during operation. Such changes are associated most commonly with episodes of intraoperative hypotension, hypertension or tachycardia; the last two occur most frequently in response to noxious stimuli, e.g. tracheal intubation, surgical incision. The drugs used, and the manner in which they are employed by the anaesthetist, influence the incidences of both intraoperative ischaemia and perioperative MI. Regional anaesthesia is not associated with a reduction in risk when major surgery is undertaken.

Reduction of risk

The incidence of perioperative MI may be reduced by:

1. *Identification of patients at risk*. Elective surgery should be postponed if possible until at least 3 months after a previous MI.
2. *Treatment of risk factors*. Cardiac failure, hypertension and arrhythmias should be controlled before surgery. If necessary, the operation should be postponed until control is achieved. Coronary artery bypass grafting or aortic valve replacement may be required in patients with severe coronary artery disease or aortic stenosis respectively, before other major abdominal or thoracic surgery is undertaken.
3. *Avoidance of ischaemia*. The anaesthetic technique and postoperative management should ensure adequate oxygenation of the myocardium and should minimize myocardial oxygen demand (see Chapter 40).
4. *Monitoring*. ECG must be monitored throughout anaesthesia, including induction, in all patients at risk; the CM5 electrode configuration (see Fig. 20.3) is suitable for detection of ischaemic changes. Arterial pressure should be monitored regularly, and continuously in patients undergoing major surgery. Monitoring of right and left atrial pressures by central venous and pulmonary artery catheterization, and prompt treatment of abnormalities which occur during operation and in the first 72 h postoperatively, reduce substantially the incidence of perioperative MI.

Diagnosis

Perioperative MI may be difficult to diagnose. It occurs most commonly on the third postoperative day. The classical distribution of pain is present in only 25% of patients.

The diagnosis should be considered in any patient at risk who develops an arrhythmia or becomes hypotensive in the postoperative period. Premature ventricular contractions occur in 90% of patients who experience an MI; sinus bradycardia and the development of any degree of atrioventricular conduction defect are also common. There is often a pyrexia of up to 39°C. The diagnosis is confirmed by changes in serial ECG recordings and/or cardiac enzymes.

OTHER MAJOR POSTOPERATIVE COMPLICATIONS

Deep venous thrombosis (DVT)

The main factors postulated by Virchow as contributing to the formation of venous thrombi are:

1. Changes in the composition of blood.
2. Damage to walls of blood vessels.
3. Decreased blood flow.

However, the exact trigger mechanism which initiates thrombosis remains unknown.

Risk factors

A higher incidence of DVT has been reported in patients with:

1. Extensive trauma.
2. Infection.
3. Heart failure.
4. Blood dyscrasias.
5. Malignancy.
6. Metabolic disorders.

DVT is commoner after hip, pelvic and abdominal surgery than other types of surgery. There is a well-established association between spontaneous DVT and oestrogen, and DVT may occur in women who take the oral contraceptive pill. The number of women who develop this complication is small. However, the incidence increases if surgery is performed while the patient is currently taking the drug. The risk is reduced but not abolished if a low-oestrogen (50 μg or less) preparation is used. There is no evidence of increased risk among post-menopausal women who take hormone replacement therapy.

Diagnosis

Approximately 70% of patients with a DVT have neither symptoms nor signs. Fifty per cent of patients with calf pain and tenderness on dorsiflexion of the foot do not have a DVT. Often there is mild pyrexia.

Investigations

Venography. This is an effective method for demonstrating most thrombi of clinical importance.

Radioactive fibrinogen uptake. Iodine-labelled fibrinogen is taken up preferentially by a growing thrombus. The investigation is quick to perform and may detect small thrombi in the calf vessels. Its main disadvantage is that it cannot be used to detect iliac and pelvic vein thrombi, although most thrombi in surgical patients occur in the calf. It does not correlate well with either venography or the development of pulmonary embolism and is associated with a high incidence of false-positive results.

Ultrasonography. This is non-invasive and simple to perform. However, it is insensitive and is useful only for confirming the diagnosis of a major thrombus.

Prophylaxis

Elimination of stasis. The efficacy of early ambulation after operation in reducing the incidence of DVT is not clear. Attempts directed at preventing stasis, including physiotherapy, elastic stockings and elevation of the feet, may reduce the incidence of DVT but have not been shown to influence the incidence of pulmonary embolism.

Two methods are currently used for increasing venous return from the lower limbs during surgery:

1. *Electrical stimulation of the calf muscles.* A low-voltage current is applied across the calf to contract the muscles every 2–4 s.

2. *Pneumatic compression of the calves.* The legs are encased in an envelope of plastic material, which is inflated and deflated rhythmically, thus squeezing the calves intermittently. This technique may be continued postoperatively.

Although the incidence of DVT is substantially reduced by these techniques, there is no reduction in the incidence of, or mortality from, pulmonary embolism.

Alteration of blood coagulability

Platelet aggregation. Various drugs which interfere with different aspects of platelet function have been investigated. These include dextran 70, dipyridamole, aspirin and chloroquine. There is no evidence to suggest that dipyridamole or aspirin prevents DVT. Infusion of dextran during and after surgery may reduce the incidence of fatal postoperative pulmonary embolism but its role in the prevention of peripheral venous thrombosis is undetermined.

The coagulation mechanism. Oral anticoagulant instituted before operation is the only well-substantiated method of reducing venous thrombosis. However, there is a risk of increased surgical haemorrhage. Low-dose heparin, 5000 units subcutaneously 2 h before operation and subsequently at 8- or 12-h intervals until the patient is mobile, is the most promising regimen for prevention of DVT and carries little risk of major haemorrhage. If DVT does occur, it is more likely to be confined to the calf if heparin has been given. Subcutaneous heparin reduces the incidence of fatal pulmonary embolism. There is evidence that low-molecular-weight-heparins (dalteparin, enoxaparin and tinzaparin) are more effective antithrombotics than standard heparin in orthopaedic surgery, and that they are as effective and safe in other types of surgery. They have a longer duration of action, and are therefore more convenient.

Pulmonary embolism

This term covers a range of events from sudden circulatory collapse and death, through minor episodes of pleurisy and haemoptysis, to the long-standing disability of patients with chronic thromboembolic pulmonary hypertension. The acute forms of pulmonary embolism are encountered after anaesthesia and surgery. In the elderly, multiple small pulmonary emboli may be mis-diagnosed as bronchopneumonia.

The common sites of origin for thrombi which result in pulmonary embolus are the veins of the pelvis and lower extremities. The most common time for presentation of a postoperative pulmonary embolism is during the second week. In some patients, predisposing factors may have existed preoperatively for some time, and the whole time-scale of events may be shifted; the embolus may occur at the time of, or shortly after, surgery.

Diagnosis

Presenting features. The principal features are circulatory collapse and sudden dyspnoea, often associated with chest pain. If the embolus is large, the pulmonary artery outflow is blocked and sudden death results. If the embolus involves more than 50% of the main pulmonary arteries, it is termed massive.

Physical signs. A low cardiac output state develops. Tachypnoea and central cyanosis are usual. There is arterial hypotension, sinus tachycardia and constricted peripheral circulation. The jugular venous pressure is elevated. A fourth heart sound is usually present on auscultation.

Investigations

ECG (Fig. 23.10). This reflects acute right ventricular strain, with features that often include right axis deviation, T-wave inversion in leads V1–V4 and sometimes right bundle branch block. The classical S1–Q3–T3 pattern is less common.

Chest X-ray. This is often unremarkable but may show areas of oligaemia reflecting pulmonary vascular obstruction.

Arterial blood gases. There is usually hypoxaemia because of ventilation–perfusion imbalance, and hypocapnia resulting from hyperventilation.

Perfusion and ventilation lung scans. The perfusion scan shows uneven circulation, with perfusion defects delineating the emboli. A simultaneous ventilation scan is usually normal.

Pulmonary angiography. This provides a definitive diagnosis of major obstruction in the pulmonary circulation. This investigation is particularly useful if the patient is critically ill and the diagnosis is in doubt, and is essential if pulmonary embolectomy is planned. However, it is invasive and normally requires transfer of the patient to the X-ray department.

Treatment

DVT. The mainstay of therapy is anticoagulation. Initially, i.v. heparin is infused in a dose of 40 000 units per day. At the same time, oral anticoagulant therapy is started. Warfarin is used most commonly. Heparin may be discontinued after 48 h. Oral anticoagulants are continued for at least 3 months.

Pulmonary embolism. Immediate treatment consists of administration of oxygen in a high concentration and i.v. heparin. Digoxin is often

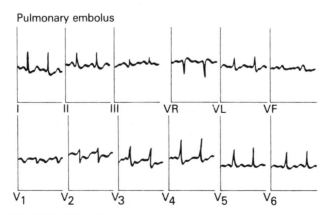

Fig. 23.10   Typical electrocardiogram changes in pulmonary embolism.

useful. Sometimes it is necessary to use additional inotropic support for the circulation. Heparin is continued for 5–6 days. Oral anticoagulant therapy is started as soon as possible and is continued for at least 6 months.

Massive pulmonary embolus which does not respond to the above measures may warrant the use of thrombolytic agents, e.g. streptokinase. The risk of haemorrhage with these agents is considerably higher than with heparin. If the cardiovascular effects of the embolism are life-threatening, open pulmonary embolectomy under cardiopulmonary bypass may be considered.

Postoperative renal dysfunction

The kidney is vulnerable to a wide range of drugs and chemicals. It is particularly susceptible to toxic substances for the following reasons:

1. Large blood flow per unit mass.
2. High oxygen consumption.
3. Non-resorbable substances concentrated by tubules.
4. Permeability of tubular cells.

All anaesthetic techniques depress renal blood flow and, secondary to this, interfere with renal function. Provided that prolonged hypotension is avoided, the effects are temporary. However, there is the potential for some anaesthetic agents to produce permanent renal damage.

Methoxyflurane

The administration of this volatile anaesthetic agent was associated with a relatively high incidence of renal dysfunction. Clinically, the defect was characterized by failure of the concentrating ability of the kidney. In certain instances this progressed to high-output renal failure. The nephrotoxicity of methoxyflurane was dose-dependent, and was caused by inorganic fluoride ions produced during its metabolism. Administration of methoxyflurane in combination with other nephrotoxic drugs, e.g. aminoglycosides, was particularly hazardous.

Large quantities of fluoride ion are also produced during metabolism of enflurane and sevoflurane, although a much smaller proportion of these drugs (2–3%) is metabolized in comparison to methoxyflurane (45%). Concentrations of fluoride ion in blood following administration of sevoflurane may exceed the value associated with renal impairment after anaesthesia with methoxyflurane. However, there has been no evidence to suggest that either enflurane or sevoflurane is associated with renal impairment related to the production of fluoride ions. The reason is probably related to the fact that the very soluble methoxyflurane continued to be metabolized for some days, resulting in prolonged production of fluoride ions, whereas the peak concentrations associated with the use of enflurane and sevoflurane are of short duration because of their relative insolubility in tissues.

Postoperative hepatic dysfunction

There are many causes of postoperative hepatic dysfunction (Table 23.8). Most patients show no evidence of hepatic damage after anaesthesia and surgery. If it occurs, it is usually attributable to one of the causes shown in Table 23.8. However, if other causes are excluded, consideration should be given to the possibility of hepatotoxicity from anaesthetic drugs.

Table 23.8 Causes of postoperative hepatic dysfunction

Increased bilirubin load	Hepatocellular damage	Extrahepatic biliary obstruction
Blood transfusion	Pre-existing liver disease	Gallstones
Haemolysis and haemolytic disease	Viral hepatitis	Ascending cholangitis
Abnormalities of bilirubin metabolism	Sepsis	Pancreatitis
	Hypotension/hypoxia	Surgical misadventure
	Drug-induced hepatitis	
	Congestive heart failure	

Chloroform was the first anaesthetic agent to be suspected of causing hepatic damage. In large doses, chloroform is a direct hepatotoxin, and after anaesthesia a hepatitis-like syndrome, with histological evidence of centrilobular hepatic necrosis, occurred occasionally. Methoxyflurane was also associated with hepatic damage, causing a syndrome clinically similar to viral hepatitis. Two of the volatile agents in current use have been implicated in cases of postoperative hepatic dysfunction.

Halothane

Attention was focused first on halothane-associated hepatitis in the early 1960s. Numerous case reports prompted institution in 1969 of the largest retrospective anaesthetic study ever undertaken (United States National Halothane Study). The incidence and causes of fatal hepatic necrosis occurring within 6 days of anaesthesia were reviewed. The overall incidence was 1 in 10 000; that associated with halothane was 1 in 35 000, and was no greater than the incidence associated with other anaesthetic agents. However, it is believed at present that there is a small number of patients who develop postanaesthetic jaundice in which halothane is the aetiological agent.

The histological picture of halothane-associated hepatitis is similar to that seen in type-A viral hepatitis. Clinically, there is hepatocellular jaundice, with elevation of the aminotransferase enzymes. The exact mechanism of liver damage is not known. At present, there are two main hypotheses:

1. Metabolites of reductive halothane metabolism bind covalently to hepatocyte macromolecules, causing hepatocellular damage.
2. Halothane or its metabolites react with hepatocyte proteins to form antigenic compounds, against which the body mounts an immune response that results in hepatocellular damage.

Antibodies to halothane have been demonstrated in patients who have suffered hepatic damage after administration of the drug. At present, this is the most promising method for evaluating the aetiology of a condition which has been a source of great controversy in recent years.

The following groups of patients are believed to be at the greatest risk of developing hepatic dysfunction after halothane anaesthesia:

1. Patients subjected to repeated halothane anaesthetics, especially within a 3-month period.
2. Patients who have developed unexplained pyrexia or jaundice after a previous halothane anaesthetic
3. Obese patients, particularly women.

Enflurane

A number of causes of unexplained jaundice have been reported after the use of enflurane.

OTHER COMPLICATIONS (Table 23.9)

Local vascular complications

Haematoma formation is probably the commonest complication of i.v. injection. This usually results from inadequate pressure at the injection site after removal of the needle. Phlebitis, thrombosis or thrombophlebitis may occur after the use of some i.v. induction agents. Etomidate, propanidid and methohexitone are probably the most troublesome, although some studies have shown little difference between the various in-

Table 23.9 Minor morbidity resulting from anaesthesia

Nausea and vomiting
  Related to operation site
  Females > males
Sore throat
  Up to 70% of patients
Hoarseness
Laryngeal granulomata
Headache
  Up to 60% of patients
Backache
Discomfort from catheters, drains, nasogastric tubes
Anxiety
Muscle pains
  Up to 100% of those who receive suxamethonium
Shivering
Drowsiness
Anorexia
Disorientation
Thrombophlebitis at injection site
Bruised or cut lip
Chipped teeth
Corneal abrasions

duction agents. Intravenous diazepam is a potent cause of phlebitis, although the formulation of diazepam in a fat emulsion (Diazemuls) has overcome this problem.

Intravenous infusions commonly cause thrombophlebitis. The incidence is related to the duration of infusion, and this is more important than the type of cannula used. Thrombophlebitis is rare if the infusion site is changed every 12 h. If it is changed every 72 h, the incidence of thrombophlebitis is 70%. Cannulae constructed from polytetrafluorethylene (Teflon) appear to be the least thrombogenic of those available.

Arterial cannulation is commonly performed to permit continuous monitoring of systemic arterial pressure during major surgery. Unfortunately, it is not without adverse sequelae. Intimal damage may lead to thrombosis and occasionally aneurysm formation. Recannulation of the vessel generally occurs, even when the vessel has been completely occluded. Nevertheless, gangrene of the extremities is an occasional complication, particularly if the brachial artery is used rather than the radial. Ischaemia of the hand or fingers may occur after radial artery cannulation if there is inadequate collateral circulation.

It has been suggested that a modified Allen's test should be performed to assess the adequacy of the collateral circulation through the ulnar artery before radial artery cannulation. The patient is asked to clench the fist, and radial and ulnar arteries are compressed by the examiner. The patient is subsequently instructed to unclench the fist; the examiner releases the ulnar artery and observes the palm of the hand. If there is adequate collateral flow, prompt return of colour to the palm is seen; if there is little or no return of colour within 15 s, the collateral flow is poor. However, there is some doubt about the relationship between the results of Allen's test and the incidence of ischaemic episodes after radial artery cannulation.

The incidence of thrombosis after arterial cannulation is reduced by the use of a cannula made of Teflon and of a diameter that is small relative to the size of the artery. A 20-gauge cannula is appropriate in the adult, and a 22- or 24-gauge in children. Arterial damage is also reduced by avoiding multiple punctures of the artery during cannulation. The incidence of radial artery thrombosis is highest in the presence of sepsis, low cardiac output states and when the duration of cannulation is prolonged beyond 24 h.

Nausea and vomiting

Although often regarded by medical and nursing staff as only a minor complication of anaesthesia and surgery, nausea and vomiting are frequently the cause of great distress to patients. In severe cases, fluid and electrolyte imbalance may result. In some circumstances, e.g. after intraocular surgery, vomiting may prejudice the result of the operation.

Many studies have been undertaken to investigate nausea and vomiting after anaesthesia and surgery. The incidence varies from 14 to 82%, the wide range resulting partly from differences in design of studies. Several factors contribute to the aetiology of postoperative nausea and vomiting:

1. *The patient.* Some individuals are particularly susceptible to sickness after the most minor events. Those who are prone to motion sickness are more likely to vomit postoperatively. Women are more likely to vomit than men, and children more so than adults.

2. *Perioperative drugs.* All the opioids possess marked emetic properties. The use of an anticholinergic, especially hyoscine, for premedication reduces the incidence of postoperative vomiting caused by opioids.

3. *Anaesthetic agents.* Ether, cyclopropane and trichloroethylene were associated with high incidences of postoperative vomiting. However, there is little difference in this respect between the volatile anaesthetics used currently, or between techniques in which the patient breathes spontaneously compared with those in which a relaxant and IPPV are used. Propofol appears to have specific antiemetic properties.

4. *Site of operation.* Vomiting is more likely after abdominal procedures than those in most other areas. Middle-ear surgery is associated with a high incidence of vomiting, presumably because of the proximity of the vestibular apparatus. Surgery for correction of strabismus is associated with more vomiting than other ocular procedures. Dilatation of the cervix may also cause postoperative emesis.

5. *Other factors.* The duration of surgery is related to the incidence of postoperative vomiting. Gastric dilatation, e.g. caused by inflation of the stomach with anaesthetic gases, may result in emesis in the postoperative period. Intraoperative or postoperative hypoxaemia may cause vomiting. Hypotension during regional anaesthesia induces vomiting, as does the administration of ergometrine, e.g. during Caesarean section. Premature resumption of oral fluids may make emesis worse.

Prevention and treatment

The incidence of postoperative vomiting may be reduced by careful selection of drugs in the perioperative period, and the prophylactic use of antiemetic agents (see Chapter 13).

Headache

The reported incidence of severe headache after anaesthesia and surgery ranges from 12 to 35%, but up to 60% of patients complain of some headache. Individuals who are susceptible to headaches caused by stress, etc. are more likely to complain of postoperative headache. Most investigations have failed to identify any single agent as being responsible for postoperative headache.

Sore throat

Up to 80% of patients complain of sore throat after anaesthesia and surgery. Some of the common causes include:

1. *Trauma during tracheal intubation.* Damage to the pharynx and tonsillar fauces may be caused by the laryngoscope blade.
2. *Trauma to the larynx.* This is more likely if a red rubber tracheal tube is used rather than a plastic disposable tube. A poorly stabilized tube causes more frictional damage to the larynx than one which is securely stabilized
3. *Trauma to the pharynx.* This may occur during passage of a nasogastric tube or insertion of an oropharyngeal airway, and is particularly common when a throat pack has been used. Sore throat is likely if a nasogastric tube remains in situ during the postoperative period.

4. *Other factors.* The mucous membranes of the mouth, pharynx and upper airway are sensitive to the effects of unhumidified gases; the drying effect of anaesthetic gases may cause postoperative sore throat. The antisialagogue effect of anticholinergic drugs may also contribute to this symptom.

The use of topical local anaesthetics does not reduce the incidence of sore throat. Lubrication of the tracheal tube is effective in reducing the incidence, although there is no difference in this respect between plain or local anaesthetic jellies. However, there is little difference in the incidence of sore throat between an anaesthetic technique in which tracheal intubation is employed and one in which only an oropharyngeal airway is used.

In the absence of a nasogastric tube, postoperative sore throat is usually of short duration; most patients are symptom-free within 48 h.

Hoarseness

This should not be confused with sore throat. It is almost always associated with tracheal intubation, and is caused predominantly by prolonged abduction of, and pressure on, the vocal cords.

Laryngeal granulomata

These may occur after tracheal intubation, and arise from areas of ulceration, usually on the posterior aspect of the vocal cords. The ulcers are caused by pressure and consequent ischaemia. Granulomata are reported most frequently after thyroidectomy.

If hoarseness persists for longer than 1 week, indirect laryngoscopy should be performed. If ulceration is present, complete voice rest is indicated. Any granulomata present should be excised; untreated granulomata may grow to such a size as to obstruct the airway.

Dental trauma

This is the commonest cause of litigation against anaesthetists. Damage usually occurs during laryngoscopy, especially if tracheal intubation is difficult. Loose teeth, crowns, caps and bridges are particularly susceptible to damage. Preoperative enquiry and examination should alert the anaesthetist to the possibility of damage.

Ocular complications

Carelessness is the commonest cause of damage to the eyes; corneal abrasion is the most frequent lesion. The eyes are often allowed to remain open during anaesthesia. The cornea is thus exposed and vulnerable to the irritant effects of skin preparations, dust and surgical drapes. This type of damage is easily prevented by securing the eyelids in a closed position with adhesive tape.

Retinal infarction has occurred on rare occasions as a result of pressure on the eyeball from a face mask. It can also occur if patients are placed in the prone position in such a way that pressure is exerted on the eye, e.g. by a horseshoe head-rest.

Muscles

Problems associated with inadequate reversal of neuromuscular blocking drugs have been discussed above. The detection and treatment of malignant hyperpyrexia are described in Chapter 22; it is important to appreciate that this condition may present during recovery.

Shivering

This is a common complication in the recovery room. It may occur in patients who are hypothermic as a result of prolonged surgery and during injection of local anaesthetic solution into the extradural space. However, in most patients, the onset of shivering is not related to body temperature, and there is evidence from electromyography that the characteristics of postoperative (or postanaesthetic) shivering differ from those of thermoregulatory shivering. The incidence and severity of shivering are increased in patients who have received an anticholinergic premedication, and women are more likely to shiver in the luteal than the follicular phase of the menstrual cycle.

Shivering increases oxygen consumption and carbon dioxide production, and may result in hypoxaemia and hypercapnia if the response of the respiratory centre to carbon dioxide is impaired by drugs. Oxygen should be administered. A small dose of pethidine is frequently effective in aborting postoperative shivering.

Suxamethonium pains

Muscle pains after suxamethonium are very common, occurring in at least 50% of patients who receive the drug. The muscles involved most frequently are those of the shoulder girdle, neck and thorax. The pain is similar in nature to that caused by viral-related myositis. The incidence is influenced by the following factors:

1. *Age*. Suxamethonium pains are unusual in young children and the elderly.
2. *Gender*. Women are more susceptible than men. The incidence is reduced during pregnancy.
3. *Type of surgery*. There is an increased incidence after minor procedures, when early ambulation is likely.
4. *Physical fitness*. The incidence is higher in individuals who are physically fit.
5. *Repeated doses*. The incidence is increased if repeated doses of suxamethonium are administered.

The exact cause of muscle pains after suxamethonium is unknown, although it is thought that fasciculations produced by depolarization of the motor nerve end-plate are involved in the pathogenesis. However, the visible extent of fasciculations does not correlate with the severity of subsequent pain. Myoglobinuria occurs after administration of suxamethonium, demonstrating that muscle cell injury does occur.

After minor surgery, the patient may be disturbed by the muscle pains to a greater extent than the discomfort caused by the operative procedure.

It is possible to reduce, but not to eliminate, the incidence of suxamethonium pains by pretreatment with one of the following agents:

1. A small dose of non-depolarizing muscle relaxant (usually 10% of the normal dose) 2–3 min before induction of anaesthesia.
2. A small dose of suxamethonium (0.1 mg.kg^{-1}).

3. Lignocaine 1 mg.kg^{-1}.
4. Diazepam 0.15 mg.kg^{-1} i.v. before induction of anaesthesia.
5. Dantrolene 2 h preoperatively.

Surgical considerations

During the recovery period, a number of surgical complications may occur. These include haemorrhage, blockage of drains or catheters and soiling of dressings. Prosthetic arterial grafts may block, resulting in ischaemia of the limbs. Recovery ward nurses and anaesthetists must be aware of potential surgical complications, as rapid surgical intervention may be required.

The recovery period may also be used to institute orthopaedic traction before the patient returns to the ward.

FURTHER READING

Frost E A M 1996 Postanaesthesia care. In: Aitkenhead A R, Jones R M (eds) Clinical Anaesthesia. Churchill Livingstone, Edinburgh, pp. 619–635

Frost E A M, Goldiner P L 1990 Postanesthetic care. Appleton & Lange, Norwalk

Hindmarch I, Jones J G, Moss E (eds) 1987 Aspects of recovery from anaesthesia. Wiley, Chichester

24. Postoperative pain

Pain is an extraordinarily complex sensation which is difficult to define and equally difficult to measure in an accurate objective manner. It has been defined as the sensory appreciation of afferent nociceptive stimulation which elicits an affective (or autonomic) component; both are subjected to rational interpretation by the patient. It may be represented as a Venn diagram (Fig. 24.1), the shaded area of which represents the quantum of suffering experienced by the patient. The advantage of describing pain by means of the Venn diagram is that it may be seen instantly that the sensation of pain differs among individual patients; the emotional component may vary according to the patient's psychological composition and the rational component varies with the patient's previous experience, insight and motivation.

Postoperative pain differs from other types of pain in that it is usually transitory, with progressive

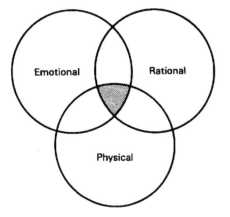

Fig. 24.1 The interrelationship between emotional, rational and physical components of pain. Perceived pain is represented by the area of intersection of all three components.

improvement over a relatively short time-course. Typically, the affective component tends towards an anxiety state associated with diagnosis of the condition and fear of delay in provision of analgesic therapy by attendants. In contrast, chronic pain is persistent, frequently with fluctuating intensity, and the affective component contains a greater depressive element. Thus, acute pain is more easily amenable to therapy than chronic pain.

The traditional management of postoperative pain comprises the prescription of a standard dose of an opioid, to be given i.m. on demand by a nurse when the patient's pain threshold has been exceeded. This leads to poor control of postoperative pain for the following reasons:

1. Responsibility for management of pain is delegated to the nursing staff who err on the side of caution in the administration of opioids. They tend to give too small a dose of drug too infrequently because of fears of producing ventilatory depression or addiction.

2. Because the administration of drugs is left entirely to the discretion of the nursing staff, the degree of empathy between nurse and patient affects analgesic administration. This explains the common observation that the mean dosage of morphine given for a standard operation varies among hospitals and even among wards in the same hospital.

3. Because the measurement of pain is difficult, it is seldom possible to adjust the dosage of drug to match the extent of pain.

4. There are enormous variations in the extent of analgesic requirements depending upon the type of surgery, pharmacokinetic variability, pharmacodynamic variability, etc.

Causes of variation in analgesic requirements

Using patient-controlled analgesic apparatus (see below), it has been shown that there is marked interindividual variation in analgesic requirements. Thus after cholecystectomy some patients may require no morphine within the first 24 h, whereas others may require as much as 120 mg. Unfortunately, there is no way of predicting in advance the extent of opioid requirements of an individual patient. In clinical practice, requirements are assessed on a trial-and-error basis; anaesthetists are therefore in an ideal position to be involved in prescribing postoperative analgesia, as they obtain a 'feel' for dose requirements during management of anaesthesia.

Site and type of surgery

In general, upper abdominal surgery produces greater pain than lower abdominal surgery, which in turn is associated with greater pain than peripheral surgery. This generalization is not entirely accurate; operations on the richly innervated digits may be associated with quite severe pain.

The type of pain may differ with different types of surgery. Operations on joints are associated with sharp pain; in contrast, abdominal surgery is associated with two types of pain: a continuous dull nauseating ache (which responds well to morphine) and sharper pain induced by coughing and movement (which responds poorly to morphine). Pain associated with surgery on the digits may respond relatively poorly to opioids but well to non-steroidal anti-inflammatory drugs.

Table 24.1 provides an approximate guide to the duration and severity of postoperative pain.

Age, gender and body weight

The analgesic requirements of males and females are identical for similar types of surgery. However, there is a reduction in analgesic requirements with advancing age. Consequently, it is essential that the anaesthetist reduces the dosage of opioid drugs in elderly patients.

The established anaesthetic practice of prescribing the potent opioid drugs on a mg or µg

Table 24.1 Duration and severity of postoperative pain

Site of operation	Duration of opioid use (h)	Severity of pain (0–4)
Abdominal:		
upper	48–72	3
lower	up to 48	2
inguinal	up to 36	1
Thoracotomy	72–96	4
Limbs	24–36	2
Faciomaxillary	up to 48	2
Body wall	up to 24	1
Perineal	24–48	2
Hip surgery	up to 48	2

per body weight basis lacks scientific validity. There is no evidence to suggest that variations in body weight in the adult population affect opioid requirements.

Psychological factors (Table 24.2)

The patient's personality affects pain perception and response to analgesic drugs. Thus, patients with a low anxiety and low neuroticism score on a personality scale exhibit less postoperative pain and require smaller doses of opioid than patients who rate highly on these scales. Patients with high scores may exhibit a higher incidence of postoperative chest complications.

The extent of a patient's anxiety also affects pain perception; increased anxiety results in a greater degree of perceived postoperative pain and increased opioid requirements.

These psychological factors help to explain the efficacy of preoperative psychotherapy. Anxiety and postoperative analgesic requirements are re-

Table 24.2 Psychological factors which influence postoperative analgesic requirements

Personality
– more pain if high neuroticism/extraversion
Social background
Culture
Motivation
Preoperative psychotherapy

duced if the preoperative visit by the anaesthetist includes an explanation of forthcoming perioperative events and details regarding the provision of pain relief.

Pharmacokinetic variability

After the intramuscular injection of an opioid, there is a three- to seven-fold difference between patients in the rate at which peak plasma concentrations of the drug occur and a two- to five-fold difference in the peak plasma concentration achieved. This is illustrated in Figure 24.2, which shows the mean change in plasma concentration after the first and second, and seventh and eighth injections. The variability in the plasma concentration is reflected by the large standard deviation of the mean. In addition, average concentrations increase after each of the first few injections; oscillation around a steady mean concentration does

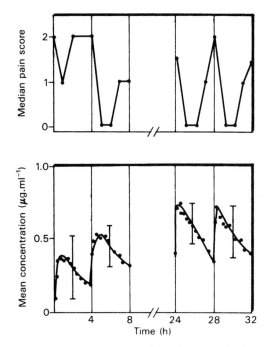

Fig. 24.2 Blood concentrations of pethidine and pain score after surgery; a pain score of 0 indicates no pain. Doses of pethidine 100 mg have been given 4-hourly. Mean blood concentration of pethidine continues to rise for 24 h before a plateau is reached. Little pain relief is provided by the first dose. Even after 24 h, significant pain is present 3 and 4 h after each injection, as blood concentrations decline.

not occur until after approximately the fourth injection.

This pharmacokinetic variability helps to explain the relatively poor response to a single intramuscular injection given in the postoperative period.

Pharmacodynamic variability

Although there are widespread pharmacokinetic variations between patients in response to administration of opioids, the major reason for variation in opioid sensitivity is pharmacodynamic, i.e. a difference in the inherent sensitivity of opioid receptors.

Using continuous infusions of opioids to achieve equilibrium between receptor drug concentration and plasma concentration, it is possible to define a steady-state plasma concentration of opioid at which analgesia is produced. This is termed the minimum effective analgesic concentration (MEAC); values of MEAC for the commonly available opioids are shown in Table 24.3. MEAC levels vary four- to five-fold between individual patients and are affected by age and differences in psychological profile.

METHODS OF TREATING POSTOPERATIVE PAIN (Table 24.4)

Conventional administration of opioids

Intramuscular administration of opioids on a *pro re nata* (p.r.n.; as required) basis is the method used most commonly for prescribing postoperative analgesia. However, for the reasons noted above, this leads frequently to inadequate pain relief. Almost 60% of patients report dissatis-

Table 24.3 Minimum effective analgesic concentration (MEAC) in blood for a number of analgesic drugs. Note the wide range of values for each agent

Drug	MEAC (ng.ml^{-1})
Fentanyl	1–3
Alfentanil	100–300
Pethidine	300–650
Morphine	12–24
Methadone	30–70

Table 24.4 Methods of treating postoperative pain

Conventional administration of opioid
Intramuscular on-demand bolus

Opioid agonist/antagonist drugs

Parenteral administration of opioid
Bolus intravenous administration
Continuous intravenous infusion
Patient-controlled analgesia
  Bolus   } intravenous/intramuscular/
  Bolus + infusion } subcutaneous/extradural

Non-parenteral administration of opioid
Buccal/sublingual
Oral
Rectal
Transdermal
Nasal
Inhalation
Intra-articular opioids

Local anaesthetic techniques

Spinal/extradural opioids

Non-steroidal anti-inflammatory drug (NSAIDs)

α₂-adrenergic agonists
Systemically
Extradurally

Non-pharmacological methods
Cryotherapy
Transcutaneous electrical nerve stimulation (TENS)
Acupuncture
Psychological methods

Table 24.5 Advantages and disadvantages of intramuscular p.r.n. administration of opioids

Advantages	Disadvantages
Familiar practice	Fixed dose not related to pharmacovariability
Gradual onset of side-effects	I.m. administration causes profound pharmacovariability
Nursing assessment before administration	Painful injections
Inexpensive	Fluctuating plasma concentrations Delayed onset of analgesia

Table 24.6 Drugs used systemically for postoperative pain relief and antiemesis

Drug	Dose i.m. (healthy adult)
Opioids	
Morphine	10 mg 4-hourly
Papaveretum	20 mg 4-hourly
Pethidine	100 mg 3-hourly
Buprenorphine (sublingual)	0.4 mg 6-hourly
Moderate analgesics	
Ketorolac	10–30 mg 6-hourly
Dihydrocodeine	50 mg 4-hourly
Antiemetics	
Prochlorperazine	12.5 mg 6-hourly
Perphenazine	5 mg 6-hourly
Cyclizine	50 mg 6-hourly
Metoclopramide	10 mg 6-hourly
Ondansetron	4 mg i.v.

faction with the quality of postoperative analgesia administered in this way.

Intramuscular injection results in variable absorption, particularly in patients with hypothermia, hypovolaemia or hypotension. In addition, there is inevitably a considerable delay between request for analgesia and subsequent administration while controlled drugs are checked and drawn into a syringe. Although it is customary to prescribe opioids on a 4-hourly p.r.n. basis, there are frequently much longer periods between injections and this may lead to considerable 'breakthrough' pain.

The commonest cause of postoperative nausea and vomiting is the administration of opioids either intraoperatively or in the postoperative period. It should therefore be standard practice to prescribe antiemetic drugs regularly for administration with opioids.

Regular administration of i.m. opioids provides improved analgesia, although care must be taken

to avoid overdosage in debilitated patients and those at the extremes of age.

The advantages and disadvantages of repeated p.r.n. administration of opioids are listed in Table 24.5. Drugs used commonly for postoperative pain and antiemesis are listed in Table 24.6; their pharmacological properties are discussed fully in Chapters 10 and 13.

Properties of morphine and morphine-like drugs

1. Analgesia. Morphine produces analgesia by binding with opioid receptors which are present in high concentrations in the periaqueductal area and limbic system of the brain and in the region of the substantia gelatinosa of the spinal cord.
2. Ventilatory depression.
3. Sedation.
4. Cough suppression.
5. Vasodilatation.

6. Release of histamine.
7. Constipation.
8. Nausea and vomiting.
9. Pupillary constriction.
10. Biliary spasm.
11. Urine retention.
12. Tolerance.
13. Physical dependence.

The most important side-effects of morphine are ventilatory depression and nausea and vomiting. Morphine should not be administered to patients with biliary or renal colic (occasionally it may precipitate pain in patients with gall-bladder disease when administered as premedication) and should be avoided in patients with head injury and perhaps in asthmatics.

Alternative drugs are described in Chapter 10. Despite manufacturers' claims to the contrary, there is no evidence that any of the opioid agonist/antagonist drugs produce analgesia equivalent to that of morphine with lesser degrees of ventilatory depression. Some of the newer drugs produce a higher incidence of side-effects such as nausea, vomiting and sedation than equianalgesic doses of morphine.

Buprenorphine is a particularly interesting drug. By virtue of its very high lipid solubility it is absorbed readily across membranes and can be administered by the sublingual route. However, it undergoes a high degree of first-pass metabolism in the gut wall and liver; thus the drug is largely inactivated if the tablet is swallowed. Buprenorphine is a partial agonist with a much higher affinity for μ receptors than morphine. In low doses it displaces morphine from the receptors, thereby apparently 'antagonizing' the morphine. In slightly higher doses it produces excellent analgesia in its own right. Sublingual buprenorphine 0.4 mg 6-hourly provides reasonable analgesia after abdominal surgery. A major disadvantage of buprenorphine is the greater degree of sedation compared with that produced by morphine and this accounts for its relative unpopularity for patients who are mobilized rapidly after surgery (e.g. herniorrhaphy). Because of its high receptor affinity it is recommended that the use of buprenorphine should not be combined with that of morphine.

Parenteral routes of opioid administration

Bolus i.v. administration

It is possible to improve the quality of analgesia in the postoperative period by giving small incremental doses of opioid i.v. when required. However, this carries the risk of rapid induction of ventilatory depression and in the majority of hospitals cannot be undertaken by nursing staff. In general, this technique is employed only by anaesthetists in the immediate recovery period.

Continuous i.v. infusion (Table 24.7)

This technique is employed to provide analgesia in patients receiving artificial ventilation in ITU. An infusion rate designed to exceed MEAC in all patients is clearly safe and ventilatory depression is an advantage in this situation.

Continuous infusions have been used in general surgical wards for the provision of postoperative analgesia in spontaneously breathing patients. The dosage rate is determined by the medical attendant on a trial-and-error basis and a fixed infusion rate prescribed. However, this carries great risks of producing ventilatory depression and cannot be recommended in spontaneously breathing patients outside a high-dependency or intensive therapy unit.

Patient-controlled analgesia (PCA)

The main problem with continuous i.v. infusion is that there is no way of predicting an individual patient's MEAC. With PCA, the patient determines the rate of i.v. administration of the drug, thereby providing feedback control.

PCA equipment comprises an accurate source

Table 24.7 Advantages and disadvantages of continuous i.v. infusions

Advantages	Disadvantages
Rapid onset of analgesia	Fixed dose not related to pharmacodynamic variability
Steady-state plasma concentrations	Errors may be fatal
Painless	Expensive fail-safe equipment required May result in less frequent assessment by nursing staff

Table 24.8 Advantages and disadvantages of patient-controlled analgesia (PCA)

Advantages	Disadvantages
Dose matches patient's requirements and therefore compensates for pharmacodynamic variability	Technical errors may be fatal
	Expensive equipment
Doses given are small and therefore fluctuations in plasma concentrations are reduced	Requires ability to cooperate and understand
Reduces nurses' workload	
Painless	
Placebo effect from patient autonomy	

of infusion, coupled to an i.v. cannula and controlled by a patient-machine interface device. Safety features are incorporated to limit the preset dose, the number of doses which may be administered and the 'lock-out' period between doses. Accidental triggering of the patient control is prevented usually by a requirement for the patient to make two successive presses on a hand control within 1 s.

Advantages and disadvantages of PCA are listed in Table 24.8.

The drug that has been most commonly used with PCA is morphine. The size of the demand dose is usually 1–2 mg with a lockout period of between 5–10 min. Although there may be some theoretical advantage in the use of a continuous low-dose infusion on which the patient may superimpose demand bolus administrations, in practice several clinical investigations have failed to reveal any advantage. Because of the slightly increased risk of overdosage, therefore, it is generally recommended that PCA apparatus be used in the 'bolus alone' mode.

Intravenous PCA is now a standard method of providing postoperative analgesia in many hospitals worldwide. It provides better pain relief than conventional intermittent intramuscular administration. It is essential that monitoring of the patient is not reduced as respiratory depression may occur with this technique and many patients will require antiemetics for nausea. If the pump is being used to deliver morphine via an intravenous infusion it is essential that a one-way valve be incorporated between the PCA equipment and the infusion giving set in order to prevent morphine collecting in the giving set which may then be delivered as a large bolus at a later time, with possible lethal effects.

PCA equipment is usually provided in hospitals where an acute pain service exists involving pain nursing staff and pharmacists; provision is necessary for the correct prescription, storage and exchange of syringes containing large amounts of morphine (50–100 mg).

Non-parenteral opioid administration

Sublingual opioids

Sublingual administration requires cooperation. With buprenorphine, good analgesia can be provided without the necessity for painful injections, making this route popular with patients and convenient for nursing staff.

This route is confined largely to buprenorphine. Combination with morphine may result in dysphoria and withdrawal phenomena. If this route is chosen, it is preferable to use buprenorphine as the sole opioid in the perioperative period.

Oral route

In the immediate postoperative period there is invariably a reduction in the rate of gastric emptying (caused mainly by the intraoperative or preoperative use of opioids). For this reason, opioids should not be used orally for pain relief in the immediate postoperative period because:

1. Absorption is delayed, with poor analgesia.
2. If opioids have been given orally on a regular basis, there is a danger of a large dose being dumped into the upper gastrointestinal tract when gastric motility returns to normal, resulting in overdosage and ventilatory depression.

Oral administration of opioids may be used in the late postoperative period. However, it is more customary to use less potent drugs such as dihydrocodeine or paracetamol because the severity of the pain is generally declining by this time.

All the opioids undergo extensive metabolism in the gut wall and liver (first-pass metabolism) and therefore the bioavailability is relatively low (e.g. 20–30% for morphine).

The rectal route

The rectal route may be used as a means of delivering morphine but there is marked variability in the plasma concentrations achieved. Venous blood from the lower part of the rectum drains directly into the systemic circulation, but the upper part drains into the portal circulation. Thus, bioavailability varies according to the site of a suppository within the rectum. However, this route avoids the problems of reduced gastrointestinal motility. Probably the best indication for the rectal route is the treatment of chronic intractable pain particularly where there is dysphagia.

Transdermal

Because of the high lipid solubility and high potency of fentanyl, this drug may be absorbed across the skin in sufficient quantities to produce effective plasma concentrations. Because of the difficulty in matching transdermal patches of differing strengths to the pharmacodynamic variability between different patients, this technique is not suitable for management of acute pain. However, several centres are currently investigating transdermal administration of fentanyl using a rate-controlled delivery system for management of chronic pain associated with terminal malignancy.

Local anaesthetic techniques

Many local anaesthetic techniques, administered for the purpose of operative surgery or during the course of general anaesthesia, may provide excellent analgesia in the early postoperative period. However, it is usually necessary for the anaesthetist to administer an opioid to the patient before the block regresses to reduce the likelihood of severe pain when the block wears off.

Many local anaesthetic techniques may be used for the primary purpose of providing analgesia in the early postoperative period. However, a major disadvantage is that the duration of blockade with a 'single-shot' technique is relatively short. Bupivacaine (0.25% or 0.5%) is the drug of choice and may produce peripheral nerve blockade lasting for 8–12 h and occasionally for as long as 18 h. The duration of action for extradural nerve block is 4–6 h.

Adrenaline may be added to a local anaesthetic solution to prolong the block, although this produces relatively little effect on the duration of analgesia produced by bupivacaine. The most effective means of prolonging the block is by the use of a catheter to permit either repeated bolus doses or a continuous infusion of local anaesthetic to be administered.

Local anaesthetic blocks in common use are described in Chapter 25. The following blocks represent those which are employed most usefully for postoperative analgesia.

Spinal nerve block

Subarachnoid analgesia rarely lasts more than 3–4 h with the drugs currently available and is therefore of limited use for postoperative analgesia. Although the insertion of a catheter into the subarachnoid space is employed in the United States, this is not a popular manoeuvre in the United Kingdom.

Extradural block

Extradural block is popular for postoperative analgesia because of familiarity with the technique and ease of insertion of a catheter. Repeated injections may be made through the catheter or a dilute solution of local anaesthetic infused continuously. Initially, bupivacaine produces analgesia lasting up to 4 h, but by 24–48 h some tolerance develops and single-bolus administrations may last for only 2 h.

Bupivacaine 0.25% injected at L2/3 provides good analgesia after lower abdominal or perineal surgery, e.g. hysterectomy or transurethral resection of prostate. Upper abdominal procedures require a higher block; 15 ml of bupivacaine 0.5% produces analgesia up to T7.

For thoracic surgery, an extradural catheter may be inserted in the thoracic region between T6 and T8 and volumes of bupivacaine of 6–12 ml may provide excellent postoperative analgesia.

It is recommended that extradural catheter techniques should be employed only when the patient is nursed in an intensive therapy or high-dependency unit, because of the risks of hypotension after extradural injections and total spinal block if the catheter migrates into the subarachnoid space.

Caudal block

Caudal administration of local anaesthetic drugs is useful for child day-case surgery, e.g. circumcision, or in patients undergoing anal or perineal surgery. It is customary to administer only a single dose of local anaesthetic; catheter techniques are unpopular in the United Kingdom because of the risk of infection. Suitable dosage of local anaesthetic solution for use by the caudal route are shown in Table 24.9.

Other regional blocks used for postoperative analgesia

1. *Intercostal nerve blockade.* Blocks from T4 to T8 or 9 provide satisfactory analgesia for pain relief after subcostal incision for cholecystectomy. Intercostal blocks may be repeated at regular intervals; the use of catheters for repeated administration has been employed. Bilateral blockade should not be carried out because of the risk of pneumothorax.

2. *Paravertebral block.* This may be used to provide analgesia after thoracic or abdominal surgery. Local anaesthetic solution is injected into the region of the paravertebral space to block the dorsal sensory nerve roots as they emerge from the vertebral foramina. This technique may be performed using single or repeated injections or with an indwelling catheter.

3. *Femoral nerve block* may be performed during anaesthesia for analgesia after arthroscopy of the knee but is not very effective.

Spinal and extradural opioids (see also p. 167)

In recent years there has been great interest in the use of opioids by the subarachnoid or extradural routes. After injection of opioid into the CSF drug is taken up in the region of the sub-

stantia gelatinosa within the dorsal horn. It is thought that opioids act predominantly on the presynaptic enkephalin receptors, although opioid is absorbed from the CSF into the circulation. After extradural administration of opioids, the drug diffuses through the dura into CSF and produces analgesia by the same mechanism as that associated with subarachnoid injection. However, there is more rapid uptake of opioid into the circulation via the rich network of blood vessels in the extradural space. Consequently, there is a rapid increase in both CSF and blood concentrations of the drug after extradural administration.

Uptake into the dorsal horn, and rate of passage through the dura, are dependent upon lipid solubility. Thus the more highly lipid-soluble drugs (e.g. fentanyl) have a more rapid onset and a shorter duration of action. The less lipid-soluble drugs (e.g. morphine) have a slower rate of onset of action; in addition there is a greater dispersion within the CSF because of reduced uptake into spinal cord and the drug may reach the medulla to cause delayed ventilatory depression.

Subarachnoid opioids

This route is less popular than the extradural route of administration for opioids because of the production of spinal headache. However, smaller doses are required than when the extradural route is used and therefore systemic concentrations are lower. The quality of analgesia is not as good as that achieved with subarachnoid local anaesthetic drugs.

Extradural opioids

The administration of extradural opioids is more popular because spinal headache is avoided and a catheter technique may be employed. It is possible to achieve analgesia without the motor or autonomic block produced by local anaesthetic injected into the extradural space. Thus, postural hypotension and changes in heart rate do not occur. Early ventilatory depression may occur as a result of systemic absorption (e.g. within the first 1–2 h) but late ventilatory depression (8–20 h) is a result of rostral spread of opioid within the CSF to the medulla. Prolonged duration of action

Table 24.9 Doses of bupivacaine (0.25% plain) for caudal analgesia

Adult	Child
0.3–0.4 ml.kg^{-1}	0.5–0.7 ml.kg^{-1} (or 0.1 ml.year^{-1} for each segment to be blocked)

N.B. Dosage of bupivacaine should *never* exceed 2 ml.kg^{-1}.

of analgesia is produced by a single injection (up to 24 h).

Side effects of extradural opioids

1. Early ventilatory depression – occurs more commonly with lipid-soluble agents.

2. Late ventilatory depression – occurs more commonly with agents of lower lipophilicity.

3. Coma – occurs relatively late, usually in association with late ventilatory depression and can be reversed by naloxone.

4. Urinary retention.

5. Itching – this is reversed only partially by naloxone.

6. Nausea and vomiting.

Inhalation of volatile or gaseous anaesthetics

Although volatile anaesthetics were used in the past, the only agent in current use is N_2O. This is administered in the form of Entonox (premixed 50% N_2O, 50% O_2) usually via a demand valve and face mask. Entonox is used extensively in obstetric analgesia, in the field situation (e.g. by ambulance personnel to provide analgesia at the site of an accident) or occasionally in the wards during change of surgical dresings.

Non-steroidal anti-inflammatory drugs (NSAIDs)

With increasing knowledge of the role of inflammatory mediators in the genesis of pain at the site of surgery, the use of NSAIDs has become very popular in recent years. These drugs may be given orally, rectally (e.g. diclofenac 100 mg), i.m. or i.v. (e.g. ketorolac). NSAIDs may be used as the sole method of analgesia for some types of minor surgery and their use reduces the requirements for opioids after major surgery. Aspirin is contraindicated in children under 12 years and a history of gastric ulceration or renal impairment may be contraindications to the use of NSAIDs.

Non-pharmacological methods

Cryotherapy

This may be applied to intercostal nerves exposed during a thoracotomy. The nerve is surrounded by an iceball produced by intense sub-zero temperatures at the end of a probe. The neuronal disruption produced by this method is temporary and sensation returns after some months, although it may be accompanied by unpleasant paraesthesiae and occasionally by persistent neuralgia.

Transcutaneous electrical stimulation

A small alternating current is passed between two surface electrodes at low voltage and at a frequency between 0.2 and 200 Hz. It is thought that the technique acts by increasing CNS concentrations of endorphins. Acupuncture may work in a similar manner. The technique produces only moderate analgesia.

PRE-EMPTIVE ANALGESIA

Experimentally, it has been shown that nociceptive stimulation causes functional changes in the spinal cord which leads to enhancement and prolongation of the sensation of pain. It has also been shown that prior administration of analgesics may inhibit the development of the hyperexcitability within the spinal cord. Unfortunately, however, in clinical practice, prior administration of analgesics (pre-emptive analgesia) has not been shown to have an important effect on postoperative pain.

BALANCED (COMBINED) ANALGESIA

The concept of balanced analgesia is analogous to that of balanced anaesthesia. It is possible to block the development of pain by the use of a combination of different drugs acting at different sites: peripherally, on somatic and sympathetic nerves, at spinal cord level, and centrally. The benefit of this technique is that not only may superior analgesia be achieved by a combination of drugs but their individual doses may be reduced, thereby decreasing the incidence of side-effects.

Pain transmission may be blocked clinically at the following sites:

1. Inhibition of peripheral nociceptor mechanisms using NSAIDs, steroids or opioids.

2. Blockade of afferent neuronal transmission

using peripheral, extradural or spinal local anaesthetic administration.

3. Interference at both spinal cord level and higher centres using systemic opioids.

The technique of balanced analgesia has been shown to provide optimum analgesia in major bowel surgery.

Typically, for minor surgery, e.g. hernia repair on a day-case basis, the anaesthetist may employ balanced analgesia in the form of:

1. Preoperative administration of a mild oral analgesic, e.g. paracetamol or an NSAID.

2. Administration of fentanyl intraoperatively.

3. Local anaesthetic block using ilioinguinal and iliohypogastric nerve blocks and wound infiltration.

4. The use of NSAIDs in the form of a diclofenac suppository 100 mg.

With this technique, patients frequently do not require supplementary opioids postoperatively and may be managed on a day-case basis using simple oral analgesics in the postoperative period, e.g. paracetamol.

FURTHER READING

Ogilvy A J, Smith G 1994 Postoperative pain. In: Nimmo W S, Rowbotham D J, Smith G (eds) Anaesthesia, 2nd edn. Blackwell Scientific Publications, Oxford

25. Local anaesthetic techniques

The efficacy of local anaesthetic techniques has increased greatly within the past two decades as a result of advances in drugs, equipment and the anatomical approaches to nerve blocks. This chapter outlines the basic principles of patient management and the methods employed in the performance of a variety of blocks which are commonly undertaken by the trainee anaesthetist.

Regional techniques for obstetrics and dental surgery are described in other chapters.

FEATURES OF LOCAL ANAESTHESIA

In some circumstances, regional anaesthesia may have distinct advantages over general anaesthesia, as for example in the use of axillary block for hand surgery in a respiratory cripple. However, rather than view a local anaesthetic technique as a rival to general anaesthesia, it is more useful to consider it as part of an individually selected technique which may include the use of sedative or centrally acting anaesthetic drugs. Although the trainee may consider local anaesthesia as having advantages and disadvantages, it becomes apparent with experience that an advantage in one situation may be a disadvantage in another.

Preservation of consciousness is often considered to be an advantage of regional anaesthesia. For example, the patient undergoing Caesarean section is able to protect her own airway and experience the birth of the child. However, patients who require other forms of surgery may be unhappy at the prospect of being awake; in this situation the combination of a regional block and light general anaesthesia may be valuable.

One benefit of a regional block is the quality of early postoperative analgesia, but this may carry disadvantages. Some patients are distressed by the accompanying numbness, although correct preoperative explanation should minimize this concern; in addition, it is important that nursing staff are aware of the risk of trauma to the blocked segments.

Other features of regional anaesthesia include simplicity of administration, sympathetic blockade, attenuation of the stress response and minimal depression of ventilation. Some studies have suggested that the net effect of these features may be a reduction in the incidence of major postoperative complications, but this is controversial.

COMPLICATIONS OF LOCAL ANAESTHESIA

The incidence of complications may be minimized by ensuring adequate supervision and training in local anaesthetic techniques, and by exercising care in the performance of each block. Sufficient expertise and equipment must always be available to deal with potential complications. Complications common to many techniques are discussed in this section; more specific problems are considered later.

Local anaesthetic toxicity

This usually results from accidental intravascular injection, an excessive dose of local anaesthetic or faulty technique, particularly during performance of Bier's block.

Features and treatment

These are described in Chapter 14.

Prevention

Correct technique, careful and repeated aspiration and the use of a test dose are important, but the main safety measure is *slow injection* of the local anaesthetic. This prevents rapid production of very high plasma concentrations even if the injection is intravascular. By this means, toxicity may be diagnosed early, the injection discontinued and a major reaction avoided. Fast injection of local anaesthetic is not necessary for the performance of any block.

Test dose

This may be used before administration of the main dose of local anaesthetic drug. It is particularly indicated for extradural block, where it should be capable of demonstrating inadvertent intravenous (i.v.) or subarachnoid injection. A test dose of 4 ml of 2% plain lignocaine is sufficient to cause mild symptoms in most patients after accidental i.v. injection and any features of local anaesthetic blockade 2 min after injection are good evidence of accidental subarachnoid block. No test dose is infallible; slow administration of the main dose is the most important factor in avoiding local anaesthetic toxicity.

Hypotension

There are several possible mechanisms by which a local anaesthetic technique may cause hypotension. The anaesthetist must always remember that surgical factors may be responsible.

Sympathetic blockade

A limited sympathetic block may be produced by peripheral nerve anaesthesia, but only central blocks are likely to produce hypotension by this mechanism.

Total spinal blockade

This is discussed on page 460. It occasionally occurs during subarachnoid block if excessive spread of local anaesthetic solution occurs, and is a recognized complication of extradural block if

the dura has been penetrated. Apnoea may occur if local anaesthetic solution reaches the cerebrospinal fluid (CSF) during interscalene brachial plexus block, or the ventricular system during retrobulbar nerve block.

Vasovagal attack

This is particularly likely to occur in an anxious patient with a rapidly ascending spinal block. Pallor, nausea and bradycardia are associated with the hypotension. The supine position is no guarantee against this complication. Rapid resolution results from placing the patient head-down and the administration of i.v. ephedrine 5–6 mg. Cautious i.v. sedation (e.g. midazolam 1–2 mg) may be helpful.

Anaphylactoid reaction

This is very rare with amide local anaesthetics.

Local anaesthetic toxicity

This is considered above and in Chapter 14.

Motor blockade

To avoid unnecessary distress, patients must be warned of the possibility of lower limb weakness or paralysis which may persist for some time after operation.

Pneumothorax

This is a potential hazard of supraclavicular brachial plexus, intercostal and paravertebral blocks. The possibility of its occurrence is an absolute contraindication to the use of these techniques in outpatients and also to the performance of these blocks bilaterally.

Urinary retention

This may follow the use of central blocks. It is important to avoid overhydration, as bladder distension may require catheterization.

Neurological complications

Carefully performed blocks rarely result in neurological complications.

Neuritis with persisting sensory changes and/or weakness may result from trauma to the nerve, intraneural injection or bacterial, chemical or particulate contamination of the injected solution. Injection of the incorrect solution has caused some of the most severe neurological complications. To avoid this serious error, all drugs must be checked personally by the anaesthetist immediately before injection.

Anterior spinal artery syndrome may follow an episode of prolonged, severe hypotension and results in painless permanent paraplegia. *Adhesive arachnoiditis* has been described after subarachnoid and extradural blockade and may lead to permanent pain, weakness and bladder or bowel dysfunction. It is suspected that this complication results from injection of the incorrect solution. *Haematoma* or *abscess* formation in the spinal canal after subarachnoid or extradural anaesthesia results in weakness and sensory loss below the level of spinal cord compression. It is associated with intense back pain and is a neurosurgical emergency which demands immediate decompression to avoid permanent disability.

Equipment problems

Needles are most likely to break at the junction with the hub and therefore should never be inserted fully. Catheters may also break, but exploratory surgery to find small pieces of catheter is inappropriate, as complications are very unlikely.

GENERAL MANAGEMENT

Patient assessment and selection

Careful preoperative evaluation is as important before a local anaesthetic as it is before general anaesthesia, and the same principles of preoperative management apply. Therapy to improve the patient's condition before surgery should be instituted if appropriate. It is inappropriate to proceed with surgery under local anaesthesia for the sake of convenience in the poorly prepared patient. A decision on the need for immediate surgical intervention should be made before the anaesthetic technique is chosen.

The preoperative visit should be used to establish rapport with the patient. A clear description of the proposed anaesthetic should be given in simple terms, but there is rarely a need for excessive detail. Occasionally patients require some explanation of the reasons for selecting a regional technique before accepting it, but there should be no attempt at coercion.

Potential problems related to the intended block should be sought. Anatomical deformities may render some blocks impractical. A history of allergy to amide local anaesthetics is rare, but is an absolute contraindication, as is infection at the site of needle insertion. For most blocks, anticoagulant therapy and bleeding diatheses are also absolute contraindications, and the use of major blocks in patients with distant infection or receiving low-dose subcutaneous (s.c.) heparin requires careful consideration. Sympathetic blockade with consequent vasodilatation may lead to profound hypotension in patients with aortic or mitral stenosis because of the relatively constant cardiac output. Hypovolaemia must be corrected before contemplating subarachnoid or extradural anaesthesia.

There is no evidence that neuromuscular disorders or multiple sclerosis are adversely affected by local anaesthetic techniques, but most anaesthetists use regional anaesthesia in such patients only if there are obvious benefits to be gained; any perioperative deterioration in the neurological condition is often associated by the patient with the local anaesthetic procedure. Raised intracranial pressure is a contraindication to central blockade.

Selection of technique

Local anaesthetic drugs may be administered by:

1. Single dose.
2. Intermittent bolus:
   a. repeated injections.
   b. indwelling catheter for repeat administration.
3. Continuous infusion (with optional bolus doses) via a catheter.

If regional anaesthesia has been selected primarily to provide analgesia during and after surgery under general anaesthesia, a distal technique is appropriate and is associated with the fewest complications.

Because a local anaesthetic technique renders only part of the body insensible, it is essential that the method employed is tailored to, and sufficient for, the planned surgery. Account must be taken of the duration of surgery, its site (which may be multiple, e.g. the need to obtain bone grafting material from the iliac crest), and the likelihood of a change of procedure in mid-operation. The problem of multiple sites of surgery may be met by one block which covers both sites, or by more than one regional procedure. The duration of anaesthesia may be tailored to the anticipated duration of surgery by selection of an appropriate local anaesthetic agent, or may require the use of a technique which allows further administration of drug.

Premedication

Manipulation of fractures and other short emergency procedures are often carried out using a local anaesthetic technique in the unpremedicated patient, as rapid recovery is desirable. However, premedication is helpful before inpatient elective or emergency surgery. An oral benzodiazepine allays anxiety, but an opioid (e.g. morphine) alleviates the discomfort of prolonged immobility which may be required during a long procedure. Preoperative analgesia may be required before definitive fixation. A nerve block may be useful in these circumstances, e.g. to alleviate the pain from a fractured femur, but often the administration of opioids, preferably i.v. in a controlled manner, is more appropriate at this time.

Patients should be fasted for all but the most minor peripheral nerve blocks.

Timing

It is essential that sufficient time is allowed to perform the block without undue haste on the part of the anaesthetist. This is largely a matter of organization, and the experienced practitioner seldom causes delay to an operating list. Any preoperative delay is compensated for by the ability to return the patient to bed immediately after completion of surgery.

Resuscitation equipment

A full range of resuscitative equipment must be in working order and immediately available. This includes:

1. An anaesthetic breathing system through which oxygen may be administered under pressure via a face mask or tracheal tube.
2. A laryngoscope with two sizes of blade, a range of tracheal tubes and an introducer.
3. A table which can rapidly be tilted head-down.
4. Suction apparatus.
5. Intravenous cannulae and fluids.
6. Thiopentone to control convulsions.
7. Drugs to treat hypotension, especially atropine, ephedrine and methoxamine.

A cannula must be inserted intravenously before *any* local anaesthetic block is performed in case emergency therapy is required.

Regional block equipment

Regional anaesthesia may be employed with basic equipment, but some special items increase the success rate and reduce the risk of complications.

Needles

Very fine spinal needles (26 G) have significantly reduced the incidence of post-spinal headache. 29 G Needles are now readily available, but confident and successful use of these needles requires greater expertise than is needed for the use of larger needles.

Pencil-point 24 G needles are associated with a reduced incidence of post-spinal headache. Disposable prepacked spinal and extradural needles ease preparation and ensure sterility. Short-bevelled needles (Fig. 25.1) reduce the likelihood of nerve damage and are recommended for plexus and peripheral nerve blockade. Sheathed needles are valuable for use with nerve stimulators.

Immobile needle technique

For plexus and major nerve blocks, local anaes-

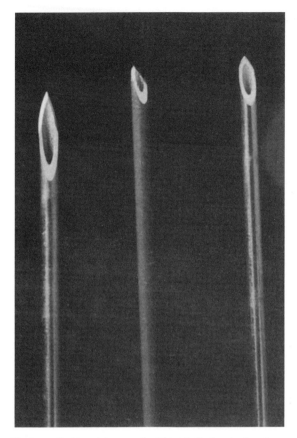

Fig 25.1 Left to right: standard-bevelled, sheathed and unsheathed short-bevelled needles.

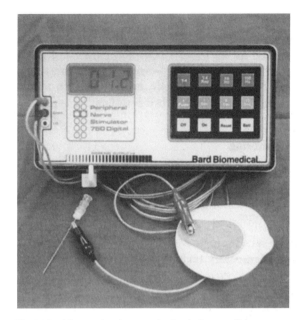

Fig 25.2 Nerve stimulator and stimulating needle.

thetic drug is drawn into labelled syringes and connected to the block needle by a short length of tubing (see Fig. 25.14). This allows the anaesthetist to hold the needle steady while aspiration tests are performed and syringes changed. The system must be primed to avoid air embolism.

Catheters

Continuous administration of local anaesthetic drugs has been made possible by the development of high-quality catheters, which are introduced through a needle and left in position for many hours.

Nerve stimulators

Many anaesthetists prefer to elicit paraesthesiae when performing a major nerve block. However,

a nerve stimulator (Fig. 25.2) is a useful aid, especially for the beginner. It is important to explain to the patient the sensation elicited by stimulation.

Stimulators that deliver a constant current and give a digital display of the current used are readily available. One lead is attached to an electrocardiogram (ECG) electrode on the patient's skin, and the other to the shaft of the needle. After skin puncture, the stimulator is set to a frequency of 1 Hz and an initial current of 3 mA. As the nerve is approached, motor fibre stimulation causes muscle movement. This procedure is not painful unless the nerve is touched, when paraesthesiae result.

The current is gradually reduced until movement is still present at a current of, optimally, less than 1 mA. At this point, an aspiration test is performed and 2 ml of local anaesthetic solution injected. Movement should cease immediately. If it does not, and an unsheathed needle is being used, the tip may be beyond the nerve; the needle should be withdrawn slightly and the procedure repeated. Severe pain on injection suggests intraneural injection and the needle should be repositioned. When the correct position has been found, the remainder of the anaesthetic solution should be injected slowly with repeated aspiration tests.

Asepsis

A 'no-touch' technique is essential. Drapes should be used for all major blocks and gloves and gown worn by the beginner. Gown and gloves are advisable for all central blocks, even with a 'no-touch' technique, especially when a catheter is inserted.

Monitoring

It is essential that the anaesthetist remains with the patient. Monitoring equipment should be appropriate to the anaesthetic and surgical procedure.

Supplementary techniques

A local anaesthetic may be the only drug administered to the patient, or it may form part of a balanced anaesthetic technique. During surgery, patients may be awake, or sedated by i.v. or inhalational means. Propofol, midazolam or low concentrations of nitrous oxide are commonly employed. General anaesthesia may be used as a planned part of the procedure. Experienced anaesthetists use a combination of regional and general anaesthesia to obtain advantages from both.

When a surgical tourniquet is used, the chosen block must extend to the tourniquet site unless the procedure is brief. Discomfort from prolonged immobility on a hard table is relieved by the administration of an opioid either as a premedicant or i.v. during surgery; this type of discomfort is not relieved by sedative drugs, which often result in the patient becoming confused and uncooperative.

Aftercare

Clear instructions should be given to the nurses caring for the patient.

After day-case surgery, the patient must be in a safe condition at the time of discharge. Plexus blockade with a long-acting agent is inappropriate because of the risk of the patient injuring the anaesthetized limb, but is suitable for postoperative pain relief in supervised inpatients. Patients who have received central blockade should have routine nursing observations at least until the block has worn off.

Continuous infusion techniques are only suitable for use by experienced anaesthetists. When used correctly, administration by infusion is safer than repeated bolus injection of drug, but regular observations are essential and the nursing staff must have an adequate level of knowledge to appreciate possible complications. An anaesthetist must be available within the hospital at all times.

INTRAVENOUS REGIONAL ANAESTHESIA (IVRA)

Ideally, IVRA (Bier's block) should be the first local anaesthetic technique learnt by a trainee, because its technical simplicity allows him or her to concentrate on acquiring the skills of patient management. Bier's block is simple, safe and effective when performed correctly using an appropriate drug in correct dosage. Deaths from IVRA have resulted from incorrect selection of drug and dosage, incorrect technique and the performance of the block by personnel unable to treat toxic reactions. The drug involved in these deaths, bupivacaine, was not the most suitable agent and is no longer recommended. The lessons to be learned from these deaths are applicable to all local anaesthetic techniques, and emphasize that expert guidance is essential even when learning the most basic blocks.

Indications

IVRA is suitable for short procedures when postoperative pain is not marked, e.g. manipulation of Colles fracture or carpal tunnel decompression. Recovery is rapid, and the technique is appropriate for outpatient surgery. Premedication may delay patient discharge and a reassuring visit preoperatively from the anaesthetist is usually sufficient in these circumstances.

Method (Fig. 25.3)

IVRA involves isolating an exsanguinated limb from the general circulation by means of an arterial tourniquet and then injecting local anaesthetic

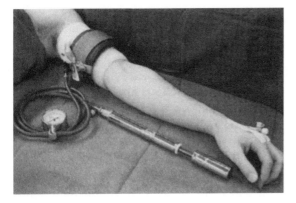

Fig 25.3 Tourniquet and intravenous cannulag for Bier's block

solution intravenously. Analgesia and weakness rapidly occur and result predominantly from local anaesthetic action on peripheral nerve endings.

An orthopaedic tourniquet of the correct size is applied over padding on the upper arm. All connections must lock, and the pressure gauge should be calibrated regularly. A cannula is inserted intravenously in the contralateral arm in case administration of emergency drugs is required. An indwelling cannula is inserted into a vein of the limb to be anaesthetized; scalp vein needles are best avoided as they are liable to penetrate the vein during exsanguination. A vein on the dorsum of the hand is preferred; injection into proximal veins reduces the quality of the block and increases the risk of toxicity. Exsanguination by means of an Esmarch bandage improves the quality of the block and increases the safety of the technique by reducing the venous pressure developed during injection. In patients with a painful lesion (e.g. Colles' fracture), elevation combined with brachial artery compression is adequate. The tourniquet should be inflated to a pressure 100 mmHg above systolic arterial pressure.

In an adult, 40 ml of prilocaine 0.5% is injected over 2 min with careful observation that the tourniquet remains inflated. Analgesia is complete within 10 min, but it is important to inform the patient that the feeling of touch is often retained at this time. The anaesthetist must be ready to deal with toxicity or tourniquet pain throughout the surgical procedure. The tourniquet should not be released until at least 20 min after injection,

even if surgery is completed. This delay allows for diffusion of drug into the tissues so that plasma concentrations do not reach toxic levels after release of the tourniquet. The technique of repeated reinflation and deflation of the cuff during release has little effect on plasma concentrations, and is not necessary.

Reinstitution of the block within 30 min of tourniquet release is possible using 50% of the initial dose, because some drug is retained within the limb. Bilateral blocks may be performed without exceeding the maximum recommended doses, but it is preferable to do this consecutively rather than concurrently.

Tourniquet pain

This may be troublesome if the cuff remains inflated for longer than 30–40 min. It is sometimes alleviated by inflating a separate tourniquet below the first on an area already rendered analgesic by the block; the first cuff is then deflated. Failing this, light general anaesthesia is preferable to administration of large and often ineffective doses of opioids and sedatives.

Choice of drug

The agent of choice for this procedure is prilocaine 0.5% plain. It has an impressive safety record with no major reactions reported after its use, although minor side-effects such as transient light-headedness after release of the tourniquet are not uncommon. The drug has distinct pharmacokinetic advantages in IVRA (see Chapter 14). Methaemoglobinaemia does not result from the doses employed for IVRA.

Lower limb

IVRA of the foot can be produced using the same dose of prilocaine and a calf tourniquet carefully positioned to avoid compression of the common peroneal nerve on the neck of the fibula.

CENTRAL NERVE BLOCKS

Spinal anaesthesia is a term that may be used to denote all forms of central blockade, although it usually refers to intrathecal administration of local anaesthetic. The term subarachnoid block (SAB) avoids ambiguity. The technique of SAB is basically that of lumbar puncture, but a knowledge of factors which affect the extent and duration of anaesthesia, and experience in patient management, are essential. Extradural (also termed epidural) nerve block may be performed in the sacral (caudal block), lumbar, thoracic or cervical regions, although lumbar block is employed most commonly. Local anaesthetic solution is injected through a needle after the tip has been introduced into the extradural space.

Physiological effects of SAB

Differential nerve blockade

As spinal anaesthetic solutions spread away from the site of injection, the concentration of the solution declines as mixing occurs with CSF. A differential blockade of fibres occurs because small fibres are blocked by weaker concentrations of local anaesthetic solution. Sympathetic fibres are blocked to a level two segments higher than the upper segmental level of sensory blockade. Motor blockade tends to extend to within two segments caudal to the upper level of sensory block. Thus, sensory levels of spinal anaesthesia to T3 are associated with total blockade of the T1–L2 sympathetic outflow.

Respiratory system

Low spinal block has no effect on the respiratory system and the technique is used frequently for patients with chest disease.

Motor blockade extending to the roots of the phrenic nerves (C3–5) causes apnoea.

Blocks which reach the thoracic level cause loss of intercostal muscle activity. This has little effect on tidal volume (because of diaphragmatic compensation), but there is a marked decrease in vital capacity resulting from a significant decrease in expiratory reserve volume. A thoracic block may lead to a reduction in cardiac output and pulmonary artery pressure, and increased ventilation/perfusion imbalance, resulting in a decrease in arterial oxygen tension (Pa_{O_2}). Awake patients

with a high spinal block should always be given oxygen-enriched air to breathe.

Cardiovascular system

The cardiovascular effects are proportional to the height of the block and result from denervation of the sympathetic outflow tracts (T1–L2). This produces dilatation of resistance and capacitance vessels and results in hypotension. In awake patients, compensatory vasoconstriction above the height of the block may compensate almost completely for these changes, thereby maintaining arterial pressure, but general anaesthetic agents may reduce this compensatory response, with consequent profound hypotension.

Hypotension is augmented by:

1. The use of head-up posture.
2. Any degree of hypovolaemia — pre-existing or induced by surgery.

Prevention of hypotension

Both the incidence and the degree of hypotension are reduced by limiting the height of the block and, in particular, by keeping it below the sympathetic supply to the heart (T1–5). Many authorities advise that all patients who receive subarachnoid or extradural block should be placed in a slight head-down position (5–10°) throughout the procedure. This small degree of tilt has little effect on distribution of block, but has a significant effect on venous return.

It is common practice to attempt to minimize hypotension during SAB or extradural anaesthesia by preloading the patient with 500–1000 ml of crystalloid solution i.v. before or during the institution of the block. These volumes are usually ineffective even in the short term, may risk the development of pulmonary oedema in susceptible individuals either during the procedure or when the block wears off, and may lead to postoperative urinary retention. Appropriate fluid should be given to replace blood and fluid losses and prevent dehydration.

Bradycardia may occur because of:

1. Neurogenic factors in awake patients, i.e. vasovagal syndrome.

2. Block of the cardiac sympathetic fibres (T1–4).

Careful patient positioning, maintenance of a normal circulating volume and the use of pharmacological agents (see later) if required should minimize the incidence of hypotension.

SAB has no direct effect on the liver or kidneys, but reductions in hepatic and renal blood flow occur in the presence of hypotension associated with high spinal blocks.

Gastrointestinal system

The vagus nerve supplies parasympathetic fibres to the whole of the gut as far as the transverse colon. Spinal blockade causes sympathetic denervation (proportional to height of block) and unopposed parasympathetic action leads to a constricted gut with increased peristaltic activity. This is regarded by some as advantageous for surgery.

Nausea, retching or vomiting may occur in the awake patient and is often the first symptom of impending or established hypotension.

If nausea or retching occurs, the anaesthetist must measure arterial pressure and heart rate immediately and take appropriate measures.

Physiological effects of extradural block

The physiological effect of extradural blockade are similar to those following SAB. However, there may be important differences resulting from the much larger volumes of anaesthetic solutions used, as there is appreciable systemic absorption of local anaesthetic and adrenaline if an adrenaline-containing solution is used.

Indications for SAB

Blockade is produced more consistently and with a lower dose of drug by the subarachnoid route than by extradural injection. It is not customary in the UK to use a catheter in the subarachnoid space and the duration of analgesia is therefore limited to 2–4 h. SAB is most suited to surgery below the umbilicus and in this situation the patient may remain awake. Surgery above the umbilicus using SAB is less appropriate and would necessitate a general anaesthetic in addition, in order to abolish unpleasant sensations from visceral manipulation resulting from afferent impulses transmitted by the vagus nerves.

Types of surgery

Urology. SAB is well-suited to urological procedures such as transurethral prostatectomy, but it should be remembered that a block to T10 is required for surgery involving bladder distension. Perineal and penile operations may be carried out more conveniently under peripheral blockade or caudal anaesthesia.

Gynaecology. Minor procedures such as dilatation and curettage may be performed reliably with a block to T10. For major intra-abdominal gynaecological procedures and for diagnostic laparoscopy, light general anaesthesia is usually necessary in addition.

Obstetrics. The rapid onset of SAB may be advantageous in some circumstances, but this should be weighed against the high incidence of post lumbar puncture headache in this group of patients. The introduction of the pencil-point spinal needle with a reduction in the incidence of post lumbar puncture headache has led to an increased use of SAB in obstetric practice.

Any surgical procedure on the lower limbs or perineum. For patients with medical problems, low SAB may be the anaesthetic technique of choice:

1. *Metabolic disease.* Diabetes mellitus, thyrotoxicosis.

2. *Respiratory disease.* Low SAB has no effect on ventilation and obviates the requirement for anaesthetic drugs with depressant properties, but there is little evidence that spinal anaesthesia reduces the incidence of postoperative chest infections, as is commonly believed.

3. *Cardiovascular disease.* Low SAB may be valuable in patients with ischaemic heart disease or congestive cardiac failure, in whom a small reduction in preload and afterload may be beneficial. SAB is effective in preventing cardiovascular responses to surgery (e.g. hypertension, tachycardia) which are undesirable, particularly in patients with ischaemic heart disease.

Indications for extradural blockade

The indications for extradural anaesthesia are widespread because it is an extremely versatile technique which can be tailored to suit a variety of situations. The duration of analgesia may be prolonged as necessary by means of an indwelling catheter and the use of intermittent top-ups or a continuous infusion. Bupivacaine is the drug of choice when one of these continuous techniques is employed. The pharmacokinetic properties of bupivacaine are such that, with the doses necessary to maintain adequate blockade, systemic accumulation of the drug is slow and the risk of toxicity is small. Either local anaesthetic drugs or opioids may be used extradurally, but the latter are most suited to provision of postoperative analgesia and are inadequate for surgery in most circumstances. Almost all opioids have been tried by the extradural route with success.

Contraindications to SAB and extradural anaesthesia

Most contraindications are relative, but are best regarded as absolute by the trainee.

1. Bleeding diathesis.
2. Hypovolaemia.
3. Sepsis close to site of lumbar puncture.
4. Severe stenotic valvular heart disease. The patient may be unable to compensate for vasodilatation because of a fixed cardiac output.
5. Pre-eclamptic toxaemia. Extradural block has been used with great benefit in this condition, but a platelet count of less than 100×10^9 litre^{-1} usually precludes extradural or subarachnoid anaesthesia.

Performance of SAB

Intravenous access

An intravenous infusion must be instituted before lumbar puncture is performed.

Positioning the patient

Lumbar puncture for SAB may be performed with the patient sitting or in the lateral decubitus position (Fig. 25.4). If it is anticipated that lumbar puncture may be difficult, the midline is usually more discernible with the patient in the sitting position. The technique of lumbar puncture for the patient in the lateral position is described in the next section.

Technique of lumbar puncture

For the right-handed anaesthetist, the patient is positioned on the operating table in the left lateral position. The patient's back should lie along the edge of the table and must be vertical (Fig. 25.5A). A curled position opens the spaces between the lumbar spinous processes. An assistant stands in front of the patient to assist with positioning and to reassure the patient. The anaesthetist must inform the patient before performing each part of the procedure.

A line between the iliac crests lies on the fourth lumbar spinous process or interspace; lumbar puncture should be performed at the third or fourth space. A full sterile technique (with gown, gloves and surgical drapes) is adopted. All drugs should be drawn into syringes directly from sterile ampoules using a filter needle to prevent the injection of glass particles into the subarachnoid

Table 25.1 Techniques of subarachnoid block

Type of block	Upper level of analgesia	Position during lumbar puncture	Volume of solution
Saddle block	S1	Sitting 5 min	1 ml hyperbaric solution
Low thoracic	T10–12	Sitting/lateral decubitus	3–4 ml*
High thoracic	T4–6	Lateral decubitus Sitting (immediately supine)	2–3 ml hyperbaric solution
Unilateral	Not possible with hyperbaric solutions which eventually affect both sides after the patient is placed supine. Hypobaric solutions, e.g. amethocaine in water, may be used when the patient can remain with the operative side uppermost throughout, e.g. hip replacement surgery		

*Plain bupivacaine is slightly hypobaric at body temperature and the eventual block height is difficult to predict. Plain amethocaine, available in some countries, is truly isobaric, gives a more predictable height of block and is often used in volumes of 2 ml to achieve low thoracic blockade.

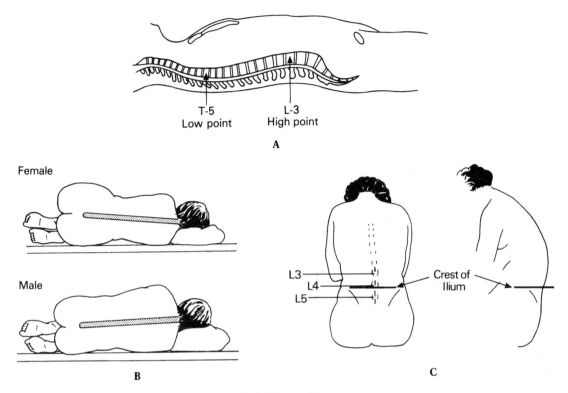

Fig 25.4 Spinal curvature in: **A** supine; **B** lateral; **C** sitting positions.

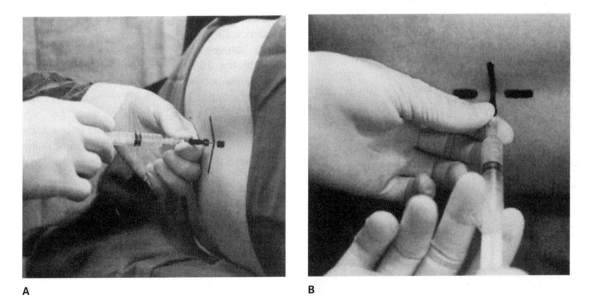

Fig 25.5 Injection of local anaesthetic solution into the subarachnoid space. Note that the needle is horizontal. The third lumbar interspace is marked.

space. A selection of spinal needles (22–26-gauge) should be available.

The skin and subcutaneous tissues are infiltrated with local anaesthetic using a small needle. The spinal needle is inserted in the midline, midway between two spinous processes. In the well-positioned patient, the needle is directed at right angles to the skin. Passage through the interspinous ligament and ligamentum flavum into the spinal canal is easily appreciated with a 22-gauge needle. With some practice these structures are usually discernible with a 26-gauge needle or 24 G pencil-point needle, which all anaesthetists should aspire to use. The use of an introducer (19-gauge needle) is advisable to brace the 26-gauge needle, which is very flexible. A Quincke point spinal needle should be inserted with the bevel facing laterally to minimize the risk of postspinal headache. When the needle tip has entered the spinal canal, the stilette is withdrawn from the needle and the hub is observed for flow of CSF; a needle with a transparent hub makes this easier. A gentle aspiration test should be performed if a free flow of CSF is not observed.

The three most common reasons for difficulty are poor patient position, failure to insert the needle in the midline and directing the needle laterally. This last fault is seen most easily from one side (Fig. 25.6), and is usually apparent to

onlookers, but not to the anaesthetist, who looks only along the line of the needle.

When CSF is obtained, the syringe containing the local anaesthetic solution should be firmly attached to the needle. Gentle aspiration confirms the needle position and the solution is injected at a rate of 1 ml every 5 s. Aspiration after injection confirms that the needle tip has remained in the correct place. Needle and introducer are withdrawn and the patient placed supine.

Factors affecting spread (Table 25.2)

The most important factor which affects the height of block in SAB is the baricity of the solution, which may be made hyperbaric (i.e. denser than CSF) by the addition of glucose. The specific gravity (SG) of CSF is 1.004. The addition of glucose 5% or 6% to a local anaesthetic produces a solution with SG of 1.024 or greater. A patient who assumes the sitting position for 5 min after injection of 1 ml of hyperbaric solution develops a saddle block which affects the perineum only. Conversely, a patient placed supine immediately after injection develops a block to the mid-thoracic region. Slightly larger volumes are advisable

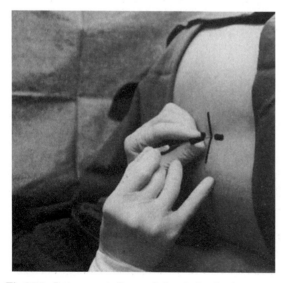

Fig 25.6 Incorrect needle angulation during lumbar puncture for subarachnoid block.

Table 25.2 Factors influencing spread of hyperbaric spinal solutions

Factor	Effect
Position of patient	Sitting position produces perineal block only, provided that low volumes are used
Spinal curvature	With standard volumes (2–3 ml) the block often spreads to T4. With low volumes (1 ml) the block may affect only the perineum even when the patient is placed supine immediately
Dose of drug	Within the range of volumes usually employed (2–4 ml), increasing the dose of drug increases the duration of anaesthesia rather than the height of the block
Interspace	Minor factor affecting height of block
Obesity	Minor factor affecting height of block. Obese patients tend to develop higher blocks
Speed of injection	Rapid injection makes the height of block more variable
Barbotage	No longer employed. Makes the height of block more variable

to ensure spread above the lumbar curvature (Fig. 25.4).

Within the range normally used for SAB (2–4 ml), the volume of solution has only a minor effect on spread. Obesity, pregnancy and a high site of injection are minor factors which increase the height of the block; lower volumes may be desirable in these situations. Barbotage and rapid injection may produce high blocks, but increase the unpredictability of spread.

Factors affecting duration

The duration of anaesthesia depends on the drug used and the dose of drug employed. Vasoconstrictors added to the local anaesthetic solution significantly increase the duration of action of amethocaine (tetracaine), which is widely used in the USA, but this is not so for other agents.

Agents

Only three agents are readily available for SAB in the UK. Plain bupivacaine 0.5% is slightly hypobaric at body temperature and may very occasionally have an unpredictable spread and produce an inadequate block. It is used in volumes of 3–4 ml and lasts 2–3 h. Hyperbaric bupivacaine 0.5% is much more predictable and consistently produces a block to the umbilicus (and usually to T5) in supine patients. As with all hyperbaric solutions, hypotension is encountered more frequently because of higher levels of sympathetic blockade. Volumes of 2–3 ml are used and a duration of 2–3 h is usually assured. Plain lignocaine 2% usually provides analgesia of the lower limbs and perineum. Volumes of 3–4 ml are used and duration is approximately 1 h.

Complications

Acute

1. *Hypotension.* Significant hypotension should be anticipated with SAB. Changes in position, e.g. turning the patient from the supine to the prone position, may result in a sudden increase in the height of block, with consequent extension of sympathetic blockade. This may occur even after 15–20 min. Treatment (Table 25.3) may not

Table 25.3 Management of hypotension

5° head-down tilt	
Maintain blood volume	
Heart rate:	
<60 beat.min^{-1}	Atropine 0.3 mg
60–80 beat.min^{-1}	Ephedrine 3 mg
>80 beat.min^{-1}	Methoxamine 2 mg

be necessary; moderate hypotension may help to reduce operative blood loss and is tolerated well by most patients. Severe or unwanted hypotension may be treated by i.v. fluids or drugs. The use of large volumes of crystalloid or colloid in this situation is not recommended as urinary retention may occur postoperatively or circulatory overload may result when the block wears off. However, it is essential that operative blood losses are replaced promptly, and when blood losses are expected (e.g. Caesarean section) it is wise to administer fluid in advance of the loss. Hypotension commonly is associated with bradycardia and ephedrine 5–6 mg i.v. is the most appropriate treatment. Atropine may be useful, but sympathomimetic drugs are usually more effective than vagolytics.

2. *Oversedation.* This may occur when sedative drugs have been administered before performance of SAB. When the block is established the previously satisfactory level of sedation may become excessive, with the attendant risks of respiratory obstruction or aspiration. Reports of cardiac arrest associated with SAB may be related to hypoxaemia produced in this manner.

Postoperative

1. *Headache.* This is more common in young adults and particularly in obstetric patients. It may occur up to 2–7 days after lumbar puncture, and may persist for up to 6 weeks. Characteristically, it is worse on sitting, occipital in distribution and very disabling. The incidence is reduced by using small-gauge or pencil-point needles and ensuring that the bevel of the needle penetrates the dura in a sagittal plane. Simple analgesics may be the only treatment required, but occasionally an extradural blood patch is necessary. The incidence of post-spinal headache is not reduced by keeping the patient supine for 24 h; the patient

should remain supine only until the anaesthetic has worn off and the risk of postural hypotension is minimal. If headache is severe and persistent, an extradural blood patch may be performed by removing 20 ml of the patient's own blood under aseptic conditions and injecting it extradurally at the same interspace as SAB was performed. Injection should be stopped if discomfort is experienced. This is an effective cure for lumbar puncture headache and appears to be remarkably free from adverse effects.

2. *Urinary retention.* This may be associated with the surgical procedure. Large volumes of i.v. fluids may increase the frequency of this complication.

3. *Labyrinthine disturbances.*

4. *Cranial nerve palsy.* Sixth nerve palsy may occur and is usually temporary. This complication is more common with larger needles.

5. *Meningitis and meningism.*

6. *Transverse myelitis* and *cauda equina syndrome* resulting from adhesive arachnoiditis. Fortunately these conditions, giving rise to permanent neurological damage or paraplegia, are extremely rare.

Extradural block

By virtue of its great versatility, extradural analgesia is probably the most widely used regional technique in the UK. It may be used for procedures from the neck downwards and the duration of analgesia can be tailored to meet the needs of surgery and postoperative pain relief by using a catheter system.

The major differences between SAB and extradural block are summarized in Table 25.4. Further expansion of the technique has taken place with the advent of extradural administration of opioids (see Chapter 10).

Equipment

Extradural anaesthesia is usually performed using a Tuohy needle (Fig. 25.7). The needle is marked at 1-cm intervals and has a Huber point which allows a catheter to be directed along the long axis of the extradural space. Disposable catheters are available with a single end-hole or with a sealed tip and three side-holes distally.

Table 25.4 Differences between subarachnoid and extradural block

	Subarachnoid	Extradural
Dose of drug employed	Small: minimal risk of systemic toxicity	Large: possibility of systemic toxicity after intravascular injection or total spinal blockade after subarachnoid injection
Rate of onset	Fast: 2–5 min for initial effect 20 min for maximum effect	Slow: 5–15 min for initial effect 30–45 min for maximum effect
Intensity of block	Usually complete anaesthesia	Often not complete anaesthesia for all segments
Pattern of block	May be dermatomal for first few minutes, but rapidly develops appearance of cord transection	Dermatomal
Addition of vasoconstrictor	Reliably prolongs block with amethocaine, but not with other drugs	Reliably prolongs block with lignocaine. May prolong block with bupivacaine, but not in all patients

Technique

Extradural block may be performed at any level of the spinal cord to provide segmental analgesia over an area that can be predetermined with reasonable success. Initial experience should be gained in the lumbar region before progressing to sites above the termination of the spinal cord.

The pressure in the extradural space is usually subatmospheric, particularly in the thoracic region, because of communications by valveless veins between the extradural and intrathoracic spaces. Some older methods of identifying the extradural space (e.g. Odom's indicator, Macintosh's balloon) relied on detection of the subatmospheric pressure in the extradural space. However, methods which depend on loss of resistance to injection of air

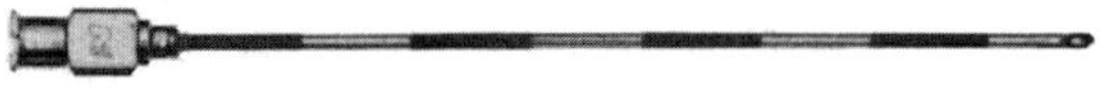

Fig 25.7 16-Gauge Tuohy extradural needle.

or saline as the tip of the needle penetrates the ligamentum flavum and enters the extradural space have become more popular. A midline approach is described here, using loss of resistance to saline to detect the extradural space.

The patient is positioned as for SAB and the vertebral level is identified from the iliac crests. The skin and subcutaneous tissues of the third lumbar interspace are infiltrated with local anaesthetic solution in the midline. A sharp needle is used to puncture the skin and the Tuohy, round-ended extradural needle is introduced through the skin puncture, subcutaneous tissue and supraspinous ligament. The common reasons for difficulty are the same as those for SAB. When inserted into the interspinous ligament, the unsupported needle remains steady. The stilette is withdrawn and a 20-ml plastic syringe filled with saline is attached and advanced using firm but gentle pressure on the plunger. The needle must be gripped tightly at all times (Fig. 25.8) to prevent sudden forward movement. When the needle penetrates the ligamentum flavum there is a sudden loss of resistance to pressure on the plunger, but the needle must not be allowed to advance further. The needle must not be rotated after its tip has entered the extradural space, as this increases the risk of penetration of the dura.

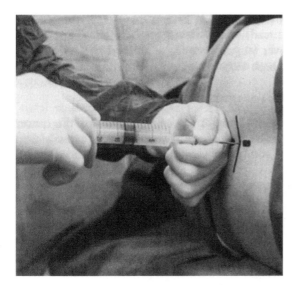

Fig 25.8 Loss-of-resistance technique to identify the extradural space. See text for details.

Single-dose technique

The syringe containing local anaesthetic is connected to the extradural needle, and after aspiration a test dose is administered to detect intravascular or subarachnoid placement. After an appropriate pause, the remainder of the solution is injected at a rate not exceeding 10 ml.min^{-1} while verbal contact is maintained with the patient.

Catheter insertion

An extradural catheter should pass freely through the needle into the extradural space. If the catheter does not thread easily, the needle should be repositioned, as forcing the catheter into the extradural space makes intravascular placement more likely. When a sufficient length of catheter (2–3 cm) is in the space, the needle is carefully withdrawn over the catheter. After ensuring that there is no flow of blood or CSF down the catheter, the hub is attached, and an aspiration test performed; if blood or CSF is obtained, the catheter should be reinserted in an adjacent space. A filter is connected and a test dose given. If this is satisfactory, the catheter is fixed to the patient's back with adhesive strapping and the main dose is administered.

Factors affecting spread

Extradural spread is variable and the initial dose depends on the clinical situation. The volume of solution has a relatively minor effect on spread, and increasing the dose of local anaesthetic is more likely to prolong the duration of the block than to increase spread. Posture has a minimal effect on spread, but patients who are pregnant or aged over 60 years may have an increased likelihood of a high block with a given dose of local anaesthetic.

Factors affecting onset

Onset time is reduced by increasing the concentration of the local anaesthetic and by the addition of adrenaline 1 : 200 000.

Factors affecting duration

The choice of local anaesthetic agent has a major effect on the duration of anaesthesia. The concentration of the drug also has an effect; the higher concentrations of bupivacaine produce a more prolonged block. To some extent this is a reflection of increased dose, which is known to increase the duration of anaesthesia. The addition of adrenaline 1:200 000 to lignocaine increases duration.

Agents

Lignocaine. This drug is used in concentrations of 1.5–2% with or without adrenaline 1 : 200 000. Without adrenaline, the duration of action is approximately 1 h; a duration of approximately 2–2.5 h may be expected when solutions containing adrenaline are used.

Bupivacaine. This agent is available in concentrations of 0.25%, 0.5% and 0.75%. The 0.75% concentration is no longer recommended for obstetric use. Increasing the concentration results in a faster onset, a denser block, more profound motor block (and therefore muscle relaxation) and increased duration of anaesthesia. A block lasting more than 4 h may be achieved with 0.75% solution. The addition of adrenaline 1 : 200 000 prolongs analgesia with 0.75% bupivacaine; the block may last for 6–8 h.

Complications

Intraoperative

1. Dural tap. The incidence should be less than 0.5% in experienced hands. It usually occurs with the needle rather than the catheter and is immediately obvious because of the free flow of CSF. Puncture of the dura with a large extradural needle leads to a high incidence of headache. If this occurs, extradural block should be instituted at an adjacent space, and 0.9% saline 40 ml.h^{-1} should be infused extradurally for 36 h after surgery or labour to reduce the likelihood of headache. Simple analgesics may suffice if headache occurs; if not, an extradural blood patch should be performed. Accidental total spinal anaesthesia (see below) is rare because the dural tap is usually obvious.

2. Total spinal anaesthesia. This may occur if the large volume of solution used for extradural anaesthesia is injected into the subarachnoid space. The consequences may be:
   a. Profound hypotension.
   b. Apnoea, unconsciousness and dilated pupils secondary to local anaesthetic action on the brain stem.

Paralysis of the legs should alert the physician to the possibility of subarachnoid injection. When using a test dose, motor function should be tested by asking the patient to raise the whole leg and not merely to wiggle the toes; movement of the toes may not be abolished for 20 min after SAB, if at all. It should be noted that relatively large volumes of local anaesthetic solution, e.g. 10 ml of bupivacaine 0.25%, may be injected into the subarachnoid space without total spinal anaesthesia occurring.

Provided that skilled resuscitation is undertaken rapidly, a total spinal should be followed by complete recovery. Appropriate personnel and equipment should be present before extradural analgesia is instituted and whenever top-up injections are administered.

3. Massive extradural block and subdural block. A very high block may occur in the absence of subarachnoid injection. This may be associated with Horner's syndrome.

4. Intravenous toxicity (see Chapter 14).

5. Hypotension.

6. Shivering.

7. Nausea/vomiting. This may result from hypotension or visceral manipulation in the awake patient.

Postoperative

1. Headache following dural tap.

2. Extradural haematoma. The spinal canal acts as a rigid box and an expanding haematoma within the canal compresses the spinal cord, resulting in loss of neurological function unless the compression is relieved surgically at a very early stage. Decompression within 6 h is completely effective in virtually all patients, but after 12 h is almost totally ineffective.

3. Neurological complications.

Anticoagulants and SAB or extradural anaesthesia

1. *Oral anticoagulants.* Anticoagulation should be stopped at an appropriate time before surgery if SAB or extradural anaesthesia is planned. The degree of anticoagulation most appropriate for the patient depends on a balance between the risk of withholding anticoagulation and the nature of the surgery, in particular the associated risk of bleeding.

2. *Platelets.* The platelet count should ideally be in excess of 150×10^9 litre^{-1}.

3. *Heparin.* The half-life of heparin given i.v. is 58–160 min, depending on dose. When given s.c. blood concentrations vary widely; in some patients plasma concentrations are in the anticoagulant range. At present it is regarded as imprudent to use SAB or extradural analgesia with 'minihep' regimens.

4. *Intraoperative heparinization.* Extradural analgesia and SAB offer advantages for major vascular surgery but the routine use of heparin introduces the theoretical risk of haemorrhage if an extradural catheter is in place. The precise risk is unknown, as prospective trials would require in excess of 10 000 cases. Some large series (3000 patients) have been conducted under extradural analgesia without haematoma formation.

Caudal anaesthesia

Caudal block involves injection of local anaesthetic into the extradural space through the sacral hiatus to obtain anaesthesia of sacral and coccygeal nerve roots. Injection of very large volumes to obtain anaesthesia of lumbar and thoracic roots is seldom practised in adults because there is a high incidence of side-effects and failure to achieve a sufficiently high block. With appropriate volumes, caudal blockade affects the lower limbs infrequently, does not cause sympathetic blockade and has a low risk of dural puncture. The anatomy is variable and difficulty is experienced in approximately 5% of subjects.

Indications

Caudal anaesthesia is suitable for perineal operations, e.g. haemorrhoidectomy. Regional anaes-

thesia for circumcision is better achieved with a penile block.

Method

Caudal blockade may be performed with the patient in the prone position, but the left lateral position is usually more acceptable to the patient. Palpation down the sacral spine leads to the depression of the sacral hiatus at S5, flanked by the sacral cornua, through which the needle is inserted. A 21-gauge hypodermic needle is introduced through skin and sacrococcygeal ligament in a cephalad direction at 45° to the skin (Fig. 25.9). When the membrane is penetrated, the needle hub is depressed toward the natal cleft, and the needle inserted 2–3 mm along the sacral canal; it must be remembered that the dura may extend to S3. Lignocaine 2% with or without adrenaline or bupivacaine 0.5% are suitable agents. In an adult, 10 ml of solution blocks anal sensation consistently.

In conjunction with light general anaesthesia, caudal anaesthesia provides smooth operating conditions and good postoperative analgesia. With this combined technique it is preferable to perform caudal block before induction of general anaesthesia because:

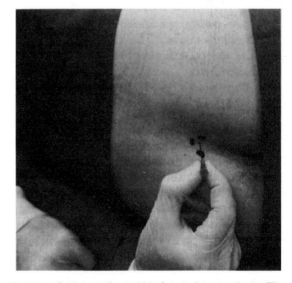

Fig 25.9 Initial needle position for caudal anaesthesia. The sacral hiatus is marked.

1. The patient does not need to be lifted while anaesthetized.
2. Subperiosteal injection is reported by the patient.
3. Accidental i.v. injection may be detected before the full dose is given.

Avoidance of complications

Misplaced needle. Injection into subcutaneous tissue causes a swelling with fluid, or surgical emphysema with 2–3 ml of air. Intraosseous or subperiosteal injection results in marked resistance to injection. Penetration of rectum and fetal head (in obstetric practice) have been reported but should not occur if the technique is performed carefully.

Dural tap. This is rare, but the procedure should be abandoned if CSF is aspirated.

PERIPHERAL BLOCKS

Head and neck blocks

These are mostly specialized blocks which are used in ophthalmic and plastic surgery. Only the technique of local anaesthesia for awake intubation is described here. Blocks used in ophthalmic surgery are discussed in Chapter 28.

Awake intubation

This may be the safest option in a patient with upper airway obstruction or a history which suggests difficulty with intubation. Sedation with midazolam or a combination of fentanyl and droperidol is desirable if this is not likely to exacerbate airway obstruction. A fibreoptic or rigid technique of laryngoscopy may be employed, but considerable experience is necessary with the former.

The patient sucks a benzocaine lozenge, or the mouth and pharynx are sprayed with lignocaine 1%. The laryngoscope blade and tube are smeared with 4% lignocaine gel. This may suffice in sick patients, but in robust subjects a cricothyroid injection is necessary. A 25-gauge needle is advanced through the cricothyroid membrane (Fig. 25.10) and air is aspirated to confirm the position. Two millilitres of lignocaine 2% are injected and the

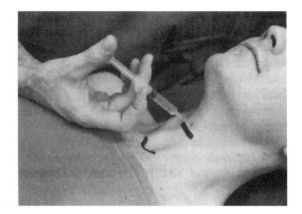

Fig 25.10 Cricothyroid injection. The sternal notch and cricoid cartilage are marked.

needle is withdrawn immediately. A vigorous cough results and spreads the solution. The total dose of lignocaine must be kept as low as possible because absorption from mucous membranes is rapid.

Upper limb blocks

The upper limb is well-suited to local anaesthetic techniques, as it is possible to block almost the whole arm with a single injection. Percutaneous approaches to the brachial plexus were first described in 1911, but approaches based on the concept of a sheath surrounding the brachial plexus are more effective.

Anatomy of the brachial plexus

The nerve supply of the upper limb is mainly derived from the brachial plexus, which is formed from the anterior primary rami of the fifth to eighth cervical and first thoracic nerve roots. The roots of the plexus divide repeatedly and recombine to form trunks, divisions, cords and terminal nerves (Fig. 25.11). The roots emerge from the intervertebral foramina and combine into three trunks above the first rib. Each trunk separates above the clavicle into anterior and posterior divisions; anterior divisions supply the flexor structures of the arm and posterior divisions the extensor structures. The divisions recombine into three cords, which surround the second part of the axillary artery behind the pectoralis minor and then form the terminal nerves (Fig. 25.12).

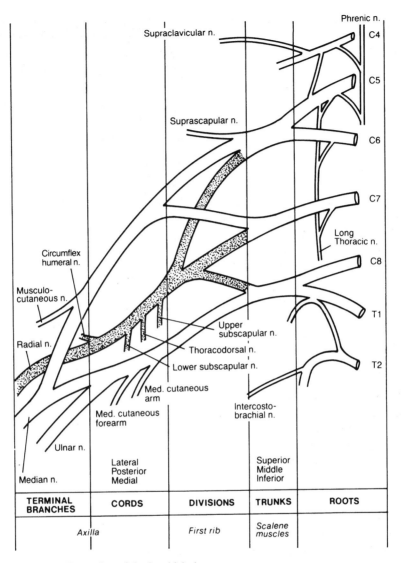

Fig 25.11 Formation of the brachial plexus.

The roots lie between the anterior and middle scalene muscles and are invested in a sheath, derived from the prevertebral fascia, which splits to enclose the scalenes. This fascial covering extends into the axilla and causes solution injected anywhere within the sheath to spread along the line of the plexus. The cutaneous and deep nerve supplies of the upper limb are depicted in Figure 25.13.

Part of the cutaneous nerve supply of the upper limb is not derived from the brachial plexus; the upper medial part of the arm is supplied by the intercostobrachial nerve (T2) and has to be blocked separately if a tourniquet is to be used for a prolonged period. The reader is referred to standard texts for a more detailed anatomical description.

Axillary block

Positioning. The patient lies supine with the arm to be blocked abducted to no more than 90° and the elbow bent to 90° (Fig. 25.14). Further abduction with the hand placed behind the

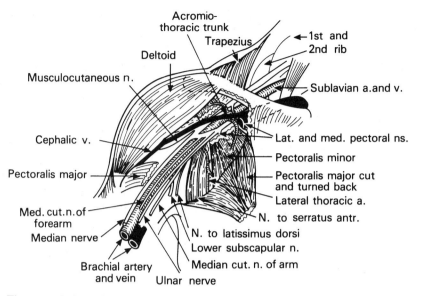

Fig 25.12   Relationship of the brachial plexus to adjacent structures.

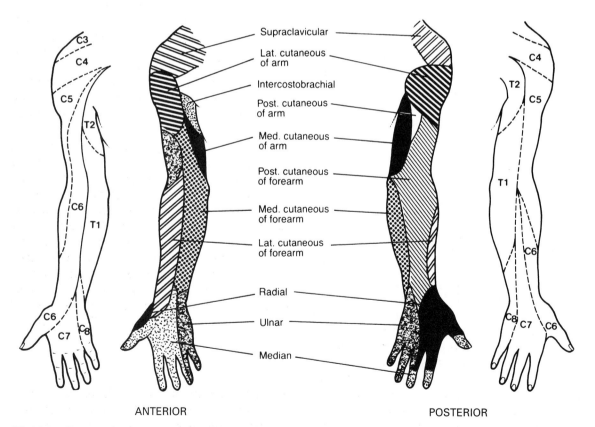

Fig 25.13   Dermatomal innervation of the upper limb. Outer: innervation of the skin. Inner: innervation of deep structures.

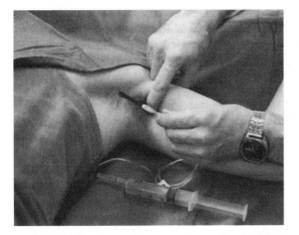

Fig 25.14 Correct position and approach for axillary block. The axillary artery is marked.

head is convenient but the axillary vessels become stretched and distorted, and performance of the block is more difficult.

Method. The axillary artery is palpated and followed as far medially as possible. A skin wheal is raised with local anaesthetic at this point just above the palpating finger. A short-bevelled block needle is introduced through this wheal after puncturing the skin with a standard 19-gauge needle. A nerve stimulator is attached and the needle is directed towards the apex of the axilla at an angle which places it alongside, but does not penetrate, the axillary artery. A click may be felt as the needle enters the sheath. Stimulation causes flexion or extension at the wrist or elbow. When this is produced by a suitably low current, the local anaesthetic is injected.

Forty millilitres of solution are required in an adult to achieve consistent blockade of the musculocutaneous and axillary nerves which leave the sheath at the level of the coracoid process. Digital pressure should be applied just distal to the needle during and immediately after injection to promote proximal flow of solution; a venous tourniquet is ineffective for this purpose. After completion of injection, the arm should be returned to the patient's side and digital pressure maintained. This manoeuvre may allow further spread of local anaesthetic beyond the humeral head.

The intercostobrachial nerve is blocked using 5 ml of solution. This can be performed without further skin puncture by redirecting the needle in the subcutaneous tissues around the medial side of the arm.

Disadvantages and complications. The onset time may be as long as 30–40 min. If the musculocutaneous nerve is not blocked, there is no analgesia on the lateral border of the arm. Puncture of the axillary artery is rarely a problem, but may lead to haematoma formation or inadvertent intravascular injection. The block should not be abandoned if the axillary artery is punctured; local anaesthetic solution is injected after penetrating the posterior wall of the artery and performing a careful aspiration test. Nerve damage occurs rarely, and usually results from malposition of the anaesthetized limb or failure to recognize a compression syndrome postoperatively.

Supraclavicular block

Supraclavicular approaches to the brachial plexus are favoured by many anaesthetists and the relatively recent description by Winnie (1984) of the subclavian perivascular approach has increased the safety of this technique.

Advantages. Onset time may be as short as 10–15 min, analgesia of the whole arm is more likely and 25–30 ml of solution is sufficient in an adult.

Disadvantages. The risk of pneumothorax is always present, but is very small in experienced hands. Phrenic nerve paralysis is probably common, but is usually asymptomatic. However, axillary block is the method of choice if there is diminished respiratory reserve. If bilateral blocks are intended, one should be performed by the axillary route. Recurrent laryngeal nerve block may result in hoarseness. Sympathetic block is relatively common, and results in Horner's syndrome. Subarachnoid or extradural spread of local anaesthetic solution is possible, but rare.

Interscalene block

This is the highest approach to the brachial plexus and may be the most suitable block for proximal procedures on the arm. Block of the C8 and T1 roots may prove difficult, and this approach is therefore less suitable for hand surgery. Complications are similar to those for supraclavicular blocks. Vertebral artery puncture and direct intraspinal injection are also possibilities.

Agents

Lignocaine or prilocaine 1.5–2% with or without adrenaline 1: 200 000 or bupivacaine 0.375–0.5% are suitable. The more dilute solutions are necessary when larger volumes are required.

Blocks in the trunk

Intercostal and paravertebral blocks have potentially important roles in abdominal and thoracic surgery, but there is a significant risk of pneumothorax when they are performed by unskilled personnel. Paravertebral block is a relatively difficult procedure. These methods are only suitable for the more experienced anaesthetist and are not considered further here.

Field block for inguinal hernia repair

The main nerves which supply the groin are the subcostal (T12), iliohypogastric (L1) and ilioinguinal (L1). Their blockade produces good postoperative analgesia, but supplementary infiltration, especially around the internal ring and hernial sac, is usually necessary during surgery if this is the only anaesthetic employed.

A needle is inserted 1.5 cm medial and inferior to the anterior superior iliac spine. Using a regional block needle the external oblique aponeurosis is readily appreciated as the needle is advanced. 15 ml of local anaesthetic are injected deep to the aponeurosis, down to the inner surface of the ilium between the abdominal muscle layers. A further 5 ml of solution are deposited superficial to the external oblique aponeurosis medially from this point. Bupivacaine 0.5% is a suitable agent for postoperative analgesia.

Local infiltration is employed routinely as the sole anaesthetic in some centres and may be the method of choice in the unfit patient or in the day-case unit, but only when surgeons are experienced with this technique.

Penile block

The dorsal nerves to the penis are derived from the pudendal nerves and are blocked with 5–10 ml of local anaesthetic solution injected inferior to the symphysis pubis in the midline at a depth of 3–4 cm. Care must be taken to avoid intravascular injection in this area and vasoconstrictors *must not* be used. Plain bupivacaine 0.5% is suitable. The base of the penis is innervated by the genital branch of the genitofemoral nerve, which may be blocked if necessary by s.c. infiltration around the penis.

Penile block is quick and simple, produces a limited effect and is the block of choice for circumcision or other minor penile surgery such as meatotomy. It is commonly used in combination with light general anaesthesia and provides good postoperative pain relief. However, a simpler technique is to smear lignocaine jelly over the wound on a regular 4–6-hourly basis in the postoperative period.

Lower limb blocks

Lower limb blocks are practised less frequently than upper limb blocks for three reasons:

1. It is not possible to block the whole of the lower limb with one injection.
2. Subarachnoid or extradural anaesthesia may prove simpler.
3. There is an impression among anaesthetists that lower limb blocks are difficult and unreliable.

However, new approaches to the peripheral nerves of the lower limb have simplified the subject and the blocks considered below are appropriate for the junior anaesthetist.

Sciatic nerve block

Anatomy. The sciatic nerve (L4, 5, S1–3) arises from the sacral plexus, passes through the great sciatic foramen and descends in the posterior thigh to the popliteal fossa, where it divides into the tibial and common peroneal nerves. In the thigh it supplies muscles and the hip joint. The posterior cutaneous nerve of the thigh (S1–3) may run with the sciatic nerve or separate from it proximally; this nerve supplies the skin of the posterior thigh and upper calf. The tibial and common peroneal nerves, together with the saphenous nerve, supply all structures below the knee.

Method. There are four approaches to the sciatic nerve; the supine approach described by Raj is the most straightforward. After leaving the pelvis the sciatic nerve lies in a groove between the greater trochanter and the ischial tuberosity covered only by skin, subcutaneous tissue and gluteus maximus. The patient lies supine with both the hip and knee of the leg flexed to 90°. This manoeuvre stretches the nerve and holds it firmly in the groove while making the gluteus maximus thinner. After infiltration of the skin, a short-bevelled 3-in (7.5 cm) needle is inserted midway between the greater trochanter and the ischial tuberosity, at right angles to the skin (Fig. 25.15). A nerve stimulator simplifies this technique; stimulation should cause plantar or dorsiflexion of the foot.

This block has a high success rate with few complications. In combination with femoral nerve block, it is suitable for operations below the knee. The posterior cutaneous nerve is not blocked if it does not run with the sciatic.

Lignocaine 1.5–2% with or without adrenaline 1 : 200 000, prilocaine 1.5–2% or bupivacaine 0.375–0.5% are suitable agents. Fifteen to 20 ml of solution are necessary. The more dilute solutions are required when other blocks are performed concurrently.

Femoral nerve block

Anatomy. The femoral nerve (L2–4) arises from the lumbar plexus and runs between psoas and iliacus to enter the thigh beneath the inguinal ligament, 2–3 cm lateral to the femoral artery, and at a slightly greater depth. Branches of the anterior division include the intermediate and medial cutaneous nerves of the thigh and the supply to the sartorius. The posterior division supplies the quadriceps, the hip and knee joints and terminates as the saphenous nerve, which supplies the skin of the medial side of the calf as far as the medial malleolus and sometimes the medial side of the dorsum of the foot.

Method. The patient lies supine and the inguinal ligament and femoral artery are identified. The skin is anaesthetized just lateral to the femoral artery, 1 cm below the inguinal ligament. A short-bevelled needle is inserted parallel to the artery in a slightly cephalad direction (Fig. 25.16). Patellar twitching is observed when the femoral nerve is stimulated. Care should be taken not to confuse this movement with the movement obtained by direct stimulation of the sartorius. Ten to 15 ml of solution are required.

Femoral nerve block is usually combined with

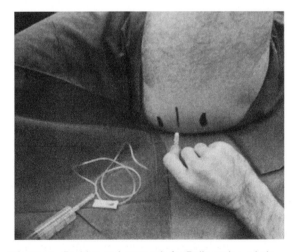

Fig 25.15 Position and approach for Raj's supine sciatic nerve block. The ischial tuberosity and medial border of greater trochanter are marked.

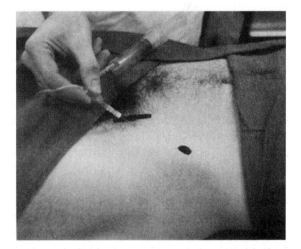

Fig 25.16 Position and approach for femoral nerve block. The anterior superior iliac spine and femoral artery are marked.

sciatic block for operative procedures. Analgesia after femoral fracture or knee surgery may be satisfactory with femoral nerve block alone.

The inguinal perivascular technique of lumbar plexus anaesthesia (three-in-one block) provides anaesthesia in the distribution of the femoral, lateral cutaneous and obturator nerves from a single injection and is an extension of the femoral nerve block technique. Twenty to 30 ml of solution are necessary and digital pressure is applied below the needle to encourage cephalad spread of the solution between iliacus and psoas.

Suitable local anaesthetic agents for femoral or three-in-one block are the same as for sciatic nerve block.

Mid tarsal block

In comparison with the traditional ankle block, mid-tarsal block has the advantages of clear landmarks, a supine position and reliability. If performed after induction of light general anaesthesia, it provides good postoperative analgesia and is ideal for operations such as removal of metatarsal heads.

Anatomy. Five nerves supply the forefoot. The medial and lateral plantar nerves are the terminal branches of the tibial nerve and enter the foot posterior to the medial malleolus; they supply deep structures within the foot and all of the sole. The common peroneal nerve divides into deep and superficial branches; the deep peroneal nerve supplies the web space between first and second toes, and the superficial branch supplies the dorsum of the foot. The saphenous nerve may supply a variable area of skin on the medial side of the dorsum of the foot. The sural nerve is a branch of the tibial nerve; it runs posterior to the lateral malleolus and supplies skin over the lateral side of the foot and fifth toe.

Method. The posterior tibial artery is palpated as far distally as possible. Injection of 3 ml of local anaesthetic to each side of it, below deep fascia, blocks medial and lateral plantar nerves. Injection of 2 ml of local anaesthetic to each side of the dorsalis pedis artery, below deep fascia, blocks the deep peroneal nerve. The saphenous, superficial peroneal and sural nerves are blocked by s.c. infiltration at the level of the ankle joint in a line

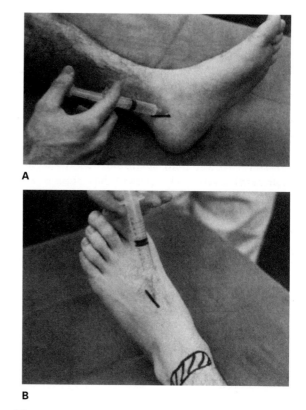

Fig 25.17 Mid tarsal block. The posterior tibial and dorsalis pedis arteries are marked. The area of subcutaneous infiltration is outlined.

extending from a point anterior to the medial malleolus to a point posterior to the lateral malleolus as for a classical ankle block (Fig. 25.17). A complete block of the foot requires 15 ml of solution; bupivacaine 0.375–0.5% is most suitable for postoperative analgesia. It is probably advisable to avoid this block when the circulation to the foot is impaired.

Special situations

Paediatric techniques

Most blocks employed in adult practice are suitable for use in children, but because of the nature of most paediatric surgery and the understandable difficulties that may be experienced with patient co-operation, only a limited number of techniques are commonly used. Many of these are used for postoperative analgesia and are performed after induction of light general anaesthesia; they should only be performed by experienced anaesthetists.

The disposition of local anaesthetic agents in children differs from that in adults. Recent work suggests that, in children of less than 1 year of age, and particularly in the neonate, very high plasma concentrations of local anaesthetic may ensue after standard doses based on weight. In children over 1 year of age, plasma concentrations are consistently lower than would be expected from adult data.

Agents and doses for paediatric blocks are shown in Table 25.5.

Topical anaesthesia

The introduction of Emla (eutectic mixture of local anaesthetics) cream allows anaesthesia of intact skin. The cream must remain in contact with the skin for at least 1 h and is held in place with an occlusive dressing. This technique is particularly useful before venepuncture in children.

Table 25.5 Agents and doses of local anaesthetics used in paediatric practice

Caudal anaesthesia
0.25% Bupivacaine

0.5 ml.kg^{-1}	Sacral block
1.0 ml.kg^{-1}	Low thoracic block

0.19% Bupivacaine (three parts bupivacaine 0.25% : one part saline)

1.25 ml.kg^{-1}	Mid thoracic block

Penile block
0.5% Bupivacaine *plain*

Body weight	Dose
2.5 kg	0.5 ml
10 kg	1.0 ml
20 kg	2.0 ml
40 kg	4.0 ml

Axillary block
0.25% Bupivacaine

Body weight	Dose
10 kg	6 ml
20 kg	12 ml
30 kg	18 ml
40 kg	24 ml

FURTHER READING

Arthur D S, McNicol L R 1986 Local anaesthetic techniques in paediatric surgery. British Journal of Anaesthesia 58: 760

Cousins M J, Bridenbaugh P O 1980 Neural blockade in clinical anesthesia and management of pain. Lippincott Philadelphia

Ellis H, Feldman S 1983 Anatomy for anaesthetists, 4th edn. Blackwell Scientific Publications, Oxford

Eriksson E 1979 Illustrated handbook in local anaesthesia. Lloyd-Luke, London

Murphy T M, Fitzqibbon D 1996 Local anaesthesia techniques. In: Aitkenhead A R, Jones R M (eds) Clinical Anaesthesia. Churchill Livingstone, Edinburgh, pp. 557–593

Sharrock N E, Waller J F, Fierro L E 1986 Midtarsal block for surgery of the forefoot. British Journal of Anaesthesia 58: 37

Wildsmith J A W, Armitage E N 1993 Principles and practice of regional anaesthesia, 2nd edn. Churchill Livingstone, Edinburgh

Winnie A P 1984 Plexus anesthesia, vol I. Perivascular techniques of brachial plexus block. Churchill Livingstone, New York

26. Anaesthesia for gynaecological, genitourinary and orthopaedic surgery

Of the many surgical specialties encountered by the trainee anaesthetist, gynaecological, genitourinary and orthopaedic surgery are often chosen as a testing ground for the novice.

When first exploring the world of anaesthesia for specialty surgery, it is important to remember some rules which apply equally to all these areas.

1. Minor surgery does not mean minor anaesthesia – procedures such as D & C or cystoscopy require a very carefully managed anaesthetic.

2. Know your operation – it is impossible to prepare a proper anaesthetic plan without knowing something about the procedure to be performed. If in doubt, ask.

3. Never allow yourself to be hurried. A long list of short procedures may tempt the anaesthetist to cut corners in order to increase throughput, especially if encouraged by an enthusiastic surgeon. Nowhere is the old adage, 'more haste, less speed' more appropriate than in the field of anaesthesia for minor surgery.

Posture

A common feature of the specialties covered by this chapter is that many of the procedures require postures other than the standard supine position. Whatever posture is to be assumed for surgery, it is important that anaesthesia is induced with the patient in the supine position and that at the end of surgery the patient is either lying laterally or can rapidly be turned on to one side. These precautions are necessary so that, should regurgitation of stomach contents occur at induction or recovery, steps can be taken immediately to minimize the risk of aspiration.

Full lithotomy or Lloyd-Davies positions are most commonly used for gynaecology and urological surgery. Both postures involve flexion and abduction of the hips and flexion at the knees, more pronounced in lithotomy. When these postures are to be used, it is important to ensure at the preoperative visit that there is no limitation of movement of these joints, particularly caused by osteoarthritis in the older patient. Pre-existing lumbar back pain may be worsened by extended periods in the lithotomy position and a small lumbar support may be used to maintain the lumbar lordosis. During positioning, the assistant pulls the patient down the table before elevating the legs. The anaesthetist should support the patient's head carefully and ensure that there is sufficient slack in the hoses of the breathing system to avoid accidental extubation or disconnection. The arms should not be forgotten as they may fall from the table as the patient is moved. Legs should be elevated and lowered together to avoid stressing the spinal ligaments. In the lithotomy position, the legs are placed inside the supporting poles; this may result in the common peroneal nerve being compressed against the head of the fibula. To avoid this and the resultant foot drop, the poles must be well padded and the legs should not be overabducted. Finally, the sacrum should be supported and padded.

Head-down tilt or Trendelenburg position is often used, with or without the legs elevated, for laparoscopic procedures. Positioning the patient in this way rarely causes problems although, if supports are used against the shoulders to prevent the patient sliding, these should be well padded to avoid damage to the accessory nerve. In both lithotomy and Trendelenburg positions, there is a tendency to splinting of the diaphragm by abdominal contents, making spontaneous ventilation more difficult, especially over prolonged periods. This situation is considerably worsened if pneumoperitoneum has been induced for laparoscopy; this, along with the increased risk of regurgitation of stomach contents, is discussed later in this chapter. Venous return to the heart is, of course, enhanced in these postures. This may become relevant when the legs are lowered at the end of an operation during which fluid replacement has been inadequate; hypovolaemia may suddenly become manifest as a falling blood pressure and tachycardia, especially if subarachnoid or extradural anaesthesia has been used. This is particularly common during transurethral resection of the prostate (TURP) and is discussed later.

The lateral position is often employed during hip or renal surgery. Turning a patient requires skilled assistance. The anaesthetist should concern himself primarily with controlling the head during positioning. Once positioned, attention should be paid to the head to avoid excessive lateral flexion of the neck, to the lower arm and leg to minimize compression, to the upper arm and leg to prevent them flopping across the front of the patient and to the hips and shoulders to ensure that the thoracolumbar spine is not stressed. Stability is often a problem in this position and supports may be used against the front and back of the pelvis. These should be well padded and care should be taken in male patients to ensure that the penis is not trapped between the support and the abdominal wall. Spontaneous breathing is quite possible in the lateral position, although it is difficult to maintain an airtight seal with a face mask and a laryngeal mask airway should therefore be used if there is no indication for tracheal intubation.

The prone position may be used during renal and spinal surgery. Although spontaneous breathing is possible, positive pressure ventilation is strongly recommended and an armoured tracheal tube should be used to minimize the risk of kinking. The tube should be fixed very firmly to the face with a fabric tape such as Elastoplast and the eyes taped shut and padded. Confirmation of the position of the tube should be sought by auscultation and with a carbon dioxide analyser whenever the posture is altered after intubation. Patients should be 'log rolled' on to the operating table from the trolley with at least two people to roll and two to catch. The anaesthetist should control the head throughout to prevent excessive rotation. Rolling is best done with as few wires and tubes attached to the patient as possible, as tangling is easily achieved and sorted out only with difficulty. Monitoring should be removed (for as brief a time as possible) and the breathing system should be disconnected briefly to avoid traction on the tracheal tube.

Bolsters should be used to support the upper chest and pelvis; this leaves the abdominal wall uncompressed and thus allows easy diaphragmatic excursion. A further bolster should be placed under the ankles to prevent forced extension and pressure on the dorsal aspect of the feet. The head should be turned gently to one side to allow clearance for the tracheal tube and to prevent pressure on the eyes. Finally, the arms may be left at the sides but are often best managed by rotating them forward at the shoulder before bringing them to lie at either side of the head on an arm board. The elbows should be flexed to prevent overabduction of the shoulder and padded to protect the vulnerable ulnar nerve.

GYNAECOLOGY

The patient

Patients who present for gynaecological surgery tend to be younger and fitter than those encountered in many other specialties. However, those undergoing continence and cancer surgery are particularly likely to be elderly and, of course, intercurrent disease can be a problem in any patient.

A preoperative visit is particularly important as these patients are especially likely to be apprehensive about their forthcoming surgery. For many, it will be their first experience of anaesthesia and surgery. A reassuring chat with a sympathetic anaesthetist is often greatly appreciated and can often obviate the need for heavy premedication before minor surgery.

There is considerable evidence to show that women undergoing gynaecological surgery are more prone than the general population to suffer from postoperative nausea and vomiting (PONV). Any previous history of PONV or significant travel sickness should be sought and susceptible individuals should be given an antiemetic prophylactically. Even after minor surgery, particularly involving dilatation of the cervix, it is a wise precaution to prescribe postoperative antiemetic drugs.

Many gynaecological procedures are carried out to treat menorrhagia and preoperative measurement of haemoglobin concentration should therefore be mandatory in all but the most straightforward of cases. Older women undergoing pelvic surgery are especially prone to deep venous thrombosis (DVT) and prophylactic measures should be used. Pre- and postoperative low-dose heparin and graduated compression stockings are commonly used to prevent DVT. Many of the younger patients take the oral contraceptive pill and this increases the risk of DVT in proportion to the oestrogen content of the preparation. Current advice is that oral contraceptives containing oestrogen should be stopped 6 weeks preoperatively if pelvic or lower limb surgery is to be carried out; this precaution is unnecessary if minor gynaecological procedures such as D&C or laparoscopic sterilization are to be performed.

Minor procedures

Dilatation and curettage (D&C), evacuation of retained products of conception (ERPOC) and suction termination of pregnancy (STOP) are minor operations performed in the lithotomy position and last usually for 5–15 min. Dilatation of the cervix is a surgically stimulating procedure and anaesthesia must be surprisingly deep to prevent movement and/or laryngospasm. This is particularly true during D&C and STOP, where the cervix must be dilated from a fully closed state. The need for a brief period of deep anaesthesia may present a problem, as all currently used volatile agents cause dose–dependent uterine relaxation; this may result in persistent vaginal bleeding after ERPOC or STOP. Inspired concentrations equivalent to 1.5 MAC or less have little effect on the uterus when used for 20 min or less, but many anaesthetists employ small

boluses of an induction agent to maintain anaesthetic depth for these procedures. Propofol is an ideal agent for this purpose but should be used with caution in ERPOC if significant haemorrhage has occurred.

Towards the end of ERPOC and STOP procedures, the gynaecologist usually asks for a uterine stimulant to be administered. Syntocinon is normally used and may cause a brief episode of hypotension. Ergometrine is a more powerful stimulant, but is best avoided unless absolutely necessary as it is a potent emetic and may cause vomiting as the anaesthetic is lightened, potentially very hazardous if the patient is still in the lithotomy position. Ergometrine can cause a significant increase in blood pressure due to vasoconstriction and is therefore contraindicated in patients with pre-existing cardiovascular disease.

Cervical dilatation may cause postoperative pain although, if a short-acting opioid has been used intraoperatively, a non-steroidal drug such as diclofenac or ketorolac usually suffices. Emergence from anaesthesia may be accompanied by profound emotional upset after ERPOC or STOP and recovery staff should be prepared to deal with the patient sympathetically.

Laparoscopy

The problems of the Trendelenburg and Lloyd-Davies positions have already been alluded to but during laparoscopy they are compounded by the need to induce a pneumoperitoneum by insufflating gas (usually carbon dioxide) into the abdominal cavity. This splints the diaphragm (making ventilation more difficult), raises intragastric pressure (increasing the risk of regurgitation) and causes diffusion of carbon dioxide into the bloodstream (raising arterial $P\mathrm{CO_2}$). For these reasons, although some experienced practitioners employ a laryngeal mask during laparoscopy, tracheal intubation and IPPV are strongly recommended, especially for the novice.

Reversal of neuromuscular blockade can present a problem as a quick gynaecologist can complete laparoscopic examination or sterilization within 15 min. A moderate dose of atracurium or vecuronium is appropriate in these circumstances, with monitoring of neuromuscular transmission to ensure adequate reversal. Intermittent administration of suxamethonium may also be employed but is associated with potential hazards and is best left to the anaesthetist experienced in its use.

The degree of postoperative pain following laparoscopic clip sterilization often takes the novice anaesthetist by surprise and is probably due to compression of the Fallopian tubes. An opioid should be prescribed and is often required postoperatively. Concomitant non-steroidal analgesics can also be very effective.

Even in the best hands, laparoscopy may sometimes go seriously wrong. The insufflating trochar may perforate bowel, bladder or blood vessel, necessitating urgent laparotomy. Inadvertent intravascular gas insufflation results in hypotension, tachycardia and a massive increase in ventilation–perfusion mismatch which is manifest as a sudden fall in end-tidal carbon dioxide concentration. Early detection is the most important way of reducing morbidity and close attention should be paid to the monitors during insufflation. If misplacement of the insufflating needle is suspected, the surgeon should be warned immediately; nitrous oxide should be discontinued, as this diffuses into and expands the volumes of gas already in the vascular tree. Turning the patient into the left lateral position to trap gas in the right side of the heart has been suggested but is probably of limited use as, by the time the problem has been detected, the gas will have passed into the pulmonary circulation. Fortunately, carbon dioxide is absorbed rapidly by tissues and the consequences of carbon dioxide embolism are usually less serious than those associated with other gas emboli.

All the procedures so far described may be carried out as day cases. The subject of day-case anaesthesia is discussed in Chapter 30, which should be consulted in conjunction with this chapter.

Major procedures

Major pelvic and perineal procedures in gynaecology range from abdominal hysterectomy and prolapse surgery to radical vulvectomy and pelvic exenteration. The latter procedures and others used in the radical treatment of malignancy are often associated with extensive blood loss; this should be taken into account during preoperative preparation, establishment of intravenous access and decisions regarding monitoring. Blood loss should be monitored carefully and the preoperative haemoglobin concentration should be taken into account when planning replacement, as these patients often have pre-existing anaemia. Postoperative pain is often severe unless treated adequately; many experienced practitioners opt for an intraoperative combination of general and extradural anaesthesia. With adequate supervision, an extradural block may be used postoperatively but failing this, regular doses of opioids are essential, preferably given via a PCA system.

Emergency surgery

Apart from ERPOC, which has already been discussed, the commonest gynaecological emergency is ectopic pregnancy. Presentation may range from a normovolaemic patient with mild abdominal pain to a severely shocked woman with major internal haemorrhage. An ectopic pregnancy may rupture and bleed at any time and an apparently stable patient can suddenly deteriorate; the severity of this condition should never be underestimated. Crossmatched blood should be available in the operating theatre in all but the direst emergencies, as induction of anaesthesia can reveal a previously well-compensated hypovolaemia. At least one large-bore cannula should be established in a good vein and rapid sequence induction commenced with the gynaecologist standing by. If hypovolaemia is anticipated, agents such as etomidate or ketamine should be used to avoid excessive cardiac depression. In the worst cases, when major haemorrhage has resulted in a collapsed patient, tracheal intubation and surgery are part of the resuscitative process and should not be delayed whilst hopeless attempts are made to stabilize the cardiovascular system.

In many centres, it is routine practice to undertake laparoscopy in patients with a suspected ectopic pregnancy. If haemorrhage has occurred, the induction of the pneumoperitoneum may impede venous return to the heart, causing a sudden fall in blood pressure. If this occurs, the surgeon should be advised to proceed immediately to laparotomy.

Once the abdomen has been opened, it is usually not long before haemostasis is achieved and blood loss can then be replaced in a more measured fashion. The propensity for patients with gynaecological haemorrhage to develop disseminated intravascular coagulation (DIC) should not be overlooked and coagulation screens should be performed regularly until bleeding has ceased and the situation is completely under control.

Recent developments

In common with many specialties, the laser is being used more frequently in gynaecology. Strict regulations exist regarding the wearing of eye protection in an environment in which the laser is being used and these should be followed. The use of explosive anaesthetic agents should, of course, be avoided but this is rarely a problem in modern practice. The gynaecological anaesthetist does not have the concerns of colleagues in the ENT theatre, where the proximity of the laser beam to the tracheal tube can cause ignition or rupture of the cuff.

Endometrial resection is becoming a popular procedure as an alternative to hysterectomy for menorrhagia and is performed endoscopically using either diathermy or laser. Apart from the fact that patients undergoing this procedure are generally younger and fitter, there are many similarities between endometrial resection and transurethral resection of the prostate (TURP) from the anaesthetist's point of view. Unexpectedly large blood loss may occur which, because it is diluted by irrigation fluid, may be difficult to measure. Absorption of irrigation fluid may result in hyponatraemia, a decrease in serum osmolality and pulmonary oedema and hypothermia may occur due to continuous lavage with cold fluids. These problems are discussed on page 476.

In the ever-expanding subspecialty of fertility surgery, anaesthesia may be required for long laparoscopic or open procedures. In vitro fertilization (IVF) techniques call for oocyte retrieval from patients in whom ovulation has been stimulated artificially. This is performed under ultrasound control, usually transvaginally and often in conditions of subdued lighting, as fluorescent light has been shown to inhibit oocyte function. A brief anaesthetic may be required some days later for embryo insertion, after which the patient is usually recovered lying on her back with steep head-down tilt to increase the chances of successful implantation.

GENITOURINARY SURGERY

The patient

In contrast to gynaecology, the patient presenting for genitourinary surgery is typically male and elderly and frequently suffers from intercurrent illness. The most common procedures performed by urologists are cystoscopy and transurethral resection of the prostate (TURP). The cystoscopy patient is often being checked for recurrence of bladder tumour and may be attending as frequently as every 6 months. Prostatic hypertrophy is a condition of old age and is rarely symptomatic below the age of 55 years.

Patients undergoing renal surgery, and to a lesser extent those who suffer from long-term ureteric reflux or outflow obstruction, may have impaired renal function. This should be assessed carefully before operation. Renal disease may be associated with hypertension and antihypertensive treatment should be optimized before surgery. The possibility of concomitant ischaemic heart disease should be considered.

Insulin-dependent diabetics may present for renal procedures or surgery for impotence. Preoperative control should be established using a dextrose and insulin infusion on a sliding scale (see p. 680). Autonomic balance is often disturbed in this group of patients and excessive swings in blood pressure may occur during induction and surgical stimulation.

Cystoscopy

Patients who present for cystoscopy are often elderly. A long list of patients for cystoscopy, many admitted on the day of surgery and usually relaxed and blasé because of multiple previous attendances, may lull the unsuspecting anaesthetist into a false sense of security. Careful inspection of the notes is often rewarding, as previous anaesthetists will have left useful information about successful (or less successful) techniques as well as specific problems that they have encountered. Preoperative assessment should not be stinted in these patients; regular medication should have been taken, vital signs recorded and necessary preoperative investigations performed. Just because a patient was well 6 months ago does not mean that the same applies now. Premedication is rarely required for the regular attender and, if given unnecessarily, may interfere with early discharge.

Anaesthetic technique requires a level of anaesthesia deep enough to permit tolerance of urethral instrumentation but without resulting in a prolonged recovery time. Induction with propofol is ideal for fit subjects but a more cardiostable drug such as etomidate should be used for patients with cardiovascular disease. Whatever agent is used, it should be remembered that elderly patients have a slower arm–brain circulation time and often require smaller doses to induce sleep. Bolus doses should therefore be given slowly and an adequate time allowed for circulation before a further dose is administered.

It is important to avoid obstruction to expiration as this raises abdominal pressure and may interfere with bladder dilatation; consequently the laryngeal mask airway (LMA) is a very useful adjunct. A small dose of a short-acting opioid may facilitate LMA insertion. Postoperative pain is rarely a problem and simple analgesics usually suffice.

Transurethral resection of prostate (TURP)

This cystoscopic technique has all but replaced retropubic prostatectomy and the modern anaesthetist will rarely see the older operation, characterized by sudden and often torrential haemorrhage during the blunt dissection of the prostate.

TURP is not without its problems, however, the most important of which is the so-called 'TURP syndrome'. During the procedure, the operator must irrigate the bladder constantly with a solution infused at pressures of around 70 cmH$_2$O. The solution used must be non-conductive and of neutral visual density; glycine 1.5% is used most commonly but distilled water is sometimes employed. As much as 4–5 litre of this fluid can enter the circulation via the prostatic bed, the exact amount being dependent upon the pressure used for infusion, the venous pressure in the prostate, duration of operation and surgical technique; the average amount is 1–1.5 litre. Some idea of the quantity absorbed can be obtained by comparing the volume infused with the volume retrieved, but this may be very inaccurate.

The syndrome is characterized by fluid overload; this may lead to raised blood pressure, acute left ventricular failure and pulmonary and cerebral oedema. The oedema may be worsened by:

1. *Dilutional hyponatraemia.* This is pathognomonic of TURP syndrome, with sodium levels of 120 mmol.litre^{-1} or less. As well as exacerbating pulmonary and cerebral oedema, hyponatraemia may prolong the effects of non-depolarizing muscle relaxants;

2. *Haemolysis.* Although this may occur purely as a result of a fall in serum osmolality, it is more common when distilled water is used as the irrigant solution. Haemolysis may lead to anaemia, renal failure and prolonged coagulation times with persistent bleeding from the prostatic bed.

Signs and symptoms of TURP syndrome are usually detected earlier in the awake patient who may complain of difficult breathing or headache. Nausea, vomiting and confusion are also common. The first signs in the anaesthetized patient are usually increases in blood pressure and heart rate and, if IPPV is being used, an increase in airway pressures.

If TURP syndrome is suspected, the surgeon should be alerted, surgery discontinued as soon as practicable and the intravenous infusion slowed. Serum electrolyte and haemoglobin concentrations should be checked. Postoperatively, administration of a loop diuretic aids excretion of excess water. In severe cases, intravenous hypertonic saline may be infused in conjunction with careful monitoring. In milder cases, saline 0.9% should be infused until the serum sodium concentration approaches normal; glucose solutions should not be employed. Patients with pulmonary or cerebral oedema may require a period of mechanical ventilation on the intensive care unit.

Blood loss during TURP is often difficult to assess as the blood is heavily diluted by the irrigating fluid and the inexperienced anaesthetist often underestimates total losses. Generally, blood loss is related to surgical experience and duration of procedure and the anaesthetist should be guided by clinical signs, advice from experienced theatre staff and judicious haemoglobin checks, if necessary. The possibility of hypothermia resulting from the use of large volumes of cold irrigating fluid should not be overlooked.

Although no specific anaesthetic technique has ever been shown consistently to be superior, the earlier diagnosis of TURP syndrome in the awake patient probably makes subarachnoid block the method of choice. To be effective, the block should extend from the sacrum up to T10. This is best achieved by using a hyperbaric local anaesthetic solution with the patient sitting. An injection of 2.5–3.0 ml of bupivacaine 0.5% should be used. After placing the patient in the supine position, any tendency for the block not to extend high enough can be overcome by reducing the lumbar lordosis with hip flexion or by carefully introducing a degree of head-down tilt. A large intravenous preload is rarely necessary or advisable as it may increase the risk of TURP syndrome. Recent studies have suggested that the incidence of postspinal headache after TURP surgery is higher than had been suspected previously. If Quincke-type needles are to be used, then they should be 26 gauge or smaller, but it may be better and simpler to use a larger pencil point (e.g. Sprotte) needle.

If general anaesthesia is to be used, tracheal intubation and IPPV are recommended. TURP may take an hour or longer and it is difficult for an elderly, anaesthetized patient to maintain adequate spontaneous ventilation for so long in the lithotomy position. Care should be taken to avoid high airway pressures as they may result in increased bleeding from the prostatic bed.

Postoperative analgesia may be needed after TURP, particularly if the indwelling catheter irritates the raw prostatic bed. Doses of opioids should be scaled down for frail, elderly patients. Continuous bladder irrigation may be used to prevent blood clotting in the catheter; this fluid should ideally be warmed and the volumes checked regularly to ensure that large amounts are not being absorbed.

Renal surgery

Although laparoscopic techniques have been used for renal surgery, open procedures are much more common. Classically, the patient is placed in the lateral position and the operating table is 'broken', thus lowering the trunk and legs and stretching the skin over the flank. This is an extremely unnatural position and may interfere with diaphragmatic excursion and venous return. The inevitable lateral flexion of the lower thoracic and lumbar spine can cause significant postoperative backache.

Patients recovering from renal surgery are likely to have considerable pain. This is amenable to regional analgesia and either epidural or intercostal blocks are commonly used for intra- and postoperative pain relief. The intercostal block is particularly appropriate for the unilateral incision of renal surgery; 2–3 ml of bupivacaine 0.5% infiltrated beneath the inferior border of each of the lower six ribs provides excellent analgesia for up to 10 h. Pneumothorax is an ever-present risk when using this technique and may become manifest up to 24 h later; some practitioners insist on an immediate chest X-ray, although this is not helpful if collapse of the lung is delayed. It should be remembered that pneumothorax may also occur as a result of renal surgery.

Other procedures

Extracorporeal shock wave lithotripsy (ESWL) is a non-invasive technique for treatment of renal calculi and involves the use of focused ultrasound shock waves applied to a patient suspended in a water bath. The technology has now advanced to the point where the patient can tolerate the treatment with intravenous sedation and analgesia. In some units, regional analgesia, normally epidural, is still employed and general anaesthesia may occasionally be required. There are unique problems of access, monitoring and positioning; anaesthesia for this procedure is best left to an experienced anaesthetist.

Circumcision is commonly performed as a

day-case procedure, especially in children. Some form of regional block should be used for post-operative analgesia; although a caudal injection is usually effective, the accompanying motor block of the legs may delay discharge. Block of the dorsal nerve of the penis is a sensible alternative, although this may miss fibres supplying the ventral aspect of the prepuce.

ORTHOPAEDICS

The patient

A wide range of patients require orthopaedic surgery. Many patients are young and fit, but a significant proportion are not. Concomitant cardiovascular and respiratory diseases need careful preoperative assessment. Particular attention must be paid to the effects of osteo- or rheumatoid arthritis in patients with disease of the joints. Both forms of arthritis may affect the cervical spine; this may result in instability of the atlantoaxial joint, with the attendant risk of dislocation during intubation or positioning. The anaesthetist should be very wary of the patient in whom neck extension causes paraesthesiae in the arms and any doubts should lead to preoperative X-rays in flexion and extension with an expert radiological opinion. Patients with confirmed instability are best managed under regional block and tracheal intubation should be attempted only by an experienced anaesthetist, preferably with the patient awake. Other joints should be checked for range of movement, particularly those which will be affected when the patient is positioned. Systemic effects of rheumatoid arthritis such as renal and pulmonary involvement should be sought and drug therapy, particularly steroids, should be noted. Many of these patients take non-steroidal anti-inflammatory drugs and should be questioned regarding symptoms of gastric irritation. These patients often have atrophied skin with little subcutaneous fat and pressure areas may need particularly careful attention.

Management of the patient with multiple trauma is discussed elsewhere in this book (Ch. 31), but particular mention should be made of the frail, elderly (usually female) patient who presents with fractured neck of femur following a fall. There is evidence to suggest that the best outcome is achieved if these patients are operated upon within a few hours of admission and the anaesthetist may be presented with a confused and dehydrated patient with little past history available. Although excessive delay should be avoided, it is reasonable to wait until at least basic resuscitation has been performed and the results of investigations are known before proceeding to theatre. The mortality rate among these patients is high and careful attention to detail is probably the most effective method of improving the likelihood of survival.

Patients undergoing joint replacement or internal fixation are particularly prone to deep venous thrombosis and it is important that prophylaxis in the form of low-dose heparin is started before surgery.

Joint replacement

These procedures are carried out under strictly aseptic conditions and the anaesthetist should take care to observe the precautions in effect in the local unit. Operations are often carried out under a laminar flow hood with the anaesthetist and equipment outside the boundary. Prophylactic antibiotics are invariably prescribed and the anaesthetist should check that these have been given.

Hip replacement, the commonest of the joint replacement procedures, is carried out in a modified lateral position and particular care should be taken in positioning the arthritic patient. Although it is possible for these procedures to be performed under regional anaesthesia alone, the duration of the procedure, posture-related discomfort and the noise of the operation make a combination of light anaesthesia and extradural block probably the best compromise. The epidural minimizes the stress response to surgery and reduces blood loss and postoperative pain.

Blood loss during these procedures is usually enough to warrant transfusion. Patients undergoing hip replacement bleed throughout the procedure, especially when the femur and the acetabulum are being prepared; during knee replacement, a substantial volume of blood is lost at the end of the operation when the tourniquet is removed.

Postoperatively, patients who have undergone hip replacement are recovered for the first 24 h in the supine position with the legs abducted to minimize the risk of dislocation. Pain after surgery is more of a problem following knee replacement; these patients often benefit from PCA. The regular use of non-steroidal anti-inflammatory drugs has a significant sparing effect on opioid requirements.

Two topics that need further discussion with respect to joint replacement are tourniquets and bone cement.

Tourniquets

A tourniquets is commonly applied prior to surgery on the arm or leg to provide a blood-free operative field. The tourniquet should be thoroughly padded, especially in thin patients, and inflation pressure should not exceed 100 mmHg above systolic pressure (50 mmHg above systolic pressure is usually sufficient for the upper limbs). Two hours is considered an upper limit for tourniquet time; if surgery is to be prolonged beyond this time, the tourniquet should be temporarily deflated before continuing.

When regional or local anaesthesia is being used, the pressure of the tourniquet can cause considerable pain. It is important to ensure that the tourniquet site as well as the operative site is adequately blocked (see below).

The occlusion of one or more limbs by a tourniquet may cause circulatory problems. Exsanguination of the limb decreases the size of the intravascular compartment and so has a similar effect to that of a large fluid bolus. This causes blood pressure to rise and may even precipitate left ventricular failure in susceptible individuals. In practice, this rarely happens unless tourniquets are applied to both legs simultaneously. Removal of the tourniquet causes reactive hyperaemia of the affected limb and a temporary 'loss' of circulating volume. Release of a tourniquet after prolonged occlusion results in the products of anaerobic metabolism entering the circulation. The subsequent decrease in pH and increase in serum potassium concentration may cause arrhythmias in susceptible patients. Intracranial pressure may also increase; this is of importance in patients who have sustained a recent head injury.

Finally, if neuromuscular blocking agents are used in a patient with a tourniquet it is best to avoid drugs such as atracurium which degrade spontaneously. Once the preliminary dose has worn off, further boluses (although effectively paralysing the rest of the patient) will have no effect on the isolated limb, which will continue to move throughout the procedure, embarrassing the surgeon and anaesthetist alike!

Bone cement

Prosthetic joints may be fixed to natural bone with methylmethacrylate cement. Application and hardening of the cement are often accompanied by a sudden fall in blood pressure in a previously stable patient. This is noticeable particularly during insertion of cement into the femoral shaft during hip replacement. This response may be due to air embolus following the exothermic reaction of the cement with its hardener or may be a direct effect of cement particles entering the circulation. Whatever the cause, hypovolaemia should be corrected scrupulously before application of cement and blood pressure should be monitored carefully. The incidence and severity of hypotension may be reduced if the surgeon uses a vent to allow air to exit the femoral shaft during cementing.

Fractured neck of femur

Patients who require repair of a fractured neck of femur are usually very elderly and frail and management is directed primarily at early ambulation. It may be necessary to induce anaesthesia with the patient in bed.

Many anaesthetists employ achieved with spinal anaesthesia in combination with light intravenous sedation and oxygen supplementation. Following a small dose of midazolam (1 mg is usually sufficient), the patient may be turned gently into the lateral position with the affected limb uppermost. It is often easier to use a paramedian approach for the spinal needle as this avoids the frequently calcified interspinous ligaments and can be performed without optimum flexion on the part of the patient. A dose of 2–2.5 ml of bupivacaine 0.5% plain usually produces an acceptable block and further small increments of midazolam may be given during the procedure, if necessary.

General anaesthesia is an appropriate alternative. Cardiac depressant drugs should be avoided; etomidate is usually the induction agent of choice.

These patients are usually more comfortable after surgery than before; postoperative analgesia should not be excessively sedative as early mobilization is an important factor in minimizing morbidity.

Regional anaesthetic techniques

Orthopaedic surgery particularly lends itself to the use of regional blocks. Spinal and epidural anaesthesia are appropriate for lower limb surgery, but the upper limb is also very amenable to local anaesthesia. Minor procedures below the elbow include excision of ganglion, manipulation of fractured wrist and simple hand surgery. These procedures can be performed using intravenous regional anaesthesia (IVRA, Bier's block). This method is discussed more fully in Chapter 25 but several points should be stressed.

1. The safety of IVRA depends entirely upon a correctly inflated tourniquet. This should be tested before use, regularly maintained and monitored throughout the procedure.

2. Intravenous access should be established in the non-isolated arm before administration of the local anaesthetic.

3. The patient should be fully fasted.

4. At least 20 min should be allowed to pass after local anaesthetic administration before the tourniquet is deflated, even if surgery is completed very quickly.

5. Bupivacaine should *never* be used for IVRA.

IVRA is most successful when the limb has been fully exsanguinated first. Although an Esmarch bandage is commonly used, this can prove uncomfortable when treating a fracture. In this case, exsanguination is best achieved by elevating the

arm and compressing the brachial artery with the thumb while inflating the tourniquet.

The tourniquet may become uncomfortable if the procedure lasts longer than 20 min. Double cuff tourniquets are available in which the proximal cuff is used whilst establishing the block and the distal cuff inflated (over a now anaesthetized area) for the procedure itself.

For procedures above the elbow or more complex lower arm operations, a brachial plexus block may be used. The axillary approach is advocated widely but this may miss the musculocutaneous nerve which innervates the radial aspect of the forearm; tourniquet pain is also likely to be a problem. A supraclavicular or interscalene approach is more likely to result in a complete block suitable for tourniquet application.

Other procedures

Spinal surgery represents a considerable challenge to the anaesthetist. Patients often have severe kyphoscoliosis with respiratory embarrassment and may have limited neck movements or an unstable cervical spine. Sitting, knee–chest or deckchair positions may be used and deliberate hypotension is often employed to minimize bleeding. During correction of kyphoscoliosis, the patient may need to be wakened to test peripheral nerve function.

Minor orthopaedic manipulations are often carried out in the accident and emergency department. These usually involve reduction of a fracture or dislocation and may be performed after a single bolus of intravenous induction agent. It is important, however, to avoid taking shortcuts with these minor procedures. Full anaesthetic facilities must be available, the anaesthetist should have the undivided services of a trained assistant and the patient should have been fasted, allowing for delayed gastric emptying consequent upon trauma.

FURTHER READING

Azar I 1988 Transurethral prostatectomy syndrome. Abstracts of scientific papers, ASA Annual Refresher Course 126: 1

Martin J T 1978 Posturing in anesthesia and surgery. WB Saunders, Philadelphia

Roberts C J, Goodman N W 1990 Gastro-oesophageal reflux during elective laparoscopy. Anaesthesia 45: 1009

Wedel D J 1993 Orthopedic anesthesia. Churchill Livingstone, New York

27. Anaesthesia for ENT surgery

Two hundred and seventy thousand ear, nose and throat operations are performed in the United Kingdom each year, accounting for approximately 5% of the workload of an anaesthetic department. Patients are usually young and healthy and the average hospital stay is short (less than three days). Many operations are performed as day cases, thereby reducing the need for inpatient admission.

Children and young adults are frequently apprehensive and require reassurance. Some may have an atopic history which influences the choice of premedication and anaesthetic technique. Older patients may have hypertension or ischaemic heart disease and require careful preoperative assessment.

Smooth anaesthesia and a clear airway are essential as coughing and straining result in venous congestion which may persist during surgery and cause increased bleeding. Partial obstruction of the airway may lead to hypoxaemia, hypercapnia and unduly light anaesthesia.

THE SHARED AIRWAY

Special problems are caused when the airway is shared by both anaesthetist and surgeon. If bleeding is anticipated, the airway *must* be protected by the use of a tracheal tube and the oropharynx packed to obviate contamination of the larynx with blood, pus and other debris. Techniques which rely on insufflation of anaesthetic vapours to an unintubated, unprotected trachea are no longer in common use and are not described here.

Sometimes, a Boyle Davis gag may compress the tracheal tube and cause partial airway obstruction. During IPPV this is detected by a decrease in compliance and increased inflation pressure and in the spontaneously breathing patient by decreased movement of the reservoir bag.

At the end of the procedure the pack must be removed and the pharynx cleared of blood and debris before the trachea is extubated with the patient in a head-down lateral position.

TONSILLECTOMY

Each year 80 000 adenotonsillectomies are performed in the UK with a rate of 8 per 1000 children under the age of 15. This frequency is 40% of that 15 years ago. In 1968 there were 6 deaths, a mortality rate of 1 in 28 000, but this has now been reduced to less than 1 in 100 000.

It has been customary to prescribe a premedication prior to tonsillectomy. This is administered most conveniently to the younger child as a syrup (trimeprazine 1.5 mg.kg^{-1} or diazepam 0.2 mg.kg^{-1}). Many anaesthetists combine this with atropine 20 μg.kg^{-1} to a maximum of 600 μg given orally (except in hot weather) to decrease secretions intraoperatively. Increasing numbers of children are attending for surgery on the day of operation and premedication may not be practical for these children.

Most children are given an i.v. induction following the application of a patch of EMLA cream; some children, however, may prefer an inhalation induction and inhalation induction is still necessary in the child with poor venous access. Oral intubation is facilitated by suxamethonium or performed under deep inhalation anaesthesia; on occasions it may be difficult to maintain a patent airway because of respiratory obstruction produced by the enlarged tonsils.

Relaxation provided by suxamethonium may

assist the surgeon who guillotines (as opposed to dissects) tonsils before achieving haemostasis.

Analgesia should be given at the end of surgery, if none has been given previously, so that the child awakens in a pain-free state. Tracheal extubation is performed with the patient slightly head-down in a lateral position after suction has ensured that the pharynx is free from blood. The trachea may be extubated either under deep anaesthesia or when fully awake; with 'deep extubation' the anaesthetist must continue to take responsibility for protecting the airway. Postoperative vomiting occurs frequently.

Blood loss during tonsillectomy is not usually measured but may be deceptively large. Increasing numbers of children under three (15 kg) are presenting for tonsillectomy for sleep apnoea syndrome. Particular care is required in this group as blood transfusion is required after 100 ml blood loss. Many of these children should have an intravenous infusion until they are ready to take oral fluids.

The postoperative bleeding tonsil

Diagnosis is made usually on the basis of clinical signs of hypovolaemia – tachycardia, pallor and sweating. Swallowing is not uncommon, followed by vomiting of a large quantity of blood. Anaesthesia for such a child is difficult and the assistance of an experienced anaesthetist must be sought.

An i.v. infusion is essential and blood transfusion is required. After resuscitation, the patient is placed head-down in a lateral position and suction apparatus is positioned within grasp. After preoxygenation, a small dose of thiopentone (2–3 mg.kg^{-1}) is given followed by suxamethonium 1 mg.kg^{-1} and cricoid pressure applied, although this may make laryngoscopy difficult. Alternatively, a gaseous induction with halothane in oxygen may be used and pharyngeal suction and tracheal intubation undertaken under deep halothane anaesthesia. When bleeding has been controlled surgically the stomach is emptied with a nasogastric tube. At the end of the procedure the trachea is extubated with the child in a lateral position.

It should be emphasized that induction of anaesthesia with thiopentone must *never* be attempted before adequate resuscitation has been undertaken and the intravascular volume restored.

ADENOIDECTOMY

Adenoidectomy is often combined either with tonsillectomy or examination of the ears under anaesthesia. Premedication is similar to that for tonsillectomy and anaesthesia is induced either by inhalation or by the i.v. route. Oral tracheal intubation is advisable either under deep anaesthesia or facilitated by suxamethonium. A Boyle Davis gag is inserted, the adenoids are curetted and the postnasal space is packed to achieve haemostasis. After 3 min, this pack is removed, the patient is turned into the lateral position and the trachea extubated.

Increasingly adenoidectomy in the absence of tonsillectomy is being performed as a day-case procedure. For these patients rectal paracetamol may be an appropriate analgesic.

MICROLARYNGOSCOPY

The operating microscope revolutionized the treatment of laryngeal disorders. The Kleinsasser laryngoscope is supported on the chest by rests and the operating microscope allows detailed examination and assessment of the larynx.

Premedication with pethidine and promethazine has been suggested if there is no evidence of airway obstruction. The most popular technique uses a Coplan's microlaryngoscopy tube (5 mm i.d., 31 cm long, constructed from soft plastic, with a 10-ml cuff volume). Anaesthesia is induced with thiopentone followed by a non-depolarizing muscle relaxant; the vocal cords are sprayed with 3 ml lignocaine 4% to assist smooth anaesthesia and to minimize the possibility of postextubation laryngospasm. Alternatively, the cords may be 'painted' with 3% cocaine at the end of the procedure, which has the added advantage of reducing bleeding from biopsy sites. The Coplan's tube is passed either orally or nasally. The lungs are ventilated artificially with 66% N_2O in O_2 supplemented either with a volatile agent or analgesic drug. The small-diameter tube does not impede the surgeon's view and allows good access to the larynx. The cuff prevents contamination of the trachea with blood or debris.

At the end of the procedure, the pharynx is cleared with suction under direct vision, muscle relaxants are antagonized and tracheal extubation performed in a lateral position. Oxygen is administered to minimize the risk of hypoxaemia if laryngeal stridor occurs.

Other techniques used for microlaryngoscopy include:

1. Topical analgesia to the larynx with insufflation of N_2O/O_2 and halothane via a fine catheter.
2. Neuroleptanalgesia combined with topical analgesia.
3. Venturi ventilation with O_2 using a catheter and a Sanders injector. Hypnosis is maintained with increments of a rapidly metabolized induction agent.

In children, microlaryngoscopy is performed using spontaneous ventilation via an oral tracheal tube one size smaller than would be used normally. The larynx should be sprayed with a measured quantity of lignocaine in an attempt to prevent postoperative laryngospasm. Occasionally the surgeon requests that he observe the larynx without a tracheal tube in situ; in these circumstances the tube is removed during deep anaesthesia, allowing examination to take place during emergence or during Venturi ventilation via the operating laryngoscope.

LARYNGECTOMY

The incidence of carcinoma of the larynx is 3–4 per 100 000 population. Many tumours may be treated with radiotherapy and therefore surgery is relatively uncommon for this condition. Airway obstruction by tumour is the major anaesthetic problem; alcohol and smoking are aetiological factors which may influence anaesthesia.

Respiratory function should be assessed preoperatively although this is difficult to measure accurately if there is airway obstruction. Chest physiotherapy should always be prescribed since it aids clearance of secretions pre- and postoperatively.

When respiratory obstruction is present, opioid or sedative premedication should always be avoided. If awake intubation is contemplated, successful topical anaesthesia of the mouth and pharynx requires an anticholinergic agent in addition. There is a risk of mechanical obstruction on induction of anaesthesia; consequently, if an i.v. agent is used, it should be given slowly in minimal dosage until consciousness is lost. If subsequently the patient's lungs can be inflated using a face mask, suxamethonium may be given to facilitate tracheal intubation; if not, anaesthesia is deepened slowly with nitrous oxide and halothane in oxygen until laryngoscopy is possible. If there is any doubt regarding the patient's ability to maintain a patent airway after loss of consciousness, the anaesthetist must *not* use an i.v. induction even with the smallest dose of thiopentone. Instead, an inhalational technique should be used; if there is progression to severe respiratory tract obstruction, awake intubation should be employed. A selection of non-cuffed tracheal tubes should be available as the lumen of the trachea may be narrowed at the level of the cords or subglottically. Tracheal intubation may be more difficult if preoperative radiotherapy has reduced the mobility of the floor of the mouth.

Monitoring of ECG and arterial pressure should be instituted in the anaesthetic room before induction of anaesthesia, which is maintained using controlled ventilation with nitrous oxide in oxygen supplemented by a volatile agent or opioid analgesic. Induced hypotension is often used to facilitate dissection of the neck (see Ch. 36). When the larynx has been dissected free, it is important to check that a sterile tracheal tube and compatible connections are available before the trachea is divided. The patient's lungs are ventilated with 100% oxygen for 2 min, the tracheal tube is withdrawn into the larynx, the trachea is divided and a second tracheal tube is placed rapidly in the trachea and secured firmly. This tube should be positioned carefully within the shortened trachea to prevent inadvertent one-lung anaesthesia.

At the end of surgery, residual neuromuscular blockade is antagonized and the tracheal tube changed for a laryngectomy or tracheostomy tube. Adequate humidification is essential postoperatively. Enteral nutrition is provided via a nasogastric tube.

PHARYNGOLARYNGECTOMY

Pharyngolaryngectomy is performed for tumours of the postcricoid region. The pharynx and larynx are removed and the stomach mobilized and anastomosed in the neck behind the tracheostomy. There are two surgical approaches: in one, after initial laparotomy, the stomach is passed through a mediastinal tract which is formed by blunt dissection; in the other more common procedure the stomach is mobilized via a thoracoabdominal incision to be anastomosed in the neck. Thus several problems may arise:

1. Difficulty in intubation.
2. Temperature loss resulting from a large surgical incision, a prolonged operative procedure and extensive blood loss.
3. Pneumothorax if the pleura is damaged during dissection.
4. Rupture of the trachea causing difficulty in ventilation and mediastinal emphysema.

LASER SURGERY

The laser is used to strip polyps or tumours from the vocal cords accurately and with immediate control of bleeding. There are two anaesthetic problems:

1. *Damage to the tracheal tube.* It has been found that in the presence of oxygen PVC microlaryngoscopy tubes may be ignited by the intensity of the laser beam. The use of an aluminized PVC tube does not remove this threat completely. The introduction of cuffed flexible stainless steel tubes for nasal or oral use has essentially solved this problem. For added safety the cuffs should be filled with water.
2. *Retinal damage.* The DOH recommends that all personnel wear protective spectacles to prevent retinal damage.

NASAL OPERATIONS

Preparation of the nose with local anaesthetic

In 1942 Moffatt described a method of topical anaesthesia of the nose using cocaine as an alternative to spraying or packing the nose. There were three advantages of his method: minimal patient discomfort during preparation, a low risk of cocaine toxicity and a bloodless surgical field. In 1952 Curtiss simplified Moffatt's method as follows:

The patient lies supine with his head extended fully over the end of a trolley and supported by an assistant. A round-ended angulated needle is inserted with its tip directed along the floor of the nose. When the angle of the needle is reached, the tip is directed towards the roof of the nose and 2 ml of solution deposited when the tip has made contact. The procedure is repeated in the second nostril. The patient remains in this position for 10 min and is advised not to swallow any solution which may have trickled into the pharynx. Then he sits upright and spits out any residual solution.

Analgesia is produced by accumulation of cocaine in the region of the sphenopalatine ganglion, thereby blocking most of the sensory supply to the nose, including the anterior ethmoidal nerve. The columella is not affected and requires a separate injection. Arterial blood supply to the nose accompanies the nerve supply, and is therefore constricted by the cocaine, producing good haemostasis.

Preparation of the nose in this manner enables any operation to be performed and dispenses with the need to use hypotensive techniques to control surgical bleeding.

In the anaesthetized patient Moffatt's prescription can be further modified by diluting it into 20 ml of solution. 10 ml is instilled into each nostril with the head extended, after placement of a gauze throat pack. The pack holds the solution in the nose for maximum effect. This method has the advantage of requiring less precise placement of the solution.

Anaesthetic technique for nasal operations

Adequate premedication is essential and may be given either orally or i.m. A smooth induction is desirable to avoid coughing and straining. Suxamethonium or a non-depolarizing muscle relaxant may be used to facilitate tracheal intubation. The larynx is not sprayed with local anaesthetic before intubation so that full laryngeal reflexes return as soon as possible after surgery.

Anaesthesia may be maintained using either spontaneous or controlled ventilation, depending on the duration of surgery. It is important to use a non-kinking tracheal tube and to pack the pharynx with 2-inch ribbon gauze so that blood, pus or debris does not contaminate the larynx. The presence of the pack should be marked in writing on the strapping which secures the tube to remind the anaesthetist to remove it at the end of the operation.

The patient is positioned 10° head-up and all breathing system connections are checked before surgery begins. An ECG should be used to detect the presence of arrhythmias which occur commonly during operations on the face. When surgery has been completed, the pack is removed, the pharynx cleared and the patient is turned into a lateral position for tracheal extubation.

A Guedel airway is placed in position before the tracheal tube is removed to provide a patent airway in the presence of surgical nasal packing. The advent of cannulated nasal packs has improved the patient's airway, but not all procedures are suitable for these packs.

Most anaesthetics for nasal procedures are delivered via a preformed oral tracheal tube in order to remove connections from the operative field.

Epistaxis

Surgical intervention may be necessary to control bleeding from the nose and may involve packing the nose or postnasal space or ligation of the maxillary artery.

The patient is often elderly and may be hypertensive. It is essential that the blood volume is restored before induction of anaesthesia. The problems inherent in haemorrhage from the upper airway and a stomach containing swallowed blood are similar to those of the bleeding tonsil and the anaesthetic technique used is similar.

The sinuses

Bacterial infection of the paranasal sinuses occurs when the self-cleansing mechanism becomes impaired and mucus accumulates and stagnates. Antral washouts and intranasal antrostomies are performed to aid restoration of normal mucosal activity. In a Caldwell Luc operation a radical antrostomy is performed via a buccal incision above the canine tooth.

In all these procedures, the airway is protected by means of an oral tracheal tube and pharyngeal pack. Ethmoidectomy may require hypotensive anaesthesia.

Maxillectomy

Excision of the maxilla for tumour is a major procedure and hypotensive anaesthesia is used to reduce bleeding; ECG monitoring using a CM_5 lead is advisable. Accurate measurement of arterial pressure requires radial artery cannulation. A pack or obturator is inserted into the maxillectomy cavity at the end of surgery; first a mould is fashioned from a rapidly setting plastic compound in situ and additional debris may be deposited in the pharynx as a result. Usually, the patient is anaesthetized on a second occasion one week later to insert the permanent prosthesis.

EARS

Myringotomy

Examination of the ears together with myringotomy and insertion of grommets is carried out commonly in children who have secretory otitis media. This operation is increasingly performed as an outpatient. Either inhalation or i.v. induction, following the application of EMLA cream, may be used and anaesthesia is maintained with spontaneous ventilation via a face mask for myringotomy alone; if adenoidectomy is performed also, oral tracheal intubation is essential. The use of nitrous oxide increases middle ear pressure significantly, especially when combined with IPPV, and this may alter the appearance of the tympanic membrane.

Middle ear surgery

Relative hypotension is required to produce a bloodless field in the field of the microscope. Smooth anaesthesia is essential for operations on the middle ear. Coughing, straining or bucking increase venous pressure and produce oozing which may persist for some time. Premedication may be given orally. After induction of anaesthesia with thiopentone, suxamethonium is used to facilitate intubation with a non-kinking oral tracheal tube; the trachea and larynx are sprayed with lignocaine to aid tolerance of the tube. The hypertensive response to intubation may be attenuated with alfentanil. Often, sufficient reduction in arterial pressure is obtained using nitrous oxide in oxygen with halothane, enflurane or isoflurane in combination with a non-depolarizing muscle relaxant and IPPV. Small doses of a β-blocker to reduce heart rate are often effective adjuvants. A 10° head-up tilt aids venous drainage. When induced hypotension is used, ECG and accurate arterial pressure monitoring are essential. Labetolol, glyceryl trinitrin or sodium nitroprusside can be used as infusions for relative hypotension.

The middle ear is a closed cavity and nitrous oxide diffuses rapidly into the middle ear causing an increase in pressure. The maximum pressure is reached approximately 40 min after induction. There is concern that this may cause grafts to become dislodged. Such complications have led some authors to suggest that O_2/N_2 should be used in place of O_2/N_2O gas mixtures.

Bandaging the ear at the end of surgery involves movement of the head. This should be anticipated and supervised by the anaesthetist to prevent undue movement which may lead to gagging on the tracheal tube. If labyrinthine function has been disturbed, an antiemetic may be necessary to control postoperative vertigo and vomiting.

FURTHER READING

Chambers W A 1994 ENT anaesthesia. In: Nimmo W S, Rowbotham D J, Smith G (eds) Anaesthesia, 2nd edn. Blackwell Scientific Publications, Oxford

Hospital Inpatient Inquiry Series MB4, 27. DHSS Office of Population Censuses and Surveys, Welsh Office, ENT Microfiches 24, 25

Hunton J, Oswal V H 1985 Metal tube for ear, nose and throat carbon dioxide laser surgery. Anaesthesia 40: 1210

Morrison J D, Mirakhur R K, Craig H J L 1985

Anaesthesia for eye, ear, nose and throat surgery, 2nd edn. Churchill Livingstone, Edinburgh

Puttick N, Van der Walt J H 1987 The effect of premedication on the incidence of postoperative vomiting in children after ENT surgery. Anaesthesia and Intensive Care 15: 158

Van der Spek A L, Spargs P M, Norton M L 1988. The physics of lasers and implications for their use during airway surgery. British Journal of Anaesthesia 60: 709

28. Anaesthesia for ophthalmic surgery

Patients who present for eye surgery are frequently at the extreme ends of the age spectrum. Both neonatal and geriatric anaesthesia have their special problems. Repeated anaesthetics at short intervals are often necessary. The anaesthetic technique may influence intraocular pressure (IOP) and the skilled administration of either local or general anaesthesia contributes directly to the successful outcome of the surgery. Close co-operation and clear understanding between surgeon and anaesthetist are essential. Risks and benefits must be assessed carefully and the anaesthetic technique selected accordingly.

Ophthalmic surgery can be categorized into subspecialties and intraocular or extraocular procedures may be performed (Table 28.1); each has different anaesthetic requirements.

Table 28.1 Categorization of ophthalmic surgery

Ophthalmology subspecialties
Paediatric
Oculoplastic
Retinovitreous
Anterior segment
Glaucoma
Neuro-ophthalmology

Extraocular operations
Globe and orbit
Eyebrow and eyelid
Lacrimal system
Muscles
Conjunctiva
Cornea, surface

Intraocular operations
Iris and anterior chamber
Lens and cataracts
Vitreous
Retina
Cornea, full thickness

CHOICE OF ANAESTHESIA

Many ophthalmic procedures can be carried out under either local or general anaesthesia. The type of surgery and planned duration influence the choice (Table 28.2). In general, local anaesthesia is preferred for older patients. The stress response to surgery is less and complications such as post-operative confusion, nausea, vomiting and urinary retention are eliminated. Younger patients do not tolerate local anaesthesia well and are mostly managed with general anaesthesia.

CONDITIONS FOR INTRAOCULAR SURGERY

For most intraocular operations the eye must be immobile and pain-free. Except for glaucoma surgery, the pupil should be dilated and the intraocular pressure reduced.

Widespread use of the operating microscope has

Table 28.2 Preferred anaesthetic technique for common surgical procedures in ophthalmology

Local anaesthesia
Cataract
Glaucoma techniques
Minor extraocular plastic surgery
Laser dacryocystorhinostomy
Minor anterior segment procedures

General anaesthesia
Paediatric surgery
Squint surgery
Major oculoplastic surgery
Dacryocystorhinostomy
Perforating keratoplasty
Orbital trauma repair
Perforating eye injuries
Retinovitreous surgery

enabled the surgeon to place finer and stronger sutures with more precision than previously. The risk of wound dehiscence following postoperative Valsalva-type manoeuvres has been reduced.

Intraocular pressure (IOP)

There is a diurnal variation in IOP, but a mean pressure of 15 mmHg above atmospheric pressure is normal. Resting pressure greater than 22 mmHg is considered abnormal. In the presence of raised IOP, sudden reduction in pressure on incision of the globe may lead to the expression of the contents. On rare occasions, a disastrous expulsive haemorrhage may result in the loss of the entire contents of the eyeball.

Control of intraocular pressure

Factors controlling IOP are similar to those which influence intracranial pressure, as both involve manipulation of a volume contained in a semirigid container. These factors include external pressure, volume of arterial and venous vasculature (choroidal volume) and the volumes of the aqueous and vitreous humour (Fig. 28.1).

External pressure

Pressure from squeezing the eyes closed or the injection of a volume of local anaesthetic into the orbit is transmitted to the eyeball and increases the IOP. During general anaesthesia, pressure from the anaesthetic mask, retractors, etc. should be avoided.

Venous pressure

Venous congestion increases vascular volume within the eye and reduces aqueous drainage

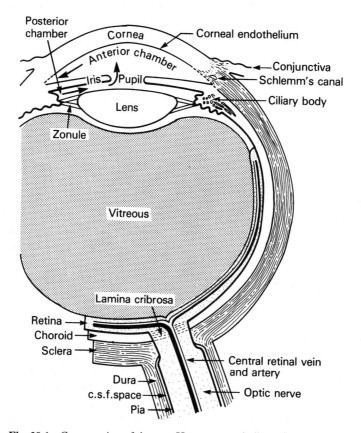

Fig. 28.1 Cross-section of the eye. Heavy arrows indicate flow of aqueous.

through the canal of Schlemm, causing an increase in IOP. During anaesthesia, venous pressure is influenced mainly by posture and transmitted intrathoracic pressure. A 15° head-up tilt causes a significant decrease in IOP.

Coughing, retching and airway obstruction cause an instant increase in venous pressure which is reflected immediately in the IOP. Intermittent positive pressure ventilation (IPPV) produces a small increase in venous pressure secondary to the elevation in the mean intrathoracic pressure, but is compensated for by the control of arterial P_{CO_2}.

Arterial blood gases

Arterial P_{CO_2} is an important determinant of choroidal vascular volume and IOP. A reduction in Pa_{CO_2} constricts the choroidal vessels and reduces IOP. Elevation of Pa_{CO_2} results in a proportional and linear increase in IOP. Increases in Pa_{CO_2} may also raise central venous pressure. Hypoxaemia produces intraocular vasodilatation and an increase in IOP.

Arterial pressure

Stable values of blood pressure within the physiological range maintain normal IOP. Sudden increases in systolic arterial pressure above the normal autoregulatory range increase choroidal blood volume and consequently IOP. Reduction in blood pressure below normal physiological levels reduces IOP, but the response is unpredictable in old age when arterial capacitance is reduced.

Aqueous and vitreous volumes

A decrease in either aqueous or vitreous volume reduces IOP. Osmotic diuretics are sometimes used to reduce vitreous volume and acetazolamide reduces the production of aqueous.

Haelon (sodium hyaluronate)

Sodium hyaluronate is now used as a soft viscous retractor during surgery. It can augment the effect of general anaesthesia by controlling vitreous bulge and compensates for small changes in IOP. Sodium hyaluronate is an expensive, large molecular weight, clear viscoelastic polysaccharide and should not be confused with the enzyme hyaluronidase. The two are incompatible. Injected by the surgeon at the time of incision, it helps to maintain the shape of the anterior chamber and the work space.

Effect of anaesthetic drugs on IOP

Premedication

Drugs used for premedication have little effect on intraocular pressure and the commonly used anxiolytic and antiemetic drugs may be used as preferred.

Induction agents

Most of the intravenous induction agents, with the exception of ketamine, reduce the intraocular pressure and can be used as indicated clinically. Ketamine is best avoided if intraocular surgery is planned.

Muscle relaxants

Suxamethonium increases intraocular pressure, with a maximal effect 2 min after injection, but the pressure returns to baseline values after 5 min. This effect is thought to be caused by the increase in tone of the extraocular muscles and intraocular vasodilatation. Pretreatment with a small dose of a non-depolarizing muscle relaxant does not obtund this response reliably. The problems involved with the use of suxamethonium in the patient with penetrating eye injury are discussed below.

Non-depolarizing muscle relaxants have no significant direct effects on IOP

Volatile anaesthetic agents

Halothane, enflurane and isoflurane all decrease intraocular pressure. Nitrous oxide has no effect on intraocular pressure in the absence of air or sulphur hexafluoride in the globe (for further explanation see the discussion on retinal surgery below).

Opioids

Opioids cause a moderate reduction in IOP in the absence of significant ventilatory depression. They contribute to postoperative nausea and vomiting and are rarely necessary for postoperative analgesia following eye surgery.

Techniques of general anaesthesia

Premedication

A short-acting benzodiazepine is frequently given orally as premedication to anxious patients, but premedication is not required in day-case patients. Benzodiazepines should be used with caution in the elderly as they may result in confusion. Premedication by injection should be avoided in children, particularly if more than one anaesthetic is required. Anticholinergic agents are generally not given with premedication. They are more likely to be needed in strabismus or retinal surgery, but can be given intravenously after induction if necessary.

Induction

Short-acting opioid analgesics such as fentanyl or alfentanil may precede induction. They reduce dose requirements of induction and maintenance agents and modify the cardiovascular response to tracheal intubation. Propofol is used widely because of its short duration of action, pleasant induction and reduced postoperative nausea. Etomidate is useful in elderly or unfit patients because of its cardiostability, IOP reduction and rapid recovery. Frequent pain on injection and involuntary movements offset these advantages. Thiopentone is a satisfactory alternative in both adults and children.

Airway management and maintenance of anaesthesia

Most anaesthetists elect to employ IPPV for intraocular surgery. Moderate hyperventilation reduces the Pa_{CO_2} and provides excellent operating conditions. Additionally, a 15° head-up tilt may be used. Breath-by-breath monitoring of the end-tidal CO_2 concentration and the use of a peripheral nerve stimulator virtually guarantee that no coughing or straining occurs while the eye is open. Less anaesthetic is used and the patient should wake up rapidly at the end of surgery. Spontaneous ventilation is not used commonly as deeper levels of anaesthesia are required. CO_2 retention, hypotension and slow recovery may result.

Tracheal intubation was used routinely for intraocular surgery until recently. Non-depolarizing muscle relaxants are required for intubation and maintenance but coughing and straining at extubation are problems for which there is no easy solution. Continuation of the volatile agent until reversal of residual neuromuscular blockade, or the use of i.v. lignocaine, have been recommended to overcome this problem.

More and more anaesthetists now use the laryngeal mask, muscle relaxants and IPPV for eye surgery. Insertion is easier and the problems associated with postoperative coughing, straining and laryngospasm are virtually eliminated. The laryngeal mask should be positioned accurately to give unobstructed ventilation. An armoured tube laryngeal mask may be preferable. Care should be taken to maintain sufficiently deep anaesthesia and muscle relaxation so that the laryngeal mask is not rejected. The laryngeal mask is unsuitable for patients at risk of aspiration; a cuffed tracheal tube should be used to protect the airway. This group includes the morbidly obese, those with gastro-oesophageal reflux and patients with hiatus hernia.

Penetrating eye injury

The anaesthetic management of the patient with a penetrating eye injury and a full stomach creates a dilemma. Rapid sequence induction with tracheal intubation is advisable but the use of suxamethonium is theoretically contraindicated as it produces an increase in IOP which could expel the ocular contents. It may be possible to delay surgery for a few hours but following trauma gastric emptying is not assured in the usual time scale. Drugs which facilitate gastric emptying such as metoclopramide may help. In choosing a muscle relaxant for tracheal intubation, the risks of further damage to the eye must be weighed against the life-threatening dangers of pulmonary aspiration. If it is anticipated that tracheal intubation will be uneventful, a large dose of non-depolarizing muscle relaxant (rocuronium may be the most appropriate for this purpose) can be substituted for suxamethonium in the usual crash induction technique. Care should be taken not to exert pressure on the injured eye with the face mask during preoxygenation. If intubation is difficult and ventilation with a face mask is not efficient, the resulting hypoxaemia and hypercapnia can cause more damage to the eye than a single dose of suxamethonium.

Anaesthetic management during surgery conforms to the pattern used for other intraocular procedures. Extubation should be performed with the patient in the lateral position and almost awake.

Retinal surgery

General anaesthesia is used for most retinal surgery. Patients are often in younger age groups and the procedures may take longer than anterior segment surgery. Patients are liable to become uncomfortable and restless if required to lie still on a hard operating table for too long. Local anaesthesia is an option which should be considered in the medically compromised patient or for retinal procedures of short duration. Cautious monitoring is needed as the oculocardiac reflex is not blocked reliably by local anaesthetic. The surgeon can readily top up the local anaesthetic if it starts to wear off.

As fundal examination, vitrectomy and laser therapy are carried out in the dark, the anaesthetist must ensure that there is sufficient lighting to conduct anaesthesia safely. Goggles *must* be worn by all theatre staff during laser therapy.

Traction on the extraocular muscles and distortion of the eyeball by banding with a scleral buckle can cause severe vagal bradycardia or even asystolic cardiac arrest. The oculocardiac reflex is more pronounced in young people. Prophylactic atropine or glycopyrrolate may be needed. The surgical stimulus must be suspended until the heart rate has recovered. An audible heart rate monitor which the surgeon can hear is useful.

Towards the end of a retinal detachment procedure, the surgeon often injects a bubble of sulphur hexafluoride (SF_6) or perfluoropropane (C_3F_8) into the eye to tamponade the retina. Some minutes before this is done, the anaesthetist must discontinue administration of nitrous oxide but continue to anaesthetize the patient with air, oxygen and additional volatile agent. The use of a continuous intravenous propofol technique is a suitable alternative. If the nitrous oxide is not eliminated beforehand, it equilibrates with the tamponading gas during the operation but at the end of the anaesthetic the nitrous oxide diffuses out and reduces the pressure in the gas bubble. The inhaled anaesthetic gas mixture at the time of injection of SF_6 or C_3F_8 should approximate as nearly as possible to normal room air. As soon as there is sufficient recovery from anaesthesia, the patient is turned to the prone position so that the bubble exerts upward pressure on the area of the retinal detachment.

The use of silicone oil as a heavy medium to roll the retina back into position following specific types of detachment or giant retinal tears has largely eliminated the need for 360° longitudinal rotation of the patient during surgery. This technique, using gas instead of silicone, may be used on rare occasions in institutions equipped with special rotating operating tables. The surgical and anaesthetic implications are considerable.

Patients with intraocular tamponading gas bubbles are in danger from the bubble expanding if subsequent nitrous oxide anaesthesia is administered for purposes other than surgery on the same eye. The ophthalmologist should be consulted beforehand.

LOCAL ANAESTHESIA

Serious reactions to local orbital anaesthesia are rare but have been well documented. The need to monitor patients closely is now well recognized. Better quality of patient care, quicker turn around times and excellent operating conditions can be achieved by the skilled anaesthetist trained in local orbital anaesthesia techniques. A detailed knowledge of the anatomy of the eye is a prerequisite (Fig. 28.2).

Applied anatomy of the orbit

Squeezing and closing the eyelids are controlled

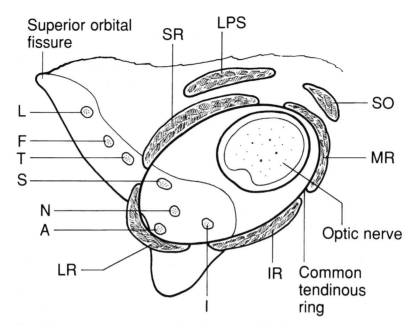

Fig. 28.2   Anatomy of the right orbit: relationship of the four rectus muscles and apex of the cone to orbital nerve supply.

Muscles
LPS = Levator palpebrae superioris
SO = Superior oblique
SR = Superior rectus
MR = Medial rectus
IR = Inferior rectus
LR = Lateral rectus

Nerves
L = Lacrimal V
F = Frontal V
T = Trochlear IV
S = Superior division of oculomotor III
N = Nasociliary V
I = Inferior division of III
A = Abducent VI

by the zygomatic branch of the facial nerve (VII), which supplies the motor innervation to the orbicularis oculi muscle. This nerve emerges from the foramen spinosum at the base of the skull, anterior to the mastoid and behind the earlobe. It passes through the parotid gland before crossing the condyle of the mandible, then passes superficial to the zygoma and malar bone before its terminal fibres ramify in the orbicularis oculi.

Movement of the globe is controlled by the six extraocular muscles. The motor nerves which control these muscles emerge from the skull through the superior orbital fissure. The common tendinous ring forms the fibrous origin of the four rectus muscles at the apex of the orbital cone. The trochlear nerve (IV) emerges through the superior orbital fissure *outside* the common tendinous ring and supplies the superior oblique muscle. All the other motor nerves to the extraocular muscles pass *inside* the common tendinous

ring and are situated inside the cone. The ophthalmic division of the oculomotor nerve (III) divides into superior and inferior branches before emerging from the superior orbital fissure. The superior branch supplies the superior rectus and the levator palpebrae superioris muscles. The inferior branch divides into three to supply the medial rectus, the inferior rectus and the inferior oblique muscles. The abducent nerve (VI) emerges from the superior orbital fissure beneath the inferior branch of the oculomotor nerve to supply the lateral rectus muscle.

Sensation to the eyeball is supplied through the ophthalmic division of the trigeminal nerve (V). Just before entering the orbit, it divides into three branches, lacrimal, frontal and nasociliary. The nasociliary nerve is sensory to the entire eyeball. It emerges through the superior orbital fissure between the superior and inferior branches of the oculomotor nerve and passes *through* the common tendinous ring. Two long ciliary nerves give branches to the ciliary ganglion and, with the short ciliary nerves, transmit sensation from the cornea, iris and ciliary muscle. Some sensation from the lateral conjunctiva is transmitted through the lacrimal nerve and from the upper palpebral conjunctiva via the frontal nerve. Both nerves are outside the cone.

The cone is the area between the four rectus muscles and the posterior surface of the globe. The muscles arise from a fibrous ring which bridges over the superior orbital fissure. Through this common tendinous ring pass the optic nerve, the ophthalmic artery, the two divisions of the oculomotor nerve, the nasociliary nerve and the abducent nerve. The superior and inferior ophthalmic veins may also pass through the ring. A thin membrane envelops the eyeball from the optic nerve to the sclerocorneal junction, separating it from the orbital fat and forming a socket in which it moves. The sheaths of the rectus muscles interconnect in the perimysium in a complex and variable manner and form the walls of the cone. Well-defined expansions laterally and medially form the check ligaments and inferiorly a hammock-like expansion forms the suspensory Lockwood's ligament.

Selection of patients for local anaesthesia

Most older patients accept the idea of local anaesthesia if the procedure is explained when first seen by the ophthalmologist and they may prefer it to general anaesthesia. The young, the mentally unstable and those with physical disabilities that prevent them from lying still are usually unsuitable. Warfarin therapy is not considered an absolute contraindication to local anaesthesia provided that preoperative INR values are in the therapeutic range. There are some patients whose chronic illness poses too severe a risk for general anaesthesia, but whose quality of life may be improved by the proposed surgery. The chance of having surgery under local anaesthesia need not be denied to this group. Operating conditions may not be ideal. Surgery of brief duration may have to proceed with the patient semi-sitting and the surgeon standing.

Premedication is not usually necessary. If appropriate, it should be given well in advance of surgery so that the patient's sedation is stable. Caution should be exercised with the dose of benzodiazepines in the elderly. There is a danger that the oversedated patient may fall asleep during the surgery, only to wake up suddenly and in confusion and try to sit up. A small dose (0.1 mg.kg^{-1}) of morphine 30–60 min before surgery is an appropriate alternative. With this dose, patients are quiet and withdrawn, can lie still more comfortably and coughing is suppressed. Nausea is not usually a problem and any meiotic central effect of morphine is counteracted by the ciliary ganglion block

Axial length and eye movements

It is good practice at the time of the preoperative visit to check the axial length of the eyeball. All patients scheduled for fitting of an intraocular lens will have an ultrasound scan and this measurement will have been recorded. There is an increased danger of global perforation in the high myope and patients with an axial length in excess of 25 mm should be treated with caution. Patients scheduled for glaucoma surgery are not usually scanned preoperatively, but rarely have a long axial length. The extraocular movements and facial nerve function should be checked and recorded. It is not unknown for a patient with a pre-existing Bell's palsy to try to implicate a subsequent facial nerve block. Myopathy of one or more of the extraocular muscles following the inadvertent injection of local anaesthetic into the muscle has been recorded.

Conditions for performing local eye blocks

The patient should be prepared in the same way as for general anaesthesia and should be in optimal health. The staff should establish friendly rapport with the patient, who should be allowed to keep dentures and hearing aids in place.

Intravenous access should be established in all patients. It is essential that full cardiopulmonary resuscitation equipment is immediately available and that the medical personnel who undertake these blocks are familiar with resuscitation techniques. Monitoring with pulse oximetry, three lead ECG and non-invasive blood pressure is strongly recommended both before the block is given and during surgery. Occasionally, intravenous sedation is necessary in the management of the panicky patient.

Local anaesthesia techniques for intraocular surgery

Topical anaesthesia with 1% amethocaine eyedrops or other topical local anaesthetic agents can be used for minor surgery to the conjunctiva if akinesia of the globe is not necessary. It is also used to anaesthetize the conjunctiva before perconjunctival injections are made.

Extraconal or intraconal anaesthesia

Many different techniques and ingredients may be used to achieve akinesia and analgesia of the eyeball. The anaesthetist must learn a suitable technique under the supervision of an experienced practitioner.

Essentially, two different methods are practised: extraconal or peribulbar anaesthesia and intraconal or retrobulbar anaesthesia. The percutaneous or periconjunctival approach may be used in either of these methods. In some ways, the two techniques are analogous to epidural and subarachnoid anaesthesia. Intraconal anaesthesia places the injectate in the fatty compartment which surrounds the nerve to be blocked, whereas extraconal techniques rely on variable diffusion across a fascial layer. Periconal techniques were introduced more recently in the expectation that the incidence of complications would be reduced but this expectation has not been realized. Periconal anaesthesia takes longer to achieve the same degree of akinesia and analgesia than intraconal anaesthesia.

All orbital blocks should be performed with the patient looking straight ahead in the primary gaze position. This ensures that the optic nerve is out of the direct line of approaching needles.

Injections should be no deeper than 31 mm from the orbital margin as this ensures that the needle does not approach the apex of the orbit; the mean distance from the temporal border of the orbital margin to the optic foramen is 50 mm.

The chances of penetrating the optic nerve or damaging other important structures increase with the depth of the injection.

The gauge of needle should be the finest that can be used comfortably. In practice, this means a 25 or 27 gauge needle, as finer needles are difficult to manipulate and larger needles can cause more pain and damage. Sharp needles are used because blunt needles are painful to insert and cause vasovagal syncope. The operator should consistently use the same volume syringe with the same gauge needle, as it is then possible to feel the resistance to the injection. A correctly placed injection has minimal resistance.

The operator should make sure that the hand used to hold the syringe and needle in a pen fashion stays in firm contact with the patient's cheek. By so doing, any unexpected movement by the patient will not displace the needle.

Hyaluronidase and local anaesthetics

Many studies have confirmed that the addition of hyaluronidase to the local anaesthetic used for orbital blocks improves their efficacy. With hyaluronidase, an injectate placed more anteriorly (and therefore more safely) in the orbit diffuses to the apex to block the relevant nerves as they emerge. A dose of hyaluronidase 5 units in each 1 ml of local anaesthetic is optimal.

The addition of adrenaline 1:400 000 to the injectate is acceptable as it improves the solidity and duration of the block and may reduce the incidence of haemorrhage. It may be omitted for medical reasons.

High concentrations of local anaesthetic improve the diffusion and efficacy but at the expense of an increased risk of generalized systemic toxicity and local myotoxicity. High concentrations are necessary for effective periconal anaesthesia.

For short procedures, lignocaine 2% with hyaluronidase and adrenaline is acceptable but usually a longer acting local anaesthetic is added. A suitable combination for periconal anaesthesia comprises equal volumes of bupivacaine 0.75% and lignocaine 4%, whereas for intraconal anaesthesia, equal volumes of bupivacaine 0.5% and lignocaine 2% are sufficient. Lignocaine is less toxic and speeds the onset of the block; bupivacaine increases the duration and provides postoperative analgesia.

Freshly prepared, preservative-free anaesthetic mixtures are better than the pre-prepared combinations.

Following orbital injection, gentle digital pressure and massage help to disperse the anaesthetic and reduce IOP. Extraocular volume is further reduced by the application of a pressure-reducing device such as Honan's balloon. It is important that this is applied for a period of at least 20 min and at a pressure of no greater than 35 mmHg. At this pressure, blood supply to the eyeball is assured. The balloon should be removed just before the operation. The low IOP facilitates surgery but the effect lasts only for a short time.

Extraconal peribulbar anaesthesia

These techniques rely on the placement of relatively large volumes and high concentrations of local anaesthetic outside the cone. The anaesthetic mixture takes time to diffuse through the connective tissue layers of the cone. Spread of the anaesthetic superficially ensures that the terminal fibres of the facial nerve are blocked as they enter the orbicularis oculi. Most peribulbar methods require two initial injections, each of about 5 ml of local anaesthetic. The volume injected depends on the shape of the orbit. The injections are made to a depth of no more than 31 mm using a fine 25 gauge or smaller needle. The safest sites for the injections are in the inferotemporal quadrant and just medial to the medial canthus. The superonasal quadrant should be avoided as injection at this site may damage the trochlear apparatus or cause haemorrhage. After the injections, a pressure-reducing device should be applied to the eye for 10 min before checking again for akinesia. Additional injections may be necessary.

Intraconal retrobulbar anaesthesia

Facial nerve block

Most anaesthetists prefer to block the facial nerve first as this weakens the orbicularis oculi muscle so that the intraconal injection can be inserted without its squeezing action. The facial nerve can be blocked anywhere along its course to the orbit and many different methods have been described. The simplest method is to use the most prominent part of the zygoma, midway between the tragus of the ear and the lateral orbital margin, as the landmark. A 25 gauge 30 mm needle on a 5 ml syringe containing the local anaesthetic mixture is inserted perpendicularly down to the zygoma, withdrawn from the periosteum and aspirated. A volume of 3–5 ml is injected lateral to the lateral orbital margin. Gentle massage to the weal that is raised helps to spread the local anaesthetic and ensures that there is no bleeding.

Intraconal injection

Once the facial nerve block has been completed, the intraconal injection can be inserted (Fig. 28.3). With the patient looking straight ahead, the anaesthetist uses one index finger to palpate the groove between the eyeball and the inferolateral orbital margin and gently displaces the eyeball superiorly. A fine retrobulbar needle on a 5 ml syringe of local anaesthetic is inserted perpendicularly until the point is safely past the equator of the globe. The point is then directed superomedially and floats into the cone with minimal resistance. After aspiration, 3–4 ml of local anaesthetic are injected very slowly. The syringe and needle are then withdrawn in the reverse direction to which they were inserted. The last 1–3 ml of local anaesthetic are injected just under the orbicularis oculi muscle, where it spreads to block the terminal fibres of the facial nerve and enhance the facial nerve block. A single-shot local anaesthetic with intraconal and suborbicularis injection is effective in patients who do not have marked blepharospasm.

HAEMORRHAGE

Haemorrhage is a serious complication of both intraconal and extraconal anaesthesia and occurs with a frequency of between 0.1% and 3%. It is more likely to occur in patients who have acquired vascular disease. Despite this, eventual visual outcome after surgery is not significantly worse than in patients who have uncomplicated anaesthesia. The haemorrhage can be either venous or arterial in origin and may be concealed or revealed.

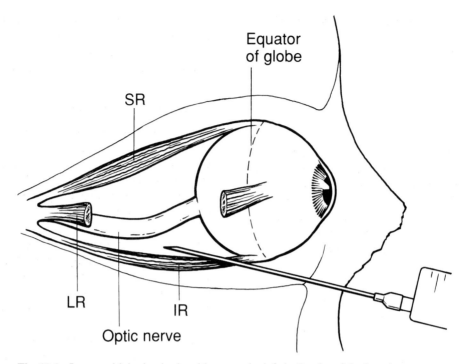

Fig. 28.3   Intraconal injection is placed between the inferior border of the lateral rectus muscle and the inferior rectus. SR = superior rectus; LR = lateral rectus; IR = inferior rectus.

Extravasation of blood into the periorbital tissues increases the tissue volume and pressure. This is transmitted to the globe, raising the intraocular tension and creating difficult and dangerous conditions for intraocular surgery.

Venous haemorrhage usually presents as markedly bloodstained chemosis and raised intraocular pressure. It may be possible to reduce the intraocular pressure by digital massage and the cautious applications of an intraocular pressure-reducing device to such an extent that surgery can proceed safely. Before the decision is made to proceed with surgery or postpone it for a few days, it is advisable to measure and record intraocular pressure.

Arterial haemorrhage is a more serious complication and urgent measures must be taken to stop the haemorrhage and reduce the seriously elevated intraocular pressure. Firm digital pressure usually stops the bleeding and, once it has been arrested, consideration must be given to reducing the intraocular pressure so that the blood supply to the retina is not jeopardized. Lateral canthotomy, intravenous acetazolamide, intravenous mannitol or even paracentesis may need to be considered in consultation with the ophthalmologist.

Prevention of haemorrhage

Patients with elevated blood pressure are more likely to bleed and optimum control of hypertension should be achieved before surgery is attempted. The fewer injections that are made into the orbit, the less is the chance of damaging a blood vessel. Cutting and slicing movements at the needle tip should be avoided. Fine needles are less traumatic than thicker ones. Deep intraorbital injections are more likely to cause haemorrhage than is a shallow injection. The inferotemporal quadrant has fewer blood vessels and is less hazardous. Blunt Atkinson-type needles have been recommended but are painful to insert, cause vasovagal syncope and can still damage blood vessels. A technique of producing a liquid stilette of local anaesthetic in front of the advancing needle by slow injection also has its advocates. The addition of adrenaline to the injectate may reduce the incidence of haemorrhage. It is advisable to apply firm digital pressure to the orbit as soon as the needle is withdrawn after any intra-orbital injection, as this reduces any tendency to ooze.

CENTRAL SPREAD

Mechanism

The cerebral dura mater provides a tubular sheath for the optic nerve as it passes through the optic foramen. This sheath fuses to the epineurium of the optic nerve and is continuous with the sclera, providing a potential conduit for local anaesthetic to pass subdurally to the brain. Central spread occurs if the needle tip has perforated the optic nerve sheath and injection is made. Even a tiny volume injected under the optic nerve sheath may pass to the central nervous system and/or cross the optic chiasma to the opposite eye and may cause life-threatening sequelae. The time of onset of symptoms is variable, but any major sequelae usually develop in the first 15 min after the injection. It is advisable that the patient's face is not covered up on the operating table for at least this interval after the block has been inserted.

Another mechanism for central spread may occur on rare occasions if an orbital artery is cannulated by the needle tip. The local anaesthetic is injected in a retrograde fashion up the artery until it meets a branch, where it can then flow in a cephalad direction. The onset of central nervous system toxicity is almost instantaneous if this mechanism is invoked; in addition, orbital haemorrhage usually occurs.

Signs and symptoms of central spread

The symptomatology of central spread is varied and depends upon which part of the central nervous system is affected by the local anaesthetic. Due to the anatomical proximity of the optic nerve to the midbrain, it is usual for this area to be involved. A range of different signs and symptoms has been described, including the cardiovascular and respiratory systems, temperature regulation, vomiting, temporary hemiplegia, aphasia and generalized convulsions. Palsy of the contralateral oculomotor and trochlear nerves with amaurosis

(loss of vision) is pathognomonic of central nervous system spread and should be sought in any patient whose response to questions following block are not as crisp as they were beforehand.

Treatment of central spread

The treatment is symptomatic throughout the duration of effect of the local anaesthetic drug. With longer acting local anaesthetic agents, treatment may be required for 60–90 min. The patient must be monitored intensively. Bradycardia requires treatment with an anticholinergic drug. Asystole has been reported rarely but if it occurs, intravenous adrenaline and sustained cardiac massage are required. Respiratory depression or apnoea necessitate ventilatory support and administration of supplementary oxygen. Convulsions are treated conveniently with intravenous sodium thiopentone and conversion to general anaesthesia. When the vital signs are stable, it may be feasible to continue with the proposed surgery under general anaesthesia in the knowledge that the patient will need continuing intensive support until the local anaesthetic action has worn off.

Prevention of central spread

Intraconal or extraconal injections should always be made with the patient looking straight ahead in the primary gaze position (Fig. 28.4). The optic nerve is then slack and out of the way of the advancing needle. If the needle encounters the optic nerve in this position, it is unlikely to damage or perforate its sheath as slackness in the structure allows the nerve to be pushed aside. If the eyeball is directed away from the primary gaze position in any other extreme direction, the optic nerve is stretched. When stretched, the nerve cannot be easily pushed aside. The most dangerous position is when the patient looks upward and inwards as this presents the stretched nerve to a needle directed from the inferotemporal quadrant. As in the prevention of haemorrhage, injections should not be made too deeply into the orbit where the optic nerve is tethered to its sheaths as it emerges through the optic foramen. It is good practice to withdraw the needle by 1 mm from its maximum depth before injection is made. If the tip had been

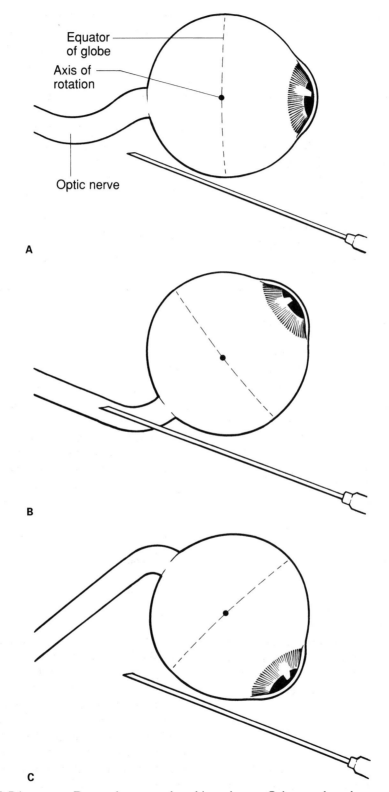

Fig. 28.4 **A** Primary gaze; **B** upwards or upwards and inwards gaze; **C** downwards or down and out movement.

resting against the optic nerve sheath, this manoeuvre will withdraw the tip to a safer position.

Puncture of the eyeball

Global puncture is a serious complication of local anaesthesia for eye surgery. It has been reported following both intraconal and extraconal injections and even following local anaesthesia for more minor procedures such as eyelid surgery. With appropriate care, it should be a very rare complication. The sclera is a tough structure and in most cases is not perforated easily.

Puncture of the eyeball is most likely to occur in patients with high myopia, previous retinal banding, posterior staphyloma or a deep sunken eye with a narrow orbit (Fig. 28.5).

Not all eyeballs are the same length and not all orbits are the same shape. In most patients who present for cataract surgery, an ultrasound measure is made of the axial length of the eyeball to calculate the power of the intraocular lens. Normal eyeballs have an axial length of 20–24 mm. High myopes have much longer axial lengths of 25–35 mm and extreme caution should be exercised in these patients. The axial length in patients for glaucoma surgery is not usually measured.

Global puncture is often a double puncture of the posterior segment of the eyeball; the tip of the needle is in the orbit at the time of injection and the local anaesthetic block may be good. Puncture is usually recognized at the time of surgery and presents as an exceptionally soft eye. In cataract surgery, if the block is good the surgeon should be encouraged to proceed with the lensectomy but to stitch up the eye with twice as many sutures as normal. Without lensectomy it may not be possible to observe the damage to the posterior segment of the eye. It can be expected that the needle track through the vitreous will form a band of scar tissue. If this is not excised, it will contract and detach the retina, sometimes causing sudden total blindness in the affected eye.

Optic nerve damage

Fortunately, this is a rare complication which results usually from obstruction of the central retinal artery. This artery is the first and smallest branch of the ophthalmic artery, arising from that vessel as it lies below the optic nerve. It runs for a short distance within the dural sheath of the optic nerve and about 35 mm from the orbital margin, pierces the nerve and runs forward in the centre of the nerve to the retina. Damage to the artery can cause bleeding into the confined space of the optic nerve sheath, compressing and obstructing blood flow. If the complication is recognized soon enough, it may be possible to perform surgical decompression of the optic nerve.

Myopathy of the extraocular muscles

The inadvertent injection of a long-acting local anaesthetic into any extraocular muscle body can result in prolonged weakness of the muscle. An injection site well away from these muscles should be selected.

Vasovagal syncope

This is more likely to occur in young and anxious patients when eye blocks are administered. Painful injection with a blunt Atkinson needle may cause this response. It is important that vascular access is secured before any block is given. Treatment is symptomatic and should include administration of oxygen, intravenous injection of an anticholinergic agent and head-down positioning. Differentiation from central spread should be made by testing vision and extraocular movements in the opposite eye.

EXTRAOCULAR PROCEDURES

Squint surgery

Squint surgery is best carried out under general anaesthesia. A laryngeal mask or tracheal tube can be used to secure the airway and either spontaneous breathing or mechanical ventilation may be employed. Traction on the extraocular muscles or pressure on the globe may provoke bradycardia via the oculocardiac reflex. The audible pulse rate monitor should be sufficiently loud so that the surgeon is warned. The treatment for the bradycardia is temporary cessation of the

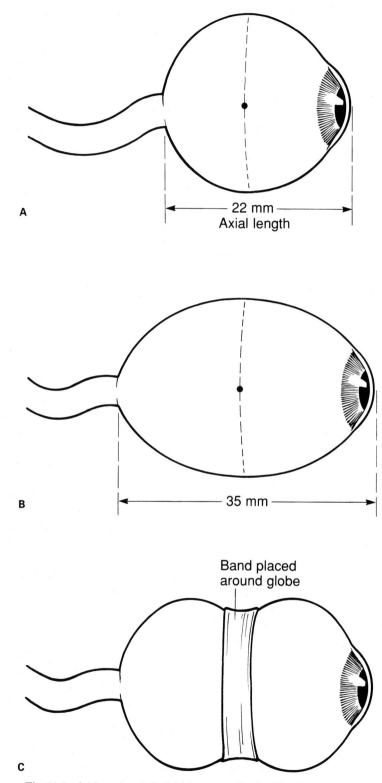

Fig. 28.5 **A** Normal eyeball; **B** high myope; **C** scleral buckle.

stimulus and the administration of i.v. atropine. Strabismus surgery is associated with a high incidence of postoperative nausea and vomiting and administration of a prophylactic antiemetic is advisable. Drugs with a prolonged action on muscle tone should be avoided when squint repair with postoperative adjustable sutures is planned.

Squint and ptosis are presenting signs of the progressive external ophthalmoplegia syndrome (PEO). Patients with this syndrome may have marked cardiac and respiratory decompensation and pose a significant hazard for anaesthesia. Preoperative pulmonary function testing is advisable in these patients. Myasthenia gravis may also present with ptosis and strabismus.

Injection of botulinum toxin is used occasionally in the treatment of strabismus. Ketamine is a suitable anaesthetic for children scheduled to undergo this procedure as it does not reduce muscle power; the surgeon tests muscle power intraoperatively.

Examination under anaesthesia (EUA)

Children may require repeated examinations under anaesthesia. If the purpose of the EUA is to measure the IOP, as may be the case in neonates with congenital glaucoma, then the method of anaesthesia must be discussed with the surgeon. Inhalation anaesthesia by mask is often satisfactory but the surgeon may wish to measure IOP while the patient is still lightly anaesthetized, before IOP is reduced by the effects of anaesthetic drugs. Painless preoperative intravenous access using EMLA local anaesthetic cream has made i.v. induction a practical choice for most children. The use of the laryngeal mask is ideal. Ketamine does not lower the IOP, but it is a long-acting anaesthetic and may cause hallucinations and nightmares postoperatively. It should be reserved for special cases.

Dacryocystorhinostomy (DCR)

Open DCR is usually carried out under general anaesthesia because the operation is frequently bilateral and may be complicated by haemorrhage. It is necessary to use a tracheal tube and throat pack because blood can trickle down the naso-pharynx. The nostril(s) should be packed with cocaine paste or another suitable vasoconstrictor before operation. The operation site may be infiltrated with adrenaline by the surgeon and caution is necessary with the use of halothane.

The use of lasers for DCR has largely eliminated haemorrhage and local anaesthesia is preferable if open surgery is not planned.

DRUG INTERACTIONS

Patients with eye disease often use systemic or topical medications which may pose potential problems for the anaesthetist. Systemic absorption of potent eyedrops is reduced if the lacrimal puncta are occluded digitally while the drops are being inserted.

Cyclopentolate is an antimuscarinic with an action of up to 24 h; 1% drops are used to dilate the pupil and paralyse the ciliary muscle before surgery. Excessive systemic absorption causes toxic effects similar to those associated with an overdose of atropine. The young and the very old are particularly susceptible.

Phenylephrine is a direct-acting α-adrenergic stimulant and has weak β-effects; 2.5% or 10% drops are used to dilate the pupil. Systemic effects may cause an increase in myocardial irritability and hypertension. Dangerous interactions with monoamine oxidase inhibitors may occur.

Adrenaline is used intraoperatively in a diluted solution by the surgeon to reduce excessive bleeding. Systemic absorption may be significant. Caution is necessary with halothane.

Timolol or other β-blocking agents are used topically to treat glaucoma. Systemic absorption may be significant. Asthma and chronic obstructive airways disease may be exacerbated. Precautions as for systemic β-adrenergic blocking drugs should be observed.

Ecothiopate iodide (phospholine iodide) is a potent anticholinesterase and is used rarely in the treatment of glaucoma. It depletes pseudocholinesterase and thus prolongs the action of suxamethonium.

Botulinum toxin A is an effective treatment in a variety of neuromuscular conditions including strabismus. It causes a decrease in skeletal muscle power by binding irreversibly to receptor sites on the cholinergic nerve terminal. Function does not return until new motor endplates have formed. When injected locally into the extraocular muscle(s), the toxin binds rapidly and firmly to the tissue; in the doses used normally, it should not cause systemic side-effects.

Mannitol is an osmotic diuretic which reduces the volume of the vitreous humour. Infusions in doses of up to 1.5 g.kg^{-1} are given before surgery over a period of 30–45 min. There is an initial increase in circulating blood volume followed by a diuresis and decrease in blood volume. When combined with the induction of general anaesthesia, haemodynamic instability may occur. Particular caution must be exercised in patients with cardiovascular disease. A urinary catheter should be inserted preoperatively if patients are to receive mannitol in this way.

Acetazolamide, a carbonic anhydrase inhibitor, is used in the medical treatment of glaucoma. Its main actions are to reduce the production of aqueous humour and to facilitate drainage. It is of questionable value during surgery because it results in increased intrachoroidal vascular volume. Congenital glaucoma is treated with acetazolamide and repeated surgery. Metabolic acidosis may be a serious consequence of this treatment and the neonate presenting for anaesthesia for glaucoma surgery must be treated with special care. Any respiratory depression caused by sedatives, opioids or anaesthesia reduces the compensatory respiratory alkalosis. It may be advisable to perform blood gas analysis before anaesthesia.

FURTHER READING

Todd J G 1994 Anaesthesia for ophthalmic surgery. In: Nimmo W S, Rowbotham D J, Smith G (eds) Anaesthesia, 2nd edn. Blackwell Scientific Publications, London

29. Anaesthesia for radiology, radiotherapy and psychiatry

Recent advances in radiology and new expensive equipment requiring specialized environments have led to an increase in anaesthesia outside the operating room.

General considerations

Many problems encountered in the radiology department, radiotherapy suite and psychiatric hospital are similar:

1. In most hospitals, radiology, radiotherapy and ECT suites have not been designed with anaesthetic requirements in mind. Anaesthetic apparatus often competes for space with bulky equipment and in general, conditions are less than optimal.

2. Monitoring equipment may not be available readily and is often the oldest in the hospital. Clinical observation may be limited by poor lighting.

3. Preparation of the patient may be inadequate because the patient comes from a ward in which staff are unfamiliar with preoperative protocols. Mentally disturbed patients may fail to comply with fasting instructions. Consequently, the patient may have a full stomach and may not be premedicated.

4. Anaesthetic assistance and maintenance of anaesthetic equipment may be less than ideal. Consequently, the anaesthetist must be particularly vigilant in checking the anaesthetic machine, changing empty gas cylinders (only the most modern suites have piped gases) and ensuring the presence of spare laryngoscope blades and batteries if required.

5. Communication between radiologist, radio-therapist or psychiatrist and the anaesthetist may be poor, with failure to recognize the other's requirements.

6. Often, recovery facilities are inadequate and anaesthetists may have to recover their own patients. Consequently, they must be familiar with the siting of suction apparatus and supplementary oxygen supply within the recovery area.

ANAESTHESIA FOR RADIOLOGICAL PROCEDURES

The traditional role of the radiology department has changed in recent years. Conventional use of X-rays has been augmented by the introduction of new non-invasive diagnostic imaging techniques. Magnetic resonance imaging (MRI) and computerized tomography (CT) scanning have reduced the use of angiography and pneumo-encephalography in neurodiagnosis. Whilst the main focus of clinical interest in these techniques has been centred on the brain, application has extended into delineation of thoracic and abdominal lesions. The major requirement of all these imaging techniques is that the patient remains almost motionless. Thus, anaesthesia may be necessary when these investigations are performed on children, the critically ill or the uncooperative patient.

Computerized tomography (CT scan)

General principles

Computerized tomography has become the most widely used neuroradiological procedure. A CT scan provides a series of tomographic axial 'slices' of the head and/or body. Each image is produced by computer integration of the differences in the radiation absorption coefficients between different normal tissues and between normal and abnormal tissues. The image of the structure under investigation is generated by a cathode ray tube, the brightness of each area being proportional to the absorption value.

One rotation of the gantry produces an axial slice or 'cut'. A series of cuts is made usually at intervals of 7 mm but may be larger or smaller, depending on the diagnostic information sought. The first-generation scanners took 4.5 min per cut, but the newest scanners take only 2–4 s.

Anaesthetic management

Computerized tomography is non-invasive and painless, requiring neither sedation nor anaesthesia for most adult patients. However, patients who cannot cooperate (most frequently paediatric and head trauma patients) may need general anaesthesia to prevent movement, which degrades the image. Anaesthetists may be asked to assist also in the supervision of critically ill patients from the ITU in the CT scan room.

General anaesthesia is preferable to sedation when there are potential airway problems or when control of intracranial pressure (ICP) is critical. As the patient's head is inaccessible during the CT scan, it is mandatory to intubate the trachea. The scan itself requires only that the patient remains motionless and tolerates the tracheal tube. If ICP is high, controlled ventilation is essential to induce hypocapnia and decrease cerebral blood flow.

A propofol/thiopentone, nitrous oxide, oxygen and relaxant technique with tracheal intubation and mild hyperventilation is acceptable. Anaesthetic complications include kinking of the tracheal tube (especially during extreme degrees of head flexion required for examination of the posterior fossa), hypothermia in paediatric patients and acute brain stem compression if the head is flexed excessively in the presence of an infratentorial tumour.

Computerized tomography involves exposure to ionizing radiation and access to the patient is limited. Consequently, a breathing system dis-

connection alarm, ECG display and automatic arterial pressure monitoring and pulse oximetry are essential.

Magnetic resonance imaging

General principles

Magnetic resonance imaging (MRI) is a new imaging modality that does not use ionizing radiation, but depends on magnetic fields and radiofrequency pulses for the production of its images. The imaging capabilities of MRI are similar to those of CT with the advantage that no ionizing radiation is produced.

An MRI imaging system requires a large-bore magnet in the form of a tube which is capable of accepting the entire length of the human body. A radiofrequency transmitter coil is incorporated in the tube which surrounds the patient; the coil acts also as a receiver to detect the energy waves from which the image is constructed. In the presence of the magnetic field, protons in the body align with the magnetic field in the longitudinal axis of the patient. Additional perpendicular magnetic pulses are applied by the radiofrequency coil; these cause the protons to rotate into the transverse plane. When the pulse is discontinued, the nuclei relax back to their original orientation and emit energy waves which are detected by the coil. The magnet is over 2 m in length and weighs approximately 500 kg.

MRI can differentiate clearly between white and grey matter in the brain, thus making possible the in vivo diagnosis of demyelination. It can display images in the sagittal, coronal or transverse planes and, unlike the CT scanner, is capable of detecting disease in the posterior fossa.

Anaesthetic management

The indications for general anaesthesia during MRI are similar to those for computerized tomography. However, unique problems are presented by MRI. These include relative inaccessibility of the patient and the magnetic properties of the equipment. The body cylinder of the scanner surrounds the patient totally; manual control of the airway is impossible and tracheal intubation is essential, preferably with a Rae pattern oral tube. The patient may be observed from both ends of the tunnel and may be extracted quickly if necessary. As there is no hazard from ionizing radiation, the anaesthetist may approach the patient in safety.

The magnetic effects of MRI impose some restrictions on the selection of anaesthetic equipment. Any ferromagnetic object distorts the magnetic field sufficiently to degrade the image. It is also likely to be propelled towards the scanner and held tightly against it. Of relevance to anaesthetists are such items as intravenous fluid stands, oxygen and nitrous oxide cylinders and monitoring equipment. Although laryngoscopes are non-magnetic, batteries are strongly magnetic and laryngoscopy and intubation are difficult in close proximity to the scanner. The safest approach is to avoid all metallic equipment, e.g. use pipeline gases rather than cylinders, and to substitute apparatus of plastic or nylon manufacture whenever possible.

Monitoring may be difficult. Conventional ECG monitoring is not possible. A pulse oximeter may be used provided that the sensor lead is long enough to prevent the oximeter from affecting the magnetic field and thus the image. Heart rate and ventilatory rate may be monitored with an oesophageal stethoscope, although the sounds may be obscured by the noise of the equipment. If the patient is allowed to breathe spontaneously, movement of the reservoir bag may be used as an index of ventilation. A non-invasive automated arterial pressure monitor, in which metallic tubing connectors are replaced by nylon connectors, is useful.

Hazards

The static magnetic field may prove dangerous in patients with implanted ferromagnetic devices. Patients fitted with a demand cardiac pacemaker should not be exposed to MRI because induced electrical currents may be mistaken for natural electrical activity of the heart and may inhibit pacemaker output. Metallic implants, e.g. intracranial vascular clips, may be dislodged from blood vessels. Patients with large metal implants should be monitored for implant heating. Heating of the pulse oximeter probe may result in burns.

Angiography

General principles

Computerized tomography has reduced the need for angiography in neurodiagnosis. However, angiography is indicated for the investigation of a suspected cerebral aneurysm, arteriovenous malformation or vascular tumour. Vertebral angiography is used if a posterior fossa lesion is suspected and carotid angiography is required for detection of supratentorial lesions. Direct puncture of the common carotid or vertebral arteries has been replaced almost entirely by insertion of a catheter into the femoral artery using a Seldinger technique. This allows several vessels to be investigated through a single puncture site.

Most contrast media are exceedingly hypertonic (osmolarity 2000 mosmol.litre^{-1}) and consequently produce expansion of the circulating blood volume. Injection of contrast medium causes burning pain in the face and eye and vasodilatation produces headache and flushing. Newer agents, such as metrizamide, are less hypertonic and therefore preferable.

Anaesthetic management

Angiography can usually be accomplished in the adult patient using local anaesthesia with or without sedation. Sedation to augment local anaesthesia must be avoided in the presence of intracranial hypertension as the increased Pa_{CO_2} leads to vasodilatation and a further increase in ICP; in addition, vasodilatation results in poor-quality angiography. Children will usually require general anaesthesia.

General anaesthesia for angiography is more comfortable for the patient and ensures complete immobility during X-ray exposures. A relaxant/IPPV technique with moderate hyperventilation to induce hypocapnia (Pa_{CO_2} 4.0–4.5 kPa) is used. A moderate reduction in Pa_{CO_2} causes vasoconstriction of normal vessels, slows cerebral circulation and contrast medium transit time and improves delineation of small vascular lesions. The failure of autoregulation within tumours increases blood flow relative to that in other areas because of an intracerebral steal phenomenon and allows better visualization of their vascularity.

Complications

Local. Haematoma and haemorrhage, vessel wall dissection, thrombosis, embolism of air or atheroma and the development of Horner's syndrome are all recognized complications.

General. The hypertonicity of contrast medium may exacerbate cerebral oedema and result in seizures. Transient hypotension and bradycardia on asystole can occur during cerebral angiography with contrast dye injection and usually respond to volume replacement and atropine.

Contrast encephalography

General principles

Encephalography is performed rarely in centres which possess a CT scanner. However, it is used occasionally to delineate small mass lesions in the suprasellar region and cerebellopontine angles.

These diagnostic studies are accomplished by injecting a contrast agent either into the lumbar subarachnoid space or directly into the ventricles via a burr hole and employ gravity to manoeuvre the agent so that the ventricular system is outlined. Most commonly, air or oxygen is employed as the contrast agent, although iodinated compounds are used occasionally.

Lumbar air encephalography is performed by the injection of air into the lumbar subarachnoid space with the patient in the sitting position. The air rises and by appropriate positioning of the head, it enters the cisterna magna and the ventricular system of the brain, outlining its size, shape and symmetry. The technique is contra-indicated in patients with raised ICP because medullary 'coning' may be precipitated.

Ventriculography is performed usually on patients with obstructive hydrocephalus or those with raised ICP, in whom lumbar encephalo-graphy is considered too dangerous. There is a high risk of convulsions if iothalamate (Conray) is used as contrast medium.

Anaesthetic management

Encephalography is a very uncomfortable and un-popular procedure. Although performed occa-sionally under local anaesthesia and sedation, encephalography is distressing to most patients because of the protracted nature of the investiga-tions (1–1.5 h), frequent changes of position and invariable headache and vomiting caused by the injection of air. Consequently, general anaesthesia is preferable, although there are difficulties. Ni-trous oxide diffuses into any air-filled body cavity much more rapidly than nitrogen diffuses out, because of the difference between their blood/gas solubility coefficients. Nitrous oxide anaesthesia is contraindicated if air is used as the contrast medium, as distension of the ventricular system occurs and ICP increases.

If nitrous oxide is used as the contrast agent, there is no contraindication to its use as an anaes-thetic gas. This modification reduces morbidity, as the rapid absorption of nitrous oxide from the ventricles after the procedure shortens the duration of headache. If air has been used as the contrast medium, any subsequent anaesthetic administered within one week of the study should not include nitrous oxide.

Miscellaneous procedures

Translumbar aortography (TLA)

TLA is a common investigation in the assess-ment of patients with peripheral vascular disease. Although it may be carried out under local anaes-thesia with sedation, general anaesthesia is de-sirable. The patient is placed prone and therefore tracheal intubation and controlled ventilation are essential. The patient and operating table move rapidly by up to 2 m during radiological exposure so that additional lengths of ventilator tubing and an intravenous drip extension are necessary. Serious complications are infrequent but include pneumothorax, perforation of the bowel and renal puncture. Often, patients who require TLA have generalized vascular disease and most are heavy smokers with associated pulmonary pathology; consequently, anaesthesia may be hazardous.

Bronchography

Bronchography is used mainly for the diagnosis and evaluation of bronchiectasis and its use is declining. Most bronchograms are carried out using local anaesthesia, but children and anxious adult patients require general anaesthesia.

Commonly, respiratory function in these patients is compromised and additional hypoxaemia is inevitable after inhalation of the oil-based contrast medium.

Intravenous or inhalational induction is followed by tracheal intubation without any local anaesthetic spray, so that the cough reflex returns rapidly at the end of the procedure. Spontaneous ventilation is preferred, as it allows contrast medium to be drawn gradually into the bronchi to provide even distribution; controlled ventilation tends to disperse the dye too rapidly and delineates the bronchial tree poorly. Contrast medium is instilled through a catheter passed down the lumen of the tracheal tube. The posture of the patient is altered sequentially to fill the various lobes of the lung.

As much contrast material as possible is removed at the end of the procedure by suction and physiotherapy. The tracheal tube remains in situ until there is an active cough reflex. Humidified oxygen should be given during the recovery period and the patient should be nursed in a head-down position with the healthier lung uppermost.

Intussusception

This condition occurs usually between the ages of 6 and 18 months. Commonly, the ileum invaginates into the caecum because of small bowel lymphadenopathy. General anaesthesia may be necessary in the radiology department during attempted reduction of the intussusception by instillation of rectal barium.

The major problems are those of anaesthetizing any young child in an unfamiliar environment. Precautions should be taken to minimize the decrease in body temperature. Fluid losses are always greater than expected and plasma (or substitute) may be needed to restore circulating blood volume.

Embolization procedures (vascular malformations, aneurysms, tumours)

These procedures may be painful and require sedation, regional or general anaesthesia. Adequate hydration is important as patients undergoing contrast dye procedures usually have an induced osmotic diuresis which can exacerbate pre-existing renal dysfunction.

Nausea and vomiting are common (consider prophylaxis with ondansetron) and may occur as prodromal symptoms in as many as 20% of all anaphylactoid reactions to contrast dye. The treatment of allergic reactions depends upon their severity but includes general measures such as volume expanders and oxygen, as well as specific drugs including atropine, steroids, antihistamines and adrenaline.

ANAESTHESIA FOR RADIOTHERAPY

Adults may require general anaesthesia for insertion of radioactive sources locally to treat some types of tumour. The commonest tumours to be treated in this way are carcinoma of the cervix, breast or tongue. These procedures are undertaken in the operating theatre and the anaesthetic management is similar to that for any type of surgery in these anatomical sites. However, the patients may have undergone anaesthesia recently for a diagnostic procedure and may require more than one anaesthetic for radiotherapy treatment; consequently, halothane should be avoided. In addition, the anaesthetist may be exposed to radiation and appropriate precautions should be taken.

Radiotherapy is used increasingly in the management of a variety of malignant diseases which occur in childhood. These include the acute leukaemias, Wilms' tumour, retinoblastoma and central nervous system tumours. High-dose X-rays are administered by a linear accelerator, but all staff must remain outside the room to be protected from radiation.

Anaesthesia in paediatric radiotherapy presents several problems:

1. Treatment is administered daily over a 4–6 week period and necessitates repeated doses of sedation or general anaesthesia.
2. The patient must remain alone and motionless for short periods during treatment, but immediate access to the patient is required in an emergency.

3. Monitoring is difficult as the child can be observed only on a closed-circuit television screen during treatment.

4. Recovery from anaesthesia must be rapid, as treatment is organized usually on an outpatient basis and disruption of normal activities should be minimized.

Before treatment begins, the fields to be irradiated are plotted and marked so that the X-rays can be focused on the tumour without damaging surrounding structures. This procedure requires the child to remain still for 20–40 min and takes place in semi-darkness. Radiotherapy treatment is of much shorter duration; two or three fields are irradiated for 30–90 s each, but a considerably longer period of anaesthesia is required so that the child can be positioned correctly and the radiation source focused precisely. A typical treatment session lasts 20–30 min.

Anaesthetic management

A wide range of techniques has been employed for this purpose.

Intravenous or intramuscular administration of ketamine is distressing for children. Ketamine produces excessive salivation, even if an antisialagogue is prescribed, and there is a risk of airway obstruction or laryngospasm. Tachyphylaxis occurs with repeated use and sudden purposeless movements are not infrequent. The use of ketamine as a sole anaesthetic agent is unsatisfactory.

Often, children who require repeated daily anaesthesia have a Hickman line in situ to ensure reliable i.v. access for induction of anaesthesia. If establishment of i.v. access is required daily, venepuncture becomes not only technically difficult, but also increasingly distressing for the patient, parent and anaesthetist. Inhalational induction with the child sitting on the parent's knee is an alternative technique.

When anaesthesia has been induced, the child is placed on a trolley and anaesthesia maintained with nitrous oxide, oxygen and volatile agent delivered via a laryngeal mask. Halothane remains the most suitable inhalational agent for repeated anaesthesia in children as the risk of hepatic damage is very low and airway complications are much less frequent than with enflurane or isoflurane. No analgesia is required and tracheal intubation is not necessary.

Monitoring during radiotherapy under general anaesthesia is not easy. Closed-circuit television cameras provide visual monitoring of the patient's respiratory movements. Continuous ECG and automatic arterial pressure monitoring are essential. The pulse oximeter is a useful non-invasive monitor, especially if the trachea is not intubated. Ideally a microphone transmits the audible ECG signal and the saturation-dictated pitch of the oximeter signal.

ANAESTHESIA AND PSYCHIATRIC DISEASE

Patients who require anaesthesia and surgery usually experience some degree of anxiety and apprehension. Often a professional attitude, together with a friendly and humane approach by the anaesthetist, alleviates much of this anxiety.

The management of the patient with pre-existing psychological illness requires specific anaesthetic considerations. Patients with disorders of affect may require a course of treatment with electroconvulsive therapy (ETC) and thus repeated anaesthesia. The safe management of these patients demands an understanding of potential drug interactions between anaesthetic agents and psychotropic drugs such as tricyclic antidepressants, monoamine oxidase inhibitors and lithium. The prevalence of alcoholism is increasing and the close association between alcohol consumption and acute trauma results commonly in the presentation of alcoholic patients for emergency surgery. Many patients with Down's syndrome and mentally subnormal individuals survive into late adulthood and may require anaesthesia for correction of associated medical conditions or dental care. Finally, the management of the narcotic addict is an area of increasing personal concern for the anaesthetist in view of the bloodborne transmission of hepatitis B and HIV.

Drug interactions

The concomitant administration of psychotropic drugs is frequent in psychiatric patients scheduled for anaesthesia. The drugs encountered most commonly are tricyclic antidepressants, monoamine oxidase inhibitors, phenothiazines and lithium.

Tricyclic antidepressants

Tricyclic antidepressants inhibit the reuptake of noradrenaline into the presynaptic nerve terminals. Most of these drugs have anticholinergic effects also.

Tricyclic antidepressants may produce tachycardia and arrhythmias even in therapeutic doses and the hypertensive response to directly acting sympathomimetic amines is increased dramatically. Although it has been recommended that tricyclic antidepressants are discontinued 2 weeks before anaesthesia, this may not be possible in many psychiatric patients.

Side-effects of tricyclic therapy include sedation and anticholinergic symptoms (dry mouth, blurred vision, constipation, urinary retention). Centrally acting anticholinergic drugs (atropine, hyoscine) should be avoided in premedication because the additive effect may precipitate confusion, especially in the elderly.

Monoamine oxidase inhibitors (MAOIs)

Monoamine oxidase is responsible for the intraneuronal metabolism of sympathomimetic amines. Inhibition of this enzyme by drugs such as phenelzine and tranylcypromine is responsible for their antidepressant action. Usually, these agents are used when the response to tricyclic antidepressants has been unsatisfactory.

Tyramine, a precursor of noradrenaline, is known to precipitate hypertensive crises in the presence of MAOIs. Similarly, indirectly acting sympathomimetic amines, e.g. ephedrine, result in unpredictable changes in arterial pressure. These hypertensive responses may be eliminated by withdrawal of MAOIs 2 weeks before anaesthesia but, as with tricyclic drugs, this may not always be practical in the psychiatric patient.

The interaction between MAOIs and pethidine is important also, although uncommon. Agitation, restlessness, hypertension, rigidity, convulsions and hyperpyrexia may result. Morphine appears to be safe.

Phenothiazines

Phenothiazines possess antipsychotic, antiemetic, antihistamine and sedative properties. Interactions with anaesthetic drugs are common. The central depressant actions of opioids are potentiated and opioid requirements are decreased. Central anticholinergic effects are additive with those of atropine and hyoscine, so that glycopyrronium is the preferred antisialagogue. Moderate α-adrenoceptor blockade aggravates the hypotensive effect of anaesthetic agents.

Lithium

Lithium carbonate is used predominantly in the long-term treatment of mania. Its mode of action is inhibition of the release, and increased reuptake, of noradrenaline.

As lithium tends to act as an imperfect sodium ion, potentiation of both depolarizing and non-depolarizing muscle relaxants occurs and close monitoring of neuromuscular function is necessary.

Lithium is excreted by the kidneys. Toxicity may ensue in hyponatraemic states, when there is intense renal conservation of sodium and consequently lithium. The risk may be minimized by establishing a saline infusion during the perioperative period.

Electroconvulsive therapy (ECT)

ECT is used widely in psychiatric practice, primarily for the treatment of endogenous depression when drug therapy has failed. The electrically induced grand mal seizure produced by ECT is responsible for the therapeutic effect.

Originally, seizures were induced chemically and electrical stimulation was not introduced until the late 1930s. Further advances involved the use of muscle relaxants (initially curare and later suxamethonium) to modify the convulsion. By the 1960s, the technique of using a short-acting i.v. barbiturate and a depolarizing muscle relaxant became accepted as a simple, safe regimen for modified ECT.

Administration of ECT

The electrical stimulus produced by all ECT

devices comprises short pulses of current interrupted by longer periods of electrical inactivity. The electrical transmission lasts for only a fraction of the total stimulus duration and this results in a decrease in the amount of electrical energy required to provoke a generalized seizure. Typical settings are a pulse of 60 Hz of 0.75 ms duration, with a total stimulus time of 1.25 s.

The electrical stimulus is applied to the patient's head by hand-held electrodes of low impedance. Traditionally, electrodes are placed in the bifronto-temporal region for bilateral ECT, whereas both electrodes are placed over the non-dominant hemisphere to produce unilateral ECT.

Physiological effects of ECT (Table 29.1)

Cardiovascular system. Activation of the autonomic nervous system is responsible for the profound cardiovascular changes during ECT. The autonomic disturbance consists of a para-sympathetic–sympathetic sequence; this results in an initial bradycardia followed by tachycardia and hypertension secondary to intense sympathetic stimulation. This, together with the increased muscle activity of the convulsion, increases myocardial oxygen demand and may result in myocardial ischaemia in susceptible individuals unless hypoxaemia is avoided by administration of supplementary oxygen during the convulsion.

Cerebrovascular system. Cerebral blood

flow increases dramatically to 1.5–7 times the basal level. This increased flow represents mainly a response to the increase in cerebral oxygen consumption that accompanies the seizure. There is an associated increase in ICP which may prove hazardous in patients with a space-occupying lesion.

Anaesthetic considerations

In an effort to avoid or minimize the physiological sequelae and attendant complications of ECT, a technique of modified ECT has evolved gradually in which drugs are employed to reduce the detrimental effect of ECT without the abolition of the essential beneficial effects.

Preanaesthetic assessment. All patients should receive a visit and evaluation by the anaesthetist before treatment. Special attention should be paid to cardiorespiratory function, symptoms of oesophageal reflux, allergies and previous anaesthetic experiences. The presence of loose or missing teeth should also be noted.

The patient must be fasted for a period of at least 6 h before anaesthesia. This may seem simple, but many of these patients are extremely unreliable and occasionally uncooperative, so that careful supervision is required to ensure that fasting does occur.

Premedication with sedatives or opioids is not required and may serve only to prolong the anaesthetic recovery time. The routine administration of atropine is no longer considered to be necessary.

Anaesthetic management. Anaesthetic requirements include smooth induction, autonomic stability, safety with repeated administration and rapid recovery.

Methohexitone is the induction agent used most commonly. It is a barbiturate with a rapid onset and short duration of action that decreases the duration of, and raises the threshold to, electrically induced seizures. Thiopentone offers no advantages over methohexitone and prolongs the recovery time. Propofol appears to be unsuitable as it shortens the duration of the seizure and may limit the therapeutic benefits.

The use of muscle relaxants in ECT has virtually eliminated the risk of fractures. Suxamethonium is used most commonly; the usual dose is 0.5 mg.kg^{-1},

Table 29.1 Physiological effects of electroconvulsive therapy

Cardiovascular effects	
Immediate	
Parasympathetic stimulation	Bradycardia
	Hypotension
Late (after 1 min)	
Sympathetic stimulation	Tachycardia
	Hypertension
	Arrhythmias
	Myocardial oxygen
	consumption increases
Cerebral effects	
Cerebral oxygen consumption	
Cerebral blood flow	
Intracranial pressure	
Intraocular pressure	
Intragastric pressure	

but a record should be kept of the dose and degree of modification of the seizure so that subsequent adjustments may be made if necessary.

When neuromuscular blockers are used it may be difficult to ascertain if a convulsion has occurred. The most effective way to record a seizure is by monitoring EEG activity; this is possible with modern ECT machines. Alternatively, an isolated forearm technique may be used.

After induction of anaesthesia and administration of suxamethonium, the lungs are ventilated with 100% oxygen using face mask and anaesthetic breathing system. When the limbs are flaccid, a rubber 'bite block' is inserted between the teeth before electrical stimulation is applied. During the seizure, artificial ventilation with oxygen is continued to avoid arterial desaturation and continued until adequate spontaneous ventilation has returned.

Patients should be recovered in the lateral position by trained nursing staff with equipment available immediately for treatment of any emergency.

Contraindications

There is no general agreement regarding conditions which constitute relative or absolute contraindications to ECT (Table 29.2). However, the consensus is that patients with an intracranial mass lesion, or those who have suffered a myocardial infarction or cerebrovascular accident within the last 3 months, should not undergo ECT. The decision to proceed with ECT is determined after balancing the risks of treatment

Table 29.2 Contraindications to electroconvulsive therapy

Absolute
Recent myocardial infarction (< 3/12)
Recent cerebrovascular accident (< 3/12)
Intracranial mass lesion

Relative
Angina pectoris
Congestive cardiac failure
Severe pulmonary disease
Severe osteoporosis
Major bone fractures
Glaucoma
Retinal detachment
Pregnancy

and the risks associated with progression of the psychiatric disease and long-term therapy with antidepressants.

Morbidity after ECT

Modified ECT in association with skilled anaesthetic management is safe and effective. Patients may complain of headache, muscle aches and confusion for 1–2 h after treatment, but memory disturbances may persist for several weeks. The latter are minimized by unilateral ECT over the non-dominant cerebral hemisphere.

Other mental disorders

Mental subnormality

Mentally subnormal patients should be assessed in the presence of parents or a guardian. Relevant medical history can be obtained, consent for surgery given (if the patient is unable to give this himself) and rapport with the patient established.

Pharmacological premedication is usually unnecessary. The interval between arrival in the anaesthetic room and induction of anaesthesia should be minimized and the presence of a reassuring parent may be invaluable. A flexible approach by the anaesthetist is required during induction of anaesthesia, which may have to be performed with the patient in the sitting position or even lying on the floor! Adequate help must be available to lift or restrain the patient if necessary. Induction of anaesthesia should be as smooth and rapid as possible; either an inhalational or i.v. technique may be employed. Occasionally, i.m. ketamine is required.

Poor dental hygiene and difficulty with tracheal intubation should be anticipated.

Patients must be allowed to recover undisturbed and the presence of parents in the recovery area is to be encouraged.

Down's syndrome

Down's syndrome is associated with a variety of medical abnormalities including congenital heart disease and duodenal or choanal atresia. Patients with this condition have a large tongue, small mandible and increased incidence of subglottic stenosis; consequently, airway management and tracheal intubation may prove difficult. Antibiotics are necessary in the prophylaxis of endocarditis. No abnormal responses to anaesthetic agents have been substantiated.

Alcohol withdrawal

Denial of alcohol intake in the perioperative period may result in disturbances associated with acute withdrawal. Delirium tremens is characterized by extreme disorientation, increased psychomotor activity, hallucinations, marked autonomic activity and hyperpyrexia. Usually, the syndrome lasts for 7–10 days.

Delirium tremens should be treated by correction of fluid and electrolyte imbalance and administration of vitamins, particularly thiamine. Control is achieved most readily by i.v. sedation with 0.8% chlormethiazole; barbiturates should be avoided.

A nitrous oxide, oxygen and relaxant technique with analgesic supplementation is suitable if anaesthesia is required for a surgical procedure, although maintenance of anaesthesia may require the administration of larger doses of anaesthetic agents than normal.

FURTHER READING

Casey W F, Price V, Smith H S 1986 Anaesthesia and monitoring for paediatric radiotherapy. Journal of the Royal Society of Medicine 79: 454
Edwards R, Mosher V B 1980 Alcohol abuse, anaesthesia, and intensive care. Anaesthesia 35: 474
Gaines Y G, Rees D I 1986 Electroconvulsive therapy and anaesthetic considerations. Anesthesia and Analgesia 65: 1345
Hutton P, Cooper G 1985 Psychiatry. In: Guidelines in clinical anaesthesia. Blackwell Scientific Publications, Oxford
Weston G, Strunin L, Amundson G M 1985 Imaging for anaesthetists: a review of the methods and anaesthetic implications of diagnostic imaging techniques. Canadian Anaesthetists' Society Journal 32: 552
Willatts S M, Walters F J M 1986 Anaesthesia for neuroradiology. In: Anaesthesia and intensive care for the neurosurgical patient. Blackwell Scientific Publications, Oxford

30. Day-case anaesthesia

A day-case patient is one who is admitted for investigation or operation on a planned non-resident basis. The patient occupies a bed in a ward or unit set aside for this purpose. The concept of day-case anaesthesia and surgery has existed for many years. In 1899 Ries showed that patients improved with early ambulation and suffered fewer complications. In 1900 Cushing described hernia repairs performed using cocaine as a local anaesthetic and in 1909, when Nicoll reported a series of 8988 outpatient operations in children, he stressed the need for careful selection of patients.

During the last 25 years there has been a rapid expansion in the use of day-case surgery. At the inception of day care procedures, a case was considered suitable if it took less than 90 min. Procedures that are commonly selected today are those taking less than 30 min to complete and which do not cause severe haemorrhage or produce excessive amounts of postoperative pain (Table 30.1).

To achieve the end result of a pain-free ambulant patient at the end of the day requires skilful patient selection and experienced anaesthetists and surgeons working within a day-case surgery unit.

Many anaesthetists and surgeons have indicated that day surgery represents a safe, cost-effective and efficient practice.

PATIENT SELECTION

The selection of patients for day-case surgery is of vital importance if maximum use is to be made of the resources in the day-case unit and also to facilitate smooth running of the unit. The selection of patients must take account of two separate

Table 30.1 A selection of surgical procedures commonly undertaken as day cases

Gynaecology
Dilatation & curettage, laparoscopy, vaginal termination of pregnancy, colposcopy

Plastic surgery
Dupytren's contracture release, removal of small skin lesions, nerve decompression

Ophthalmology
Strabismus correction, lacrimal duct probing, examination under anaesthesia

ENT
Myringotomy, insertion of grommets, removal of foreign bodies, polyp removal

Urology
Cystoscopy, circumcision, vasectomy

Orthopaedics
Arthroscopies, carpal tunnel release, ganglion removal

General surgery
Breast lumps, herniae, varicose veins, endoscopy

Paediatrics
Circumcision, orchidopexy, squint, dental extractions

aspects: firstly the patient's state of health and secondly his social circumstances. Patients should normally be ASA I or II, i.e. normal healthy people or those with minor systemic disease not interfering with normal activities, the latter including medical conditions that are well controlled with therapy, e.g. hypertension. An upper age limit of 65–70 years should be judged on biological rather than chronological age.

The selection of patients for day-case surgery is made at the time of outpatient consultation, where routine measurement of pulse, BP and urine analysis and other relevant investigations (e.g. sickle cell testing) are performed; these routine tests reduce problems when patients are admitted on the day of surgery. Careful attention to patient selection and consultation with anaesthetists involved in the provision of anaesthetic services to the day unit minimizes problems. Studies have demonstrated that a simple preoperative questionnaire can be very effective in screening patients to detect common medical problems. A typical preoperative questionnaire is shown in Table 30.2.

When considering children for day-case procedures, they should be healthy normally falling into ASA I or II groups. Premature babies who have not reached 44 weeks conceptual age should not be considered for day-case surgery and special consideration should be given to babies who have been on ventilatory support. The parent must be able to cope with the pre-procedure instructions and with the care of the child after treatment. The parent must agree to day treatment and be available to stay throughout the day, although there may be exceptions for older children who attend regularly. The facilities at home should be taken into account, as should travel conditions. After a general anaesthetic the use of public transport is inappropriate.

Following selection of a patient for day-case surgery, the nature of the operation and the routine of management are fully explained to the patient and the consent form is signed. Many units issue the patient with explanatory leaflets or audio cassettes explaining the procedure. A date for the operation may then be arranged and registration completed as for an inpatient admission. It is wise to book any pathological or radiological investigations that are required well in advance of the day of admission.

The patient should be given written instructions detailing the date and time of attendance at the day unit, with written instructions relating to preoperative starvation. These instructions should be written clearly in plain English, advising the patient not to eat anything from midnight for a morning list. It is advisable to ask patients who smoke to refrain from smoking for 4–6 weeks before the operation. The patients should be asked to bring with them all tablets and medicines that they take regularly.

After day-case surgery patients should be accompanied home and have a responsible adult stay with them for 24 h following the operation. They should also be advised to abstain from drinking alcohol and not to drive a car or operate machinery for 24 h.

An example of instructions for children presently in use at Leicester Royal Infirmary relating to preoperative starvation is given in Table 30.3.

ORGANIZATION OF THE DAY-CASE UNIT

The types of unit

There are three common types of day-case unit:

1. A unit within a hospital complex, but with separate wards and operating theatre. This is

Table 30.2 A typical preoperative questionnaire

Name	Date
D.o.B	Operation
Unit number	

Blood pressure (mmHg)
Pulse (bpm)
Weight (Kg)
Temperature (°C)

Please answer the following questions:

	No	Yes
Have you had anything to eat or drink in the last 4 hrs?		
Have you had any previous operations?		
Will you go home alone?		
Will you be on your own when you get home?		
Have you, or anybody in your family, ever had any problems with general anaesthetics?		
Do you have a cough or a cold?		
Have you had any serious illnesses in the past?		
Do you suffer with heart disease or high blood pressure?		
Do your ankles swell?		
Do you get breathless or have chest pain on exercise or at night		
Do you have asthma or bronchitis?		
Do you smoke?		
Do you have epilepsy (fits)?		
Do you have diabetes?		
Do you suffer from anaemia, bruise easily or bleed excessively?		
Have you ever had liver disease or been jaundiced?		
Do you drink excessive amounts of alcohol?		
Are you allergic to anything, including Elastoplast?		
Are you taking any drugs or medication from your GP?		
Do you have any loose or false teeth?		
Do you usually wear contact lenses?		
If female, are you pregnant?		

Table 30.3 Preoperative starvation instructions for children

Morning operations

Children over 4 years old
  Nothing to eat or drink after midnight on the day before the operation.

Children between 2–4 years old
  Wake the child when you go to bed and give a drink and a biscuit; after this *nothing* to eat or drink.

Children less than 2 years old
  Wake the child very early on the morning of the operation and give a milk drink (up to 1/2 pint milk). This must be completed by 6 am; after this *nothing* to eat or drink.

Afternoon operations

Children of all ages
  Nothing to eat or drink after a light breakfast before 9 am.

functionally the most flexible type as it may be adapted to the varying requirements of day-case patients.

2. A unit with a separate ward, but using the hospital's main operating theatre complex.

3. Outside the UK, it is common for a separate centre to have its own operating theatres and wards remote from a conventional hospital.

Ideally day surgical units should not be free-standing but situated on inpatient hospital sites. The ward area should be close by the theatre, to reduce portering time, particularly when short operations are to be performed. This arrangement also enables parents to accompany their children to the anaesthetic room if this is desirable.

Preferably the unit should be near to a car park and be well signposted to facilitate the prompt arrival of patients and to avoid unnecessary delays.

Facilities available

The accommodation should ideally include:

1. A reception area/play room/discharge area.
2. Anaesthetic room, fully equipped and large enough to allow free access around the patient's trolley to permit the use of local or general anaesthesia. Good lighting, scavenging, piped gases and suction equipment. Anaesthetic machine and monitoring equipment. The hazards and risks of day-stay surgery general anaesthesia are no less than for inpatient surgery; indeed, in some respects they may be greater and the facilities provided must be comparable.

3. Operating theatre. This should be of the same specification as the inpatient equivalent. A good operating light, air-conditioning and piped services are required, as well as the usual scrub-up and lay-up facilities. There is always the possibility of a minor operation developing unexpectedly into a major operation and this therefore demands that the theatre is well equipped to deal with this eventuality.

4. A fully equipped recovery room. This must always be equipped and staffed for the safe recovery of patients following general anaesthesia. Piped gas supplies and resuscitation equipment are mandatory and the full range of monitoring and ventilation equipment must be readily available.

Other facilities that should be available include:

- autoclave facilities
- office space
- nurses' station
- treatment/examination room
- equipment store/staff locker room
- a pantry to make drinks
- lavatories for patients, parents and staff
- staff room.

Admission

Patients should be admitted to the day ward in adequate time for history taking and examination. The results of any investigation requested as an outpatient should be available and noted. Patients should receive an identity bracelet and their names should be entered into the nursing record. The operation site should be marked.

ANAESTHESIA

Premedication

Most anaesthetists do not routinely prescribe premedication for day-cases, as mostly it is unnecessary. It is thought that premedication may prolong the recovery time and delay the patient's discharge from hospital.

However, Obey et al (1988) conducted a double blind study of temazepam premedication for day-cases and found effective anxiolysis in the groups that received 10 or 20 mg temazepam; there was no delay in recovery times as measured by memory test cards and all patients were discharged from the day unit 3 h after administration of general anaesthesia.

Oral midazolam has been used as a premedicant in day surgery, but it was found that it produced delay in the immediate and late recovery when compared with temazepam.

If anticholinergic agents are required they can usually be satisfactorily administered at induction of anaesthesia.

Recent clinical studies suggest that overnight fasting may not be justified in adults or children. Pulmonary aspiration usually occurs in emergency abdominal and obstetric procedures where there may be complicating factors such as recent food and fluid intake, trauma or administration of opioid analgesics. These factors do not normally apply to healthy elective day-case patients. The universal order of nil by mouth from midnight should only apply to solids. Clear fluids should be allowed until 3 h before the scheduled time of surgery.

Goodwin studied the effect of giving patients 150 ml clear fluid 2 h before general anaesthesia for termination of pregnancy. The results showed that clear fluids do not increase the incidence of regurgitation or vomiting during anaesthesia and that preoperative thirst was decreased in the clear fluid group.

General anaesthesia

Local, regional or general anaesthesia can be administered safely to day-case patients. The choice of technique should be determined by surgical requirements, anaesthetic considerations and the patient's physical status and preference.

The choice of induction agent depends upon the requirements of the patient and the preference of the anaesthetist. Any induction agent used in day-case anaesthesia should ensure a smooth induction, good immediate recovery with minimal postoperative sequelae and a rapid return to street fitness.

A number of different induction agents have been used successfully for induction of anaesthesia in day-case patients; these include methohexitone, etomidate and thiopentone. Increasingly propofol (2,6-di-iso-propylphenol in soya bean oil emul-

sion; Diprivan ICI Pharmaceuticals) is being chosen as the primary induction agent in day-case anaesthesia. One of the main advantages of propofol is the ease with which patients recover from its effects. Patients are clear-headed and have a lower incidence of nausea and vomiting. Several recent studies indicate that propofol should now be considered as the induction agent of choice for day-case anaesthesia and surgery. One disadvantage of propofol is pain on injection and there have been several studies reporting a reduction in pain on injection by addition of lignocaine to the propofol or by keeping the propofol in a refrigerator. Propofol causes cardiovascular depression and reports of bradycardia have appeared in the literature. The upper airway is easier to manage following induction of anaesthesia with propofol compared with thiopentone and Szneke showed that oropharyngeal airways are accepted more readily following induction with propofol. This indicates a fundamentally different action of these drugs on the upper airway and may explain some of the differences that are observed in clinical practice.

Recently the new inhalation anaesthetic agent desflurane has been described for use in day-case anaesthesia. Desflurane has several qualities that make it suitable for use in ambulatory surgery. It has a lower blood/gas solubility coefficient than any of the available potent volatile anaesthetics (0.42). In human volunteers and rats it produces rapid induction and recovery from anaesthesia. This may make this agent useful for inhalation induction of anaesthesia in day-case patients. Desflurane does seem to be irritant to the upper airway on induction of anaesthesia, causing a higher incidence of coughing during induction compared with the use of propofol for induction of anaesthesia.

Which technique should we use for maintenance of anaesthesia? Comparisons of recovery after enflurane and halothane techniques in patients undergoing day-case anaesthesia suggest that recovery is faster after enflurane. Times to awakening were reported not to be significantly different between isoflurane and enflurane in patients undergoing short surgical procedures. Newer techniques such as continuous infusion of propofol or the use of desflurane may confer some advantages, but these have to be balanced against the cost of these agents.

A clear airway is a fundamental requirement of safe anaesthesia. In day-case anaesthesia simple face mask anaesthesia with a Guedel airway is commonly used. Longer procedures may necessitate the use of a tracheal tube. The laryngeal mask is now being used frequently both in adults and children.

The choice of muscle relaxant depends on the anticipated duration of surgery. Suxamethonium is associated with muscle pains especially in ambulant patients and for all but the shortest of procedures is not ideal in the day-case setting. Of the non-depolarizing muscle relaxants currently available, atracurium and vecuronium have a relatively short duration of action when they are used in appropriate doses and are readily reversed after 20–30 min.

The recently introduced short-acting muscle relaxant mivacurium has a short duration of action which may make it suitable for day-case anaesthesia. It is a non-depolarizing, bis-benzylisoquinolinium muscle relaxant. It undergoes rapid hydrolysis by plasma cholinesterase. Intubating dose of 0.2–0.25 mg.kg^{-1} requires 2 min for maximum blockade to occur. It has approximately twice the duration of action of equipotent doses of suxamethonium and approximately half those of atracurium and vecuronium. Therefore its short duration of action makes it useful in day-case anaesthesia.

Spinal anaesthesia has been used for day-case anaesthesia but its use is limited by the occurrence of an unacceptable incidence of headache especially in the younger age groups. Also, slow return of motor power and difficulty with micturition may delay discharge.

Local anaesthetic blocks are an excellent choice for day-case patients, because of the low incidence of postoperative nausea and vomiting and the provision of good postoperative analgesia. For operations on the hand or arm, axillary brachial plexus block is preferable to the supraclavicular approach because of the risk of producing a pneumothorax, which may only become apparent after discharge. Intravenous regional anaesthesia (Bier's block) can be used successfully for hand operations.

POSTOPERATIVE CARE

Postoperative pain control should be started intraoperatively by supplementing intravenous or inhalation anaesthesia with a combination of short-acting opioid analgesics, a non-steroidal anti-inflammatory drug and local/regional block intraoperatively. The patient's awakening is smoother and discharge home is quicker. The most frequently used drugs to provide intraoperative analgesia are fentanyl and alfentanil; the relatively short duration of action of these drugs makes them suitable for use in day-case anaesthesia.

The provision of good postoperative analgesia is primarily the responsibility of the anaesthetist. We can do little to limit the number of patients requiring admission caused by surgical complications but we can play a major role in reducing admissions caused by pain and vomiting.

There are a variety of techniques that are available and regional techniques and local blocks are widely used. Caudal block is used to reduce pain in paediatric patients (circumcision, herniorrhaphy, hypospadias, orchidopexy) using 0.25% bupivacaine plain; this can provide excellent postoperative analgesia. Whenever a caudal block is administered for analgesia, care must be taken to ensure that motor strength is not compromised. There does not appear to be any advantage in using more concentrated solutions than 0.25% bupivacaine. Penile blocks and the local application of local anaesthetic cream are also effective. Intra-articular local anaesthetics have been found to be useful following arthroscopy.

Non-steroidal anti-inflammatory drugs, e.g. diclofenac and more recently ketorolac, have a place in the provision of postoperative analgesia in day-case patients. Ketorolac is a peripherally acting potent injectable analgesic associated with few central nervous system side-effects.

The factors contributing to postoperative nausea and vomiting are pain, opioid analgesic drugs, the choice of anaesthetic technique or agents, operative procedure, sudden movement or position change, history of motion sickness, hypotension, obesity, day of menstrual cycle and high oestrogen levels. A relationship between pain and the frequency of nausea and vomiting in the postoperative period has been established. There is controversy regarding the use of opioid analgesics in the day-case patient, because they may increase postoperative nausea and vomiting. Several studies have shown that if an opioid, nitrous oxide anaesthetic is given, the occurrence of nausea and vomiting is increased compared with an inhalation anaesthetic. In contrast there are studies which have demonstrated that an opioid supplemented anaesthetic technique results in earlier ambulation and discharge.

Postoperative nausea and vomiting can be reduced by the use of low dose droperidol $10-20 \mu g.kg^{-1}$ and more recently the selective $5HT_3$ antagonist ondansetron appears to be an effective antiemetic without causing drowsiness or extrapyramidal symptoms.

Recovery from anaesthesia is an important aspect of day-case anaesthesia. The recovery area should be provided with monitoring equipment such as pulse oximetry and ECG. The overall responsibility for assessing when patients are ready to go home is that of the clinicians involved. Often experienced nursing staff who regularly work in the day unit become very good at detecting potential problems with day-case patients. Nurses who work in day-case units must be multiskilled and able to work in all areas.

In general, discharge of the patient should not take place until the patient is able to sit unaided, walk in a straight line and stand still without swaying. Usually patients have been able to have a drink and something to eat (this also demonstrates the absence of nausea). A responsible person should be present to escort the patient home and both the responsible person and the patient should be given both verbal and written discharge instructions. The patient should be advised to refrain from activities such as driving a car, operating machinery and drinking alcohol for 24 h. Communication with the patient's general practitioner is very important and many units are now using modern telecommunications, e.g. fax machines, to ensure that the GP is aware of the operation performed and the requirements for postoperative follow-up.

FURTHER READING

Burn J M B 1979 A blueprint for day surgery. Anaesthesia 34: 790–805
Commission on the Provision of Surgical Services 1985 Guidelines for day case surgery. Royal College of Surgeons of England, London
Ogg T W 1988 A case for the expansion of day surgery. Health Trends 21: 114–117
Strunin L 1993 How long should patients fast before surgery? Time for new guidelines. British Journal of Anaesthesia 70: 1–3
Obey P A, Ogg T W, Gilks W R 1988 Temazepam and recovery in day surgery. Anaesthesia 43: 49–51

31. Emergency anaesthesia

Patients scheduled for elective surgery are usually in optimal physical and mental condition, with a definitive surgical diagnosis and with concomitant medical illness well controlled.

In contrast, the patient with a surgical emergency may have an uncertain diagnosis and uncontrolled concomitant medical illness, with consequent cardiovascular and metabolic derangements.

Thus a major principle governing the practice of emergency anaesthesia is to be prepared for all potential complications, including vomiting and regurgitation, hypovolaemia and haemorrhage and abnormal reactions to drugs in the presence of electrolyte disturbances and renal impairment.

PREOPERATIVE ASSESSMENT

The objective of emergency anaesthesia is to permit correction of the surgical pathology with the minimum of risk to the patient. This requires adequate and accurate preoperative evaluation of the patient's general condition, with particular attention to specific problems which may influence anaesthetic management.

It is essential to ascertain the likely surgical diagnosis, the magnitude of the proposed surgery and how urgently surgery is required, as these dictate both the extent of preoperative preparation and the method of anaesthesia.

A pertinent past medical and drug history is elicited. In particular, enquiry is made into the presence and severity of specific symptoms relevant to cardiopulmonary reserve: angina, productive cough, dyspnoea of effort, orthopnoea or nocturnal coughing bouts. The presence of such symptoms should provoke detailed enquiry into the cardiovascular and respiratory systems (see Ch. 18 on preoperative assessment).

Depending upon the urgency of surgery, physical examination may be selective to identify significant cardiopulmonary dysfunction or any abnormalities which might lead to technical difficulties during anaesthesia. Basal crepitations, triple rhythm and raised jugular venous pulse signify impaired ventricular function and limited cardiac reserve, which increase significantly the risk of anaesthesia. It is also important to exclude arrhythmias and heart sounds indicative of valvular disease, as these influence the patient's response to physiological change and thus anaesthetic management. Assessment of respiratory function is particularly difficult as the patient in pain (with or without peritoneal irritation) may be unable to cooperate in pulmonary function testing.

It is important to cultivate the habit of airway evaluation if a rapid-sequence induction (see p. 523) is contemplated, as contingency plans are required for management of the patient in the event of failure to intubate the trachea. Irregular dentition, limitation of mouth opening, poor range of movement at the atlanto-occipital joint and/or reduced distance between the hyoid bone and the mental symphysis are associated with difficult laryngoscopy. A history of difficult intubation is of considerable significance.

Finally, a review of any laboratory investigations is made and urgent requests are made for further tests which may influence patient management.

Assessment of volaemic status

Assessment of intravascular volume is essential as

underestimated or unrecognized hypovolaemia may lead to circulatory collapse during induction of anaesthesia, which attenuates the sympathetically mediated increases in arteriolar and venous constriction. In any patient in whom fluid is sequestered or lost (e.g. peritonitis, bowel obstruction) or in whom haemorrhage has occurred (e.g. trauma), efforts should be made to quantify the blood volume or extracellular fluid volume and to correct any deficit.

Intravascular volume deficit

Assessment of blood loss may be made from the history and any measured losses, but more commonly the anaesthetist has to rely on clinical evaluation. Useful indices include heart rate, arterial pressure (especially pulse pressure), the state of the peripheral circulation, central venous pressure and urine output. Table 31.1 describes approximate correlations between these clinical indices and the extent of haemorrhage, but it should be stressed that these refer to the 'ideal' patient. In young, healthy adults, heart rate and arterial pressure may be unreliable guides to volume status and in elderly patients with widespread arterial disease, limited cardiac reserve and a rigid vascular tree (fixed total peripheral resistance), signs of severe hypovolaemia may become evident when blood volume has been reduced by as little as 15–20%. However, as baroreceptor sensitivity decreases with age elderly patients may exhibit less tachycardia for any degree of volume depletion.

In general, hypovolaemia does not become apparent clinically until blood volume has been reduced by at least 1000 ml (20% of blood volume). A reduction by more than 30% of blood volume occurs before the classic 'shock syndrome' is produced, with hypotension, tachycardia, oliguria and cold, clammy extremities. Haemorrhage in excess of 40% of blood volume may be associated with loss of the compensatory mechanisms that maintain cerebral and coronary blood flow and the patient becomes restless and agitated and eventually comatose.

In patients with major trauma, it is valuable to compare the clinical assessment of the extent of haemorrhage with the measured or assumed loss. A marked disparity between these two estimates leads not infrequently to a diagnosis of a further concealed source of haemorrhage.

Extracellular volume deficit

Assessment of extracellular fluid volume deficit is difficult, as considerable losses must occur before clinical signs are apparent. Clinical acumen and a high index of suspicion are necessary to detect the subtle signs of lesser deficits.

Guidance is obtained from the nature of the surgical condition, the duration of impaired fluid intake and the presence and severity of symptoms associated with abnormal losses (e.g. vomiting). At the time of the earliest radiological evidence of intestinal obstruction, there may be 1500 ml of fluid sequestered in the lumen of the bowel.

Table 31.1 Clinical indices of extent of blood loss

Grade of hypovolaemia	1 Minimal	2 Mild	3 Moderate	4 Severe
Percentage blood volume lost	10	20	30	Over 40
Volume lost (ml)	500	1000	1500	Over 2000
Heart rate (beat.min^{-1})	Normal	100–120	120–140	Over 140
Arterial pressure (mmHg)	Normal	Orthostatic hypotension	Systolic below 100	Systolic below 80
Urinary output (ml.h^{-1})	Normal (1 ml.kg^{-1}.h^{-1})	20–30	10–20	Nil
Sensorium	Normal	Normal	Restless	Impaired conscious
State of peripheral circulation	Normal	Cool and pale	Cold and pale, slow capillary refill	Cold and clammy Peripheral cyanosis
CVP (cmH$_2$O)	Normal	–3	–5	–8

If the obstruction is well established and vomiting has occurred, the deficit may exceed 3000 ml. At this stage, clinical signs are minimal but evident to the skilled observer.

For convenience, extracellular fluid volume loss may be graded into four degrees of severity; in each instance, loss is expressed as the percentage of the body weight lost as a fluid. It may be seen from Table 31.2 that in minor degrees of extracellular fluid volume loss diagnosis is dependent on two highly subjective signs: diminished skin elasticity and reduced intraocular pressure. Changes in skin turgor are difficult to assess in elderly patients in whom a natural loss of subcutaneous tissue elasticity may contribute to the impression of reduced turgor. The most reliable sites for interpreting 'tenting' of the skin as a sign of tissue dehydration are the anterior thigh, the forehead, sternum, clavicle or tibia, areas where, under normal circumstances, there is little subcutaneous fat or redundant skin. Soft eyeballs resulting from lower intraocular pressure are assessed by asking the patient to close his eyes and look downwards; the examiner presses lightly on the eyeballs (above the tarsal plate) with the index finger of each hand.

It should be noted that the presence of orthostatic hypotension indicates considerable deficit which, if not corrected, may lead to severe hypotension on induction of anaesthesia. Orthostatic hypotension should be elicited with caution.

Laboratory investigations may help to confirm the extent of extracellular fluid volume deficit. Haemoconcentration results in an increased haemoglobin concentration and an increased packed cell volume. As dehydration becomes more marked, renal blood flow diminishes, reducing renal clearance of urea and consequently increasing the concentration of blood urea. Patients with moderate volume contraction exhibit a prerenal pattern of uraemia characterized by an elevation in blood urea out of proportion to any elevation in serum creatinine. Under maximal stimulation from ADH and aldosterone, conservation of sodium and water by the kidneys results in excretion of urine of low sodium content (0–15 mmol.litre^{-1}) and high osmolality (800–1400 mosmol.kg^{-1}).

After estimation of the extent of blood volume or extracellular fluid volume deficit, correction is accomplished with the appropriate fluid. Hartmann's solution (compound sodium lactate) and 0.9% saline are isotonic, remaining predominantly in the extracellular space, and are suitable for the replacement of extracellular fluid losses. Haemorrhage is treated preferably by blood transfusion, but alternative fluids may be used (see Ch. 6). The optimal time for surgical intervention is when all fluid deficits have been corrected, but if there are urgent indications for surgery (e.g. presence of gangrenous bowel), compromise is necessary. As a general rule, the demonstration of orthostatic hypotension indicates that further fluid replacement is required.

THE FULL STOMACH

Of all the hazards of emergency anaesthesia, vomiting or regurgitation of gastric contents, followed by aspiration into the tracheobronchial tree whilst protective laryngeal reflexes are obtunded, is one of the commonest and most devastating.

Vomiting is an active process that occurs in the lighter planes of anaesthesia. Consequently, it is a potential problem during induction of, or emergence from, anaesthesia, but should not occur during maintenance if anaesthesia is sufficiently deep. In light planes of anaesthesia, the

Table 31.2 Indices of extent of loss of extracellular fluid

Percentage body weight lost as water	ml of fluid lost per 70 kg	Signs and symptoms
Over 4% (mild)	Over 2500	Thirst, reduced skin elasticity, decreased intraocular pressure, dry tongue, reduced sweating
Over 6% (mild)	Over 4200	As above, plus orthostatic hypotension, reduced filling of peripheral veins, oliguria, nausea, dry axillae and groins, low CVP, apathy, haemoconcentration
Over 8% (moderate)	Over 5500	As above, plus hypotension, thready pulse with cool peripheries
10–15% (severe)	7000–10 500	Coma, shock followed by death

presence of vomited material above the vocal cords stimulates spasm of the cords, which prevents material from entering the larynx. Apnoea may persist until severe hypoxaemia occurs, at which point the vocal cords open and ventilation resumes. Thus the presence of laryngeal reflexes provides a margin of safety provided that the anaesthetist clears the oropharynx of all debris before ventilation resumes.

In contrast, regurgitation is a passive process that may occur at any time, is often 'silent' (i.e. not apparent to the anaesthetist) and, if aspiration occurs, may have clinical consequences ranging from minor pulmonary sequelae to fulminating aspiration pneumonitis. Because regurgitation occurs usually in the presence of deep anaesthesia or at the onset of action of muscle relaxant drugs, laryngeal reflexes are absent and the risk of aspiration is high.

In elective surgery, patients are usually starved of food and drink overnight or at least for 4–6 h, although the need for such absolute rules concerning clear fluids has been questioned. However, in emergency surgery, it may be necessary to induce anaesthesia urgently before an adequate period of starvation occurs. In addition, the patient's surgical condition is often accompanied by delayed gastric emptying.

The most important factors determining the extent of gastric regurgitation are the function of the lower oesophageal sphincter and the rate of gastric emptying.

The lower oesophageal sphincter

The lower oesophageal sphincter (LOS) is an area (2–5 cm in length) of higher resting intraluminal pressure situated in the region of the cardia. The sphincter relaxes during oesophageal peristalsis to allow food into the stomach, but remains contracted at other times. The structure cannot be defined anatomically but may be detected using intraluminal pressure manometry.

The LOS is the main barrier preventing reflux of gastric contents into the oesophagus and its resting tone is affected by many drugs used in anaesthetic practice. Reflux is related not to the LOS tone per se, but to the difference between gastric and LOS pressures; this is termed the barrier pressure. Drugs which increase the barrier pressure decrease the risk of reflux. Prochlorperazine, cyclizine, anticholinesterases, α-adrenergic agonists and suxamethonium increase barrier pressure. For many years it was thought that the increase in intragastric pressure during suxamethonium-induced fasciculations predisposed to reflux. However, there is an even greater increase in LOS pressure with a consequent increase in barrier pressure.

Anticholinergic drugs, ethanol, ganglion blocking drugs, tricyclic antidepressants, opioids and thiopentone reduce LOS pressure and it is reasonable to assume that these drugs increase the tendency to gastro-oesophageal reflux.

Gastric emptying

Under normal circumstances, peristaltic waves sweep from cardia to pylorus at a rate of approximately 3 per minute, although temporary inhibition of gastric motility follows recent ingestion of a meal. The rate of gastric emptying is proportional to the volume of the stomach contents, with approximately 1–3% of total gastric content reaching the duodenum per minute. Thus, emptying occurs at an exponential rate. The presence of some drugs, fat, acid or hypertonic solutions in the duodenum delays significantly the rate of emptying (the inhibitory enterogastric reflex), but both the nervous and humoral elements of this regulating mechanism are still poorly understood. Many pathological conditions are associated with a reduced rate of gastric emptying (Table 31.3). In the absence of any of these factors, it is reasonably safe to assume that the stomach is empty provided that solids have not been ingested within the preceding 6 h or fluids consumed in the preceding 2 h, and provided normal peristalsis is occurring.

Vomiting and regurgitation during induction of anaesthesia are encountered most frequently in patients with an acute abdomen or trauma. All patients with minor trauma (fractures or dislocations) must be assumed to have a full stomach; gastric emptying virtually ceases at the time of significant trauma as a result of the combined effects of fear, pain, shock and treatment with opioid analgesics. In all trauma patients, the time interval between ingestion of food and the acci-

Table 31.3 Situations in which vomiting or regurgitation may occur

Full stomach
1. Peritonitis of any cause ⎫
2. Postoperative ileus   ⎪
3. Metabolic ileus: ⎬ Absent or
   hypokalaemia, uraemia, ⎪ abnormal peristalsis
   diabetic ketoacidosis   ⎪
4. Drug-induced ileus: ⎪
   anticholinergics, those with ⎪
   anticholinergic side effects ⎭
5. Small or large bowel   ⎫ Obstructed
   obstruction   ⎬ peristalsis
6. Gastric carcinoma   ⎭
7. Pyloric stenosis   ⎫
8. Shock of any cause   ⎪
9. Fear, pain or anxiety   ⎬ Delayed gastric
10. Late pregnancy   ⎪ emptying
11. Deep sedation (opioids) ⎪
12. Recent solid or fluid intake ⎭

Other causes
1. Hiatus hernia
2. Oesophageal strictures – benign or malignant
3. Pharyngeal pouch

dent is a more reliable index of the degree of gastric emptying than the period of fasting. It is not uncommon to encounter vomiting up to 24 h after ingestion of food when trauma has occurred very shortly after the meal. Thus the 4–6 h rule is quite unreliable.

Injury from the aspiration of gastric contents results from three different mechanisms: chemical penumonitis (from acid material), mechanical obstruction from particulate material and bacterial contamination. Aspiration of liquid with a pH < 2.5 is associated with a chemical burn of the bronchial, bronchiolar and alveolar mucosa leading to atelectasis, pulmonary oedema and reduced pulmonary compliance. Bronchospasm may also be present. The claim that patients are at risk if they have more than 25 ml of gastric residue with a pH < 2.5 is based on data from animal studies extrapolated to humans and should not be regarded as indisputable fact. Day cases often have residual gastric volumes higher than 25 ml.

If aspiration of gastric contents occurs, the first manoeuvre after the airway is secured is to suction the trachea to remove as much foreign material as possible. If particulate matter is obstructing proximal bronchi, bronchoscopy may be necessary. Hypoxaemia is managed with O_2, IPPV and PEEP. Steroids are not recommended and anti-biotics should be given if the aspirated material is considered unsterile.

TECHNIQUES OF ANAESTHESIA

It is important to recognize any patient who may have significant gastric residue and is in danger of aspiration. The anaesthetic management of such a patient may be described in five phases: preparation, induction, maintenance, emergence and postoperative management.

Phase I – preparation

Whilst postponement of surgery in the emergency patient may be indicated in order to obtain investigations and institute resuscitation with i.v. fluids, there is usually no benefit to be gained in terms of reducing the possibility of aspiration of gastric contents and the risk of aspiration must be weighed against the risk of delaying an urgent procedure. However, two manoeuvres are available:

1. Although not completely effective, insertion of a nasogastric tube to decompress the stomach and to provide a low pressure vent for regurgitation may be helpful. Aspiration through the tube may be useful if gastric contents are liquid, as in bowel obstruction, but is less effective when contents are solid. Cricoid pressure is still effective at reducing regurgitation even with a nasogastric tube in situ.

2. Clear oral antacids (e.g. sodium citrate) may be used to raise the pH of gastric contents immediately before induction. However, this also increases gastric volume. Particulate antacids should not be used, as they can be very damaging to the airway if aspirated. The preoperative administration of H_2-receptor antagonists can consistently raise gastric pH and may reduce the chance of chemical pulmonary injury occurring in the event of inhalation. Although this is standard practice in obstetric anaesthesia, few anaesthetists employ these measures for emergency general surgery. The regimens which may be used are described in Chapters 13 and 32.

Phase II – induction

Rapid-sequence induction

This is the technique employed most frequently

for the patient with a full stomach, although it contravenes one of the fundamental rules of anaesthesia, namely that muscle relaxants are not given until control of the airway is assured. The decision to employ the rapid-sequence induction technique balances the risk of losing control of the airway against the risk of aspiration. It is therefore imperative to assess carefully whether or not difficulty is likely to be encountered in performing tracheal intubation. The anaesthetist must have prepared a contingency plan for management of the patient should intubation fail. If preoperative evaluation indicates a particularly difficult airway, the anaesthetist should consider alternative methods of proceeding, e.g. local anaesthetic techniques or 'awake intubation' under local anaesthesia.

For rapid-sequence induction to be consistently safe and successful it should be performed with meticulous attention to detail. The patient *must* be on a tipping trolley or table, preferably with an adjustable head piece so that the degree of neck extension/flexion may be altered quickly. Ideally, the patient's head should be in the classic 'sniffing position' with the neck flexed on the shoulders and the head extended on the neck. Failure to appreciate this point increases the likelihood of difficult intubation.

The anaesthetist *must* be aided by at least one skilled assistant to perform cricoid pressure, assist in turning the patient, obtain smaller tracheal tubes, supply stilettes for tubes, etc. High volume suction apparatus *must* be functioning and the suction catheter should be within reach of the anaesthetist's hand.

As with any anaesthetic, the machine should have been checked before starting, the ventilator adjusted to appropriate settings and all drugs drawn up into labelled syringes before induction. The patient should breathe 100% O_2 for 3–5 min while appropriate monitoring devices are attached and an i.v. infusion started (if not already in place). The optimal inclination of the operating table is debatable as some authorities recommend the reverse Trendelenburg (head-up) position (to prevent regurgitation) and some the classic Trendelenburg position (to prevent aspiration of any regurgitated or vomited material). In general, the optimum position is that in which the junior

anaesthetist has gained greatest experience in performing intubation.

Preinduction measurement of heart rate, arterial pressure (and, when appropriate, central venous pressure) and inspection of the ECG are made and a skilled assistant is positioned on the patient's right side to perform Sellick's manoeuvre (cricoid pressure). It is important that the assistant can identify the cricoid cartilage, as compression of the thyroid cartilage distorts laryngeal anatomy and may render tracheal intubation very difficult. To perform Sellick's manoeuvre correctly, the thumb and forefinger of the right hand press the cricoid cartilage firmly in a posterior direction, thus compressing the oesophagus between the cricoid cartilage and the vertebral column. Because the cricoid cartilage forms a complete ring, the tracheal lumen is not distorted (Fig. 31.1).

Opinions differ with regard to the time at which cricoid pressure should be applied. Some prefer to inform the patient and apply it just before administration of the i.v. induction agent; others apply it as soon as consciousness is lost.

With the assistant in position, a predetermined sleep dose of i.v. induction agent is given (usually thiopentone, 2–4 mg.kg^{-1} or less in the presence of hypovolaemia). Without waiting to assess the effect of the induction agent, a paralysing dose of suxamethonium (1.5 mg.kg^{-1}) is administered immediately. As soon as the jaw begins to relax, laryngoscopy is performed and the trachea intubated with the aid of a stilette. Cricoid pressure is maintained until the cuff of the tracheal tube

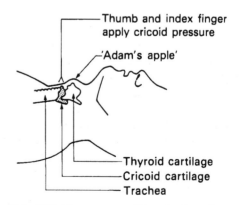

Fig. 31.1   Sellick's manoeuvre. The cricoid cartilage is palpated immediately below the thyroid cartilage.

is inflated and correct placement of the tube ascertained by auscultation of both lungs. The lungs are gently ventilated manually as excessive increases in intrathoracic pressure may have harmful effects on circulatory dynamics. One of the main disadvantages of the rapid-sequence induction technique is the haemodynamic instability which may result if the dose of induction agent is excessive (hypotension, circulatory collapse) or inadequate (hypertension, tachycardia, arrhythmia). Unfortunately, selection of the correct dose is difficult and is dependent largely upon the experience of the anaesthetist. For thiopentone, a dose of 4 mg.kg^{-1} may suffice for healthy, young patients, 2 mg.kg^{-1} for the elderly and less for the very frail. Alternatives are etomidate 0.1–0.3 mg.kg^{-1} (which is less cardiodepressant than thiopentone) and methohexitone 1–1.5 mg.kg^{-1}.

Inhalational induction

If there is reasonable doubt about the ability to perform intubation or to maintain a patent airway in a patient with a full stomach (e.g. the patient with faciomaxillary trauma or the child with epiglottitis or bleeding tonsil), an inhalational induction may be used with oxygen and halothane, followed by an attempt at tracheal intubation during spontaneous ventilation. Normally, the patient should be placed in the left lateral, head-down position, but if circumstances do not allow the lateral position then the supine posture with cricoid pressure may have to be accepted.

Awake intubation

Although blind nasal intubation is a valuable skill, the introduction of the narrow bore fibreoptic intubating laryngoscope has replaced it as the technique of choice in those patients who are likely to develop unrelievable airway obstruction when loss of consciousness occurs (e.g. trismus from dental abscess or angioneurotic oedema). Before embarking on awake fibreoptic nasal intubation it is necessary to render the nasopharynx and, to a greater or lesser extent, the upper airway insensitive, so that the introduction of a tracheal tube may be tolerated. The details of the technique differ depending on the preference of the

individual anaesthetist and one method that is employed commonly is described.

1. The nasal mucosa is anaesthetized with cocaine solution 4% (maximum 2.5 ml per 70 kg) which is sprayed into the more patent nasal passage. In addition to providing surface anaesthesia, this shrinks the nasal mucosa and reduces the chance of bleeding. A well lubricated, soft nasopharyngeal airway (size 6 or 7) is then gently inserted into the nasopharynx and left in situ for 3–5 min. Lignocaine is sprayed through the nasopharyngeal airway to anaesthetize the oropharynx and supraglottic area.

2. Anaesthesia of the tracheal mucosa below the vocal cords is accomplished best by transtracheal injection of local anaesthetic. A 21 G needle is introduced in the midline through the cricothyroid membrane. Entry into the trachea is confirmed by aspiration of air and a bolus of 3–5 ml of lignocaine 1% is injected rapidly. Invariably this results in a bout of coughing which aids spread of the local anaesthetic over the inferior surface of the vocal cords. This procedure may be omitted if the risk of aspiration is considered high, as anaesthesia of the upper airway increases the risk of pulmonary aspiration if vomiting or regurgitation occurs.

For patients in whom there is a high risk of aspiration, it is possible with experience to perform awake nasal intubation after performing only step 1 above and employing a 'spray as you go' technique, injecting aliquots of lignocaine through the suction port of the fibreoptic laryngoscope as it is advanced.

The nasopharyngeal airway is removed and with the patient's head in the 'sniffing the morning air' position, a well lubricated, soft endotracheal tube (size 6 or 7) is inserted gently into the anaesthetized nostril and advanced towards the nasopharynx. The tube should be rotated slowly between thumb and forefinger (pill-rolling movement) and a distinct 'give' is felt on entry into the nasopharynx. Whilst maintaining optimal head position the fibreoptic laryngoscope is then advanced through the endotracheal tube and the pharynx and laryngeal aperture visualized. As maximal vocal cord abduction occurs during inspiration, the scope is advanced slowly in small steps coordinated with inspiration. Even with good upper airway anaesthesia, entry into the larynx results frequently in a violent cough. Once through the larynx the position of the scope is confirmed by visual recognition of tracheal rings and the endotracheal tube is railroaded gently over the scope into the trachea. Position is again confirmed by seeing tracheal rings and the scope removed.

Although considerable practice is needed in the operation of this instrument to ensure a successful outcome, attention to the details of the technique improves the chance of success.

Regional anaesthesia

Anaesthetic expertise in the use of regional anaesthesia is lacking in many United Kingdom hospitals. This is unfortunate as local blocks are eminently suitable for emergency procedures on the extremities (e.g. to reduce fractures or dislocations).

Brachial plexus block by the axillary, supraclavicular or interscalene approach is satisfactory for orthopaedic manipulations or surgical procedures involving the upper extremity. It satisfies surgical requirements for analgesia, muscle relaxation and immobility. There is minimal effect on the cardiovascular system and there is a prolonged period of analgesia postoperatively. Similarly, i.v. regional anaesthesia is useful for orthopaedic reductions; prilocaine 0.5% plain is the drug of choice.

For regional anaesthesia of the lower extremity, techniques available include subarachnoid and extradural anaesthesia. These techniques are contraindicated if there is doubt about the adequacy of ECF or vascular volumes, as large decreases in arterial pressure may result from the associated pharmacological sympathectomy.

It is a common surgical misconception that subarachnoid or extradural anaesthetic techniques are safer than general anaesthesia for patients in poor physical condition. It must be emphasized that for the *inexperienced* anaesthetist, these techniques are invariably more dangerous than general anaesthesia for the patient with moderate/ major trauma or any intra-abdominal emergency condition.

Phase III – maintenance of anaesthesia

In emergency anaesthesia, there are strong arguments in favour of a balanced technique of anaesthesia combining:

1. anaesthesia: loss of awareness
2. analgesia to attenuate autonomic reflexes in response to the painful stimulus
3. muscle relaxation.

If a rapid-sequence induction has been performed, the patient's lungs are gently ventilated manually whilst heart rate and arterial pressure measurements are repeated to assess the cardiovascular effects of the drugs used and of the insult of tracheal intubation. Nitrous oxide 50–66% (dependent upon the patient's condition) in oxygen contributes to loss of patient awareness but does not ensure it and some anaesthetists advocate the use of either 0.5% halothane, 0.5–1% isoflurane or 0.5–1% enflurane in addition.

When there is evidence of return of neuromuscular transmission (by clinical signs or use of a nerve stimulator) as suxamethonium is degraded, a non-depolarizing myoneural blocking agent is administered. The choice is dependent upon the patient's condition and the effect of the induction of anaesthesia on the patient's cardiovascular status. Vecuronium is an appropriate drug for routine use in a dose of 80–100 μg.kg^{-1}. Pancuronium (dose 50–100 μg.kg^{-1}) is useful in patients with hypovolaemia, as it tends to increase arterial pressure and heart rate. (The tachycardia it produces is undesirable in patients with ischaemic heart disease or valvular disease.) Alcuronium (250–300 μg.kg^{-1}) is an alternative drug, but it may produce hypotension which is not usually desirable in emergency anaesthesia. Atracurium has virtually no cardiovascular effects in clinical doses and is useful if renal impairment is present.

When the muscle relaxant has been administered, the tracheal tube is connected to a mechanical ventilator and minute volume adjusted to produce normo- or slight hypocapnia. There are few accurate means of estimating ventilatory requirement, but a minute volume of 100 ml.kg^{-1}.min^{-1} at a tidal volume of 8–12 ml.kg^{-1} should be employed initially. The inspiratory flow rate should be adjusted to minimize peak airway pressure.

Before the initial surgical incision is made, analgesia may be supplemented by small incremental doses of morphine 1–5 mg, papaveretum 2–10 mg or fentanyl 25–100 µg.

The use of supplemental doses of analgesic and muscle relaxant drugs are described in Chapters 10 and 11. The trainee should be aware that during emergency anaesthesia, particularly for intra-abdominal or trauma surgery, much smaller doses of drugs are usually required. As a general rule, it is safe practice to administer half the dose which might be considered appropriate for an elective patient and to determine further doses by assessment of the subsequent response. If there are poor or inadequate recovery room facilities, it is also a good general rule to err on the side of caution in the use of i.v. drugs and consider supplementing anaesthesia with a volatile agent.

Fluid management

During emergency intra-abdominal surgery there may be large blood and fluid losses which exceed the patient's maintenance fluid replacement. These include evaporative losses from exposed gut and mesentery, blood loss on to swabs and into suction bottles and the poorly defined 'third-space losses' caused by sequestration of fluid in inflamed and traumatized tissue. Intraoperatively, maintenance requirements are supplied with Hartmann's solution (compound sodium lactate) at 2 ml.kg^{-1}.h^{-1}. An appropriate volume of replacement for third-space loss and evaporative gut loss is given in addition. This volume depends on the degree of surgical trauma but is normally in the range 2–7 ml.kg^{-1}.h^{-1}.

Haemorrhage in excess of 15% blood volume in adults or 10% in children is usually an indication for blood transfusion.

Phase IV – reversal and emergence

Any volatile agent is discontinued 5–10 min before surgery finishes. On insertion of the last skin suture, direct pharyngoscopy is performed and secretions/debris removed from the pharynx; if a nasogastric tube is in situ, it is aspirated and

left unspigoted. Atropine and neostigmine are given in one bolus of 20 µg.kg^{-1} and 50 µg.kg^{-1} respectively and ventilation is undertaken manually (with an F$_{IO_2}$ of 1.0) so that spontaneous ventilatory activity may be detected. Because the risk of aspiration of gastric contents is as great on recovery as at induction, extubation of the trachea should not be performed until protective airway reflexes are intact. To demonstrate adequacy of reflexes, both level of consciousness and neuromuscular transmission should be assessed.

Level of consciousness

The patient should be awake and respond appropriately to verbal commands, e.g. eye opening.

Neuromuscular function

The adequacy of reversal of paralysis may be determined by observing the patient's ability to sustain a head lift for 5 s and sustain a firm grip without fade (see Table 11.5). Preferably, a nerve stimulator is used to define reversal of neuromuscular transmission (see Ch. 11).

Immediately before tracheal extubation, the patient is turned to the lateral position (if possible) and asked to take a deep inspiration while gentle positive pressure is applied to the airway. At the peak of inspiration, the cuff is deflated and the tracheal tube removed as the patient exhales, thus assisting removal of any secretions which may have accumulated above the cuff. Oxygen 100% is administered until a regular ventilatory rhythm is re-established and the patient has demonstrated an ability to cough and maintain a patent airway. Breathing 40% O$_2$ the patient is transported in the lateral position to the recovery room and remains there until all vital signs are stable, postoperative shivering has ceased, core temperature is normal and there is good perfusion as judged by warm extremities and good urine output.

If there is any doubt about the adequacy of ventilation after reversal of neuromuscular blockade, the patient is taken to the recovery room with the tracheal tube in situ and this is removed from the trachea only when ventilation and gas exchange are adequate.

Phase V – postoperative management

Postoperatively the patient requires analgesics, e.g. morphine 0.2 mg.kg^{-1} i.m. 4-hourly or papaveretum 0.3 mg.kg^{-1} 4-hourly. If there is continued concern about the metabolic or volaemic state of the patient, these dosages should be reduced considerably. Fluid balance should take into account maintenance needs plus compensation for abnormal fluid loss (e.g. gastric aspirate, loss from intestinal fistulae or from surgical drains). This subject is discussed in Chapter 21.

The need for further blood replacement is assessed by regular observation of vital signs and drainage measurements and postoperative Hb or haematocrit measurements.

Prophylactic postoperative IPPV

Continuation of IPPV should be considered electively in a number of ill-defined circumstances, some of which are listed in Table 31.4.

THE ANAESTHETIST AND MAJOR TRAUMA

The management of the patient with major trauma requires a multidisciplinary team effort. Successful treatment is often dependent on the efficacy of the initial resuscitation and rapid formulation of the correct priorities.

Immediate care

As soon as the patient arrives in the Accident and Emergency Department, resuscitation, diagnosis and specific treatment are required simultaneously.

The first priority for the anaesthetist when confronted with an unconscious trauma victim is to establish the patency of the patient's airway whilst

Table 31.4 Indications for continuation of ventilatory assistance postoperatively

1. Prolonged shock/hypoperfusion state of any cause
2. Massive sepsis (faecal peritonitis, cholangitis, septicaemia)
3. Severe ischaemic heart disease
4. Extreme obesity
5. Overt gastric acid aspiration
6. Previously severe pulmonary disease

assuring immobilization of the cervical spine. If upper airway obstruction is present, the pharynx is cleared of any debris and the jaw displaced forward (jaw thrust). Neck tilt and chin lift are avoided as these manoeuvres could displace an unstable cervical spine. Early establishment of a patent airway is paramount to successful resuscitation and although unstable cervical spine injuries are relatively uncommon, all patients should be assumed to be at risk until proven otherwise. Exclusion of this injury will require cervical spine radiography and possibly computed tomography.

When the airway is clear, attention is directed to the adequacy of ventilation and the need for tracheal intubation. If the patient is apnoeic, ventilation by mask with 100% oxygen is started immediately, as good oxygenation and correction of hypercapnia should be ensured before tracheal intubation is undertaken. The possibility of a cervical spine injury does not contraindicate orotracheal intubation provided it is performed with care and in-line immobilization of the cervical spine is maintained throughout the procedure.

Patients with severe faciomaxillary trauma who are cooperative and awake despite their injuries may not require immediate tracheal intubation, but do need frequent and regular upper airway evaluation to assess the rate of progress of pharyngeal or laryngeal oedema which may proceed to complete airway obstruction with alarming rapidity.

When the airway is under control, ventilation is deemed adequate and any obvious external bleeding has been arrested, the next priority is evaluation of the cardiovascular system; this may be divided into assessment of blood volume status and pump function.

Volume status

This has been described earlier in this chapter. Patients with major trauma often require urgent restoration of circulating blood volume. At least two large-gauge (14-gauge) i.v. cannulae are inserted percutaneously into veins in one or two limbs and both cannulae are attached to blood warming coils. As soon as possible, a reliable CVP catheter is inserted. The right internal jugular vein is the preferred site for this purpose. Fluid is infused through the peripheral i.v. cannulae to produce a CVP of approximately 0–3 cmH$_2$O (manubrium being the zero reference).

Whilst whole blood is the ideal fluid for restoration of blood volume in haemorrhagic shock, substitute fluid should be given immediately while crossmatching is undertaken. If total exsanguination is imminent, type-specific blood may be given, as the chance of a reaction is less than 1% in males, but over 2% in parous females. If the patient has 20–30% blood volume depletion, 2 litres of Hartmann's solution may be infused rapidly whilst crossmatching is in progress. If this does not increase perfusion and arterial pressure significantly and blood is still not available, either plasma or a plasma substitute should be considered. Human albumin solution is very expensive and probably has little advantage over gelatin solutions. Their half-life in the circulation is approximately 4 h in the normal patient, but is shorter in the presence of shock. As 85% is excreted by the kidneys, gelatin solutions promote an osmotic diuresis and may therefore preserve urine output and renal function. Up to 1500 ml may be given initially; in most circumstances this is adequate to restore circulating blood volume until crossmatched blood is available. Warmed, stored blood is administered subsequently to maintain urine output, arterial pressure and CVP.

Pump function

The commonest cause of pump failure in major trauma is the presence of a tension pneumothorax, but other possibilities include severe myocardial contusion and traumatic pericardial tamponade.

Tension pneumothorax causes compression of the mediastinum (heart and great vessels) and presents with extreme respiratory distress, shock, unilateral air entry, a shift of the trachea towards the normal side and distension of the veins in the neck, although the last sign may not be seen in hypovolaemic shock. It may be relieved immediately by insertion of a 14-gauge cannula through the 2nd intercostal space in the midclavicular line but this should be followed by standard chest drainage. If there is any suspicion of tension pneumothorax, IPPV should not be instituted until decompression has been achieved, otherwise mediastinal compression is increased. Patients with blunt chest trauma and fractured ribs may develop a tension pneumothorax rapidly when positive pressure ventilation is commenced and consideration should be given to the prophylactic insertion of chest drains in such patients.

Definitive care

Whenever possible, hypovolaemia should be corrected before anaesthesia is induced, but if the rate of haemorrhage is likely to exceed the rate of transfusion and continued transfusion results only in further bleeding (e.g. ruptured aorta), it may be necessary to induce anaesthesia in a hypovolaemic patient.

On arrival in theatre, the patient is placed on the operating table, which is covered by a warming blanket at 37°C. One hundred per cent oxygen is given whilst at least two large-gauge cannulae are inserted (one connected to a blood warming coil), if this has not already been accomplished. In patients with major trauma, anaesthesia should be induced in theatre so that surgery can start as soon as possible. Figure 31.2 illustrates standard monitoring which is necessary for the management of major trauma. In the unconscious patient, the trachea may be intubated after administration of a paralysing dose of suxamethonium. If the patient is conscious, despite being severely hypovolaemic, a controlled rapid-sequence induction employing ketamine as the i.v. induction agent is preferred. The dose of ketamine is critical and often very small doses (0.3–0.7 mg.kg^{-1}) suffice. If the dose is misjudged, cardiovascular decompensation similar to that seen with other i.v. induction agents may occur. The depressant effects of i.v. induction agents are exaggerated because the *proportion* of the cardiac output going to the heart and brain is increased. In addition, the rate of redistribution and/or metabolism is decreased as a result of reduced blood flow to muscle, liver and kidneys and thus blood concentrations remain elevated for longer periods in comparison with healthy patients. Ketamine should not be used in patients with significant head injury. Etomidate (0.1–0.3 mg.kg^{-1}) is an alternative for normovolaemic patients with head injury, but is more likely to attenuate compensatory mechanisms. Even a single bolus dose of etomidate may interfere with adrenal function and recommendations concerning the use of this drug must be guarded.

After tracheal intubation, the lungs are ventilated at the lowest peak airway pressure consistent with an acceptable tidal volume. Pancuronium is given in small incremental doses of 1 mg to maintain relaxation. When the haemodynamic situation has stabilized and systolic arterial pressure exceeds 90 mmHg, consideration may be given to deepening anaesthesia. This should be undertaken cautiously and, in principle, agents which are rapidly reversible or rapidly excreted should be employed.

In the shock state, there is very rapid uptake of inhalational agents. As a result of chemoreceptor stimulation, the patient hyperventilates, thus accelerating the rate of increase of alveolar concentration of anaesthetic gas. Similarly, reduced cardiac output and pulmonary blood flow decrease the rate of removal of anaesthetic agent from the alveoli, producing a rapid increase in alveolar concentration. Thus the MAC value is approached more rapidly than in normovolaemic patients.

Monitoring should be comprehensive in these patients (Fig. 31.2) and should be commenced before induction of anaesthesia when feasible. Blood may be sampled from the arterial line to monitor changes in acid–base state, haemoglobin concentration, coagulation, PCV and elec-

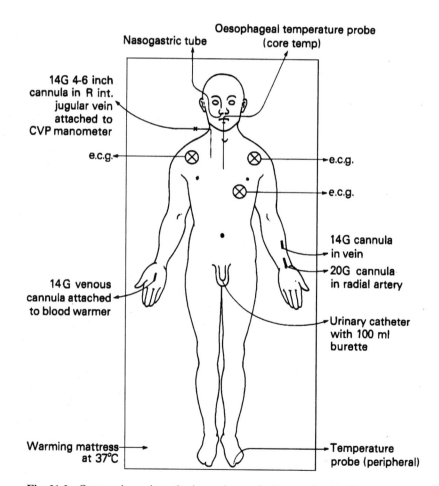

Fig. 31.2 Commonly used monitoring and resuscitation attachments in management of a patient with multiple injuries.

Table 31.5 Causes of persistent hypotension

1. Continued overt bleeding
2. Continued concealed bleeding – chest, abdomen, retroperitoneal space, pelvis, soft tissues of each thigh } Surgical or medical (check platelets and clotting screen)
3. Pump failure – haemothorax, pneumothorax, tamponade, myocardial contusion
4. Metabolic problem – acidaemia (only correct pH less than 7.1)
   hypothermia (largely preventable)
   hypocalaemia

trolyte concentrations. Requirements for further colloid replacement may be assessed from CVP measurement and urine output.

When surgical bleeding has been controlled, the patient's cardiovascular status should improve, but if hypotension persists despite apparently adequate fluid administration, other causes of haemorrhage should be sought (Table 31.5). It is important that the anaesthetist assesses the patient regularly during prolonged anaesthesia to exclude these latent complications of major trauma.

Massive transfusion

One definition states that if an amount greater than 50% of the patient's blood volume is replaced rapidly, the transfusion is deemed massive, e.g. 5 units of blood in 1 h in a 70 kg adult. Stored blood is an unphysiological solution with a pH of 6.6–7.2, serum potassium concentration of 5–25 mmol.litre^{-1} and a temperature of 4–6°C. It contains citrate as an anticoagulant. When stored for more than 5 days, it contains insignificant amounts of 2–3 DPG; consequently the oxygen dissociation curve is shifted to the left. Blood stored for more than 24 h has no functional platelets; concentrations of factors V and VIII are approximately 10% of normal and factor IX 20% of normal. Effete cells and platelets clump together forming debris that is potentially harmful when infused in sufficient quantity. Many of these disadvantages of stored blood are not clinical problems; for example, citrate is removed by metabolic conversion in the liver (forming mostly bicarbonate), the transfused cells act as a potassium 'sink' and mop up excess potassium quickly

and the post-transfusion alkalosis (resulting from citrate metabolism) may contribute to hypokalaemia in the post-transfusion period. If the transfused blood is warmed to body temperature before transfusion and a 20 micron filter is used to remove unwanted cellular debris, the commonest problem is haemostatic failure.

Transfusion of bank blood in quantities approaching the patient's blood volume causes a dilutional thrombocytopenia and some degree of clotting factor deficiency, both of which affect haemostasis adversely. These abnormalities may be detected by a platelet count, prothrombin time and partial thromboplastin time, reflecting disorders of extrinsic and intrinsic systems as a result of dilutional loss of factors V and VIII. Treatment should be directed at correcting the dilutional coagulation change and consists of fresh frozen plasma (1 unit for every 4 units of blood), platelet concentrate for severe thrombocytopenia (platelet count less than 30×10^9 platelets.litre^{-1}). Requests for these expensive blood products should be made early as there is often delay in obtaining them and it is better, if possible, to prevent the development of coagulation failure and the resulting bleeding tendency. Although diffuse pathological bleeding may be secondary to dilutional effects it is also a manifestation of tissue hypoperfusion due to shock and inadequate or delayed resuscitation. Clinically this microvascular bleeding produces oozing from mucosae, raw surfaces and puncture sites and may increase the extent of soft tissue and pulmonary contusions. It is difficult to treat and this underscores the importance of rapid and adequate resuscitation.

The rapid and effective restoration of an adequate circulating blood volume is crucial in the management of major haemorrhage, as mortality increases with increasing duration and severity of shock. The importance of the prevention of hypothermia during massive transfusion cannot be overstated. Hypothermia causes platelet dysfunction, reduced metabolism of citrate and lactate and an increased tendency to cardiac arrhythmias, which may result in a bleeding diathesis, hypocalcaemia, metabolic acidaemia and cardiac arrest. Core temperature should be measured continuously during massive transfusion and every effort must be made to prevent heat loss. Thermally insulating plastic drapes can be used to cover the patient who should be placed on a heated 'ripple' mattress. A heated water bath humidifier is more efficient than the disposable heat and moisture exchangers. Efficient systems for heating stored blood and allowing rapid infusion are available but all fluids should be warmed to body temperature if possible.

FURTHER READING

Nimmo W S, Rowbotham D J, Smith G (eds) 1994 Anaesthesia, 2nd edn. Blackwell Scientific Publications, London

32. Obstetric anaesthesia and analgesia

The profound physiological effects of pregnancy have an important role in altering the maternal response to systemically administered analgesics, anaesthetic drugs and vertebral blocks. These changes are described in detail in Chapter 5.

History

Labour is painful for the majority of mothers and extremely painful for some. Indeed, progress in labour in former years was frequently related to the degree of pain experienced by the mother. The successful outcome, the delivery of a healthy baby and survival of a healthy mother, reduced the subjective importance of the pain experienced by the mother during labour. However, not all mothers have a successful outcome. Until 1846, little could be done to relieve the distress and suffering undergone by those mothers. In that year, Simpson administered ether to a labouring mother and delivered her of a dead child. The significance of the benefits of general anaesthesia was immediately recognized, the practice spread rapidly and was welcomed in other fields of surgical practice. However, considerable resistance to its adoption in obstetrics was manifest by the conservative clergy. It says much for Simpson's strength of character and eloquence that he overcame the clergy's criticisms successfully.

Although ether was the first anaesthetic agent, chloroform was quickly adopted as the drug of choice. The importance and acceptance of general anaesthesia and analgesia by inhalational methods may be judged by the fact that chloroform was administered to Queen Victoria by Dr John Snow at the birth of her eighth child in 1853. The administration of chloroform was probably unnecessary but it was a powerful advertisement for its safety and propriety, and resistance crumbled subsequently.

Spinal anaesthesia, introduced by Bier in 1899, was popularized by Tuffier and gained widespread acceptance with astonishing rapidity. By 1907 it had been used widely in almost all branches of surgery, including obstetrics. Complications such as ventilatory failure, hypotension and the high incidence of headaches were recognized but were outweighed by the benefits. Systemic analgesics were introduced in obstetrics in 1901; morphine was employed initially but the combination of papaveretum and hyoscine (twilight sleep) became the most popular technique. The value and safety of nitrous oxide/oxygen or air mixtures were known, but early apparatus was cumbersome. It was not until 1933, when Minnitt introduced a portable nitrous oxide/air machine, that inhalational analgesia became widespread. Unfortunately, the mixture of nitrous oxide and air was hypoxic. Nevertheless, the Minnitt apparatus was used widely in the UK for many years. Extradural analgesia was not introduced to obstetric practice until 1941 and in the UK a continuous extradural analgesia service did not become available until 1964.

Innervation of the uterus and birth canal

This is depicted in Figure 32.1. Afferent nerves from the body of the uterus and the cervix are somatic sensory fibres, although they travel with sympathetic nerves. They emerge bilaterally from the uterus on each side of the cervix and pass laterally in the paracervical tissues to traverse the cervical plexus. The fibres continue in the base

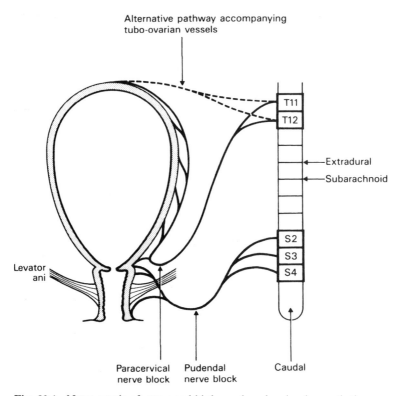

Fig. 32.1 Nerve supply of uterus and birth canal, and regional anaesthetic techniques which may be used to produce pain relief during labour and vaginal delivery.

of the broad ligament, pass through the inferior, middle and superior hypogastric plexuses and enter the sympathetic chain in the lumbar and lower thoracic regions. The central connection from the sympathetic chain is via the white rami communicantes of the 11th and 12th thoracic nerves; in some women, a proportion of nerve fibres pass through the first lumbar nerve. There may be an additional afferent pathway from the cervix to S2–4 through pelvic splanchnic nerves.

The haemorrhoidal and perineal nerves, and the dorsal nerve of clitoris, carry impulses from the vagina, vulva and perineum through the pudendal nerve bilaterally to S2–4; the pudendal nerves also provide the motor supply to levator ani. Some areas of perineal and vulval skin are innervated by the ilioinguinal, genitofemoral and posterior femoral cutaneous nerves and by cutaneous branches of S2–4.

Sympathetic (T5–L2) and parasympathetic fibres (S2–4) carry efferent impulses to the uterus and affect its motor function. Uterine contractility during labour is largely independent of these impulses, although the relationship between uterine function and neurophysiology is far from clear.

The choice of nerve block is directly related to the pain relief required. For simple outlet forceps delivery a pudendal nerve block can be adequate, but for more complicated deliveries, more extensive blocks are required.

PAIN RELIEF IN LABOUR

Pain during the first stage of labour is caused by uterine contractions and dilatation of the cervix. In the second stage, pain is caused by stretching, distension and tearing of fascia, skin and subcutaneous tissues, and by pressure on the skeletal muscle of the perineum.

This brief account of analgesia and anaesthesia in obstetrics does not deal in depth with the subject of preparation of the mother for labour, but this must not deny or diminish the importance of adequate, skilled preparation. The aspirations and expectations of each mother are different and must be taken into account in the assessment of analgesic requirements. Birth plans are a common feature now, and must be discussed in detail with the mother early in her pregnancy. However, with the increase in the popularity of shared care with the general practitioner, many mothers do not have the opportunity to discuss their aspirations. This can have a profound effect on the conduct of the mother's delivery. Many practices are in place at present in the belief that they enhance maternal safety or welfare. The proscription of food intake during labour on the basis that a general anaesthetic may be required at any time is an example. Mothers, encouraged by groups of health care professionals, are beginning to question such practices and even insist that they can have the freedom of choice regarding oral intake. It is true that there is no proof that limited oral intake would be a real hazard, but circumstantial evidence would support the restriction of oral intake to clear fluids.

The current situation emphasizes the urgent need for adequate time and facilities for discussion of the mother's aspirations and that must include the subject of pain control in labour. It is clear from many studies that the pain experienced by many mothers is extremely severe, but that the most effective method of pain relief, extradural analgesia, does not necessarily provide the greatest maternal satisfaction. Pethidine, diamorphine and Entonox have been shown to be relatively ineffective in relieving pain, but the proportion of satisfied mothers who have used these techniques are similar to that of those who receive extradural analgesia. Clearly, pain is but one element in the complex issue of the distress of labour; however, it may be treated effectively and therapy must not be withheld. Psychological preparation and sympathetic support are essential during labour.

It is impossible to predict when emergency intervention may be required in obstetrics, but if oral fluids are restricted, dehydration and thirst must be recognized and treated with an intravenous (i.v.) infusion. An infusion is mandatory if extradural analgesia is considered. Ketosis is a normal accompaniment of labour and is not necessarily related to maternal dehydration. The use of i.v. solutions that contain glucose to relieve ketosis is unnecessary and should be avoided; either saline 0.9% or compound sodium lactate should be used. Frequently, labour is augmented by i.v. Syntocinon, which is best prepared in a concentrated form and administered by syringe pump in order to limit the volume infused.

Systemic analgesics

The ideal analgesic drug should relieve pain without other effects on the mother and baby. Unfortunately, none of the available drugs is without side-effects and all opioid analgesics share similar advantages and disadvantages. The disadvantages include:

1. Transfer across the placental barrier.
2. Sedation of the baby.
3. Ventilatory depression of the mother.
4. Delay in gastric emptying.

Pethidine is probably the most popular analgesic used in British obstetric practice. It is administered most frequently by intramuscular (i.m.) injection in a dose of 100–150 mg and is most effective when given relatively early in labour, before distress is severe. There is a rapid increase in the maternal serum pethidine concentration after i.m. injection followed by a similar and parallel increase in the fetal serum pethidine concentration as the drug crosses the placenta freely. Paediatric staff should be informed if pethidine has been given within 3 h of delivery, as it may induce ventilatory depression in the neonate. Neonatal ventilatory depression resulting from opioid drugs administered to the mother may easily be reversed by naloxone (20 µg injected into the umbilical cord vein). Neurobehavioural assessment studies of neonates whose mothers have been given sedation during labour or for delivery have shown that the influence of sedative drugs can be detected for up to 48 h after delivery. The long-term significance of these effects, if any, is still not clear.

Pethidine may also be administered intravenously, either as a single bolus injection or by a patient-controlled analgesia system (see p. 439). The volume and concentration of the drug and the lock-out period are preset, thus leading to more flexible administration.

Inhalational analgesia

Entonox, a 50% mixture of nitrous oxide and oxygen, is the most widely used inhalational analgesic agent in the UK. It has the advantages of providing a high inspired oxygen concentration and rapid onset of analgesia, and is self-administered. The rapid onset is attributable to the relatively insoluble nature of nitrous oxide in blood, and is mirrored by an equally rapid elimination; consequently it is non-cumulative. The apparatus designed for its use is simple and safe, provided that the cylinders are kept at a temperature above −7°C. Nitrous oxide is not inert, but there are no physiological or biochemical consequences of note in the concentrations and durations used in obstetric practice. Entonox is usually used in conjunction with pethidine, and the majority of labours in the UK are conducted with this form of pain relief. To obtain the maximum benefit, contractions should be regular and the mother starts to inhale the gas mixture just before a contraction occurs. A gas-tight fit with the mask is essential; for mothers who prefer it, a mouthpiece is available.

Local anaesthetic techniques

Local blocks are designed to interrupt the sensory input and so are dependent on the site of injection. Apart from a pudendal block, which is suitable for outlet forceps delivery, blocks used in obstetrics are now almost exclusively confined to spinal and extradural techniques.

Pudendal block

This block is usually performed by the obstetrician. Using the vaginal approach, the pudendal nerves are blocked as they pass under and slightly posterior to the ischial tuberosity. The major disadvantage is that the block is frequently unilateral. In addition, there is a distinct risk of exceeding the maximum dose of local anaesthetic agent if the perineum is infiltrated. For this reason, prilocaine 0.5% should be used to minimize the risk of toxic

reactions. Otherwise the block is safe and is not associated with risk to the fetus. Anaesthesia is confined to the vagina; the block is suitable only for outlet or low-cavity forceps delivery. The pain of mid-cavity, rotation or Ventouse deliveries is not relieved.

Caudal block

Caudal block is rarely used in the UK, but it can be a useful technique for providing rapid relief of pain when mothers are approaching or in the second stage of labour and require vaginal anaesthesia. It provides excellent analgesia for instrumental delivery.

The sacral hiatus lies caudal to the fourth sacral tubercle, between the two sacral cornua. The anaesthetist must be familiar with and able to identify the anatomical landmarks of the sacral hiatus before undertaking the block. If the patient is particularly obese, or if the landmarks cannot be identified, the anaesthetist should not proceed with the block. Under sterile conditions, the sacral hiatus is identified, the overlying skin infiltrated with local anaesthetic and a needle (e.g. 21-gauge) is inserted at an angle of 45° to the patient's back until the sacrococcygeal ligament is pierced. The needle direction is then changed to 30° when loss of resistance is felt as the needle passes through the ligament into the extradural space. In other respects, the injection is identical to lumbar extradural analgesia and the same precautions are taken. After ensuring that neither cerebrospinal fluid nor blood is aspirated, 10–15 ml of local anaesthetic are injected slowly. If continuous caudal block is required, the needle should be replaced with a 16- or 18-gauge i.v. cannula, through which an extradural catheter is inserted. Precautions, complications and their management are similar to those of continuous lumbar extradural analgesia. Like extradural anaesthesia, the choice of local anaesthetic is usually bupivacaine 0.5% or 0.25%.

Paracervical block

Paracervical block is simple to perform and is rapidly effective. It is performed by injecting 5 ml of bupivacaine 0.25% solution, superficially, on each side of the cervix, close to the uterine artery and venous plexus. As a result of its position in relation to the venous plexus, absorption is rapid and the block is frequently associated with profound fetal bradycardia. For this reason it is rarely used in the UK.

Extradural analgesia

The introduction of continuous lumbar extradural analgesia has given mothers the opportunity to benefit from a technique that can virtually eliminate the pain of labour. Studies of the effectiveness of the blocks vary slightly, but 70–80% of mothers experience complete relief of pain in labour when bupivacaine 0.5% is used; no other technique approaches this level of success. Bupivacaine is the local anaesthetic of choice, but the optimum concentration is a matter of debate. The use of 0.25% solution produces less motor block and a lower incidence of instrumental delivery, but provides less effective analgesia than the 0.5% solution. The use of a reduced concentration has the added benefit of reducing the total mass of drug used during labour. Unless the mother wishes complete analgesia, it is probably preferable to start with bupivacaine 0.25% in a volume of 5–9 ml; the volume of injection may be increased if analgesia is inadequate, and a higher concentration may be employed if analgesia continues to be unsatisfactory. If an extradural block is ineffective, the anaesthetist should establish if any degree of block exists by mapping sensory and motor deficits; a frequent cause of failure is that the catheter does not lie within the extradural space.

The use of low concentrations of bupivacaine (0.125% or less) plus the addition of 1–2 μgm of fentanyl.ml^{-1} is proving to be increasingly popular and is now in use as the solution of choice in over 40% of the obstetric units in Scotland, the advantages being the reduced frequency and severity of muscle weakness which may reduce the proportion of instrumental deliveries.

Indications

Pain is the principal indication for extradural analgesia in normal labour. If pregnancy is com-plicated by hypertension or pre-eclampsia, the use of extradural analgesia is almost mandatory, as the resulting sympathetic block reduces arterial pressure and eliminates that element of hypertension which is a consequence of pain and distress.

Contraindications

1. Mother opposed to extradural analgesia.
2. Presence of a coagulopathy.
3. Anticoagulant therapy.
4. Sepsis in the lumbar area.
5. Pre-existing neurological deficit.

Mother opposed to extradural analgesia. In this matter, the mother's views are paramount, and while gentle persuasion may be tried in an effort to provide an informed view, the mother's distress should not be added to.

Presence of a coagulopathy. Coagulation efficacy is almost directly related to the platelet count, and it is generally agreed that if the platelet count is less than 100×10^9 litre^{-1}, extradural and spinal anaesthesia should not be administered unless there are other factors, e.g. difficult endotracheal intubation, which would alter the risk/benefit equation.

Anticoagulant therapy. If the patient is fully anticoagulated, the use of vertebral blocks is proscribed. However, if the mother is receiving low-dose heparin therapy, the position is less clear. There is considerable evidence in non-obstetric practice to suggest that extradural analgesia may be safe in patients receiving low-dose heparin. Low-dose heparin (5000 i.u. twice or three times daily) does not affect the coagulation cascade adversely as routine laboratory tests of coagulation function are usually normal. The response to low-dose heparin is unpredictable; approximately 3% of patients may bleed. If a spinal or extradural block is being considered, a coagulation profile should be obtained before insertion of the block, and if abnormal, the block should not be performed.

Aspirin occupies a similar and equally controversial position. Aspirin has been in widespread use as antiplatelet therapy as part of the management of pre-eclampsia in low doses of 75 mg daily. The results of the recent CLASP study in over 9000 women has identified the value of aspirin therapy to be in mothers with very premature infants and hypertensive disease. The administration of a single dose of aspirin permanently alters platelet function for the life of that platelet, which is approximately 10 days. Aspirin is a thromboxane A inhibitor, and thus a platelet disaggregator, which prolongs the bleeding time. The prolongation of the bleeding time, though statistically significant, is slight, and the bleeding time usually stays within normal limits. Again, if the risk/benefit ratio is sufficiently weighted in favour of the benefit, the bleeding time may be measured, and if within the normal range, the block may be given.

Technique

The insertion of a Tuohy needle into the extradural space is a tactile technique. Optimum conditions for access are essential, and thus time and patience spent in obtaining complete patient co-operation are not wasted. An i.v. cannula must be in place and secured before the block is established.

The patient may be prepared either in the sitting or lateral position; the sitting position provides better access. The back is cleaned and draped and the L2/3 interspace identified; the spinous process of L4 is level with the ischial spines. After local infiltration, a skin puncture is made, through which a Tuohy needle is passed, and advanced into the supraspinous ligament. It is essential to identify the supraspinous ligament to be certain that the needle is correctly sited. A syringe, in which the plunger moves freely, is filled with sterile saline and attached to the extradural needle. The assembly is held in the right hand, and constant pressure applied to the piston of the syringe (Fig. 32.2). The left hand, which is braced against the back, is used to advance the needle. While the point of the needle is in the ligament, injection of saline is impossible. If the point of the needle moves out of the ligament, i.m. injection is possible, but there is resistance to injection. If in doubt, the needle should be withdrawn into the supraspinous ligament, repositioned slightly, and advanced again. Ligamentum flavum is felt as increased resistance to advancement of the needle; when this is detected, the left hand should be

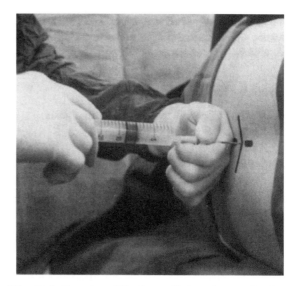

Fig. 32.2 Insertion of Tuohy needle into the extradural space using the loss-of-resistance method. See text for details.

repositioned, and the needle advanced more slowly.

Identification of the extradural space is characterized by a palpable click, felt with the left hand, and a simultaneous and unmistakable total loss of resistance to pressure on the piston of the syringe. The volume injected should be minimal, and the syringe should be disconnected from the needle immediately to ensure that accidental dural puncture has not occurred. Any fluid leaking from the hub of the needle should be allowed to drop on to the back of the gloved hand; if cold, it is likely to be saline, and final identification, in the absence of any bleeding, may be made by using a Dextrostix as saline and local anaesthetic solutions do not contain glucose. It is useful to inject 5–7 ml saline before insertion of the catheter as it makes insertion easier.

The catheter is then passed through the needle and the needle is withdrawn. A sufficient length should be left in the extradural space to allow for movement of the catheter that occurs during labour. It is recommended that 4–5 cm should be inserted; this length is sufficient to permit repositioning if a unilateral block develops and to prevent accidental removal.

If bleeding occurs during insertion of the needle or the catheter, it is essential to ensure that it has ceased before local anaesthetic solution is injected and that the catheter has not passed into a vein. I.v. insertion may be suspected by persistent bleeding into the catheter. Aspiration is not entirely reliable to confirm this, as the vein wall can be drawn against the holes in the catheter, so occluding them. If in doubt, the catheter end should be lowered to allow blood to flow gently along the catheter. If this occurs, the catheter can be advanced until it leaves the vein, or withdrawn, if sufficient catheter is in the extradural space, until the flow of blood ceases. During this manoeuvre, blood can be cleared by gentle flushing and the catheter end lowered or gently aspirated to ensure that blood has ceased to enter the catheter.

Test doses

Despite careful insertion of the extradural catheter, the position of the catheter tip cannot be known with certainty and four possibilities exist:

1. Correct siting.
2. I.v. placement.
3. Subarachnoid insertion.
4. Subdural placement.

A test dose should correctly identify subarachnoid or i.v. injection. It has been shown in a non-obstetric population that the i.v. injection of 15 µg of adrenaline will, within 30 s, cause a transient tachycardia. However, the value of this is disputed in obstetric practice as the maternal heart rate varies widely during labour and many false-positive results would be obtained.

It is essential to administer a test injection to exclude subarachnoid injection. The injection of a suitable volume and concentration of local anaesthetic results in a subarachnoid block if the catheter has pierced the dura. The test dose used to identify subarachnoid placement of the catheter must always be given by the anaesthetist. The block should be assessed to ensure that the injection has not entered the subarachnoid space before administering a top-up injection. Either 3 ml of bupivacaine 0.25% or 2 ml of bupivacaine 0.5% is adequate for the purpose.

Subdural block is difficult to detect, but occurs occasionally, and results from the catheter piercing the dura but not the arachnoid membrane. The

development of a patchy and unexpectedly high but not intense block following a top-up injection should arouse suspicion of subdural placement. This results from the catheter being inserted into the subdural space or, if a typical three-hole catheter is used, part of the catheter may enter the subarachnoid space. The subsequent block, following a top-up injection, will depend on the number of holes lying in the extradural or subarachnoid spaces, and through which holes the major proportion of the local anaesthetic volume escaped.

Management of extradural analgesia

Caval occlusion must be avoided at all times, and the mother *must* be nursed in either the lateral position or in the modified supine position using a Crawford wedge. Careful monitoring of the mother is essential after the initial injection and also after the first dose injected through the catheter, as discussed above. Occasionally, extensive sensory, motor and sympathetic blocks follow extradural injection, even when there is no apparent dural puncture.

Monitoring

1. Caval occlusion *must* be avoided.
2. Check arterial pressure at 5-min intervals if satisfactory, and more frequently if hypotension develops.
3. Check that the i.v. infusion is running satisfactorily.
4. The fetal heart should be monitored continuously.
5. The mother *must not* be left unattended.
6. The anaesthetist must be readily available.

Complications

Hypotension. The limited extradural block that follows the modest doses described above is accompanied by slight hypotension in approximately 5% of normal mothers. If the reduction in arterial pressure is more than 20 mmHg, or the systolic pressure is less than 90 mmHg, active measures should be taken to limit any further reduction. Caval occlusion must be eliminated as a cause by turning the mother to the left lateral position. The rate of the i.v. infusion should be increased. The anaesthetist must be called if the arterial pressure continues to decrease. On arrival, the anaesthetist should assess the extent of the block immediately, as it is vital to differentiate between an unusual response to extradural injection and a subarachnoid injection. If the mother can move both her arms and legs, subarachnoid injection is unlikely. If no arm weakness exists, ventilation will not be significantly impaired. Subarachnoid injection is extremely rare, but the injection of an extradural dose of local anaesthetic solution into the subarachnoid space will produce a total spinal block. Early recognition is essential and demands trained nursing and medical staff; prompt and skilled management will prevent any morbidity or mortality.

Total spinal block. Total spinal blockade occurs when a dose of local anaesthetic intended for the extradural space is injected inadvertently into the subarachnoid space. Cardiovascular support should be provided immediately with i.v. fluids and i.v. ephedrine (5–10 mg), and the systolic arterial pressure should be maintained above 90 mmHg if possible. The development of arm or hand weakness and advancing sensory loss often precedes ventilatory impairment. Before respiratory distress is marked, a standard general anaesthetic (described below) should be administered and controlled ventilation continued until recovery, which occurs usually within 45–60 min. Continual explanation to and reassurance of the mother are mandatory. Subsequent recovery may be complicated by a spinal headache which may require an extradural blood patch (see below) if it remains severe.

Dural puncture. This complicates 1–2% of extradural blocks. The frequency of the spinal headache that follows a dural puncture is related to the diameter of the needle used. Extradural needles are large (16–18-gauge) and 75% of dural punctures caused by a needle of this diameter are followed by severe headache. This low-pressure spinal headache is usually occipital initially. It is characteristically throbbing in nature, more severe when standing or sitting, and relieved by lying down. If dural puncture occurs, it is best to perform an extradural block in an adjacent inter-space; the dermatomal spread of the block should be carefully monitored after each top-up injection, as extensive blocks have been reported in patients with a dural puncture. Isotonic saline 500 ml over 24 h should be infused through the extradural catheter after delivery. The patient should remain in bed during this time, although bed rest has not been shown to be of benefit in reducing the risk of headache.

If the headache is disabling, treatment by extradural blood patch should be considered. The injection of 15–20 ml (or until the mother complains of discomfort) of autologous blood into the extradural space under sterile conditions is thought to produce a fibrinous plug that prevents further escape of cerebrospinal fluid. The headache is relieved in 90% of patients within 4–5 h.

Unilateral block and unblocked segment. An unblocked segment exists when there is evidence of a block above and below the segmental nerve root; a block is described as unilateral if it is more effective on one side. In the latter case, the dependent side usually has the most effective and profound block. Unilateral block may be eliminated by the administration of a further top-up injection after positioning the mother on her other side. Unblocked segments are relatively rare, and the cause is not always clear. A further top-up injection or withdrawal of the catheter by 1–2 cm usually effects a cure. However, if adequate pain relief is not experienced, the catheter should be resited in an adjacent interspace. If an extradural block is totally ineffective, the anaesthetist should examine the patient and map sensory and motor deficits, as the catheter may not lie in the extradural space.

Analgesia may be maintained by intermittent top-up injections when pain recurs, by continuous infusion or by patient-controlled extradural analgesia. The advantages of top-up injections are that the injection may be given when required and the volume and concentration of local anaesthetic increased or decreased as necessary. Close supervision of each top-up is required. Top-up injections should be given in divided doses; 3 ml should be injected initially, and the remainder administered 5–10 min later when assessment has been undertaken to ensure that injection into the subarachnoid space has not occurred.

Continuous injection by infusion pump appears to be an attractive solution, as top-up injections are not required and the pain experienced while waiting for a top-up injection is eliminated. However, the individual requirements of each mother for analgesia make it difficult to identify correctly the optimum concentration and infusion rate of local anaesthetic which unfailingly relieves the pain without producing too extensive a block. The objective is to provide a satisfactory block which relieves the mother's pain without further intervention by either medical or nursing staff. An effective technique is to establish an excellent block initially by injecting a bolus dose of bupivacaine 0.5% plain solution followed by an infusion of 10–14 ml.h^{-1} of bupivacaine 0.125%. Monitoring of the mother is relatively simple and consists of checking the arterial pressure every 30 min. T8 should be marked, and sensory levels checked when the arterial pressure is being taken; if the block extends above this mark, or if motor block is severe, the infusion should be stopped and the anaesthetist informed.

Patient-controlled extradural analgesia has recently been established as an equally effective method of providing good analgesia and offers the additional feature of allowing the mother to control the administration of her own analgesia; not all mothers wish to have complete relief of pain, particularly if they feel that the amount of pain experienced can be controlled. The block is established as described above with 0.5% bupivacaine plain solution and the patient-controlled extradural analgesia (PCEA) device set to deliver 3 ml of 0.25% bupivacaine plain solution with a 5 min lock-out period. This has proved to provide analgesia which is as effective as the other two methods of delivery, has fewer anaesthetic interventions and requires the administration of less bupivacaine than extradural infusions. Patients should be monitored as for midwife top-up injections after each self-administered top-up. T8 should be marked on the abdomen, the block height checked every 30 min and the mother instructed to stop administration if this height is exceeded. Occasionally the block will be above or up to this level and still not provide adequate pain relief; it is therefore essential to monitor the extent of the blockade.

Secondary complications

A number of randomized studies of the increased incidence of instrumental deliveries which are associated with epidural analgesia have attributed part of the increase to the use of epidural analgesia and not solely to the more painful and difficult labour which mothers who receive epidural analgesia frequently experience. The incidence of long-term backache and rectal and urinary incontinence, which are not as rare as originally thought, are currently being attributed to the mode of delivery and/or the epidural block, but this is rather more controversial.

Subarachnoid block

Subarachnoid block is not a suitable technique for pain relief in labour as the duration of the block produced by local anaesthetic agents is too short. The introduction of fine spinal catheters raised hopes that they would provide an effective method of producing analgesia using a small dose of local anaesthetic. However, in the USA, the cauda equina syndrome (long-term bladder and bowel dysfunction) has been reported following their use, although it is believed that this was due to the use of too concentrated a solution of local anaesthetic. Following this, the catheters were withdrawn from the market and are no longer available in the USA.

Spinal anaesthesia remains an excellent choice for Caesarean section, manual removal of placenta and for any instrumental delivery requiring a more extensive and effective block than that provided by a pudendal block if an extradural block is not in place.

The precautions taken before the administration of spinal anaesthesia are the same as for general anaesthesia as it is impossible to predict how effective the block will be, and a general anaesthetic may be required at any time.

If an extradural block is not in place for delivery, subarachnoid block is often used for a trial of forceps, where the obstetrician is not certain that the baby can be delivered vaginally and Caesarean section may be required. For this reason, it is advisable to provide a block which would be suitable for Caesarean section if it proved necessary, rather than having to administer a general anaesthetic. If the reason for instrumental deliver is fetal distress, and the obstetrician is happy that vaginal delivery will be possible, a saddle block is appropriate; the injection is performed in the sitting position, and 1.5 ml of hyperbaric bupivacaine 0.5% given slowly.

CAESAREAN SECTION

Risks of anaesthesia for Caesarean section

For the last 30 years, the triennial *Report on the Confidential Enquiry into Maternal Deaths in England and Wales* has provided a unique and invaluable service to obstetrics. It has contained an objective and detailed analysis of the causes of all maternal deaths and has played a seminal role in the development of obstetric services.

The number of maternal deaths has fallen consistently during the past 30 years, but the proportion attributable to anaesthesia has increased until the last triennium. Clearly, the causes of the reduction are multifactorial and include better maternal health, improvements in maternity care, availability of improved services of laboratories, blood transfusion and so on. It has been disappointing that general anaesthesia has proved so intractable but in the last triennium, 1988–90, the number of deaths due to general anaesthesia

was substantially less than in previous years. Although a very high proportion of deaths due to anaesthesia are associated with avoidable factors (Table 32.1), it is incorrect to assume that if the avoidable factor had not been there, then that death would not have occurred. The majority of deaths were associated with difficulties with tracheal intubation or pneumonitis resulting from aspiration of gastric contents. Most of these deaths follow anaesthesia for Caesarean section. The increased use of subarachnoid and extradural anaesthesia for Caesarean section avoids the need for tracheal intubation and its complications. It is assumed — although not proven — that local techniques reduce the risk of aspiration of gastric contents. However, regional anaesthesia is not suitable for all patients, and general anaesthesia will always have an important role in obstetric practice. In addition, there is a small risk of loss of airway reflexes in patients who inadvertently develop an unduly high extradural or subarachnoid block for Caesarean section. This risk is extremely small, and less than the 1/300 incidence of failed tracheal intubation reported in obstetric general anaesthesia. There is also the possibility that the block will not prove to be sufficiently effective, and the mother will feel pain and so require a general anaesthetic. Consequently, precautions must be taken to control the volume and pH of gastric contents in all patients who

Table 32.1 Direct causes of maternal mortality: figures in brackets represent the percentage of the total number of deaths

	England and Wales			UK	
	1982–84	1985–87	1988–90	1985–87	1988–90
Pulmonary embolism	25 (18.1)	24 (19.8)	23 (16.9)	29 (20.9)	24 (16.6)
Hypertensive disease	25 (18.1)	25 (20.7)	25 (18.4)	27 (19.4)	27 (18.6)
Anaesthesia	18 (13.0)	5 (4.1)	3 (2.2)	6 (4.3)	4 (2.8)
Amniotic fluid embolism	14 (9.0)	9 (7.4)	10 (7.4)	9 (6.5)	11 (7.6)
Abortion	11 (8.0	6 (5.0)	7 (5.1)	6 (4.3)	9 (6.2)
Ectopic pregnancy	10 (7.2)	11 (9.1)	15 (11.0)	16 (11.5)	15 (10.3)

In 1985, the UK figures were published. Note the decline in deaths due to anaesthesia, while ectopic pregnancy remains alarmingly high.

may require Caesarean section. This statement is true of *all* patients who may require a general anaesthetic in the peripartum period.

Control of gastric contents

The physiological changes of pregnancy are associated with slight slowing of gastric emptying, but the administration of opioids such as pethidine or diamorphine for pain relief in labour delays gastric emptying significantly, with an inevitable increase in the volume of acidic fluid. It is believed that if gastric fluid has a pH of less than 2.5, and a volume of more than 0.4 ml.kg^{-1}, aspiration may lead to potentially fatal pulmonary damage. The risks may be minimized by adoption of the following precautions.

Dietary restriction. The mother is allowed to suck ice during labour, but no food or drink is permitted. If fluids are required, these are administered i.v. The precautions for elective surgery are similar to those taken for general surgery; breakfast is withheld. This protocol is coming under increasing pressure in that mothers in a low-risk category want to be permitted the personal freedom at least to drink fluids of their choice, if not to eat food, during labour.

It is the belief of many anaesthetists that the substantial reduction in maternal mortality is attributable to standards that have been introduced and maintained over the last 30 years since Mendelson showed that mothers who consumed food before the administration of a general anaesthetic in obstetrics could die from inhalation of partially digested foodstuffs. In a low-risk pregnancy, the need for general anaesthesia may be slight indeed, but if the mother wishes to eat, the risks, albeit small, must be discussed. It is, however, the mother's choice to accept the consequences. These views must be expressed to the mother in a sympathetic and non-confrontational manner.

It is the author's belief that the mother should be permitted to drink only a limited amount of water during labour. Over one-third of consultant maternity units in the UK allow no food or drink at all in labour, and only 7% allow food.

Elevation of the pH of the gastric contents. This is achieved by the use of antacids and H_2-receptor antagonists. Particulate antacids were used routinely, administered every 2 h in labour, for many years, but experimental studies have shown that aspiration of particulate antacids causes a pneumonitis, and the use of magnesium trisilicate has failed to reduce mortality from aspiration of gastric contents. These observations have led to a reassessment of antacid therapy. The introduction of H_2-receptor antagonists has provided a method of controlling both the gastric volume and the pH. These drugs do not affect the volume and pH of fluid already present in the stomach. However, 6-hourly administration of ranitidine 150 mg during labour reduces the volume of subsequent gastric secretions, and increases the pH by almost eliminating production of acid. Alternatively, treatment may be given selectively only to those mothers who require delivery by Caesarean section or those who need general anaesthesia. Immediately the decision is made to deliver the mother by Caesarean section, cimetidine 200 mg is administered i.m. and 30 ml of $0.3 \text{ mol.litre}^{-1}$ sodium citrate is given orally 5 min before induction of anaesthesia. Ranitidine, which is administered i.m. or by slow i.v. injection, would be a suitable alternative to cimetidine. If surgery is being undertaken with extradural or subarachnoid anaesthesia, the sodium citrate should be administered a few minutes before surgery is started.

Cricoid pressure. The correct application of cricoid pressure reduces substantially the risk of regurgitation of gastric contents. Cricoid pressure must be applied to all obstetric patients who require general anaesthesia until the airway is secured by a cuffed tracheal tube, or while the patient is unconscious in the event that intubation proves to be impossible.

Extradural analgesia

Successful extradural blockade for Caesarean section is a rewarding experience for the mother and the anaesthetist, but is a most demanding technique. The proportion of elective Caesarean sections being undertaken with extradural analgesia is rapidly reducing following the introduction of pencil-point spinal needles and refinements of techniques for subarachnoid block. Nevertheless, extradural block remains a most valuable technique and will be described in some detail. The use of local blocks for Caesarean section continues to increase; they reduce the need for general anaesthesia and permit the mother to participate in the delivery of her child. The technique of extradural block is essentially similar to that described above, but the motor, sensory and sympathetic blocks are more extensive and thus the incidence and severity of complications are increased. Meticulous care and attention to detail are essential. Preparations for surgery begin on the previous day. The H_2-receptor antagonist ranitidine 150 mg should be administered on the evening before, and on the morning of surgery. Recent work has suggested that the formal preload of large volumes of i.v. fluids is unnecessary, but in view of its safety it seems reasonable to infuse at least 500 ml of crystalloid prior to inserting the block. The block is inserted as described above using bupivacaine 0.5% plain solution. An initial injection of 10–12 ml is made through the needle, and a catheter is inserted for administration of subsequent doses. Following institution of the block, the mother is positioned on her side (caval occlusion *must* be avoided) and the onset of the block is monitored at 5-min intervals.

Top-up injections of 7 ml are given when the level of the block can be assessed by the anaesthetist, but the precautions described for the first top-up through the catheter *must* be followed. The onset of action of bupivacaine is relatively slow; on average it is 45 min before the block is established. The block must extend from T6 to S5 to be effective. The dose required to achieve this degree of block is variable, but a total dose of 100 mg of bupivacaine at least is usually required. The extent of the block must be mapped accurately before permitting surgery to commence, and if the block is not level with the xiphisternum, additional top-up injections should be given and adequate time allowed to permit the block to spread.

Hypotension is common, and management is by judicious use of i.v. fluids and ephedrine 5–10 mg i.v., as described previously. Movement of the patient should be avoided when the block is effective to minimize the hypotensive effects of the extensive sympathetic block. During surgery, judicious use of sedatives and analgesics after delivery of the baby may make the procedure more pleasant for the mother, who should always be asked if she wishes sedation. Ergometrine must be avoided in the absence of haemorrhage, as it is associated with a 50% incidence of vomiting, and Syntocinon should be used as an alternative.

Emergency Caesarean section

The majority of emergency Caesarean sections can be undertaken with extradural anaesthesia because the majority of mothers in a unit with an extradural service and who require to be delivered by emergency Caesarean section in labour have an extradural block in place. In addition, the need for the administration of general anaesthesia for Caesarean section can be significantly reduced if the anaesthetist involved in the obstetric unit maintains close contact with both the activity in the labour suite and with obstetric colleagues. Early awareness of obstetric problems in labour, such as failure to progress, or incipient fetal distress that requires either invasive monitoring or repeated determinations of fetal acid–base status, will allow sufficient time to extend an existing and functioning extradural block. The solution of local anaesthetic used to provide pain relief in labour should be changed to bupivacaine 0.5% plain solution and top-up doses administered as described above to achieve a block from T6 to S5. Management should be identical to that above.

If time is a limiting factor, but an otherwise effective block is in place, the speed of onset may be increased by using lignocaine 2% solution with 1/200 000 adrenaline (0.1 ml of 1/1000 solution added to 20 ml of lignocaine 2% plain solution). The commercially prepared 2% lignocaine solution with 1/200 000 adrenaline should not be used as it contains preservative. An additional method of increasing the speed of onset of the extradural block is to administer the local anaesthetic as a slow, continuous single bolus injection of 20 ml over a period of 4 min. Continuous monitoring is important throughout the injection and verbal contact must be maintained with the patient in an attempt to identify inadvertent intravenous injection. Using this technique, the majority of blocks can be extended within 20 min.

Subarachnoid block

The introduction of bupivacaine for subarachnoid block and, more recently, the availability of pencil-point needles have greatly enhanced the value of this block in obstetric practice. Although bupivacaine 0.5% plain solution and bupivacaine 0.5% hyperbaric solution (with 8% glucose) have different characteristics when used in non-obstetric practice for subarachnoid block, this difference is not significant in obstetrics. However, the majority of anaesthetists prefer to use the hyperbaric solution for Caesarean section. The incidence of post-dural puncture headaches (PDPH) is higher in young patients who mobilize early, and thus is high in the obstetric population. The reported incidence has varied widely in obstetrics and has ranged from 5 to 15%. The incidence when using the currently available pencil-point needles (the Sprotte and Whitaker) is less than 2%, and if a headache occurs, it is usually mild. The needles are thought to work by parting the longitudinal fibres of the dura and ligamentum flavum without cutting them, producing a small hole that closes more readily when the needle is removed, thus preventing cerebrospinal fluid leakage. The incidence of PDPH is almost the same as that following extradural blockade, which has a dural puncture rate of approximately 1%.

Subarachnoid anaesthesia offers a number of advantages over extradural anaesthesia for Caesarean section:

1. Onset of action is much faster (10 min versus 45 min).
2. Less bupivacaine is required (12.5 mg).
3. It is arguably a simpler technique with a positive end-point — the detection of cerebrospinal fluid.
4. Patient discomfort is less during performance of the block.

The disadvantages are:

1. Hypotension is common (up to 40%) and may be severe and very rapid in onset, requiring rapid and energetic treatment.
2. Top-up doses are not possible.
3. Patients may be alarmed by the rapidity of onset of the motor and sensory block.

These disadvantages may be minimized but not eliminated. Recent work suggests that the incidence of hypotension and its severity is not modified by the infusion of large volumes of crystalloid, but in view of its safety it seems reasonable to infuse at least 500 ml in the period immediately preceding the administration of the block. An infusion of ephedrine is also effective in maintaining maternal arterial pressure. PDPH may be minimized by the use of fine-gauge spinal needles such as 25-gauge or smaller; 29- and 32-gauge needles have been used in clinical practice, but are very difficult to use. Insertion of the Quincke-type needle with the bevel parallel to the plane of the fibres has also been reported to reduce the incidence of PDPH. However, the use of 25- or 27-gauge Whitaker needles is to be preferred. Enforced bed rest is not desirable, effective or necessary after subarachnoid block.

The use of subarachnoid opioids has refined the technique. Morphine has been advocated, but its use may be associated with delayed-onset respiratory depression, which has occurred following the administration of a dose of 1 mg. Effective analgesia may be provided by the injection of 0.3 mg. Side-effects of nausea and itching may be severe, and although the risk of respiratory depression is still present, it would appear to be small. The use of a small dose of fentanyl would appear to be almost ideal, and subarachnoid injection of 10 µg (0.2 ml) has proved to be very effective. Although the ampoule is supplied in wrapping in the UK, it is not sterile, and care must be taken when preparing the solution for use; the ampoule should not be touched by the anaesthetist.

The risk of delayed-onset respiratory depression following such a small dose has not been reported. Side-effects of nausea and itching are rare, and it is now our standard practice to add fentanyl as described to all subarachnoid injections for Caesarean section.

General anaesthesia

Although there has been an increased tendency to turn to local blocks as the preferred technique for Caesarean section, general anaesthesia will always have a place. Patient preference and the inevitable — if hopefully uncommon — emergency will demand that general anaesthesia is always available. The reduction in the number of general anaesthetics being given for Caesarean section gives rise to concern, as there are, in some maternity units, insufficient cases for anaesthetists and assistants to be trained adequately. If the patient is known previously to have had failed or difficult tracheal intubation, a local block is the technique of choice.

The safe administration of general anaesthesia in obstetrics relies on proper and adequate preparation of the mother where possible, and meticulous checking of the anaesthetic machine to ensure that it is functioning properly and that the vaporizers are full. This check must be part of the routine every day, and if possible, before every anaesthetic. Anaesthetic drugs such as thiopentone, suxamethonium, Syntocinon, etc. should be freshly prepared daily and kept ready in labelled syringes in the refrigerator.

The general anaesthetic technique used for Caesarean section comprises light general anaesthesia with a muscle relaxant, and is very similar to that for most types of emergency surgery. Before anaesthesia is induced, the mother must be placed in the modified supine position with left lateral tilt to avoid caval occlusion. A secure i.v. route must be established, and cross-matched blood should be available. Appropriate antacid therapy must be administered. Adequate pre-oxygenation (5 min) is essential. Rapid-sequence induction of anaesthesia is achieved by i.v. injection of thiopentone 6–7 mg.kg^{-1}, and tracheal intubation with an 8-mm cuffed tracheal tube facilitated by administration of suxamethonium 1.5 mg.kg^{-1}. Cricoid pressure must be applied by a skilled assistant as soon as consciousness is lost, and must not be removed until the tracheal tube is in place and the cuff inflated. Positive-pressure ventilation of the lungs is started immediately after tracheal intubation, using a 50% oxygen/nitrous oxide mixture and the addition of halothane 0.5% or an equipotent concentration of another volatile agent. Ventilation should be sufficient to achieve an end-tidal carbon dioxide tension of 4 kPa. There is some evidence that the inspired concentration of the volatile agent can be increased to 2–3%, until the end-expired concentration approximates to 1 minimum alveolar concentration (MAC); the inspired concentration can then be reduced appropriately. The use of a volatile agent

analyser is essential when this technique is used. The choice of volatile agent is less important.

After delivery of the baby, the inspired oxygen concentration may be reduced to 30% and an opioid drug administered i.v. Muscle relaxation is maintained by administration of small doses of vecuronium, 3–5 mg. An appropriate concentration of volatile agent should be continued to prevent the risk of awareness.

General anaesthesia in obstetrics is unique in that two patients are being anaesthetized. The anaesthetist has to walk the tight-rope between inadequate anaesthesia that results in awareness and the administration of concentrations which anaesthetize the neonate and may cause significant uterine relaxation and consequent haemorrhage. Following the realization in the early 1970s of both the incidence of awareness and its horrors to the victim (the mother), Moir popularized the technique in which halothane 0.5% is added to the inspired gas mixture. This reduced the incidence of awareness to less than 1% without apparently affecting the neonate or the mother adversely. The 50% oxygen/nitrous oxide mixture is used as this increases neonatal oxygenation, but has the disadvantage of increasing the risk of awareness.

Failed intubation

This occurs in approximately 1 in 300 general anaesthetics in obstetrics. The anaesthetist must acknowledge failure at an appropriate time and institute a failed intubation drill. Skilled help should always be available and consultant assistance sought. All the equipment required must be available immediately:

1. A second laryngoscope.
2. A complete range of tracheal tubes of different sizes.
3. Long and short introducers.
4. Gum elastic bougie.
5. Minitracheotomy set.
6. Oesophageal obturator — combi — tube.
7. Magill forceps.
8. Range of oral airways.
9. Nasal airways.
10. Size 3 and 4 laryngeal masks.
11. Cricothyroid puncture set and i.v. cannula.

Before undertaking any general anaesthetic in which tracheal intubation is part of the procedure, an assessment of the ease or otherwise of intubation must be made. A number of schemes have been devised. Perhaps the most common is that of Mallampati, in which assessment consists of asking the patient to open the mouth wide with the tongue protruding; the grade is made on the anatomy of the pharynx that is revealed. These assessments are neither very sensitive nor specific and an additional and most useful guide is to find if the lower teeth can be moved in front of the upper teeth. If this can be accomplished with ease, intubation is likely to be straightforward.

Early admission that intubation is proving difficult is an important part of the failed intubation drill. The anaesthetist must ensure that ideal intubating conditions exist before announcing that a failed intubation has occurred. Failed intubation has important repercussions for all the medical and nursing staff in theatre. Senior help should be summoned when the decision is made to begin the failed intubation drill.

Failed intubation drill

1. Cricoid pressure must be maintained.
2. Place patient head-down in the left lateral position.
3. Maintain oxygenation with 100% oxygen; gentle insufflation of the lungs using an oropharyngeal airway may be required. The maternal oxygen saturation must not be allowed to fall below 90% if at all possible. If the airway cannot be maintained, a laryngeal mask airway may be inserted and has proved invaluable in some cases.
4. The mother should be allowed to wake up; respiratory support should be maintained until the return of spontaneous ventilation.

These difficulties are compounded by the reason for the Caesarean section. If the reason for the surgery is fetal distress, careful but rapid consideration must be given to both maternal and neonatal safety. If the airway can be maintained with the laryngeal mask and the risk of regurgitation is thought to be low, then the operation may continue using an inhalational technique. If, however, this does not prove practical, the patient should be allowed to recover and the alternatives of local blocks considered. Awake fibreoptic intubation is, in this situation, a possibility, but the equipment is not available in many UK maternity units, and relatively few anaesthetists have the required expertise. If regional techniques are impossible, local infiltration remains a possible technique, but it does not provide good operating conditions for either the mother or the surgeon.

If the decision is made to continue the anaesthetic using a volatile agent, the inexperienced anaesthetist should use the technique and volatile agents that are most familiar.

If regurgitation and/or aspiration occurs, a sample of the aspirate should be obtained for measurement of the pH; when the operation is concluded, the patient should be treated symptomatically. Intermittent positive-pressure ventilation should be administered early if respiratory failure develops and the patient should be transferred to an intensive therapy unit.

Awareness

Awareness during general anaesthesia has been a problem of increasing importance. In an effort to reduce the transfer of anaesthetic agents to the neonate, a technique of light general anaesthesia has been used, as described above. The use of unsupplemented nitrous oxide/oxygen mixtures has been associated with an awareness incidence of 17%, and it is clear from the accounts of mothers who have been aware that it can be a terrifying experience. The isolated forearm technique was developed to detect light anaesthesia, which could then be treated before awareness occurred. A sphygmomanometer cuff is placed on the patient's arm and inflated above systolic arterial pressure before the administration of muscle relaxants; the mother retains power in that forearm, and if anaesthetized lightly, could move the isolated arm in response to questioning. However, the technique has proved disappointingly non-specific. Awareness has been shown to be reduced by using an induction dose of thiopentone 5–6 mg.kg^{-1} and an initially high inspired volatile concentration as soon as intubation has been achieved successfully. The use of a volatile agent analyser is invaluable and high concentrations of 2–3 MAC can be used until the end-expired concentration approximates to 1 MAC. It may not be possible to eliminate awareness entirely, but using a suitable concentration of anaesthetic drugs should render it largely a problem of the past. The need to check the anaesthetic machine before use and at least once a day is obvious.

Choice of technique for Caesarean section

The introduction of pencil-point spinal needles and the reduction in PDPH associated with their use have transformed the proportion of elective Caesarean sections undertaken with subarachnoid block, because of the speed of onset and the quality of the block. The elimination of local anaesthetic toxicity has made spinal anaesthesia the most popular choice for elective Caesarean section, almost entirely replacing extradural analgesia for this purpose. The picture changes in the emergency as most patients have extradural analgesia in place and this can be extended rapidly for Caesarean section. For this reason, the anaesthetist must be aware of, and take part in, the activity of the labour suite and should have a knowledge of any developing problems.

The mother must be made aware of the differences between the types of block and their advantages and disadvantages. The incidence of headache following spinal and extradural anaesthesia is similar and should be less than 1%. The hypotension that often accompanies spinal anaesthesia should be borne in mind if fetal distress is severe, although the speed of onset makes it an attractive proposition. General anaesthesia will always be required in some patients, and maternal choice must be paramount if no obvious contraindications to general anaesthesia exist. The advantages of local blocks should be discussed, but no more than gentle pressure should be brought to bear on the mother. If a local technique is chosen, it must be made clear to the mother than she can be given a general anaesthetic at *any* time and at her request. In certain circumstances, general anaesthesia may be the first choice, such as:

1. Anterior placenta praevia.
2. Back sepsis.

3. The presence of a coagulopathy.
4. Maternal choice.

Extradural and spinal opioids

The identification of spinal opioid receptors opened the way for the introduction of intrathecal and extradural administration of opioids. Initial enthusiasm has been tempered by the number of undesirable side-effects associated with their use, such as itching, nausea, vomiting and, of considerably greater anxiety, the onset of delayed respiratory depression due to the rostral spread of the less soluble opioids, of which morphine is the most important example. The use of opioids alone has been disappointing but they are very effective when combined with local anaesthetic solutions. Fentanyl has proved to be the most ubiquitous and has proved of value in both spinal and extradural blocks. The addition of fentanyl 10 µg to spinal anaesthetic solutions improves the quality of the block and reduces the amount of discomfort as the block wanes and postoperative analgesia is administered. Fentanyl has also proved useful in the management of second-stage backache; 50–75 µg may be injected through the extradural catheter in 10 ml of sterile saline. The use of low concentrations of fentanyl and 0.1% or 0.0625% bupivacaine solutions can produce effective extradural analgesia with less motor block than usually associated with extradural blocks.

Spinal and extradural morphine has also proved effective but its use is associated with itching, which can be relieved by naloxone 0.1 mg, and with nausea and vomiting. The use of small subarachnoid doses of morphine 0.1 mg reduces the incidence of side-effects and is still effective although slow in onset. The real risk is the delayed onset of respiratory depression and, if morphine is used, the patient should be kept in a high-dependency unit where adequate monitoring can be performed. Respiratory depression can be reversed with naloxone; an infusion of naloxone may be required if respiratory depression is severe.

COMMON OBSTETRIC PROBLEMS

Retained placenta

Retained placenta is defined as failure to deliver

the placenta within 20 min of delivery, and may be associated with haemorrhage. If bleeding is substantial (more than 500 ml), a postpartum haemorrhage exists and efforts are directed at hastening the removal of the placenta and maintaining cardiovascular stability by rapid i.v. infusion of fluids. If haemorrhage is severe, general anaesthesia may be the preferred choice. All precautions taken for Caesarean section should be employed for the emergency induction and must include antacid therapy, preoxgenation, cricoid pressure and a rapid-sequence induction with tracheal intubation. I.v. opioid and a volatile agent should be employed; anxiety regarding the choice and concentration of volatile agent in relation to uterine relaxation and haemorrhage have probably been exaggerated, and normal concentrations should be used.

If bleeding has not occurred, a regional technique is the one of choice. If an extradural block is in place this can be extended; if not, spinal anaesthesia is suitable. The usual precautions should be taken, but the absence of the neonate diminishes anxiety about hypotension.

Failure of pregnancy

Early failure of pregnancy at 8–14 weeks' gestation is relatively common and evacuation of the uterus under general anaesthesia is undertaken. The technique is simple and generally undemanding. An i.v. induction and mask anaesthesia with a spontaneously breathing patient is the most frequently used technique. Tracheal intubation is rarely necessary, as it is unusual for such patients to require urgent surgery and the patient can be prepared adequately for theatre.

Termination of pregnancy for fetal abnormality is becoming more common as diagnostic precision in early pregnancy improves. If the diagnosis is made sufficiently early, the technique described above is suitable. In later pregnancy (greater than 16–18 weeks' gestation), termination of pregnancy is usually undertaken by the use of extra-amniotic prostaglandins. The anaesthetist is not usually involved in these cases, but a prostaglandin-induced labour may be both extremely painful and slow and the patient may be very distressed; extradural analgesia offers good relief

and should not be withheld. Sedative drugs should also be administered freely.

Pregnancy-induced hypertension

Hypertension, arbitrarily defined as a diastolic arterial pressure exceeding 90 mmHg, complicates some 5% of pregnancies; 1% of patients develop proteinuric hypertension. Fetal outcome is related to the severity of the hypertension and the gestational age of onset. The majority of mothers develop benign hypertension, frequently manifest as an increase in arterial pressure during labour. Extradural analgesia is almost mandatory for such patients, as it reduces arterial pressure and removes that element attributable to pain and distress.

Eclampsia and severe hypertension are frequently associated with a coagulopathy and, occasionally, impaired renal function, and are the third largest cause of maternal death; the most common cause is cerebral haemorrhage. It is for this reason that all obstetric departments should have a protocol prepared, agreed by all senior staff, readily available and applied to all severe cases. Judicious but effective reduction of the blood pressure is essential, as is anticonvulsant therapy; the most commonly used anticonvulsant in the UK is phenytoin, infused in a dose of 750 mg over 30 min. However, this does not always control or prevent convulsions. The definitive treatment is delivery of the baby, but attempts may be made to prolong the pregnancy if the baby is not mature. Delivery may be required urgently under general anaesthesia. Difficulties may be experienced as a result of oedema and the hypertensive response to tracheal intubation.

Haemorrhage

Haemorrhage is defined in relation to the stage of pregnancy as it may develop before, during or after labour and delivery.

Antepartum haemorrhage

Before delivery, haemorrhage is complicated by the presence of the baby. Clearly, the management of the haemorrhage is the same — resuscitation of the mother if necessary, and assessment of the cause and the condition of the baby.

Placenta praevia is diagnosed most frequently at an early ultrasound scan and the mother managed conservatively for as long as possible. The risk of bleeding is related to the position of the placenta and the extent to which it overlies the internal os of the uterus. Delivery is undertaken if bleeding becomes frequent or prolonged, or if pregnancy is near term and bleeding occurs. Fetal welfare is likely to be in jeopardy only if bleeding is severe.

Placental abruption occurs when part of the placenta separates from the wall of the uterus. It is associated with severe abdominal pain. External bleeding is not always obvious, but the degree of shock and hypotension is unrelated to the extent of external blood loss. Fetal well-being is severely compromised and Caesarean section is undertaken as soon as possible. Maternal resuscitation should be vigorous. General anaesthesia should be administered rather than a regional technique, as a coagulopathy is frequently associated with this complication of pregnancy. Laboratory assistance is essential.

Postpartum haemorrhage

Postpartum haemorrhage is said to have occurred if blood loss at or after delivery is greater than 500 ml. Severe blood loss is unusual, but vigorous management should be implemented at an early stage. If the haemorrhage is severe, it is important to alert staff that an emergency has occurred; senior help should be summoned and laboratories informed so that sufficient blood and blood products can be made available rapidly. This complication is frequently associated with a retained placenta as discussed above, or incomplete emptying of the uterus. If bleeding is slight but continuous, exploration of the uterus may be undertaken under subarachnoid anaesthesia.

FURTHER READING

Bogod D G 1995 Obstetric anaesthesia. Baillière's Clinical Anaesthesiology: International Practice and Research 9(4): 591–759

Breivik H, Bogod D G 1996 Obstetric analgesia and anaesthesia. In: Aitkenhead A R, Jones R M (eds) Clinical Anaesthesia. Churchill Livingstone, Edinburgh, pp. 329–365.

Datta S 1991 Anaesthetic and obstetric management of high-risk pregnancy. Mosby Year Book, St Louis, USA.

Moir D D, Thorburn J 1986 Obstetric anaesthesia and analgesia, 3rd edn. Ballière Tindall, London

Morgan M 1994 Obstetric anaesthesia and analgesia. In: Nimmo W S, Rowbotham D J, Smith G (eds) Anaesthesia. Blackwell Scientific Publications, London, pp 1000–1028

Ostheimer G W 1992 Manual of obstetric anaesthesia, 2nd edn. Churchill Livingstone, Edinburgh

Shnider S, Levinson G (eds) 1993 Anaesthesia for obstetrics. Williams and Wilkins, Baltimore

33. Paediatric anaesthesia and intensive care

Major differences in anatomy and physiology in the small infant have important consequences on many aspects of anaesthesia. These differences also cause different patterns of disease in small infants and children seen in the intensive therapy unit, in comparison with adult patients.

The physical disparity between the adult and child diminishes at 10–12 years of age, although major psychological differences continue through adolescence.

PHYSIOLOGY IN THE NEONATE

Respiration

At birth the alveoli are thick-walled and number only approximately 10% of the adult total. Lung growth continues by alveolar multiplication until the age of 6–8 years. The airways remain relatively narrow up to this age, resulting in high airway resistance, and leading to a high incidence of airway disease in the young.

Ventilation is almost entirely diaphragmatic with soft horizontal ribs contributing little to gas movement, in comparison with the bucket-handle movement in the adult.

The high airway resistance and low compliance result in a short time constant (Table 33.1). As a result, the ventilatory rate is rapid. The metabolic cost of ventilation is higher in the infant and may reach 15% of total oxygen consumption.

The metabolic rate in infants is almost twice that of the adult and consequently alveolar minute ventilation is also greater, while functional residual capacity (FRC) is a similar fraction of lung volume as that in the adult. Consequently, inhalational induction of anaesthesia and awakening at the termination of anaesthesia are more rapid than in the adult. Similarly, hypoxaemia occurs much more rapidly in a child.

The poor elastic qualities of the infant lung cause the closing volume (CV) to be greater than FRC until the age of 6–8 years; thus, airways closure occurs during tidal ventilation, leading to an increase in the alveolar–arterial oxygen tension difference ($A-aP_{O_2}$) and a normal arterial oxygen tension (Pa_{O_2}) in the newborn of approximately 9–9.5 kPa (70 mmHg).

Physiological dead space is approximately 30% of tidal volume ($V_d/V_t = 0.3$) as in the adult but the absolute volume is small, so that any increase caused by apparatus dead space has a disproportionately greater effect on a small child (Table 33.2). During anaesthesia, dead space should be kept to a minimum and the resistance of breathing apparatus should be kept low. Secretions resulting either from cholinergic activity or upper respiratory infection may cause respiratory difficulty.

Table 33.1 Lung mechanics of the neonate compared with the adult

	Neonate	Adult
Compliance ($ml.cmH_2O^{-1}$)	5	100
Resistance ($cmH_2O.litre^{-1}.s^{-1}$)	30	2
Time constant (s)	0.5	1.3
Respiratory rate ($breath.min^{-1}$)	32	15

Table 33.2 Respiratory variables in the neonate

Tidal volume (V_t)	$7\ ml.kg^{-1}$
Dead space (V_d)	$V_t \times 0.3\ ml$
Respiratory rate	Neonate 32 $breath.min^{-1}$
	Age 1–13 (24 − age/2) $breath.min^{-1}$

Table 33.3   Variation of heart rate (beat.min^{-1}) with age

Age	Mean value	Normal range
Neonate	140	100–180
1 year	120	80–150
2 years	110	80–130
6 years	100	70–120
12 years	80	60–100

Cardiovascular system

Following the dramatic change from fetal to adult circulation at birth, the child establishes a high cardiac output (commensurate with the high metabolic rate) of approximately 200 ml.kg^{-1}.min^{-1}, which is two to three times the adult value. The small ventricles result in poor ventricular compliance; thus increased cardiac output is produced by an increase in heart rate. Babies tolerate heart rates of up to 200 beat.min^{-1} without evidence of cardiac failure (Table 33.3).

Bradycardia may occur readily in the presence of hypoxaemia or vagal stimulation, and rapid treatment with oxygen or atropine is required. Arrhythmias are uncommon in the absence of cardiac disease, and cardiac arrest usually occurs in asystole rather than ventricular fibrillation.

Systemic arterial pressure is low at birth (approximately 80/50 mmHg) because of the low systemic vascular resistance resulting from the large proportion of vessel-rich tissues in the child. The pressure increases within the first month to approximately 90/60 mmHg and reaches adult levels of 120/70 mmHg at approximately 16 years of age.

Monitoring of the cardiovascular system

The cardiovascular system must always be carefully monitored in babies. Arterial pressure may be measured with a non-invasive monitor using an appropriate-sized cuff.

Intra-arterial monitoring is feasible even in the neonate using a 22- or 24-gauge cannula. Invasive techniques should only be used in major cases and when multiple blood samples may be required. The complication rate associated with intra-arterial monitoring is significantly increased in the very young and can lead to ischaemic damage and emboli. Retrograde flow to the carotid artery has been demonstrated following intermittent flushing of a radial artery cannula.

Central venous pressure (CVP) can be monitored via the internal jugular or subclavian vein. Insertion must be carried out with great care to avoid damage to neighbouring structures such as the pleura.

Pneumothorax has a greater significance in the small child compared to the adult. Venous thrombosis has been reported following CVP catheterization, and the technique should only be employed when required for monitoring of fluid imbalance or cardiac failure. Pulmonary artery catheterization is rarely required in children undergoing non-cardiac surgery.

Blood volume

Variations of up to ±20% of blood volume occur at birth depending on the stage at which the cord is clamped. The average blood volume at birth is 90 ml.kg^{-1}. This decreases in the infant and young child to 80 ml.kg^{-1} and attains the adult level of 75 ml.kg^{-1} at the age of 6–8 years. Blood losses of greater than 10% should be replaced if further losses are expected. Most children with a normal haemoglobin concentration can tolerate losses of up to 20%. Volume replacement with plasma proteins may avoid unnecessary blood transfusion. A haematocrit of 25% is acceptable to avoid transfusion with the attendant risks of transmitted infection and antibody formation which can cause problems later in life, particularly in female children.

Haemoglobin

At birth, 75–80% of haemoglobin is fetal haemoglobin (HbF). A decrease in blood volume and HbF occurs before adult haemoglobin (HbA) haemopoiesis is established fully at 6 months. HbF has a greater affinity for oxygen than HbA because of a lower content of 2,3-diphosphoglycerate (2,3DPG) and the dissociation curve is shifted to the left (Fig. 33.1). The greater affinity of HbF for oxygen is overcome in the tissues of the fetus because of low tissue partial pressure

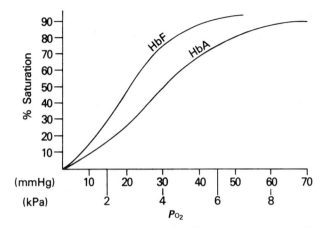

Fig. 33.1 Effects of fetal haemoglobin (HbF) on oxygen dissociation curve. HbA = Adult haemoglobin; Po_2 = partial pressure of oxygen.

of oxygen (Po_2) and a metabolic acidosis. The acidosis, which persists into infancy, and the high carbon dioxide output as a result of the high metabolic rate aid oxygen delivery to the tissues by shifting the dissociation curve to the right. Respiratory alkalosis caused by hyperventilation reduces oxygen availability and should be avoided in both the operating theatre and the intensive care unit.

Blood for transfusion should be warmed and filtered. If required in small volumes, it may be given by syringe through a tap in the intravenous (i.v.) line. This system allows rapid transfusion. In other cases, a burette type of infusion set should be used to minimize the risk of accidental overtransfusion and to permit careful monitoring of the volumes of blood administered.

As a result of the small blood volume of the neonate, haemorrhage should be carefully monitored. Swabs should be weighed, and all suction losses collected in a graduated container. Blood loss may also be measured by washing swabs and drapes in a fixed volume of fluid and measuring the haemoglobin content of the fluid.

Renal function and fluid balance

Body fluids constitute a greater proportion of body weight in the infant, particularly the premature infant, than the adult (Table 33.4).

The proportion of total body water present as extracellular fluid (ECF) exceeds that of intra-

Table 33.4 Distribution of water as percentage of body weight

Compartment	Premature	Neonate	Infant	Adult
ECF	50	35	30	20
ICF	30	40	40	40
Plasma	5	5	5	5
Total	85	80	75	65

ECF = extracellular fluid; ICF = intracellular fluid.

cellular fluid (ICF). This ratio gradually reverses with increasing age. Plasma volume remains constant — at approximately 5% body weight — throughout life.

The turnover of fluid is much greater in infants (15% total body water per day) than in adults. Thus, interruption in fluid intake in the infant rapidly results in dehydration.

The kidneys are immature at birth; both glomerular filtration and tubular reabsorption are reduced until the age of 6–8 months and, as a result, there is inability to handle excessive water loads, and overtransfusion may lead to oedema and cardiac failure. There is also diminished ability to handle sodium loads, which may occur with administration of excess sodium (e.g. sodium bicarbonate solutions).

Immature renal function may lead to cumulation and toxicity of drugs excreted by the kidneys (e.g. digoxin and penicillin). Reduced doses or increased dosage intervals may be required in the neonate.

Fluid therapy

Normal maintenance requirements of fluid increase over the first few days of life (Tables 33.5 and 33.6) and thereafter reduce more slowly.

Suitable solutions are one-quarter strength saline for the neonate and infant up to 1 year, and one-half strength saline or one-half strength compound sodium lactate thereafter. Because of the high metabolic rate, all fluids should contain at least 5% glucose to avoid hypoglycaemia. During surgery, administration of glucose-containing solutions may lead to hyperglycaemia and is not required routinely. Patients likely to suffer from hypoglycaemia should be given glucose-containing fluids. These fluids should also be used during prolonged surgery.

Clinical examination of skin turgor, tension of fontanelles, arterial pressure and venous filling may aid the estimation of hydration, but electrolyte and haemoglobin concentrations and haematocrit, urine volumes and plasma and urine osmolalities should be monitored if problems of fluid balance exist (Table 33.7).

During surgery, fluid administration should be increased by 10–20%; intake should be increased by 10% also in babies nursed under radiant heaters because of increased insensible loss, and in babies with pyrexia. Plasma proteins may require replacement (either as plasma or human albumin solution) in severe dehydration.

Calculation of replacement fluids, as opposed to maintenance fluids, should allow also for additional losses of water, protein and electrolytes which may occur with vomiting or diarrhoea. An i.v. infusion should be established for all but the briefest of procedures, to permit correction of preoperative dehydration and hypoglycaemia, to cover fluid requirements in the immediate postoperative period, and for administration of drugs.

Small doses of drugs should be given using either a 1- or 2-ml syringe or by dilution; overdilution should be avoided as excessive fluid administration may result. The drug and dilution should be labelled clearly on all syringes.

I.v. fluids should be administered using a burette type of infusion set which (in the small infant) should deliver 60 drops per millilitre (Fig. 33.2), thus allowing the rate to be controlled down to very small volumes. Drip controllers and infusion pumps of either mechanical or electrical type assist in the administration of small volumes (Fig. 33.3).

Venous access in the shocked or dehydrated infant may be difficult. Resuscitation can be carried out and blood volume restored using the intraosseous needle (Fig. 33.4). This is usually inserted into the proximal or distal ends of the tibia or distal end of the femur.

Table 33.5   Fluid requirements in the first week of life

Day	Rate
1	0
2, 3	50 ml.kg^{-1}.day^{-1}
4, 5	75 ml.kg^{-1}.day^{-1}
6	100 ml.kg^{-1}.day^{-1}
7	120 ml.kg^{-1}.day^{-1}

Table 33.6   Maintenance fluid requirements

Weight	Rate
Up to 10 kg	100 ml.kg^{-1}.day^{-1}
10–20 kg	1000 ml + 50 × [weight (kg) – 10] ml.kg^{-1}.day^{-1}
20–30 kg	1500 ml + 25 × [weight (kg) – 20] ml.kg^{-1}.day^{-1}

Table 33.7   Effects of dehydration in the young infant

	Mild	Moderate	Severe
Percentage loss of body weight	5%	10%	15%
Clinical signs	Dry skin and mucous membranes	Mottled cold periphery Loss of skin elasticity Depressed eyeballs and fontanelles Oliguria ++	Shocked Moribund Unresponsive to pain
Replacement	50 ml.kg^{-1}	100 ml.kg^{-1}	150 ml.kg^{-1}

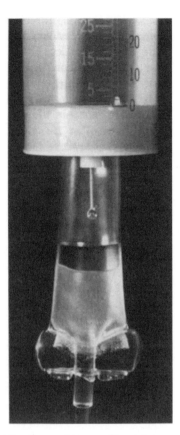

Fig. 33.2   Microburette for controlling intravenous infusion.

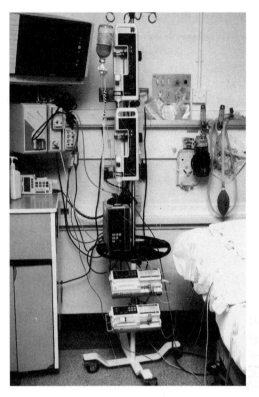

Fig. 33.3   Types of infusion controllers. Drip controller/pump and syringe pumps.

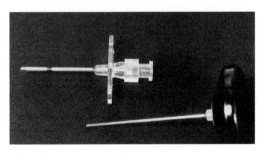

Fig. 33.4   Intraosseous needle.

Temperature regulation and maintenance

The neonate has a surface area to volume ratio 2.5 times greater than the adult, and thus a greater area for heat loss. Heat is lost by conduction, by convection and by evaporation from the skin and the respiratory tract. However, 70% of heat loss occurs by radiation to nearby surfaces, e.g. the walls of an incubator.

In a thermoneutral environment, heat loss and energy expenditure are minimal. The temperature of such an environment is 34°C for the premature infant, 32°C for the neonate and 28°C for the adult. It is important therefore to raise the environmental temperature to reduce heat loss in the very young. Infants less than 3 months old do not shiver to generate heat if exposed to cold, but depend on non-shivering thermogenesis. This is achieved by increasing metabolism of brown fat which is present in the neck and upper thoracic area, and surrounds the great vessels. This metabolism is controlled by the sympathetic nervous system. As with the muscular activity of shivering, the increase in metabolism causes an increase in oxygen consumption which may stress the immature respiratory system and may even induce respiratory failure. The control of brown fat metabolism is compromised by general anaesthesia, and so it is important to maintain body temperature by other means during surgery. A decrease in temperature may lead to respiratory depression, reduced cardiac output, prolongation of the action of drugs (especially the muscle relaxants) and increased risks of hypoventilation, regurgitation and aspiration in the postoperative period.

At birth, subcutaneous fat is minimal (almost absent in the premature) and so natural insulation is poor. Heat loss may be reduced during surgery by wrapping the limbs in orthopaedic wool or padding, or by using a space blanket or silver swaddler. The child should be placed on a heating blanket; water or heated air is preferable to an electric blanket to avoid the danger of electric shock, hot spots and interference with monitoring equipment. Overhead radiant heaters may be used (as in modern intensive care incubators) before surgery, but are inconvenient for the surgeon during surgery. Humidification and warming of inspired gases reduce heat losses from evaporation.

Malignant hyperpyrexia is extremely rare under 3 years of age, although it has been reported in a child of 5 months.

Monitoring

Temperature should be monitored, even during the shortest procedure. An axillary probe is normally adequate. For longer surgery and in the intensive care area, core temperature should be monitored using a rectal, nasopharyngeal or oesophageal probe. The external auditory meatus should not be used in children because of the danger of damage to the tympanic membrane. If heating apparatus is in use, the temperature of the skin adjacent to the heating apparatus should be closely monitored and gradients of more than 10°C must be avoided at all temperatures to prevent burning. The core–skin temperature gradient is a useful monitor of cardiac output in the intensive care area. Decreases in cardiac output increase the gradient above the normal 3–4°C.

PHARMACOLOGY IN THE NEONATE

Central nervous system

At birth, the neurones are developed, but myelination is incomplete. In spite of this, the majority of body fat is contained within the central nervous

Table 33.8 Minimum alveolar concentration (%) of anaesthetic agents

Age	Halothane	Enflurane	Isoflurane	Desflurane
0–3 years	1.08	2.0	1.35	9.0
3–10 years	0.9	1.9	1.3	8.0
Adult	0.76	1.7	1.15	7.0

system. Thus lipid-soluble drugs (e.g. anaesthetics) reach high levels in the central nervous system more rapidly than in the adult. The blood–brain barrier is more permeable in the newborn period, allowing the passage of drugs (including opioids), which should therefore be given with caution and in small doses. Antibiotics cross more readily, which is advantageous in the treatment of meningitis, but bilirubin also crosses the blood–brain barrier, leading to brain damage (kernicterus). The immaturity of the central nervous system (associated with the high metabolic rate) may be responsible for the increase in the minimum alveolar concentration (MAC) of the inhalational anaesthetic agents in young children (Table 33.8).

Liver

The liver is partly immature at birth but rapidly becomes the centre of protein production and drug detoxification. In the neonate, there is a quantitative and qualitative difference in the plasma proteins with a reduction in plasma albumin. There is therefore less protein binding in the neonate, allowing more drug to remain active. Some drugs (e.g. diazepam and vitamin K) may displace bilirubin from protein and increase the likelihood of kernicterus in the neonate.

The enzymes responsible for glucuronidation are immature; as a consequence the opioids (and chloramphenicol) are metabolized slowly, with an increased risk of toxicity.

The immaturity of the liver microsomal enzymes may be responsible for the extreme rarity of halothane-related hepatic damage in patients under 10 years of age. By the age of 1–2 years, the liver is twice the volume relative to body weight as in the adult. This may result in local anaesthetics being safer in youth than in later years.

Specific drugs in relationship to paediatric anaesthesia

Inhalational agents

The greater alveolar ventilation in relation to FRC, and the preponderance of vessel-rich tissues, lead to more rapid increases in alveolar and brain concentrations of inhalational anaesthetics than in the adult. Induction is therefore more rapid, as is excretion of the agent at the termination of anaesthesia. The rapid increase in levels of depressant agents (e.g. halothane or enflurane) may lead to dramatic decreases in arterial pressure and cardiac output, particularly during controlled ventilation.

The minimum alveolar concentrations of inhalational anaesthetics are increased in the young (Table 33.8). This results in a more restricted therapeutic range between surgical anaesthesia and cardiovascular and respiratory depression. Great care should therefore be exercised in their use and the patient must be monitored closely.

Nitrous oxide. Nitrous oxide is used as a carrier gas and supplement for most inhalational anaesthetics. Because of the low solubility of nitrogen, an increase in the volume of air-containing spaces occurs during induction with a gas mixture which contains nitrous oxide. In the neonate this is important in lesions of the lung, especially pneumothorax and congenital lobar emphysema. Expansion of the bowel in diaphragmatic hernia, exomphalos or gastroschisis may increase diaphragmatic splinting after surgical correction. In necrotizing enterocolitis, the gas within the bowel wall may expand and worsen the condition.

Halothane. Halothane is the most commonly used agent in paediatric anaesthesia. It produces smooth, rapid induction of anaesthesia. The cardiovascular-depressant properties are not normally marked in clinical anaesthesia, but are severe in the presence of cardiac failure. There is an increased tendency for laryngeal spasm to occur during tracheal intubation or extubation at light levels of anaesthesia; tracheal intubation should be undertaken at the level of surgical anaesthesia and the patient should be awake before extubation. However, extubation under deep anaesthesia is preferable in some circum-stances, e.g. after intraocular surgery. Hepatic dysfunction after repeated halothane anaesthesia has been reported in children; however, the incidence is extremely small compared with that in adults. At present, halothane remains the drug of choice for emergency inhalational induction of anaesthesia in conditions such as acute epiglottitis or post-tonsillectomy haemorrhage.

Enflurane. This does not produce as smooth an induction as halothane and may induce breath-holding, coughing and laryngospasm. The high MAC value of enflurane in children, and particularly in infants, renders the drug of less value as a sole anaesthetic agent. Ventilatory and cardiovascular depression may occur. Central nervous system excitation occurs on electroencephalogram (EEG) recordings and epileptiform seizures have been reported some hours after enflurane anaesthesia; thus the drug should not be used in children with a history of epilepsy.

Isoflurane. Isoflurane possesses cardiovascular and respiratory-depressant properties similar to those of halothane. Recovery occurs more rapidly because of its lower blood/gas solubility coefficient. Unfortunately, isoflurane is an irritant and thus inhalational induction is slow; breath-holding, coughing and laryngeal spasm may occur, particularly in the unpremedicated child. Laryngospasm occurs less commonly on extubation than after halothane.

Sevoflurane. Sevoflurane is a possible successor to halothane as a smooth and rapid induction agent in children. There is a small incidence of excitement in some cases on induction. The low blood/gas solubility coefficient which allows rapid induction also results in rapid recovery. Adequate analgesia must be ensured prior to recovery to avoid excitement at this stage.

Sevoflurane is metabolized to fluoride. Metabolism is around 3%. This does not result in blood concentrations likely to lead to nephrotoxicity.

Desflurane. This is another modern agent with low blood solubility. Unfortunately it is very irritant and causes laryngospasm in up to 30% of patients. It is of little value as an induction agent in children. The low boiling point requires a special temperature-controlled and pressurized vaporizer. These disadvantages are likely to limit its use in paediatric anaesthesia.

Intravenous agents

Thiopentone is still the most frequently used i.v. induction agent for children. Very young infants are extremely sensitive to barbiturates, but older children are less sensitive, and a dose of 5–6 mg.kg^{-1} is required.

Methohexitone 1 mg.kg^{-1} may cause pain on injection; this can be abolished by adding lignocaine (1 mg.ml^{-1}) to the solution before injection. Methohexitone may also cause central nervous system excitation which results in muscular twitching, and the drug should be avoided in patients with epilepsy.

Barbiturates may be given rectally in increased dosage (e.g. thiopentone 30 mg.kg^{-1}, methohexitone 25 mg.kg^{-1}) as 10% solutions. Onset of sleep is pleasant but slow, taking 5–10 min, during which time the child must be closely observed for signs of respiratory obstruction or depression.

Propofol can be used as an induction agent or for total i.v. anaesthesia by continuous infusion. The latter technique is not frequently used in paediatric anaesthetic practice. The induction dose for children is higher than that used for adults. Infants require a larger dose than older children (2.5–4 mg.kg^{-1}).

The incidence of pain on injection is higher in children than in adults but can be prevented by adding lignocaine to the drug before injection. The rapid awakening seen in adult practice is of value for day surgery but the difference between propofol and thiopentone is less marked in children, particularly those under 5 years of age.

Propofol should not be used as a sedative for children in intensive care.

Etomidate has a rapid action and causes little cardiovascular or respiratory depression but does cause pain on injection. Involuntary movements and coughing are common. Because of its rapid metabolism, it has been advocated as a suitable agent for total i.v. anaesthesia. This technique is not frequently used in children because of rapid fluctuations in depth of anaesthesia and the volume of infusion required.

Ketamine may be used i.v. in a dose of 2 mg.kg^{-1}, or intramuscularly (i.m.) in a dose of 10 mg.kg^{-1}. In the very young, increased doses are required as a consequence of poor cortical development.

Following i.v. induction, respiratory depression may occur, and breath-holding is not uncommon. There is a risk of aspiration at this time. The presence of secretions or an airway in the mouth may cause laryngospasm because of increased airway reflex activity.

The psychic phenomena associated with emergence from ketamine anaesthesia in adults are less common in children and may be further reduced by premedication with diazepam and provision of a quiet, undisturbed recovery period. The analgesia and catatonia provided by ketamine are useful for skin grafting of burns and allow exposed skin grafts to become adherent while the child remains immobile after surgery. Ketamine tends to maintain or slightly increase intraocular pressure and can be used for examination of the eye under anaesthesia if the intraocular pressure is to be measured. Intracranial pressure is increased by ketamine and its use should be avoided if there is any possibility of pre-existing elevation of intracranial pressure.

Relaxants (see Appendix IXb)

Although it has been stated that the neonate is particularly sensitive to non-depolarizing neuromuscular blockers, this is probably related to the more marked effect of small doses of relaxant on respiration because of poor respiratory reserve and dependence on the diaphragm, rather than a myasthenic response of neonatal neuromuscular function. Recent work shows a greater variation amongst neonates in their response to non-depolarizing relaxants than occurs in the older child and adult, but the conclusion is that for surgical relaxation a scaled-down adult dose should be used initially. Subsequent top-up doses should be restricted to one-tenth of the initial dose. Residual paralysis or difficulty in reversal at the end of surgery is likely to be associated either with acid–base abnormalities or hypothermia, correction of which restores muscle activity to normal.

Curare (0.5 mg.kg^{-1}) causes much less hypotension in the child than the adult. Histamine release does occur; thus there is a relative contraindication to the use of curare in the asthmatic child.

Pancuronium (0.1 mg.kg^{-1}) is similar in action

to curare, but has the advantage of causing less histamine release. The tachycardia caused by pancuronium is a disadvantage in children, who normally have a rapid heart rate.

Atracurium (0.5 mg.kg^{-1}) causes rapid onset of relaxation. The duration of action (approximately 30 min) is particularly appropriate for many paediatric surgical procedures. Release of histamine occurs, and anaphylactic reactions have been reported in children.

Vecuronium (0.1 mg.kg^{-1}) has a similar onset and duration of action as those of atracurium. The incidence of histamine release is less. Vecuronium may be the muscle relaxant of choice for procedures that last 20–30 min. When given by infusion, vecuronium may be used for longer surgical procedures or in the intensive therapy unit.

Rocuronium has a short duration of action and may be of value for short procedures or for administration by infusion, as the rate of recovery is rapid, regardless of the dose or duration of infusion. The short time for full relaxation following the initial dose makes this a particularly useful agent for intubation. As with other muscle relaxant drugs, the initial dose in children is greater compared with that in adults.

Suxamethonium is rapidly distributed throughout the ECF following injection. The relatively greater ECF volume in infants requires larger doses on a body weight basis to be used in children and may be the cause of the apparent resistance to suxamethonium seen in infants. Intubation in the neonate requires 2 mg.kg^{-1} and in the infant it is recommended that a dose of 3 mg.kg^{-1} is used. The bradycardia following injection of suxamethonium can be prevented by the prior use of atropine.

ANAESTHETIC MANAGEMENT

Preoperative preparation

Every patient should be visited by the anaesthetist prior to surgery. The procedures involved in anaesthesia should be explained to the patient, in the presence of a parent if possible, and in suitable language if the child is old enough to understand. Older children may express a preference for the type of induction and this should be used if possible.

Table 33.9   Estimates of children's weights

Age	Body weight (kg) (approximate average values)
Neonate	3
4 months	6
1–8 years	2 × age + 9
9–13 years	3 × age

The patient should be assessed for fitness for anaesthesia. Upper respiratory infections are common, as are other viral infections, e.g. measles, mumps or chickenpox. These are a contraindication to anaesthesia for non-essential operations, but not for a more urgent procedure. The presence of pyrexia may indicate infection and is a contraindication to non-urgent surgery. The patient's weight should be noted, as this is the most reliable and simple guide to drug dosage (Table 33.9). Veins should be examined with regard to i.v. induction and the establishment of i.v. infusions.

Preoperative fasting

Morbidity and mortality due to aspiration of gastric contents are rare in children. Prolonged periods of starvation and dehydration can result in hypoglycaemia and hypovolaemia, particularly in the very young infant with the rapid turnover of fluids and high metabolic rate.

It is important to reduce the preoperative fasting time to a safe minimum on humane grounds as well as from the safety point of view. Single guidelines are not appropriate for all age groups.

The increase in day surgery makes it imperative that guidelines are clear for parents and that the importance of preoperative starvation is understood by those involved in day surgery as well as for inpatients. Appropriate fasting times are as follows:

1. No food, milk or bottle feeds for 6 h preoperatively.
2. Breast-fed infants should not be fed for 4 h preoperatively.
3. Clear fluids can be given up to 3 h preoperatively and should be actively encouraged up to that time.

Premedication

Premedication should be prescribed according to the needs of the patient. The advent of cutaneous local anaesthetic creams has reduced the requirement for sedative premedication, particularly in day cases.

Secretions may contribute to respiratory obstruction in small airways and premedication with an antisialagogue may be required. Hyoscine ($15\,\mu g.kg^{-1}$) is an effective drying agent with sedative and antiemetic properties. Atropine ($20\,\mu g.kg^{-1}$) is a most effective drug for prevention of arrhythmias from cardiovagal stimulation resulting from the oculocardiac reflex or tracheal intubation, but is more useful for this purpose when given i.v. at the induction of anaesthesia. Atropine should not be given i.m. to patients with pyrexia, but may be used i.v. at induction. Glycopyrronium bromide is a suitable alternative in children; in a dose of $10\,\mu g.kg^{-1}$ i.v. it causes less tachycardia than atropine $20\,\mu g.kg^{-1}$.

If analgesia is required preoperatively, an opioid premedication (morphine $0.2\,mg.kg^{-1}$ or papaveretum $0.3\,mg.kg^{-1}$) may be prescribed. However, the resultant respiratory depression may impede inhalational induction of anaesthesia.

The majority of older children require only sedation. The drugs used most frequently are trimeprazine $3\,mg.kg^{-1}$, diazepam $0.2-0.4\,mg.kg^{-1}$ or droperidol $0.2-0.4\,mg.kg^{-1}$ administered orally.

Induction

Parents should be allowed to be present during induction of anaesthesia if they so wish.

Anaesthesia may be induced by inhalation, i.v., i.m. or rectal administration of drugs. I.v. induction is associated with decreased oxygen saturation in a significant proportion of children. Inhalational induction may be rapidly accomplished with halothane or sevoflurane; these may be administered directly by mask or by placing the T-piece in the anaesthetist's hands. The latter technique reduces anxiety in the patient, but causes greater pollution of the atmosphere.

There is no place for the use of gas mixtures containing less than 30% oxygen to increase the rapidity of induction. If laryngeal spasm occurs, the small reserves of oxygen are depleted further by such mixtures and very severe hypoxaemia may result.

The child should be monitored throughout an inhalational induction using pulse oximetry and a precordial stethoscope.

The use of transcutaneous local anaesthetic agents can allow virtually painless intravenous induction in children. These agents require a certain duration of contact to be effective; for EMLA, the time is a minimum of 1 h and more usually 1.5–2 h. Newer formulations of amethocaine act within an hour.

Modern cannulae down to 24-gauge in size make cannulation of small veins possible. Venous access can be difficult in the chubby infant of 6 months to 2 years. The veins of small children are very mobile but can be stabilized by stretching the skin tightly. A trained assistant is required to hold and squeeze the arm, to distract the child and to prevent sudden movements that can dislodge the cannula.

Rectal induction is slow, taking up to 15 min, and requires supervision for a prolonged period, during which the patient is at risk of developing respiratory depression and obstruction.

Airway management

The physiological dead space of the young infant is small but the V_d/V_t ratio is the same throughout life (0.3). Any increase in dead space from anaesthetic apparatus is more significant in the infant, and therefore must be kept to a minimum.

The Rendell-Baker-Soucek mask is specifically designed to minimize dead space in infants. When holding the mask, it is important not to press (Fig. 33.5) upwards on the tongue below the mandible as this may occlude the airway totally by pushing the tongue against the posterior pharyngeal wall. The chin should be supported by pressure on the mandible alone (Fig. 33.6).

Modern clear anaesthetic masks such as the Rendell-Baker-Soucek or those with pneumatic cushions (Fig. 33.7) are less intimidating than the older black masks for children. They also permit close monitoring of respiration during induction.

The use of Ayres T-piece apparatus reduces dead space to a minimum and also has the ad-

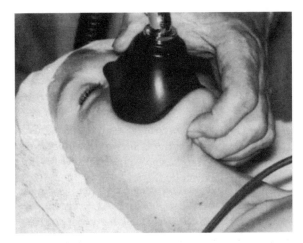

Fig. 33.5   Incorrect way of holding a paediatric face mask.

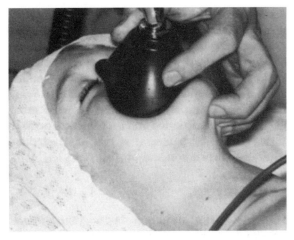

Fig. 33.6   Correct way of holding a paediatric face mask.

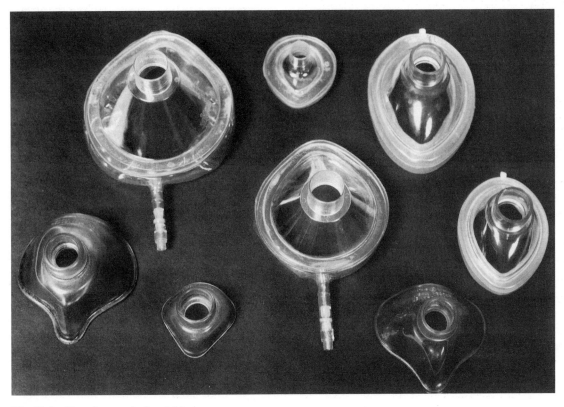

Fig. 33.7   Clear face masks for children.

vantage of a low resistance to expiration because of the absence of valves. The T-piece may be used for anaesthesia using spontaneous ventilation, but only for short periods in the very young as even the small increase in dead space causes an unacceptable level of rebreathing. The fresh gas flow should be calculated as 2.5 times the predicted minute volume.

Jackson Rees modified the T-piece by the addition of an open-ended reservoir bag, and this allows the apparatus to be used for controlled ventilation. Alternatively, a ventilator may be attached to the expiratory limb for controlled ventilation. In this mode, a fresh gas flow rate of (1000 ml + 100 ml.kg^{-1} body weight) per minute results in an arterial partial pressure of carbon dioxide (P_{CO_2}) of 4.8–5.3 kPa (35–40 mmHg). A minimum gas flow of 3 litre.min^{-1} is required to operate the system satisfactorily.

The size of the small baby causes difficulty in maintenance of the airway during surgery with a mask. Most infants require tracheal intubation. The reduction in cross-sectional area of the airway caused by a 3.5 or 5.0 mm tube in a small infant causes an increase in resistance of approximately 16 times, compared with a threefold increase in an adult with a 9.5 mm tracheal tube. Thus, controlled ventilation should always be undertaken in an infant subjected to tracheal intubation. The laryngeal mask airway (LMA) allows many shorter operations to be carried out in children without tracheal intubation and the consequent risks of extubation spasm or stridor related to the trauma of intubation. Operations such as squint correction can be performed as day cases using the LMA. It is not appropriate to ventilate the lungs of small children using the LMA. The relatively short oesophagus and the possibility of inappropriate positioning of the LMA can lead to gaseous gastric distension and resultant regurgitation.

The very young are obligate nose-breathers and secretions caused by upper respiratory infection may lead to respiratory difficulty, particularly in the postoperative period. Enlarged tonsils and adenoids may cause difficulty with airway maintenance, especially in the older child. This may be overcome by the use of an oropharyngeal airway.

Atmospheric pollution

The Ayres' T-piece is a low-dead space, low-resistance apparatus, frequently used for paediatric anaesthesia, but it requires high gas flows for spontaneous respiration and is difficult to scavenge. Scavenging of waste gases can be carried out but must avoid the dangers of obstruction to the expired gases. Alternative breathing systems such as the Bain, Humphrey ADE or small disposable closed circuits can be used for older children in order to reduce gas flows and subsequent pollution problems.

Tracheal intubation

The anatomy of the infant may cause difficulties in tracheal intubation. Infants have a relatively large head, short neck and large tongue. The mandible may be underdeveloped.

The larynx is higher in the neck (C3–4) than in the adult (C5–6) and is placed more anteriorly. The epiglottis is large, floppy and U-shaped and is not easily elevated using the conventional Macintosh laryngoscope in the vallecula (Fig. 33.8). Intubation in the very young is easier if the epiglottis is elevated using a laryngoscope with a straight blade.

The internal diameter of a tracheal tube for a child may be calculated from the formula:

$$\frac{Age}{4} + 4\,mm$$

The tube should be small enough to allow a leak during the application of positive pressure, otherwise pressure on the tissues of the glottis or cricoid may lead to oedema following extubation. This may cause stridor up to 8 h later and require reintubation. For this reason, intubation, although not entirely contraindicated, should be avoided if possible in outpatients or day cases. Tracheal tubes with shoulders (e.g. the Cole) may cause glottic oedema from pressure of the shoulder on the lax tissues of the glottis.

The tracheal tube should be firmly secured to avoid accidental extubation or bronchial intubation during anaesthesia. If adhesive tape is used,

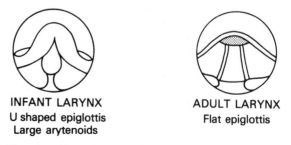

INFANT LARYNX
U shaped epiglottis
Large arytenoids

ADULT LARYNX
Flat epiglottis

Fig. 33.8 The infant and adult larynx.

the tube should be secured to the maxilla and not the mandible, which is extremely mobile in small children (except where this is not feasible, e.g. cleft lip and palate surgery).

The trachea of the infant is short (4 cm) at birth. Both lung fields must be auscultated to confirm correct positioning of the tracheal tube. Although the angles between the main bronchi and trachea are more nearly equal than in the adult, a tracheal tube still tends to enter the right main bronchus. Preformed tracheal tubes (e.g. the RAE or Oxford) have the disadvantage of a fixed length, which may result in bronchial intubation.

The narrowest part of the airway of the child is the cricoid ring. Because this is circular (unlike the diamond-shaped glottic opening, which is the narrowest part of the adult airway) a cuff on the tracheal tube is unnecessary if the correct size has been selected. Thus, in children up to 5–6 years of age, a tube of the same diameter may be used for either nasotracheal or orotracheal intubation.

Monitoring

Direct observation of the patient is the most important single method of monitoring. The anaesthetist may see changes in the patient's colour (cyanosis or pallor). Movement or lacrimation may be detected if anaesthesia is too light, or a change in respiratory pattern if respiratory obstruction occurs. A clear plastic drape permits observation of the patient during head and neck surgery when normal drapes totally obscure the small patient (Fig. 33.9).

The stethoscope, precordial or oesophageal, is the single most valuable monitoring device available to the paediatric anaesthetist and should always be attached before induction. It allows continuous monitoring of heart sounds for rate, rhythm and intensity. In the infant, the intensity of sound varies with the stroke volume, and acts as a qualitative monitor of cardiac output. The stethoscope should always be used to check both lungs following intubation to confirm that bronchial intubation has not taken place and it continues to give an indication of changes in ventilation during anaesthesia (Fig. 33.10).

The electrocardiogram (ECG) provides less information than the stethoscope but may demonstrate arrhythmias. An arterial pressure cuff and temperature probe should always be attached before induction.

Pulse oximetry is considered a mandatory monitor during anaesthesia, sedation and for postoperative care. It is a valuable instrument but the probes available for very small infants and babies are still not completely reliable and may

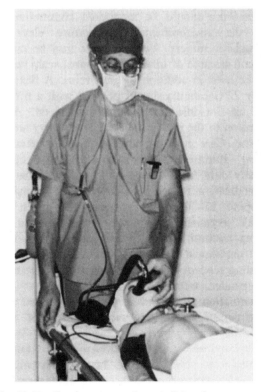

Fig. 33.10 Continuous use of precordial stethoscope.

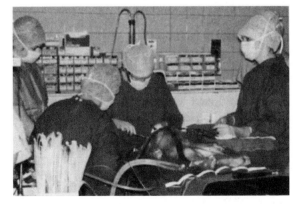

Fig. 33.9 Use of plastic surgical drapes to permit observation of child.

give erroneous readings due to movement, theatre lighting and pressure from towels, instruments and surgical assistants. It is vital to keep a close eye on the patient's clinical condition at all times.

It is important to have an i.v. infusion established, all monitoring apparatus attached and the patient correctly positioned before draping, as access to the patient may be extremely limited during surgery.

Day surgery

Many of the surgical procedures carried out on small children can be carried out as day cases. This has the major advantage for the child that parental separation is virtually eliminated. The majority of patients will be American Society of Anesthesiologists' (ASA) classes I or II, but occasional patients who are ASA III or even IV can be treated as day cases. Selection of patients must take into account postoperative pain in addition to the surgical condition.

The use of long-acting local anaesthetics such as bupivacaine allows excellent postoperative analgesia. Intraoperative rectal diclofenac or oral paracetamol administered in the early postoperative period can be used to supplement analgesia before the effects of any local anaesthetic wear off, thus allowing prolonged analgesia; it is prudent to inform parents about the proposed use of analgesic suppositories to prevent misunderstandings. Social conditions and travelling distance must also be considered. A community nurse attached to the unit can extend the number of patients who can benefit from treatment as day cases. Clear instructions must be given to parents regarding preoperative starvation and postoperative care appropriate to the particular procedure.

NEONATAL ANAESTHESIA

Additional problems are associated with anaesthetizing the neonate because of size and immaturity. Temperature maintenance mechanisms are immature, and the patient must be kept warm during transport, induction and anaesthesia. The temperature should be monitored continuously, and the environmental temperature elevated throughout surgery. Venous access may be more difficult because of small mobile veins; scalp veins can be used in addition to limb veins. A flexible 24- or 22-gauge cannula should be used with a three-way tap for injection of drugs or blood. Any extension to the i.v. line should have a very small volume. Care must be taken to avoid over-transfusion. Burette infusion sets should be filled initially only to a volume of 10 ml.kg^{-1}. Sedative premedication is not required for the neonate. Atropine 15–20 µg.kg^{-1} i.m. may be given to reduce secretions and prevent vagal stimulation during tracheal intubation and surgery. Vitamin K$_1$ 1 mg should be given to reduce the neonatal bleeding tendency resulting from lack of vitamin K-dependent factors.

Ventilation by face mask should be carried out with extreme care to avoid inflation of the stomach.

The anatomy of the neonate may render tracheal intubation difficult. In the very small, weak or premature neonate, it is customary to perform intubation before induction of anaesthesia. This reduces the likelihood of aspiration of gastric contents and the need to ventilate by mask, with subsequent gastric distension. In addition, the baby is able to breathe if attempts to intubate fail. The disadvantages of awake intubation are that it is often traumatic and it may be more difficult to see the larynx than in the anaesthetized child.

A normal neonate requires a 3.5 mm tube, and a premature child a 3.0 mm or rarely a 2.5 mm tube.

Drugs should be prepared before anaesthesia and given from 1- or 2-ml syringes to avoid excessive administration of fluid. Cardiovascular monitoring must be continuous. Non-depolarizing relaxants may be given in scaled adult doses initially (atracurium 0.5 mg.kg^{-1}, vecuronium 0.2 mg.kg^{-1}) but subsequent doses should be only one-tenth of the initial dose.

The neonate should not be allowed to breathe spontaneously under anaesthesia for any length of time; the inefficient respiratory system is easily depressed and the presence of a small tracheal tube greatly increases resistance. Controlled ventilation is preferably carried out by hand so that changes in compliance or resistance may be detected early.

Many neonatal surgical procedures affect pulmonary function. The major airways may be totally obstructed in the repair of tracheo-oesophageal fistula, or compliance greatly reduced following the treatment of exomphalos or diaphragmatic hernia.

Bradycardia is usually a sign of hypoxaemia and should be treated by ventilation with 100% oxygen. Supplements of inhalational agents (halothane, enflurane or isoflurane) should be used in small doses to avoid hypotension, and should be discontinued several minutes before the end of anaesthesia to avoid residual depression. Sevoflurane and desflurane are associated with much more rapid recovery even after prolonged anaesthesia, and administration should be continued until surgical stimulation has stopped.

Relaxants should be antagonized by neostigmine and atropine. If there is any doubt with regard to the quality of reversal, the temperature should be carefully checked and any abnormality in acid–base status treated appropriately. Any child whose ventilation may be compromised after surgery should receive pulmonary ventilation electively. Opioid analgesics should be avoided postoperatively as they cause severe depression of ventilation. Local anaesthetic techniques may provide excellent analgesia after many procedures in the neonate.

SPECIFIC OPERATIONS IN THE NEONATE

Pyloric stenosis

This usually occurs in babies of 3–8 weeks of age. In mild cases, the child may be well-nourished and hydrated, but if severe, extreme dehydration and electrolyte imbalance are present, with hypokalaemia and severe metabolic alkalosis. Surgical treatment by pyloromyotomy is not an emergency and fluid and electrolyte imbalances should be corrected before anaesthesia. The child may have had a barium swallow, and a nasogastric tube should always be passed and aspirated before induction; the patient should nevertheless be treated as though he or she has a full stomach. If an i.v. infusion is in progress, i.v. induction should be used, the trachea intubated after suxamethonium ($1.5–2$ mg.kg^{-1}) and paralysis maintained with a non-depolarizing muscle relaxant or intermittent

suxamethonium. Hyperventilation should be avoided to prevent worsening of the pre-existing alkalosis which may lead to slow onset of ventilation at the termination of anaesthesia. The nasogastric tube should be aspirated before tracheal extubation.

Tracheo-oesophageal fistula and oesophageal atresia

The commonest form of this disorder is oesophageal atresia with a fistula between the trachea and the lower part of the oesophagus. The diagnosis may be made if the child aspirates secretions continually or chokes on feeding. The presence of a fistula may be detected by persistent pulmonary problems as a result of aspiration from the stomach. A large tube should be placed in the upper oesophageal pouch to aspirate secretions. Anaesthesia is similar to that for other neonates but particular problems are associated with intubation of the fistula and inflation of the stomach. The position of the tracheal tube must be checked by auscultation.

During surgery, large airways may be kinked or clamped accidentally and surgical retraction may cause dramatic decreases in cardiac output by compression of the left and right atria or vagus nerve. Respiratory and cardiovascular systems should be monitored closely. The respiratory problems resulting from aspiration through the fistula do not resolve until after surgery but tracheobronchial toilet should be performed both before and after surgery, and postoperative elective ventilation may be required.

Diaphragmatic hernia

The usual presentation is that of severe acute respiratory distress and cyanosis, with a flat or scaphoid abdomen. Chest X-ray is usually diagnostic. Resuscitation should be initially by tracheal intubation and controlled ventilation. Positive-pressure ventilation must not be carried out using bag and mask, as expansion of the viscera in the hernia further compresses the contralateral lung and heart. Nitrous oxide should be avoided to prevent gas distension. Arterial or capillary blood gases should be monitored.

If the lungs expand well, the trachea may be extubated postoperatively when blood gases are normal. Some infants have a hypoplastic lung on the side of the hernia—usually the left. If the hernia occurred early in fetal life, there may be some hypoplasia of the contralateral lung also; thus there may be insufficient pulmonary tissue to maintain life. Some of these children may survive after treatment in the intensive therapy unit with controlled ventilation and a pulmonary arterial vasodilator, e.g. tolazoline. Bilateral chest drains should be inserted, as there is a danger of pneumothorax if high ventilatory pressures are required.

Babies with severe physiological compromise are initially resuscitated before surgery. Techniques that are used include extracorporeal membrane oxygenation and the administration of nitric oxide to overcome pulmonary hypertension. Patients are stabilized in the intensive therapy unit before surgery.

Exomphalos and gastroschisis

In these conditions there is herniation of the abdominal contents through the anterior abdominal wall. In exomphalos, the sac of the hernia is within the umbilical cord. In gastroschisis the hernia is lateral to the umbilicus and the bowel usually lacks any covering. If the defect is large, there is a likelihood of dramatic loss of heat and fluid from exposed bowel. It may not be possible to return the bowel to the small abdominal cavity; the bowel may be initially protected in a Silastic pouch and gradually replaced into the abdomen over a few days.

Bowel obstruction

Obstruction may be the result of an atresia at any point from duodenum to anal canal. Malrotation, volvulus and reduplication of bowel may cause obstructive symptoms. Meconium ileus, a premonitory sign of cystic fibrosis, may cause neonatal obstruction, although the associated respiratory problems are not usually of significance in the neonate. The major anaesthetic problems are those of fluid and electrolyte imbalance and danger of regurgitation and aspiration.

Myelomeningocoele

This is a defect resulting from the failure of the neural tube to close in the fetus. If the defect is large, there may be severe problems of heat and fluid loss during surgery, and blood loss may be difficult to estimate because of mixture with cerebrospinal fluid (CSF).

Hydrocephalus

Hydrocephalus may result from the closure of a myelomeningocoele or the associated Arnold–Chiari syndrome. A shunt procedure to drain CSF into the right atrium or peritoneal cavity may be required. Problems may be encountered in relation to raised intracranial pressure (ICP). In the very young with open fontanelles, tapping of the lateral ventricle may help to reduce acute increases in pressure. Ketamine and volatile agents must be avoided. Hypertension resulting from raised ICP may disappear rapidly when ICP is reduced. Hypercapnia should be avoided at all stages. Blood loss is not usually a problem during shunt surgery.

Cleft lip and palate

This may cause airway problems which lead to difficult intubation, especially in association with the Pierre Robin syndrome. Some surgeons treat these conditions during the neonatal period but it is more common to repair the cleft lip at 2–3 months and the palate at 18 months to 2 years.

Atropine 20 µg.kg^{-1} should be given, as secretions may be a problem. The airway should be monitored closely, as the tracheal tube may be kinked or compressed by the gag used during cleft palate repair. A throat pack is inserted before surgery; its insertion and removal should be recorded. In some cases of Pierre Robin syndrome or mild micrognathia, closure of the soft palate may cause airway difficulty postoperatively, requiring tracheal intubation for a day or two. Blood transfusion may be required for cleft lip or palate surgery, but losses do not usually exceed 15% of blood volume. Congenital heart disease is a commonly associated disorder in patients with cleft lip or palate.

The airway may be compromised after cleft

palate closure and analgesic drugs must be given in reduced doses. The child should be admitted to the intensive therapy unit or a 24-h recovery area overnight.

Associated abnormalities

Many congenital disorders have associated abnormalities, such as cardiac or renal defects. These should be suspected and diagnosed before surgical intervention. Ultrasonic examination can detect the majority of such problems in a rapid and non-invasive manner.

The premature and post-premature baby

Improved neonatal care has led to an increased number of very premature infants (<32 weeks) surviving. These infants have an increased likelihood of hernia which may require surgery if obstruction is to be avoided. General anaesthesia, although safe in the appropriate centres, has been shown to lead to postoperative respiratory complications, particularly apnoeic spells. Alternative techniques such as spinal or caudal anaesthesia can be used. These infants also have an increased incidence of patent ductus arteriosus which may require surgical closure. Cryotherapy is also required in an increasing number of cases of retinopathy of the premature. All such infants should only be anaesthetized where appropriate neonatal intensive care facilities exist.

The very premature infant is subject to the complications associated with prematurity up to 60 days post-conceptual age and cannot be treated as a normal child until that time. These babies are therefore not suitable for surgery as day cases.

POSTOPERATIVE CARE

When adequate ventilation has been re-established after recovery from anaesthesia, the child should be nursed in the lateral position and the airway, cardiovascular system and temperature closely monitored in an adequately equipped postoperative recovery area (see Chapter 23). Oxygen should be administered during transfer from the operating theatre, and until the child awakens in the recovery area. The patient should be awake before return to the ward. Recovery from ketamine anaesthesia should take place in a quiet undisturbed manner. Diazepam 0.2 mg.kg^{-1} may be required if there is evidence of psychological upset.

Laryngeal spasm

Laryngeal spasm is a relatively frequent complication of paediatric anaesthesia, particularly after volatile agents have been used. Treatment comprises ventilation with 100% oxygen under positive pressure by bag and mask. If bradycardia occurs, the trachea should be reintubated rapidly and the lungs inflated with 100% oxygen. Laryngeal spasm may be avoided by extubating the trachea either when the patient is totally awake or when surgically anaesthetized. Extubation should not be carried out when the patient is only lightly anaesthetized or just beginning to cough. The pharynx should be cleared of all secretions under direct vision as these may precipitate this particularly dangerous hazard.

Postoperative pain

Postoperative pain has been an area of neglect in paediatric surgery, largely through anxiety concerning the respiratory depression associated with opioid agents and the perceived requirement for intramuscular injections. A considerable amount of recent work has demonstrated that techniques such as patient-controlled analgesia (PCA) can be used in children from the age of 5 years. Below that age, nurse-controlled analgesia is feasible. Alternatives are subcutaneous and i.v. infusions of opioids. Safe dosage regimens have been established but the need for trained nurses and adequate monitoring, including pulse oximetry, must be stressed. The recommended dose of morphine by infusion is 20 µg.kg^{-1}.h^{-1}. Continuous epidural infusions of local anaesthetics with or without the addition of an opioid require intensive care facilities. Non-steroidal analgesics such as diclofenac 1 mg.kg^{-1} given as a suppository and paracetamol 10–15 mg.kg^{-1} orally or rectally are effective in prolonging analgesia if given prior to a local anaesthetic wearing off. They are also of value for mild analgesia when opioids are not required.

These techniques of analgesia are appropriate even in small neonates provided that adequate monitoring facilities are available.

Local anaesthesia

Blocks which are suitable include extradural (thoracic or lumbar) block with or without a catheter, and caudal, intercostal, ilioinguinal and penile blocks. For the upper limb, axillary block, and for the lower limb, femoral, lateral cutaneous nerve of thigh, or sciatic nerve block may be useful. A local block can be used as the sole technique of anaesthesia in the severely ill child, or in circumstances in which it may be desirable to avoid the metabolic upset associated with general anaesthesia, e.g. the severely dehydrated child with pyloric stenosis. Caudal anaesthesia has been shown to be useful in the neonate with a low imperforate anus. Local techniques should only be performed on the young child by experienced anaesthetists.

INTENSIVE THERAPY

The total reliance of the newborn on the diaphragm for adequate ventilation may result in a requirement for prolonged controlled ventilation if the diaphragm is paralysed or splinted by high intra-abdominal pressure. This may occur after surgery for gastroschisis or exomphalos, where abdominal growth is not adequate to contain the entire bowel. Severe splinting may also occur with distension of the bowel as a result of necrotizing enterocolitis, bowel obstruction or gastroenteritis.

Controlled ventilation may be required for babies with cardiac or respiratory failure. Institution of controlled ventilation may be necessary irrespective of blood gas values because of a clinical diagnosis of exhaustion.

The newborn tolerates relatively high ventilatory and intrathoracic pressures without a decrease in cardiac output because of the large right ventricle, which regresses slowly following the change from fetal to adult type of circulation. However, there is a danger of lung rupture leading to pneumothorax.

The immature respiratory system with small, easily obstructed airways is the factor responsible for the majority of admissions to the intensive therapy unit. The child has little respiratory reserve and any increase in airway resistance or decrease in compliance may require respiratory support or assistance.

The method of choice for maintenance of the airway is nasotracheal intubation in preference to tracheostomy except when very prolonged airway control is required or a severe anatomical disorder of the upper airway or trachea is present. Narrow nasal tubes require meticulous care and attention to detail, including fixation to prevent kinking or dislodgement of the tube and ulceration of the nares as a result of pressure. Humidification is of paramount importance if obstruction by secretions (requiring reintubation under emergency conditions) is to be avoided. If necessary, the patient should be sedated to assist toleration of the tracheal tube. Aspiration of secretions should be carried out regularly using soft atraumatic catheters no larger than half the diameter of the tracheal tube. The duration of suction should be limited to a few seconds to prevent hypoxaemia. As with patients undergoing anaesthesia, a child should not be allowed to breathe through a small tracheal tube for prolonged periods without support either by positive-pressure ventilation or continuous positive airways pressure (CPAP). Particular attention should be paid to adequate hydration of the patient, in addition to humidification of inspired gas. The environmental temperature should be kept close to the neutral thermal environment to minimize oxygen requirements.

Respiratory distress syndrome (hyaline membrane disease)

This occurs particularly in the premature as a result of absence of pulmonary surfactant. This defect allows the alveoli to collapse, causing a decrease in compliance and tachypnoea. Respiration is grunting in nature as the child breathes out against a closed glottis in an attempt to maintain alveolar patency. Mild cases may recover if the hypoxaemia is treated with humidified oxygen, and the acidosis is corrected. The arterial partial pressure of oxygen (Pa_{O_2}) should be maintained at a minimum of 9.5 kPa (70 mmHg). More severe cases require mechanical assistance to keep the alveoli patent either with spontaneous ventilation using nasal catheters or tracheal intubation to induce CPAP. The most severe cases require intermittent positive-pressure ventilation with positive end-expiratory pressure.

Acute epiglottitis

This condition results from bacterial infection, usually by *Haemophilus influenzae*. The child usually presents between the ages of 2 and 7 years. There is a rapid onset of severe respiratory obstruction and dysphagia resulting from glottic swelling. The patient cannot swallow saliva and has to sit to avoid choking. Toxaemia is usually present. Treatment is by tracheal intubation under general anaesthesia, and antibiotic therapy. An i.v. infusion should be started and atropine 20 μg.kg^{-1} given i.v. to avoid the effects of vagal stimulation when the inflamed epiglottis is stimulated during intubation. Anaesthesia is induced by inhalation of 100% oxygen with halothane, with the child in the sitting position. Induction may be difficult and protracted in the presence of respiratory obstruction. Intubation may be extremely difficult because of the swollen epiglottis. An ear, nose and throat surgeon should be standing by to perform emergency tracheostomy if total respiratory obstruction occurs. An oral tube should be used initially, but this may be changed subsequently for a nasal tube when a clear airway has been established. Extubation is normally possible after antibiotic therapy for 24–48 h.

Laryngotracheobronchitis

This may be bacterial or, more commonly, viral in origin and is the most frequent cause of croup in children. It is a disorder of the larger airways. In mild conditions it may be treated with well-humidified oxygen, but if severe, the trachea should be intubated. If hypoxaemia is present, intermittent positive-pressure ventilation may be necessary. Stridor and an increase in the work of breathing leading to physical exhaustion may necessitate tracheal intubation and mechanical ventilation on purely clinical grounds before the establishment of biochemical evidence of hypox-

aemia. Profuse viscid secretions are a major problem. Humidification is of the utmost importance, and additional quantities of water should be instilled into the airways before the aspiration of secretions to maintain patency of the tube. If the cause is viral, the course of the disease runs for 10–14 days, during which time airway support may be required.

Bronchiolitis

This is a viral disorder of the smaller airways causing expiratory wheeze. Hypoxaemia tends to occur early and secretions are a problem. Tracheal intubation and mechanical ventilation are frequently required in this condition.

Cardiac arrest and resuscitation in children

The commonest causes of cardiac arrest in children are as follows:

1. Hypoxaemia.
2. Hypovolaemia.
3. Electrolyte imbalance.
4. Overdose of drugs.

Prevention of cardiac arrest and its sequelae may be achieved to a great extent by ensuring that all seriously ill children are well-oxygenated, the circulating volume is maintained and electrolyte imbalances are continuously monitored and treated when appropriate. Meticulous care should be taken with the doses of all drugs.

Cardiac arrest in children is associated more commonly with asystole than ventricular fibrillation. Thus, treatment with adrenaline (1 in 10 000) should be used early, as acidosis reduces the effectiveness of catecholamines.

Resuscitation

Children requiring resuscitation in the absence of adequate i.v. access can receive drugs by other routes. The tracheal route is straightforward and rapid. This is a suitable route for administration of adrenaline, atropine, lignocaine and naloxone. The intraosseous route is also of value for fluid administration in addition to drug therapy. Appropriate drug doses are shown in Table 33.10.

Table 33.10 Paediatric resuscitation chart

	Age and weight						
	Neonate 3.5 kg	3 months 5 kg	1 year 10 kg	3 years 15 kg	6 years 20 kg	8 years 25 kg	12 years 40 kg
Tracheal tube							
Size (4 + age/4); mm	3.0	3.5	4.0	5.0	5.5	6.0	7.0
Length (oral); mm	9	10	11	13	14	15	17
Length (nasal); mm	11	13	14	16	19	20	22
Adrenaline 1:10 000 i.v./i.o./e.t.* 0.1 ml.kg^{-1} repeated as necessary	0.5 ml	0.5 ml	1 ml	1.5 ml	2 ml	2.5 ml	4 ml
Sodium bicarbonate 8.4% 1 ml.kg^{-1} i.v.	3 ml	5 ml	10 ml	15 ml	20 ml	25 ml	40 ml
Atropine 500 μg in 5 ml 0.2 ml.kg^{-1} i.v./e.t.	1 ml	1 ml	2 ml	3 ml	4 ml	5 ml	8 ml
Calcium chloride 10% 0.1 ml.kg^{-1} i.v.	0.5 ml	0.5 ml	1 ml	1.5 ml	2 ml	2.5 ml	4 ml
Defibrillation (J) 4 J.kg^{-1}	10	20	40	60	80	100	160
Colloid volume (ml) 10 ml.kg^{-1} × 2–3 as necessary	35	50	100	150	200	250	400

i.v. = intravenous; i.o. = intraosseous; e.t. = endotracheal.
*For endotracheal administration, give 10 times i.v. dose.
N.B. All drugs and fluids may be administered via the intraosseous route.

Drug infusions
Adrenaline: 0.03 mg.kg^{-1} in 50 ml glucose 5%; start at 2 ml.h^{-1}.
Dopamine: 3 mg.kg^{-1} in 50 ml glucose 5%; 3–20 ml.h^{-1}.
Dobutamine: 3 mg.kg^{-1} in 50 ml glucose 5%; 5–20 ml.h^{-1}.
Isoprenaline: 0.25 mg.kg^{-1} in 50 ml glucose 5%; 1–4 ml.h^{-1}.

FURTHER READING

Arthur D S, McNicol L R 1986 Local anaesthetic techniques in paediatric surgery. British Journal of Anaesthesia 58: 76

Brown T C K, Fisk G C 1991 Anaesthesia for children. Blackwell Scientific Publications, Oxford

Cote C J, Ryan J F, Todres I D, Goudsouzian N G 1993 A practice of anesthesia for infants and children. W B Saunders, Philadelphia

Gregory G A 1989 Pediatric anesthesia. Churchill Livingstone, New York

Hatch D, Sumner E 1986 Neonatal anaesthesia and perioperative care. Edward Arnold, London

Katz J, Steward D J 1987 Anesthesia and uncommon pediatric diseases. W B Saunders, Philadelphia

Lloyd Thomas A R 1990 Pain management in paediatric patients. British Journal of Anaesthesia 64: 85–104

Morton N S, Raine P A M (eds) 1994 Paediatric day case surgery. Oxford Medical Publications, Oxford

Rylance G 1981 Clinical pharmacology. Drugs in children. British Medical Journal 181: 50

Winter R W 1973 The body fluids in paediatrics. Little, Brown, Boston

34. Dental anaesthesia

Anaesthesia and dentistry have a long historical association. Some of the first anaesthetics given were for dental extractions and the use of anaesthesia was quickly taken in to dental practice in the late nineteenth century. Dental anaesthetic techniques have evolved in parallel with the changes in practice in other aspects of anaesthesia. The days of single operator anaesthetists and the 'black gas' induction (100% nitrous oxide) are now long gone. For many years dental anaesthesia has been practised in a variety of sites varying from within dental schools to remote dental practices, with the anaesthesia having been provided by anaesthetists, medical practitioners or indeed dentists.

Anaesthesia and dentistry cover three main types of surgery. First, outpatient anaesthesia for simple extractions of teeth, mainly in children ('dental chair anaesthesia'); second, day-case anaesthesia for straightforward extractions of molars or for minor oral surgery and third, inpatient treatment for more complicated extractions or oral surgical procedures. These three areas of anaesthetic practice will be covered in this chapter. In addition, sedation techniques are described as they are likely to become of increasing importance as a result of the future changes in dental anaesthetic practice in the UK.

The provision of dental anaesthetic and sedation services has been the subject of a recent report (DoH 1991). The recommendations of this working party have far-reaching consequences on the provision of dental anaesthetic services and will affect anaesthetists as well as dentists. The recommendations within this report covered general anaesthesia, sedation and resuscitation. With regards to general anaesthesia, the report stated that the use of general anaesthesia should be avoided wherever possible and the same standards in respect of personnel, premises and equipment should apply wherever the anaesthetic is being administered. It further recommended that all anaesthetics should be administered by an accredited anaesthetist and that anaesthetic training should include specific experience in dental anaesthesia. It made further recommendations on the standard of equipment, techniques and facilities and these will be referred to in the text. With regards to sedation, the report started by stating that sedation should be used in preference to general anaesthesia wherever possible. It made further recommendations on training in sedation techniques and on the drugs and techniques to be used. These will be referred to in the text. The report made strong emphasis on the teaching, training and assessment of resuscitation skills and resuscitation facilities within dental practices. The majority of the recommendations from this working party have been accepted by the General Dental Council and the Department of Health.

OUTPATIENT DENTAL ANAESTHESIA

The use of general anaesthesia for outpatient dental extractions (exodontia) has decreased steadily in England and Wales from over 2 million per year in the mid–1950s to around 1.2 million per year in 1970 and down to less than 200 000 per year in 1990. This steady decrease reflects several factors including a general improvement in dental hygiene, a decreased number of practices providing general anaesthetic services and the increased use of local anaesthetic and sedation techniques. The use of general anaesthesia for dental extractions is much more common in the UK than elsewhere in Europe or North America. Within the past few years some centres have shown an increase in the numbers attending for outpatient general anaesthesia. This probably reflects the change in practice with more dental practitioners not providing an anaesthetic service and referring patients requiring general anaesthesia to a central resource. Implementation of the recommendations of the DoH report will make this more likely to occur with centres such as dental schools or medical centres providing the general anaesthetic outpatient dental service for an area.

Patient selection

The selection of patients presenting for dental chair anaesthesia should be the same as those for patients undergoing any outpatient procedure. That is, only healthy ASA grade I and II patients are appropriate. The preoperative screening of patients may be particularly difficult in a dental practice but this is the situation in which careful selection of patients is of greatest importance. It is essential that the dental practitioners involved have some understanding of the anaesthetic implications of common medical conditions and be able to exclude patients with significant cardiac or respiratory disease, renal or hepatic impairment, bleeding disorders or a potentially difficult airway from referral as outpatients. Patients who do not meet these criteria should be referred on to a specialist centre which has back-up facilities and not treated in a dental surgery.

The majority of patients are children between the ages of 4 and 10 years presenting for extraction of carious teeth. This group has a low incidence of systemic disease but a high incidence of respiratory tract infections. Dental problems requiring general anaesthesia are relatively uncommon under the age of 3 years. In adults the indications for general anaesthesia are fewer and include situations where local analgesia is ineffective such as dental abscesses. A further indication for general anaesthesia is for patients who are unable to cooperate with treatment under local analgesia because of mental impairment or physical disability. It is important that this group receive a full preoperative assessment in view of coexistent disease and concurrent medication which may influence anaesthesia. The use of general anaesthesia as an option in adults who do not like dental treatment under local analgesia should be discouraged in favour of the use of sedation techniques (see below).

It is important that the nature of the dental surgical procedure undertaken is appropriate for a day case. This implies that the surgery should be of short duration and not so extensive that it is difficult to provide adequate postoperative analgesia.

The patient's social circumstances must be taken into account when offering them outpatient treatment. The patient must be accompanied before and after the surgery and supervised by an adult for 24 h. Some patients may need time to make appropriate domestic arrangements.

Equipment

The site at which outpatient dental anaesthesia is administered should be equipped to the standards required in the day-case anaesthesia report and the DoH report. That is, the facilities for the anaesthetist and a surgeon should match those that would be provided in an inpatient theatre setting. For an anaesthetist this is best dealt with under the areas of anaesthetic equipment, monitoring and resuscitation equipment.

The equipment necessary would include an anaesthetic machine which is capable of delivering a fast flow of 100% oxygen should this be necessary. Other facilities should include nitrous oxide and a vaporizer, an anaesthetic breathing system with which it is easy to provide assisted ventilation if required. If the patients regularly include children, a low resistance circuit is required. Some older anaesthetic machines included on-demand breathing circuits. These were developed to minimize anaesthetic gas use when the anaesthetist carried gas cylinders from practice to practice and there is no indication for their current use. Modern machines such as those using a Quantiflex flowmeter provide a range of gas flows with mixtures ranging from 30 to 100% oxygen in nitrous oxide. Other equipment should include a variety of nasal and facial masks, oral and nasal airways, laryngoscopes with a variety of blades, including paediatric, and a range of oral and nasal endotracheal tubes. A high pressure suction unit should be available, preferably separate from the suction used by the dentist. The chair should be capable of head-down tilt and should be movable even in the event of power failure.

The minimum standards for monitoring during anaesthesia should be met. The DoH report specifically states that pulse oximetry, ECG and a method for non-invasive measurement of arterial pressure should be available at any site in which an anaesthesic is given (Fig. 34.1). Although most of the procedures in dental practice are short, it is very important that monitoring is used in each case. There is a high potential for airway obstruction resulting in hypoxaemia and also a relatively high incidence of cardiac arrhythmias especially where halothane is used. In practices where tracheal intubation is used a capnograph is required.

A full range of resuscitation equipment must be available; this should include a defibrillator, an emergency drug pack (Table 34.1), facilities for intubation and full delivery of high flow oxygen with positive pressure if necessary e.g. an Ambu or Laerdal bag. The DoH report recommends that the anaesthetist, dentist and dental nurse are all trained in resuscitation and attend regular refresher courses. It also recommends that they practise resuscitation procedures as a team.

Potential preoperative problems

1. Presentation of poorly prepared or inappropriate patients requiring dental treatment.

2. High proportion of patients are children who may have URTI.

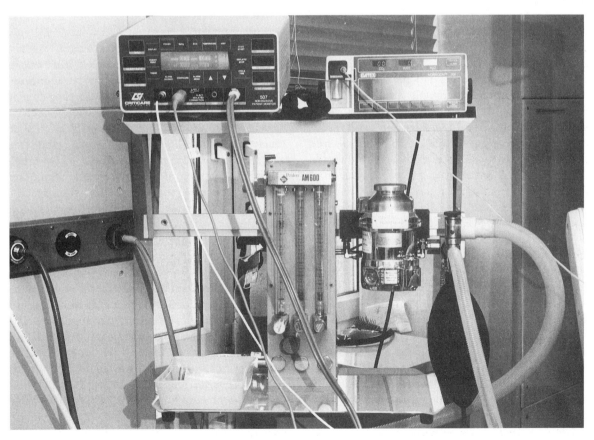

Fig. 34.1 Anaesthetic machine and monitoring suitable for dental anaesthesia.

Table 34.1 List of emergency drugs to be available in dental practices

Oxygen
Adrenaline
Lignocaine 1%
Atropine
Calcium chloride
Sodium bicarbonate
Glyceryl trinitrate (tabs or spray)
Aminophylline
Salbutamol inhaler
Chlorpheniramine
Dextrose 50%
Hydrocortisone
Midazolam
Dextrose/saline infusion bag
Colloid infusion bag
Flumazenil*
Naloxone*

* Only if practice provides i.v. sedation

Table 34.2 Induction of anaesthesia for dental extractions using halothane, enflurane or isoflurane. 50 children in each group (data based on Simmons et al 1989)

	Halothane	Enflurane	Isoflurane
Induction time (min)	2.4	2.8	3.5
Respiratory problems (%) (cough, breath-holding, laryngospasm)	12	12	42
Ventricular arrhythmias (%)	14	0	0
Mean maximum increase in heart rate (%)	22	25	48
Mean maximum fall in SAP (%)	17	15	4

3. Dental abscesses may lead to a difficult airway.

4. Site may have inadequate facilities or equipment.

Induction of anaesthesia

Anaesthesia may be induced by the inhalational or intravenous route. Traditionally, the inhalational route has been used for young children and the intravenous route for older children and adults. The introduction of EMLA cream has allowed the intravenous route to be used more frequently. However, EMLA cream needs to be placed at least 1 h before anticipated cannulation. For many years methohexitone was the drug of choice for induction of anaesthesia for dental outpatient practice. In the past few years this has largely been replaced by propofol.

Inhalational induction has been described using all three agents in common use. Halothane is still very widely used as it has advantages of ease of induction compared with enflurane and isoflurane which are more irritant, particularly isoflurane which may be associated with high incidence of coughing and laryngospasm (Table 34.2). However, halothane is also associated with a high incidence of cardiovascular disturbances, particularly arrhythmias. Arrhythmias are particularly common with halothane in the presence of a raised Pa_{CO_2} which can occur with respiratory depression or if the airway is compromised. The technique of inhalational induction with halothane followed by maintenance with enflurane has been described and this may have advantages because of ease of induction with halothane and limitation of the cardiovascular effects by subsequent use of enflurane.

Induction of anaesthesia in younger children may be difficult if they become frightened or uncooperative. The risk of this can be minimized by a friendly explanation of what is going to happen and the use of some visual aid such as a well know cartoon character breathing into an anaesthetic mask. The induction can be made into a game such as blowing up a balloon (reservoir bag). It is often helpful to have one of the child's parents present during induction, having first explained to the parent the sequence of events and what is expected of them. The management of a screaming child who will not cooperate with either inhalational or i.v. induction is difficult. There is little to be gained and a lot of potential problems in holding the child down with a mask on the face. This is very distressing for the child, the parents and all the staff involved. The potential for problems during induction is high in a child who has a blocked nose and secretions from crying and is distressed and tachycardic before the procedure starts. It is best in this situation to delay anaesthesia until the child is calm. This can usually be done by allowing the parents and the child to sit quietly for half an hour to discuss the problem. In the worst cases it may

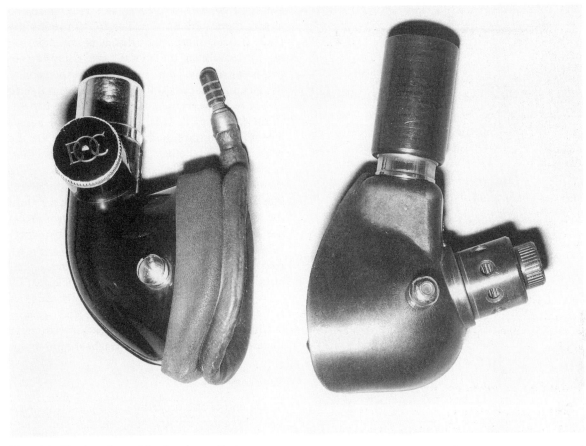

Fig. 34.2   Nasal masks used for dental anaesthesia.

be better to bring the child back on another day, perhaps following oral premedication.

Following either intravenous or inhalational induction, anaesthesia is usually maintained by spontaneous respiration of an inhalational agent, nitrous oxide and oxygen by nasal mask (Fig. 34.2). The use of incremental bolus doses of propofol to maintain anaesthesia during dental anaesthesia has been described and is used in some centres. Several studies have shown the benefits of using 50% inspired oxygen concentration in preference to 30% as this has been shown to decrease the number and severity of hypoxaemic episodes.

The operation

The sequence of events is induction of anaesthesia, stabilization of the airway with a nasal mask (Fig. 34.3), positioning of the gag or bite

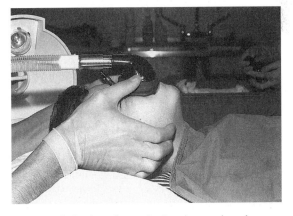

Fig. 34.3   Induction of anaesthesia using nasal mask over mouth and nose.

block by the dentist or anaesthetist, placement of a mouth pack to prevent debris from extracted teeth falling in to the airway (Fig. 34.4), extraction

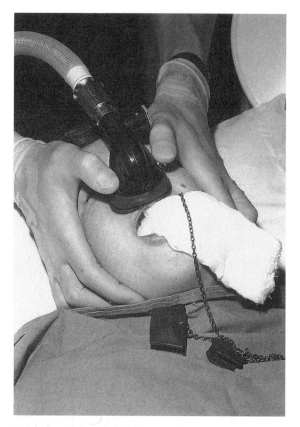

Fig. 34.4 The nasal mask has now been moved to cover the nose only and a gag and mouth pack inserted.

of teeth (Fig. 34.5), if necessary changing sides with repositioning of the bite block and pack, finishing the operation, turning the patient on to the side and recovery from consciousness.

As the airway is shared by the dentist and anaesthetist, it is important that both know the requirements of the other. The dentist requires, in turn, access to all four quadrants of the mouth and also some resistance to the pressure required for extraction of some teeth. In particular, in extraction of teeth from the lower jaw, the downward pressure required can potentially compromise the airway (Fig. 34.5). The anaesthetist needs to maintain the airway throughout the procedure using the nasal mask. This implies that the anaesthetist needs access to the upper half of the face to place the thumb on the nasal mask and the airway is maintained by forward lift of the lower jaw with the fingers (Fig. 34.3). In placing the mouth gag it is important not to use too large a size to over-open the jaw as this may make the airway more difficult to maintain. In placing the pack, it is also important that it is not sited too far posteriorly in the mouth and compromises the nasal airway (Fig. 34.4). The responsibility for placing the pack and gag varies from centre to centre between the anaesthetist or the dentist. Whoever places it, it is important that a patent airway is re-established after placement of the pack and gag, before any operative procedure starts. If at any point throughout the procedure there is a problem with the airway it is important that the anaesthetist can interrupt surgery until the airway is restored. At the end of the procedure, the packs are usually placed across the sockets to absorb any continuing bleeding and the gags removed, the patient placed in the left lateral position and given 100% oxygen to breathe.

As in any general anaesthetic procedure it is important that full resuscitative and support facilities are available immediately, in particular suction and facilities for oral tracheal intubation.

Recovery

At the end of the procedure, the patient is given 100% oxygen to breathe until return of consciousness. The recovery facilities must provide space for the patient to recover in the supine position. A nurse should be there to supervise the recovery.

Peroperative problems

The potential problems associated with the peroperative period include:

1. Difficulty in induction of anaesthesia in an uncooperative child who will not tolerate a mask or insertion of an i.v. cannula.

2. Airway problems occurring – during induction due to irritant gases or airway obstruction, during placement of the gag and pack, during extractions or during early recovery.

3. Obstruction of the airway by bleeding or bits of broken tooth.

4. Cardiac arrythmias.

Fitness for discharge

There are several methods of assessing the patient's

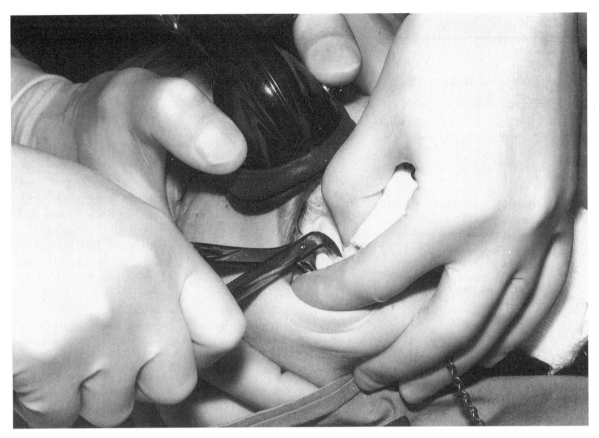

Fig. 34.5 Extraction of tooth from lower jaw. The dental pack is pushed to the left by the operator and the anaesthetist maintains the airway by upward lift of the lower jaw to counteract the downward pressure exerted by the dentist.

fitness for discharge from the recovery room. It is important that the patients are assessed by the medical practitioner before discharge to identify any problems or potential problems which may arise. Assessment includes several clinical observations or the use of sophisticated tests of recovery. Clinical assessments include testing that the patient is alert and orientated and is able to stand and walk unassisted; simple scoring systems include the Steward's score and the Aldrete score.

Postoperative analgesia

It is usual to give postoperative analgesics during outpatient dental extraction procedures. The amount of pain experienced postoperatively varies with the number of teeth extracted and the difficulty encountered in extraction. That is, if there has been a difficult extraction of a tooth that has produced trauma to the gums, there is considerably more pain than simple extraction of, for example, a single upper incisor. Postoperative analgesia is usually provided with non-steroidal anti-inflammatory agents (NSAIDs) given orally in recovery or in the early postoperative period. The use of NSAIDs is ideal for postoperative dental pain as some of the pain comes from the tissue swelling and these agents act in part by decreasing swelling. More recently the use of suppositories which are placed while the patient is anaesthetized has been described. Drugs given in this manner include paracetamol and diclofenac. It is vital to discuss the use of analgesic suppositories with the patient or patient's parents preoperatively. Inability to control postoperative pain is one reason for admitting the patient postoperatively. Likewise, if it is anticipated that the surgery or extractions may produce considerable pain, the procedure may be deemed more appropriate for inpatient treatment.

Postoperative problems

The potential problems associated with the postoperative period can be classified under the headings of immediate or longer term:

Immediate

1. Hypoxaemia – secondary to diffusion hypoxaemia or airway problems.
2. Airway problems – caused by laryngeal spasm, bleeding or debris in the airway.
3. Vomiting.

Long term

1. Continued bleeding.
2. Postoperative pain and swelling.
3. Nausea and vomiting.

DAY-CASE ANAESTHESIA

Recent developments in provision of day-case facilities have allowed some dental procedures to be undertaken on a day-case basis. This differs from the outpatient dental chair anaesthesia in that the patient goes through a formal admission to the hospital but is discharged home later in the day. The procedures for which this is appropriate are limited dental extractions such as those of wisdom teeth and minor oral surgical procedures including laser treatment.

Patient selection

These patients are usually adults and should be of ASA grade I or II and should comply with the standard criteria for selection of day-case patients. It is important to consider also the extent of the surgery involved and that a limitation may be the availability to provide adequate analgesia for the patient who is being discharged home. Therefore, caution should be shown in undertaking extensive oral surgical procedures or difficult extractions of wisdom teeth. It is important that the patient is assessed formally by the anaesthetist at some time before the anaesthetic so that appropriate investigations may be made. This will avoid unnecessary delays or cancellation on the day of surgery. Ideally, the patients should be assessed at a preoperative anaesthetic clinic.

Anaesthetic technique

The patient should arrive early on the morning of surgery, fasted and accompanied. If appropriate the patient can be given an oral premedicant, such as temazepam, to take at home before coming into hospital and this could be arranged at a preoperative assessment visit. The majority of patients, however, do not receive premedication. A full admission clerking of the patient should be made and also preoperative assessment by the anaesthetist.

The nature of the surgery involved dictates that the majority of these patients require nasotracheal intubation. As the majority of the patients involved are young, healthy and are mobilized early, the potential for post-suxamethonium muscle pains is high and the use of suxamethonium is perhaps best avoided. The advantages of suxamethonium in speed of intubation and in controlling the airway have to be weighed against these potential disadvantages. There are several methods of reducing the incidence of postoperative suxamethonium pains using pretreatment with a non-depolarizing relaxant, dantrolene or benzodiazepines. Many of these techniques have been shown to reduce the incidence of muscle pain but none completely abolishes it. The alternatives for achieving nasal tracheal intubation would be to use a non-depolarizing relaxant or, following intravenous or inhalational induction, take the patient to a deep plane of anaesthesia breathing a volatile agent spontaneously. If the anaesthetist is satisfied that there is no preoperative indication of a difficult intubation the use of a non-depolarizing relaxant is probably the easiest.

Following intravenous induction and placement of the nasotracheal tube, the anaesthetist should place the throat pack in the back of the mouth, around the tracheal tube to prevent any blood or debris falling into the back of the larynx. It is extremely important that the tail of the throat pack is brought out of the mouth and secured in some way to make sure that it is removed at the end of surgery. If nasotracheal intubation has been achieved using a non-depolarizing relaxant it is obvious that maintenance is with intermittent positive pressure ventilation with nitrous oxide, oxygen and a volatile agent. If suxamethonium has been used there is a choice between spontaneous respiration following recovery from blockade or continuation with a non-depolarizing relaxant. If an inhalational method has been used to achieve tracheal intubation it is possible to maintain anaesthesia with the patient breathing spontaneously. As the patient has to be at a relatively deep plane of anaesthesia for nasotracheal intubation and because the nasotracheal tube is narrow due to the airway dimensions, this technique should only be used for short procedures as carbon dioxide retention may occur. In the presence of halothane this technique has a high potential for producing arrythmias. If for any reason the trachea cannot be intubated successfully using the nasal route, for example because of a deviated septum or previous nasal injury, orotracheal intubation can be used. While this is not ideal for allowing the dentist access to the operation site, it is an acceptable technique and the orotracheal tube can be carefully moved from one side of the mouth to the other, in turn, to allow access to the appropriate quadrants.

At the end of surgery the patient should be turned to the left lateral, head-down position before tracheal extubation.

Extubation

The trachea may be extubated while the patient is still quite deep or when the patient is very light. In view of the potential for blood and secretions to drain into the larynx it is recommended that the trachea is extubated during light anaesthesia and that the airway is maintained until that time using the nasotracheal tube.

Peroperatively small doses of short-acting opioids may be used to provide analgesia for particularly painful procedures. It is also common practice to introduce an NSAID peroperatively, such as intramuscular diclofenac, to produce postoperative analgesia. Many dental surgeons recommend

the use of a small dose of dexamethazone given peroperatively to help reduce the swelling and hence pain. If the surgery is limited to one or two quadrants it is appropriate to perform a local analgesic block during or at the end of surgery to help provide postoperative analgesia. However, it is not appropriate to produce local analgesic blocks in all four quandrants as this would create difficulties in swallowing secretions and in talking.

The patient should be recovered in a supine position and when appropriate, allowed to sit up and then to gradually mobilize. It is appropriate that discharge does not occur until the patient is fully recovered and should take place a minimum of two hours postoperatively. It is important that the patient is assessed by a medical practitioner before discharge and that the patient has good pain control, has no evidence of continuing bleeding and is fully orientated. On discharge the patient should be accompanied and should be given a set of written instructions for the postoperative period with regards to operating machinery, drinking alcohol and being accompanied. It is important that should there be any problems the patient has a contact telephone number to seek advice. As with all day-case procedures, should a problem arise per- or postoperatively, such as continued bleeding or persistent uncontrolled pain, there must be an easily implemented procedure which would allow overnight admission of the patient to hospital.

INPATIENT DENTAL ANAESTHESIA

Some more invasive surgical procedures are managed more appropriately on an inpatient basis. These procedures include impacted wisdom teeth where considerable surgery is anticipated or where all four wisdom teeth are to be extracted at one go and also include oral surgical procedures on the gums and jaw. In this latter group the anaesthetist must be particularly aware of the potential for difficulty in achieving tracheal intubation produced by limitation of jaw movement. It is very important in the preoperative assessment to make a full assessment of the airway. Limitation of jaw movement produced by pain or swelling cannot always be relied upon to decrease following blockade with a muscle relaxant.

In general, inpatient dental cases are managed with nasotracheal intubation following intravenous induction. However, if difficulty is anticipated with the airway an awake fibreoptic intubation or an inhalational induction should be considered. Following nasotracheal intubation a throat pack is placed by the anaesthetist around the tracheal tube. Some oral surgical procedures use lasers and a laser-protected tracheal tube may be required.

These operations can be painful and the peroperative use of short-acting opioids and NSAIDs is recommended. Postoperatively the patients may require i.m. or i.v. opioids with a PCA. Most dental surgeons request the use of dexamethazone peroperatively to help minimize swelling.

SEDATION

The move away from the use of general anaesthesia for dental procedures has been accompanied by increasing use of sedative techniques to permit dental procedures to be carried out under local analgesia in patients who are either anxious or who are having more invasive procedures carried out. Although dentists receive training in the use of sedation, it is likely that with its increasing use, anaesthetists will be called on to provide sedation for patients undergoing dental procedures. The DoH report defined sedation as:

A carefully controlled technique in which a single intravenous drug, or a combination of oxygen and nitrous oxide, is used to reinforce hypnotic suggestion and reassurance in a way which allows dental treatment to be performed with minimal physiological and psychological stress, but which allows verbal contact with the patient to be maintained at all times. The technique must carry a margin of safety wide enough to render unintended loss of consciousness unlikely. Any technique of sedation other than as defined above would be regarded as coming within the meaning of dental general anaesthesia.

The important aspects of this definition are that it states that a *single* i.v. drug is used, that it is only part of an overall technique of reassurance for the patient, that verbal contact is maintained throughout the procedure and that a wide safety margin from loss of consciousness is essential. These definitions imply that the use of a benzo-

diazepine in combination with an opioid for a surgical procedure is regarded as general anaesthesia and not as sedation.

There are two techniques which are used: intravenous use of small doses of benzodiazepines and, less commonly, inhalation of low concentrations of nitrous oxide in oxygen (termed *relative analgesia*).

Intravenous sedation

The aim of this technique is to have a patient who is feeling no anxiety, is cooperative although drowsy but is easily rousable. The procedure starts with intravenous cannulation and attachment of a pulse oximeter. Increments of benzodiazepine, usually midazolam, are given and the amount titrated to the patient's response. Midazolam has largely replaced diazepam as the benzodiazepine used for these procedures as it has the advantage of a shorter half-life and no active metabolites. This implies the patient has less postoperative sedation and is ready for discharge more promptly. The endpoint for titration of midazolam and diazepam may be the onset of Verrill's sign, which is drooping of the eyelids (ptosis). This is thought by some authors to be too deep a level of sedation and they use an endpoint where the patient starts to have a delayed response to verbal command. It is important that verbal contact is not lost at any stage.

The use of intravenous sedation with midazolam can occasionally be associated with the occurrence of dreams which may be of a sexual nature. These may be very distressing to the patient and can lead to misunderstandings with the operator. There are two recommendations which should be followed to minimize this risk: first, the dose of midazolam should be limited to $0.1 \, mg.kg^{-1}$ and second, the operator should always be accompanied throughout the procedure by another person, usually the practice nurse.

The titration of midazolam should be done slowly and it must be remembered that there is a lag time before the onset of its sedative effect. When the appropriate level of sedation has been reached, local analgesia can be placed in the usual manner and the procedure can start. The initial dose of midazolam produces amnesia which may persist for 10–15 min and a longer period of anxiolysis. As the anxiolysis is the main reason for administering the drug, top-up doses should not be required too frequently. The patient should be monitored continuously using the pulse oximeter and it is important that the operator communicates regularly with the patient to assess their degree of awareness and comfort. At the end of the procedure the patient should be given adequate time to recover before discharge. Flumazenil should be used only in the situation of accidental overdosage of benzodiazepines and not as a routine method of reversing sedation. The criteria for fitness discharge that would apply to a patient receiving a general anaesthetic should also apply to those who receive intravenous sedation; that is, they should be accompanied home and should not operate machinery for the first 24 h.

Inhalational sedation

Inhalational sedation involves the use of low inspired concentrations of nitrous oxide in oxygen and is also termed *relative analgesia*. The technique has been used in both adults and children but requires a degree of cooperation from the patient and significant input from the operator to make the technique work. The aim of the technique is to titrate a dose of inspired nitrous oxide which produces a light level of sedation and mild analgesia. This allows procedures to take place under subsequent local anaesthetic block.

This technique may be useful in patients who have 'needle phobia' for local analgesic injections in the mouth. It is important for this procedure that the patient has been selected appropriately and that the patient understands what is involved. A nasal mask which can be clipped round the head is used and an initial concentration of 5–10% nitrous oxide in oxygen is used. This is stepped up in 5% increments to a maximum of 30% to provide an appropriate level of sedation and cooperation. The use of higher concentrations of nitrous oxide can lead to restlessness and occasionally aggression in the patient. A Quantiflex flowmeter is very useful for administration of nitrous oxide for this technique as when the initial flow has been set, the relative concentrations of nitrous oxide and oxygen can be varied using a single dial. During onset of sedation it is important that the operator maintains verbal communication and assists in establishing anxiolysis to allow placement of the local block and commencement of the procedure. Recovery from this technique is rapid and it has the advantage compared with intravenous sedation that, following a short recovery period, the patient is ready for discharge early and there is less restriction on mobility in the first 24 h.

Relative contraindications to the use of relative analgesia include a blocked nose, deafness, inability to cooperate either through physical or mental disability, active neurological disease or severe respiratory disease.

FURTHER READING

Church J A, Pollock J S S, Still D M, Parbrook G D 1991 Comparison of two techniques for sedation in dental surgery. Anaesthesia 46: 780–782

Commission on the Provision of Surgical Services 1985 Guidelines for day case surgery. Royal College of Surgeons of England, London

Department of Health 1991 Report on an expert working party on general anaesthesia, sedation and resuscitation in dentistry. Department of Health, Dental Division, London

Rood J P, Healy T E J 1990 The dental day case unit. Clinical Anaesthesiology 4: 799–806

Seward G R 1990 The use of nitrous oxide–oxygen inhalation sedation with local analgesia as an alternative to general anaesthesia for dental extractions in children. British Dental Journal 168: 467–470

Simmons M, Miller C D, Cummings G C, Todd J G 1989 Outpatient paediatric dental anaesthesia. A comparison of halothane, enflurane and isoflurane. Anaesthesia 44: 735–738

35. Anaesthesia for plastic, endocrine and vascular surgery

PLASTIC SURGERY

The term 'plastic surgery' is used to describe procedures which involve reconstitution of damaged or deformed tissues, removal of cutaneous tumours or cosmetic alteration of body features. Tissue may be deformed as a result of trauma, burns, infection or congenital abnormality. Division or removal of the abnormality often results in skin cover defects. Major plastic surgery includes the formation and repositioning of free and pedicle grafts and the movement of skin flaps.

General considerations

There are several important features common to many of these operations. The patient may be deformed grossly as a result of previous trauma or serious disease and attention should be directed to the patient's psychological state, which is influenced by long periods of confinement and rehabilitation, concern over disfigurement or loss of limb function and occasionally chronic pain. Preoperative drug therapy should be controlled carefully and attention paid to removal of local or generalized infection, state of nutrition and haematocrit, which are important factors in the outcome of this form of surgery. Cosmetic surgery of the face, tattoo removal, breast augmentation and removal of unwanted adipose tissue are performed usually on healthy patients.

Haemorrhage is a common occurrence during plastic surgery and all but the most minor operations may necessitate blood transfusion. Operations (especially vascular reconstruction) may last many hours and care must be taken to position the patient in such a way that ligament strain and pressure on skin over bony prominences are avoided. The use of lumbar support and soft padding minimizes these risks. When surgery has been completed, wound dressing and bandaging may be lengthy procedures. It is common for bandages to be applied round the trunk and the patient must be lifted carefully to avoid injury. Finally, there may be severe postoperative pain, especially from donor skin graft sites.

Head and neck

Tracheal intubation is mandatory for surgery in this area and a reinforced tube should be used. It is important to protect the eyes from pressure, the ears from blood and other fluids and the teeth and anaesthetic tubing from dislodgement. It may be difficult to monitor chest movement and access to the arms may be impossible. An i.v. infusion with extension tubing is essential; there should be access to a three-way tap for injection of drugs. A foot should be exposed to allow the anaesthetist to monitor colour, capillary filling and arterial pulse. Venous drainage is improved in surgery on the head or neck if the patient is positioned in a 10–15° head-up tilt and this reduces surgical bleeding.

The anaesthetist should anticipate difficulties in tracheal intubation and a complete range of equipment should be available. Tumours or scarring of the neck, deformity of facial bones and cleft palate make tracheal intubation particularly difficult. Use of muscle relaxants in such patients may be unwise before intubation; the anaesthetist should consider the use of local anaesthesia for awake intubation or an inhalational technique. The method of maintenance should be determined by the condition of the patient, the type and duration of surgery and the experience and preference of the anaesthetist. Hypotensive techniques are employed frequently (see Ch. 36).

Trunk

Problems encountered in surgery on the trunk include the adoption of unusual postures and their attendant risks, haemorrhage, prolonged operation and restrictive dressings applied after surgery.

Limbs

Local anaesthesia may be an advantage for surgery on upper or lower limbs. However, Bier's block is of limited value as the surgeon often requires cuff deflation to identify bleeding points. The duration of some plastic operations may preclude local anaesthetic techniques, although prolonged neural blockade may be achieved by repeated injection (e.g. through an extradural catheter) or by employing an agent with a prolonged duration of action (e.g. bupivacaine). Sedative drugs or light general anaesthesia may be required to help the patient to remain motionless on the operating table. Specific nerve blocks may be useful, e.g. blockade of the femoral and lateral cutaneous nerve of thigh provides analgesia for skin graft donor sites during and after operation.

Surgical techniques of reimplantation and microsurgical repair of the limbs are well established and make specific demands upon the anaesthetist. These include maintenance of general anaesthesia for up to 24 h, control of vascular spasm and provision of optimum conditions for postoperative recovery.

Anaesthesia should be administered using humidified gases in a warmed theatre environment. Nitrous oxide may produce marrow depression with prolonged exposure and should be avoided. If a volatile agent is required, isoflurane is regarded by some as the agent of choice as it undergoes little biotransformation (0.2%), is eliminated rapidly and in normovolaemic patients produces vasodilatation which may be beneficial to the outcome of the operation. Fluid balance should be maintained scrupulously. Pressure areas should be protected by a ripple mattress. An arterial cannula

should be inserted for measurement of arterial pressure and sampling of blood as a check that normocapnia is maintained. Measures should be taken to prevent DVT formation.

Vascular spasm in an isolated limb may be prevented by preoperative i.v. regional sympathetic blockade using guanethidine 15–20 mg, heparin 500 units and prilocaine 0.5% to a suitable volume. Normocapnia, normotension, adequate analgesia and maintenance of body temperature are important. Local anaesthetic blockade of nerve plexuses in the neck, axilla and groin provides vasodilatation and this may be prolonged using a catheter technique.

Burns

Hypoxaemia is the principal cause of rapid death in victims of fire. This may result either from a reduction in inspired oxygen concentration in a smoke-filled atmosphere or poisoning by products of combustion. Carbon monoxide has an affinity for haemoglobin over 200 times greater than that of oxygen and high concentrations cause reduced oxygen carriage in the blood. The oxygen dissociation curve is distorted and shifted to the left resulting in reduced oxygen delivery to the tissues. In addition, there may be direct thermal injury to the airway with ciliary damage, mucosal oedema, loss of surfactant and epithelial destruction. These may result in mucosal sloughing and alveolar oedema. Ventilation/perfusion mismatch is thus a serious problem in these patients.

The aim of immediate treatment is to secure the airway and administer 100% oxygen; this may require tracheal intubation and IPPV until Pa_{O_2} is adequate. Such patients require humidification of inspired gas, physiotherapy and bronchial suction. Bronchodilators and PEEP may be necessary.

Burning of flesh produces rapid fluid shifts and formation of tissue oedema, particularly during the first 36 h. The resulting depletion of intravascular volume is greatest in the first few hours and it is essential that a fluid replacement regimen is started as early as possible in order to avoid acute renal failure. Fluid regimens based on that of Muir and Barclay are still widely used (Table 35.1).

The volume requirements calculated should be

Table 35.1   Fluid regimen for burned patients

1. Estimate/measure weight
2. Estimate percentage area of burns using 'rule of nines' for adults and 'rule of tens' for children
3. Proceed with i.v. regimen if > 15% burns (adults) or > 10% burns (children)
   Measure:
      haematocrit
      haemoglobin
      electrolytes
      heart rate and arterial pressure
4. Give fluid replacement (at least 50% as human albumin solution) – weight in kg × % burns (ml) in each of the following six periods from time of burning:
      1. 0–4 h
      2. 4–8 h
      3. 8–12 h
      4. 12–18 h
      5. 18–24 h
      6. 24–36 h
5. If extensive full-thickness burns are present, some of the above fluid must be given as whole blood.

modified appropriately in response to alterations in urine output, plasma deficit, osmolality, vital signs and body temperature. The use of treatment algorithms is well suited to this aspect of burns management and these may be found in specialist journals.

The hormonal response to burning results in a hypercatabolic state with tachycardia, hyperpnoea and hyperpyrexia.

After the eschar has formed, there is loss of pure water from the body surface with a resultant increase in plasma concentration of aldosterone. The patient is at risk from water depletion and relative sodium overload. In addition, there is a rapid increase in serum potassium and urea concentrations (caused by cellular disruption in damaged tissue) and haemolysis and these are accentuated by acidosis caused by infection. In the natural course of recovery, kalliuresis and anaemia result from continuing haemolysis of red cells.

Sepsis frequently develops in severely burned patients and is a major cause of mortality. The picture of clinical sepsis includes fever, haematological and metabolic derangement leading to multiorgan failure. The excessive inflammatory response to trauma and infection is associated with cytokine activity, notably tumour necrosing factor α, interleukin-1 and interleukin-6. The latter can be used to predict outcome in that patients with continuously raised IL-6 levels tend not to survive.

The anaesthetist's involvement with burn victims may commence at an early stage when hypoxaemia is life-threatening and basic resuscitation is required. If sepsis and multiorgan failure develop the patient must be admitted to an intensive therapy unit. Thereafter, general anaesthesia may be required for:

1. Early excision of damaged tissue from 72 h after the burn.
2. Excision of granulation tissue and grafting.
3. Changes of dressing.
4. Reparative plastic procedures to relieve contractions, permit limb function or remove unsightly deformity.

Recovery from burns trauma may be protracted. The anaesthetist must be aware of the probable requirement for multiple administrations of general anaesthesia, frequent use of opioid analgesics in the early stages and the importance of psychological support throughout the patient's hospitalization.

Anaesthetic problems

1. *Airway.* Thermal damage to the head and neck of a patient may provide the anaesthetist with a severe test of his ability. In the initial stages, raw, painful tissues may prohibit application of a face mask, while a rapid-sequence induction using a depolarizing muscle relaxant drug may be inadvisable (see below). Later, as soft tissues fibrose and distort, the range of movement in the neck and temporomandibular joints may become grossly restricted and render laryngoscopic intubation impossible (Fig. 35.1). Tracheostomy is regarded generally as undesirable because of the risk that infection may spread to damaged skin. Awake intubation may be necessary.

It may be difficult to secure the tracheal tube in place. Several ingenious methods have been devised, such as suspension of the anaesthetic breathing system from the ceiling, the use of umbilical tape to tie the tube in place and wiring the tube to the upper teeth.

In the early stages of the patient's treatment, and after prolonged surgery, it is wise to examine

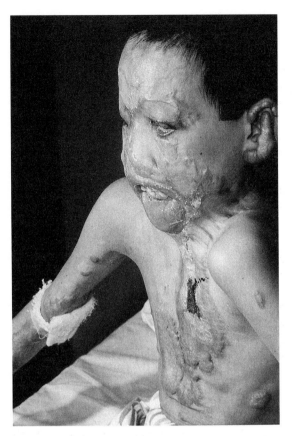

Fig. 35.1 Severe scar formation and contractions caused by burns to the thorax and neck.

the pharynx closely before tracheal extubation. Oedema may form in the soft tissues around the base of the tongue and cause respiratory obstruction when the tracheal tube is removed.

2. *Ventilation.* Mechanical ventilation should be employed in the severely burned patient and careful monitoring of ventilation is required. Metabolic rate may be doubled in a patient with 40% burns; this results in large increases in oxygen consumption and carbon dioxide production; i.v. alimentation increases the latter. Inhalational injury causes increased scatter of $\dot{V}/\dot{Q}$ ratios. A sophisticated ventilator, capable of providing PEEP and minute volumes up to 30 litre.min^{-1}, is required. There should be continuous monitoring using a pulse oximeter and capnograph, with regular blood/gas analysis.

3. *Fluid balance.* In addition to the fluid balance problems mentioned above, the modern practice of early tissue excision is accompanied by extensive and rapid blood loss. Crossmatched blood must be available before the operation is started, and it is wise to have two large-gauge venous cannulae in situ and facilities for warming infused fluids.

4. *Temperature loss.* Heat loss is increased from a burned area by evaporation and inability of cutaneous vessels to constrict and prevent radiation. This loss is offset partly by the increased heat production which results from the raised metabolic rate, but the anaesthetist should minimize heat loss during anaesthesia and surgery by use of a warming blanket, foil blanket, blood warmer, gas humidifier and an ambient theatre temperature and humidity of 27°C and 50% respectively.

5. *Choice of anaesthetic agent.* This is governed by personal preference and the knowledge that repeated administration of some volatile agents may result in hepatic damage. Ketamine is useful; it may be used also as an infusion for analgesia during burns dressings. However, it is not safe to assume that the airway is preserved during ketamine anaesthesia and it is wise to premedicate the patient with an antisialagogue. Diazepam may control the emergence hallucinations suffered by some patients who receive ketamine.

Suxamethonium should be avoided in burned patients. In the presence of muscle damage its administration may cause release of potassium into the circulation in concentrations sufficient to cause cardiac arrest. It is thought that the most dangerous period in this respect is between 4 days and 10 weeks after thermal injury.

SURGERY FOR TUMOURS OF THE ENDOCRINE SYSTEM

APUD (amine precursor uptake and decarboxylation) cells are thought to originate from neuro-ectoderm and are distributed widely throughout the body. They are able to synthesize and store neurotransmitter substances including serotonin, ACTH, calcitonin, MSH, glucagon, gastrin and vasoactive intestinal polypeptide. Neoplastic change within these cells produces the group of tumours termed apudomas, for example carcinoids, pancreatic islet cell tumours, pituitary and thyroid adenomas, medullary carcinoma of thyroid and small cell carcinoma of the lung. These may be orthoendocrine or paraendocrine; the former produce amines and polypeptides associated normally with the constituent cells, while the latter secrete substances produced usually by other organs. There are two orthoendocrine apudomas which may produce significant difficulty for the anaesthetist.

Carcinoid tumour

Carcinoid tumours arise in the enterochromaffin cells of the intestinal tract, are commonly benign and are found most often in the appendix (Table 35.2). However, they may occur at any site in the gut and, rarely, in the gall-bladder or bronchus. Malignant change occurs in 4% and may give rise to hepatic secondaries which are potentially resectable.

Carcinoid tumours secrete over 20 substances with a variety of effects on vascular, bronchial and gastrointestinal smooth muscle activity. Kallikrein is an enzyme which acts on circulating plasma kininogen to produce bradykinin. This is a potent vasodilator which causes flushing, bronchospasm, increased intestinal motility and contributes to hypotension and oedema. Adrenergic stimulation and alcohol ingestion increase the production of bradykinin. The treatment of bronchospasm in a patient with carcinoid syndrome should therefore be with aminophylline and not adrenaline.

Serotonin (5-hydroxytryptamine; 5-HT) is responsible for abnormal gut motility and diarrhoea and possibly for endocardial fibrosis which may result in pulmonary and tricuspid stenosis. Left-sided valvular lesions of the heart may be caused by the secretions of a bronchial carcinoid tumours.

The amine secretions of a carcinoid tumour are metabolized normally in the liver. It is only when they escape the portal circulation (hepatic metastases, bronchial primary) that the clinical

Table 35.2 Distribution of carcinoid tumours

Midgut	73% (appendix 45%; ileum 28%)
Rectum	16%
Bronchus	10%

Table 35.3 Symptoms, signs and causal agents in carcinoid syndrome

Symptoms and signs	Causal agents
Cutaneous flushing	Bradykinin, histamine, prostaglandin
Diarrhoea	Bradykinin, serotonin, prostaglandin
Bronchospasm	Bradykinin, histamine, prostaglandin
Cardiac valvular lesions	Serotonin
Telangiectasia	Vasoactive peptide
Glucose intolerance	Serotonin
Arthropathy	Serotonin
Hypotension	Serotonin

picture of carcinoid syndrome (Table 35.3) is seen.

Diagnosis is confirmed by high urinary excretion of 5-hydroxyindoleacetic acid (5-HIAA), a metabolite of 5-HT (a total of more than 27 mg.day^{-1} is diagnostic). Liver scan may show filling defects caused by secondary tumours.

Treatment

While patients may be receiving drug therapy to alleviate the symptoms of diarrhoea and flushing, the definitive treatment of carcinoid tumours is surgical removal. To control the effects of secretion release in the perioperative period, patients are now managed with octreotide, a somatostatin analogue.

Somatostatin is a universal inhibitor of both exocrine and endocrine secretions, muscle contractions and cell growth. It has an enormous variety of actions throughout the body and specifically inhibits release of growth hormone, TSH and prolactin. Because the compound has only a short half-life of 1–3 min, it is of limited clinical use. However, its octapeptide analogue, octreotide, has a much longer half-life of 45 min and may be given i.v. or s.c. It has a high potency, low clearance and a minimal effect on glucagon and insulin. Unfortunately its long-term use is associated with the formation of gall stones.

Conduct of anaesthesia

Acute attacks of carcinoid syndrome may be

precipitated by fear, hypotension and handling of the tumour. The anaesthetist should be aware of the following factors:

1. Hypovolaemia and electrolyte imbalance may occur in patients with diarrhoea.

2. Adequate preoperative sedation with minimal cardiovascular disturbance is essential. A sedative with antihistamine properties, e.g. promethazine, is suitable.

3. Techniques which may cause hypotension, including extradural and subarachnoid block, should be avoided.

4. Sudden bronchospasm, arrhythmias and extreme fluctuations in arterial pressure may occur. Continuous monitoring of ECG and arterial pressure are mandatory. Bronchospasm may be particularly resistant to treatment.

5. Drugs which release histamine (e.g. curare or morphine) should be avoided. Volatile anaesthetics may prolong recovery time and their use may be hazardous in the presence of valvular lesions.

Promethazine, diazepam or droperidol are appropriate premedicants. Anaesthesia is induced most safely by an opioid agent such as fentanyl and muscle relaxation may be achieved with vecuronium. After tracheal intubation, nitrous oxide and oxygen should be administered and additional fentanyl given as required. IPPV should be delivered by a ventilator of the flow-generator type which is capable of delivering the inspired gases at high pressure if bronchospasm develops. Monitoring should include ECG, direct arterial and central venous pressure measurement, pulse oximetry and capnography. IPPV may be required after operation, but in any event the patient should be observed in a high-dependency or intensive therapy unit.

Phaeochromocytoma

Ninety-four per cent of these rare tumours arise in the phaeochromocytes of the adrenal medulla; the remainder are associated with the paravertebral sympathetic ganglia. They produce adrenaline and noradrenaline, the hormones which cause the symptoms and signs of phaeochromocytoma (Table 35.4).

Table 35.4 Clinical symptoms and signs associated with phaeochromocytoma

Symptoms	Signs
Headache	Hypertension, paroxysmal or sustained
Palpitations	Increased basal metabolic rate
Excessive sweating	Haemoconcentration
Weight loss	Renal pathology
Pallor	Increased blood glucose, lactic acid and FFA concentrations
Visual disturbance	Cardiomyopathy

The presentation of the disease and its subsequent management depend on the total output of catecholamines and the relative proportions of adrenaline and noradrenaline.

Tachycardia, tachyarrhythmias and high-output cardiac failure are characteristic findings when the tumour secretes adrenaline predominantly; those which secrete predominantly noradrenaline result in a reduced circulating blood volume.

Diagnosis is confirmed by measurement of high plasma concentrations of catecholamines and high urinary excretion rates of catecholamines and their metabolite 3-methoxy-4-hydroxymandelic acid. It may be more practical to measure excretion of the intermediary metanephrines; increased concentrations in combination with the clinical findings and demonstration of raised circulating concentrations of catecholamines are diagnostic. Localization of a tumour may be undertaken by selective venous catheterization with sampling for raised catecholamine concentrations. Computerized tomography may be used to identify tumours greater than 1 cm in diameter. Uptake of [131I]*meta*-iodylbenzylguanidine (MIBG), monitored by gamma camera, is now the most specific test to identify and localize the position of tumours.

Treatment

The aim is to control the effects of the tumour with drugs and then to remove it surgically. Pharmacological control is achieved by α-adrenergic blockade to counteract the increased peripheral vascular resistance and reduced circulating volume. Phenoxybenzamine, phentolamine and prazosin have all been used successfully. A β-adrenergic antagonist may be required subsequently to control tachycardia but this may precipitate cardiac failure and acute pulmonary oedema if introduced without α-adrenergic blockage and appropriate fluid replacement. Propranolol, metoprolol and atenolol are useful agents if β-blockade is required. Labetalol is favoured by some physicians. Synthesis of catecholamine may be suppressed actively by administration of methyl-*p*-tyrosine, a tyrosine hydroxylase inhibitor. This drug may be very successful in controlling the disease, but may cause severe side-effects including diarrhoea, fatigue and depression.

Preoperative preparation of the patient by α-blockade with phenoxybenzamine may be accomplished by oral administration of increasing dosage of the drug over a period of weeks. In this event, expansion of the capacitance system occurs gradually with normal oral intake of fluid. Alternatively, phenoxybenzamine may be given by i.v. infusion (frequently on a daily basis for the 3 days preceding surgery). In this event, it is necessary to monitor intravascular volume by measurement of CVP and to maintain a normal volume by i.v. infusion of colloids.

Conduct of anaesthesia

Sudden and large fluctuations in arterial pressure occur during surgery for phaeochromocytoma, especially when tumour tissue is handled. Monitoring of ECG, central venous pressure and direct arterial pressure must be instituted *before* induction of anaesthesia.

Premedication should provide sedation and agents used for induction and maintenance should be selected on the basis of cardiovascular stability (Table 35.5).

Table 35.5 Drugs to avoid in patients with phaeochromocytoma

Atropine	Droperidol
Suxamethonium	Morphine
Gallamine	Halothane
d-Tubocurarine	
Atracurium	
Pancuronium	

Anaesthesia may be induced by slow administration of thiopentone or etomidate and maintained with nitrous oxide in oxygen, supplemented by either enflurane or isoflurane. A lipid-soluble opioid, e.g. fentanyl, reduces the risk of excessive hypertension during tracheal intubation and skin incision. Release of catecholamines occurs commonly when the tumour is mobilized and an arterial vasodilator such as sodium nitroprusside is usually required to control arterial pressure. Arterial pressure may decrease after removal of the tumour, although this is uncommon if preoperative preparation has been adequate.

Invasive monitoring should be continued for 12–24 h after surgery and the patient must be nursed in a high-dependency or intensive care unit.

MAJOR VASCULAR SURGERY

Anaesthesia for major vascular surgery is a complex subject. Only the more important features of four vascular operations are described here: elective and emergency repair of abdominal aortic aneurysm, bypass of abdominal aortoiliac occlusion and carotid artery surgery.

Patients presenting for major vascular surgery have a high incidence of coexisting disease and many exhibit the features of one or more of the following:

1. Hypertension
2. Ischaemic heart disease
3. Renal disease
4. Congestive cardiac failure
5. Diabetes mellitus
6. Pulmonary disease.

It is vital that such conditions are treated preoperatively and that the patient presents for surgery only when no further improvement might be expected. The risks of morbidity and death after these operations are increased greatly by the presence of cardiac failure, recent myocardial infarction, hypertension and arrhythmias (see Chs 18 and 40).

Recent general anaesthesia for arteriography should be noted and evidence sought of renal dysfunction following injection of large volumes of radio-opaque dye. Physical examination should include Allen's test on both wrists because radial artery cannulation will be required during anaesthesia for measurement of systemic arterial pressure and sampling of blood for acid–base and blood/gas status.

Abdominal aortic aneurysm

These vascular abnormalities occur in 3% of the population over the age of 50 years. It has been suggested that when the aneurysm exceeds 5.5 cm in diameter, there is a very much increased risk of rupture. There is an overall mortality of 90% from ruptured aortic aneurysm and in those patient who survive until emergency surgical repair can take place, the mortality is still 50%. Consequently there are now more screening programmes which will identify those patients with small asymptomatic aneurysms. They will be followed up and offered surgical repair before the risk of rupture is significant.

Elective repair

Consideration should be given to the collection and storage of the patient's own blood in the weeks preceding surgery. This may then be used as autologous blood transfusion per- and postoperatively.

It is normal practice to prescribe a sedative premedication. Atropine should be avoided if there is evidence of ischaemic heart disease.

On arrival in the anaesthetic room, the patient should be placed on a warming blanket, arterial pressure measured and an oximeter attached. In patients with myocardial disease, direct intra-arterial pressure and ECG monitoring should be instituted before induction of anaesthesia. Preoxygenation of the lungs is followed by induction of anaesthesia by slow injection of thiopentone or propofol. After muscle relaxation, the trachea is intubated (see below) and IPPV continued using humidified gases.

The following procedures are performed before surgery starts:

1. A suitable vein or veins are cannulated with at least one 14-gauge cannula for infusion of warmed fluids.

2. Cannulation of a radial artery.

3. Central venous catheterization for measurement of right atrial pressure.

4. An oesophageal or tympanic membrane temperature probe is inserted for measurement of temperature.

5. The bladder is catheterized for monitoring of urine output.

Three specific stimuli may give rise to cardiovascular instability in patients undergoing aneurysm repair:

1. *Tracheal intubation.* The increase in systemic arterial pressure which accompanies tracheal intubation may be of considerable magnitude and must be minimized to avoid myocardial ischaemia. Attenuation of this response may be produced by the i.v. administration of a β-blocker or a high dose of a lipid-soluble opioid (e.g. alfentanil 500–600 μg) before intubation. Topical anaesthesia to the larynx is not effective.

2. *Crossclamping of the aorta.* Clamping of the aorta causes a sudden increase in systemic vascular resistance (afterload). This increases cardiac work and may result in myocardial ischaemia, arrhythmias and left ventricular failure. It may be necessary to administer vasodilators (e.g. sodium nitroprusside or glyceryl trinitrate) during this period to obviate these problems.

While the aorta is clamped, the large bowel and lower limbs suffer variable degrees of hypoxia during which inflammatory mediators are released from white blood cells, platelets and capillary endothelium. These mediators include oxygen radicals, neutrophil proteases, platelet activating factor, cyclo-oxygenase products and cytokines including the interleukin series.

3. *Aortic declamping.* Declamping of the aorta causes a sudden decrease in afterload with reperfusion of the bowel, pelvis and lower limbs. The inflammatory mediators are swept into the systemic circulation causing vasodilatation, metabolic acidosis, increased capillary permeability and sequestration of blood cells in the lungs. Mannitol has a positive effect in countering these deleterious pulmonary effects.

Bleeding is a problem throughout the operation but may be particularly severe at this time as the adequacy of vascular anastomoses is tested.

All these factors may result in severe hypotension unless circulating volume has been well maintained and transfusion is continued to maintain an adequate CVP. If relative hypervolaemia is produced during the period of clamping by infusion of fluids to produce a CVP of 10–12 cmH$_2$O (and perhaps administration of SNP), declamping hypotension is not a problem and metabolic acidosis is avoided.

Many patients undergoing this operation are elderly and have a low metabolic rate. Consequently they are unable to tolerate the large heat loss which occurs through the extensive surgical exposure, which necessitates displacement of the bowel outside the abdominal cavity. All possible measures must be taken to minimize heat loss. These include:

1. Warming of infusion fluids.
2. Warming and humidification of anaesthetic gases.
3. Use of a warming blanket under the patient.
4. Wrapping the bowel in a clear plastic bag.
5. Use of a warm, humid ambient atmosphere in the operating theatre.

In the more compromised patient, e.g. ischaemic heart disease and poor left ventricular function, the use of a pulmonary artery catheter is indicated. This permits measurement of cardiac output and monitoring of left ventricular preload during the more dangerous stages of the operation. Preservation of an optimal left ventricular preload reduces the incidence of precipitous decreases of arterial pressure after declamping of the aorta.

The postoperative period

Repair of abdominal aortic aneurysm should only be conducted in hospitals with adequate facilities. Postoperatively the patient should be transferred rapidly to a high dependency or intensive care unit, where full monitoring is resumed and ventilation continued with oxygen enriched humidified air. IPPV is required until body temperature has increased to normal levels, the consequent vasodilatation treated with i.v. fluids and adequate analgaesia achieved. After weaning, attention is paid to renal function and signs of continued blood loss from oozing.

Emergency repair

The principles of management are similar to those discussed above. However, the patient is likely to be grossly hypovolaemic and often arterial pressure is maintained only by the tone of the abdominal muscles acting on the abdominal capacitance vessels. The patient is prepared and anaesthetized on the operating table in theatre. While 100% oxygen is administered by mask, all monitoring lines and two large-gauge i.v. cannulae are inserted under local anaesthesia. The surgeon then prepares and towels the patient ready for surgery and it is only at this point that anaesthesia is induced. When muscle relaxation occurs, systemic arterial pressure may decrease precipitously and immediate laparotomy and aortic clamping may be required. Thereafter, the procedure is similar to that for elective repair.

The prognosis is poor for several reasons. There has been no preoperative preparation and the patient may be suffering from concurrent disease. There may have been a period of severe hypotension, resulting in impairment of renal, cerebral or myocardial function. Massive blood transfusion, which in itself carries significant risks is usually required. In addition, postoperative jaundice is common because of haemolysis of damaged red cells in the circulation and in the large retroperitoneal haematoma which usually develops after aortic rupture.

Bypass of aortoiliac occlusion

Patients suffering from atherosclerotic arterial disease may present with ischaemic pain in a limb. Many are heavy smokers and suffer from pulmonary disease which results in dyspnoea, productive cough and polycythaemia. They will commonly be taking drug therapy, for example β-blockers, calcium channel blockers, nitrates and antihypertensives. Aortic bifurcation grafting is performed to overcome occlusion in the aorta and iliac arteries and to restore flow to the lower limbs. It must be assumed that all patients have widespread arterial disease, even in the presence of a normal ECG. Anaesthetic management is similar to that required for surgery of aortic aneurysm. Where possible, it is normal surgical practice to side-clamp the aorta, maintaining some peripheral flow, and to declamp the arteries supplying the legs in sequence. The metabolic changes and hypotension are thus less severe than those seen during aneurysm surgery.

Peripheral arterial surgery

The commonest peripheral arterial grafts inserted are those between axillary and femoral, or femoral and popliteal, arteries. Because of the prolonged nature of these operations, an IPPV/relaxant anaesthetic technique should be used. Extradural anaesthesia is a useful adjunct, although heparin is often administered i.v. during vascular operations (see below) and this may increase the risk of an extradural haematoma if a catheter has been introduced. There may be considerable postoperative blood loss through the walls of open-weave grafts. In patients who have undergone an axillofemoral graft, it is important to monitor cardiovascular status closely for the first 12 h so that such loss is observed and adequate replacement instituted.

Carotid artery surgery

Patients are selected for carotid artery surgery if symptoms are thought to result from cerebral ischaemia secondary to obstruction in the carotid arteries. The underlying pathology is usually atherosclerosis, which presents typically in elderly hypertensive patients. Cerebral autoregulation is deficient and cerebral blood flow tends to be proportional to systemic arterial pressure. The perioperative mortality varies with the severity of the presenting symptoms (Table 35.6).

The main risk of operation is the production of a neurological deficit which was not present

Table 35.6 Mortality rates for patients with differing neurological states on presentation for carotid artery surgery

Symptoms	Mortality
Frank stroke with neurological deficit	6%
Transient cerebral ischaemia	
Chronic cerebral ischaemia	↓
Asymptomatic carotid bruit	0%

before surgery and/or an increase in pre-existing symptoms.

The carotid artery is clamped during surgery. The adequacy of cerebral blood flow during the period of clamping must be assessed at an early stage before proceeding with the endarterectomy. This can be achieved by one of the following methods:

1. Transcranial Doppler ultrasonography of the middle cerebral artery.
2. Determination of the arterial pressure in the occluded distal carotid segment (the 'stump' pressure).
3. Neurological assessment in the awake patient following clamping under local anaesthesia.
4. Monitoring the EEG.
5. Recording somatosensory evoked potentials.
6. Measurement of jugular venous oxygen tension.

Cerebral perfusion is dependent on collateral circulation and maintenance of an adequate blood flow is the primary aim of the anaesthetic technique. A moderately high systemic arterial pressure (up to 170 mmHg systolic), a high PaO_2 and normocapnia are desirable. These may be achieved by ventilation of the lungs using an inspired oxygen concentration of 50% in nitrous oxide (100% inspired oxygen produces cerebral vasoconstriction) with isoflurane and the administration of pancuronium or vecuronium to achieve muscle relaxation. An arterial cannula is mandatory for pressure monitoring and sampling for blood gas analysis. Under no circumstances should hypotension be allowed to develop. Cerebral ischaemia may be overcome during the period of clamping by insertion of a temporary shunt which bypasses the site of obstruction. In this way carotid arterial flow is uninterrupted and may even be improved.

After surgery, early assessment of cerebral function is required and residual anaesthetic effects may confuse the diagnosis of intraoperative embolism or ischaemic change. Approximately 30% of patients require control of postoperative hypertension, which may otherwise compromise the graft or cause intracranial haemorrhage. An infusion of trimetaphan, hydralazine or sodium nitroprusside may be required for this purpose.

Heparin

Centres in the UK differ in their use of heparin during vascular surgery. In units where it is used systemically, a dose of 100 units.kg^{-1} is given i.v. after preclotting the graft (where material such as Dacron is used) and at least one circulation time should elapse before arterial clamping begins. Some vascular surgeons rely solely on the local use of heparinized saline. If i.v. heparin has been employed the anaesthetist may be asked to antagonize the heparin with protamine (0.5 mg per 100 units heparin) before the termination of surgery.

CARDIOVERSION

DC cardioversion is an effective treatment for some re-entrant tachyarrhythmias which may produce haemodynamic instability and myocardial ischaemia and which do not respond to other measures. Atrial fibrillation, atrial flutter, supraventricular tachycardia and ventricular tachycardia may be converted to sinus rhythm, although maintenance of sinus rhythm depends usually on the subsequent use of drugs. The technique is not useful in atrial tachycardias (with or without block) or in digitalis-induced tachyarrhythmias.

Cardioversion is a simple and immediate therapy with a low incidence of side-effects or complications. It has little effect on contractility, conductivity or excitability of the myocardium.

Patients may present with a chronic arrhythmia for elective cardioversion or as an emergency with an arrhythmia which is life-threatening.

Preanaesthetic assessment

Patients may have serious pre-existing cardiovascular pathology such as rheumatic disease, arteriosclerotic heart disease, myocardial infarction, congestive cardiac failure or cerebrovascular occlusive disease. Digitalis therapy predisposes to post-cardioversion arrhythmias; in some centres, it is withheld for a least 24 h before cardioversion. Accurate knowledge of the medical and drug history, and thorough clinical examination, are essential before selecting the method of anaesthesia. Preanaesthetic sedation reduces circu-

lating endogenous catecholamine concentrations. Atropine should be avoided.

Cardioversion

DC electrical discharge passed through the heart depolarizes all excitable myocardial cells and interrupts abnormal pathways and foci. The attendant physician sites the electrodes anterolaterally with the patient supine or anteroposteriorly with the patient in the lateral position. The paddles should not be sited over the scapula, sternum or vertebrae and the skin must be protected with electrolyte jelly, saline-soaked gauze or any type of conducting pad.

The ECG monitoring lead chosen should demonstrate a clear R wave in order to synchronize the discharge away from the T wave and thus reduce the risk of development of ventricular fibrillation. If the arrhythmia does not convert after the first 50 J discharge, further shocks are given using an increased energy discharge of up to 200 J.

Despite the use of synchronized discharge, ventricular fibrillation may be produced in the present of hypokalaemia, ischaemia, digitalis intoxication and Q–T prolongation (caused by quinidine, tricyclic antidepressants or hyperalimentation). There is a risk of embolic phenomena in patients with:

1. Mitral stenosis and atrial fibrillation of recent onset.
2. A history of embolic phenomena.
3. A prosthetic mitral valve.
4. Congestive cardiac failure.

Patients with these conditions should receive prophylactic anticoagulants.

Anaesthesia

Treatment should be carried out only in areas specifically designed for the purpose and with a full range of drugs, resuscitation and monitoring equipment available. These must be checked by the anaesthetist before every list. Patients should be prepared as for a surgical procedure.

Insertion of a cannula into a vein and preoxygenation, together with institution of ECG monitoring, oximetry and measurement of arterial pressure, should precede induction of anaesthesia with an i.v. agent. The choice of agent is determined by the cardiovascular stability and recovery period required.

As soon as the patient is insensible, the airway is secured and oxygenation maintained with a suitable breathing system. If repeated shocks are required incremental doses of the anaesthetic may be given (e.g. propofol or etomidate).

The patient should be monitored carefully both during anaesthesia and after recovery of consciousness, with particular regard to evidence of hypotension, cardiac dilatation and pulmonary oedema, or systemic or pulmonary embolism.

FURTHER READING

Muir I F K, Barclay T L, Settle J A D 1987 Burns and their treatment. Butterworth, London

Nimmo W S, Rowbotham D J, Smith G (eds) 1994 Anaesthesia, 2nd edn. Blackwell Scientific Publications, Oxford

Vickers M D, Jones R M (eds) 1989 Medicine for Anaesthetists, 3rd edn. Blackwell Scientific Publications, Oxford

36. Hypotensive anaesthesia

The justification for using induced hypotension, which may be defined as the deliberate reduction of systemic arterial pressure in order to reduce bleeding and facilitate surgery, remains one of the greatest causes for debate among anaesthetists. Since a decrease in bleeding, not hypotension per se, is the prime aim for the majority of routine situations, well-conducted anaesthesia avoiding hypercapnia with a degree of circulatory depression is more than adequate. If a surgeon prefers to operate under normotensive conditions, this must be respected or haemostasis may be inadequate. Hypotension is seldom an absolute requirement for surgery. However, a reduction in systemic arterial pressure can confer several advantages and because of this, the technique has retained a place in modern anaesthesia (Table 36.1).

BLEEDING

A normal haemostatic response is incapable of controlling bleeding from a surgical incision. The flow from a damaged arteriole is related to the size of the cut vessel and its intraluminal pressure. The pressure can be lowered by reducing vascular resistance, cardiac output or both. In addition, if the operative site is raised above heart level, the inflow to vascular beds is reduced (postural ischaemia) and the drainage improved. There is a decrease in systemic pressure of approximately 2 mmHg per 2 cm vertical height in sites elevated above heart level. Tachycardia increases arterial bleeding, probably because there is less time for arteriolar run-off.

Venous bleeding is a major component of surgical haemorrhage and may be reduced by eleva-

Table 36.1 Indications and rationale for induced hypotension

1. **Microsurgery** where small quantities of blood may obscure the operative field:
   ENT surgery, e.g. mastoid, middle ear
   Ophthalmic, e.g. intraocular tumours, lacrimal, oculoplastic, orbital surgery

2. **Major cancer surgery** where a bloodless field facilitates clearance of tumour tissue.
   Head and neck, e.g. laryngectomy, radical neck dissection, maxillofacial tumours

3. **Reduction in major blood loss** when it is desirable to reduce the need for blood transfusion.
   Pelvic surgery, e.g. cystectomy, radical vulvectomy
   Orthopaedic surgery, e.g. spinal surgery, hip arthroplasty
   Jehovah's witness
   Neurosurgery, e.g. A-V malformation, meningiomas

4. **Reduction in intraocular pressure (IOP).** Controlled arterial hypotension is the most effective method of maintaining a very low IOP.
   Ophthalmic, e.g. lens extraction, vitrectomy

5. **Reduction of aneurysmal wall tension** to diminish the risk of rupture during dissection.
   Neurosurgery, e.g. clipping of intracranial aneurysm

tion of the wound to improve venous drainage and pooling of blood away from the operative site. When a head-up posture is used, venous pooling in dependent areas (enhanced by vasodilating agents) leads to a reduction in venous return and hence cardiac output. IPPV also reduces venous return by increasing mean intrathoracic pressure.

Obstruction to venous flow by poor patient positioning, surgical retraction or excessive rises in intrathoracic pressure (e.g. cough, straining) must be avoided. A reduction in Pa_{CO_2} during controlled ventilation results in low levels of circulating catecholamines. These factors are summarized in Table 36.2.

Table 36.2   Factors which help to reduce surgical haemorrhage

Normal haemostatic response
Arterial hypotension
   reduction in systemic vascular resistance
   reduction in cardiac output
Decreased venous pressure
   wound elevation
   avoidance of venous obstruction
   low intrathoracic pressure
Avoidance of tachycardia

GENERAL CONSIDERATIONS FOR THE INDUCTION OF SAFE HYPOTENSION

As blood pressure is reduced, blood flow within the brain, myocardium and kidney is maintained by autoregulatory vasodilatation. In the coronary and cerebral circulations, maximum vasodilatation is reached when mean arterial pressure (MAP) falls to 50–60 mmHg and further reductions in pressure result in parallel decreases in organ blood flow. Renal perfusion and glomerular filtration are reduced when MAP is lowered to similar levels. Oliguria occurs but a long-standing deleterious effect is not seen.

Standard quotes for the limits of autoregulation are based on experimental hypotension induced by haemorrhage and resulting in intense sympathetic stimulation. In contrast, during well-managed controlled hypotension, myocardial oxygen demand is reduced and coronary blood flow is preserved to lower pressures. In addition, the cerebral vasculature is relaxed by vasodilating hypotensive agents, maintaining the oxygen supply to the brain. Anaesthetic agents reduce cerebral metabolism and are considered to confer a degree of cerebral protection in hypoperfused states.

Since the compensatory mechanisms in the heart and brain take time to develop, the blood pressure must be reduced slowly. Sudden swings in pressure must be avoided because autoregulation is impaired by vasodilators. Avoid tachycardia, as this increases oxygen demand and reduces coronary filling.

The techniques for interfering with the physiological control of arterial pressure may be classified under three major headings.

1. Intravascular volume may be reduced by haemorrhage. This technique is dangerous and is of historical interest only.

2. Peripheral resistance may be reduced by blocking part of the negative feedback loop.

3. Cardiac output may be reduced.

REDUCTION OF PERIPHERAL RESISTANCE

The sympathetic reflex arc may be blocked at six discrete sites (Fig. 36.1).

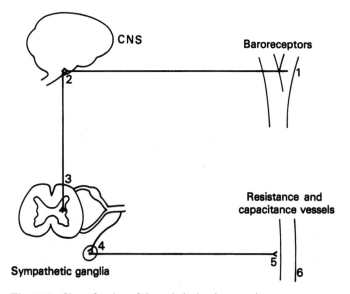

Fig. 36.1   Sites of action of drugs inducing hypotension.

1. Baroreceptors

A decrease in arterial pressure results normally in an increase in heart rate, mediated by the baroreceptor reflex. The baroreceptors operate over a discrete range of arterial pressure and the sensitivity to changes in pressure may be reduced by the volatile anaesthetic agents. Therefore, lower levels of arterial pressure may be achieved without reflex tachycardia, especially if halothane is used.

2. Vasomotor centre

All general anaesthetics depress the vasomotor centre, resulting in a reduction in sympathetic outflow and a decrease in arterial pressure.

3. Preganglionic sympathetic nerves

The preganglionic sympathetic nerve fibres (which leave the spinal cord from T1–L2) may be blocked by subarachnoid or extradural anaesthesia. Blockade of all or part of the sympathetic outflow results in vasodilatation of both resistance and capacitance vessels, the latter promoting venous pooling which enhances the decrease in arterial pressure. The advantages of a regional technique over a purely general technique, in terms of blood loss and transfusion requirements, have been confirmed for many procedures including total hip replacement, prostatic, gynaecological and abdominal surgery.

4. Sympathetic ganglia

The ganglion blockers (e.g. trimetaphan, hexamethonium, pentolinium) decrease the excitability of the postganglionic neurone by competing with acetylcholine for the postsynaptic receptor sites. The competitive ganglion blockers have more affinity for the nicotinic sites in the ganglia than in the neuromuscular junction. They have little affinity for the muscarinic sites.

Trimetaphan camsylate (TMP) is the only commonly used ganglion blocker. It has a rapid onset of action (1–3 min) and its potency is increased by additional direct vasodilator action and α-adrenergic blockade. Histamine release, which occurs when the drug is given, does not play an important part in its haemodynamic effect but is a contraindication to its use in asthmatic patients. Other side-effects include the potentiation of muscle relaxants, paralytic ileus, retention of urine and increased sensitivity to insulin. A further disadvantage of TMP is that the mydriasis caused by ciliary ganglion blockade prevents the pupil being used as an indicator of cerebral perfusion and anaesthetic depth.

Hypotension is produced primarily through arteriolar vasodilatation, but venodilatation with blood pooling also contributes and the ganglion-blocked patient is very sensitive to postural changes. Although ganglion blockade obtunds the sympathetic and renin–angiotensin responses to hypotension, tachycardia and resistance to reduction of blood pressure still occur because of vagal blockade and vasopressin release.

5. Adrenergic antagonists

The chemical transmitters at postganglionic sympathetic nerve endings may be antagonized by drugs which act at α- and β-adrenergic receptors. Phentolamine is a short-acting competitive α-antagonist which has an additional direct vasodilator action. Although phentolamine is used occasionally to achieve rapid control of pressure, tachycardia reduces its usefulness in controlled hypotension. Phenoxybenzamine produces more prolonged blockade and its main use is in anaesthesia for phaeochromocytoma surgery.

The actions of labetalol, a mixed antagonist, at β-receptors are up to seven times greater than its effect at α-receptors. The overall effect is a rapid reduction in blood pressure without concomitant tachycardia. Repeated increments can lead to bradyarrhythmias and a delay in recovery of blood pressure for several hours but despite this, labetalol is very useful on its own or as an adjuvant to sodium nitroprusside (SNP).

6. Vessel wall

Several drugs which act as direct vasodilators may be used to induce hypotension. Some have actions which affect predominantly resistance vessels (e.g. SNP), whilst others dilate capacitance vessels (e.g. glyceryl trinitrate; GTN). The more commonly employed agents are:

Hydralazine

Hydralazine dilates predominantly resistance vessels, producing a reduction in vascular tone which develops relatively slowly over 15–20 min. In addition to its use as an adjuvant in induced hypotension (i.v. boluses of 5–10 mg at 20–30 min intervals), hydralazine has a place in the treatment of postoperative hypertension.

Isoflurane

In concentrations of up to 1.9 MAC, isoflurane produces little change in cardiac output but induces a dose-related reduction in blood pressure by lowering systemic vascular resistance. It is mainly excreted unchanged in the lungs and, like other volatile anaesthetics, inhibits the baroreceptor pathways so that reflex tachycardia is obtunded. These factors make it suitable as a sole agent for induced hypotension.

There have been concerns that isoflurane may lead to 'coronary steal' with ischaemic myocardial changes. This now appears to be no more common than with enflurane or halothane and much less common than with non-anaesthetic arterial vasodilators.

Cerebral blood flow is usually maintained at normal levels during isoflurane-induced hypotension. Since cerebral oxygen consumption is markedly reduced, isoflurane has advantages over halothane, TMP, SNP, GTN and adenosine for induced hypotension in neurosurgery.

Sodium nitroprusside

Sodium nitroprusside (SNP) is a powerful, rapidly acting, smooth muscle relaxant. This property is attributed to the nitroso radicals which combine with the sulphydryl groupings on the cell membrane of the vessel wall. This interaction stabilizes the membrane and prevents the flux of ionized calcium which is necessary to activate the contractile mechanism in the smooth muscle. SNP acts predominantly upon small resistance vessels, the fourth order arterioles. Its evanescent action requires administration by continuous intravenous infusion. Once prepared, the solution is unstable and should be protected from light.

General vasodilatation aids tissue perfusion and cardiac output is well maintained even at low arterial pressures. Dilatation of cerebral vessels may cause an increase in intracranial pressure in the presence of pre-existing intracranial hypertension. Rebound hypertension has been reported and this has been attributed to the release of renin during the period of hypotension. Reflex tachycardia is marked and may require the use of a β-blocker.

Several deaths have been reported in association with the use of SNP, usually after the administration of excessive quantities. Figure 36.2 shows the possible routes of elimination of SNP from the body. If the rate of breakdown of SNP to cyanide exceeds the rate of removal of cyanide from the

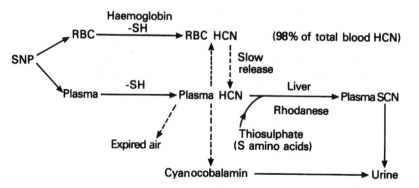

Fig. 36.2 Diagram of nitroprusside metabolism. At the end of the infusion about 98% of the cyanide liberated from the SNP is found in the red cells, from which it is slowly released. The half-life of the plasma cyanide is about 30 min.

plasma, cyanide concentration increases, cellular respiration is impaired and histotoxic hypoxia results. The total dose of SNP given acutely should be limited to 1.5 mg.kg^{-1} body weight to avoid this complication. During chronic use, the rate of administration should not exceed 4 µg.kg^{-1}.min^{-1}. Various drug combinations have been used to limit the dose of SNP. These include captopril, β-blockers and a 1:5 mixture of SNP with trimetaphan.

Glyceryl trinitrate

Glyceryl trinitrate (GTN) causes direct relaxation of vascular smooth muscle by reacting with sulphydryls to produce nitric oxide. Its action is more pronounced on capacitance vessels. The onset of action and half-life are both approximately 2 min and the effects are usually reversed within 10 min of discontinuing the infusion. The rate of onset of action is slower than with SNP and there is less risk of overshoot and rebound hypertension. GTN is the agent of choice in patients with ischaemic heart disease. Cerebral blood flow is maintained by direct cerebral vasodilatation but, as with SNP, the increased venous volume may lead to an increase in intracranial pressure.

Adenosine and adenosine triphosphate

Adenosine and adenosine triphosphate (ATP) are naturally occurring purines which at present are not licensed for use in induced hypotension although there is much interest in their potential in this field. Adenosine is the active purine which causes arteriolar dilatation. However, it is unstable and ATP is preferred, as it is degraded rapidly to adenosine in the circulation. ATP produces similar effects to those seen with SNP, except that tachycardia does not occur and tachyphylaxis and rebound hypertension are minimal.

REDUCTION IN CARDIAC OUTPUT (CO)

Safety in hypotensive anaesthesia is most dependent on maintaining the oxygen supply to the brain and techniques which primarily reduce CO are best avoided. When hypotension is produced

by arteriolar dilatation, CO is well maintained or even increased, provided that the patient is not positioned so as to produce excessive pooling of blood in the capacitance vessels. By contrast, hypotension induced purely by myocardial depressants, including β-blocking drugs and volatile anaesthetics, causes a reduction in CO and may compromise organ blood flow.

β-Adrenergic blockade

Premedication with a β-blocker modifies renin and catecholamine release in response to SNP-induced hypotension, reduces SNP dosage and suppresses reflex tachycardia and rebound hypertension. Oral propranolol, atenolol, metoprolol and oxprenolol premedications all have similar effects. There is, however, an increased risk of bradyarrhythmias after induction of anaesthesia and some anaesthetists prefer to use a cardio-specific drug intravenously during hypotensive anaesthesia only if reflex tachycardia is troublesome.

Esmolol, a β$_1$-adrenoreceptor antagonist, has the advantage over other β-blockers of having a short elimination half-life (9 min) and is a useful adjuvant in controlled hypotension to prevent tachycardia and rebound hypertension.

Volatile anaesthetic agents

Halothane and enflurane have quantitatively similar cardiovascular effects. Both are powerful direct myocardial depressants and produce dose-related decreases in arterial pressure. During controlled ventilation with hypocapnia, excessive cardiovascular depression, associated with a severe bradycardia, can occur. Halothane or enflurane should not be used as the sole agents for hypotensive techniques, but are useful adjuvants in low concentrations.

Isoflurane, when employed in high concentrations (> 2 MAC), significantly impairs cardiac output.

Calcium channel blockers

Calcium antagonists are used primarily in the treatment of angina and hypertension but they have been used during hypotensive anaesthesia.

Table 36.3 Drugs used for inducing hypotension

Drug	Formulation	Dosage	Duration of action
Trimetaphan	500 mg powder in 500 ml 5% glucose	I.v. infusion of 0.1% solution starting at 20–50 μg.kg^{-1}.min^{-1}	5–15 min
Sodium nitroprusside	50–200 mg in 500 ml of 5% glucose, protected from light	I.v. infusion of 0.01–0.04% solution. Initial dose 0.2–0.5 μg.kg^{-1}.min^{-1}	1–2 min
Nitroprusside/ trimetaphan mix	50 mg nitroprusside + 250 mg trimetaphan in 500 ml of 5% glucose	I.v. infusion, commence at 2–3 ml.h^{-1}	2–10 min
Glyceryl trinitrate	10–40 mg in 100 ml saline	I.v. infusion of 0.01–0.04% solution. Start at 10–20 μg.min^{-1} and increase at 2 min intervals	1–5 min
Labetalol	100 mg in 20 ml	I.v. bolus of 10–20 mg every 5 min to max of 100 mg	β-block effect 90 min α-block effect 30 min
Hydralazine	20 mg powder in 10 ml sterile water	I.v. bolus of 5–10 mg, repeat at 20–30 min intervals	3–4 h

A single bolus dose of verapamil has been used to produce hypotension without tachycardia and of diltiazem to reduce dose requirements in SNP hypotension. Nicardipine infusions induce comparable hypotensive conditions to SNP but are associated with slower recovery of blood pressure. Nifedipine was found to be a suitable alternative to GTN when used to lower arterial pressure during coronary artery surgery. Their use in hypotensive anaesthesia may increase in the future.

A summary of the main drugs used for inducing hypotension is shown in Table 36.3.

PREOPERATIVE ASSESSMENT

The need for an induced hypotensive technique must be weighed against the value of the technique with regard to the operative procedure and the likely benefit to the patient before the final decision can be agreed with the surgeon. However, there are a number of absolute contra-indications to any reduction of blood pressure in the anaesthetized patient.

1. Carotid artery stenosis; previous cerebrovascular accident.
2. Uncontrolled hypertension.
3. 'Fixed' cardiac output e.g. left ventricular failure, aortic stenosis, cardiomyopathy.
4. Angina; myocardial infarction within past 6 months.
5. Pregnancy.
6. Hypovolaemia.

Induced hypotension may be undertaken in patients with the following relative contra-indications, but careful assessment of the cardiovascular, pulmonary and cerebrovascular systems must be made.

1. *Treated hypertension.* Anaesthetic drugs and short-acting hypotensive agents act synergistically with the antihypertensive treatment and additional care is needed.

2. *Coronary artery disease.* Autoregulation is impaired and coronary perfusion is reduced in induced hypotension. In addition, coronary 'steal' can be precipitated by the use of pure arterial vasodilators. If the patient is considered fit for anaesthesia in relation to the proposed operative procedure then the response of the patient to general anaesthesia itself is a good indication of whether it is wise to lower the blood pressure. Careful ECG monitoring is essential.

3. *Respiratory disease.* Induced hypotension is accompanied by decreased arterial oxygen tension and it is understandable that greater decreases are likely in patients with respiratory dysfunction. The most important factors for assessment are the age of the patient and the preoperative arterial oxygen tension. Intraoperative monitoring of arterial blood gases in addition to oxygen saturation (pulse oximeter) are essential in patients with asthma, chronic obstructive airways disease and structural deformities of the chest wall (e.g. scoliosis and kyphosis).

4. *Insulin-dependent diabetes mellitus.* Careful

monitoring and adjustment of blood sugar is essential. Ganglion blockers and β-adrenergic antagonists are contraindicated as both potentiate hypoglycaemia. Cerebral autoregulation may be impaired in insulin-dependent diabetes and pressure reduction should be limited.

ANAESTHETIC TECHNIQUE

Induced hypotension must not be a substitute for good anaesthesia. An anxiolytic and analgesic premedication is useful in obtunding the early catecholamine response to preoperative anxiety, pain and tracheal intubation. Vagolytic agents should be avoided as the increase in heart rate is detrimental to the production of a good haemostatic field.

Thiopentone is the preferred induction agent. Tracheal intubation is mandatory. Following muscle relaxation with a non-depolarizing agent such as vecuronium, the larynx is sprayed with 4% lignocaine. Classically, d-tubocurarine was the relaxant of choice, but the effect on the blood pressure is unpredictable, depending on the degree of ganglion blockade and histamine release. The long duration of action reduces flexibility in relaxant control.

Maintenance is by IPPV with at least 50% oxygen in nitrous oxide and ventilation adjusted to give a Pa_{CO_2} of approximately 4 kPa (30 mmHg). Analgesia is provided by systemic opioids and, where possible, local or regional nerve blockade. No single hypotensive technique has been shown to be superior in all circumstances but isoflurane (up to 2%) is simple to use and has the advantage of helping to maintain adequate anaesthetic depth. Enflurane (0.75–1%) is the volatile agent of choice if direct-acting vasodilators or ganglion blockers are being administered intravenously. β-blockers may be required if tachycardia results.

The importance of correct positioning, so that the operation site is elevated, cannot be overemphasized. Local hypotension ('postural ischaemia') is promoted and the requirement for systemic hypotension reduced.

MONITORING

In addition to standard monitoring of the patient,

apparatus and breathing system, several areas are of special importance.

ECG

Continuous monitoring of the ECG, to detect bradyarrhythmias from β-blockade, reflex tachycardia or signs of myocardial ischaemia, is essential. A CM5 configuration, where the positive electrode is placed at V5 and the negative at the manubrium, is most likely to show evidence of myocardial ischaemia when a bipolar lead is used. Multilead systems increase sensitivity and allow the display of ST segment trends. It is important to spend time preparing the skin before placing the electrodes and securing the leads.

Arterial blood pressure

Automated oscillometric devices (e.g. Dinamap), set to give readings at 1 minute intervals, are suitable for mild hypotensive procedures in which significant blood loss is not a consideration and isoflurane is used to control the blood pressure. Direct arterial pressure monitoring is indicated whenever evanescent agents are used to titrate pressure, if hypotension is likely to be prolonged or when large blood losses or pressure swings are anticipated. An indwelling arterial cannula also permits measurements of blood gas and acid–base status.

Gas exchange

Capnography and pulse oximetry are essential. Capnography acts as a disconnection alarm and as an indicator of air embolism but its value as an index of arterial carbon dioxide tension is limited because of the increase in alveolar dead space during hypotension. Pulse oximetry allows appropriate adjustment of the inspired oxygen concentration to compensate for $\dot{V}/\dot{Q}$ mismatch secondary to hypotension and the direct effects of the hypotensive agents.

Cerebral blood flow

Monitoring the adequacy of cerebral perfusion during general anaesthesia is difficult and various methods have been employed with limited success. Historically, spontaneous ventilation was considered to be a sign of adequate perfusion of vital centres, but this view is no longer held. Analysis of cerebral electrical activity can indicate ischaemia. There is an increase in EEG slow wave activity and a decrease in evoked potential responses at a cerebral perfusion pressure (CPP) of 50 mmHg (CBF of approximately 20 ml.min^{-1}.100 g^{-1}). The EEG becomes flat and the evoked responses disappear at a CPP of 30 mmHg (CBF of approximately 15 ml.min^{-1}.100 g^{-1}).

POSTOPERATIVE CARE

The patient must be observed closely in the recovery room and attention paid to the ECG, blood pressure, respiratory rate, oxygen saturation, urine output and wound drainage until stability is achieved. The recovery staff must maintain a clear airway, administer supplemental oxygen and analgesia and realize that the patient may be slower to regain consciousness after a hypotensive anaesthetic, especially if high concentrations of isoflurane have been used. If rebound hypertension occurs, treatment with hydralazine and a degree of head-up tilt reduce the risk of cerebral oedema. Propping the patient up too soon can result in orthostatic hypotension, especially if there is residual sympathetic blockade from a regional or ganglion blocker technique. Myocardial ischaemia and arrhythmias can occur. Postoperative reactionary haemorrhage will result from inadequate haemostasis and may be aggravated by rebound hypertension or clotting disorders.

It is difficult to assess the increase in morbidity and mortality associated with induced hypotension, due to a lack of large controlled studies. Smaller ones have failed to show any increase in either morbidity or mortality with properly applied hypotensive techniques. Careful selection of patients is essential as those with pre-existing hypertension, cerebrovascular and cardiac disease, hypovolaemia and anaemia are more likely to suffer complications. The anaesthetist must be aware of the advantages and disadvantages of the technique and endeavour to keep any period of hypotension as short as possible.

FURTHER READING

Enderby G E H (ed) 1985 Hypotensive anaesthesia. Churchill Livingstone, Edinburgh

MacRae W R, Wildsmith J A W (eds) 1991 Monographs in anaesthesiology: induced hypotension. Elsevier Scientific Publishers, Amsterdam

McLintic A J, Todd J G 1995 Induced hypotension. In: Healy T E J, Cohen P J (eds) Wylie and Churchill-Davidson: A practice of anaesthesia, 6th edn. Edward Arnold, Sevenoaks

37. Neurosurgical anaesthesia

Neurosurgical procedures include elective and emergency surgery of the central nervous system, its vasculature and the cerebrospinal fluid (CSF), together with the surrounding bony structures, the skull and spine. Almost all require general anaesthesia. Apart from a conventional anaesthetic technique which pays meticulous attention to detail, the essential factors are the maintenance of cerebral perfusion pressure and the facilitation of surgical access by minimizing blood loss and preventing increases in central nervous tissue volume and oedema.

APPLIED ANATOMY AND PHYSIOLOGY

The skull is a rigid closed 'box', except in neonates and infants before the various component bones have fused together. The skull contains the brain, cerebral blood supply and CSF, and an increase in the space occupied by one of these components must be compensated for by a decrease in volume of one of the others. Failure of this mechanism leads to a rise in intracranial pressure. The normal brain weighs about 1400 g, and the total intracranial volumes of CSF and blood are 100 ml and 150 ml respectively. The most important factors producing a rise in intracranial volume and therefore pressure are: for the brain, cerebral tumours, cysts and abscesses; for the vasculature, traumatic haematomas and vasodilatation caused by an elevated Pa_{CO_2}; and for the CSF, obstruction to the normal circulation leading to hydrocephalus.

Cerebrospinal fluid

The brain and spinal cord are surrounded by three meningeal layers: the pia, the arachnoid and the dura mater. The first of these layers is closely applied to the brain and between it and the arachnoid is the subarachnoid space containing the circulating CSF. This space is enlarged in parts of the brain to form ventricles, which contain both CSF and areas for secretion of this fluid, the choroid plexuses. CSF circulates in the subarachnoid space surrounding both the brain and the spinal cord and is reabsorbed by the arachnoid villi which lie in the superior sagittal sinus over the surface of the brain. It is essential that circulation of CSF is unimpeded because obstruction to the foraminae leading to and from the ventricles or to the aqueduct of Sylvius causes local accumulation of CSF and hydrocephalus.

In the normal adult there are 120 ml of CSF, of which about 50 ml are in the spinal subarachnoid space. Its composition is similar to protein-free plasma and it is formed at the rate of 0.3–0.5 ml.min^{-1}. The functions of CSF are both to buffer the brain against movements of the skull and to surround certain parts of the brain with a fluid capable of fluctuation in its concentration of ions, e.g. sodium, potassium and bicarbonate. Changes in CSF bicarbonate concentration are responsible for alterations in respiratory rate and volume mediated by the chemoreceptors. Some drugs can pass into CSF while others cannot, since its formation is one of selective secretion. The normal CSF pressure is about 120 mmH$_2$O in the recumbent position.

Intracranial pressure

With normal cerebral compliance, the intracranial pressure (ICP) is 100–150 mmH$_2$O in the horizontal position. In the erect posture, ICP falls

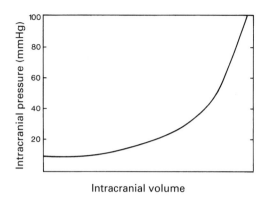

Fig. 37.1 The intracranial pressure/volume relationship.

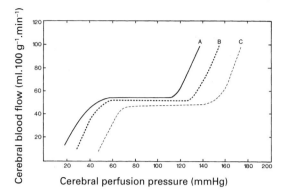

Fig. 37.2 Autoregulation of cerebral blood flow.
Key: A = Drug-induced vasodilatation; B = Normal;
C = Hypertension or haemorrhagic hypotension.

initially, but then, due to a decrease in reabsorption, the pressure returns to normal. ICP is related directly to intrathoracic pressure and has a normal respiratory swing. It is increased by coughing, straining and positive end-expiratory pressure. In cases of reduced cerebral compliance, small changes in cerebral volume produce large changes in intracranial pressure and such critical changes can be induced by anaesthetic drugs (e.g. halothane, isoflurane and sodium nitroprusside — see below), elevations in Pa_{CO_2} and posture, as well as by surgery and trauma (Fig. 37.1).

Cerebral blood flow

The brain is dependent for its blood supply on four main arteries — the internal carotids and the vertebrals, the latter joining to form the basilar artery. These vessels anastomose at the base of the brain, forming the circle of Willis which then gives off the anterior, middle and posterior cerebral arteries. Because of this anastomotic link, the brain can survive with occlusion of one or even two of its main arteries. Under normal conditions, the brain receives about 15% of the cardiac output, which corresponds to a cerebral blood flow (CBF) of 50 ml per 100 g tissue or 600–700 ml.min^{-1}. The cerebral circulation is able to maintain a constant blood flow between mean arterial blood pressures of 60 and 140 mmHg by the process of autoregulation. This is mediated by a primary myogenic response involving local alteration in the diameter of blood vessels in response to changes in transmural pressure. Above and below these limits, or in the traumatized

brain, autoregulation is impaired or absent, so that cerebral blood flow is related directly to cerebral perfusion pressure (CPP) (Fig. 37.2). This effect is also seen in association with cerebral hypoxia and hypercapnia, in addition to acute intracranial disease and trauma.

As CPP falls due to systemic hypotension or an increase in ICP, CBF is maintained until the ICP exceeds 30–40 mmHg. The Cushing reflex increases CPP in response to this rise in ICP by producing reflex systemic hypertension and bradycardia, despite these compensatory mechanisms also producing an increase in ICP. In the treatment of closed head injuries, where both ICP and mean arterial blood pressure are being monitored, it is essential to control the resultant CPP by vasopressor therapy where cerebral perfusion is borderline since even transient absence of flow to the brain may produce focal or global ischaemia with corresponding infarction.

Figure 37.2 also demonstrates that haemorrhagic hypotension associated with excess sympathetic nervous activity results in a loss of autoregulation at a higher CPP than normal, while the use of vasodilators to induce hypotension shifts the curve to the left, maintaining flow at lower levels of perfusion pressure. Vasodilators also differ in their effect, so that autoregulation is preserved at a lower CPP with sodium nitroprusside than with trimetaphan.

Cerebral metabolic rate also affects cerebral blood flow; the increased electrical activity associated with convulsions produces an increase in lactic acid and other vasodilator metabolites. This, together with an increase in CO_2 production mediated possibly via changes in CSF pH, produces an increase in CBF. Conversely, cerebral metabolic depression, in association with either deliberate or accidental hypothermia or induced by drugs, reduces cerebral blood flow.

Cerebral metabolism

The overall energy consumption of the brain is relatively constant, whether during sleep or in the awake state, and represents approximately 20% of the oxygen consumption at rest, or 50 ml.min^{-1}. Cerebral metabolism relies on glucose supply via the cerebral circulation as there are no stores of metabolic substrate. This is why the brain can tolerate only short periods of hypoperfusion or circulatory arrest before irreversible neuronal damage occurs. The brain also metabolizes amino acids, including glutamate, aspartate and γ-amino-butyric acid (GABA), together with release and subsequent inactivation of neurotransmitters.

The energy production of the brain is related directly to its rate of oxygen consumption, and the cerebral metabolic rate for oxygen ($CMRO_2$) is used to measure this index of cerebral activity. By the Fick principle, $CMRO_2$ is equal to the cerebral blood flow multiplied by the arterio–venous oxygen difference. Although this is a quantitative measurement, where there is failure of oxygen or glucose supply and ATP production is less than its utilization, an alteration in $CMRO_2$ does not indicate the nature or extent of the problem.

Although barbiturates have been used to reduce cerebral metabolic rate, propofol and benzodiaze-pines have a similar, although less profound, effect. All are used in the sedation of patients with head injury and postoperative neurosurgical patients, and the choice is related more to the anticipated duration of sedation than to differences in the effects of the drugs, with the exception of prolonged barbiturate coma induced by infusion of thiopentone.

Effects of oxygen and carbon dioxide on cerebral blood flow

Carbon dioxide is physiologically the most im-

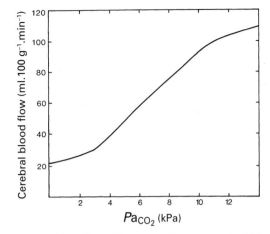

Fig. 37.3   The effect of increasing Pa_{CO_2} on cerebral blood flow.

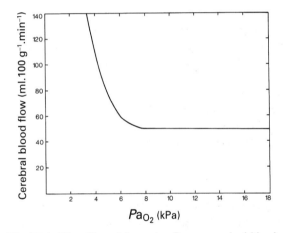

Fig. 37.4   The effect of decreasing Pa_{O_2} on cerebral blood flow.

portant cerebral vasodilator. Even small increases in Pa_{CO_2} produce significant increases in cerebral blood flow and therefore intracranial pressure. There is virtually a linear relationship between Pa_{CO_2} and cerebral blood flow (Fig. 37.3). Over the normal range, an increase of Pa_{CO_2} by 1 kPa increases cerebral blood flow by 30%. Conversely, hyperventilation to a Pa_{CO_2} of 4 kPa produces cerebral vasoconstriction and a decrease in intra-cranial pressure, although this is compensated for by an increase in CSF production over a more prolonged period of hyperventilation, such as that used in the treatment of head injuries. This is why there is no advantage in aggressive hyperventila-tion regimens in head injury management; indeed, the vasoconstriction induced may be detrimental to the recovery of a severely compromised brain. Hyperventilation below a Pa_{CO_2} of 4 kPa has little acute effect on ICP and 2.5 kPa should be regarded as the absolute minimum, since below this level, the vasoconstriction induced leads to a fall in jugular bulb oxygen saturation. At a Pa_{CO_2} above 10 kPa, the increase in cerebral blood flow becomes less marked.

Unlike the acute effects of carbon dioxide, alterations in Pa_{O_2} have little effect on cerebral blood flow over the normal range. It is only when Pa_{O_2} falls below about 7 kPa that cerebral vasodilatation occurs and further reductions are associated with dramatic rises in cerebral blood flow (Fig. 37.4).

ANAESTHESIA FOR ELECTIVE INTRACRANIAL SURGERY

General principles

Most intracranial operations involve a craniotomy, i.e. removal of a flap of bone to gain access to the brain substance beneath. Operative treatment may range from the removal of either an intracerebral or extracerebral tumour to the clipping of an arterial aneurysm in the region of the circle of Willis, but anaesthesia for all these operations has many important factors in common. A smooth, uncomplicated technique is essential, avoiding increases in either venous blood pressure, carbon dioxide concentration or arterial blood pressure while at the same time avoiding a decrease in cerebral oxygenation.

Most anaesthetists use a technique of intra-operative analgesia with either fentanyl or phenoperidine, neuromuscular blockade with either vecuronium or pancuronium, and IPPV. Low inspired concentrations of volatile anaesthetic agents, particularly isoflurane, are also used frequently, although particular care must be taken before the skull is open since, by inducing cerebral vasodilatation, they inevitably produce a rise in intracranial pressure. Many of these patients, particularly those with an intracerebral tumour, already have a markedly reduced cerebral compliance and a further increase in ICP may compress the brain severely (Fig. 37.1).

Patients with raised intracranial pressure are prone to nausea and vomiting and for this reason some anaesthetists intubate the trachea using a 'rapid sequence induction' technique to avoid possible regurgitation.

It is extremely important to ensure adequate fixation of the tracheal tube and intravascular cannulae and to protect the eyes, because access to the head and limbs is severely restricted during the operation. Continuous monitoring of the electrocardiograph and vascular pressures are essential; direct arterial blood pressure and central venous pressure monitoring are normally used, together with continuous measurement of oxygen saturation and end-tidal carbon dioxide concentration.

It is important to ensure that the patient is transferred to the recovery room with no residual neuromuscular blockade or opioid-induced respiratory depression, as either may produce critical increases in ICP related to hypercapnia and hypoxaemia (Figs 37.3 & 37.4).

Preoperative assessment and premedication

Intracranial tumours

The preoperative condition of patients who present for craniotomy varies enormously. The level of consciousness ranges from completely awake and orientated to comatose; some patients are confused, disorientated, euphoric or aggressive. The anaesthetist must always assume that any abnormal behaviour is related to their condition and not place too much reliance on what the patient says if it appears to conflict with previous history. In particular, apparently unrelated medical conditions may be forgotten, such as diabetes and hypertension, and patients may fail to mention previous anaesthetic problems.

Patients with intracranial tumours are usually taking steroids (normally dexamethasone 4 mg every 6–8 h), which may in turn precipitate a latent diabetic state, requiring insulin during the acute episode. Most patients have some symptoms of raised intracranial pressure, such as headache, nausea, vomiting or visual disturbances. Anticonvulsant therapy, usually with phenytoin or carbamazepine, will have been prescribed to patients who have presented with fitting or who are thought to be at risk. Some patients may be frankly dehydrated, but it is important to avoid aggressive preoperative fluid therapy since this may elevate intracranial pressure further. Many patients are extremely anxious, often exacerbated by mild confusion, and premedication with temazepam or diazepam, together with metoclopramide, is usually appropriate.

Vascular lesions

These include intracranial aneurysms, arteriovenous malformations and meningiomas. Congenital lesions are frequently seen in young and previously fit patients. Arteriosclerotic aneurysms occur in the older age group and may be associated with other, more widespread cardiovascular disease. Subarachnoid haemorrhage is now graded from 1 (in which the patient is symptom-free) to 5 (in which the patient is unconscious). Although clipping should prevent the risk of further bleeding, significant perioperative morbidity and mortality result from vasospasm, which may occur pre- or postoperatively. The current trend is to undertake emergency cerebral angiography and clipping of aneurysms in Grade 1 and 2 patients, but to wait the conventional 10-day period in the remainder. Vasospasm is reduced or prevented by intravenous infusion of the calcium channel blocker nimodipine, which is started preoperatively in most patients.

Patients with intracerebral haemorrhage range from complete lucidity to confusion and the preoperative assessment must take this into account. Those in the older age group may be receiving drugs with cardiovascular effects and are also frequently treated with aspirin, which may be a contraindication to urgent craniotomy. Those with a meningioma should be treated like patients with any intracranial space-occupying lesion. Benzodiazepine and antiemetic premedication is again appropriate in almost all patients, many of whom are quite aware of the severity of their condition.

Effects of drugs and anaesthetic techniques

Induction of anaesthesia

With appropriate preoperative care, assessment and premedication, most patients arrive in the anaesthetic room sedated and without a grossly elevated ICP. Intravenous induction should always be used whenever possible, even in difficult children where a stormy inhalational induction might be detrimental to a pre-existing high ICP. An intravenous infusion of an isotonic electrolyte solution should be started through a large bore intravenous cannula before induction.

Both thiopentone and propofol reduce ICP and are suitable induction agents. The intravenous anaesthetic should be given with an appropriate dose of short-acting opioid and a neuromuscular blocking agent to facilitate a smooth induction and tracheal intubation, avoiding hypoxaemia and hypercapnia. It is equally important to remember that cerebral perfusion may be reduced in association with a raised ICP, and therefore an induction technique which produces significant hypotension may critically reduce cerebral perfusion in patients with a space-occupying lesion (SOL) or intracranial and subarachnoid haemorrhage associated with vasospasm.

Appropriate techniques for reducing the hypertensive response to laryngoscopy and intubation, such as supplementary thiopentone, intravenous lignocaine ($1-2$ mg.kg^{-1}) or a β-adrenoceptor blocker, are particularly appropriate when acute hypertension might precipitate secondary rupture of an aneurysm. Tracheal intubation should be preceded by topical anaesthesia of the trachea and larynx with lignocaine and should be with an armoured latex tracheal tube. Careful positioning of the tube is vital because any intraoperative flexion of the neck may result in intubation of the right main bronchus if the tube is initially too close to the carina. Nasogastric intubation is also used in patients in whom gastric aspiration may be needed and a pharyngeal pack is necessary if pharyngeal bleeding may occur, e.g. during transsphenoidal hypophysectomy.

Positioning

Many neurosurgical operations are long, and positioning of the patient to facilitate optimum access, while preventing hypothermia and pressure sores or peripheral nerve injury, is very important. Supratentorial cranial surgery involving the frontal or frontotemporal areas is performed with the patient supine, while parietal and occipital craniotomies are carried out in the lateral or three-quarters prone (park-bench) position. In all cases, care must be taken to avoid neck positions which impede venous drainage, because this may elevate intracranial venous pressure, while arterial compression, particularly in the elderly, may precipitate vertebrobasilar insufficiency.

In the full prone position which is used for surgery of the foramen magnum and cervical spine, the patient is supported on chest and iliac crest blocks or a purpose-built frame, both of which allow unimpeded respiratory movements and avoid abdominal compression. The use of 'jelly packs' on top of the support blocks greatly reduces the incidence of pressure damage, which can be serious in the frail and elderly. In the prone position, pressure areas can develop over the facial bones, particularly around the eyes; again, careful padding is vital. Eye protection is usually effected by taping, adhesive foam padding and the use of polyfax eye ointment together with meticulous care to prevent skin cleaning solutions applied by the surgeon from entering the eyes. The head is shaved either partly or totally, usually under anaesthesia, and the skin cleaned before transferring the patient to the operating theatre. Prevention of infection is essential because postoperative intracranial sepsis, although rare, is difficult to treat and can be fatal.

Active methods of protection against deep venous thrombosis (DVT), such as subcutaneous heparin or an infusion of dextran 70, are not usually employed despite the significant risk of DVT in this group of patients. The risks of perioperative haemorrhage tend to outweigh the advantages in the majority of patients, but the use of thromboembolism (TED) stockings is a useful compromise.

Heat loss

Prevention of heat loss during prolonged surgery, and particularly in children, is accomplished by using either a 'space blanket' or wrapping the patient in 'bubble wrap' through which a small operative window is cut. Intravenous fluids are warmed and inspired gases are humidified. A warming blanket is also effective unless the patient is prone and supported on blocks. It may be advantageous to allow the patient to cool a little in cases where a reduction in cerebral metabolism would be beneficial.

Maintenance of anaesthesia

The basis of anaesthesia for neurosurgery is mild hyperventilation with 66% nitrous oxide in oxygen to a Pa_{CO_2} of 3.5–4.0 kPa, supplemented with fentanyl 2–3 μg.kg^{-1} and isoflurane 0.5–1.0%. The choice of neuromuscular blocking agent should take account of the length of operation and the relative need for normo- or elective hypotension; while pancuronium may be useful, particularly in elderly patients lying prone, it may be prudent to use an alternative agent to prevent excessive hypertension in, for example, aneurysm surgery. The advantage of longer acting drugs is that neuromuscular blockade wears off gradually, minimizing the risk of intraoperative coughing and straining. A nerve stimulator is important if shorter acting drugs are used intermittently or by infusion, to avoid difficulty in reversal or recurarization and consequent hypoventilation in the recovery period.

The initial part of a craniotomy is painful, but once the bone flap is reflected and intracranial surgery begins, pain is not an important feature again until closure of the wound. For this reason, supplementary intraoperative opioids in large doses are unnecessary and the use of a low concentration of isoflurane is sufficient to maintain anaesthesia. The use of isoflurane also prevents any possible awareness and consequent hypertensive reaction.

Reflex vagal stimulation can occur, particularly following stimulation of the cranial nerve roots or during vascular surgery around the circle of Willis and the internal carotid artery. This may necessitate immediate anticholinergic therapy with atropine to avoid severe bradycardia or even asystole.

Maintenance of normal blood pressure is important in all patients, but can be a particular problem during induction in elderly patients who are turned lateral or three-quarters prone. Hypotension, with the consequent reduction in cerebral perfusion, should be treated by infusion of a moderate volume of fluid, but it is advisable to administer a vasopressor such as ephedrine at an early stage.

The use of air/oxygen mixtures in place of nitrous oxide is advocated by a number of neurosurgical anaesthetists. There are obvious contraindications to the use of nitrous oxide, for example pneumocephalus, intracranial cysts and following air encephalography (rarely performed since the advent of CT and MRI scanners). In addition, some anaesthetists believe that nitrous oxide should be avoided in situations where air embolism is a possibility, e.g. posterior fossa surgery.

Continuous total intravenous anaesthesia with propofol and alfentanil infusions is also gaining in popularity because it allows rapid postoperative recovery and assessment, avoids shivering and reduces the incidence of postoperative nausea and vomiting. It is particularly valuable in situations where the patient is required to wake up and move to command intraoperatively, e.g. during spinal surgery and trigeminal nerve radiofrequency lesion generation (see below). There are potential difficulties with hypotension and hypoventilation in such patients, but in expert hands, these are not major problems.

Fluid replacement therapy

Most patients who present for elective intracranial operations are satisfactorily hydrated preoperatively. The main exceptions are those with high intracranial pressure associated with nausea and vomiting, and patients with general debility and cachexia. The main intraoperative distinctions between patients are related to the underlying pathology. Cerebral tumours are associated with oedema and raised ICP, and therefore such patients require moderate fluid restriction, e.g. 1.5 litres daily for a 60 kg female or 2 litres daily for a 70 kg male.

Cerebrovascular surgery is associated with vasospasm and therefore blood flow is the prime prerequisite. A normal circulating blood volume is essential if the perfusion pressure is to be maintained, and although a slight fall in haematocrit to about 0.30 is optimal for perfusion, adequate colloid replacement must be given. Patients who have undergone aneurysm surgery do not require fluid restriction; indeed, some are given a volume expansion regimen using a mixture of low and high molecular weight colloids (Haemaccel and Hespan) together with crystalloid to improve perfusion which may be limited by vasospasm.

Supplementary drug therapy

In addition to the normal anaesthetic drugs, care must be taken to continue or even supplement specific neurological drug therapy. Patients with a tumour or some vascular lesions may already be receiving anticonvulsants (usually phenytoin or carbamazepine) but others may require intravenous phenytoin perioperatively, depending upon the site of surgery. Patients receiving high-dose steroids need peri- and postoperative dexamethasone; the normal dose is 4 mg 6-hourly with 8–12 mg as an intraoperative bolus. Perioperative antibiotics are administered to all patients; a common choice is cefuroxime 1.5 g, which may need to be repeated during long operations.

Monitoring during neurosurgical anaesthesia

Monitoring should be instituted before induction; in patients in whom cardiovascular instability may be a problem, this should include invasive vascular monitoring.

Electrocardiographic (ECG) monitoring and measurement of oxygen saturation, together with non-invasive blood pressure monitoring, are essential in all patients.

It may be desirable to set up *direct arterial pressure monitoring* via a radial artery cannula under local anaesthesia prior to induction, although this may already have been established in acutely traumatized and head-injured patients. Arterial cannulation is now employed routinely in all intracranial operations, for surgery of the cervical spine, and in other situations in which rapid fluctuations in blood pressure may occur. It also facilitates arterial sampling for blood gas and acid–base balance measurements.

Central venous pressure measurement should be used where major blood loss is expected, and during posterior fossa or cervical spine surgery, in which air embolism can occur (see below).

Accurate placement of the tip of the catheter in the right atrium is important if aspiration of air is likely to be attempted.

Temperature monitoring (either oesophageal or rectal) is employed during many cases, particularly those which may be prolonged.

Oxygen saturation and end-tidal carbon dioxide concentration are monitored continuously in all patients. The latter has made a dramatic difference to the safety and quality of neurosurgical anaesthesia because alterations in carbon dioxide tension have such a profound effect on cerebral blood flow and intracranial pressure.

A precordial or oesophageal stethoscope can be used to auscultate cardiac and respiratory sounds and also abnormal flow murmurs produced by air embolism. An oesophageal stethoscope is used more frequently in children.

Mechanisms for reducing intracranial pressure

The methods used commonly to limit increases in intracranial pressure or electively to reduce it include drugs, ventilation, posture and drainage. The use of diuretics such as 10–20% mannitol or frusemide is designed to deplete the intravascular fluid volume and subsequently reduce CSF production. Direct drainage of CSF may be accomplished either by lumbar puncture or by direct puncture of the cisterna magna or lateral ventricles. Hypercapnia must be prevented by the use of IPPV, while moderate hyperventilation produces cerebral vasoconstriction and a reduction in cerebral blood volume. Volatile anaesthetic agents such as isoflurane and other vasodilators (e.g. sodium nitroprusside) must be used cautiously, particularly before the skull is open.

Elective hypotension

Although elective hypotension was formerly one of the mainstays of cerebrovascular surgery, its use has diminished considerably in recent years, because of the increasing appreciation that cerebral perfusion is all-important. Most aneurysm surgery in now carried out at normotension; indeed, if the patient has an element of cerebral vasospasm, any reflex hypertension should be maintained. This concept has been made easier to implement by the simultaneous use of nimodipine.

If elective hypotension is required, the choice of technique is determined by the anticipated duration of induced hypotension. The main indications are to facilitate dissection and clipping of a difficult and inaccessible aneurysm or arteriovenous malformation, in which case a low pressure is needed for only a short period and sodium nitroprusside is the drug of choice. To reduce continuous and excessive blood loss in, for example, spinal surgery, moderate hypotension induced by isoflurane in increasing concentration or an autonomic ganglion blocker such as trimetaphan is more suitable; the emphasis must be on perfusion because spinal cord oxygenation is also critical and excessive hypotension may lead to anterior spinal artery thrombosis. The dose of sodium nitroprusside should be limited to 10 μg.kg^{-1}.min^{-1} or 1.5 mg.kg^{-1} as a total intraoperative dose. Tachyphylaxis is occasionally a problem with sodium nitroprusside, but frequently occurs with trimetaphan.

Special problems

Cerebrovascular surgery

Although aneurysm surgery is the largest component in this group, arteriovenous malformations and intracranial–extracranial anastomotic operations are also important. Meningiomas are formed from abnormal blood vessels and tend to produce symptoms related to a space-occupying lesion, rather than specific vascular problems. Nevertheless, their extreme vascularity, combined with difficult access, may make severe haemorrhage and blood volume replacement a significant factor.

The current trend in cerebrovascular surgery is for the maintenance of a normal cerebral perfusion pressure in all situations, which, combined with nimodipine, will produce adequate cerebral blood flow. Although fluid replacement therapy may be all that is required, mild peripheral vasoconstriction with ephedrine may be necessary in the often prolonged interval between induction and incision. Thereafter, induced hypotension is seldom employed and a colloid/crystalloid perfusion regimen to an optimal haematocrit of 0.30

is ideal (see above). Nimodipine therapy interacts with inhalational anaesthetic agents, particularly isoflurane, to enhance their hypotensive effects and may need to be discontinued temporarily during induction until surgery has started. Post-operative nimodipine therapy is continued for several days until the risks of vasospasm are past and this is often also the case with removal of arteriovenous malformations.

Blood entering the CSF either as a result of the initial haemorrhage or during operation is an extreme irritant. Its presence may cause large increases in plasma catecholamine concentrations with corresponding hypertension and vaso-spasm. Blood which clots in the aqueduct of Sylvius causes obstruction to CSF flow and non-communicating hydrocephalus, necessitating temporary ventricular drainage or ventriculo-peritoneal shunt.

Pituitary surgery (hypophysectomy)

The pituitary fossa is approached either through a frontotemporal craniotomy in the case of large suprasellar tumours, or through the nose or ethmoid sinus for smaller lesions. The importance of pituitary surgery lies in the endocrine abnor-malities such as acromegaly, which may be caused by an adenoma, or those which result from surgi-cal hypophysectomy, such as diabetes insipidus. In addition, pituitary ablation may be used in the treatment of hormone-dependent tumours such as ovarian or breast neoplasms; in these condi-tions, the patients may be frail, cachectic and anaemic as a result of disseminated carcinoma.

Glucocorticoid replacement is all that is required in the immediate perioperative period; mineralo-corticoid requirements increase only slowly over the subsequent days. Diabetes insipidus can pre-sent in the immediate postoperative period and requires stabilization with vasopressin until the degree of the imbalance is known.

Acromegalic patients who present for pituitary surgery may pose considerable difficulties in tracheal intubation and venous access. If the transoral, nasal or ethmoidal approaches are used for surgery, a pharyngeal pack must be inserted and the airway protected meticulously to prevent aspiration of blood and CSF.

CSF shunt insertion and revision

The majority of patients who present for insertion or revision of ventriculo-peritoneal shunts are children with congenital hydrocephalus, usually resulting from spina bifida. Some patients require a permanent shunt after intracranial haemorrhage or head injury, particularly the elderly. The major anaesthetic considerations lie in the presentation of a patient with severely raised intracranial pres-sure who may be drowsy, nauseated and vomiting, with resultant dehydration. Compensatory sys-temic hypertension to maintain cerebral perfusion may also be present.

Rapid sequence induction may be indicated to avoid aspiration; the increase in ICP due to suxamethonium is of secondary importance. Arti-ficial ventilation to control Pa_{CO_2} is essential to prevent further increases in ICP, and volatile anaesthetic agents should be used sparingly for the same reason. When the ventricle is first drained, a rapid decrease in CSF pressure can result in an equally rapid reduction in arterial blood pres-sure, which no longer needs to be elevated to maintain cerebral perfusion. Adequate venous access is then important to allow rapid resuscita-tion in response to this severe but temporary hypotension.

The distal end of the shunt is usually introduced intraperitoneally, particularly if infection is a potential problem. Ventriculo-atrial shunts have largely been superseded because of arrhythmias during their insertion. When a ventriculo-atrial shunt is inserted, the anaesthetist may be asked to confirm correct positioning of the distal end by priming it with saline and attaching an ECG lead to observe changes in waveform during advancement of the catheter.

Relief of chronic pain

Although peripheral nerve blocks are normally performed in the pain clinic, severe intractible pain is sometimes relieved only by dorsal cordo-tomy or rhizotomy. Both techniques involve upper thoracic laminectomy to expose the spinal cord, with the patient prone as for decompressive sur-gery. Some patients are extremely frail, and posi-tioning them to avoid pressure sores is particularly important. A number also have an element of autonomic neuropathy, with resultant cardiovascular instability. Neurological ablation produces intense temporary stimulation and adequate anaesthesia and analgesia are particularly important during the process of nerve section.

Treatment of trigeminal neuralgia

This extremely debilitating condition is usually treated medically with large doses of carbamazepine. However, surgical lesions of the trigeminal ganglion are performed when the side-effects of medical treatment become unacceptable. Lesions of the ganglion are achieved by radiofrequency or injection of either phenol or alcohol. All of these techniques are very painful and require general anaesthesia. Current techniques involve anaesthetizing the patient while the ganglion is identified radiologically, waking the patient up to identify correct placement of the needle, and then re-anaesthetizing the patient during generation of the lesion or neurolytic injection. Propofol and alfentanil anaesthesia using a laryngeal mask provides optimal conditions. If the CSF is entered during localization of the ganglion, nausea frequently occurs and vomiting with the patient in the supine position should be anticipated.

A recent development in the treatment of trigeminal neuralgia has been the demonstration of an abnormal vascular loop compressing the trigeminal nerve in the posterior cranial fossa. A small craniotomy and decompression of the nerve is extremely successful in curing the symptoms; the problems of anaesthesia and surgery in this area are highlighted below.

Posterior fossa craniotomy

Surgery in the posterior cranial fossa involves lesions of the cerebellum and fourth ventricle. In addition, this position facilitates operations on the foramen magnum and upper cervical spine.

In the past, some surgeons favoured the sitting position because this produced superb venous drainage, relative hypotension and excellent operating conditions. The patients were frequently allowed to breathe a volatile anaesthetic agent, usually trichloroethylene, spontaneously so that changes in their respiratory pattern could be used to monitor the progress of fourth ventricular surgery in the region of the respiratory centre. This posed several major anaesthetic problems. Patients in the sitting position are prone to hypotension, which results inevitably in poor cerebral perfusion. Air embolism is also a severe potential problem because, when the skull is opened, many of the veins within the bone are held open and, if the venous pressure at this point is subatmospheric, air may enter the veins, leading to systemic air embolism.

For these reasons, the sitting position is no longer used other than in exceptional circumstances and posterior fossa surgery is carried out in the 'park-bench' position; operations on the cervical spine are performed with the patient prone and supported on blocks (see above). Although this change has diminished the risks of cerebral hypoperfusion and consequent hypoxia, air embolism is still a potential problem. The operative site, particularly with a moderate head-up tilt, is still above the level of the heart and the veins are still held open by the surrounding structures.

Detection and treatment of air embolism. The mainstay of detection is vigilance and a high index of suspicion. The main period of risk is when the posterior cervical muscles are cut and the craniectomy is being performed. Bone is usually removed as a craniectomy in the posterior fossa rather than by raising a bone flap. Although the incidence of major air embolism is vastly less than when the sitting position was used, small amounts of air still enter the circulation quite frequently. The severity of the problem depends upon the volume of air entrained and the fact that air bubbles expand in the presence of nitrous oxide.

The main practical method of detection is by end-tidal carbon dioxide monitoring, because the air-lock produced in the pulmonary circulation results in a rapid reduction in CO_2 excretion (together usually with a fall in oxygen saturation). Arterial blood pressure decreases and cardiac arrhythmias are frequently seen. The use of an oesophageal stethoscope permits auscultation of the traditional 'mill-wheel' murmur with large quantities of air, but requires continuous listening.

Doppler ultrasonography is probably the most accurate method of early detection, before the embolus leaves the heart, but frequently suffers from interference.

In practice, provided that the sitting position is not used, large air emboli are uncommon. Treatment consists of preventing further entry of air by telling the surgeon, who immediately floods the operative field with saline, lowering the level of the head and increasing the venous pressure by jugular compression to raise intrathoracic pressure. Ideally, the air should be trapped in the right atrium by placing the patient in the left lateral position; it is then occasionally possible to aspirate air through a central venous catheter, which is commonly inserted in posterior fossa explorations. Vasopressors are sometimes required until the circulation is restored; occasionally full cardiopulmonary resuscitation is necessary.

Recovery from anaesthesia and postoperative analgesia

The majority of patients are allowed to wake up as usual at the end of operation in a dedicated neurosurgical recovery room. It is essential to avoid hypercapnia or hypoxaemia, both of which may increase intracranial pressure; cerebral compliance following surgical intervention is often critical, particularly following removal of a space-occupying lesion or traumatic haematoma.

Complete reversal of non-depolarizing neuromuscular blockade must be achieved and judicious use of intraoperative opioids should remove the need for administration of naloxone. Doxapram may be used, although its cardiovascular side-effects also increase intracranial pressure. After major procedures or when severe oedema is likely, elective postoperative ventilation may be necessary.

ANAESTHESIA FOR EMERGENCY INTRACRANIAL NEUROSURGICAL PROCEDURES

The main indications for emergency intracranial surgery are bleeding as a result of trauma, which may be exacerbated in patients on anticoagulant drugs, including aspirin. Intracranial haematomata may arise either extradurally, subdurally or intra-

cerebrally and may accumulate either rapidly or slowly. Many patients who present for anaesthesia are unconscious or semiconscious and irritable as a result of raised intracranial pressure and cerebral compression. The anaesthetic maintenance technique is similar to that used for elective intracranial surgery, consisting of a short-acting intravenous opioid, neuromuscular blockade with vecuronium and IPPV to a Pa_{CO_2} of 4 kPa, preceded by emergency intubation with suxamethonium to avoid regurgitation and CO_2 retention in a patient with a potentially full stomach and raised intracranial pressure. Although suxamethonium has been shown to increase intracranial pressure in the normal brain, its effect in a non-compliant situation is less certain; more importantly, the risk of aspiration far outweighs that of a transient increase in ICP.

If the patient is unconscious, the initial anaesthetic requirements may be small. In the past, decompression of an intracranial haematoma through burr holes was often conducted under local anaesthesia. This method of treatment has been superseded by a full craniotomy and evacuation of the haematoma, because, if necessary, the bone flap can be left out or allowed to 'float' free, providing a method of decompression in the case of severe oedema. Burr holes are usually performed under local anaesthesia for the diagnosis and treatment of chronic sub- and extradural haematomata.

As the patient's brain is decompressed, the level of consciousness may lighten considerably and it may be necessary to deepen anaesthesia to prevent the patient becoming aware. It is important to avoid long-acting opioid analgesics because these may mask the eye signs and the level of consciousness, which are used to follow the progress of cerebral trauma postoperatively. Virtually all patients with head injury have had an emergency CT scan as part of their initial treatment. Many have undergone tracheal intubation and ventilation of the lung for this procedure and are subsequently kept anaesthetized and taken straight to the operating theatre for surgery to decompress the brain. It is important to remember that, with an expanding intracranial haematoma, speed is of the essence if cerebral damage is to be minimized or avoided. While adequate anaesthetic time must be taken to ensure safety, excessive delays may seriously affect the overall result of decompression and make the difference between a good, or only a moderate, recovery.

The maintenance technique selected is influenced to an extent by the decision either to wake the patient immediately postoperatively (usually considered appropriate only in the case of an acute extradural haematoma in a young patient), or to use elective postoperative ventilation for 24 h. In the former case, the usual conditions mentioned earlier for elective neurosurgery apply; in the latter, generous short-acting opioid administration and neuromuscular blockade will prevent ICP increases in an intubated patient, particularly during transfer to the intensive care unit, or by ambulance to another hospital.

MANAGEMENT OF THE HEAD-INJURED PATIENT

Head injuries and their subsequent treatment and rehabilitation represent a considerable proportion of neurosurgical practice. The immediate management must involve meticulous attention to the prevention of any secondary brain injury; little can be done about the primary insult to the brain or spinal cord. In recent years, the awareness of both the medical profession and the general public has had a profound effect on general resuscitation simply by improving airway management in the unconscious patient. The basic rules of head injury care are as follows:

1. *Initial airway maintenance*, remembering that oxygenation is initially more important than tracheal intubation.

2. *Assessment of any craniofacial injury*, together with the possibility of associated damage to the cervical spine. When in doubt, assume that the neck is unstable.

3. *Immediate assessment of other injuries*, particularly thoracoabdominal, with appropriate emergency treatment.

4. *Further airway management*, including tracheal intubation. This must be accomplished without excessive neck manipulation and should be performed by an experienced person. It is important to make intubation as atraumatic as

possible; consequently, sedation and neuromuscular blockade should be used irrespective of the level of consciousness, except in the most severe situation. The benefits of suxamethonium far outweigh the potential risks. Nasotracheal intubation is contraindicated in patients with a potentially fractured base of skull.

5. *Sedation and analgesia*, and neuromuscular blockade.

6. *Detailed assessment of thoracic, abdominal and limb injuries* and appropriate therapy to stabilize the patient's cardiovascular and respiratory systems before transfer to the CT scanner and X-ray room.

7. *Invasive arterial blood pressure monitoring*, together with ECG, end-tidal CO_2 and pulse oximetry. All of these are important in the early detection of deterioration in intracranial pressure, cardiovascular stability or respiratory function. A contused, oedematous and non-compliant brain tolerates only minimal changes in oxygen supply or carbon dioxide tension before intracranial pressure rises still further.

8. *After CT scan*, many patients are transferred directly to the neurosurgical operating theatre for evacuation of haematoma or insertion of an intraventricular catheter or extradural pressure monitor. Some patients who are scanned in peripheral hospitals have their scans 'Imtran'ed' to the main neurosurgical centre. The patient is then transferred directly by ambulance to the neurosurgical operating theatre, but both cardiovascular and neurological stability must be achieved before the journey. Realistically, this means the transfer of a sedated, intubated and ventilated patient, pretreated with mannitol to minimize acute increases in intracranial pressure.

Intensive care of head-injured patients

The main benefits of intensive care are in the provision of optimal conditions to allow recovery from the primary cerebral injury while minimizing any secondary damage. In practice this means:

1. *Sedation*. This is best achieved with an infusion of either propofol or midazolam together with an opioid (usually morphine or alfentanil). Thiopentone may be beneficial in cases of severely compromised cerebral blood flow and metabolism (see above).

2. *Ventilation*. It is particularly important in patients suffering from multiple trauma, especially with the combination of head and chest injuries, to ensure optimal oxygenation in the face of pulmonary contusion. This is normally achieved by the use of IPPV and may involve the use of positive end-expiratory pressure, the effects of which on the non-compliant brain are probably not as severe as in the normal situation, whereas the damage caused by hypoxaemia could be fatal. There is no evidence to suggest that severe hyperventilation improves outcome, and the main benefits of ventilation are therefore the prevention of hypercapnia and the provision of adequate cerebral oxygenation.

3. *Detailed neurological assessment*. This centres on the Glasgow coma scale, which is based upon eye opening, and verbal and motor responses (Table 37.1). Each response on the scale is assessed numerically; the lower the number, the more impaired is the response. The numbers are summated to produce a score. The lowest score is 3 and the highest 15.

4. *Intracranial pressure monitoring*. It is very helpful to be able to monitor the effectiveness of therapy against intracranial pressure, and in particular to demonstrate an effective cerebral perfusion pressure. ICP increases in response to stimulation, physiotherapy, tracheal suction, etc.,

but should return to the pre-stimulation value within 5–10 min. Frequent and prolonged increases in ICP demonstrate a low cerebral compliance and the need for further sedation and ventilation. If weaning from mechanical ventilation is started and ICP rises and remains elevated, the patient should be resedated and the lungs ventilated for a further 24-h period.

It is beneficial to nurse head-injured patients in a 15° head-up tilt to assist in ICP reduction, provided that coexisting conditions permit.

5. *Adequate fluid therapy and nutrition*. Although otherwise fit patients with an isolated head injury have very low metabolic requirements, many fail to absorb from the gastrointestinal tract because of the effects of sedative and opioid drugs or simply secondary to head trauma; associated hypoxaemia exacerbates the problem. It is sometimes necessary to introduce parenteral nutrition, particularly in patients who are catabolic from coexisting injuries. As in elective patients at risk from elevated ICP due to cerebral oedema, head-injured patients are also at risk from excessive intravenous fluid therapy. Fluid restriction to a similar degree is appropriate, and if large amounts of fluid have been given during initial resuscitation, a gentle drug-induced diuresis with frusemide to create an overall negative fluid balance (or at least to prevent a positive balance) may be appropriate. Fluid overload also impairs oxygenation further in potentially hypoxic patients with combined head and chest injuries, or following aspiration at the time of head injury. The use of mannitol 20% tends to be reserved for the emergency treatment of raised ICP rather than the treatment of simple fluid overload.

6. *High-dependency nursing care*. Provision of appropriate care for the unconscious patient, even when breathing spontaneously, is difficult, and demands a high intensity of nursing care. Intensive or high-dependency care centralizes nursing, medical and monitoring resources to provide optimal care of the head-injured patient.

Table 37.1 The Glasgow coma scale.

Clinical sign	Response	Score
Eyes open	Spontaneously	4
	To verbal command	3
	To pain	2
	No response	1
Best motor response to verbal command or to painful stimulus	Obeys	6
	Localizes pain	5
	Flexion withdrawal	4
	Abnormal flexion (decorticate rigidity)	3
	Extension (decerebrate rigidity)	2
	No response	1
Best verbal response	Orientated, converses	5
	Disorientated, converses	4
	Inappropriate words	3
	Incomprehensible sounds	2
	No response	1
Total	Minimum 3, maximum 15	

ANAESTHESIA FOR NEURORADIOLOGICAL PROCEDURES CT AND MRI SCANNING

This is discussed in detail in Chapter 29.

SURGERY OF SPINE AND SPINAL CORD

Many neurosurgical procedures involve surgery in the region of the spinal cord, usually either for the decompression of nerves as a result of a prolapsed intervertebral disc or degenerative arthritis, or for the decompression of the cord when the spinal canal is occupied by tumour.

Anaesthesia for cervical spine surgery

The cervical spine can be approached from either the anterior or posterior route, depending largely upon the site of cord compression. Although the posterior approach is less likely to damage any vital structures, the patient must lie prone, and hypotension, blood loss and access, particularly in a large individual, may all cause problems.

Preoperative assessment is perhaps one of the most important in neurosurgical anaesthetic practice, because an unstable cervical spine is a major reason for the proposed surgery. In many patients, the neck is relatively unstable as soon as it is either flexed or extended, and the patient may be in a cervical collar or even neck traction. Bony degeneration from rheumatoid or osteoarthritis produces severe cord compression. However, with regard to tracheal intubation, the neck tends to be unstable in flexion and relatively stable in extension in most patients. It is essential to assess the range of neck movement fully with the collar removed, either in the ward or anaesthetic room, in addition to the assessment of the ease of tracheal intubation. It is doubly unlucky to have a difficult intubation in a patient with an unstable neck! If problems are anticipated, the normal 'difficult intubation' drill should be followed, using the methods with which the anaesthetist is most familiar. Severe ankylosing spondylitis involving the neck probably presents the most awkward problem, related to the rigid immobility of the cervical spine. Additional factors which apply particularly in rheumatoid patients include anaemia, steroid therapy, fragile skin, and renal and pulmonary problems.

Anterior cervical decompression with or without fusion (Cloward's operation)

This technique involves exposing the anterior aspect of the cervical vertebral bodies and their interposing discs through a collar incision and drilling out a cylinder of bone and disc down to the posterior longitudinal ligament. The cord is decompressed microscopically through this hole, which is then filled with a bone dowel from the hip to produce a fusion. Single or multiple levels are involved, but the neck may be quite rigid for future intubation if several adjacent fusions are carried out.

Apart from the potential problems of tracheal intubation and the need to use an opioid-relaxant–IPPV technique, anaesthesia is relatively straightforward, although pneumothorax is a potential problem with operations at the C7–T1 level. Retraction of the oesophagus and more particularly the carotid sheath and sinus may produce severe temporary cardiovascular disturbance (usually sinus bradycardia), which can be prevented by surgical instillation of local anaesthetic around the carotid artery.

Posterior cervical laminectomy

When these operations were performed in the sitting position, all the problems associated with posterior fossa surgery in this position also occurred. Patients are now placed prone, with the neck flexed, and in a slightly head-up posture to reduce haemorrhage. Nevertheless, bleeding from the nuchal muscles is often a problem and air embolism is still a potential risk. The main difficulties, as in all spinal surgery in the prone position, arise from epidural venous bleeding, and the waveform of IPPV can have a significant effect. It is important to have an intrathoracic pressure of zero for the majority of the expiration phase (a difficulty with some pressure-generators such as the Manley). In addition, prolonged cord compression can result in an autonomic neuropathy which may produce significant hypotension both at induction and when the patient is turned into the prone position.

Cervical laminectomy is often accompanied by posterior fusion with either bone or metal. Many permanent designs such as the Ransford loop or Halifax clamp are used, and all produce immediate postoperative stability.

Anaesthesia for thoracolumbar decompressive surgery

In most instances, patients are placed in the prone

position, either supported on chest and iliac crest blocks or in the 'jack-knife' position. A technique employing IPPV is essential because these procedures often take a long time. However, because raised intracranial pressure is not a problem it is often sufficient to ventilate the lungs with a volatile anaesthetic agent unless this causes a decrease in systemic blood pressure. An opioid-relaxant sequence is normally quite satisfactory, with the proviso that many patients, particularly the elderly, become hypotensive when placed prone. Considerable vagally-mediated bradycardia can arise from nerve root stimulation during surgery, and pancuronium is particularly useful in both these situations. Vecuronium may be too short-acting for spinal surgery unless given by infusion.

As the spine is an extremely vascular area, hypotensive anaesthesia is occasionally used to decrease bleeding, and particularly the venous ooze in the operative field. This is also considerably reduced if the operative site can be placed above the level of the heart — another advantage of the patient lying prone. The magnitude of blood loss during bony surgery involving laminectomy is often sufficient to require blood transfusion and is very different from the peaceful conditions associated with lumbar microdiscectomy in the young, fit adult!

Thoracic discs and tumours such as neuro-fibromata are occasionally approached by the transthoracic route, involving thoracotomy and a combined approach with the patient in the lateral position. Endobronchial intubation and one-lung anaesthesia may be needed to facilitate access in this situation.

LASERS

While lasers are used increasingly for tissue dissection and cautery, particularly in neurosurgery, their use demands specialized anaesthetic techniques because the laser beam burns through most substances, including tracheal tubes. The beam is reflected off impermeable structures such as retractors, producing damage in its path. Theatre staff must wear eye protection during laser surgery, even when they are remote from the beam, which usually passes through the operating microscope. Lasers must not be used in the presence of inflammable gases or vapours because

the heat generated may ignite the gas, producing an explosion.

POSTOPERATIVE NEUROSURGICAL CARE

Although many patients who have undergone spinal or intracranial surgery are awake and conscious in the immediate postoperative period, some still require active, intensive treatment. This is important particularly in patients who have raised intracranial pressure (or when ICP is liable to rise), and in those who have undergone cerebral aneurysm surgery, when postoperative vasospasm may be a problem. Elective postoperative ventilation to control cerebral oxygenation and to produce a mild decrease in intracranial pressure is often employed, with continuous monitoring of both arterial and intracranial pressures. If vasospasm is present, specific vasodilator therapy with nimodipine is continued, together with a hyperperfusion regimen as described earlier, to prevent local areas of cerebral ischaemia which may result in hemiplegia. In general, postoperative opioids are avoided following craniotomy or upper cervical spine surgery, intramuscular codeine phosphate being used most commonly to provide analgesia, together with an antiemetic, e.g. metoclopramide, to treat the nausea which occurs frequently.

Surgery of the thoracic and lumbar spine, particularly involving fusion with an autologous bone graft, is associated with significant postoperative pain. Intramuscular opioids, non-steroidal anti-inflammatory drugs and patient-controlled analgesia have all been used to good effect. Systemic rather than regional analgesia is preferable because the graft donor site is often the most painful area. Urinary retention is a frequent neurological problem, which is exacerbated by anaesthesia, and temporary or intermittent catheterization may be required.

If the spine is stable postoperatively, early mobilization is encouraged unless there is a major neurological deficit which prevents it. Patients with unstable spinal conditions are nursed on a variety of special purpose-built beds and frames for significant periods. In this situation, the risks of hypostatic pneumonia, deep venous thrombosis and pulmonary embolism are considerable.

FURTHER READING

Frost E A M 1991 Clinical anesthesia in neurosurgery. 2nd edition. Butterworths, Boston

Mini-Symposium 1990 The brain. Current Anaesthesia and Intensive Care 1: 72–105

Mini-Symposium 1994 The brain. Current Anaesthesia and Intensive Care 5(1)

Newfield D, Cottrell J E 1991 Neuroanesthesia handbook of clinical and physiologic essentials, 2nd edition. Little Brown

Walters F J M, Ingram S, Jenkinson J 1994 Anaesthesia and Intensive Care for the Neurosurgical Patient, 2nd edition. Blackwell Scientific Publications, Oxford

38. Anaesthesia for thoracic surgery

In the early 20th century, thoracic surgery was predominantly confined to the treatment of tuberculosis and empyema. Advances in anaesthetic practice permitted thoracoplasty, and subsequently lung resection and pneumonectomy, to be performed with increasing safety. With the introduction of antibiotics and antituberculosis agents, surgical intervention has become progressively less common for pulmonary tuberculosis and bronchiectasis. The most common conditions presenting currently for thoracic surgery are carcinoma of bronchus, carcinoma of oesophagus, metastatic disease and a variety of benign processes.

PREOPERATIVE ASSESSMENT

General assessment of the preoperative patient is considered in Chapter 18. In this section, only factors specific to thoracic surgery are discussed.

History

Dyspnoea

This common symptom may indicate disease of lungs or airways, cardiac disease or anaemia. Attempts should be made to relate dyspnoea to a specified degree of activity, e.g. climbing a flight of stairs, walking on the level, etc. The degree of dyspnoea in an individual may vary considerably, particularly if it is associated with disease of small airways, e.g. asthma or chronic bronchitis, when it may be accompanied by wheezing. Dyspnoea may also result from mucosal oedema, secretions, premature small airways closure, or alveolar fibrosis and infiltration.

Cough

A dry cough usually indicates irritation of the large airways, but if persistent may be caused by serious pathology, e.g. compression of the trachea or main bronchi by glands. A productive cough is of greater importance, as material in the bronchial tree may spread infection, or cause obstruction and collapse of areas of lung. Sputum should be obtained for bacteriological examination.

Haemoptysis

Large haemoptyses are uncommon, but have important anaesthetic implications, as the area responsible may require isolation using a technique of bronchial intubation in order to prevent contamination of the entire respiratory tree. Bronchiectasis and cavitating tuberculosis may cause severe haemoptysis, as may some tumours, particularly after biopsy. Minor degrees of haemoptysis are common in inflammatory and neoplastic disease of the lung.

Dysphagia

Severe dysphagia has two important sequelae — the patient rapidly becomes malnourished and cachectic, and the oesophagus above the lesion dilates and may contain large volumes of previously ingested food which may be regurgitated when the patient becomes unconscious.

Examination

Careful examination of the respiratory system

is essential in patients presenting for thoracic surgery.

Cyanosis may be present, either centrally because of severe pulmonary disease, or peripherally in the distribution of superior vena caval drainage if that vessel is obstructed. Asymmetry of chest wall movement should be noted, together with any deviation of the trachea. If an intercostal drain is in place, the presence of an air leak should be noted, and its magnitude assessed. Stridor may be present if there is major obstruction of the trachea.

Percussion may demonstrate the presence of a pleural effusion or a major area of lung collapse.

Auscultation may reveal mild tracheal stridor, or partial obstruction of a main or lobar bronchus. More generalized airways obstruction is indicated by widespread rhonchi, often heard only during expiration. Fine crepitations suggest disease of peripheral airways or alveoli; coarse crepitations are more usually associated with secretions in large airways, and may disappear after coughing.

The mouth and neck should be examined carefully. Features which suggest difficulty in tracheal intubation are likely to result in severe hindrance to the introduction of a bronchial or double-lumen tube. Loose, prominent or capped teeth may interfere with, or be damaged during, rigid bronchoscopy or oesophagoscopy.

Preoperative investigations

Routine

Full blood count, serum urea and electrolyte concentrations, and blood glucose estimation are requested normally. A coagulation screen and liver function tests may be indicated. An electrocardiogram (ECG) is essential.

Radiological

Good-quality posteroanterior and lateral X-rays of chest are helpful in demonstrating localized disease of the lungs, and distortion of the tracheobronchial tree. Tomography provides more detailed information on a lesion or malformation of the bronchial anatomy. Computed tomography (body scan), magnetic resonance imaging and radionuclide scanning are used increasingly.

Bronchography, using radio-opaque contrast medium to display the tracheobronchial tree, is particularly employed in patients with bronchiectasis. A barium swallow is required to define lesions of the oesophagus.

Pulmonary function tests

Objective assessment of pulmonary function is essential to assess the extent of impairment of lung function and as an aid in predicting the ability of a patient to survive pneumonectomy.

Reduction in forced vital capacity (FVC) indicates a restrictive defect. A low forced expiratory volume in 1 s (FEV_1), reduced FEV_1/FVC ratio, and decreased peak expiratory flow rate (PEFR) suggest the presence of obstructive disease of the airways. Additional information may be obtained by displaying flow–volume loops (see Chapter 120). Reversibility of airways obstruction should be ascertained by repeating these tests after administration of a bronchodilator, e.g. salbutamol. Measurement of gas transfer using carbon monoxide, and in particular, calculation of the gas transfer coefficient (gas transfer per unit of ventilated lung volume) provides information on gas exchange which may be useful in predicting the extent of postoperative hypoxaemia. Arterial blood gas analysis is necessary in all patients with moderate or severe lung disease in order to select an appropriate inspired oxygen concentration during and after surgery, and to detect patients with hypercapnia, in whom excessive inspired oxygen concentrations may reduce respiratory drive.

Regional lung function is assessed using radioisotope techniques, and aids decisions concerning pulmonary resection; overall lung function is unlikely to be significantly impaired if the resectable area has poor function.

Interpretation of lung function tests is not always easy, particularly with regard to prediction of postoperative problems. It is important to consider measurements in comparison with those predicted for a patient on the basis of height and weight (see Appendix VIIIb). In general, if the FVC, FEV_1/FVC and gas transfer are less than 50% of predicted values, prognosis after pneumonectomy is poor. If PEFR is less than 70% of predicted, or FEV_1/FEV less than 60%, complications may be anticipated after any form of pulmonary surgery. However, many factors not amenable to measurement are likely to influence the outcome, including motivation of the patient, coexisting non-pulmonary disease and the occurrence of surgical complications.

PREPARATION FOR SURGERY

If possible, patients should stop cigarette smoking in order to reduce bronchial secretions. Antibiotics may be required if infected sputum is present. Bronchodilator drugs, preferably inhaled, may reduce airway obstruction considerably. Occasionally, corticosteroids may be required to reduce bronchospasm.

Preoperative physiotherapy is used to help clear bronchial secretions, and to encourage all patients to practise breathing exercises which are required in the postoperative period.

Rehydration, electrolyte correction and intravenous (i.v.) nutrition are often necessary in patients with oesophageal obstruction. Oesophageal lavage may be advisable in patients with a grossly dilated oesophagus.

Perioperative digitalization is used in a number of centres for older patients undergoing thoracotomy. Low-dose heparin therapy has become popular to reduce the incidence of deep venous thrombosis and its sequelae.

An explanation should be given to the patient of the procedure which is to be undertaken, and of the postoperative environment. In particular, it is wise to warn the patient of the presence of chest drains and postoperative pain.

Premedication

The choice of premedication, if any, is one of personal preference, although an anticholinergic agent is advisable before bronchial instrumentation.

DIAGNOSTIC PROCEDURES

Fibreoptic bronchoscopy

The fibreoptic bronchoscope (Fig. 38.1) may be introduced through the nose, injecting local anaesthetic solution through the injection port under direct vision as the instrument is advanced. In the anaesthetized patient, the bronchoscope may be introduced through a tracheal tube by insertion through a diaphragm (Fig. 38.2) which minimizes leakage of gas during ventilation. Artificial ventilation should be maintained throughout bronchoscopy. Ventilation is significantly impaired unless the internal diameter of the tube is more than 2 mm larger than the diameter of the bronchoscope. Techniques of ventilation using jet devices may be dangerous if expiration through the tracheal tube is impeded by the presence of the bronchoscope, resulting in very high pressures

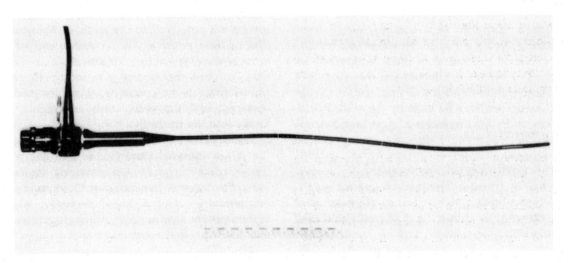

Fig. 38.1 The fibreoptic bronchoscope.

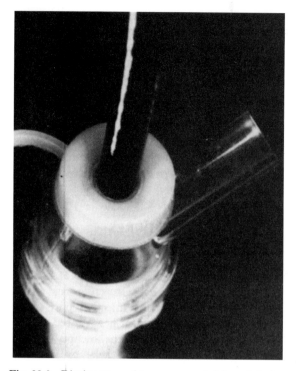

Fig. 38.2 Diaphragm used to ensure an airtight seal during fibreoptic bronchoscopy in patients receiving intermittent positive-pressure ventilation.

in the lower trachea and bronchi with the risk of alveolar rupture, tension pneumothorax and massive surgical emphysema.

Rigid bronchoscopy

Although fibreoptic bronchoscopy has become popular, the rigid bronchoscope remains the preferred instrument of many thoracic surgeons for location of bronchial tumours and for removal of foreign bodies or dilatation of strictures. Although this instrument may be used by the skilled practitioner under local anaesthesia, rigid bronchoscopy is carried out more commonly during general anaesthesia.

The rigid bronchoscope is essentially a long, tapered metal tube. The most commonly used is the Negus. An appropriate-sized bronchoscope is chosen, and the patient's head positioned on one pillow with the neck slightly flexed. The head is extended on the neck. A gauze swab is placed on the patient's upper teeth or gums, and the middle finger of the bronchoscopist's left hand positioned

on the patient's upper left second incisor (or the corresponding position in the edentulous patient). The bronchoscope is held in the right hand and introduced into the mouth alongside the operator's left middle finger, ensuring that the instrument is in the midline at the alveolar margin. The index finger and thumb of the left hand support the bronchoscope as it is advanced, keeping it clear of the teeth. The bronchoscope is passed backwards in the mouth until the uvula is visualized. The tip of the bronchoscope and the portion at the alveolar margin are now both in the midline. Maintaining this midline position, the proximal end of the bronchoscope is angled downwards, thus lifting the tip, until the epiglottis is seen. The tip is passed beneath the epiglottis, then forwards and upwards until the vocal cords are visible, and finally into the trachea.

The head of the table may now be lowered, or the pillow removed carefully, so that the whole trachea comes into view. On advancing the instrument, the carina is seen. To pass the bronchoscope into one of the main bronchi, the head is rotated to the opposite side in order to bring the bronchus into line with the mouth. The appearance of the carina and main bronchi as seen through a bronchoscope is shown in Figure 38.3.

Rigid bronchoscopy may induce bronchospasm or cardiac arrhythmias, and interfere with ventilation. Thus, the anaesthetic technique should provide adequate analgesia and muscle relaxation to permit introduction of the instrument and abolish reflexes from stimulation of the respiratory tract. Adequate gas exchange must be maintained. Rapid recovery is desirable to enable the patient to cough up secretions or blood.

Topical analgesia is used occasionally, the technique being similar to that described for tracheal intubation in Chapter 31.

Inhalational anaesthesia using halothane is used by some anaesthetists for rigid bronchoscopy in children. The child is anaesthetized deeply using the volatile agent, and bronchoscopy performed with the patient breathing air spontaneously through the instrument. The depth of anaesthesia lightens progressively, and the bronchoscope may have to be removed intermittently to allow the level of anaesthesia to be deepened.

More commonly, i.v. anaesthesia is used. Fol-

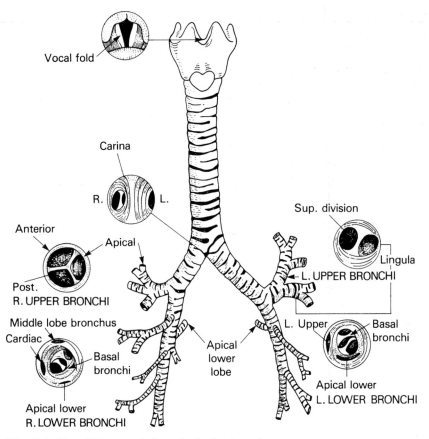

Fig. 38.3 Bronchial tree and views obtained at bronchoscopy.

lowing preoxygenation, light narcosis is induced using an i.v. anaesthetic agent, e.g. propofol. Suxamethonium is used to provide muscle relaxation. The lungs are inflated with oxygen by face mask, and bronchoscopy undertaken. Incremental doses of i.v. anaesthetic agent and suxamethonium are given as indicated. Artificial ventilation is usually achieved using an injector, which produces a high-pressure jet of gas down the bronchoscope. Either oxygen or Entonox may be used as the driving gas. The jet of gas entrains air and produces inflation of the lungs. Expiration occurs through and round the bronchoscope. An appropriate size of jet must be selected (Table 38.1). High-frequency positive-pressure ventilation (HFPPV), at rates of 100–300 breath.min^{-1}, may be used during bronchoscopy. This technique eliminates air entrainment and allows ventilation with an undiluted anaesthetic gas mixture.

Table 38.1 Appropriate sizes, and typical maximum inflation pressures, with Venturi bronchoscope injectors

Patient	Size (s.w.g.)	Pressure (cmH$_2$O)
Adult (poor compliance)	14	50
Adult	16	25
Child (over 12 years)	17	20
Child (under 12 years)	19	15

Oesophagoscopy

Fibreoptic oesophagoscopy is normally undertaken in the sedated patient. The rigid oesophagoscope is inserted under general anaesthesia. Features of importance to the anaesthetist are the potential for regurgitation on induction of anaesthesia, and the risk of damage to teeth or the cervical spine as the instrument is introduced. A rapid-sequence induction technique should be used, and ventilation controlled after tracheal intubation. The cuff of the tracheal tube may temporarily require deflation to enable the oesophagoscope to pass through the cricopharyngeal sphincter.

The most serious complication of oesophagoscopy is perforation of the oesophagus, and a chest X-ray is required after the procedure before any fluids are allowed by mouth.

Mediastinoscopy

This procedure permits direct inspection and biopsy of mediastinal lesions, in particular lymph nodes. The mediastinoscope is introduced through a small suprasternal incision. Complications include haemorrhage (occasionally catastrophic), pneumothorax, haemothorax, air embolism and recurrent laryngeal nerve damage. The most commonly used anaesthetic technique employs tracheal intubation and controlled ventilation.

Bronchography

The commonest indication for bronchography is investigation of the extent of bronchiectasis. The patient may already have compromised respiratory function and copious infected sputum.

Bronchography is usually performed using the oil-based radio-opaque contrast medium propyliodine (Dionosil) to outline the tracheobronchial tree. The procedure may be undertaken in the conscious patient under local anaesthesia, either by injecting contrast medium through a catheter placed in the trachea, or by allowing it to trickle over the back of the tongue. General anaesthesia is required for children and unco-operative adults. The anaesthetic management of patients undergoing bronchography is described in Chapter 29.

CHEST WALL INTEGRITY

If chest wall integrity is lost, as a result of either trauma or surgical intervention, abnormal chest wall movement and gas distribution occur. In the patient with a damaged chest wall, e.g. crush injury, paradoxical movement of the chest wall is seen, with inward movement of the rib cage during inspiration and the reverse during expiration. During inspiration, the lung on the unaffected side expands, but fills with gas partly from the trachea, and partly from the lung on the abnormal side, which deflates. During expiration, the normal lung deflates, but part of the expired gas passes into the lung on the affected side, which expands. This pattern of ventilation, termed pendulum breathing or pendelluft, results in progressive hypoxaemia and hypercapnia. A similar pattern occurs if the chest wall is opened surgically. Thus, spontaneous ventilation is inappropriate if integrity of the chest wall is lost, and positive-pressure ventilation must be employed.

ONE-LUNG ANAESTHESIA

Distribution of ventilation and perfusion

In the awake, spontaneously breathing subject in the lateral position, the dependent lung is better perfused than the upper lung because of the effects of gravity. The dependent diaphragm is pushed higher than the upper during expiration by the weight of the abdominal contents. As a result, it contracts more efficiently, so that ventilation of the dependent lung is also better than that of the upper lung. Thus, ventilation and perfusion are reasonably well-matched in both lungs. However, in the anaesthetized patient, functional residual capacity (FRC) is reduced and the upper lung receives greater ventilation, whereas perfusion remains better in the lower lung. Similarly, during controlled ventilation, the upper lung is ventilated preferentially as the compliance of the dependent lung is reduced by the weight of the abdominal contents and mediastinum. Perfusion of the upper lung may be greater than during spontaneous ventilation in the lateral position because the higher intra-alveolar pressure in the dependent lung diverts blood to the upper lung. Nevertheless, there is increased ventilation/perfusion mismatch whether ventilation is controlled or not.

In order to improve surgical access, the upper lung may be allowed to collapse, whereupon it acts as a source of true shunt because it still receives a proportion of the right ventricular output, but no ventilation. The dependent lung receives the major portion of pulmonary blood flow, and the entire minute ventilation. Ventilation and perfusion are unlikely to be matched perfectly throughout the dependent lung, and the total calculated intrapulmonary shunt therefore varies from 25 to 40% when the upper lung is collapsed. Paradoxically, higher values tend to be found in patients with normal lungs, because a diseased lung, even if it contains a focal lesion, tends to have a reduced blood supply. During pulmonary surgery, the more diseased lung is uppermost, and the dependent lung receives an increased proportion of total pulmonary blood flow. In contrast, a patient undergoing oesophageal surgery may have two healthy lungs, and intrapulmonary shunt during one-lung anaesthesia may be very high.

Increased intrapulmonary shunting causes a decrease in arterial oxygen tension. Although there is no degree of hypoxaemia which may be regarded as safe, it is generally felt that an arterial partial pressure of oxygen (Pa_{O_2}) of approximately 9 kPa is acceptable; this results in an oxygen saturation of approximately 90%. In order to achieve this or a higher Pa_{O_2} during one-lung ventilation, a number of techniques may be employed. It is generally recommended that an inspired oxygen concentration of 40% be provided initially on switching to one-lung anaesthesia. Higher concentrations may be necessary if there is clinical or blood gas evidence of hypoxaemia. However, concentrations of oxygen in excess of 60% are unlikely to produce a substantial increase in Pa_{O_2}, and may, unexpectedly, increase intrapulmonary shunt by decreasing the normal hypoxic vasoconstriction in poorly ventilated areas of the dependent lung. Although blood flow to the unventilated lung decreases because of an increase in vascular resistance, this does not occur to a significant extent in the first few hours after lung collapse, and a large intrapulmonary shunt persists throughout the course of one-lung anaesthesia.

Blood flow through the collapsed lung may be reduced by restricting intra-alveolar pressure, thereby encouraging blood flow through the dependent lung. Thus, positive end-expiratory pressure (PEEP), which might be expected to improve arterial oxygenation by increasing FRC in the dependent lung, may increase shunt by diverting blood to the unventilated lung. In some patients, it may be necessary to supply oxygen under a small positive pressure (0.3–0.5 kPa; 3–5 cmH$_2$O) to the unventilated lung. This permits diffusion

oxygenation of the blood perfusing that lung, and reduces arterial hypoxaemia.

Because of the increased inspired oxygen concentration required to prevent arterial hypoxaemia, only 40–60% nitrous oxide must be administered. In order to ensure adequate anaesthesia, this must be supplemented with a volatile agent or i.v. anaesthetic agent (e.g. propofol) as well as an opioid. Opioids may be administered through an extradural catheter to provide intraoperative analgesia, although a volatile or i.v. anaesthetic agent should be used in conjunction with nitrous oxide in order to prevent awareness.

Although the ratio of dead space to tidal volume may diminish when one-lung ventilation starts, the increase in intrapulmonary shunt results in impaired carbon dioxide excretion. The net result is that carbon dioxide elimination remains essentially unchanged if tidal volume and minute ventilation are kept constant on changing to one-lung ventilation.

A scheme for one-lung ventilation is shown in Table 38.2.

Apparatus for one-lung anaesthesia

Bronchial blockers

A bronchial blocker is simply a suction catheter with an inflatable balloon at its distal end. It is used to isolate, and to permit aspiration of secre-

Table 38.2 A scheme for one-lung ventilation

Maintain two-lung ventilation until pleura is opened

Dependent lung
$F_{I_{O_2}}$ = 1.0
TV = 10 ml.kg^{-1}
RR = so that Pa_{CO_2} = ~5 kPa (37 mmHg)
PEEP = 0–5 mmHg

If severe hypoxaemia occurs:
Check position of double-lumen tube with fibreoptic
  bronchoscope
Check haemodynamic status
Non-dependent lung CPAP
Dependent lung PEEP
Intermittent two-lung ventilation
Clamp pulmonary artery ASAP (for pneumonectomy)

$F_{I_{O_2}}$ = Fractional concentration of oxygen; TV = tidal volume; RR = respiratory rate; PEEP = positive end-expiratory pressure; CPAP = continuous positive airways pressure; ASAP = as soon as possible.

tions from one lung or lobe. After introduction through a bronchoscope, the balloon is inflated, and a tracheal tube inserted to permit ventilation of the unblocked areas of lung. Bronchial blockers are seldom used now, having been superseded by double-lumen tubes, but they have occasional indications, e.g. for control of haemorrhage.

Single-lumen bronchial tubes

Some single-lumen bronchial tubes may be introduced blindly into position, while others are designed to be inserted under direct vision over a bronchoscope. These latter types are useful if bronchial anatomy is distorted. A single-lumen tube is passed into the main bronchus of the non-operated lung. This lung may be isolated by inflation of the balloon at the distal end of the tube, or both lungs may be ventilated, although unequally, by deflation of this balloon, and inflation of the tracheal cuff.

In infants, bronchial intubation may occasionally be required, and can be achieved by the use of a tracheal tube cut 1 cm longer than normal, and of the same diameter or 1 mm smaller than would be used normally for tracheal intubation.

Double-lumen tubes

Double-lumen tubes (Fig. 38.4) are the commonest type of endobronchial apparatus in current use. Their purpose is to provide separate channels for ventilation and suction of both lungs. The lumen on one side is shaped at its distal end to enter and occupy one or other main bronchus, while the second lumen ends in the trachea. In order to permit clamping and transection of the main bronchus during pneumonectomy, a right-sided tube is used for operations on the left lung, although it may occlude the upper lobe bronchus despite the slit in the bronchial cuff (Fig. 38.5), because the location of the right upper lobe bronchus is variable. A left-sided tube is used when surgery of the right lung is planned, or when non-pulmonary surgery is undertaken. Double-lumen tubes may be awkward to introduce through the larynx, and may not enter the desired bronchus if the anatomy is distorted. However, when correctly positioned, they permit access to both

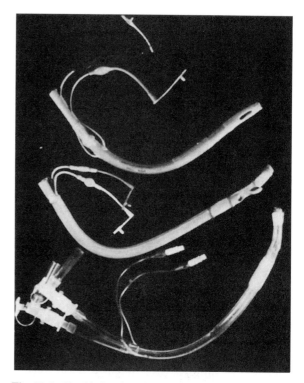

Fig. 38.4 Double-lumen tubes. Top to bottom: right-sided Robertshaw, Carlen (left-sided, with carinal hook), left-sided Bronchocath (disposable, polyvinyl chloride).

lungs, provide even ventilation, and are less likely to be dislodged than a single-lumen tube. The double-lumen tube is inserted through the larynx with the bronchial curve facing anteriorly. The tube is then rotated through 90° so that the distal curve is angled towards the intended bronchus. The tube is advanced until significant resistance is encountered. The tracheal cuff is inflated, as in a conventional tracheal tube, and the lungs are ventilated. The chest is auscultated to ensure that there is air entry to all lobes of both lungs. Each lumen is occluded in turn and, using observation and auscultation, it can be established whether the correct bronchus has been intubated. The position of the tube should then be checked using a fibreoptic bronchoscope inserted through the bronchial lumen to ensure that the tip lies in the main bronchus, and not in one of the lobar bronchi; disposable double-lumen tubes have a long bronchial segment, which often extends into the lower lobe bronchus. When the correct position has been confirmed, the endobronchial cuff

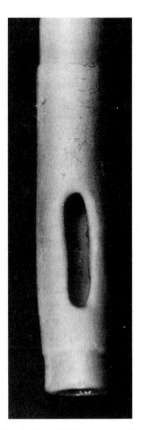

Fig. 38.5 Orifice in bronchial lumen of right-sided Robertshaw double-lumen tube to permit ventilation of right upper lobe.

is inflated gently; it is seldom necessary to use more than 1–2 ml of air.

When the patient has been positioned on the operating table, the correct position of the double-lumen tube should be confirmed, as there is a risk of dislodgement as the patient is moved.

THORACOTOMY

Anaesthetic technique

(Modifications to the technique described here are required in the presence of a bronchopleural fistula, empyema, lung cyst or pneumothorax. These modifications are detailed in the appropriate sections of this chapter.)
Induction of anaesthesia may be achieved using an appropriate i.v. agent. Although some anaesthetists prefer to use suxamethonium if a double-lumen tube is to be introduced, others use a large dose of non-depolarizing relaxant (e.g. vecuronium 0.1 mg.kg^{-1}), as comparable relaxation ensues in 2–3 min, and thoracotomy is seldom of shorter duration than that of the relaxant.

A large-gauge i.v. cannula is essential for infusion of fluids and blood (which is usually required).

Maintenance of anaesthesia is normally achieved using a combination of nitrous oxide/oxygen, i.v. opioid and volatile or i.v. anaesthetic. The choice may be influenced by the need for one-lung anaesthesia. The depth of anaesthesia required is comparable to that for abdominal surgery.

Monitoring

Monitoring of ECG, heart rate, arterial oxygen saturation and arterial pressure is mandatory. Arterial pressure may be measured indirectly with an oscillometer, although in the lateral position pressure recordings from the dependent arm may be unreliable because of compression by the thorax. Direct arterial pressure measurement using an intra-arterial cannula is indicated in the poor-risk patient, or if severe haemorrhage or mediastinal retraction is anticipated. This technique also allows sampling for blood gas analysis, and is useful if severe hypoxaemia is expected. The need for blood gas analysis has been reduced by continuous monitoring of arterial oxygen saturation using the pulse oximeter. Central venous pressure monitoring may be necessary when major surgery, associated with heavy bleeding, is planned. Monitoring of temperature is important in children, or if prolonged surgery is anticipated in adults. In these situations, a warming blanket and blood warmer should be used, and inspired gases require warming and humidification.

Position

Pulmonary surgery is normally undertaken with the patient in the lateral position (Fig. 38.6), with the diseased side uppermost. Care must be taken to avoid nerve damage in the upper arm by avoiding excessive traction, and a pillow should be placed between the legs to prevent pressure damage.

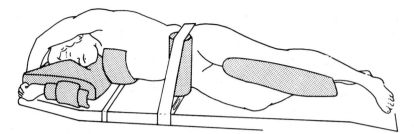

Fig. 38.6   Patient in lateral position for thoracic surgery.

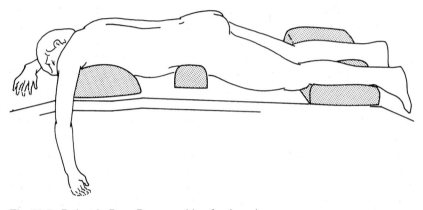

Fig. 38.7   Patient in Parry Brown position for thoracic surgery.

Some surgeons prefer the patient to be positioned prone, in the Parry Brown position (Fig. 38.7). The shoulders and pelvis are supported to prevent pressure on the abdomen, which increases intra-abdominal pressure, impairs expansion of the lung bases and reduces venous return to the heart. The arm on the operated side hangs over the edge of the operating table so that the scapula is pulled away from the site of surgery. This position allows drainage of secretions from the diseased lung towards the trachea without soiling the other lung.

Oesophageal surgery is usually undertaken with the patient in the lateral or semilateral position.

At the end of thoracotomy, the pleural cavity is drained (although not always after pneumonectomy) to ensure that air or fluid does not accumulate in the postoperative period. If the lung has been collapsed, it is reinflated before the thorax is closed so that re-expansion may be confirmed under direct vision. After closure of the thorax, the drains are connected to an underwater seal, which permits drainage of air or fluid with minimal resistance, and allows measurement of volumes of drained fluid or blood. As intermittent positive-pressure ventilation (IPPV) is continued, air is expelled from the pleural space, and the lung expands to fill the cavity.

It is usual to allow patients to breathe spontaneously after thoracotomy, and residual effects of neuromuscular blocking drugs are therefore antagonized. Secretions are aspirated via a suction catheter passed through the tracheal tube. When adequate spontaneous ventilation has returned, and the patient has regained control of reflexes, pharyngeal secretions are aspirated and the tracheal (or double-lumen) tube removed.

Postoperative care

Pulmonary function may be considerably reduced after thoracotomy. The lungs may be affected by chronic disease, a lobe or lung may have been excised, and the remaining lung tissue has been manipulated and retracted, resulting in patchy oedema and contusion, and an increase in pulmonary secretions. Blood or infected material from a resected area may contaminate the remaining lung. Pain from the incision and chest drain sites inhibits chest wall movement, and, together with any accumulation of fluid or air in the pleural cavity, may reduce expansion and encourage atelectasis and collapse.

Although mechanical ventilation in the postoperative period permits expansion of the lungs, aspiration of secretions and adequate analgesia and sedation (without fear of ventilatory depression), there are disadvantages, particularly after pulmonary surgery. Air leaks from the surface of the lung or from the resected bronchial stump may be augmented by IPPV. Continued tracheal intubation may result in increased risk of chest infection. However, elective mechanical ventilation is occasionally necessary in debilitated patients after oesophageal resection, and in patients with severely impaired lung function following pulmonary surgery.

In all patients, adequate oxygenation and ventilation should be ensured. An increased inspired oxygen concentration of 40% (unless the patient is chronically hypercapnic) is advisable to prevent arterial hypoxaemia, together with humidification of the inspired gases to prevent inspissation of secretions, and physiotherapy to aid lung expansion and coughing. Effective analgesia is essential. An opioid analgesic administered intermittently by the intramuscular route is easy to prescribe, but provides sporadic and often ineffective analgesia, and may cause depression of ventilation. Patient-controlled i.v. infusions of opioid analgesic drugs provide more continuity of analgesia. Blockade of the intercostal nerves during thoracotomy either with a local anaesthetic agent or using cryoanalgesia reduces the requirements for systemic analgesic drugs. Paravertebral or extradural nerve block with a local anaesthetic agent is extremely effective, while extradural or intrathecal opioids may provide profound analgesia with virtually no cardiovascular complications, although there is a risk of late respiratory depression. Extradural catheter techniques permit administration of repeated doses of drug and provide optimum analgesia, but require careful monitoring, and

should be contemplated only if the patient is nursed in a high-dependency or intensive care area.

THORACOSCOPY

Indications

Thoracoscopy may be used for diagnostic purposes. It facilitates examination of the intrathoracic cavity, and is used in the diagnosis of pleural and parenchymal disease, to determine the aetiology of recurrent pleural effusions and to help establish the staging of suspected tumours. In recent years, the development of endoscopic video systems and specialized instrumentation has resulted in increasing use of operative thoracoscopy. Virtually all thoracic surgical procedures have been undertaken using thoracoscopy, which causes much less systemic disruption to the patient than does thoracotomy. Thoracoscopy is particularly useful for biopsy of intrathoracic structures, peripheral wedge and sublobar resections, lobectomy, removal of cysts, drainage of abscesses and closure of persistent air leaks from abnormal lung. In addition, the technique is used by vascular surgeons to undertake cervical sympathectomy.

Technique

A small incision is made in the lateral thoracic wall, usually at the level of the sixth intercostal space, and the thoracoscope is introduced into the pleural cavity. Additional small incisions are made to insert instruments, if necessary. If large structures are resected, a small subcostal incision is made towards the end of the procedure in order to remove the resected tissue.

Partial collapse of the lung on the operated side occurs when air enters the pleural cavity. It is unnecessary, and potentially very dangerous, to insufflate gas under pressure, particularly if the lung on the operated side is not collapsed using a double-lumen tube; if the lung continues to be ventilated, then very high intrathoracic pressures are generated during inspiration, causing mediastinal distortion and the risk of cardiovascular collapse.

Anaesthetic technique

General anaesthesia is usually employed, although

the technique can be undertaken using local anaesthesia. When thoracoscopy is performed under general anaesthesia, a double-lumen tube should be used; the anaesthetic technique is therefore similar to that described above for thoracotomy. As with all endoscopic operative procedures, there is a risk that the surgeon will encounter difficulties, and that open thoracotomy will be required. Consequently, similar monitoring should be employed as that used for thoracotomy.

In the postoperative period, pain is very much less than that associated with thoracotomy. Intercostal blocks may be inserted at the level of the incision and at two intercostal spaces above and below. Commonly, a chest drain is not inserted; a small residual pneumothorax may be present, and the risk of development of a larger pneumothorax should always be considered.

SURGERY RELATED TO THE LUNG

Removal of inhaled foreign body

Inhalation of foreign bodies is not uncommon in children. Obstruction of the larynx results in acute obstruction, but smaller objects wedge more distally and may result in valvular obstruction with emphysema of the affected lobe or segment, or more commonly in total obstruction leading to distal consolidation and collapse. Eighty per cent of foreign bodies lodge in the right lung. There may be considerable reaction and oedema at the site of obstruction, particularly when an irritant object, e.g. a peanut, has been inhaled.

The patient may have a degree of respiratory obstruction, pulmonary infection and hypoxaemia. An inhalational induction is preferable in children, particularly if respiratory obstruction is present, and a selection of tracheal tubes should be available. Removal of the foreign body is performed through a rigid bronchoscope, and may be extremely difficult, particularly if bronchial oedema is present. Laryngeal stridor is not uncommon during recovery, and the patient must be observed closely for at least 12 h.

Lobectomy

The usual indications for lobectomy are:

1. *Bronchial neoplasm.*

2. *Bronchiectasis.* Lobectomy is indicated if haemoptyses occur repeatedly or infection cannot be controlled.
3. *Infection.* Although it is now relatively rare, tuberculosis is the most common infective condition under this heading.

Lobectomy may be a straightforward procedure with few surgical problems, but it may be difficult and result in severe haemorrhage in the presence of invading tumour, chronic infection or pleural adhesions. In many centres, isolation of the affected lung is achieved using a single- or double-lumen bronchial tube in the healthy lung. This permits aspiration of secretions, deflation of the affected lung when required, and reflation of the remaining lobes before closure of the chest. When the lobe has been removed, the bronchus is clamped and divided, and the remnant either sutured or stapled. The pleural cavity may be filled with saline, and inflation of the affected lung to a pressure of 3–4 kPa (30–40 cmH$_2$O) is undertaken to ensure that no significant air leak exists. Depending on the experience and requirements of the surgeon, bronchial division and closure may not require cessation of ventilation of the affected lung for any significant period of time, and a standard tracheal tube may be satisfactory unless there is a need to protect the healthy lung from secretions, or sleeve resection of the main bronchus is anticipated because of tumour close to the origin of the lobar bronchus.

Pneumonectomy

Bronchial carcinoma not confined to a single lobe is the normal indication for this operation. Pneumonectomy may be performed either in the prone or lateral position. Bronchial intubation is usually selected if the lateral position is used. Mediastinal manipulation may result in arrhythmias, and haemorrhage may be considerable. The main bronchus is divided and sutured, and tested for air leaks as described above.

After pneumonectomy, the pleural space fills with serosanguineous fluid, and this is allowed to accumulate. Thus, the pleural cavity is not always drained. If a drain is inserted at operation, it is connected to an underwater seal, and left open to drain air and fluid while the patient is returned to the supine position. After a chest X-ray has confirmed that the mediastinum is central, the drain is clamped, but the clamps are removed for a short period every hour during the 24 h following surgery to ensure that neither air nor excess fluid is accumulating.

If the pleural space is not drained, the following procedure is undertaken when the patient has been returned to the supine position at the end of surgery; a needle is inserted through the chest wall, connected to a three-way stopcock and manometer, and air removed or injected until the intrapleural pressure is normal, indicating that the mediastinum is central. The risks of leaving the cavity undrained are that air may accumulate under pressure if the bronchial stump leaks, and that massive haemorrhage may go unrecognized. Drainage may, however, increase the risk of infection.

Normally, the empty pleural space fills gradually with serosanguineous fluid, and fibrosis occurs subsequently, pulling the diaphragm into the thorax and the mediastinum across to the operated side. If fluid accumulates too rapidly, mediastinal distortion and compression of the remaining lung result in a combination of hypotension, right ventricular failure and hypoxaemia. Central venous pressure is often high because of mediastinal distortion, although the patient is usually hypovolaemic because of fluid loss. Mediastinal displacement causing cardiorespiratory distress may also occur if the space fills too slowly with fluid as air is absorbed.

Sputum retention and respiratory failure are not uncommon after pneumonectomy; mortality is significantly increased if mechanical ventilation is required. Arrhythmias and pericarditis are also frequent complications, probably because of mediastinal manipulation. The incidence of supraventricular arrhythmias is reduced if the patient is digitalized during the perioperative period.

Other complications of major surgery, e.g. myocardial infarction and renal failure, may occur. The mortality after left pneumonectomy is 7–10%, and may be as high as 20% after excision of the larger right lung.

Bronchopleural fistula

A connection between the tracheobronchial tree and the pleural cavity may result from trauma, neoplasm, rupture of an intrapulmonary cavity (e.g. abscess), or from breakdown of a bronchial stump or anastomosis after surgery. Bronchopleural fistulae are almost always complicated by the collection of infected fluid in the pleural cavity. This results in a number of problems of importance to the anaesthetist. The patient may be cachectic and dehydrated, and pulmonary function may be considerably impaired. Careful preoperative assessment is essential, although surgical intervention may be urgent. In addition to factors related to the general condition of the patient, two specific dangers exist:

1. The remaining healthy lung is at risk of contamination by the infected contents of the pleural space.
2. Positive pressure applied to the affected bronchial tree may result either in passage of the inspired gas out through the chest drain, resulting in little or no effective alveolar ventilation or, if the drain is only partially patent, in an increase in intrapleural pressure with the danger that infected material may be squeezed into the tracheobronchial tree with consequent pulmonary contamination.

Only anticholinergic premedication is prescribed. The patient is placed in a semisitting, semilateral position with the affected side dependent. Bronchial intubation is essential if possible. The optimum method of induction of anaesthesia is controversial. Some anaesthetists feel that an inhalational induction is the safest technique, as spontaneous ventilation is maintained until the bronchial or double-lumen tube is in position and the damaged lung isolated. However, deep anaesthesia is required, and this may have cardiovascular complications in the semirecumbent position. In addition, prolonged attempts at intubation may result in coughing, which increases intrapleural pressure and may spread infected material through the lungs. Consequently, many anaesthetists who are practised at bronchial intubation prefer to preoxygenate the lungs, induce anaesthesia with an i.v. agent, and produce muscle paralysis with suxamethonium. Intubation is carried out when spontaneous ventilation has ceased.

When the tube is in position, the healthy lung is ventilated, and infected material from the affected bronchial tree aspirated. A non-depolarizing muscle relaxant is administered, and one-lung anaesthesia maintained as described above. After surgery, attempts are made to restore spontaneous ventilation, although this may be precluded by the patient's position.

Drainage of empyema

An empyema is a collection of purulent material in the pleural cavity. It is usually associated with an infective process in the lung, although it may also occur after oesophageal perforation or as a complication of thoracotomy. Initial treatment is with appropriate antibiotics and drainage through an intercostal drain. This is inserted under local anaesthesia. Drainage may be incomplete, however, and a chronic empyema may develop with fibrosis of the surrounding pleura. Resection of one or more ribs may be required in order to obtain satisfactory drainage. An empyema is often accompanied by a bronchopleural fistula, and this determines anaesthetic management (see above).

Lung cysts and bullae

These are thin-walled, air-filled cavities within the lung which may be congenital, the consequence of previous infection or the result of emphysema. Their connection with the bronchial tree may be valvular. Large cysts may present problems during unrelated surgery. IPPV may result in rupture of a thin-walled cyst. Enlargement of the cyst may occur if a valvular connection is present. Nitrous oxide may also enlarge a cyst because nitrogen is less soluble in blood.

Rupture of a cyst rapidly results in respiratory distress. Gross enlargement of a cyst may produce a similar effect. The two may be indistinguishable clinically, and a chest drain should be inserted if respiratory distress occurs. A persistent air leak is likely to develop if an enlarged cyst is drained, and may also follow rupture of a cyst.

During anaesthesia for resection of a lung cyst, attention must be given to prevention of rupture of the cyst, in addition to the problems associated with thoracotomy. Bronchial blocking or intubation permits selective ventilation of the normal lung, although tracheal intubation and gentle

positive-pressure ventilation are regarded by some anaesthetists as a satisfactory technique.

Lung abscess

The majority of lung abscesses are amenable to treatment with antibiotics, and usually rupture into a bronchus from which the contents are expectorated, or into the pleura, resulting in an empyema and bronchopleural fistula. Surgery for an abscess may result in its rupture during anaesthesia. A double-lumen tube should be used to ensure that contamination of the unaffected lung does not take place, and so that infected material can be aspirated.

Pleurectomy and pleurodesis

Pleurectomy is performed through an antero-lateral thoracotomy. Pleurodesis is achieved by the introduction of iodized talc through a thoracoscope, or by abrasion of the pleura with a gauze swab through a small thoracotomy incision. The usual indication for these procedures is repeated spontaneous pneumothorax.

The patient presenting for pleurectomy may have a pneumothorax, and may have underlying pulmonary disease. If the pleural cavity is not drained, the pneumothorax may be increased in size by nitrous oxide, or by IPPV if an air leak is present or a lung cyst ruptured. However, the time period between induction of anaesthesia and exposure of the pleural cavity is short. It is seldom necessary to avoid the use of nitrous oxide, and gentle IPPV may be used until the chest wall is open. A double-lumen tube is not necessary unless a large air leak is present. Haemorrhage may be considerable, and postoperative pain is severe.

NON-PULMONARY SURGERY

Diaphragmatic hernia

Anaesthesia for repair of a congenital diaphragmatic hernia in the neonate is discussed in Chapter 33. A congenital hernia may present in adults, but the condition is more commonly associated in adult life with trauma. It may be possible to repair the hernia from the abdomen, but thoracotomy is often necessary. The lung may be compressed by distended bowel, and pulmonary function impaired as a result. Electrolyte abnormalities may be present because of intestinal obstruction. If the stomach has herniated into the thorax, the risk of reflux of gastric contents is increased.

Repair of hiatus hernia

A hiatus hernia may require repair using a thoracic approach through a left thoracotomy or using thoracoscopy. The patient may be obese. It should be assumed that regurgitation of gastric contents may occur because of incompetence of the lower oesophageal sphincter. Antacids should be continued preoperatively, and H_2-antagonists may be given with premedication to increase the pH of the gastric contents. Preoxygenation of the lungs should be carried out before induction of anaesthesia, and cricoid pressure applied until the airway is secure. A tracheal tube is usually adequate, and is easier and faster to position than a double-lumen tube. However, in some centres a left-sided double-lumen tube is used and the left lung deflated to permit better surgical access; this is essential if thorascopic repair is planned. One-lung anaesthesia in the patient with normal lungs may result in severe hypoxaemia (see above).

Oesophageal myotomy

Oesophageal myotomy (Heller's operation) is indicated in the presence of achalasia. This disorder of oesophageal motility results in gross dilatation of the oesophagus and the collection in it of large volumes of undigested food. The patient may have pulmonary disease as a result of repeated aspiration of oesophageal contents. The principal risk during anaesthesia is that of aspiration, and the anaesthetic management is similar to that described for repair of hiatus hernia.

Surgery for carcinoma of oesophagus

Inoperable carcinoma of the esophagus causes progressive obstruction, eventually resulting in complete dysphagia. Insertion of an oesophageal tube may provide some palliation. Bypass of the tumour may be accomplished by mobilization of the stomach through a laparotomy and, after passing the stomach behind the sternum, anastomosis to the upper oesophagus in the neck.

Tumours of the middle and lower thirds of the oesophagus may be resectable. This is a major procedure, undertaken in a patient who may be cachectic, hypoproteinaemic and anaemic. In addition, pulmonary function may be impaired by repeated aspiration of oesophageal contents. Preoperative nutrition, either enteral or parenteral, may be advisable in the cachectic patient. Premedication should be appropriate for the nutritional state of the patient.

Carcinoma of the lower third of the oesophagus is resected through a left thoracoabdominal incision. If the lesion is in the middle third, the operation may be performed in two stages; initially, abdominal organs are mobilized through a laparotomy, and the patient is turned into the left lateral position in order that the resection can be completed, and the anastomosis performed, through a right thoracotomy. Irrespective of the surgical approach, a left-sided double-lumen tube is used and the lung on the side of the thoracotomy collapsed intermittently to allow surgical access to the oesophagus. Haemorrhage may be considerable, and cardiovascular problems may result from retraction of the vena cava or heart. An indwelling arterial cannula and central venous catheter are required. The procedure is often of prolonged duration, and precautions should be taken to prevent hypothermia. Postoperatively, there is a high incidence of pulmonary complications, and effective analgesia is essential. Fluid balance must be maintained meticulously, and admission to a high-dependency or intensive care unit is strongly recommended. Disruption of the anastomosis occurs in 5–10% of cases, and results in severe mediastinitis, with a high mortality; the first sign is often green or yellow discoloration of the fluid in the chest drains.

FURTHER READING

Gothard J W W (ed) 1994 Thoracic anaesthesia, 2nd edn. Clinical anaesthesiology: international practice and research. Baillière-Tindall, London

Gothard J W W 1996 Thoracic surgery. In: Aitkenhead A R, Jones R M (eds) Clinical Anaesthesia Churchill Livingstone, Edinburgh, pp. 239–265

Kaplan J A (ed) 1992 Thoracic anesthesia, 2nd edn Churchill Livingstone, New York

39. Anaesthesia for cardiac surgery

The cardiac surgical theatre, with its profusion of personnel, monitors and support equipment, is often intimidating to the trainee anaesthetist. However, the principles of anaesthetic care are similar to those elsewhere, the principal difference being that essential organ perfusion is achieved artificially when the heart itself is the object of surgery. Operations are termed 'open heart' when the functions of the heart and lungs are assumed by an extracorporeal pump and gas exchange unit (cardiopulmonary bypass or CPB). During 'closed' operations, cardiac and pulmonary functions remain intact and anaesthetic management is similar to that for thoracic surgery.

Excluding the insertion of pacemakers, more than 25 000 cardiac operations are undertaken each year in the UK in NHS hospitals. These include approximately 3500 for congenital abnormalities, 5000 for acquired valvular disease and 16 000 for ischaemic heart disease.

Congenital cardiac abnormalities

These occur at a rate of 6–8 per 1000 live births. Correction of almost a third may be undertaken by closed operation but the remainder, including septal defects, valve abnormalities and cyanotic lesions such as Fallot's tetralogy, require CPB.

Acquired valvular disease

This type of cardiac lesion has become less common as the incidence of rheumatic fever has fallen. Stenosis or incompetence occur and most commonly involve the mitral and aortic valves. Surgery usually comprises replacement with an artificial valve. This may be a mechanical prosthesis with a tilting disc or a tissue valve (usually a pig valve) specially mounted and prepared (heterograft). Prosthetic valves are reliable but necessitate the patient receiving anticoagulants for life. This is not usually necessary when porcine heterografts are used but reoperation is common due to valve failure after about 10 years.

Ischaemic heart disease

The concept of revascularizing ischaemic myocardium was introduced nearly 25 years ago with the insertion of a portion of saphenous vein from aorta to coronary artery distal to a stenosis (Fig. 39.1). Since then, coronary artery bypass grafting has become the most commonly performed cardiac operation. The internal mammary artery is increasingly used as a graft conduit.

Indications for the operation remain controversial. Although angina is relieved in 80–90% of patients, life expectancy is not increased in all groups when compared with medical treatment. Short-term prognosis is improved by surgery only in patients with left main or triple vessel disease or with impaired left ventricular function, but this improvement is not sustained.

Extracorporeal circulation (ECC)

The essential components of ECC comprise:

1. pumps
2. an oxygenator
3. connecting tubes and filters
4. fluid prime of these components.

These are normally arranged as shown in Figure

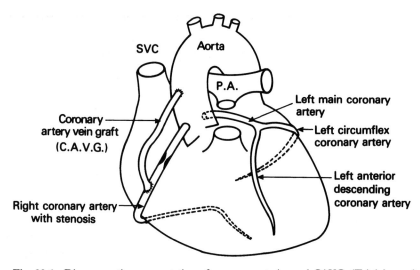

Fig. 39.1 Diagrammatic representation of coronary arteries and CAVG. 'Triple' vessel disease includes right, left circumflex and left anterior descending arteries.

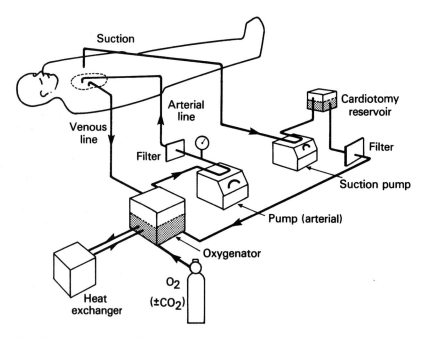

Fig. 39.2 Components of extracorporeal circuit.

39.2. Blood from the venous side of the circulation, usually from the venae cavae, is drained by gravity to a venous reservoir and thence to a gas exchange unit (oxygenator) where oxygen is delivered to, and carbon dioxide removed from, the blood. The 'arterialized' blood is pumped into the arterial side of the circulation, usually into the ascending aorta. The heart and lungs are thus 'bypassed' or isolated and their function maintained temporarily by mechanical equipment remote from the body. Most systems include a heat exchanger in the oxygenator to vary the temperature of blood rapidly and suction to drain redundant or spilled blood in or around the bypassed heart and return it to the venous reservoir for oxygenation and thence to the circulation.

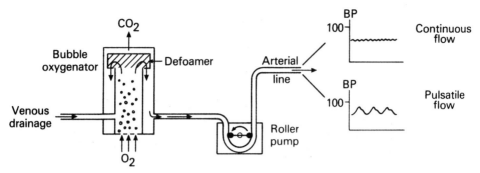

Fig. 39.3 Diagrammatic representation of oxygenator and arterial pump.

Pumps

Roller pumps (Fig. 39.3) displace blood around the circuit by intermittent compression of the circuit tubing during each sweep. By intermittent acceleration of the roller head, a 'pulsatile' waveform may be achieved but there is little evidence that this more physiological flow improves outcome.

Oxygenator

There are two types of oxygenator.

1. Bubble oxygenators

In these devices, oxygen is bubbled through venous blood. They are relatively cheap but cause damage to red cells and platelets and consumption of coagulation factors. Their use is limited to a few hours as the extent of damage is time-dependent.

2. Membrane oxygenators

These comprise a semipermeable membrane which separates gas and blood phases and through which gas exchange occurs. In comparison with bubble oxygenators, damage to blood components is reduced.

Connecting tubes, filters, manometer, suction

These must be sterile and non-toxic and should damage blood as little as possible. A filter should also be incorporated in the arterial line to remove

gas emboli which would pass directly to the aorta. Suction pumps are supplied to vent blood collecting in the pulmonary circulation or left ventricle during bypass and also to remove spilled blood from the pericardial sac. The blood is collected in the 'cardiotomy' reservoir, filtered and returned to the main circuit. This suction also causes damage to blood components.

Fluid prime

Originally it was anticipated that connection of the circulation to an external circuit would necessitate the extracorporeal circuit being filled with anticoagulated whole blood. This increases exposure to donor blood and may lead to incompatibility reactions. However, it became clear that this was unnecessary as the body tolerates a relatively low haematocrit. When CPB is commenced and the patient's blood mixed with an ECC comprising clear fluid (fluid prime), the haematocrit decreases to approximately 20–25%. Although oxygen content is reduced, availability may be increased by improved organ blood flow resulting from reduced blood viscosity. In some patients (low body weight, children or those with a low preoperative haemoglobin in whom dilution would reduce the haematocrit to below 20%), blood may be added to the prime. In the normal adult, 'clear' primes are used almost exclusively (usually compound sodium lactate solution). Most units have individual recipes for addition to the prime (e.g. plasma, dextran, mannitol, sodium bicarbonate and potassium) to achieve an isosmolar solution of physiological pH.

PREOPERATIVE ASSESSMENT

Most patients presenting for cardiac surgery have undergone comprehensive cardiological investigation and are taking medications. In addition to the routine investigations undertaken prior to any operation, specialized techniques are employed to assess the cardiac lesion and degree of resultant dysfunction. The results of these investigations permit the anaesthetist to identify patients at particular risk in whom extra care and monitoring are required.

Exercise electrocardiography

Various stress protocols are employed whereby a standard exercise test is used to provoke ischaemic changes and symptoms. Changes in rhythm, rate, arterial pressure and conduction are recorded. The anaesthetist identifies the most useful ECG leads to monitor during surgery and notes the rate–pressure product (heart rate × systolic arterial pressure) at which evidence of ischaemia occurs.

Cardiac catheterization

Considerable information may be obtained from catheterization.

1. Evidence of failing function or of gradients across stenosed valves may be identified by pressure monitoring.
2. Oximetry of blood at different sites indicates if shunts are present (Fig. 39.4).
3. Cardiac output may be measured.
4. The injection of radio-opaque dye into aorta or ventricles assesses incompetence of valves and the efficiency of ventricular contraction (ejection fraction) and wall motion.
   The ejection fraction (EF) =
$$\frac{\text{End-diastolic volume} - \text{end-systolic volume}}{\text{End-diastolic volume}}$$
5. Injection of dye into coronary arteries defines the anatomy of the coronary circulation and the degree of patency or sites of stenosis.

Echocardiography

Ultrasound is used to identify myocardial motion and valvular function. Preoperatively, this may

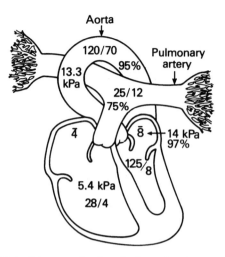

Fig. 39.4 Diagram of catheterization values in a normal adult: pressures (mmHg), oxygen saturations (%) and tensions (kPa).

be performed using a transthoracic or trans-oesophageal approach. The latter involves passing an ultrasound probe into the oesophagus under sedation. The proximity of the heart and oesophagus allows high quality 'real time' images of the anatomy and function of the heart. Doppler techniques allow recognition of the direction and velocity of blood flow and are valuable in the diagnosis of acute valvular disease, e.g. failure of a prosthetic valve.

Radionuclide imaging

By imaging the activity of an appropriate radio-isotope as it passes through the heart or into the myocardium, ventricular function and myocardial perfusion may be assessed. Technetium images blood volume and may be used to demonstrate abnormal wall motion and EF. Thallium, which is taken up by the myocardium, may be used to assess regional blood flow. These techniques may be employed before and after exercise and/or therapy.

Preoperative drug therapy

β-Blocking agents

Continued administration of these drugs up to the time of surgery is desirable as discontinuation may increase the risk of preoperative infarction.

Calcium antagonists

These drugs have a negative inotropic effect but, as with the β-blockers, it is preferable to continue therapy throughout the perioperative period.

Other drugs

Nitrates should be continued and may be included in the premedication if indicated.

Digitalis. Most centres discontinue digoxin 24–48 h before surgery to diminish digoxin-associated arrhythmias after surgery.

Diuretics should be continued until the day before surgery.

Anticoagulants, including aspirin, are usually stopped several days before surgery to permit coagulation to return towards normal. If a high risk of embolism is present, anticoagulants should be continued and coagulation defects treated postoperatively with transfusion of blood products.

Angiotensin-converting enzyme (ACE) inhibitors are increasingly prescribed for hypertension and cardiac failure. They should be given on the day of operation but may produce significant vaso-dilatation and hypotension intraoperatively.

Other investigations prior to surgery

Haemoglobin

Haemoglobin should be adequate (> 11 g.dl^{-1}) to prevent excessive haemodilution on bypass.

Coagulation

Prothrombin time should be measured prior to surgery. Specific defects require correction before surgery or alternatively the appropriate blood products should be made available.

Electrolytes

Serum potassium concentration should be within normal limits.

Urea and creatinine

Raised concentrations indicate an increased risk of renal failure postoperatively. Adequate urine output should be ensured after operation.

Liver function tests

Abnormal values may indicate congestive cardiac failure.

ASSESSMENT OF RISK

The mortality rate associated with cardiac surgery is diminishing but is still significant. Several units have achieved a mortality rate of 1–2% with un-complicated coronary vein grafts but valve surgery is usually associated with a mortality of 4–5%. When more extensive surgery is undertaken, e.g. multiple valve replacement or coronary artery vein graft (CAVG) plus valve replacement, mortality rate increases.

Patients with an increased risk of perioperative complications may be identified during pre-operative assessment. Patients who are classified as the New York Heart Association's functional Class III or IV, in which symptoms occur with minimal activity or at rest, may be expected to experience problems. Increased risk is associated with the following factors:

1. Age > 65 years.
2. Female sex.
3. Unstable angina.
4. Emergency surgery or reoperation.
5. Poor left ventricular function as shown by:
   a. left ventricular end-diastolic pressure > 18 mmHg
   b. ejection fraction $< 30\%$
   c. cardiac index < 2 litre.min^{-1}.m^{-2}
   d. dyskinetic wall motion.
6. Raised pulmonary artery pressures.
7. Evidence of right ventricular failure.
8. Other system disease, e.g. diabetes mellitus.

MONITORING

Extensive and accurate monitoring is essential throughout the perioperative period for the safe practice of cardiac surgery. The same standards of minimum monitoring apply to the patient undergoing cardiac surgery as to all other surgical patients and so a capnograph and pulse oximeter should be used in all cases.

ECG

ECG should be monitored throughout the perioperative period. The ideal system is one which allows simultaneous multiple lead monitoring or at least switching between leads II and V5, for accurate identification of ischaemia. Rate and rhythm should also be observed.

Systemic arterial pressure

Arterial cannulation is mandatory, and not only permits direct measurement but also facilitates sampling of arterial blood for analysis. The preferred site is a radial artery.

Central venous and left atrial pressures

Right-sided filling pressure should be monitored by a cannula placed into the superior vena cava.

Controversy exists regarding the necessity to monitor left heart filling pressure in all patients. A direct left atrial line can be inserted at surgery as an aid to terminating bypass and improving postoperative care but it is sometimes desirable to insert a flow-directed pulmonary artery catheter at or before induction to measure pulmonary capillary wedge pressure (PCWP). In the USA there is enthusiasm for commencing full invasive monitoring prior to anaesthesia but most anaesthetists in the UK undertake this only in poor-risk patients.

Cardiac output (CO)

CO may be measured by thermodilution using a pulmonary artery catheter. Calculation of cardiac output and cardiac index together with the derivatives of stroke work, pulmonary and systemic vascular resistances and tissue oxygen flux permits the most accurate assessment of cardiological therapy.

Echocardiography

During anaesthesia, transoesophageal echocardio-graphy may be valuable. Abnormal motion of the ventricular wall detected in this way is a reliable index of myocardial ischaemia and can guide drug therapy or indicate the need for further surgical revascularization. Doppler techniques may be useful during valvular surgery.

EEG

A simple guide to cerebral activity and perfusion may be obtained from the various forms of processed EEG monitor. Interpretation is difficult in the hypothermic patient and the value of this technique is uncertain. Similar caveats apply to the monitoring of evoked potentials.

Temperature

Core temperature should be monitored from the nasopharynx. Core–peripheral temperature gradients may give some guide to peripheral perfusion.

Biochemical and haematological analysis

Facilities should be available for immediate analysis of blood gases, acid–base balance, serum potassium and blood glucose concentrations.

Measurement of packed cell volume and coagulation status should also be available. Activated clotting time (ACT) can be measured quickly in the operating theatre using the Haemochron apparatus (normal = 100–120 s) but access to the haematology laboratory should be rapid for assessment of a full clotting screen. Thrombo-elastography – the assessment of viscoelastic changes in blood during clotting – is increasingly used to assess haemostatic function in theatre. Its place in the management of cardiac surgery patients awaits clarification.

Display

ECG, pressure waveforms and a digital output of heart rate and pressures should be displayed clearly on a screen visible to both surgeon and anaesthetist. The facility to produce a hard copy of ECG and pressures is necessary for records and accurate diagnosis.

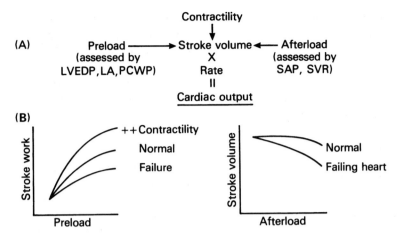

Fig. 39.5 Important aspects of mechanical function.

PATHOPHYSIOLOGICAL CONSIDERATIONS

The anaesthetist should have a clear understanding of the fundamental principles of cardiac physiology. Accurate monitoring reveals alterations in cardiac function and permits the anaesthetist to manipulate factors which ensure adequate pump output (Fig. 39.5) and myocardial blood supply.

Preload and contractility determine the amount of work that the heart can perform. In the failing heart, the afterload determines how much work is expended in overcoming pressure compared with that used to provide forward flow. Thus cardiac output may be increased either by in-

creasing preload or contractility, or by reducing afterload. However, oxygen consumption is raised by increasing heart rate, contractility, preload or afterload. Augmentation of cardiac output by increasing preload or contractility may thus have a detrimental effect on oxygen balance. However, reduction of afterload may increase cardiac output while simultaneously reducing oxygen demand.

Adequate coronary perfusion demands maintenance of diastolic aortic pressure at adequate levels. Oxygen supply to the myocardium occurs predominantly in diastole and is dependent on the gradient between diastolic aortic pressure and intraventricular pressure, and on the diastolic time. The portion of myocardium most at risk of

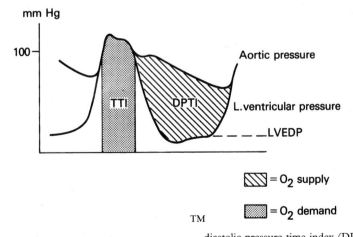

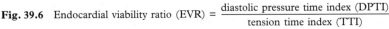

Fig. 39.6 Endocardial viability ratio (EVR) = $\dfrac{\text{diastolic pressure time index (DPTI)}}{\text{tension time index (TTI)}}$

developing ischaemia is the left ventricular endo-cardium. The endocardial viability ratio (EVR) (Fig. 39.6) is a useful index of oxygen balance. Normally, the EVR exceeds 1 but if the ratio decreases below 0.7, ischaemia may develop. Thus, care of the patient suffering from ischaemic heart disease necessitates attempts to reduce oxygen demand and maintain oxygen supply.

Care of the patient with valvular heart disease depends on the valvular lesion. Abnormal heart rates are not tolerated well by a heart with a dis-eased valve. Incompetent valves tend to perform better if afterload is maintained at a low level as this reduces the regurgitant fraction and increases forward flow. Patients with valvular stenosis re-quire adequate preload and do not tolerate rapid reduction in peripheral resistance. This is most true of patients with aortic stenosis where most of the afterload to left ventricular ejection is caused by the stenosed valve itself. This afterload is fixed and cannot be reduced by lowering periph-eral resistance. Vasodilatation produces marked hypotension and results in failure of perfusion of the hypertrophied myocardium with no increase in forward flow through the stenosed valve.

ANAESTHETIC TECHNIQUE

There is no single preferred anaesthetic technique for cardiac surgery. The choice of a specific agent is less important than the care with which the drug is administered and its effects monitored.

Premedication

The most important preoperative preparation comprises a full explanation to the patient of what is about to occur and the development of rapport with, and confidence in, the nursing and medical staff.

Most patients (particularly those with poor cardiovascular reserve) may be sedated preopera-tively with an oral benzodiazepine (lorazepam 2–4 mg or temazepam 20–40 mg). In the parti-cularly anxious patient, heavy sedation may be required to prevent increases in heart rate and arterial pressure before operation. A combination of an oral benzodiazepine and an intramuscular opioid is satisfactory.

Atropine is best avoided in cardiac patients because of its potent chronotropic effects. Patients receiving glyceryl trinitrate (GTN) may benefit from its administration as a skin paste at the time of premedication.

Induction

All drugs and equipment should be ready and the theatre and bypass circuit available for immediate use before the patient arrives in the anaesthetic room.

Before induction, ECG electrodes should be applied and the ECG trace displayed. Arterial and large gauge venous cannulae should be in-serted under local anaesthesia. The lungs should be preoxygenated.

Induction may be undertaken with the standard agents in small doses (e.g. thiopentone 1–3 mg.kg^{-1}, etomidate 0.05–0.2 mg.kg^{-1}) or the use of large doses of opioids (e.g. morphine 1–4 mg.kg^{-1}, fentanyl 10–100 µg.kg^{-1}) with benzodiazepines to obtain unconsciousness. Exponents of the latter technique claim greater cardiovascular stability, especially if nitrous oxide is avoided, and this may be valuable in the poor-risk patient. A com-bination of these techniques may be used; con-sciousness is obtunded by an opioid in moderate dose and hypnosis then produced by a small dose of an induction agent.

As consciousness is lost, a muscle relaxant is administered and ventilation supported when necessary. Atracurium or vecuronium may be associated with bradycardia, especially in the β-blocked patient. Pancuronium is preferred. The objective is to undertake tracheal intubation with-out cardiovascular stimulation and thus adequate analgesia/anaesthesia is required. A low-pressure high-volume cuffed tracheal tube should be used. Positive pressure ventilation is continued, usually with 50% nitrous oxide in oxygen.

Percutaneous cannulation of a subclavian or internal jugular vein is performed, using a multi-lumen catheter to allow monitoring and infu-sion. Nasopharyngeal and peripheral temperature probes are applied and a urinary catheter inserted. Mechanical ventilation is continued with a breath-ing system containing a humidifier and bacterial filter.

Previously identified 'poor risk' patients may require more extensive monitoring of pressures and cardiac output before induction and these are established under local anaesthesia. Induction should be undertaken in theatre with the full team ready for immediate surgery. Adequate sedation must be provided during insertion of invasive monitoring lines.

Maintenance – prebypass

During this period, surgical procedure involves preparation of the patient, skin incision, sternotomy and insertion of arterial and venous bypass cannulae. Anaesthetic management is designed to maintain stability of heart rate and arterial pressure, particularly at moments of profound stimulation, notably skin incision and sternotomy. Additional i.v. analgesic drug or inhalational anaesthetic should be given before stimulation. Large doses of opioids may be required; supplementation with volatile anaesthetic agents is effective, although their negative inotropic actions may be undesirable in those with poor ventricular function. The importance of 'coronary steal' (the diversion of blood *away from* ischaemic muscle) with isoflurane remains unclear. Two large studies have failed to demonstrate any influence of primary anaesthetic agent (including isoflurane) on outcome. Recently, the intravenous infusion of propofol 10 mg.kg^{-1}.h^{-1} during this period, in combination with fentanyl, has been described.

The alternative to deepening anaesthesia/analgesia is to counteract hypertension with vasodilators (phentolamine 1–2 mg or infusion of sodium nitroprusside 1–5 µg.kg^{-1}.min^{-1} or glyceryl trinitrate 0.5–5 µg.kg^{-1}.min^{-1}) and to treat tachycardia with a β-blocker.

Arterial blood gases, serum potassium concentration, haematocrit and the activated clotting time (ACT) should be measured when surgery is under way and conditions are stable. Before cannulation for bypass lines, heparin (300 units.kg^{-1}; 3 mg.kg^{-1}) should be injected into a secure central line of proven patency. In some units, the surgeon injects heparin directly into the left atrium before cannulation. ACT measurement should be repeated 5 min after injection of heparin; the value should exceed four times normal. Cardioplegia should be prepared and stored at 4°C.

When preparations are complete, the bypass pump commences and circulation is assumed by the extracorporeal circuit.

Maintenance – on bypass

Two factors complicate the provision of anaesthesia during cardiopulmonary bypass. Firstly, the dilutional effect of the crystalloid prime reduces the concentration of drugs administered previously. Secondly, by shortcircuiting the lungs, bypass prevents inhalational anaesthesia. Techniques therefore include the administration of bolus doses of opioids or benzodiazepines, administration of a volatile agent into the gas flow of the oxygenator or continuous intravenous infusion of propofol 3–6 mg.kg^{-1}.h^{-1}. The last of these is increasingly popular. Additional doses of muscle relaxant may also be given. When full pump oxygenator flow is reached and ventricular ejection ceases, ventilation is suspended.

Surgery is usually preceded by cross-clamping the aorta to isolate the heart and prevent backflow. In the case of valvular surgery, the appropriate valve is exposed, excised and a new valve sutured in place. During coronary artery vein grafting, the distal anastomoses are usually completed first and, following release of the cross-clamp to permit restoration of myocardial perfusion, the proximal anastomoses are constructed using a portion of the aorta isolated by a side-clamp (Fig. 39.7).

Myocardial preservation

Most surgical techniques on the heart require an immobile heart. On bypass, the aorta is cross-clamped between the aortic cannula and the aortic valve, thus isolating the heart from the flow of oxygenated blood. During aortic cross-clamping, ischaemic damage to the myocardium can be minimized by attempts to reduce myocardial oxygen consumption. Currently, techniques of myocardial preservation include hypothermia to reduce basal metabolic rate and cardiac arrest to reduce oxygen requirements to a minimum, the latter achieved by injecting 500–1000 ml of crystalloid cardioplegic solution around the coronary arteries. Many cardioplegic solutions are available; the majority contain potassium and a

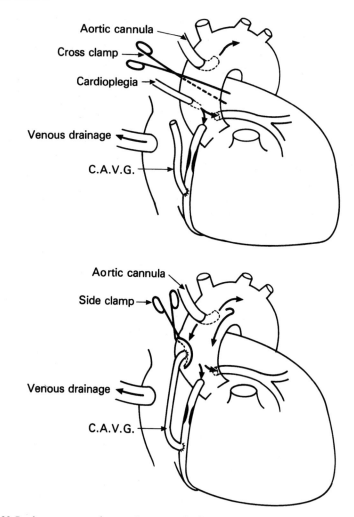

Fig. 39.7 Arrangement of cross-clamp, cardioplegia and anastomoses.

membrane stabilizing agent, e.g. procaine. Recently, continuous infusion of warm bloodbased cardioplegic solutions has been used by some centres to minimize ischaemic and reperfusion injuries and improve delivery of oxygen and other substrates to the myocardium.

Cooling is achieved by the use of ice-cold cardioplegia and by pouring cold fluid (4°C) into the pericardial sac and into the heart chambers if they have been opened. If the heart is cooled to 15°C it withstands total ischaemia for approximately 1 h. The technique used most commonly at present involves moderate hypothermia of the body to 28–32°C and local cooling of the myocardium to a temperature of 15–18°C. If cross-clamping times are prolonged, cardioplegic cooling must be repeated if evidence of spontaneous cardiac contraction is seen or the temperature of the heart increases above 18°C.

Perfusion on bypass

At normothermia, a pump flow of 2.4 litre. $min^{-1}.m^{-2}$ of body surface area is required to prevent inadequate perfusion of the tissues. The pressure achieved within the vascular system is dependent on pump output and systemic vascular resistance. Controversy exists regarding optimum perfusion pressure as essential organs, particularly the brain, may be damaged if mean arterial pressure is < 45 mmHg.

Following the institution of bypass, there are

usually marked decreases in peripheral resistance and arterial pressure, which in most instances resolve spontaneously in 5–10 min. If this does not occur, arterial pressure may be increased by raising systemic resistance with a sympathomimetic agent, e.g. methoxamine 1–5 mg. Frequently, systemic vascular resistance increases during and after bypass as a result of increasing plasma concentrations of catecholamines. If the mean arterial pressure exceeds 100 mmHg, vasodilators may be required.

Perfusion is difficult to assess clinically, especially in the hypothermic patient. Urine output and the cerebral function monitor may give some guidance.

Coagulation control

Adequate anticoagulation must be maintained during CPB; ACT should be measured every 30 min and extra heparin administered if it decreases below 480 s.

Oxygen delivery

Arterial blood samples should be obtained regularly and blood gases and haematocrit measured. Oxygen carriage is dependent on haemoglobin concentration in addition to adequate oxygen tension. Haematocrit may be permitted to decrease to 20% but further reduction should be prevented by the addition of packed cells or blood to the bypass circuit.

Acid–base balance

The development of metabolic acidosis suggests that perfusion is inadequate and if necessary (base deficit > 6–8 mmol.litre^{-1}), sodium bicarbonate may be administered.

Serum potassium

Serum potassium concentration should be maintained at approximately 4.5 mmol.litre^{-1} by the administration of potassium chloride (10–20 mmol) as required.

Restoration of spontaneous heart beat

When the cross-clamp has been removed, oxygenated blood again flows into the coronary arteries, washing out cardioplegia and repaying the oxygen debt. Usually, the heart regains activity spontaneously. In a minority of patients it starts to beat in sinus rhythm but reverts usually to ventricular fibrillation; internal defibrillation is required to convert fibrillation to sinus rhythm and is successful only if pH, serum potassium concentration, oxygenation and temperature are approaching normal values. The heat exchanger in the oxygenator is used to raise the temperature of blood but peripheral temperature is often depressed for some time. If a spontaneous heart beat cannot be maintained, pacing wires should be attached to the epicardium to initiate activity artificially.

At this stage, full bypass is maintained and although the heart is beating, there is little ejection from the ventricles. It is wise at this time to pause, ensure that all air has been vented from the heart chambers, wait until core temperature exceeds 36°C and rest the heart before it is required to pump again.

Termination of bypass

When body temperature exceeds 36°C, metabolic indices are normal and a regular heart beat present, the establishment of spontaneous cardiac output is attempted. An increasing volume of venous return is diverted into the right atrium past the extracorporeal cannulae by constricting the venous return line to the pump. Blood is now passing again through the pulmonary circulation and mechanical ventilation should be restarted. 100% oxygen is given, as the gas-exchanging efficiency of the lung is unknown at this stage and any air bubbles which have not been vented enlarge in volume if nitrous oxide is introduced.

Any output or ejection from the left ventricle gives a 'blip' on the arterial pressure trace after a QRS complex. If the myocardium is contracting satisfactorily, pump flow is reduced cautiously and the heart, now receiving all the venous return, achieves normal output. At this time small doses of ephedrine, adrenaline or calcium chloride may provide a temporary inotropic stimulus.

Arterial pressure is the most easily measured index of successful termination of bypass but is a derivative of cardiac output and peripheral resistance. If there is doubt regarding pump efficiency, cardiac output should be measured and peripheral resistance derived. Peripheral resistance is increased consistently during bypass and much of the subsequent care of many patients is directed towards producing peripheral dilatation and perfusion.

If CPB is discontinued successfully, preload should be optimized (left atrial pressure 12–15 mmHg) by infusion of as much as possible of the residual fluid contained in the pump circuit. This is facilitated by the administration of vasodilators, e.g. sodium nitroprusside (SNP) or glyceryl trinitrate (GTN). If cardiac output is inadequate, the circulation is reassumed by the extracorporeal pump and the heart allowed more time to recover.

Low output

If the heart is unable to generate sufficient output to maintain body perfusion after preload has been optimized, further action is required. An increase in contractility is produced by inotropic drugs. The simplest is a bolus of calcium chloride but the most commonly employed drugs are dobutamine or dopamine $(2–20\ \mu g.kg^{-1}.min^{-1})$ by infusion. Adrenaline $(0.05–0.2\ \mu g.kg^{-1}.min^{-1})$ or, if heart rate is slow, isoprenaline $(0.02–0.2\ \mu g.kg^{-1}.min^{-1})$ may be indicated in some patients.

All these drugs tend to precipitate tachyarrhythmias; adrenaline and dopamine also cause vasoconstriction in high doses. They all increase myocardial oxygen demand and may precipitate infarction in patients with ischaemic heart disease.

An alternative approach is to assist output by reducing the afterload with vasodilators. As described previously, reduced afterload not only reduces oxygen demand but also, in the failing ventricle, augments forward flow into the aorta. Diastolic pressure must not be reduced excessively if oxygen supply to the ventricle is not to be jeopardized. Infusion of fluid may be required during dilatation to maintain preload at adequate levels. In acute low output syndromes, vasodilators are usually prescribed in addition to inotropic

agents and the drugs may have a cumulative effect in raising cardiac index, permitting a reduction in the dosage of inotropic agents. SNP reduces both preload and afterload but may cause a 'steal' from areas of ischaemic myocardium. GTN is largely a venous dilator, but also reduces myocardial ischaemia by coronary and collateral vasodilatation. In higher doses it may cause arteriolar dilatation and reduce blood pressure. Both drugs inhibit hypoxic pulmonary vasoconstriction and may aggravate hypoxaemia.

More recently a group of drugs combining inotropic and vasodilating activity has been introduced. These drugs act by inhibiting cardiac phosphodiesterase III, thus reducing the breakdown of cyclic AMP. Milrinone and enoximone are the most commonly used examples. They improve cardiac performance and are potent arterial and venous dilators. Used alone, they can improve myocardial oxygen balance in the failing ventricle but are more effective if combined with a catecholamine as the two groups of drugs have complementary actions.

If these pharmacological methods fail to produce an adequate cardiac output, the intra-aortic balloon pump (IABP) may be used.

Intra-aortic balloon pump. The principle of the IABP is illustrated in Figure 39.8. If the balloon in the aorta is inflated immediately after systole, diastolic filling pressure is augmented and myocardial oxygen balance improved. Inflation also displaces blood from the aorta and increases peripheral flow. The balloon is deflated immediately before systole and this creates a low pressure in the aorta as ventricular output commences, reducing afterload (and thus oxygen consumption) and at the same time augmenting output. It is remarkably successsful in some patients with a persistent low output syndrome.

Coagulation control

When the bypass cannulae have been removed, residual effects of heparin are antagonized with protamine. Protamine 1 mg (or less) is given for each 100 units of heparin; the dosage may be titrated using the ACT. The drug should be given slowly, especially if there is residual hypovolaemia or raised pulmonary vascular resistance.

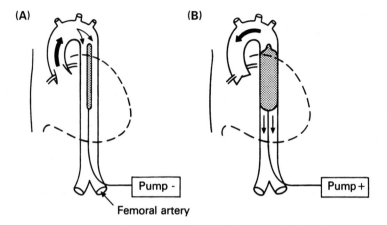

Fig. 39.8   Intra-aortic balloon pump (IABP) : **A** systole; **B** diastole.

Protamine may produce systemic hypotension rapidly, as a result of peripheral vasodilatation, but may also cause pulmonary vasoconstriction. In excessive dosage, it has anticoagulant effects.

Heparin is not the only factor which may cause bleeding during and after bypass. Contact of blood with foreign surfaces in the bypass circuit and suction tubing causes consumption of clotting factors and of platelets. Thus, if heparin appears to have been reversed satisfactorily and unexplained bleeding persists, a full clotting screen should be performed, including estimation of platelet numbers. Clotting factors may be replaced by the infusion of fresh frozen plasma and/or cryoprecipitate and platelet concentrate should be infused if the platelet count is less than 60×10^9 litre^{-1}.

Surgically, the period following termination of bypass is concerned with prevention of haemorrhage and closure of the chest with drains in situ. In addition to the maintenance of unconsciousness, the anaesthetist must ensure the efficiency of myocardial performance, oxygen balance and peripheral perfusion together with correction of metabolic, biochemical, haematological or temperature abnormalities.

CONTROL OF THE CIRCULATION AFTER BYPASS

Despite measures to protect the myocardium during bypass, the heart suffers some deterioration in function and its contractility is reduced for several hours. Thus, it operates on a lower Frank–Starling curve (see Fig. 39.5) and requires a higher preload to produce the same output. Usually, a left atrial pressure of 12–15 mmHg is optimal. The contractility of the myocardium improves in the first 3–4 h after bypass and this increased efficiency permits a reduction in preload.

In addition, the peripheral circulation remains vasoconstricted for several hours postoperatively. In patients with reasonable ventricular function, hypertension often occurs after bypass, especially in operations involving the aortic valve or revascularization. The increased afterload results in additional myocardial oxygen consumption and tends to reduce cardiac output.

Reduction of peripheral resistance and systemic arterial pressure by a vasodilator (e.g. SNP or GTN) protects suture lines from damage, decreases oxygen demand, increases cardiac output if preload is not reduced excessively, improves peripheral perfusion and accelerates warming.

Other aspects of maintenance after bypass

In addition to maintaining cardiac function and oxygen supply to the tissues during this period, the anaesthetist should ensure that normality is regained as soon as possible, and maintained, in respect of the following.

1. Temperature

Core temperature is raised easily on bypass via the

oxygenator. However, the efficiency of rewarming the peripheral tissues depends on the patient's weight, total flow rate and peripheral perfusion. After bypass, there is often a decrease in core temperature (afterdrop).

2. Biochemical monitoring

Essential monitoring includes blood gases, acid–base balance, serum potassium concentration and haematocrit.

3. Cardiac rhythm

Heart block. Epicardial pacing lines should be inserted if AV dissociation occurs, traditionally to allow ventricular pacing. Atrial pacing (for brady-cardia) or AV sequential pacing (for heart block) ensure that the atrial contribution to ventricular filling is not lost. Infusion of isoprenaline may improve ventricular rate as a temporary measure.

Supraventricular arrhythmias. Direct current cardioversion is the most convenient treatment when the chest is open. After chest closure, options include digoxin, β-blockade, verapamil, amiodarone or adenosine.

Ventricular arrhythmias. The threshold for arrhythmias is reduced by hypokalaemia and serum potassium concentration should be maintained above 4.5 mmol.litre^{-1}. If ventricular arrhythmias persist, lignocaine is the drug of first choice.

Transfer to postoperative ITU

It is normal to prolong the same level of support and monitoring undertaken during surgery into the postoperative period. The duration of this care depends on the individual patient's response to surgery and speed of recovery.

Transfer of the patient from theatre to the intensive care unit may involve journeys along corridors and into lifts. It is essential that con-trolled ventilation is continued and ECG, arterial oxygen saturation and arterial pressure monitored during transfer. Battery-powered infusion pumps are essential to allow uninterrupted vasoactive drug infusions during transfer. A bolus dose of opioid may be required before transfer; alterna-tively, an infusion of propofol may be continued.

POSTOPERATIVE INTENSIVE THERAPY

The facilities and staff used to treat patients after cardiac surgery vary considerably. Some hospitals nurse these patients in a general ITU while others have specialist cardiac ITUs. Attempts have recently been made in some centres to circumvent the problem of limited numbers of ITU beds by admitting patients to cardiac surgery recovery areas and aiming for early extubation with a rapid reduction in dependency level.

Regardless of location, there should be a well-practised routine for the care of patients after surgery. Usually, ventilation of the lungs and full cardiovascular monitoring are recommenced immediately. The principles of care in this phase are similar to those described for the period of anaesthesia after termination of bypass.

Haemodynamic care

On return to ITU, attention is directed towards achieving vasodilatation, reduction of afterload and maintenance of preload. Blood transfusion is required if the haematocrit is less than 35%. Urine output may be maintained with diuretics but usually a spontaneous diuresis occurs in re-sponse to the crystalloid load received in theatre. Serum potassium concentration must be moni-tored carefully and abnormalities corrected.

The majority of patients stabilize and regain adequate peripheral perfusion over the succeeding 3–4 h, permitting the level of cardiovascular support to be reduced.

In a minority of patients, low cardiac output requires the continued use of inotropic agents, vasodilators and, if necessary, IABP for some time.

Blood loss

This should be measured accurately. If excessive (300–400 ml.h^{-1}), it may be necessary to reoperate on the patient. Attention to the coagulation system is required and additional protamine or coagulation factors prescribed as necessary. The most sinister complication of excessive bleeding is cardiac tamponade which requires rapid thora-cotomy and evacuation of blood from the chest.

If deterioration is rapid, thoracotomy must be undertaken in the ITU.

Ventilation

In the 1960s, morphine anaesthesia for valve surgery in patients with poor ventricular function dictated postoperative ventilation for 18–24 h. Later, the aims of postoperative ventilation were to avoid shivering following hypothermic bypass and to prevent hypoxaemia and hypercapnia during the period of haemodynamic instability which is common in the first few postoperative hours. These aims were generally achieved by assisting ventilation for 4–12 h and this remains current practice in many units. Thus, when the patient's arterial pressure, peripheral perfusion and core and peripheral temperatures are satisfactory, urine output is good, blood loss less than 100 ml.h^{-1}, the patient is conscious and can maintain satisfactory blood gases with an inspired oxygen concentration of 50% or less, a trial of spontaneous ventilation is indicated. If respiratory volumes are adequate and the patient is not distressed, the trachea may be extubated.

However, advances in anaesthetic, surgical and perfusion techniques have prompted some centres to aim for earlier extubation. The trachea is extubated either on the operating table or within 2 h of surgery, provided that the criteria for extubation detailed above are met. This demands changes in the practices of all those caring for cardiac surgery patients. Cross-clamp and bypass times must be brief. Intermittent cross-clamping with fibrillation rather than cold cardioplegia and systemic hypothermia may be necessary. Active vasodilator therapy during rewarming minimizes temperature afterdrop following cardiopulmonary bypass. Anaesthetic techniques include the use of relatively small doses of fentanyl (1.5–15 µg.kg^{-1}) or its substitution with alfentanil, substitution of pancuronium by atracurium or vecuronium and the use of inhalational agents or propofol infusion for maintenance of anaesthesia. Haemodynamic stability is more difficult to achieve and these techniques are currently not for the inexperienced.

Unfortunately, some patients still require prolonged ventilation after cardiac surgery. Principles of their care are as detailed in Chapter 41.

Analgesia

The anaesthetic technique employed determines the timing of administration of postoperative analgesia. Even after high-dose opioid techniques, patients usually show some response in the first 2–3 h after surgery and it is useful to assess cerebral function at this stage in case damage has occurred. Pain relief is achieved most commonly with i.v. opioids either by bolus dose or continuous infusion. This has traditionally been supplemented with a benzodiazepine, but low-dose propofol infusion (1–2 mg.kg^{-1}.h^{-1}) is increasingly common. Recovery is rapid after the infusion is stopped and this may facilitate early extubation. Regional analgesic techniques are not popular because coagulation defects are common, but the use of prebypass intrathecal opioids and postoperative extradural analgesia has been reported.

As important as pharmacological support is the human rapport which should be achieved between staff and patient.

FURTHER READING

Gothard J W W 1987 Anaesthesia for cardiac surgery. Blackwell Scientific Publications, Oxford

Kaplan H A (ed) 1993 Cardiac anesthesia, 3rd edn. Grune and Stratton, New York

Hensley F A, Martin D A (eds) 1990 The practice of cardiac anesthesia. Little, Brown, Boston

Nimmo W S, Rowbotham D J, Smith G (eds) 1994 Anaesthesia, 2nd edn. Blackwell Scientific Publications, Oxford

Thomas S J, Kramer J L (eds) 1993 Manual of cardiac anaesthesia, 2nd edn. Churchill Livingstone, Edinburgh

40. Intercurrent disease and anaesthesia

Many patients presenting for surgery suffer from unrelated disease, for which they may be receiving drug treatment. The course of this disease may be modified by anaesthesia and surgery, while the disease process itself may influence the effects of anaesthesia.

The aims of anaesthetic management in such patients are:

1. To assess the extent of the medical problem.
2. To ensure that the patient's condition is optimized in the time available before surgery (this may vary widely between emergency and elective surgery).
3. To conduct anaesthesia and postoperative care using drugs and techniques which have the least detrimental effect on the medical condition.

To achieve these aims, all patients who present for surgery require a full clinical history and examination. A past medical history, including previous anaesthesia, drug and allergy history and examination of previous anaesthetic records (if available) may be particularly important. In addition, special investigations may be necessary depending on the age and fitness of the patient and the nature of the surgery (see Chapter 18).

CARDIOVASCULAR DISEASE

General principles

Anaesthesia for patients with cardiovascular disease involves the application of a number of basic principles:

1. Adequate oxygenation must be maintained throughout.

2. Cardiac output must be maintained at a level commensurate with adequate tissue perfusion.
3. Systemic arterial pressure must be adequate to maintain major organ perfusion, and in particular to maintain cerebral, coronary, renal and hepatic blood flow.
4. The balance of myocardial oxygen supply and demand must be preserved, thus minimizing the risk of perioperative ischaemia and infarction (Table 40.1).

This demands a knowledge of the physiological mechanisms governing cardiac output, myocardial oxygen availability and consumption, and the adjustments that occur in disease states. An

Table 40.1 Factors affecting myocardial oxygen supply and consumption

Supply
Coronary perfusion pressure (diastolic pressure – LVEDP)
Arterial oxygen tension
Haemoglobin concentration
Coronary vascular resistance
  Intraluminal obstruction
  External compression
    Heart rate
    LVEDP
  Autoregulation – dependent on myocardial oxygen consumption

Consumption
Heart rate
Contractility
Wall tension
  LVEDP
  Arterial pressure
  Contractility
External work
  Cardiac output
  Arterial pressure

LVEDP = Left ventricular end-diastolic pressure.

understanding of the effects of intravenous (i.v.) and volatile anaesthetic agents, and muscle relaxants, allows a choice to be made of appropriate drugs and techniques. Reversible risk factors (e.g. cardiac failure or hypertension) must be detected and treated preoperatively.

Preoperative assessment

History

Symptoms which suggest cardiovascular disease include dyspnoea, chest pain, palpitations, ankle swelling and intermittent claudication. Severity of symptoms assessed by a history of exercise tolerance is the most useful estimate of severity of cardiovascular disease.

Past medical history and previous medical records usually reveal the nature and severity of disease. A number of factors relating to history, clinical examination and proposed surgery are associated with an increased risk of perioperative cardiac complications, such as myocardial infarction (see Table 18.4). For example, the date of a previous myocardial infarction must be noted and elective surgery should not be performed within 6 months of that date. Unstable angina may also be associated with an increased risk of perioperative infarction, and should be investigated and treated before elective surgery. This may necessitate coronary arteriography. Previous thromboembolic disease necessitates prophylactic measures, e.g. low-dose heparin or intermittent calf compression.

Concurrent drug treatment

Digoxin. The dose should be assessed on the basis of age, weight and renal function, and reduced in the elderly, in patients with impaired renal function or if the plasma digoxin concentration exceeds the therapeutic range. Serum potassium concentration should be measured, especially when there is concurrent diuretic therapy, and symptoms of digoxin toxicity, e.g. nausea and vomiting, should be sought. Heart rate and rhythm require assessment. In excessive dosage, especially with concurrent hypokalaemia, ventricular arrhythmias or heart block may occur.

Diuretics. Serum potassium concentration should always be measured, and hypokalaemia corrected.

Anticoagulants. Where long-term therapy is indicated, perioperative control must be monitored closely. Warfarin should be stopped 48 h preoperatively, and the prothrombin time monitored daily; it should not be greater than 1.5 times control at the time of surgery. If prolonged, administration of vitamin K is indicated, while for emergency surgery, or if undue bleeding occurs, fresh frozen plasma should be given. After minor surgery, warfarin may be restarted on the first postoperative day; after major surgery, a heparin infusion may be used to maintain anticoagulation (with control by thrombin time estimations) until warfarin therapy is restarted. This allows rapid reversal of anticoagulation with protamine 1 mg for every 100 units of heparin if bleeding occurs. Protamine should be administered slowly to avoid hypotension and, if given in excessive dosage, is itself an anticoagulant.

β-Adrenergic blockers. In most instances, β-blockade should be maintained throughout the perioperative period, although the dose of β-blocker should be reduced if undue bradycardia (heart rate less than 55 beat.min^{-1}) is present. Sudden preoperative cessation may be associated with rebound angina, myocardial infarction, arrhythmia or hypertension perioperatively. Intravenous atropine or glycopyrrolate may be given prior to induction or, if undue bradycardia occurs, intraoperatively. β-Blockers may contribute to and mask the signs of hypoglycaemia. Most patients are now treated with long-acting cardioselective agents taken once daily, such as atenolol or bisoprolol.

Calcium-channel blockers. These drugs (Table 40.2) block the slow influx of calcium ions which contribute to depolarization. *Verapamil*, which acts predominantly on the atrioventricular (AV) node, is used in the management of supraventricular tachyarrhythmias, angina, hypertension and hypertrophic obstructive cardiomyopathy. As

Table 40.2 Calcium-channel blockers

Mostly vasodilator: nifedipine, nicardipine, amlodipine
Vasodilator, negative chronotrope: diltiazem
Negative inotrope and chronotrope, vasodilator: verapamil

it increases AV block, concurrent use with digoxin or β-blockers should be avoided, as should halothane and enflurane anaesthesia. *Nifedipine*, which acts predominantly on vascular smooth muscle, is used in the management of angina, hypertension and in Raynaud's phenomenon. *Diltiazem* lies between verapamil and nifedipine in terms of its effect. There is some evidence that the risk of myocardial ischaemia is increased as a result of coronary steal when isoflurane is used in patients receiving nifedipine. *Nimodipine* is predominantly a cerebral vasodilator, and is used to prevent vasospasm associated with subarachnoid haemorrhage.

Angiotensin-converting enzyme (ACE) inhibitors. These drugs produce vasodilatation by inhibiting conversion of angiotensin I to angiotensin II, a potent vasoconstrictor and stimulant of aldosterone secretion. Their main uses are in the treatment of cardiac failure, in which reduction of afterload improves left ventricular function and cardiac output, and in hypertension. They may predispose to renal failure, particularly in the presence of renovascular disease or if hypotension occurs, and can cause hyperkalaemia.

The presence of vasodilator or heart rate-limiting drugs of whatever type, whether alone or in combination, has an adverse effect on the patient's ability to tolerate the effects of anaesthetic agents or acute hypovolaemia.

Examination

Preoperative cardiovascular examination should include measurement of heart rate and rhythm, arterial pressure, assessment of peripheral perfusion and detection of signs of cardiac failure. The presence of a third heart sound or an elevated JVP have been shown to have prognostic significance for perioperative cardiac morbidity. Hypertension and cardiac murmurs are not infrequently a chance finding, and require further assessment before surgery. The murmur most commonly encountered as an incidental pre-operative finding is an aortic systolic murmur. This may represent aortic sclerosis or stenosis. It is particularly important to define whether significant stenosis exists. A normal-character pulse, normal pulse pressure and normal second heart sound suggest that aortic stenosis is less likely.

Investigations

In addition to routine haematological and biochemical investigations, an electrocardiogram (ECG) is important as a baseline before surgery for the diagnosis of arrhythmias, to provide confirmatory evidence of ischaemic heart disease and to assess the severity of cardiac disease, e.g. hypertension, cor pulmonale and valvular heart disease. However a normal ECG is common in ischaemic heart disease, and exercise testing may disclose ischaemia in these patients. While Holter 24-h ECG monitoring is useful in revealing transient ST segment changes or arrhythmias.

Chest X-ray provides information on heart and chamber sizes, the state of the pulmonary vasculature and evidence of pulmonary oedema and infection.

Echocardiography is used to diagnose valve lesions, to detect intracardiac thrombus and pericardial effusion, and to assess global or segmental cardiac function. Cardiac Doppler examination allows assessment of pressure gradients across valves.

Cardiac catheterization and coronary angiography are rarely indicated before routine non-cardiac surgery.

Preoperative treatment

Cardiac failure, arrhythmias, hypertension and angina should be controlled before surgery. The conventional treatment of cardiac failure with diuretics has been augmented by the use of ACE inhibitors such as enalapril. This has been shown to improve symptoms and reduce mortality in patients with left ventricular dysfunction (New York Heart Association, grades III and IV). Anaemia should be treated — if necessary with blood transfusion — at least 48 h before surgery; supplementary diuretic cover may be necessary during transfusion. Haemoglobin concentration should be greater than 10 g.dl^{-1} before surgery.

Premedication

In ischaemic heart disease and hypertension, premedication should be adequate to allay anxiety. A benzodiazepine such as temazepam is usually satisfactory. In patients with low or fixed cardiac output states (e.g. mitral or aortic stenosis, constrictive pericarditis) or congestive cardiac failure, premedication should be light, and in poor-risk patients, it may be preferable to omit premedication altogether. The patient's usual cardiac medications should normally be continued and be included in the premedication.

Anaesthesia

In practical terms, this involves maintenance of a normal heart rate, and an arterial pressure adequate to maintain coronary perfusion and oxygenation without increasing cardiac work and thus myocardial oxygen requirements. Excessive myocardial depression should be avoided.

The high-risk periods during anaesthesia are:

1. *Induction.* Most induction agents are cardiovascular depressants, and in patients with low or fixed cardiac output, hypertension or hypovolaemia, hypotension may occur. Of the agents currently available, etomidate has the least depressant effect on the cardiovascular system; propofol or thiopentone may cause significant hypotension due to direct myocardial depression and reduction of systemic vascular resistance. Of the numerous neuromuscular blocking drugs, atracurium and vecuronium produce least (and negligible) cardiovascular effects. The administration of a short-acting opioid such as alfentanil or fentanyl before induction allows reduction in induction dose and may limit the hypertensive response to intubation.

2. *Intubation.* Tracheal intubation is commonly associated with hypertension and tachycardia.

3. *Postoperative period.* Rebound hypertension occurs commonly in association with pain and peripheral vasoconstriction. Good analgesia is necessary, as is careful attention to optimisation of intravascular volume.

Careful monitoring is essential and must always include heart rate, arterial pressure and ECG. It should be instituted before induction, and maintained throughout the immediate postoperative period (if necessary in the intensive therapy unit (ITU). The common ECG configuration used for anaesthetic monitoring is standard limb lead II. Whilst this is useful for differentiating arrhythmias, myocardial ischaemia occurs most commonly in the left ventricle and is detected more sensitively

with a CM_5 configuration (see Fig. 20.3). The use of pulse oximetry is mandatory to avoid periods of desaturation, while end-tidal carbon dioxide monitoring allows ventilation to be set to maintain normocapnia and gives early warning of acute haemodynamic disturbances. In high-risk patients undergoing major surgery, intra-arterial cannulation and central venous pressure (CVP) measurements are indicated. Placement of a pulmonary artery flotation catheter (PAFC) is indicated in patients with severe ischaemic heart disease, left ventricular failure or shock, and in those scheduled for more major vascular or cardiac surgery. The PAFC allows measurement of pulmonary artery pressure, pulmonary artery occlusion pressure (PAOP; wedge pressure) and cardiac output, and sampling of pulmonary artery blood for mixed venous oxyhaemoglobin saturation (Svo_2) The PAOP reflects left ventricular end-diastolic pressure (LVEDP), a major determinant of myocardial oxygen supply and demand, while cardiac output determines tissue oxygen delivery. Fibreoptic pulmonary artery catheters allow continuous monitoring of Svo_2, which closely reflects cardiac output in low-flow states and may be of most practical use in theatre. Use of a PAFC may greatly aid preoperative optimisation of cardiac function in patients with severe cardiac dysfunction.

Hypertension

Untreated hypertension is associated with increased perioperative morbidity and mortality, and increased risk of cerebrovascular accident and myocardial infarction. Even mild hypertension has an important effect on long-term mortality. Because arterial pressure increases with age, an acceptable maximum pressure is difficult to define, but elective surgery should rarely be undertaken when the resting diastolic pressure exceeds 110 mmHg. Control of hypertension is usually achieved using a thiazide diuretic, with the possible addition of a β-blocker and/or a vasodilator, such as a calcium-channel blocker, e.g. nifedipine or amlodipine. β-Blockers are often contraindicated in the presence of obstructive airways disease, left ventricular dysfunction, peripheral vascular disease and bradyarrhythmias, and in these situations a peripheral vasodilator calcium-channel blocker would be preferred. ACE inhibitors may be used if left ventricular dysfunction or failure is present.

If hypertension is an unexpected preoperative finding, surgery should be delayed, if possible, until investigations are performed and treatment started. Endocrine and renal causes should be excluded. Complications of hypertension (e.g. myocardial ischaemia, cardiac failure and renal impairment) should be sought, and unstable angina and cardiac failure controlled before surgery. Appropriate investigation might include chest X-ray, ECG, echocardiography and renal ultrasound. Antihypertensive therapy should be continued throughout the perioperative period, although the dose of β-blocker may need to be reduced depending upon resting heart rate.

Anaesthesia

Premedication should be generous. Anaesthetic management should be directed towards avoidance of hypotension and, more particularly, hypertension. Close monitoring of arterial pressure and ECG is required from before induction through anaesthesia and the postoperative period. Blood loss should also be monitored carefully, and deficits replaced promptly. Hypertensive patients are particularly vulnerable to the development of hypotension following induction of anaesthesia or following establishment of subarachnoid or extradural blockade. Etomidate has least cardiovascular effects, but thiopentone is acceptable if administered carefully. Propofol may produce excessive hypotension. Ketamine is contraindicated in anaesthetic dosages. Pancuronium should be avoided in severe hypertension; atracurium and vecuronium are suitable relaxants. Tracheal intubation may cause hypertension, tachycardia and arrhythmias. Administration of a rapidly acting opioid (fentanyl 3–5 μg.kg^{-1} or alfentanil 20 μg.kg^{-1}) before induction attenuates this response, and also reduces the requirements for the induction agent.

For maintenance of anaesthesia, a nitrous oxide/oxygen/opioid/relaxant technique is appropriate in many instances. Volatile agents possess marked cardiovascular depressant effects, and require careful administration. However, they are suitable for minor procedures with a spontaneous breathing technique. Intraoperatively, nodal arrhythmias occur commonly, especially with halothane, and may produce a decrease in cardiac output. Depending on heart rate, i.v. atropine or glycopyrrolate or a decrease of the inspired halothane concentration may be effective in treating arrhythmias. The reduced left ventricular compliance and more rigid vascular tree found in hypertensive patients makes them more vulnerable to small changes in blood volume. Furthermore, β-blockers prevent the physiological heart rate response to intraoperative blood loss, while vasodilators prevent vasoconstriction. Thus, careful monitoring of blood and fluid loss, and of CVP, is important, and prompt replacement of fluid deficits is necessary to avoid undue hypotension. Local anaesthetic preparations containing catecholamine vasoconstrictors should be avoided.

Postoperative hypertension occurs frequently, partly as a result of inadequate analgesia, and partly because of peripheral vasoconstriction which occurs during prolonged surgery with associated heat loss and bleeding. Plasma adrenaline concentrations may be increased markedly. Hypertension increases myocardial work and oxygen demand, and may cause subendocardial ischaemia or infarction in patients with left ventricular hypertrophy or enlargement. Good analgesia is essential, and continuous extradural analgesia is safe in treated hypertensive patients if monitored closely.

Hypertension should be treated promptly; labetalol titrated in 10–20 mg i.v. bolus doses, followed if necessary by an infusion, is usually effective. In the presence of peripheral vasoconstriction, a vasodilator (e.g. glyceryl trinitrate 1–5 mg.h^{-1} or hydralazine by 5–10 mg bolus) is usually effective. Nifedipine may be administered using the sublingual route until there is reliable restoration of gastrointestinal function.

If the patient has been managed preoperatively with oral β-blockers, a long-acting agent, e.g. atenolol or bisoprolol, should be given before surgery, and oral treatment recommenced on the day after surgery. In some instances, nasogastric administration or i.v. infusion may be necessary. Labetalol is an appropriate agent for infusion.

All hypotensive therapy requires careful arterial pressure monitoring, with a low threshold for intra-arterial measurement.

Ischaemic heart disease

Five per cent of patients over 35 years of age have asymptomatic ischaemic heart disease. In patients who have had a previous myocardial infarction, anaesthesia and surgery within 3 months of infarction carries a 40% risk of perioperative reinfarction. This rate decreases to 15% at 3–6 months and 5% thereafter. Recent work suggests that with intensive perioperative monitoring much lower rates of reinfarction can be achieved (at less than 3 months and at 3–6 months). Mortality from postoperative infarction is 40–60%. Elective surgery should generally be postponed until 6 months after infarction unless it is urgent.

Unstable angina is particularly associated with an increased risk of perioperative myocardial infarction. Low-dose aspirin (enteric-coated 300 mg or soluble 150 mg once daily) and systemic heparinisation decrease the incidence of acute myocardial infarct in this situation. Angina should also be controlled with β-blockade and i.v. nitrate infusion before surgery. There is no evidence that the incidence of postoperative infarction is reduced by using local or regional anaesthetic techniques.

Factors which precipitate further infarction are those which increase myocardial work and thus oxygen requirement, or which decrease coronary blood flow (Table 40.1).

Anaesthesia

Preoperatively, left ventricular failure should be treated with diuretics ACE inhibitors and nitrates. Anaemia should be corrected. Premedication should be adequate to allay anxiety. Oxygen therapy may be considered appropriate with premedication in some patients. The demands of anaesthetic management are similar to those which apply in the hypertensive patient: close monitoring, avoidance of tachycardia and bradycardia, maintenance of normotension or slight hypotension and careful choice of anaesthetic agent. β-blockade should be maintained, and this necessitates care in fluid replacement and concurrent drug administration.

Halothane depresses contractility and myocardial oxygen consumption, but coronary blood flow is depressed to a proportionately lesser extent;

thus, halothane is tolerated well in low concentrations. However, high concentrations of halothane may produce excessive myocardial depression with a profound decrease in cardiac output, increased LVEDP and myocardial ischaemia. These effects may be potentiated by β-blockade.

Enflurane dilates the peripheral circulation in addition to depressing myocardial contractility. Overall, it causes a decrease in arterial pressure comparable with that resulting from administration of halothane.

Isoflurane causes less reduction in cardiac output than enflurane or halothane. It is a potent vasodilator and has been implicated as a cause of coronary steal in patients with myocardial ischaemia. Although there is some dispute about the importance of this effect at high doses, it is likely that low concentrations of isoflurane (<0.5%) do not cause coronary steal. Desflurane increases heart rate and may cause increased activity in the sympathetic nervous system. Although it does not cause coronary steal, there is concern about its use in patients with ischaemic heart disease because of its chronotropic effect.

Sevoflurance appears to be satisfactory for use in patients with ischaemic heart disease, provided that hypotension is avoided.

Interactions between calcium-channel blockers and volatile anaesthetic agents may cause serious hypotension (Table 40.2).

Normocapnia should be maintained, because hypercapnia may provoke arrhythmias, while hypocapnia causes peripheral and coronary vasoconstriction and shifts the oxyhaemoglobin dissociation curve to the left. Postoperative monitoring, management of analgesia and control of arterial pressure must be meticulous.

Cardiac failure

Anaesthesia and surgery in patients with cardiac failure carry an increased risk of morbidity and mortality. The cause of heart failure should be elucidated, and treatment instituted before surgery.

Left heart failure causes pulmonary congestion and oedema, and decreases pulmonary compliance; respiratory work is increased and hypoxaemia occurs. Signs of failure include tachycardia, gallop rhythm, mitral regurgitation, cyanosis, tachypnoea, crepitations and wheeze. Causes include ischaemic heart disease, hypertension, rheumatic heart disease and congestive cardiomyopathy. It may be precipitated by arrhythmias, e.g. atrial fibrillation.

Treatment involves delivery of a high inspired oxygen concentration (with mechanical ventilation in severe cases), diuretic, opioid and nitrate (by infusion if failure is severe). The aim of treatment is to optimize both the left ventricular filling pressure and cardiac output. If failure is precipitated by arrhythmias, these should be treated, avoiding negatively inotropic drugs.

Right ventricular failure generally results from pulmonary hypertension. This is usually secondary either to left heart failure or to chronic lung disease (cor pulmonale). ECG evidence of right atrial enlargement and ventricular hypertrophy raises the suspicion of pulmonary hypertension. Hypoxaemia in such patients causes an exaggerated increase in pulmonary vascular resistance, provoking right ventricular failure. Acute right heart failure occurs commonly when patients with chronic obstructive airways disease suffer an acute infective exacerbation with hypoxaemia. Preoperative treatment of infection is important, and intra- and postoperative maintenance of the airway and avoidance of hypoxaemia are imperative.

The clinical features of biventricular failure may also be associated with salt and water overload and hypoalbuminaemia, e.g. in renal or hepatic disease.

Low subarachnoid or extradural block may be useful in some patients with cardiac failure, as the sympathetic block produces venodilatation and reduction in preload; however, a high block should be avoided.

Shock

Surgery should not be undertaken until adequate resuscitation of the patient has been undertaken. In cases of severe haemorrhage, only initial resuscitation may be possible before surgery, and resuscitation continued during operation until bleeding is controlled. Such patients require adequate oxygenation and ventilation, guided by regular blood gas measurements. Monitoring required during resuscitation and anaesthesia includes direct arterial pressure, heart rate, CVP and urine output. Core–peripheral temperature gradient is generally recommended as a useful measure of peripheral perfusion in shock. However, it is of no value in septic shock where vasoregulation is lost, and it is of limited value either as a measure of volume status in hypovolaemic shock or of cardiac output in cardiogenic shock. Pulmonary artery catheterization for measurement of PAOP, cardiac output and oxygen transport variables is essential to direct appropriate fluid and vasoactive drug therapy in cardiogenic and septic shock which proves not to be readily reversible with volume resuscitation.

Anaesthesia in shock

Adequate venous access with large-gauge cannulae (at least two; 14G or pulmonary artery catheter introducer) should be ensured before induction of anaesthesia. Minimal doses of induction agent should be employed. Etomidate is associated with least cardiovascular disturbance, but other agents, e.g. thiopentone, may be used with care in very low dosage. A nitrous oxide/oxygen/opioid/relaxant technique, using vecuronium (or pancuronium), is usually appropriate. In theatre, maintenance of oxygen saturation and an adequate mean arterial pressure are prime objectives. It may not be practicable to institute full haemodynamic monitoring preoperatively but this should be achieved as soon as possible, and continued into the intensive care unit postoperatively. Where hypotension is difficult to reverse, adrenaline by small bolus injection or infusion is appropriate first-line therapy. The management of shock is discussed in Chapters 31 and 41.

Arrhythmias (see also Chapters 15, 13 and 22)

Arrhythmias which are present preoperatively should be treated before surgery (which should be postponed if necessary). The most commonly occurring arrhythmia is probably atrial fibrillation, which is usually caused by ischaemic heart disease, mitral valve disease, hypertensive heart disease or thyrotoxicosis. The ventricular rate should be controlled with digoxin. If the ventricular rate is normal, digoxin should usually be started preoperatively to prevent an increase in ventricular rate during surgery.

Intraoperative arrhythmias

Approximately 12% of patients undergoing anaesthesia develop arrhythmias but this frequency increases to 30% in patients with cardiovascular disease. Treatment may not be required, depending on the nature of the arrhythmia and its effect on cardiac output. Single supraventricular or ventricular ectopic beats, and slow supraventricular rhythms, do not require treatment unless cardiac output is compromised.

Factors affecting intraoperative arrhythmias include:

1. *Spontaneous ventilation.* Raised arterial carbon dioxide tension (Pa_{CO_2}) may cause ventricular extrasystoles.

2. *Hypoxaemia.* Initially this causes tachycardia, then bradycardia.

3. *Anaesthetic agents.* Cyclopropane and halogenated hydrocarbons, e.g. halothane, are associated with an increased incidence of ventricular arrhythmias, especially if Pa_{CO_2} is raised.

4. *Catecholamines.* Local anaesthetic preparations containing adrenaline may provoke ventricular arrhythmias, especially in patients anaesthetized with halothane in the presence of a raised Pa_{CO_2}. A maximum of 100 µg of adrenaline (10 ml of 1:100 000 solution) may be injected over any 10-min period (maximum 300 µg in one hour). Enflurane is less likely to be associated with adrenaline-induced arrhythmias, and isoflurane does not sensitise the myocardium to catecholamines.

5. *Hypokalaemia* may be associated with ventricular arrhythmias, especially in the presence of digoxin. Hyperkalaemia delays ventricular conduction, with eventual cardiac arrest.

6. *Reflex arrhythmias* tend to occur during light anaesthesia as a result of sympathetic or parasympathetic stimulation. They include tachyarrhythmias, e.g. in response to laryngoscopy and intubation (diminished by β-blockers), ventricular arrhythmias following dental extraction (partially blocked by local anaesthetic infiltration) and bradyarrhythmias, e.g. the oculocardiac reflex, or in response to peritoneal traction (prevented or

Table 40.3 Diagnostic features of ventricular tachycardia

Clinical
Cannon waves in JVP means VT
Variable first heart sound means VT
Often recent MI or IHD

ECG
Rate usually 120–250 beat.min^{-1}, usually regular
Broad complexes usual in VT
Independent atrial activity: P waves dissociated from QRS
Fusion beats
Capture beats
Practical point: 12-lead ECG may be necessary for diagnosis

JVP = Jugular venous pulse; VT = ventricular tachycardia; MI = myocardial infarction; IHD = ischaemic heart disease; ECG = electrocardiogram.

treated by atropine or glycopyrrolate). Reflex arrhythmias in general are prevented by deepening anaesthesia. The treatment of intraoperative arrhythmias depends on the nature of the arrhythmia and the haemodynamic decompensation caused. Supraventricular (SVT) and ventricular tachycardias (VT) differ in their clinical significance and treatment, and should be distinguished (Table 40.3)

Treatment of SVT under GA consists of:

1. Carotid sinus massage.
2. Adenosine 3–12 µg i.v.
3. Direct current (DC) cardioversion (25–50 J) if haemodynamic decompensation is present. This requires general anaesthesia. Synchronized DC shock is also indicated for atrial flutter.
4. If no decompensation, verapamil 5 mg, titrated i.v.
5. In sepsis-related or refractory SVT, volume loading plus amiodarone 300 mg i.v. by infusion over 20 min, then 900 mg over 24 h.
6. If thyrotoxic or phaeochromocytoma, β-blocker (in the latter case, not before α-blockade).

Intravenous verapamil should not be given to patients already receiving β-blockers as it may cause refractory asystole. The role of adenosine intraoperatively is, as yet, undefined. It is used as treatment for SVT and in diagnosis of regular broad complex tachycardia.

VT usually responds to i.v. lignocaine 50–100 mg followed by an infusion, but if unsuccessful, bretylium or amiodarone may be tried. DC shock should be employed early, particularly if VT is associated with decompensation. Other measures include correction of hypercapnia, hypoxaemia or hypokalaemia, and reduction of the inspired halothane concentration.

Heart block

The extent of the conduction deficit should be determined preoperatively from a 12-lead ECG or 24-h tape if no clear evidence is seen on ECG. If the patient has syncopal attacks, or is in cardiac failure, long-term pacing is indicated.

If the patient with heart block presents for surgery without a pacemaker in situ, preoperative insertion of a temporary pacing line is usually indicated in:

1. Complete heart block.
2. Second-degree heart block, of Mobitz type 2 variety.
3. First-degree heart block with bifascicular block (right bundle branch block with left anterior or posterior hemiblock).
4. Sick sinus syndrome (see below).

A decision on whether long-term pacing is indicated or not may be made by a cardiologist after the immediate postoperative period. During anaesthesia, ECG should be monitored continuously, a standby pacemaker should be available and care should be taken to avoid undue blood loss or vasodilatation as heart rate is unable to increase in compensation.

Diathermy should be avoided if possible because it may interfere with pacemaker function. Where unavoidable, the diathermy plate should be sited as far away as possible from the pacemaker generator, or bipolar diathermy should be used. Temporary generators and demand permanent generators are most often affected. Demand pacemakers should be converted to fixed-rate before surgery if the use of diathermy is essential. During transurethral prostatectomy, the 'cutting' current may affect the pacemaker, while the 'coagulation' current has no effect. With some pacemakers, the reverse may occur. Diathermy should be used in short bursts only and pacemaker threshold should be checked postoperatively. If first-degree heart block only is present, not necessitating temporary

pacing, drugs which slow AV conduction should be avoided, e.g. β-blockers, digoxin, verapamil, halothane.

Sick sinus syndrome

This term covers a number of conduction defects which affect the sinoatrial node, ranging from sinus bradycardia to sinus arrest. Sinoatrial block may be associated with runs of SVT (so-called tachycardia–bradycardia syndrome). Long-term pacing is indicated if the patient has syncopal episodes. Sinus bradycardia usually responds to atropine, while in complete sinoatrial block, atropine accelerates nodal escape rhythm. In the tachycardia–bradycardia group, temporary pacing is indicated to cover anaesthesia and surgery, because treatment of tachycardia with, for example, β-blocker, calcium-channel blocker or digoxin, may provoke severe bradycardia.

Valvular heart disease

In both aortic and mitral stenosis there is a low, fixed cardiac output, which leaves no reserve to compensate for changes in heart rate or vascular resistance.

Aortic stenosis

Isolated aortic stenosis is associated most commonly with calcification, often on a congenital bicuspid valve. In rheumatic heart disease, aortic stenosis occurs rarely in the absence of mitral disease, and is usually combined with regurgitation. The diagnosis is suggested by the findings of an ejection systolic murmur, low pulse pressure, and clinical and ECG evidence of left ventricular hypertrophy. Aortic systolic murmurs in elderly patients are frequently ascribed to aortic sclerosis, and an assessment of the degree of stenosis rests on examination. A slow-rising low-volume pulse with reduced pulse pressure, reduced intensity of the second heart sound and the presence of a click are suggestive of stenosis, and evidence of left ventricular hypertrophy on ECG usually indicates severe stenosis. Echocardiography with Doppler flow monitoring aids diagnosis and assessment. On chest X-ray, heart size is normal until late in the disease, while symptoms of angina, effort syncope and left ventricular failure indicate advanced disease.

Perioperative mortality is increased in patients with aortic stenosis; arrhythmias are common and are associated with precipitous decreases in cardiac output. The myocardial oxygen balance is upset by the decreases in coronary perfusion pressure and subendocardial blood flow, and the increase in ventricular afterload. Successful management demands precise maintenance of heart rate, arterial pressure and myocardial contractility. Bradycardia causes a decrease in cardiac output because stroke volume is fixed; tachycardia decreases the time available for coronary filling, and therefore both should be avoided.

Vasodilatation causes severe hypotension because cardiac output cannot increase significantly; coronary perfusion pressure is reduced if hypotension occurs.

All anaesthetic induction agents must be used with extreme caution. Etomidate is the agent of choice. The relaxant of choice is atracurium or vecuronium. Volatile agents which depress ventricular contractility (halothane, enflurane) may also seriously decrease cardiac output; in addition, halothane predisposes to arrhythmias. Isoflurane produces vasodilatation and causes decreases in diastolic pressure and coronary perfusion pressure. An opioid/relaxant technique is the best anaesthetic option. Replacement of blood must be prompt. Intensive monitoring is important and should include measurement of intra-arterial pressure and, in severe disease, PAOP measurement.

Mitral stenosis

This is usually a manifestation of rheumatic heart disease. Characteristic features include atrial fibrillation, arterial embolism, pulmonary oedema, pulmonary hypertension and right heart failure. Acute pulmonary oedema may follow the onset of atrial fibrillation.

Patients with mitral stenosis who present for surgery are frequently receiving digoxin, diuretics and anticoagulants. Preoperative control of atrial fibrillation, treatment of pulmonary oedema and management of anticoagulant therapy (see Chapter 61) is necessary. During anaesthesia, control of heart rate is important. Tachycardia reduces diastolic ventricular filling and thus cardiac output, while bradycardia also results in a decreased cardiac output because stroke output is limited. As with aortic stenosis, drugs which produce vasodilatation may cause severe hypotension.

As a result of pre-existing pulmonary hypertension, patients are particularly vulnerable to hypoxaemia, including transient episodes. Both hypoxaemia and acidosis are potent pulmonary vasoconstrictors and may produce right ventricular failure. Thus, opioid analgesics should be prescribed cautiously, and airway obstruction avoided.

Aortic regurgitation

Acute aortic regurgitation resulting, for example, from infective endocarditis, causes rapid left ventricular failure and requires emergency valve replacement, even in the presence of unresolved infection.

Chronic aortic regurgitation is asymptomatic for many years. Left ventricular dilatation occurs, with eventual left ventricular failure.

Patients with mild or moderate aortic regurgitation without left ventricular failure or massive ventricular dilatation tolerate anaesthesia well. A slightly increased heart rate of approximately 100 beat.min^{-1} is desirable because this reduces left ventricular dilatation. Bradycardia causes ventricular distension and should be avoided. Vasodilator therapy increases net forward flow by decreasing afterload, and is useful in severe aortic regurgitation; isoflurane anaesthesia may be beneficial. Careful monitoring is required, preferably with PAOP measurement, if severe hypotension is to be avoided.

Mitral regurgitation

Acute mitral regurgitation commonly results from infective endocarditis, or myocardial infarction with papillary muscle dysfunction or ruptured chordae tendineae. Acute pulmonary oedema results, and urgent valve replacement is required. Left ventricular failure with ventricular dilatation may cause functional mitral regurgitation.

Chronic mitral regurgitation is commonly associated with mitral stenosis. In pure mitral regurgitation, left atrial dilatation occurs with a minimal increase in pressure. The degree of regurgitation may be reduced by reducing the size of the left ventricle and the impedance to left ventricular ejection. Thus, inotropic agents and vasodilators may be useful. A slight increase in heart rate is desirable unless there is concomitant stenosis.

Infective endocarditis

This is caused predominantly by the *viridans* group of streptococci, occasionally by Gram-negative organisms or enterococci and also by staphylococci, especially after cardiac surgery or in drug addicts. *Coxiella burnetii* also accounts for a few cases. Patients with rheumatic or congenital heart disease, including asymptomatic lesions, e.g. bicuspid aortic valve, are at risk. Infection is caused by transient bacteraemia, most frequently after dental extraction or genitourinary investigation or surgery.

Antibiotic cover should be given for all surgical procedures in at risk patients. Appropriate regimens are detailed in Appendix IIIc. Flucloxacillin or an alternative antistaphylococcal agent should be included in regimens for cardiac surgery.

Role of local and regional anaesthesia

In appropriate patients with cardiovascular disease, local infiltration, peripheral nerve blocks or plexus blocks provide satisfactory anaesthesia with low risk of side-effects. However, local anaesthetic preparations which contain adrenaline may produce tachycardia and should be avoided in patients with severe cardiovascular disease.

Patients undergoing lower abdominal, pelvic or lower limb surgery may be managed satisfactorily with low subarachnoid or extradural anaesthesia. With higher blocks, sympathetic block produces vasodilatation, reducing preload and afterload. While controlled vasodilatation may have beneficial effects in ischaemic heart disease, hypertension and cardiac failure, patients anaesthetized with subarachnoid or extradural block must be managed very carefully in respect of posture, fluid preloading and replacement to avoid undue hypo-

tension. This may pose a particular problem in patients with untreated hypertension, low cardiac output states, constrictive pericarditis, severe valvular disease or a fixed heart rate resulting from heart block or β-blocker therapy. However, patients with congestive cardiac failure may benefit from the preload reduction caused by sympathetic block, and patients with peripheral vascular disease may benefit from peripheral vasodilatation.

High subarachnoid or extradural block is contraindicated in patients with cardiovascular disease.

In general, anaesthetists with limited experience in regional anaesthesia should avoid subarachnoid and extradural blocks in patients with severe cardiac disease.

RESPIRATORY DISEASE

Successful anaesthetic management of the patient with respiratory disease is dependent on accurate assessment of the nature and extent of functional impairment, and an appreciation of the effects of surgery on pulmonary function.

Assessment

History

Of the six cardinal symptoms of respiratory disease (cough, sputum, haemoptysis, dyspnoea, wheeze and chest pain), dyspnoea provides the best indication of functional impairment. Specific questioning is required to elicit the extent to which activity is limited by dyspnoea. Dyspnoea at rest or on minor exertion clearly indicates severe disease. A cough productive of purulent sputum indicates active infection. Chronic copious sputum production may indicate bronchiectasis. A history of heavy smoking or occupational exposure to dust may suggest pulmonary pathology.

A detailed drug history is important. Long-term steroid therapy within 3 months of the date of surgery necessitates augmented cover for the perioperative period and may cause hypokalaemia and hyperglycaemia. Bronchodilators should be continued during the perioperative period. Patients with cor pulmonale may be receiving digoxin and diuretics.

Examination

A full physical examination is required, with emphasis on detecting signs of airway obstruction, increased work of breathing, active infection which can be treated preoperatively, and evidence of right heart failure. The presence of obesity, cyanosis or dyspnoea is noted. In addition, a simple forced expiratory manoeuvre may reveal prolonged expiration, and a simple test of exercise tolerance may be useful.

Investigations

Chest X-ray. The preoperative chest X-ray is a poor indicator of functional impairment but is important for several reasons:

1. As a baseline for assessing postoperative radiographs.
2. To discover any localized disease of lungs and pleura not detected on clinical examination, e.g. neoplasm, collapse, consolidation, effusion.
3. To reveal underlying generalized lung disease in patients presenting with acute pulmonary symptoms, e.g. pulmonary fibrosis, emphysema.

ECG. This may indicate right atrial or ventricular hypertrophy (P pulmonale in II; dominant R wave in III, V_{1-3}) while associated ischaemic heart disease is common.

Haematology. Polycythaemia occurs secondary to chronic hypoxaemia, while anaemia aggravates tissue hypoxia. Leukocytosis may indicate active infection.

Sputum culture. Sputum culture is essential in patients with chronic lung disease or suspected acute infection.

Pulmonary function tests (see Appendix VIII). Peak expiratory flow rate, forced expiratory volume in 1 s (FEV_1), and forced vital capacity (FVC) may be measured easily at the bedside. The FEV_1 : FVC ratio is decreased in obstructive lung disease and normal in restrictive disease. In the presence of obstructive disease, the test should be repeated 5–10 min after administration of a bronchodilator aerosol to provide an indication of reversibility.

Fuller investigation involves measurement of FRC, residual volume and total lung capacity but these are rarely of value in determining clinical management.

Blood gas measurement. This is indicated in patients with chronic respiratory disease undergoing significant surgery and also if there is acute suspected acute hypoxaemia. It is also advisable when pulmonary function tests are markedly abnormal, for example, in obstructive disease where the FEV_1 is less than 1.5 litre. A raised Pa_{CO_2} is a prognostic indication that pulmonary complications are likely to develop postoperatively. With a Pa_{CO_2} of 6.7 kPa (50 mmHg) or greater, elective postoperative ventilation may be required after all but minor surgery. The combination of a low preoperative arterial oxygen tension (Pa_{O_2}) and dyspnoea at rest is associated with a high likelihood of the need for elective ventilation after abdominal surgery.

Effects of anaesthesia and surgery

Fitness for anaesthesia and surgery in patients with respiratory disease depends on the type and magnitude of surgery. The effects of anaesthesia alone on respiratory function are generally minor and short-lived, but may tip the balance towards respiratory failure in patients with severe disease. These effects include mucosal irritation by anaesthetic agents, ciliary paralysis, introduction of infection by aspiration or tracheal intubation and respiratory depression by relaxants, opioid analgesics or volatile anaesthetic agents. In addition, anaesthesia is associated with a decrease in FRC, especially in the elderly and in obese patients, which leads to basal airways closure and shunting of blood through underventilated areas of lung, an effect which is magnified by inhibition of the hypoxic pulmonary vasoconstrictor reflex.

Following recovery from anaesthesia, residual concentrations of anaesthetic agents inhibit the hyperventilatory responses to both hypercapnia and hypoxia, so that without close monitoring, e.g. with pulse oximetry, serious hypoxaemia and hypercapnia may occur.

Following thoracic and upper abdominal surgery, the decrease in FRC is more profound and persists for 5–10 days after surgery, with a parallel increase in alveolar–arterial oxygen difference $(A–a)P_{O_2}$; see Fig. 23.3). Complications including atelectasis and pneumonia occur in approximately 20% of these patients. Clearly, patients with preexisting respiratory disease are at much greater risk following upper abdominal surgery than after limb, head and neck or lower abdominal surgery.

Laparoscopic surgery

The use of laparoscopic techniques for cholecystectomy, fundoplication and other abdominal procedures has markedly reduced postoperative pulmonary morbidity, with the result that patients with severe pulmonary disease can usually undergo these procedures without the need for postoperative ventilatory support. The reasons for reduced morbidity include the relative lack of postoperative pain, and the preservation of lung volumes postoperatively. These techniques should be encouraged in patients with chronic pulmonary disease. Nevertheless cardiopulmonary function may be considerably compromised intra-operatively, and judicious use of invasive monitoring has been recommended in patients with severe cardiorespiratory disease.

Chronic obstructive airways disease

Chronic bronchitis is characterized by the presence of productive cough for at least 3 months in two successive years. Airways obstruction is caused by bronchoconstriction, bronchial oedema and hypersecretion of mucus. In the postoperative period, pulmonary atelectasis and pneumonia result if sputum is not cleared. Chronic airways disease may be classified into two groups: the bronchitis group (blue bloaters) and the emphysematous group (pink puffers), although in practice most patients have mixed pathologies. The former group is characterized by hypoxaemia, hypercapnia and right ventricular failure, while patients in the latter group are usually markedly dyspnoeic.

Preoperative management

This should include the following:

1. *Detection and treatment of active infection.*

Amoxycillin, co-amoxiclav or cefuroxime are usually appropriate, the common infecting organisms being *Streptococcus pneumoniae* and *Haemophilus influenzae*. Sputum for culture and sensitivies should be obtained to allow appropriate choice of antibiotic. Chest physiotherapy and humidification of inspired gases aid expectoration.

2. *Treatment of airway obstruction.* Some patients respond to bronchodilator therapy, either β_2-agonist (e.g. salbutamol), anticholinergic agent (e.g. ipratropium bromide) or phosphodiesterase inhibitor (e.g. aminophylline). Existing bronchodilator therapy should be continued perioperatively, while in patients receiving no bronchodilator, a trial of oral aminophylline (Phyllocontin) 225 mg b.d. and salbutamol 200 µg or ipratropium 40 µg (two puffs) by inhalation may decrease airways obstruction. Steroids may occasionally improve airways obstruction.

3. *Chest X-ray* examination to exclude spontaneous pneumothorax or emphysematous bullae.

4. *Assessment of the patient's ventilatory response* to carbon dioxide can be made by serial blood gas estimation with different levels of fractional concentration of oxygen ($F_{I_{O_2}}$). Patients dependent on a hypoxic stimulus can thus be recognized preoperatively.

5. *Treatment of cardiac failure.* Biventricular failure resulting from concurrent ischaemic heart disease and cor pulmonale frequently complicate chronic pulmonary disease. Diuretics are indicated, while nitrates or digoxin may have a role.

6. *Weight reduction* should be encouraged before elective surgery in obese patients with respiratory disease.

7. Ideally, *smoking* should be stopped for at least 6 weeks before elective surgery.

Premedication. Opioids should be avoided if severe disease exists. Atropine is useful if copious secretions are present. Temazepam is satisfactory to allay anxiety.

Regional anaesthesia

Regional anaesthesia for operations on head, neck or limbs offers freedom from respiratory side-effects, while avoiding the complications of general anaesthesia. For brachial plexus blockade, the axillary route is prefered in these patients to avoid the possible complications of pneumothorax associated with the supraclavicular route and phrenic nerve blockade with the interscalene approach. Low subarachnoid or extradural anaesthesia for lower abdominal and pelvic surgery have a similar advantage. However, if the block is sufficiently high to affect the intercostal muscles, peak expiratory flow rate is reduced and the ability to expectorate is impaired. Overall, the morbidity resulting from general anaesthesia for such operations is low, and it is only, perhaps, in the respiratory cripple that any significant advantage accrues from the use of a regional technique. In these patients, sedation should be kept to a minimum.

In upper abdominal and thoracic surgery, where changes in respiratory function are more profound and prolonged, there is no evidence that extradural anaesthesia is associated with lower morbidity than general anaesthesia. The advantages accruing from avoidance of volatile anaesthetics, muscle relaxants and opioids are balanced by the effect of extradural blockade on expiratory muscles, decreasing vital capacity. However, the use of extradural analgesia postoperatively allows pain-free coughing and clearing of secretions. Furthermore, it may reduce postoperative hypoxaemia by diminishing the decrease in FRC, and its use may result in fewer pulmonary complications.

General anaesthesia

Two approaches may be taken in the presence of severe chronic obstructive disease.

1. *Elective spontaneous ventilation.* This involves using minimal sedation, avoiding opioid analgesics and maintaining spontaneous ventilation, usually with a face mask or laryngeal mask airway. Tolerance to tracheal intubation is improved by spraying the larynx with local anaesthetic solution. Analgesia is best provided by a local or regional technique.

2. *Elective mechanical ventilation.* A deliberate decision is made to undertake intermittent positive-pressure ventilation (IPPV) during anaesthesia and for a variable period after operation, at least until elimination of muscle relaxants and anaesthetic agents has occurred. This also permits optimal provision of analgesia without fear of opioid-induced depression of ventilation. This technique is usually preferred if the preoperative Pa_{CO_2} is greater than 6.7 kPa (50 mmHg) or if major thoracic or abdominal surgery is planned. Intravenous fluid should be administered with care during the perioperative period. After surgery, salt and water retention occur and, in combination with over-enthusiastic fluid administration, and perhaps a decrease in cardiac output, may result in an increase in lung water which in turn may cause small airways closure, and hypoxaemia.

There is an increased risk of pneumothorax, especially if high inflation pressures are used.

Postoperative care

Postoperative care of the patient with severe chronic obstructive airways disease should be conducted in a high-dependency unit (HDU) or intensive care unit (ICU).

Elective postoperative controlled ventilation allows adequate oxygenation, analgesia without respiratory depression, clearance of secretions by physiotherapy, tracheal suction and, if necessary, fibreoptic bronchoscopy. Cardiac output and peripheral perfusion may be optimized and fluid overload corrected before restoration of spontaneous ventilation. Unless there is pre-existing pulmonary infection, a period of 24 h of elective controlled ventilation is usually adequate. Institution of analgesia by regional (e.g. paravertebral or extradural) blockade often allows earlier return to spontaneous ventilation when the respiratory-depressant effects of anaesthetics and relaxants have terminated.

Oxygen. With spontaneous ventilation, controlled oxygen is required using a 24% or 28% Ventimask with frequent checks on arterial blood gases to ensure an adequate Pa_{O_2} (<8 kPa) without excessive carbon dioxide retention (Pa_{CO_2} < 7.5–8 kPa). Using a pulse oximeter, the $F_{I_{O_2}}$ can be titrated to achieve an Sp_{O_2} of around 90%. Hypoxaemia may seriously aggravate existing pulmonary hypertension, and precipitate right ventricular failure.

Analgesia. Simple, non-opioid analgesics and/or local and regional techniques should be used if possible. Non-steroidal anti-inflammatory drugs such as diclofenac and ketorolac are useful in reducing the opioid requirements following major surgery, and may be adequate on their own after minor surgery. Fifty per cent nitrous oxide in oxygen (Entonox) is useful for physiotherapy and painful procedures. Opioid analgesics are best administered, where necessary, in small i.v. doses, e.g. morphine 2 mg, under direct supervision, or using patient-controlled analgesia. Physiotherapy, bronchodilators and antibiotics should be continued postoperatively. Doxapram by infusion $(2 \text{ mg.kg}^{-1}$ over a period of 30 min to 4 h) may decrease marginally the extent of postoperative alveolar collapse and infection, although the evidence for this is controversial.

A technique of percutaneous cricothyroid puncture and insertion of a small-diameter tube into the trachea (minitracheotomy) permits aspiration of secretions while preserving the ability of the patient to cough and speak. However, a number of potentially serious complications, including severe haemorrhage, have been reported and enthusiasm for the technique has diminished.

The application of continuous positive airways pressure (CPAP) via a close-fitting face mask in the spontaneously breathing patient increases functional residual capacity (FRC) and reduces the incidence of atelectasis in postoperative patients with pulmonary disease. It may reduce the need for mechanical ventilation, although it is not tolerated by many patients.

Restrictive lung disease

This category includes a wide range of conditions which affect the lung and chest wall. Lung diseases include sarcoidosis and fibrosing alveolitis, while lesions of chest wall include kyphoscoliosis and ankylosing spondylitis. Pulmonary function tests reveal a decrease in both FEV_1 and FVC with a normal $FEVI_1/FVC$ ratio and a decreased FRC and total lung capacity (TLC). Small airways closure occurs during tidal ventilation, with resultant shunting and hypoxaemia. Lung or chest wall compliance is decreased; thus, the work of breathing is increased and the ability to cough and clear secretions impaired. There is an increased risk of postoperative pulmonary infection.

Anaesthesia causes little additional decrease in lung volumes, and is tolerated well provided that hypoxaemia is avoided. Postoperatively, however, inadequate basal ventilation and retention of secretions may occur, partly as a result of pain, opioid analgesics and the residual effects of anaesthetic agents. High concentrations of oxygen may be used without risk of respiratory depression. A short period of mechanical ventilation may be necessary in patients with severe disease to allow adequate analgesia and clearing of secretions. High extradural anaesthesia should be avoided in these patients since it causes a further reduction in vital capacity.

Bronchiectasis

The patient should be admitted several days before surgery and regular postural drainage carried out. Appropriate antibiotics, based on sputum culture, should be prescribed. Disease localized in one lung should be isolated using a double-lumen tube.

Bronchial carcinoma

Patients with bronchial carcinoma frequently suffer from coexisting chronic bronchitis. In addition, there is frequently infection and collapse of the lung distal to the tumour. Patients with bronchial carcinoma may have myasthenic syndrome (see p. 68), while oat-cell tumours may secrete a number of hormones, among the commonest being adrenocorticotrophic hormone (ACTH), producing Cushing's syndrome, and antidiuretic hormone (ADH), producing dilutional hyponatraemia (syndrome of inappropriate ADH secretion; SIADH).

Tuberculosis

Tuberculosis should be considered in patients with persistent pulmonary infection, especially if associated with haemoptysis or weight loss. If active disease is present, all anaesthetic equipment should be sterilized after use to avoid cross-infection of other patients.

Bronchial asthma

This common disease, which affects all age groups,

is characterized by recurrent generalized reversible airways obstruction, caused by bronchial smooth-muscle spasm, mucus plugs and bronchial oedema. Asthma may be classified into two types: *extrinsic*, where an external allergen is demonstrable, and *intrinsic*. Intrinsic asthma tends to occur in adults, is more chronic and continuous and often requires long-term steroid therapy.

Preoperative management

The current state of the patient's disease is assessed by:

1. *History*. Frequency and severity of attacks, factors provoking attacks, drug history.
2. *Examination*. Presence or absence of wheeze, prolonged expiratory phase, overdistension, evidence of infection.
3. *Pulmonary function tests*. PEFR or FEV_1/FVC before and after inhalation of bronchodilator. Blood gas analysis may be required in severe disease.

Elective surgery should not be undertaken until asthma is well-controlled. This involves the use of one or more of a number of drugs: (1) inhaled β_2-adrenoceptor agonists, e.g. salbutamol; (2) steroids, systemic or inhaled; (3) oral phosphodiesterase inhibitors, e.g. aminophylline. In patients already on theophyllines, the plasma level should be checked. Pulmonary infection requires treatment where appropriate. A suitable bronchodilator regimen in the preoperative period comprises salbutamol 200 µg (two puffs) 4–6-hourly by inhaler, possibly in combination with oral aminophylline (Phyllocontin) 225 mg b.d. Patients with intrinsic asthma sometimes respond well to ipratropium bromide, an anticholinergic agent, 40 µg (two puffs) by inhaler. A dose of bronchodilator should be given with the premedication 1 h before induction of anaesthesia.

Patients with severe asthma who are receiving topical or systemic steroid therapy, or not responding to conventional bronchodilator therapy, require systemic steroid therapy to cover the anaesthetic and postoperative periods. Prednisolone 40–100 mg daily may be given preoperatively, with hydrocortisone 100 mg four times daily for the first postoperative day. An equivalent dose

Table 40.4 Equivalent doses of glucocorticoids

Glucocorticoid	Dose
Betamethasone	3 mg
Cortisone acetate	100 mg
Dexamethasone	3 mg
Hydrocortisone	80 mg
Methylprednisolone	16 mg
Prednisolone	20 mg
Prednisone	20 mg
Triamcinolone	16 mg

of oral prednisolone (Table 40.4) should be substituted when oral intake is resumed, and the dose gradually reduced as the severity of asthma permits.

Premedication should consist of a sedative agent, e.g. diazepam, with atropine to block vagal reflex-induced bronchospasm. Pethidine and promethazine are also satisfactory premedicants.

Anaesthesia

All volatile anaesthetic agents are bronchodilators, and are therefore well-tolerated. Bronchoconstriction may be triggered by tracheal intubation or by surgical stimulation during light anaesthesia. The larynx and trachea should be sprayed with local anaesthetic and adequate depth of anaesthesia maintained. Drugs which are associated with histamine release (atracurium and morphine) are best avoided; vecuronium and pethidine or fentanyl are preferable. β-Blocking drugs should also be avoided. With controlled ventilation, a prolonged expiratory phase is required if there is evidence of severe airways obstruction; the inspiratory time should be adequate to avoid unduly high inflation pressures. Pneumothorax is a possible complication and requires early detection and prompt drainage. Humidification is necessary if ventilation is prolonged.

If bronchospasm occurs, it may be due to easily remedied causes such as light anaesthesia or endotracheal tube irritation, and these should be corrected. If bronchospasm persists, aminophylline 125–250 mg or salbutamol 125–250 µg should be administered by slow i.v. injection under ECG monitoring. The dose should be reduced if the patient is receiving oral theophylline. Thereafter, an infusion of aminophylline, up to $0.5–0.8$ mg.kg^{-1}.h^{-1}, or salbutamol, possibly in combination with nebulized salbutamol by positive-pressure ventilation (solution of $50–100$ μg per ml of water) should be maintained until improvement occurs. I.v. hydrocortisone 200 mg should be given simultaneously, although it has no immediate effect. I.v ketamine has also been used with success when other agents have failed to relieve acute bronchospasm.

Postoperative management consists of close respiratory monitoring, treatment of bronchospasm and provision of adequate analgesia, humidified oxygen and physiotherapy. Salbutamol is best administered by nebulization (2.5 mg in 2.5 ml saline 4–6-hourly) and aminophylline by i.v. infusion ($0.5–0.8$ mg.kg^{-1}.h^{-1}). The dose should be reduced if the patient is receiving oral theophylline. There is no loss of carbon dioxide responsiveness in asthmatic patients, and high inspired oxygen concentrations are tolerated well.

GASTROINTESTINAL DISEASE

Dysphagia

Patients with dysphagia resulting from oesophageal stricture tumour or achalasia may be severely malnourished and fluid-depleted. Fluid and electrolyte depletion should be corrected preoperatively, and anaesthetic drug doses should be appropriately reduced to avoid hypotension at induction of anaesthesia. There may be a considerable quantity of food debris in the oesophagus, and the standard precautions should be taken to avoid regurgitation and aspiration at induction.

Hiatus hernia

There is a risk of regurgitation and inhalation of gastric contents, especially in the obese patient and in the lithotomy position. In addition to the usual measures to avoid aspiration, administration of a histamine H$_2$-receptor antagonist, e.g. ranitidine (150 mg on the night before surgery, followed by 150 mg with premedication) together with 0.3 mol.litre^{-1} sodium citrate 30 ml 5 min before induction may decrease the risk of pneumonitis if aspiration occurs.

Intestinal obstruction

The principal anaesthetic problems in these patients are extreme fluid and electrolyte depletion with consequent risk of cardiovascular collapse on induction of anaesthesia, and increased risk of vomiting and inhalation of gastric contents. A large nasogastric tube should be used to empty the stomach as effectively as possible before induction. A rapid-sequence induction with cricoid pressure is mandatory, but the dose of induction agent (etomidate) requires fine judgement. The nasogastric tube should arguably be removed to allow effective cricoid pressure to be applied.

Patients who have severe vomiting and diarrhoea also pose problems in relation to fluid and electrolyte depletion. All such patients undergoing surgery require appropriate fluid and electrolyte replacement preoperatively; the volume and composition depend on blood urea and electrolyte measurements and CVP monitoring.

Subarachnoid and extradural anaesthesia should be avoided if significant fluid depletion is suspected.

LIVER DISEASE

Anaesthesia and surgery may affect liver function adversely even in previously normal patients. Pre-existing liver dysfunction may have effects on the conduct of anaesthesia, for example on the metabolism of anaesthetic drugs.

Preoperative assessment should be directed towards detection of jaundice, ascites, oedema and signs of hepatic failure (encephalopathy with flapping tremor). Routine preoperative investigations should include a coagulation screen, measurement of haemoglobin concentration, white cell and platelet counts, and concentrations of serum bilirubin, alkaline phosphatase, transaminases, urea, electrolytes, proteins (including albumin) and blood sugar. Blood should also be taken to screen for viral hepatitis. Appropriate measures must be taken to protect theatre staff from possible contamination.

Particular problems relevant to the anaesthetist include the following:

1. *Acid–base and fluid balance.* Many patients are overloaded with fluid. Hypoalbumin-

aemia results in oedema and ascites, and predisposes to pulmonary oedema. Secondary hyperaldosteronism produces sodium retention (even though plasma sodium concentration may be low) and hypokalaemia. Diuretic therapy, often including spironolactone, may also affect serum potassium concentration. In hepatic failure, a combined respiratory and metabolic alkalosis may occur, which shifts the oxygen dissociation curve to the left, impairing tissue oxygenation.

2. *Hepatorenal syndrome.* This can be defined as acute renal failure developing in patients with pre-existing chronic liver failure. Jaundiced patients are at risk of developing postoperative renal failure. This may be precipitated by hypovolaemia. Prevention involves adequate preoperative hydration, with i.v. infusion for at least 12 h before surgery, and close monitoring of urine output, intra- and postoperatively. I.v 20% mannitol 100 ml is recommended immediately preoperatively, and is indicated postoperatively if the hourly urine output falls below 50 ml. Close cardiovascular monitoring is essential.

3. *Bleeding problems.* Production of clotting factors II, VII, IX and X is reduced as a result of decreased vitamin K absorption. Production of factor V and fibrinogen is also reduced. Thrombocytopenia occurs if portal hypertension is present. Vitamin K should be administered preoperatively and fresh frozen plasma given to provide clotting factors during surgery, with regular checks made on coagulation. Infusion of platelet concentrate is indicated to cover surgery in cases of severe thrombocytopenia (platelet count $< 50 \times 10^9$ litre^{-1}) or if there is overt bleeding in a thrombocytopenic patient.

4. *Drug metabolism.* Impairment of liver function slows elimination of drugs, including anaesthetic induction agents, opioid analgesics, benzodiazepines, suxamethonium, local anaesthetic agents and many others. Since the duration of action of many of these drugs is determined initially by redistribution, prolongation of action may not become apparent until a subsequent dose has been given. Altered plasma protein concentrations affect drug binding, and may account for resistance to *d*-tubocurarine and pancuronium in liver failure.

In addition, a large number of drugs have toxic effects on the liver. Rarely, halothane is associated with postoperative hepatitis, usually when administered more than once within a period of a few weeks. The mechanism appears to be induction of reductive enzymes in the liver, which, in the presence of hypoxia, causes an increase in hepatotoxic reductive metabolites. A single halothane anaesthetic is safe in patients with liver disease provided that cardiac output and hepatic blood flow are not depressed unduly. Halothane should not be employed within 3 months of a previous halothane anaesthetic, or if there is a history of unexplained jaundice or abnormal liver function tests after any previous halothane anaesthetic. If postoperative jaundice occurs, other causes should be sought before accepting a diagnosis of halothane hepatitis.

5. *Hepatic failure.* In such patients, all sedative drugs should be administered with extreme care, as they aggravate encephalopathy. All opioids and benzodiazepines are eliminated by the liver. Benzodiazepines are probably the best sedatives to use in small doses, with midazolam being first choice. Patients with hepatic failure require management in an ICU, including invasive haemodynamic monitoring with a pulmonary artery catheter, and close metabolic, fluid and electrolyte monitoring. Hypoglycaemia, which occurs as a result of depleted liver glycogen stores, should be avoided by the administration of glucose infusion, and sodium intake should be restricted. Amino acids, fat emulsions and fructose should be avoided. Patients are very vulnerable to infective complications and close bacteriological surveillance should be maintained. Mechanical ventilation is often required, and this diminishes the risks of sedative administration. In hepatic coma, ventilation is mandatory and intracranial pressure monitoring should be considered even in the presence of coagulopathy. *N*-acetyl cysteine may be of value even when given late in paracetamol-induced hepatic failure, and there is preliminary evidence for its efficacy in other forms of fulminant hepatic failure.

Conduct of anaesthesia

If liver function is severely impaired, no premedication should be given. Otherwise, a light benzodiazepine premedication is suitable.

The liver is particularly vulnerable to hypotension and hypoxia. During anaesthesia, cardiac output should be kept as stable as possible. Blood loss should be replaced promptly, and overall fluid balance maintained with CVP monitoring. Drugs which depress cardiac output or blood pressure, including volatile anaesthetic agents and β-blockers, should be used with caution to avoid decreasing hepatic blood flow unduly.

Vecuronium and atracurium are the muscle relaxants of choice because of their cardiovascular stability and short duration of action; atracurium may be preferable because its elimination is independent of liver and renal function. Opioid analgesic drugs should be administered with caution unless ventilatory support is planned postoperatively. Pethidine may be preferable to morphine, and is best titrated initially against pain in small i.v. doses, e.g. 20 mg, in the immediate postoperative period. Non-steroidal anti-inflammatory agents should be avoided.

Controlled ventilation to a normal Pa_{CO_2} is important, as hypocapnia is associated with decreased hepatic blood flow. Hypoxaemia should be avoided throughout, and oxygen saturation should be monitored (with blood gas analysis if necessary), into the postoperative period.

RENAL DISEASE

Renal dysfunction has a number of important implications for anaesthesia, and therefore full assessment is required before even minor surgical procedures are contemplated.

Measurement of blood urea and electrolyte concentrations should be undertaken before all major surgery and in all elderly or potentially unhealthy patients; a raised blood urea demonstrated preoperatively may be the first indication of renal disease. Severity of renal dysfunction may be assessed further by measurement of serum creatinine concentration and creatinine clearance, urinary : plasma osmolality ratio and urinary urea and electrolyte excretion (Table 40.5).

Preanaesthetic assessment of the patient should be directed to a number of specific problems which require correction before embarking on anaesthesia:

1. *Fluid balance.* In acute renal failure, fluid overload may develop suddenly and is uncompensated. In chronic renal failure, overload may be controlled with diuretic therapy or dialysis. Biventricular cardiac failure and hypertension may result from overload, and must be treated before induction of anaesthesia. This may require dialysis or haemofiltration.

In patients with nephrotic syndrome, hypoalbuminaemia results in oedema and ascites. Circulating blood volume in these patients is often decreased, and care should be taken at induction of anaesthesia to avoid hypotension.

2. *Electrolyte disturbances.* Sodium retention occurs in renal failure, and through increased secretion of ADH is associated with water retention, oedema and hypertension.

Hyponatraemia is also common in renal disease. It is the result either of sodium losses through the kidney or gastrointestinal tract, or of water overload causing dilutional hyponatraemia. The renal tubules may have a reduced ability to conserve sodium (e.g. in pyelonephritis, analgesic nephropathy or recovering acute renal failure) or else sodium may be lost through diuretic therapy, vomiting or diarrhoea. Dilutional hyponatraemia is due either to inappropriate fluid administration (glucose 5%) or inappropriate ADH secretion or both. Following transurethral prostatectomy, hyponatraemia may result from absorption of glycine irrigation fluid. Diagnosis of the cause of

Table 40.5 Urinary measurements in prerenal and renal failure

Variable	Prerenal	Renal
Specific gravity	High > 1.020	1.010–1.012
Sodium	Low < 20 mmol.litre^{-1}	High > 40 mmol.litre^{-1}
U:P urea ratio	High > 20	Low < 10
U:P creatinine ratio	High > 40	Low < 10
U:P osmolality ratio	High > 2.1	Low < 1.2

U = Urine; P = plasma

hyponatraemia involves measurement of urinary osmolality and sodium concentration.

Hyperkalaemia occurs typically in renal failure, frequently in association with metabolic acidosis. It causes delayed myocardial conduction and, if untreated, leads to asystolic cardiac arrest.

Hyperkalaemia should be treated promptly when the serum potassium concentration exceeds 6 mmol.litre^{-1} or when ECG changes are evident.

a. Calcium chloride 10% up to 10–20 ml to antagonize the cardiac effects of hyperkalaemia, under ECG guidance.
b. Glucose 50%, 50 ml with 12 units of soluble insulin followed by an infusion of 20% glucose with insulin as required, depending on BM-test blood sugarestimation.
c. Sodium bicarbonate to correct the metabolic acidosis partly.
d. Haemodialysis or haemofiltration. The former is more effective in lowering serum potassium concentration rapidly, but haemofiltration may be more easily set up as an emergency in a general ICU.
e. An ion exchange resin (e.g. calcium polystyrene sulphonate 15 g t.i.d. orally or 30 g retention enema) provides longer-term control in chronic renal failure.

Suxamethonium should be avoided in hyperkalaemic patients in view of its effect of releasing potassium from muscle cells. An increase of up to 0.6 mmol.litre^{-1} may be expected in normal dosage.

Hypokalaemia occurs commonly in patients receiving diuretic therapy. These patients require preoperative measurement of serum potassium concentration, and replacement if necessary. Hypokalaemia is associated with ventricular irritability, notably in patients taking digoxin.

Retention of phosphate and vitamin D depletion (1:25 dihydroxycholecalciferol) in chronic renal failure lead to hyperparathyroidism. The development of a parathyroid adenoma leads to hypercalcaemia (tertiary parathyroidism).

3. *Cardiovascular effects.* Hypertension may occur for a number of reasons. A raised plasma renin concentration secondary to decreased perfusion of the juxtaglomerular apparatus results in hypertension through increased secretion of angiotensin and aldosterone.

Fluid retention also causes hypertension by increasing the circulating blood volume. Conversely, hypertension from other causes results in renal impairment. The precise cause of hypertension in these patients should be sought and the hypertension treated. Anaesthesia for hypertensive patients is discussed on page 655.

Both pulmonary and peripheral oedema may occur from a combination of fluid overload, hypertensive cardiac disease and hypoproteinaemia. Cardiac failure should be treated preoperatively. Uraemia may cause pericarditis and a haemorrhagic pericardial effusion, which may embarrass cardiac output and require aspiration. Good control of blood urea with haemodialysis or haemofiltration will often prevent this complication and is essential for its resolution.

4. *Neurological effects.* Uraemia causes drowsiness and eventually coma. Electrolyte disturbances and rapid fluid shifts, e.g. during dialysis, may also affect conscious level by causing cerebral oedema. Sedative drugs including morphine should be used with care in these patients as renally excreted metabolites accumulate. In addition, a combined motor and sensory peripheral neuropathy may occur in uraemic patients.

5. *Haematology.* Patients with chronic renal failure suffer from normochromic anaemia, which results from marrow depression, partly as a result of erythropoietin deficiency. They also have an increased incidence of gastrointestinal bleeding and so an iron-deficiency component may be present. These patients are usually well-compensated, with an increased cardiac output; excessive preoperative blood transfusion should be avoided.

6. *Other factors.* Patients with chronic renal failure are frequently undernourished. They tend to be vulnerable to infection. Patients who have received a renal transplant and are immunosuppressed are particularly vulnerable to opportunistic pathogens, e.g. *Pneumocystis carinii.* Patients undergoing chronic haemodialysis are occasionally carriers of hepatitis B antigen, and, if so, appropriate precautions should be taken by theatre staff.

7. *Drug treatment.* Many patients with renal disease are receiving diuretics, antihypertensive therapy including β-blockers and digoxin. The doses of drugs excreted renally (e.g. digoxin and

aminoglycoside antibiotics) should be reduced; monitoring of plasma concentrations is essential in determining appropriate dosage.

The widespread use of non-steroidal anti-inflammatory drugs both as analgesics and for arthritis has considerable implications for renal function. They inhibit vasodilator prostaglandin production in the kidney and thus reduce glomerular blood flow and sodium excretion, which may be critical in septic or shocked patients, or those undergoing surgery associated with major blood loss. Their use should be restricted in such high-risk patients.

ACE inhibitors dilate the post-glomerular arterioles in the kidney and thus reduce glomerular filtration pressure. They may therefore precipitate renal failure in hypotensive patients. Patients receiving these agents should be monitored carefully and fluid should be replaced adequately to avoid hypotension. ACE inhibitors may also cause hyperkalaemia, particularly in patients with renal dysfunction.

Anaesthesia

A light premedication with benzodiazepine or opioid analgesic is satisfactory. Minor procedures, e.g. to establish vascular access for dialysis, are carried out most satisfactorily under regional anaesthesia: brachial plexus block for upper limb and combined femoral and sciatic block for lower limb.

Patients who suffer from acute renal failure, and those on long-term dialysis for chronic renal failure, may require dialysis before surgery to correct fluid overload, acid–base disturbances and hyperkalaemia. Ideally, there should be some delay before surgery to allow correction of anti-coagulation.

The i.v. cannula for induction and fluid infusion should be sited in the contralateral limb from the arteriovenous shunt or fistula (in patients undergoing dialysis) and care should be taken to protect the fistula during the operation. Careful monitoring of arterial pressure and ECG is required, and CVP measurement is indicated in patients who are clinically overloaded with fluid. I.v. fluid administration should be cautious, and in some instances titrated against CVP measurements.

Excessive sodium administration should be avoided, and potassium-containing solutions completely avoided in renal failure. If the patient is anaemic preoperatively, intraoperative blood loss should be replaced promptly.

Drugs excreted primarily via the kidneys should be used with caution in renal failure. In anaesthetic practice, the principal drugs involved are the muscle relaxants. Atracurium (elimination of which is independent of kidney and liver function, and which has minimal cardiovascular effects) is the relaxant of choice. All other relaxants depend to some extent on renal elimination, and should be avoided. In addition, many drugs, including morphine, are conjugated in the liver before excretion in the urine. Depending on the activity of the conjugated metabolite, these drugs may have adverse effects following repeated doses. Morphine-6-glucuronide, an active metabolite of morphine, accumulates in renal failure and may result in prolongation of clinical effects after administration of morphine.

Enflurane is partly metabolized to fluoride ion, which affects the concentrating ability of the kidney through an effect on the distal tubule, and should be used with caution in patients with severe renal impairment. Isoflurane, which undergoes minimal metabolism in the body, is currently the volatile agent of choice in renal disease, although desflurane, which is metabolized even less, is also suitable.

Postoperative renal failure

This is not infrequently a problem in patients undergoing major surgery which involves large blood loss, in surgery following trauma and in septic patients. Avoidance of renal failure in these patients involves close monitoring of the cardiovascular state, including CVP and urinary output, avoidance of hypotension and adequate fluid and blood replacement. In many instances, for example in patients with pre-existing renal dysfunction, shock, sepsis or liver disease, a pulmonary artery catheter is required to optimize cardiac output and oxygen delivery, and to guide vasoactive drug therapy. Low-dose (2–5 $\mu g.kg^{-1}.min^{-1}$) dopamine is frequently recommended to prevent renal failure in such situations, but its efficacy is unproven, and its use may confuse the situation by inducing diuresis through stimulation of dopaminergic receptors in the renal tubules. The only proven therapy in the prevention and early treatment of acute renal failure is adequate fluid resuscitation titrated against PAOP, and maintenance of an adequate cardiac output (cardiac index 4.5 litre.min^{-1}.m^{-2}) and mean arterial pressure (80 mmHg).

Other measures, such as use of an osmotic diuretic (mannitol 100 ml of 20% solution over 15 min) or loop diuretic (frusemide by bolus or infusion), are of doubtful value. Mannitol continues to be recommended in jaundiced patients at risk of developing the hepatorenal syndrome, and in patients with rhabdomyolysis. In some cases of oliguric acute renal failure where resuscitation has failed to achieve diuresis, frusemide i.v. does appear to 'kick start' a urine output which is then maintained.

Postoperative oliguria may also be the result of postrenal causes. Patients with prostatic enlargement are particularly liable to develop acute urinary retention. Examination to exclude a full bladder, and catheterization, should always be carried out in the anuric postoperative patient. Abdominal ultrasound may be useful in more complicated cases.

CONNECTIVE TISSUE DISORDERS

Rheumatoid arthritis

Rheumatoid arthritis is a multisystem disease, with a number of implications for anaesthesia which must be considered at the time of preoperative assessment.

1. *Airway problems.* The arthritic process may involve the temporomandibular joints, rendering laryngoscopy and intubation difficult. The cervical spine may be fixed, or subluxed, and thus unstable, especially when the patient is anaesthetized and paralysed. Cricoarytenoid involvement should be suspected if hoarseness or stridor is present.

2. *Respiratory function.* Costochondral involvement causes a restrictive defect with reduced vital capacity. Pulmonary involvement with interstitial fibrosis produces ventilation/perfusion ($\dot{V}/\dot{Q}$) abnormalities, a diffusion defect and thus hypoxaemia.

3. *Cardiovascular system.* Endocardial and myocardial involvement may occur. Coronary arteritis, conduction defects and peripheral arteritis are other uncommon features. Immobility caused by arthritis may mask symptoms of cardiorespiratory disease.

4. *Anaemia.* A chronic anaemia, hypo- or normochromic, but refractory to iron, occurs. Pre-operative transfusion to a haemoglobin concentration of approximately 10 g.dl^{-1} is advisable before major surgery. Treatment with salicylates or other non-steroidal anti-inflammatory drugs may cause gastrointestinal blood loss.

5. *Renal failure*, or nephrotic syndrome, may occur as a result of amyloidosis or drug treatment.

6. *Steroid therapy.* Many patients are receiving long-term steroid therapy and require augmented steroid cover for the perioperative period (see p. 676). They are more vulnerable to postoperative infection.

Routine preoperative investigation should include full blood count, urea and electrolytes, chest X-ray, cervical spine X-ray and ECG. Other investigations, e.g. pulmonary function tests, may be required in some instances.

Conduct of anaesthesia

Particular care should be taken with venepuncture and placing of i.v. infusions because of atrophy of skin and subcutaneous tissues and fragility of veins. Careful positioning of the patient on the operating table is required because these patients may have multiple joint involvement. Padding may be required to prevent pressure sores.

The anaesthetist should be prepared for difficult intubation; spinal, extradural or regional techniques are useful for many limb or lower abdominal operations because they obviate the need for tracheal intubation. Where intubation is essential, an awake fibreoptic-assisted intubation may be the technique of choice.

Other connective tissue diseases

Connective tissue diseases can present in many ways. Their manifestations include vasculitis, glomerulonephritis, pulmonary fibrosis, arthropathies and myocarditis or pericarditis. The diffuse nature of the vasculitis may also result in neurological involvement. Steroid and immunosuppressive therapy are other potential problems.

Scleroderma

Scleroderma (systemic sclerosis) is characterized by many of the above features, including restricted mouth opening, lower oesophageal involvement with increased risk of regurgitation, pulmonary involvement, renal failure, steroid therapy and peripheral vascular disease.

Systemic lupus erythematosus

Anaemia, renal and respiratory involvement may be severe. Cardiac involvement may include mitral valve disease. Steroid therapy is usual.

Ankylosing spondylitis

The rigid spine makes intubation difficult, and spinal and extradural anaesthesia may be technically impossible. Costovertebral joint involvement restricts chest expansion.

Marfan's syndrome

This is a disorder of connective tissue of autosomal dominant inheritance, which is characterized by long, thin extremities, high arched palate, lens subluxation and aortic and mitral regurgitation. Regurgitation may be severe, and the valve lesions may be complicated by infective endocarditis. Antibiotic cover is necessary for dental and other surgical procedures.

NUTRITIONAL PROBLEMS

Obesity

Obesity poses a number of problems to the anaesthetist and surgeon.

1. *Cardiovascular function.* Obesity is associated with increased blood volume, increased cardiac work, hypertension and cardiomegaly. Atherosclerosis and coronary artery disease are common. Diabetes may coexist.

2. *Respiratory function.* Vital capacity and FRC are decreased. Closing volume is increased. As a result, increased shunting occurs through underventilated, dependent lung regions, with consequent hypoxaemia. These changes, brought about by abdominal splinting of the diaphragm, are accentuated in the supine, Trendelenburg and lithotomy positions. Total thoracic compliance is decreased, the work of breathing increased, and increased oxygen consumption and carbon dioxide production cause hyperventilation.

3. *Other factors.* There may be difficulty in achieving venous access, and blood pressure measurement may be inaccurate unless the appropriate size of cuff is used. Assessment of volume state is generally more difficult. Surgery is technically more difficult, with heavy blood loss, and increased incidences of wound infection and wound dehiscence. Hiatus hernia with risk of regurgitation is more common, and maintenance of the airway and tracheal intubation may be more difficult.

Obese patients require careful preoperative respiratory and cardiovascular assessment (see Chapter 18). The inspired oxygen fraction should be increased to 0.4. Fluid balance should be monitored carefully. Elective postoperative ventilation should be considered, especially after abdominal surgery. Pulmonary, thromboembolic and wound complications are more common, and appropriate prophylactic measures and/or early recognition and treatment are important.

Pickwickian syndrome

Pickwickian syndrome is characterized by a combination of obesity, episodic somnolence and hypoventilation with cyanosis, polycythaemia, pulmonary hypertension and right ventricular failure. Avoidance of hypoxia is important, and elective postoperative ventilation may be necessary, especially after abdominal surgery.

Malnutrition

As a result of persistent anorexia, dysphagia or vomiting, malnourished patients may have severe depletion of fluid and electrolytes. Anaemia and hypoproteinaemia are common. The anaemia may be due to iron, vitamin B_{12} or folate deficiency, and if megaloblastic in nature, may be associated with thrombocytopenia.

Preoperative correction of fluid and electrolyte deficits is required, with CVP monitoring in severe cases. Infusion of albumin may be advisable in some instances to raise the colloid osmotic pressure. A multivitamin preparation should be administered in view of probable thiamine deficiency. Induction agents should be administered carefully to avoid hypotension, while smaller doses of relaxants are required; vecuronium and atracurium are the agents of choice.

ENDOCRINE DISEASE

Pituitary disease

The clinical features of pituitary disease depend on the local effects of the lesion and its effects on the secretion of pituitary hormones. Local effects include headache and visual field disturbances. The effects on hormone secretion depend on the cells involved in the pathological process.

Acromegaly

Acromegaly is caused by increased secretion of growth hormone from eosinophil cell tumours of the anterior pituitary gland. If this occurs before fusion of the epiphyses, gigantism results. Problems for the anaesthetist include the following.

1. Upper airway obstruction may result from an enlarged mandible, tongue and epiglottis, thickened pharyngeal mucosa and laryngeal narrowing. Maintenance of a clear airway and intubation may be difficult, and postoperative care of the airway must be meticulous.

2. Cardiac enlargement, hypertension and congestive cardiac failure occur commonly and require preoperative treatment.

3. Growth hormone increases blood sugar. Hyperglycaemia should be controlled perioperatively.

4. Thyroid and adrenal function may be impaired because of decreased release of thyroid-stimulating hormone (TSH) and ACTH. Thyroxine and steroid replacement may be required.

Treatment involves hypophysectomy, which requires steroid cover preoperatively, and steroid, thyroxine and possibly ADH replacement thereafter.

Cushing's disease

Cushing's disease results from basophil adenomas, which secrete ACTH (see below).

Hypopituitarism (Simmonds disease)

Causes include chromophobe adenoma, tumours of surrounding tissues (e.g. craniopharyngioma), skull fractures, infarction following postpartum haemorrhage and infection. Clinical features include loss of axillary and pubic hair, amenorrhoea, features of hypothyroidism and adrenal insufficiency, including hypotension, but with a striking pallor, in contrast to the pigmentation of Addison's disease (see p. 676).

The fluid and electrolyte disturbances are not as marked as in primary adrenal failure as a result of intact aldosterone production, but may be unmasked by surgery, trauma or infection. Anaesthesia in these patients requires steroid cover (p. 676), cautious administration of induction agent and volatile anaesthetic agents, and careful cardiovascular monitoring. Vecuronium and atracurium are preferable to other relaxants.

Diabetes insipidus

This is caused by disease or damage affecting the hypothalamic–posterior pituitary axis. Common causes are pituitary tumours, craniopharyngiomas, basal skull fracture, infection, or as a sequel to pituitary surgery. In 10% of cases, diabetes insipidus is renal in origin.

Dehydration follows excretion of large volumes of dilute urine. Patients require fluid replacement and treatment with vasopressin (DDAVP — desmopressin 2–4 µg i.m. daily or 1 µg i.v. in the acute situation).

Thyroid disease

Goitre

Thyroid swelling may result from iodine deficiency (simple goitre), autoimmune (Hashimoto's) thyroiditis, adenoma, carcinoma or thyrotoxicosis.

Nodules of the thyroid gland may be 'hot' (secreting thyroxine) or 'cold'.

The goitre may occasionally cause respiratory obstruction. Retrosternal goitre may in addition cause superior vena caval obstruction. The presence of a goitre should alert the anaesthetist to the possibility of tracheal compression or displacement. A preoperative X-ray of neck and thoracic inlet may be useful, and a selection of small-diameter, armoured tracheal tubes should be available. Preoperative assessment of thyroid function is essential.

Thyrotoxicosis

This is characterized by excitability, tremor, tachycardia and arrhythmias (commonly atrial fibrillation), weight loss, heat intolerance and exophthalmos. Diagnosis is confirmed by measurement of total serum thyroxine, tri-iodothyroxine (T_3) and TSH.

Elective surgery should not be carried out in hyperthyroid patients; they should first be rendered euthyroid with carbimazole or radioactive iodine. However, urgent surgery and elective subtotal thyroidectomy may be carried out safely in hyperthyroid patients using β-adrenergic blockade alone or in combination with potassium iodide to control thyrotoxic symptoms and signs. Emergency surgery carries a significant risk of thyrotoxic crisis. Control is best achieved in these circumstances by i.v. potassium iodide and a broad-spectrum β-blocker (e.g. propranolol). If patients are unable to absorb oral medication, i.v. infusion is indicated (for propranolol, the daily i.v. dose is approximately one-tenth of the oral dose).

The doses of sedative drugs for premedication, and of anaesthetic agents, should be increased to compensate for faster distribution and elimination. Larger doses of sedative drugs than normal are required to avoid anxiety when procedures are carried out under regional anaesthesia.

Preparation for thyroidectomy. Previous conventional management involved at least 6–8 weeks' administration of carbimazole to render the patient euthyroid, followed by potassium iodide 60 mg t.i.d. for 10 days to decrease the vascularity of the gland.

Many anaesthetists now use β-blockers to prepare the hyperthyroid patient for thyroidectomy. Propranolol 160–480 mg daily for 2 weeks preoperatively and a further 7–10 days postoperatively provides adequate control in most patients. However, control with β-blockers depends on maintaining an adequate plasma concentration of the drug. Since β-blockers, in common with other drugs, are cleared more rapidly than normal in thyrotoxic patients, propranolol should be prescribed more frequently (e.g. four times daily). Alternatively, a long-acting β-blocker, e.g. atenolol once daily (including the morning of surgery), provides satisfactory control, and avoids the problem of impaired drug absorption immediately after operation. A combination of β-blocker and potassium iodide 60 mg t.i.d. provides reliable control in even the most severely thyrotoxic patient.

Hypothyroidism

This may result from primary thyroid failure, Hashimoto's thyroiditis, as a consequence of thyroid surgery, or secondary to pituitary failure. The diagnosis is suggested by tiredness, cold intolerance, loss of appetite, dry skin and hair loss. It may be confirmed by the finding of a low serum thyroxine concentration, associated, in primary thyroid failure, with a raised serum TSH concentration.

Basal metabolic rate is decreased. Cardiac output is decreased, with little myocardial reserve, and hypothermia may be present. Treatment is with thyroxine, which should be started in a small dose of 25–50 µg daily. Rapid correction of hypothyroidism may be achieved using i.v. T_3, but this is inadvisable in elderly patients and those with ischaemic heart disease, which is common in hypothyroidism, as the sudden increase in myocardial oxygen demand may provoke infarction. ECG monitoring is advisable during treatment. Elective surgery should be avoided in myxoedematous patients, but if emergency surgery is necessary, close cardiovascular, ECG and blood gas monitoring is essential. Drug distribution and metabolism are slowed, and thus all anaesthetic agents must be administered in reduced doses.

Disease of the adrenal cortex

Clinical symptoms are associated with increased or decreased secretion of cortisol or aldosterone.

Hypersecretion of cortisol (Cushing's syndrome)

Most instances are caused by pituitary adenomas which secrete ACTH and thus cause bilateral adrenocortical hyperplasia (Cushing's disease). In 20–30% of patients, an adrenocortical adenoma or carcinoma is present. Rarely, an oat-cell carcinoma of bronchus, secreting ACTH, is the cause. ACTH and corticosteroid therapy present similar pictures. Clinical features include obesity, hypertension, proximal myopathy and diabetes mellitus. Biochemically, there is a metabolic alkalosis with hypokalaemia. Depending on the cause, treatment may involve hypophysectomy or adrenalectomy.

Anaesthetic management of these patients involves preoperative treatment of hypertension and congestive cardiac failure, and correction of hypokalaemia. Intraoperative management is directed towards careful monitoring of arterial pressure, and maintenance of cardiovascular stability, with careful choice and administration of anaesthetic agents and muscle relaxants. Etomidate and atracurium or vecuronium would be an appropriate choice of induction agent and relaxant. Postoperative steroid cover is required for hypophysectomy and adrenalectomy (see below). Fludrocortisone 0.1–0.3 mg daily is required after bilateral adrenalectomy.

Primary hypersecretion of aldosterone (Conn's syndrome)

Conn's syndrome is caused by an adenoma of the zona glomerulosa of the adrenal cortex and presents with hypertension, hypernatraemia, hypokalaemia and oliguria. Anaesthetic management involves preoperative treatment of hypertension, the administration of spironolactone and potassium replacement; meticulous intra- and postoperative monitoring of arterial pressure is essential.

Adrenocortical hypofunction

Primary adrenocortical insufficiency (Addison's disease) may be caused by an autoimmune process, tuberculosis, amyloid, metastatic carcinoma, or following bilateral adrenalectomy. Haemorrhage into the glands during meningococcal septicaemia may cause acute adrenal failure in association with septic shock. Secondary failure results from hypopituitarism or prolonged corticosteroid therapy. In secondary failure resulting from pituitary insufficiency, aldosterone secretion is maintained, and fluid and electrolyte disturbances less marked.

Clinical features include weakness, weight loss, hyperpigmentation, hypotension, vomiting, diarrhoea and volume depletion. Hypoglycaemia, hyponatraemia, hyperkalaemia and metabolic acidosis are characteristic biochemical findings. The stress of infection, trauma or surgery provokes profound hypotension. Diagnosis is made by measurement of plasma cortisol concentrations, and the response to ACTH stimulation.

All surgical procedures in these patients must be covered by increased steroid administration (see below). Patients with acute adrenal insufficiency require urgent fluid and sodium replacement with arterial pressure and CVP monitoring, glucose infusion to combat hypoglycaemia and hydrocortisone 100 mg 6-hourly i.v. Antibiotics are advisable to cover the possibility that infection has provoked the crisis. In cases of primary adrenal failure, mineralocorticoid replacement with fludrocortisone is required. If emergency surgery is required in acute adrenal failure, all precautions necessary for anaesthetizing the shocked patient should be taken (p. 657).

Congenital adrenal hyperplasia (adrenogenital syndrome)

This is associated with overproduction of androgens as a result of deficiency of hydroxylase enzyme required for production of cortisol. Hydrocortisone treatment overcomes adrenal insufficiency and, by suppressing ACTH production, decreases androgen accumulation. Augmented steroid cover is required for surgery in these patients.

Steroid therapy

Replacement therapy in cases of primary adrenocortical failure and hypopituitarism is given as oral hydrocortisone 20 mg in the morning and 10 mg in the evening. Fludrocortisone 0.05–0.1 mg daily is given additionally to replace aldosterone in primary adrenocortical failure. Equivalent doses of other steroid preparations are shown in Table

40.4. Prednisolone and prednisone have less mineralocorticoid effect, while betamethasone and dexamethasone have none. Requirements increase following infection, trauma or surgery.

Corticosteroids are also prescribed for a wide range of medical conditions, including asthma and collagen diseases. Prolonged therapy suppresses adrenocortical function.

Steroid cover for anaesthesia and surgery

Indications for augmented perioperative steroid cover include the following.

1. Patients with pituitary–adrenal insufficiency, on steroid replacement therapy.
2. Patients undergoing pituitary or adrenal surgery.
3. Patients on systemic steroid therapy for more than 2 weeks before surgery.
4. Patients on systemic steroid therapy for more than 1 month in the year before surgery.

Topical fluorinated steroid preparations applied widely to the skin may be absorbed sufficiently to produce adrenal suppression. Preoperative assessment should involve appropriate fluid and electrolyte correction. Evidence of infection should be sought in patients on long-term steroid therapy.

Corticosteroid cover for operation should be given as follows.

1. *Minor diagnostic procedures.* Single dose of hydrocortisone 50 mg i.m. 1 h preoperatively.
2. *Intermediate operations* (e.g. inguinal herniorrhaphy). Hydrocortisone 50 mg i.m. with premedication; 50 mg 6-hourly for 24 h.
3. *Major surgery.* Hydrocortisone 100 mg 6-hourly for 72 h starting with premedication.

The requirements may need to be increased if infection is present, or be continued beyond 3 days if infection or the effects of major trauma persist. Oral steroid preparations may be preferred for premedication and then be resumed after 24 h.

If steroids are prescribed for asthma or other medical conditions, the perioperative dosage may require modification according to the activity of the disease.

Disease of the adrenal medulla

Phaeochromocytoma

See page 588.

DIABETES MELLITUS

Fifty per cent of all diabetic patients present for surgery during their lifetime, most commonly for ophthalmic or vascular disease or for drainage of an abscess. Perioperative morbidity and mortality are greater in diabetic than in non-diabetic patients. This may result partly from controllable factors such as regulation of perioperative blood glucose, but unavoidable complications of diabetes, such as ischaemic heart disease, autonomic neuropathy and infection may affect anaesthetic management.

The problems of managing diabetics who undergo surgery are associated with its attendant period of starvation and the metabolic effects of surgery. The aim is to minimize the metabolic disturbance by ensuring an adequate intake of glucose, calories and insulin, thus controlling hyperglycaemia and reducing proteolysis, lipolysis and production of lactate and ketones. Adequate control of blood glucose concentration must be established preoperatively and maintained until oral feeding is resumed after operation. Hypoglycaemia, which may not be detectable readily in the anaesthetized patient, must be avoided. Modern techniques for frequent monitoring of blood glucose (Dextrostix, Ames: BM-Test-Glycemie, Boehringer-Mannheim, preferably used in conjunction with a reflectance colorimeter) have simplified management considerably.

Precise management depends upon the nature of the diabetes and its treatment (insulin-dependent or non-insulin-dependent), on the magnitude of the surgery contemplated (including the estimated time to resumption of oral intake) and on the time available for control of the diabetes.

Preoperative assessment

Preoperative assessment is aimed at evaluating blood glucose control; the treatment regimen used; and the presence of complications.

Control of blood glucose

This is assessed by inspection of the patient's urine-testing or BM-testing records, by random blood glucose measurements, by a 24-h blood glucose profile in patients receiving insulin and by measurement of glycosylated haemoglobin (Hb A_{1C}). Whenever possible, blood glucose concentration should be maintained between 6 and 10 mmol.litre^{-1}, and insulin dosages should be adjusted to achieve this, with the introduction of twice-daily short and intermediate-acting insulins if necessary. Potassium may fall on institution of insulin treatment and blood urea and electrolyte concentrations should be checked.

Treatment regimens

Oral hypoglycaemic agents are of two types. The sulphonylureas stimulate release of insulin from the pancreatic islets. Chlorpropamide has a very prolonged duration of action and may cause hypoglycaemia unless it is withdrawn 48 h before surgery. A change to a shorter-acting agent such as glipizide or gliclazide is preferable.

Biguanides, which increase peripheral uptake of glucose and decrease gluconeogenesis, are used in obese maturity-onset diabetics either alone or in combination with sulphonylureas. These agents may cause lactic acidosis, usually, but not exclusively, in patients with even mild renal or hepatic impairment. This complication carries a very high mortality; consequently, metformin, the only biguanide now available, should be discontinued at least 24 h before surgery.

The last dose of oral hypoglycaemic agent should be administered 24 h before surgery and no further treatment is required until the morning of surgery if blood glucose control is satisfactory.

Insulin. Some of the newer insulin preparations in common use are listed in Table 40.6. The best control is achieved by twice-daily injections of short-acting and intermediate-acting insulin. Increasingly, younger diabetics are managed with a background once-daily ultra-long-acting preparation coupled with a pen injector delivering small doses of short-acting insulin. The type of preparation must be noted, and if a change is made in the type of insulin (bovine, porcine, human) the dose must be adjusted, because increased sensitivity to the latter two may lead to hypoglycaemia. Insulin with the human sequence of amino acids is produced biosynthetically (chain recombinant DNA technology using bacteria: CRB) or semisyntheti-

Table 40.6 Newer insulin preparations

Proprietary name	Type and source	Onset (h)	Peak action (h)	Duration of action (h)	Dosage
Humulin S	Short-acting, soluble, CRB	0.5	1–3	5–7	t.i.d. alone or b.d. + intermediate preparation
Human Velosulin	Short-acting, soluble, EMP	0.5	1–3	8	
Actrapid MC	Short-acting, soluble, porcine	0.5	2–5	8	
Humulin I	Intermediate, isophane, CRB	1.0	2–8	18–20	b.d. + short-acting preparation
Insulatard	Intermediate, isophane, porcine	1.5	4–12	24	b.d. + short-acting preparation
Semitard	Insulin zinc suspension amorphous semilente, porcine	1.5	5–10	16	b.d. + short-acting preparation
Humulin M2	Mixed 20% soluble, 80% isophane, CRB	0.5	1–8	14–16	b.d.
Mixtard 30/70	Mixed 30% soluble, 70% isophane, porcine	0.5	4–8	24	b.d.
Monotard MC	Long-acting, insulin zinc suspension, 30% amorphous, 70% crystalline, lente, porcine	2.5	7–15	22	daily or b.d.
Humulin Zn	Long-acting, insulin zinc suspension, crystalline CRB	3	6–14	20–24	daily or b.d.

CRB = chain recombinant DNA technology using bacteria; EMP = enzyme modification of porcine material.

cally (by enzyme modification of porcine material: EMP) from purified porcine insulin. The biosynthetic preparations are less expensive than purified porcine, and may become the principal commercial preparations. Insulin with the human sequence is associated with a less severe degree of antigenicity and is thus the preparation of choice for newly diagnosed diabetics and for patients requiring short-term therapy (e.g. in the perioperative period).

In well-controlled diabetics, it is not necessary to change to a short-acting insulin regimen on the day before surgery, provided that the dose of the intermediate or long-acting insulin is not excessive (40 units of long-acting or 24-unit evening dose of intermediate insulin); all too often a change of regimen results in poorer control.

The poorly controlled diabetic. Whether the patient is normally insulin-dependent or not, elective surgery should be delayed until improved control is achieved by administration of short-acting insulin three times daily. If surgery is urgent, a glucose, insulin and potassium regimen (Table 40.7) should be instituted to achieve rapid blood glucose control.

Table 40.7 Perioperative management of the maturity-onset diabetic

Preoperative
Check random glucose, urea and electrolyte concentrations:
Poor control: Start insulin (t.i.d. soluble) and delay surgery
Urgent surgery: glucose/insulin infusion (Table 40.8)
Good control: Chlorpropamide — change to a shorter-acting agent
All agents terminated 24 h preoperatively

Day of surgery
Check fasting blood glucose (BM stix, Dextrostix)
No oral hypoglycaemic agent
Minor surgery: If blood glucose < 10 mmol.litre^{-1}, no specific therapy
Major surgery: Treat as insulin-dependent diabetic (Table 40.8)

Postoperative
Check blood glucose (BM stix, Dextrostix)
Minor surgery: Restart oral hypoglycaemic agent with first meal
Major surgery: Treat as insulin-dependent diabetic (Table 40.8)
When oral diet is resumed, t.i.d. soluble insulin 8–12 units before each meal; restart oral therapy when daily requirement is less than 20 units

Complications of diabetes mellitus

1. *Cardiovascular disorders* (coronary artery, cerebrovascular and peripheral vascular) are common in diabetics, and there is an increased risk of perioperative myocardial infarction. Careful preoperative assessment of cardiovascular function, appropriate choice of anaesthetic technique and precise perioperative monitoring are essential.

2. *Renal disease.* Microvascular damage produces glomerulosclerosis with proteinuria, oedema and eventually chronic renal failure. Anaesthetic implications of renal disease are discussed on pages 668–671.

3. *Ocular problems.* Cataracts, exudative or proliferative retinopathy, vitreous haemorrhage and retinal detachment may occur. In the long term, good blood glucose control has been shown to reduce the frequency of such complications.

4. *Infection.* Diabetics are prone to infection and an increased risk of septicaemia and abscess formation. Infection is associated with increased insulin requirements, which return to normal on its eradication, e.g. after surgical drainage of an abscess.

5. *Neuropathy.* Chronic sensory peripheral neuropathies are common; mononeuropathies and acute motor neuropathies (amyotrophy) are associated with poor control of blood glucose. Loss of sensation together with peripheral vascular disease can lead to ulceration after trivial trauma; consequently, care in positioning patients in the operating theatre is important. Local anaesthetic nerve or plexus blocks should be avoided in patients with an acute neuropathy as neurological deficits may be attributed to the local anaesthetic solution.

6. *Autonomic neuropathy* may cause postoperative urinary retention or vasomotor instability, e.g. postural hypotension or hypotension during anaesthesia. IPPV or subarachnoid or extradural block may be associated with severe hypotension; adequate preoperative hydration, precise cardiovascular monitoring and careful anaesthetic management are essential.

Concurrent drug therapy

Thiazide diuretics, diazoxide, adrenergic agents (e.g. salbutamol) and corticosteroids tend to increase the blood glucose concentration. Hypotensive drugs, e.g. β-adrenergic blockers, tend to potentiate hypoglycaemia and may mask its clinical signs. Blood glucose should be monitored if any of these drugs is administered, and insulin dosage altered accordingly.

Some drugs, including phenylbutazone, displace sulphonylureas from protein-binding sites and potentiate their hypoglycaemic effect.

Perioperative diabetic management

A combination of glucose and insulin is the most satisfactory method of overcoming the deleterious metabolic consequences of starvation and surgical stress in the diabetic patient.

Although satisfactory control of blood glucose may be achieved using a no-glucose/no-insulin regimen, the raised blood urea concentration which occurs often in the postoperative period is indicative of increased protein breakdown, accompanying lipolysis and ketosis. Minor procedures may be carried out at the start of an operating list by delaying the morning dose of insulin until a late breakfast is taken after recovery from anaesthesia. A low-dose insulin infusion on its own (0.5 unit.h^{-1} by syringe pump) is effective for minor surgery, but is not adequate for major surgery.

Subarachnoid and extradural anaesthesia have some advantages in the diabetic patient; avoidance of general anaesthesia allows hypoglycaemia to be recognized, while early resumption of oral diet eases postoperative management.

Tables 40.7 and 40.8 (both of which are based on Alberti's recommendations) describe schemes for the precise management of patients receiving oral hypoglycaemic agents or insulin therapy who require minor or major surgery. Minor surgery includes endoscopic procedures and body-surface surgery.

The combination of i.v. glucose solution with insulin added to the bag is a safety precaution; one cannot be infused inadvertently without the other and thus hyperglycaemia, and more particularly hypoglycaemia, are avoided. Glucose 10% is used to provide adequate carbohydrate and energy without excessive volume. The glucose/insulin solution should be administered through an i.v. cannula separate from that used for other

Table 40.8 Perioperative management of the insulin-dependent diabetic

Preoperative
Blood glucose profile; urea and electrolytes; urine ketones
Adjust insulin therapy; most patients b.d. soluble + isophane

Poor control: change to t.i.d. soluble insulin and delay surgery

Urgent surgery: glucose/insulin infusion (see below)

Day of surgery
Check fasting blood glucose; repeat 2-hourly
No subcutaneous insulin
Start infusion of 10% glucose (500 ml) with soluble (Humulin S) insulin 10 units and KCl 10 mmol at 0800 h to run 4–6 hourly

Adjust insulin in bag as follows depending on blood glucose:
  < 4 mmol.litre^{-1}: no insulin
  4–6 mmol.litre^{-1}: insulin 5 units per 500 ml glucose 10%
  6–10 mmol.litre^{-1}: infusion as above
  10–20 mmol.litre^{-1}: insulin 15 units per 500 ml glucose 10%
  > 20 mmol.litre^{-1}: insulin 20 units per 500 ml glucose 10%

Adjust potassium dosage depending on plasma K$^+$ concentration
  < 3 mmol.litre^{-1}: add KCl 20 mmol
  > 5 mmol.litre^{-1}: omit KCl

Postoperative
Check blood glucose 2–6-hourly; check urea and electrolytes daily

Continue 4–6-hourly infusion until oral diet re-established

If delayed, change to decreased volume of 20–50% glucose with independent insulin infusion by syringe pump

When oral diet resumed, t.i.d. soluble insulin s.c.; daily dosage as preoperative

When requirements stable, restart normal regimen

i.v. fluids; it is preferable to use an infusion pump to regulate the rate of infusion.

This scheme provides 250 g of glucose (1000 kcal) and an average of 50 units of insulin over 24 h. If the patient has high insulin demands normally or is obese, additional insulin may be required (e.g. 5 units/bag more than the amount stated in Table 40.8). Patients who normally receive oral hypoglycaemic agents may be more sensitive, and require less insulin.

Blood transfusion may increase insulin requirements as the elevated citrate concentration stimulates gluconeogenesis. Ringer's lactate (Hartmann's) solution elevates blood glucose concentration for the same reason, and should be avoided.

If control is difficult to achieve with this regimen because of postoperative complications such as sepsis or as a result of steroid therapy, blood glucose may be controlled by a separate insulin infusion delivered by a syringe pump, with regulation of the insulin infusion rate determined by 2-hourly blood glucose measurements.

Emergency surgery and diabetic ketoacidosis

Diabetic ketoacidosis results from inadequate insulin dosage or increased insulin requirements, often precipitated by infection, trauma or surgical stress. Diabetics who require emergency surgery often have a grossly elevated blood glucose concentration and occasionally overt ketoacidosis. Such patients require rehydration, correction of sodium depletion, correction of subsequent potassium depletion and i.v. soluble (Humulin S) insulin by infusion at an initial rate of 4–8 unit.h^{-1}.

Initial fluid replacement should consist of isotonic (0.9%) saline: 1 litre in the first 30 min, 1 litre in the next hour and a further litre over the next 2 h. If the plasma sodium concentration is greater than 150 mmol.litre^{-1}, 0.45% saline should be used.

Progress is monitored by regular measurements of blood glucose, sodium and potassium concentrations, and arterial pH and blood gases. Correction of acidosis with bicarbonate is rarely if ever required. Cellular potassium depletion is present from the outset, but hyperkalaemia or normokalaemia may be found initially because potassium shifts out of the cells in the presence of acidosis. Potassium replacement is required as the plasma concentration begins to decrease with the correction of the acidosis. Magnesium 5–10 mmol is also required. An infusion of glucose 5% should be given when the blood glucose concentration decreases to approximately 15 mmol.litre^{-1}. When volume resuscitation is under way, and some reversal of acidosis and hyperglycaemia has been achieved, surgery may be carried out while management of the diabetes is continued intra- and postoperatively.

NEUROLOGICAL DISEASE

There are several points of significance.

1. *Medicolegal.* Perioperative alteration in neurological deficit may be attributed to anaesthesia. This may render subarachnoid or extradural anaesthesia inadvisable in some patients.

2. *Respiratory impairment.* Motor neuropathy from various causes, e.g. motor neurone disease, acute polyneuritis (Guillain–Barré syndrome), disorders of the neuromuscular junction and high-spinal-cord lesions may produce respiratory inadequacy. These patients are sensitive to anaesthetic agents, opioids and relaxants, and if intraoperative IPPV is undertaken, a period of elective postoperative ventilation may be necessary until full recovery from the effects of anaesthesia has occurred. If possible, procedures should be carried out under local or regional block. If bulbar muscles are involved, protection of the airway from regurgitation and aspiration may require prolonged tracheal intubation or tracheostomy. Surgery should be postponed if a chest infection is present preoperatively.

3. *Altered innervation of muscle, and potassium shifts.* An altered ratio of intracellular to extracellular potassium tends to produce a sensitivity to non-depolarizing, and resistance to depolarizing, relaxants. If there is widespread denervation of muscle in lower motor neurone disease, e.g. in Guillain–Barré syndrome, disorganization of the motor end-plate occurs, resulting in hypersensitivity to acetylcholine and suxamethonium, with increased permeability of muscle cells to potassium. A similar potassium efflux occurs in the presence of direct muscle damage, widespread burns involving muscle, upper motor neurone lesions, spinal cord lesions with paraplegia, and tetanus. In upper motor neurone and spinal cord lesions, the reason for this shift is less clear.

The resulting increase in serum potassium concentration after suxamethonium may be 3 mmol.litre^{-1} (in comparison with 0.5 mmol.litre^{-1} in the normal patient) and may occur from 24 h after acute muscle denervation or damage until 6–12 months later. In such patients, suxamethonium is clearly contraindicated.

4. *Autonomic disturbances* may occur as part of a polyneuropathy, e.g. diabetes, Guillain–Barré syndrome and porphyria. Sympathetic stimulation, for example during light anaesthesia, tracheal intubation or following administration of pancuronium or catecholamines, may produce severe hypertension and arrhythmias. More commonly,

blood loss, head-up posture or IPPV may be associated with severe hypotension.

5. *Increased intracranial pressure.* Elective surgery should be postponed if raised intracranial pressure is suspected, until investigation and treatment have been undertaken. Anaesthetic agents which cause an increase in cerebral blood flow must be avoided. Hypercapnia must also be avoided and controlled ventilation to a Pa_{CO_2} of approximately 4 kPa (30 mmHg) is indicated. This is discussed fully in Chapter 37.

6. *Cerebrovascular disease.* In patients with suspected widespread cerebrovascular disease, the principal aim of anaesthetic management should be to avoid hypoxaemia and to maintain normotension and normocapnia. Although hypercapnia increases cerebral blood flow, it may produce steal from ischaemic to well-perfused areas of brain. Hypocapnia decreases cerebral blood flow and is also contraindicated.

Epilepsy

Epilepsy may be associated with birth injury, hypoglycaemia, hypocalcaemia, drug withdrawal, fever, head injury, cerebrovascular disease and cerebral tumour, the most likely cause depending on the age of onset. In most patients with epilepsy, no identifiable cause can be found. Epilepsy developing after the age of 20 years usually indicates organic brain disease.

Anaesthesia

Patients should be maintained on anticonvulsant therapy throughout the perioperative period. Some anaesthetic agents, e.g. enflurane and methohexitone, have cerebral excitatory effects and should be avoided. Convulsions and abnormalities of muscle posture have been reported after operation in patients who have received propofol, and it is currently recommended that this drug should not be used in known epileptics. Thiopentone is a potent anticonvulsant and is the i.v. induction agent of choice, while isoflurane is currently the volatile agent of choice. Local anaesthetic agents may cause convulsions at lower than normal concentrations and the safe maximum dose should be reduced. The anticonvulsants phenobarbitone

and phenytoin induce hepatic enzymes and accelerate elimination of drugs metabolized by the liver.

In cases of late-onset epilepsy, where increased intracranial pressure may be present as a result of tumour, controlled ventilation is advisable to avoid any further increase in intracranial pressure.

Status epilepticus

Management is aimed at cessation of the fits while maintaining tissue oxygenation. Initial treatment should be Diazemuls, titrated intravenously in a dose of up to 10–20 mg or until fitting ceases. High-flow oxygen should be administered, and the airway maintained throughout. If the convulsions persist or conscious level diminishes to the extent of compromising the airway and ventilation, the patient should be anaesthetized, the trachea intubated and mechanical ventilation commenced.

The conventional anaesthetic induction agent employed is thiopentone. A loading dose of phenytoin ($10–20$ mg.kg^{-1} over 30–60 min) should be given. The infusion of thiopentone may be discontinued when control of the fits has been achieved.

The ventilated patient with status epilepticus should not normally be paralysed, but if so, a cerebral function monitor/electroencephalogram monitor must be used so that continued fitting is noted and treated.

Multiple sclerosis

Deterioration of symptoms tends to occur after surgery, but no specific anaesthetic technique has been implicated. It is usually advisable to avoid extradural and subarachnoid anaesthesia, but only for medicolegal reasons, as there is no evidence that these techniques affect the disease adversely; they may be used if indicated strongly, provided that a full explanation has been given to the patient, e.g. in obstetrics.

If a large motor deficit of recent onset is present, there may be increased potassium release from muscle following suxamethonium, which should be avoided.

Peripheral neuropathies

These may exhibit axonal 'dying back' degeneration or segmental demyelination. They are classified by anatomical distribution, the commonest being a symmetrical peripheral polyneuropathy.

Motor, sensory and autonomic fibres are involved. Causes include:

1. Metabolic (diabetes, porphyria).
2. Nutritional deficiency.
3. Toxic (heavy metals, drugs).
4. Collagen disease.
5. Carcinoma.
6. Infective.

Problems for the anaesthetist include the effects of autonomic neuropathy, and respiratory and bulbar involvement.

Acute inflammatory polyneuropathy (Guillain–Barré syndrome)

This polyneuropathy appears some days after a pyrexial illness. Progression is very variable, ranging from near total paralysis in 24 h to progression over several weeks. Respiratory and bulbar muscles may be affected, and if so, tracheal intubation followed by tracheostomy and IPPV are required. Autonomic neuropathy may result in hypotension following institution of IPPV. This may be minimized by adequate fluid preloading and gradual increases in minute volume. Suxamethonium should be avoided. There is evidence that either high-dose immunoglobulin therapy or plasmapheresis beneficially modifies the course of the disease.

Motor neurone disease (progressive muscular atrophy, amyotrophic lateral sclerosis, progressive bulbar palsy)

Motor neurone disease is characterized by slow onset and progressive deterioration in motor function. Several patterns of motor loss occur with both upper and lower motor neurone loss. Problems for the anaesthetist include sensitivity to all anaesthetic agents and muscle relaxants, respiratory inadequacy and laryngeal incompetence. Local anaesthetic techniques may be useful.

Hereditary ataxias

Friedreich's ataxia is the most common. Spino-

cerebellar, corticospinal and posterior columns are involved, and the course of the disease is slowly progressive. Problems for the anaesthetist include scoliosis, respiratory failure and cardiomyopathy with cardiac failure and arrhythmias.

Spinal cord lesions with paraplegia

Release of potassium from muscle cells by suxamethonium precludes its use within 6–12 months of cord injury.

Huntington's chorea

It has been reported that thiopentone may cause prolonged apnoea, while abnormal serum cholinesterase may prolong the action of suxamethonium.

Myasthenia gravis

This disease usually occurs in young adults and is characterized by episodes of increased muscle fatiguability, caused by decreased numbers of acetylcholine receptors at the neuromuscular junction. Treatment comprises an anticholinesterase (pyridostigmine 60 mg q.i.d. or neostigmine 15 mg q.i.d.) with a vagolytic agent (atropine or propantheline) to block the muscarinic side-effects. Steroid therapy is useful in some cases and thymectomy may benefit many patients considerably, especially young women with myasthenia of recent onset.

The principal problems concern adequacy of ventilation, ability to cough and clear secretions, and the increased secretions resulting from anticholinesterase therapy. If there is evidence of respiratory infection, surgery should be postponed. Serum potassium concentration should be normal, as hypokalaemia potentiates myasthenia. Local and regional anaesthesia, including low subarachnoid or extradural block, may be suitable alternatives to general anaesthesia, although the maximum dose of local anaesthetic agents should be reduced because of their neuromuscular blocking action. The minimum possible dose of induction agent should be used and relaxants should be avoided if possible. For major procedures requiring relaxation, the anticholinesterase may be omitted for 4 h preoperatively, and a small dose of relaxant may be given if necessary. Atracurium is the relaxant of choice because of its short duration of action, and should be administered in a reduced dose (10–20% of normal). Suxamethonium has a variable effect in myasthenia and is best avoided.

Postoperatively, the patient's lungs should be ventilated electively after major surgery (usually for a few hours, but in some cases for up to 48 h). Frequent chest physiotherapy and tracheal suction are required. Steroid cover is given if appropriate. If extreme muscle weakness occurs, i.v. atropine 0.6–1.2 mg and neostigmine 1–2 mg may be given. Care must be taken to titrate the doses of anticholinesterase carefully, or a cholinergic crisis, characterized by a depolarizing neuromuscular block, with sweating, salivation and pupillary constriction, may occur. An infusion of neostigmine is required if resumption of oral intake is delayed after surgery; 0.5 mg i.v. is equal to 15 mg neostigmine or 60 mg pyridostigmine orally. Edrophonium may be used to test the end-plate response to acetylcholine.

A myasthenic state may also be associated with carcinoma, thyrotoxicosis, Cushing's syndrome, hypokalaemia and hypocalcaemia. In these patients, non-depolarizing relaxants should be avoided, or used in reduced dosage.

Familial periodic paralysis

This is also associated with prolonged paralysis after administration of non-depolarizing muscle relaxants.

Progressive muscular dystrophy

Several types of muscular dystrophy exist, of varying patterns of heredity and described according to their anatomical distribution. Muscular weakness occurs, and must be distinguished from myasthenia and lower motor neurone disease. The anaesthetic complications comprise sensitivity to relaxants, opioids and other sedative and anaesthetic drugs, and liability to respiratory infection. Myocardial involvement may occur.

Dystrophia myotonica

This is a disease of autosomal dominant inherit-ance characterized by muscle weakness and muscle contraction persisting after the termination of voluntary effort. Other features may include frontal baldness, cataract, sternomastoid wasting, gonadal atrophy and thyroid adenoma. Problems which affect anaesthetic management include the following.

1. *Respiratory muscle weakness.* Respiratory function should be fully assessed before operation. Respiratory depressant drugs, e.g. thiopentone or opioids, should be used with care; there is sensitivity also to non-depolarizing relaxants. Elective IPPV may be required after surgery. Postoperative care of the airway must be meticulous because of muscle weakness. Chest infections are common.

2. *Cardiovascular effects.* There may be a cardiomyopathy and conduction defects. Arrhythmias are common, particularly during anaesthesia, and may result in cardiac failure. Careful monitoring is essential.

3. *Muscle spasm.* This may be provoked by administration of depolarizing muscle relaxants or anticholinesterases. Suxamethonium and neostigmine should thus be avoided. The spasm is not abolished by non-depolarizing relaxants.

MISCELLANEOUS DISORDERS

Carcinoid syndrome

See page 587.

Myeloma

This neoplastic condition affects plasma cells and has a number of features of significance to the anaesthetist.

1. Widespread skeletal destruction occurs and careful handling of the patient on the operating table is essential. Pathological fractures are common.
2. Bone pain may be severe and often requires large doses of analgesics. Thus, tolerance to opioids may occur.
3. Hypercalcaemia occurs as a result of bony destruction, and may precipitate renal failure.

4. Chronic renal failure may also result from myeloma directly.
5. Anaemia is almost invariable, and preoperative blood transfusion is often necessary.
6. Patients are liable to infection, including chest infection, especially during cytotoxic therapy.
7. During cytotoxic therapy, thrombocytopenia is common.
8. Increased plasma immunoglobulin concentrations may raise blood viscosity, predisposing to arterial and venous thrombosis. Drug binding may be affected, e.g. resistance to *d*-tubocurarine may occur.

9. Neurological manifestations include spinal cord and nerve root compression.

Porphyria

The porphyrias are an inherited group of disorders of porphyrin metabolism characterized by increased activity of D-aminolaevulinic acid synthetase with excessive production of porphyrins or their precursors. In the UK, *acute intermittent porphyria is* the most common type. It is characterized by acute attacks which may arise spontaneously or be precipitated by infection, starvation, pregnancy or administration of some drugs.

Table 40.9 Safety of drugs commonly used in clinical anaesthesia for patients with acute porphyrias

Drug group						
Intravenous induction agents	Propofol Midazolam	PS PS	Ketamine	C	Barbiturates Etomidate	U PU
Inhalation agents	Nitrous oxide Cyclopropane Diethyl ether	S S S	Halothane Isoflurane	C ND	Enflurane	PU
Muscle relaxants	Curare Suxamethonium Vecuronium	S S PS	Atracurium Pancuronium	ND C	Alcuronium	PU
Neuromuscular blockade reversal	Atropine Neostigmine	 S	Glycopyrronium	ND		
Local anaesthetics	Procaine Amethocaine	S PS	Lignocaine Prilocaine Bupivacaine	C C C	Mepivacaine	PU
Analgesics	Morphine Pethidine Fentanyl Buprenorphine Naloxone Paracetamol	S S S S PS S	Alfentanil Sufentanil	ND ND	Pentazocine Tilidine	U U
Anxiolytics	Temazepam Lorazepam Droperidol Phenothiazines	S PS S S	Diazepam Triazolam Oxazepam	C C C	All other benzodiazepines	U
Antiarrhythmics	Procainamide β-blockers	S S	Lignocaine Mexiletine Bretylium Disopyramide	C ND ND C	Verapamil Nifedipine Diltiazem	U U U
Other cardiovascular drugs	Adrenaline Phentolamine	S S	β-Agonists α-Agonists Sodium nitroprusside	ND ND ND	Hydralazine Phenoxybenzamine	U U
Bronchodilators	Corticosteroids Salbutamol	PS S	Hexaprenaline	ND	Aminophylline	U
Gastric – for Caesarean section	Metoclopramide Domperidone	PS S	Ranitidine	C	Cimetidine	PU

PS = Possibly safe; S = safe; C = contentious; ND = no data; U = unsafe; PU = probably unsafe.

Inheritance is Mendelian dominant and thus a family history of porphyria requires further investigation. Clinical features include the following.

1. *Gastrointestinal.* Abdominal pain and tenderness, vomiting, constipation and occasionally diarrhoea.

2. *Neurological.* A motor and sensory peripheral neuropathy is common. It may involve bulbar and respiratory muscles. Epileptic fits and psychological disturbance may occur.

3. *Cardiovascular.* Hypertension and tachycardia often occur during the attacks. Hypotension has been reported also.

4. Fever and leukocytosis occur in 25–30% of patients. Drugs which provoke the attack include alcohol, barbiturates, chlordiazepoxide, steroid hormones, chlorpropamide, pentazocine, phenytoin and sulphonamides.

Anaesthesia in such patients is directed to avoiding drugs which may provoke attacks. Induction with propofol, followed by muscle relaxation with suxamethonium, *d*-tubocurarine or vecuronium, ventilation with nitrous oxide, and oxygen and analgesic supplementation with morphine or fentanyl is satisfactory (Table 40.9). If fits occur, diazepam is a suitable anticonvulsant, while chlorpromazine, promethazine or promazine are suitable sedatives.

FURTHER READING

Alberti K G M M, Thomas B J B 1979 The management of diabetes during surgery. British Journal of Anaesthesia 51: 693

Alexander J P 1991 Management of hypertension. In: Dundee J W, Clarke R S J, McCaughey W (eds) Clinical anaesthetic pharmacology. Churchill Livingstone, Edinburgh

Bennett D H 1985 Cardiac arrhythmias. Practical notes on interpretation and treatment. Wright, Bristol

British Thoracic Society 1993 Guidelines for the management of asthma: a summary. British Medical Journal 306: 776–782

Davies S C 1991 The vaso-occlusive crisis of sickle cell disease. British Medical Journal 302: 1551–1552

Goldman L 1988 Assessment of the patient with known or suspected ischaemic heart disease for non-cardiac surgery. British Journal of Anaesthesia 61: 38

Grant I S 1994 Anaesthesia and respiratory disease. In: Nimmo W S, Rowbotham D J, Smith G (eds) Anaesthesia, 2nd edn. Blackwell, London

Hamilton W F D, Forest A L, Gunn A, Peden W R, Feely J 1984 Beta-adrenoceptor blockade and anaesthesia for thyroidectomy. Anaesthesia 39: 335

Harris K 1992 The role of prostaglandins in the control of renal function. British Journal of Anaesthesia 69: 233–235

Harrison G G, Meissner P N, Hift R J 1993 Anaesthesia for the porphyric patient. Anaesthesia 48: 417–421

Jones R M, Rosen M, Seymour L 1987 Smoking and anaesthesia. Anaesthesia 42: 1

Katz J, Benumof J, Kadis L B 1989 Anaesthesia and uncommon diseases: pathophysiologic and clinical correlations. W B Saunders, Philadelphia

Opie L H 1991 Drugs for the heart, 3rd ed. W B Saunders, Philadelphia

Reiz S, Mangano D T 1994 Anaesthesia and cardiac disease. In: Nimmo W S, Smith G (eds) Anaesthesia. Blackwell, London

Shenkman Z, Shir Y, Brodsky J B 1993 Perioperative management of the obese patient. British Journal of Anaesthesia 70: 349–359

Stoelting R K, Dierdorf S R, McCammon 1988 Anaesthesia and co-existing disease, 2nd ed. Churchill Livingstone, London

Symreng T, Karlberg B E, Kagedal B, Schildt B 1981 Physiological cortisol substitution of long-term steroid treated patients undergoing major surgery. British Journal of Anaesthesia 53: 949–953

Vickers M D, Jones R M 1989 Medicine for anaesthetists, 3rd ed. Blackwell Scientific Publications, Oxford

Wahba R W M, Beipue F, Kleiman S J 1995 Cardiopulmonary function and laparoscopic cholecystectomy. Canadian Journal of Anaesthesia 42: 51–63

Welbourn R G, Joffe S N 1977 The apudomas. Recent advances in surgery 9. Churchill Livingstone, Edinburgh

41. The intensive therapy unit

The intensive therapy unit (ITU) is the hospital facility within which the highest level of continuous patient care and treatment is provided. Approximately 1–2% of acute beds are used for this purpose and are organized usually into units of 4–8 beds, as this is considered to be the optimal size.

The nature of the patient care carried out in the ITU has led to the development of designs which differ considerably from hospital to hospital. A much greater area needs to be allocated to each bed than in ordinary wards because several nurses must treat patients simultaneously and bulky items of equipment often need to be accommodated. Each bed area is supplied with oxygen and piped suction (two outlets of each per bed), medical compressed air and sometimes nitrous oxide. At least 12 electric power sockets are required and these should be connected to the emergency standby generator. Sufficient local storage space is required to make the nurse self-sufficient for common procedures such as administration of drugs and tracheal aspiration. Each bed area should be equipped with a self-inflating resuscitation bag to enable the staff to maintain artificial ventilation in case the mechanical ventilator fails.

WHO SHOULD BE ADMITTED?

Patients admitted to the unit should be those whose lives are in imminent danger but in whom, it is believed, the immediate risk may be averted by active and often invasive therapeutic efforts. A wide range of pathological conditions may lead to such a state but all involve failure, or the threat of failure, of the respiratory and/or circulatory systems. In addition, dysfunction of one or more of the renal, gastrointestinal, hepatic, haematological and neurological systems may be present, but involvement of one of these systems alone is rarely a reason for admission to the ITU.

Patients admitted to the ITU require active and aggressive therapy for either (a) appropriate management of a diagnosed condition or (b) resuscitation while a definitive diagnosis is made. Critically ill patients usually benefit from prompt rather than delayed admission to the unit and early notification of such patients elsewhere in the hospital is to be encouraged.

The ITU is not an appropriate place for patients whose death is judged inevitable because of their acute illness or underlying pathology, e.g. the severe chronic bronchitic on maximum treatment or the terminal cancer patient. There is often pressure to admit such patients because they require high levels of nursing care. It is easier to initiate complex therapeutic and supportive effort than it is to withdraw it. Critically ill patients can rarely discuss details of their care and their relatives may also find it difficult to make an objective judgement. It is a moral responsibility of ITU staff to inform patients' relatives if it becomes clear that restoration of a patient's ability to lead an independent existence is impossible. It should be noted that it is unethical and unlawful to treat a patient against his or her volition.

STAFFING CONSIDERATIONS

The ITU consultant

Difficult therapeutic and ethical policy decisions may be required at any time in the ITU. It is essential that they are taken by one whose previous experience is such as to allow a reasonable assessment of the likely outcome and whose therapeutic expertise is likely to give the patient the optimal chance of recovery. The ITU consultant, if not physically present in the unit, must always be available by telephone and should not be involved in any activity which precludes his or her attendance there within 30 min. Because of the critical nature of ITU patients' illnesses, the ITU consultant will expect to be informed immediately of any significant change in their condition. The consultant's basic specialty is relatively unimportant.

The roles of the ITU resident

Communications

Although medical involvement with therapy in the ITU is greater than anywhere else in the hospital except the operating theatre, it should be appreciated that the majority of patient care activities are undertaken by nursing staff. The route by which complex instructions and information are transmitted between medical and nursing staff is of vital importance. A system in which a relatively junior clinician serves as a 'final common pathway' for all instructions works well in practice provided that the doctor involved is present within the unit at all times so that the nurses may obtain clarification of instructions, report changes in status and receive immediate help in emergencies. Nurses shoulder a greater degree of clinical responsibility if their confidence is sustained by a continuous medical presence and this has important consequences for maintaining therapeutic momentum. In addition, a great deal of frustration is engendered by a system in which the nurses are required to contact one or more doctors outside the unit on each occasion that an unexpected alteration occurs in a patient's condition.

Confusion is minimized if the nursing staff take orders only from the unit staff and not directly from visiting clinicians, however eminent, and even if they are nominally in charge of the patient. This is to ensure that the nurses who execute orders are able to confer with the person who wrote them in case of difficulties. In addition, many patients may be under the care of several clinical teams (e.g. multiply injured patients may be treated by a selection from the orthopaedic, general, neuro-, dental, plastic or urological surgeons), so that it is essential that one individual is available to draw attention to, and when necessary harmonize, often conflicting therapeutic regimens. The ITU resident, because of his or her continuous presence in the unit, should be better informed about the patient's recent diagnostic results, physiological status and therapeutic responses than any visiting clinician and should attempt to use current knowledge to guide treatment along rational lines. The ITU consultant must be available to support the resident if conflict occurs, as well as for clinical problems.

The department which provides the unit staff differs from hospital to hospital; units serving primarily a single specialty (e.g. cardiac surgery or neurosurgery units) are usually staffed by the specialty involved, whereas most general ITUs are staffed by the anaesthetic department, which is well used to providing round-the-clock emergency services.

Therapeutic functions

The resident is the first doctor consulted by the nursing staff. It is necessary to decide rapidly whether the problem is one which can be dealt with or if more experienced help should be obtained. The number of occasions when immediate emergency action is required should be relatively small for patients already under the care of experienced ITU nurses (e.g. unforeseen circulatory collapse, accidental tracheal extubation) but resuscitative measures are often required for patients at the time of admission to the unit. The ITU must be forewarned about likely admissions (e.g. by the ambulance service or accident department, operating theatre or wards); the resident should then have time for discussion with the ITU consultant before the patient's arrival.

Most calls to the unit are the result of alterations in measurements rather than a major catastrophe. Tracheal intubation and obtunded consciousness make direct communication with many patients extremely difficult, so that assessment of their problems is based primarily on clinical observation and interpretation of patterns of change in physiological status. The resident should remember that the majority of intensive therapy nurses (and especially the sisters and charge nurses) have an enormous amount of bedside experience with critically ill patients and considerable reliance should be placed on their observations.

ASSESSMENT OF PATIENTS

When called to a patient, the resident should begin to assess the situation by observing the patient and considering questions such as:

1. What changes have occurred since I last saw the patient?
2. Is the patient alert or inert?
3. Is the patient co-operative or confused?
4. Is the patient comfortable or distressed?
5. Is the patient pale or flushed?
6. Is the patient pink or cyanosed?

Simple observations such as these may offer the resident some insight into the severity of the patient's problem and should always be undertaken before seeking additional information from the ITU chart.

As considerable information is gathered on the patient undergoing intensive care, comprehensive charts are required for its display. The charts should be accessible easily to the nursing staff who complete them and to the medical staff who refer to them. They should provide a record of changes in physiological variables (so that significant alterations are recognized easily), precise details of drugs administered to the patient and intake and output of fluid. It is desirable that a complete record of what has happened to the patient is collected on a single, although necessarily somewhat complex chart. Medical orders, which inevitably include discretionary elements, should be charted separately. Many units record the results of laboratory tests on a separate chart because of the different time-base for these investigations.

In attempting to evaluate unit performance, information may be collected on the physiological status of patients on admission and their subsequent progress (e.g. APACHE II score) and on therapeutic activities within the unit (e.g. TISS scores). However, these scoring systems are intended to provide a basis for comparison of the performance of different units and should not be used to decide on therapy for individual patients.

CLINICAL GUIDELINES

The following sections present a set of systematic guidelines designed to help the resident in the assessment of the patient's condition. As unusual problems occur commonly during intensive therapy, the flow charts and the suggested actions are obviously not comprehensive. However, the proposed order of evaluation of the different physiological variables may prove useful as a checklist in most circumstances.

Respiratory problems

Who should receive artificial ventilation?

Patients who are unable to maintain adequate levels of oxygenation or who develop hypercapnia may be candidates for mechanically assisted ventilation, provided that their pulmonary pathology is potentially reversible. Ventilatory failure may have developed already (in which case arterial blood gas values are abnormal) or may be judged as likely to occur (when blood gas values may be normal but the patient is exhausted).

Hypoxaemia. The commonest indication for ventilation a patient's lungs artificially in the ITU is inability to maintain a satisfactory Pa_{O_2}. There are many pathological conditions which produce hypoxaemia but all have the same basic problem – an area or areas of lung with greater pulmonary blood flow than alveolar ventilation. Blood flow through areas of lung from which ventilation is absent completely is said to be 'shunted' and hypoxaemia caused by this mechanism shows little improvement when the inspired oxygen concentration is increased. Some clinical conditions which are associated frequently with hypoxaemia and common responses to therapy are listed in Table 41.1. Central cyanosis (seen best in the lips) always shows that significant hypoxaemia is present, but if moderate anaemia (Hb > 10 g.dl^{-1}) is present, as it is in many ITU patients, severe hypoxaemia (Pa_{O_2} < 6 kPa) may occur without obvious cyanosis.

Table 41.1   Some causes of hypoxaemia and usual responses to therapy

Clinical condition	Response to therapy		
	O_2 by mask	IPPV	Need for PEEP
1. Pulmonary oedema			
(a) cardiac	Fair	Good	Uncommon
(b) permeability	Poor	Fair	Often needed
2. Asthma (bronchodilators may make worse)	Good	Good but technically very difficult	Uncommon
3. Chronic bronchitis	Fair (Ventimask)	Good	Uncommon
4. Emphysema	Good (Ventimask)	Good	Rare, beware pneumothorax
5. Pneumonia			
(a) lobar	Poor	Poor	Try, often disappointing
(b) broncho-	Fair	Good	Useful
6. Pulmonary contusion	Fair	Fair	Often needed, beware pneumothorax
7. Right to left intracardiac shunts	Poor	Disastrous	Never
8. Retained secretions	Poor	Good, access for suction important	Helpful
9. 'Exhaustion'	Not accepted	Good	Uncommon

The initial treatment of hypoxaemia is the administration of oxygen by face mask. At least 40% oxygen should be given, either by means of a fixed-performance mask (e.g. 40, 50 or 60% Ventimask) or by supplying at least 6 litre.min^{-1} of oxygen to a variable-performance mask (e.g. Hudson). Low-concentration fixed-performance masks and other devices which deliver 24–35% oxygen should be reserved for use in patients with chronic lung conditions and in whom hypoxic drive may be maintaining ventilation. The dangers of oxygen therapy are overestimated and in the ITU environment, where a skilled nurse is attending the patient at all times, oxygen should be administered in a concentration which achieves a satisfactory arterial oxygen saturation. The effect of oxygen therapy should be assessed continuously by pulse oximetry and blood gas analysis should be carried out after 30 min. This gives a more reliable measure of oxygenation as well as providing information regarding the P_{CO_2} and acid–base status.

If Pa_{O_2} remains below 7 kPa in patients with previously healthy lungs, the oxygen concentration should be increased and blood gases resampled after a further 20 min. In addition, measures to combat infection, pulmonary oedema or bronchospasm should be introduced as appropriate, analgesia given if indicated and chest physiotherapy started. Mechanical ventilation is indicated if Pa_{O_2} does not remain above 7–8 kPa.

Patients who are unable to maintain adequate oxygenation often have a pulmonary problem which is associated with other pathology. Persisting inability to cough effectively because of pain and/or weakness leads to retention of secretions and progressive alveolar collapse. The prophylactic use of tracheal intubation and intermittent positive pressure ventilation (IPPV) has become common in patients who normally produce significant quantities of bronchial secretions and whose ability to cough has been impaired by injury or operation to the chest and/or upper abdomen. Patients in whom pain rather than weakness is the major defect may often be managed more conservatively if first-class pain relief is provided (e.g. by regional analgesia, injections of opioid into the extradural space or i.v. infusion of opioid), together with skilful physiotherapy. Cannulation of the trachea via the cricothyroid membrane with a small-bore tube (minitracheotomy) may help by allowing access to the tracheobronchial tree for aspiration of retained secretions.

Because of the lower intensity of nursing care provided currently on most general wards, it is often appropriate to admit such a patient to the

ITU solely to obtain the medical and nursing supervision necessary to manage the analgesic technique safely. Many surgeons regularly 'book' patients into the ITU after major operations which are associated with ventilatory problems, e.g. thoracoabdominal gastrectomy, oesophagectomy or major vascular surgery.

Hypercapnia. Carbon dioxide clearance is related directly to alveolar ventilation. Causes of inadequate ventilation together with the likely duration of the disability are listed in Table 41.2; it may be inappropriate to start IPPV in clinical situations where ventilatory insufficiency cannot be reversed by therapy. Patients whose dysfunction is described in the lower part of Table 41.2 are likely to make vigorous efforts to maintain normocapnia, while those in whom the dysfunction can be described broadly as 'neurological' are usually unable to help themselves significantly. Mechanical ventilation is required usually if Pa_{CO_2} exceeds 7 kPa in patients who habitually maintain a Pa_{CO_2} in the normal range (4.7–5.3 kPa), or if Pa_{CO_2} increases by more than 2 kPa above the patient's usual level.

Exhaustion is indicated by a laboured pattern of rapid, shallow breathing which is often accompanied by deterioration in the level of consciousness. This situation may occur in a wide range of clinical conditions, including cardiac failure and severe septicaemia, when the institution of artificial ventilation may be followed by an improvement in oxygenation, a reduction in pulse rate and reversal of a trend towards metabolic acidosis. When it occurs in conjunction with myocardial failure, a disproportionate amount of the limited cardiac output is used to maintain ventilation and institution of artificial ventilation may allow adequate perfusion of vital organs to be resumed. Mechanical ventilation is probably required if the respiratory rate remains at or above 45 breath.min^{-1} for more than 1 h.

Institution of mechanical ventilation

Tracheal intubation. To enable IPPV to be carried out effectively, a cuffed tube must be placed in the trachea either via the mouth or nose or directly through a tracheostomy. In the emergency situation, an orotracheal tube is usually inserted. If the patient is conscious, anaesthesia should be induced carefully with an i.v. induction agent and muscular relaxation produced, usually

Table 41.2 Some causes of inadequate spontaneous ventilation

Site of dysfunction	Common causes	Probable duration of inadequacy
A. Patients usually unable to increase ventilation (appear passive)		
1. Respiratory centre	Brain injury (coning)	Permanent
	Pharmacological depression (e.g. opioids, barbiturates)	Hours (depends on drug)
2. Upper motor neurones	High spinal damage (above C4)	Permanent
3. Lower motor neurones	Poliomyelitis	Weeks but may be permanent
	Polyneuritis	Months
	Tetanus	Weeks
4. Neuromuscular junction	Myasthenia gravis	Weeks or months
	Neuromuscular blockers	Minutes or hours
5. Respiratory muscles	Myopathies, dystrophies	Permanent
B. Patients who attempt to increase ventilation (appear dyspnoeic)		
6. Chest wall		
(a) deformity	Kyphoscoliosis	Permanent
	Burn eschars	Until incised
(b) damage	Rib fractures	Days or weeks
7. Lungs – reduced compliance	Pulmonary fibrosis	Permanent
	ARDS	Days or weeks
8. Airways – increased resistance	Upper airway obstruction: croup, epiglottitis	Until relieved
	Lower airway obstruction:	
	asthma	Days
	bronchitis and emphysema	Permanent

with suxamethonium. If the patient is unconscious, a muscle relaxant alone may be necessary (but not obligatory) to facilitate the passage of the tube; an i.v. induction agent and muscle relaxant should always be used in patients with severe head injury to prevent an increase in intracranial pressure during laryngoscopy and intubation. As many patients may be hypoxaemic, it is essential that 100% oxygen is administered before intubation. The tube should be inserted by the route which is associated with the least delay once muscle relaxation has been induced.

Cricoid pressure should be applied to minimize the risk of aspirating gastric contents. A sterile, disposable plastic tube with a low-pressure cuff should be used. The tube should be cut so that the top of the cuff lies not more than 3 cm below the vocal cords. The incompressible plastic connector should lie between the incisor teeth if an oral tube is used or in the external nares if nasal intubation is selected. The head should be placed in a neutral or slightly flexed position (on one pillow) after tracheal intubation and a chest X-ray taken to ensure that the tip of the tube lies at least 5 cm above the carina.

Bronchial intubation is the commonest dangerous complication during mechanical ventilation as the tracheal tube may migrate down the trachea when the patient is moved for normal nursing procedures. Intubation of the right main bronchus cannot be detected reliably by observation of chest movements or by auscultation of the chest because of the exaggerated transmission of breath sounds during IPPV, although absent or asynchronous chest movement may occur when pulmonary collapse has taken place. Bronchial intubation is one of the causes of a sudden decrease in compliance, and restlessness and coughing occur if the end of the tube irritates the carina. If this is suspected, the tube should be withdrawn gradually by up to 5 cm while lung compliance and chest expansion are observed carefully. The position of the tube should always be confirmed with a chest radiograph.

Tracheostomy is mandatory only when the upper airway or larynx is obstructed and conventional intubation is not possible (e.g. occasional cases of epiglottitis or laryngeal trauma). The operation is employed more commonly as a planned procedure to make management easier and more comfortable in patients who require ventilation for prolonged periods, e.g. tetanus, poliomyelitis and some chest injuries. In such cases, it is performed as a formal operation under general anaesthesia after the airway has been secured using a tracheal tube. Tracheostomy may be performed in the ITU if transfer of the patient to the operating theatre is felt to be an unjustifiable risk. Some units now routinely use percutaneous tracheostomy kits for this procedure. This technique should be used only by experienced staff and it is recommended that an ENT surgeon is readily available in case problems occur.

Adjusting the ventilator. There are two main types of ventilator in common use: those which deliver a preset tidal volume and those which develop a set pressure during each inspiration. In most units, volume-preset machines predominate and subsequent comments and instructions refer to this general type of ventilator. The ITU resident should become familiar with the controls and facilities of ventilators available in the unit – preferably with an experienced colleague when the machine is not attached to a patient!

The ventilator should be adjusted initially to deliver a tidal volume of 12–15 ml.kg^{-1} (approximately 1000 ml for a 70 kg patient) and a minute volume of 8–10 litre.min^{-1}. An initial inspired oxygen concentration of 40% is appropriate for most patients, but an initial concentration of 50% or more should be selected in patients who are already hypoxaemic despite oxygen therapy. If controllable, the inspiratory time should be approximately half the expiratory time. After approximately 10 min, arterial blood gases should be measured and the inspired oxygen concentration adjusted if necessary.

Management of the ventilated patient

The aims of IPPV are to maintain adequate oxygenation of the tissues with an inspired oxygen concentration of less than 50% and to maintain the Pa_{CO_2} at a satisfactory level. Most patients find the process of receiving artificial ventilation uncomfortable, principally because of irritation from the oral or nasal tracheal tube. This discomfort is accentuated by movement, particularly of the head. If hypoxaemia or hypercapnia is present, the respiratory centre stimulates ventilatory efforts which are not synchronized with those of the ventilator. In conditions with decreased lung compliance, e.g. ARDS, patients tend to breathe rapidly even when blood gases are normal and the respiratory centre is depressed with large doses of opioids.

Arterial oxygenation during IPPV. Arterial oxygenation is controlled by manipulating the inspired oxygen concentration and by varying the end-expiratory pressure. Figure 41.1 describes measures that may be employed to maintain the arterial oxygen within the desired limits (Pa_{CO_2} 10–15 kPa and $Sa_{O_2} > 95\%$). Pulse oximetry is a useful continuous monitor, but does not reliably reflect small but significant changes in Pa_{O_2}. Concentrations of oxygen exceeding 50–60% should be avoided for more than a few hours if possible

because of the risk of oxygen-induced pulmonary damage. However, in severe hypoxaemia, it may be necessary to ignore this risk.

The application of positive end-expiratory pressure (PEEP) or the use of a respiratory pattern in which the inspiratory time exceeds the expiratory time (reversed I:E ratio) are methods of increasing the functional residual capacity (FRC) and improving arterial oxygenation. Both methods have inherent dangers.

1. They raise the mean intrathoracic pressure, thereby tending to impair transpulmonary blood flow and reduce cardiac output. Consequently, oxygen delivery to vital organs may be reduced.

2. They increase peak inspiratory pressure and make rupture of alveoli more likely (see below).

The effects of PEEP on the circulation should be monitored by observing trends in arterial pres-

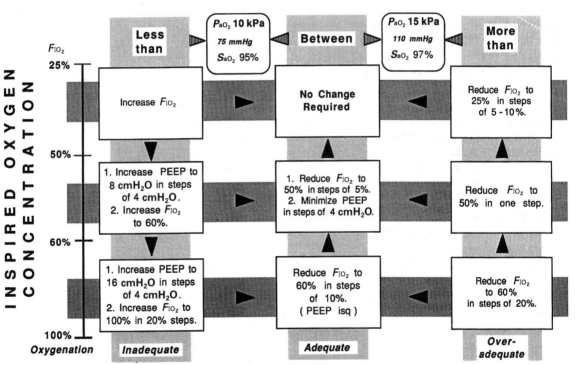

Fig. 41.1 Control of arterial oxygenation. To use this diagram: 1. Measure the inspired oxygen concentration ($F_{I_{O_2}}$) and arterial blood gases and find appropriate box on diagram. 2. Adjust $F_{I_{O_2}}$ and/or positive end-expiratory pressure (PEEP) as suggested. Where more than one action is proposed, proceed in the order described. In general, the greater the deviation from adequacy, the larger the steps required. 3. Repeat measurements after 20–30 min and readjust if necessary. NB: If P_{O_2} is measured on samples of mixed (or central venous) blood before and after adding or increasing PEEP, effect of PEEP on cardiac output and oxygen flux may be assessed (see text).

sure and by measuring changes in the oxygen concentration in mixed (or central) venous blood. The supply of oxygen available to the body (the oxygen flux) is the product of the cardiac output and the arterial oxygen content. PEEP often increases the arterial oxygen content but may depress cardiac output so that oxygen flux is reduced. If this happens and total body oxygen consumption remains unchanged, less oxygen is returned to the heart and the concentration in the mixed (or central) venous blood decreases. If venous oxygen saturation does decrease after the application of (or increase in the level of) PEEP, then:

1. PEEP should be reduced by 5 cmH_2O;
2. inspired oxygen concentration should be increased by 10%;
3. measurements of arterial and venous P_{O_2} should be repeated after 20 min.

Carbon dioxide tension. It is desirable to minimize the changes in the Pa_{CO_2} (especially if initially elevated), as a rapid reduction leads to marked decreases in cardiac output and arterial pressure. In patients with a normal or low Pa_{CO_2} before IPPV, minute volume should be adjusted to produce a Pa_{CO_2} of 4–4.5 kPa, a level at which spontaneous ventilatory efforts should be minimal. If the initial Pa_{CO_2} is high, its value should not be reduced by more than 1 $kPa.h^{-1}$ and, if raised chronically (e.g. in chronic bronchitis), it should not be reduced below 5.5–6 kPa.

If the Pa_{CO_2} is below 4 kPa, minute volume should be reduced by decreasing the respiratory rate. Because Pa_{CO_2} increases relatively slowly, at least 1 h should elapse before contemplating further changes in minute volume.

A scheme for the assessment of the patient undergoing IPPV is shown in Figure 41.2.

Fighting the ventilator. When the patient attempts to breathe out of phase with the ventilator, the first priority is to exclude and if necessary correct hypoxaemia or hypercapnia (Figs 41.1 and 41.2). When these have been excluded, two possible approaches to the problem should be considered.

Many modern ventilators allow a considerable range of adjustments so that the characteristics of the ventilatory cycle may be altered to suit the patient and reduce the need for heavy sedation. Intermittent mandatory ventilation (IMV) and its variants are modes of ventilation which are often useful in allowing the patient to continue with some spontaneous ventilatory effort whilst ensuring that a background of mechanical ventilation is continued. Sophisticated ventilators allow a range of facilities to make IMV more effective and comfortable for the patient. As the total minute volume (and hence Pa_{CO_2}) is effectively under the patient's control during IMV, it is important that muscle relaxants should have been discontinued for some hours and that only moderate doses of respiratory depressants (e.g. opioid analgesics) are being administered.

Alternatively, and especially if oxygenation is precarious, it may be necessary to inhibit spontaneous ventilatory efforts by administering central respiratory depressants (e.g. morphine in a dose of up to 20 $mg.h^{-1}$ by continuous infusion). Neuromuscular blocking drugs should be used only as a last resort to control the hypoxaemic patient who does not settle after sedation. If it is necessary to use these drugs, sedative agents *must* be given at the same time.

If patients who are improving start to fight the ventilator, it may be appropriate to wean them from IPPV.

Reassurance, analgesia and sedation. All but a few patients require some sedation or analgesia while receiving IPPV through a tracheal tube. Ideally, patients should require only light sedation, except when unpleasant or painful procedures are performed, so that they can understand and co-operate with therapy. The experienced ITU nurse explains exactly what is happening, reassures and develops methods of communication that do not distress the voiceless patient. Such explanations should be brief, as attention span is short in the sick, and should be repeated frequently because memory is impaired. A sympathetic approach by all ITU staff can often reduce sedation requirements considerably.

Analgesics. These should be given if the patient has injuries or wounds which normally merit such drugs, or complains of the tracheal tube (see above). They should be given by continuous infusion with additional boluses if painful procedures are undertaken.

Sign	Possible cause	Associated features	Suggested action
CYANOSIS YES / NO	Disconnection Oxygen failure Cardiac arrest	*Bradycardia,* *Hypotension if terminal* *ECG change, pallor*	Immediate manual ventilation with 100% oxygen External cardiac massage
CHEST EXPANSION NO / YES	Disconnection Ventilator failure Total airway obstruction Oesophageal intubation	*Airway pressure down* *Airway pressure up* *+ gastric distension*	Reconnect Manual ventilation Reintubate
AIRWAY PRESSURE LOW / HIGH	Leak from system Improved lung compliance	*Tidal and minute* *volumes down* *Tidal and minute* *volumes up*	Manual ventilation unless source of leak obvious. Check P_{aCO_2}

1. Partial airway obstruction		
(i) Tube kinked	*Suction catheter will not pass*	Reposition tube.
(ii) Tube gripped in teeth	*beyond pharynx or teeth.*	Insert oral airway
(iii) Tube in right main bronchus	*Unequal and/or asynchronous* *chest movements.*	Deflate cuff, withdraw tube 3cm, chest X-ray.
(iv) Cuff herniation	*Expiratory wheeze, overinflated* *chest, surgical emphysema* *in neck.*	Deflate cuff, reinflate until air leak just disappears. ? change tube.
(v) Inspissated secretions or blood	*Cold humidifier.*	Put 5ml saline down tube before suction, ?change tube, ?bronchoscopy.
2. Bronchospasm	*Expiratory +/- inspiratory* *rhonchi, overinflated chest.*	Bronchodilators.
3. Intrathoracic catastrophes		
(i) Pneumothorax	*Hypotension, tachycardia,* *surgical emphysema in neck,* *recent CVP lines!*	Chest drain if side obvious, chest X-ray if not.
(ii) Pulmonary oedema	*ECG changes, fine crepitations,* *copious frothy secretions.*	Increase F_{IO_2}, diuretics, treat arrhythmias.
(iii) Tamponade	*Recent cardiac surgery or trauma;* *BP & urine flow down, reduced* *loss from chest drains.*	Unblock chest drains, ?reopen chest.
4. Restlessness		
(i) Hypercapnia	*Sweating, vascular pressures up,* *pyrexia, i.v. feeding.*	Check for leaks, increase minute volume.
(ii) Hypoxia	*Cyanosis may not be present;* *falling level of consciousness.*	Increase F_{IO_2}, ?PEEP.
(iii) Coughing	*Characteristic movements.*	?tube near carina, review sedation.
(iv) Discomfort or pain	*Sweating, grimacing, vascular* *pressures up.*	Review analgesia.
(v) Stimulation of pulmonary stretch receptors	*Continuous drive to* *hyperventilate.*	Review sedation if oxygenation poor, ?IMV, ?wean.

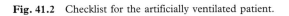

Fig. 41.2 Checklist for the artificially ventilated patient.

Sedatives. Benzodiazepines are often used to provide additional sedation in combination with analgesics. Midazolam is often used by continuous infusion ($2-10$ mg.h^{-1}), as it has a shorter action than other drugs in this group. However, it may accumulate in some patients and cause very prolonged sedation and respiratory depression. Disorientation and cardiovascular depression may also occur with these drugs.

Intravenous anaesthetic agents. Continuous infusions of anaesthetic induction agents have been used to provide sedation for long periods, but further research is required into the effects of long-term administration of these drugs before they can be recommended. At present, propofol has been shown to be effective and safe, with rapid recovery when it is discontinued.

Other drugs. Nitrous oxide may be used to provide short-term sedation and analgesia but should not be used for more than a few hours because of depressant effects on bone marrow. Isoflurane is effective in concentrations of $0.1-0.6\%$ but the effects of long-term (>24 h) administration are not known.

Complications of mechanical ventilation

While IPPV may often be a life-saving procedure, the technique is not without risk to the patient and should be employed only if appropriate and then for the minimum time required.

Pulmonary barotrauma. Rupture of alveoli may occur in any patient who receives mechanical ventilation but is most likely when high mean airway pressures are required because of poor lung compliance or because PEEP has been applied (both commonly occur together). Air is forced into the substance of the lung and then either into the pleural cavity, when a pneumothorax occurs, and/or up through the hilum and into the mediastinum. Pneumothoraces are likely particularly if there has been previous trauma to the lung, as in chest injuries, and tension develops almost inevitably if IPPV is continued. Drainage of the pleural cavity is mandatory in any patient who develops a pneumothorax while receiving IPPV.

Mediastinal emphysema is diagnosed usually on X-ray, but may appear as surgical emphysema in the neck. As there is no specific treatment for mediastinal emphysema, its significance is chiefly as a warning that a leak has occurred and that a pneumothorax may develop, although a chest drain is not yet required. Airway pressures should be reduced either by reducing PEEP (and raising F_{IO_2}), by lowering tidal volume or perhaps by switching to a high-frequency ventilator if one is available.

It should be noted that surgical emphysema appears first at a site close to the leak. Consequently, in a traumatized patient who presents initially with emphysema in the neck, particular attention should be paid to the cervical structures (larynx, pharynx, oesophagus) before assuming that the air has tracked up from the thorax.

Weaning from IPPV

Mechanical ventilation should be prolonged only for specific reasons. It should be routine to consider weaning the patient each day.

Patients who are otherwise stable should be weaned as soon as:

1. pulmonary function seems likely to be adequate during spontaneous ventilation;
2. neuromuscular strength and co-ordination seem to be sufficient to maintain an adequate minute volume and to permit coughing.

As pulmonary efficiency is usually slightly worse, at least initially, after discontinuing IPPV and because it is difficult to give an inspired oxygen concentration of more than approximately 60% through a face mask, patients whose lung function is usually normal should be able to achieve a Pa_{O_2} of more than 10 kPa with an inspired oxygen concentration of 40% or less. If the lungs are damaged permanently (e.g. in chronic lung disease), less effective oxygenation may have to be accepted both during, and particularly after, IPPV.

The indications for weaning, tracheal extubation and reinstituting IPPV are shown in Table 41.3. It is probably safer to wean patients from IPPV and to extubate the trachea early in the day rather than in the late afternoon or evening, as less medical and nursing supervision tends to be available at night.

Table 41.3 Guidelines for weaning, extubation and restarting IPPV

---

1. *When can weaning be started?*
If, when on IPPV (or IMV) and general condition stable (e.g. temperature $< 38°C$, Hb > 10 g.dl^{-1})

(a) HR < 100 beat.min^{-1} in adults (can safely be more in children)

AND (b) $Pa_{O_2} > 10$ kPa, $F_{I_O} < 0.45$ and PEEP < 5 cmH$_2$O

AND (c) $Pa_{CO_2} < 6$ kPa with minute volume < 10 litre.min^{-1} (or $V_D/V_T < 50\%$)

AND (d) Spontaneous tidal volume > 7 ml.kg^{-1}

If answers to a + b + c are YES but d is NO, start or continue IMV.

2. *When may the trachea be extubated?*
If patient co-operative and able to cough
If unconscious and tolerating tube, leave trachea intubated
If unco-operative or intolerant of tube, extubate if IPPV not required (see below)

3. *When does IPPV need to be restarted?*
(Assess patient after 5–10 min of spontaneous ventilation, then at 30 min intervals)

Restart IPPV if:

(a) RESPIRATORY RATE climbs steadily for three successive 30 min periods

OR (b) it exceeds 45 min^{-1}

OR (c) HEART RATE climbs steadily for three successive 30 min periods

OR (d) it exceeds 130 beat.min^{-1}

OR (e) HYPOXAEMIA develops ($Pa_{O_2} < 8$ kPa) (except some chronic chest failure patients)

OR (f) HYPERCAPNIA develops ($Pa_{CO_2} > 1.5$ kPa above pre-IPPV level)

OR (g) LEVEL OF CONSCIOUSNESS deteriorates.

If one of these conditions does apply, consider WHY spontaneous ventilation cannot be maintained. Bronchospasm and/or pulmonary oedema are important factors which may be overlooked

---

In general, the shorter the period of ventilation, the simpler the weaning procedures; weaning over a period of several days may be necessary after prolonged IPPV, particularly for neuromuscular disorders.

Adult respiratory distress syndrome (ARDS)

ARDS is the final common pathway of many severe pulmonary insults (e.g. shock, septicaemia, pulmonary contusion, fat embolism or aspiration of gastric contents). The syndrome is characterized by tachypnoea, cyanosis and diffuse pulmonary infiltrates visible on X-ray. The most significant pathological feature of ARDS is increased capillary permeability which permits fluid to leak into the interstitial tissues of the lung and results in severe (non-cardiac) pulmonary oedema. In severe cases, the pulmonary leak of proteinaceous fluid progresses rapidly to fibrosis over a few days and irreversible pulmonary failure ensues.

ARDS is difficult to reverse and treatment is therefore supportive and aimed at preventing further damage. Occasionally, definitive treatment may be available for the primary cause (e.g. laparotomy and drainage of intraperitoneal abscess for septicaemia), but the condition usually develops more insidiously so that curative treatment is often impossible.

Mechanical ventilation is nearly always required, although oxygen via a face mask or continuous positive airways pressure (CPAP) may be sufficient to ensure adequate oxygenation in mild cases. If IPPV is used, PEEP is usually added and may improve oxygenation dramatically by reducing interstitial oedema. High inspired oxygen concentrations and minute volumes may be required to achieve barely adequate gas exchange; however, if an inspired oxygen concentration greater than 80% is needed with more than 10 cmH$_2$O of PEEP for more than a few hours to maintain arterial oxygenation, prognosis is poor. Fluid overload must be avoided, haemodynamic status controlled and plasma oncotic pressure maintained. Pharmacological manipulations and inventive techniques of oxygenation are of value in some cases.

Despite aggressive therapy, the mortality from established ARDS remains high (over 50%). Patients with ARDS rarely die from respiratory failure as modern techniques of ventilatory support can usually (just) maintain adequate gas exchange. The pathophysiology of this condition is not confined to the lung and multisystem organ failure may develop during the days after the onset of pulmonary failure. The combination of respiratory, cardiac and renal failure carries a particularly poor prognosis.

As in many illnesses, prevention is better than cure and early diagnosis and treatment of possible precipitating causes of ARDS are likely to have a much greater effect in improving outcome than prolonged aggressive treatment of the established condition.

Cardiovascular failure

Although actual or expected ventilatory failure is the commonest reason for admission to the general ITU, cardiovascular failure is a frequent finding in the critically ill patient. When associated with pulmonary problems, the effects of cardiovascular insufficiency may be exacerbated because of reduced oxygenation of blood.

Cardiovascular failure may be acute or chronic. When it develops rapidly (e.g. heart failure after myocardial infarction or peripheral circulatory failure after haemorrhage), it is known as 'shock' and, unless the condition is corrected rapidly, admission to ITU is necessary. Chronic cardiovascular failure is one of the main *raisons d'être* of many departments of medicine (especially cardiology) and surgery (especially cardiac and vascular surgery), but patients who are receiving treatment for one of the varieties of chronic cardiovascular failure should be placed on a shortlist for ITU admission if they present with unrelated complaints or complications.

Cardiovascular monitoring

Patients are often admitted to the ITU because their cardiovascular status is unpredictable and potentially unstable, making continuous availability of information essential. All patients in the ITU should be monitored with an ECG which displays both the electrical signal and heart rate. The ECG monitoring system in the coronary care unit is often more complex and may include circuits to recognize, count and display frequency histograms of various arrhythmias and to quantify ischaemic changes in multiple lead configurations.

Arterial pressure may be measured intermittently by a conventional or automated sphygmomanometer or continuously by direct intra-arterial recording from the radial, brachial, dorsalis pedis or femoral arteries. Percutaneous arterial cannulation is used widely to monitor arterial pressure (Figs 41.3 and 41.4) and to give ready access to arterial blood samples. Enormous technical efforts are being made to design non-invasive systems (see Ch. 20) which will make invasive procedures less necessary but, at present, their accuracy and dependability are inadequate in critical situations.

Central venous pressure (CVP) may be measured from a catheter introduced into the superior vena cava or right atrium and connected to either a water or electronic manometer.

Pulmonary artery pressure may be measured using a flow-directed catheter (see Ch. 20). The information gained from measurement of pulmonary capillary wedge pressure permits distinction between pulmonary oedema from high left atrial pressure and that caused by increased permeability of pulmonary capillaries. This may be help-

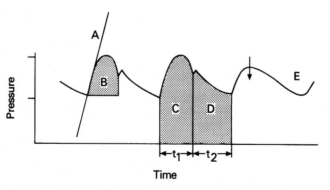

Fig. 41.3 Information to be gained from the arterial pressure signal.

Visible sign	Physiological effect
A – rate of pressure increase	Myocardial contractility
B – area under pulse pressure	Stroke volume
C – systolic pressure × time (t_1)	Myocardial oxygen consumption
D – diastolic pressure × time (t_2)	Myocardial oxygen supply
E – loss of waveform detail	Catheter occlusion (flush it!)

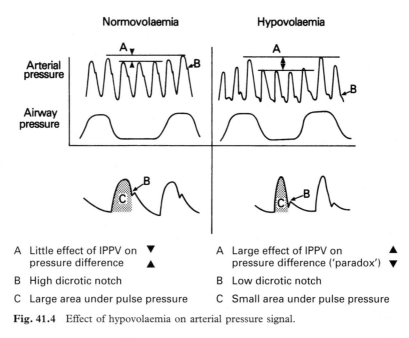

Fig. 41.4 Effect of hypovolaemia on arterial pressure signal.

ful, particularly in patients with multiple injuries and pulmonary problems, severe septicaemia or actual or incipient left ventricular failure. Pulmonary artery catheters are used also to provide information relating to other haemodynamic variables such as cardiac output and some types can also give a continuous reading of mixed venous oxygen saturation. Computerized monitoring systems can use these measurements to provide a wide range of derived parameters which may assist in resuscitation and treatment.

Cardiovascular assessment

A scheme to aid the ITU resident in assessment of cardiovascular status is shown in Tables 41.4 and 41.5. Further information which may be obtained from the arterial pressure waveform is indicated in Figures 41.3 and 41.4. A wide range of therapeutic agents, including inotropic drugs, vasodilators and antiarrhythmics, is available to modify haemodynamic status (see Appendix IIIb). These are often used singly or in combination to try to restore cardiovascular stability.

Shock (acute cardiovascular failure)

In shock, there is an acute failure of the circulatory system to supply adequate nutrients to the tissues and to remove metabolites. Under these circumstances, cell death occurs eventually as a result of impairment of vital membrane functions and abnormal cell metabolism. This sequence of events may follow severe haemorrhage (from a traumatic or surgical cause) and may occur also after loss of fluid from the gastrointestinal tract. In cardiogenic shock, the heart is unable to maintain a sufficiently high output; this occurs most commonly after severe myocardial infarction. Septic shock may complicate overwhelming infections of many types but results most frequently from Gram-negative infections.

Pathophysiology. In the early stages of circulatory insufficiency, the sympathetic nervous system is activated and constriction of veins and arteries maintains arterial pressure and perfusion of vital organs (brain, heart and kidneys). These compensatory mechanisms provide a short period during which aggressive treatment may prevent further development of the more severe and irreversible features of shock. If effective treatment is not started, poor perfusion leads to tissue hypoxia and anaerobic metabolism. The resultant acidosis causes relaxation of precapillary sphincters despite maximal sympathetic activity. However, the postcapillary sphincters remain constricted

Table 41.4 Cardiovascular checklist. Check the primary variables (systemic arterial pressure (SAP), heart rate (HR), ECG and urine flow) first. Look at (1) absolute values, (2) trends (up, down, variable), (3) relationships with one another – particularly SAP and HR. Use secondary variables (CVP/neck veins, core–peripheral temperature differences, pulmonary artery pressure (PAP) and pulmonary capillary wedge pressure (PCWP)) to distinguish between various possibilities

SAP and HR relationship	Common causes	Confirmatory findings	Suggested action
HR up, SAP up	Sympathetic activation with pain, arousal, etc.	Restlessness, CVP up, PAP up	Review sedation and analgesia
HR down, SAP down	1. Heart block	ECG change	Isoprenaline, pacemaker
	2. Severe hypoxaemia	Cyanosis	Reconnect ventilator or oxygen. Manual IPPV
	3. Response to sedative or analgesic drugs	Recent drug administration	Reduce subsequent doses of drug
HR down, SAP up	Rising intracranial pressure	Deteriorating level of consciousness, enlarging pupils	Hyperventilate, diuretics, mannitol
HR up, SAP down	1. Shock (a) hypovolaemic	CVP and urine flow down, limbs poorly perfused	Infuse colloid
	(b) septic (early)	CVP and urine flow down, limbs well perfused	Infuse colloid, release pus, give antibiotics
	2. Tamponade after heart surgery	CVP up, urine flow and lung compliance down	Unblock drains, reopen chest
	3. Pneumothorax	Restlessness, lung compliance down	Chest drain
	4. Tachyarrhythmias	ECG change, CVP up	Antiarrhythmics
	5. Pulmonary embolus	Chest pain, cyanosis, CVP up, ?ECG changes	O_2 ?Pulmonary angiography
	6. Allergic reaction	?Rash, recent drug or blood administration	Antihistamines, infuse colloid, ?steroids

and fluid becomes sequestrated in tissues. The progressive loss of intravascular volume eventually causes hypoperfusion of the previously protected vital organs; respiratory and renal failure develop, followed later by hepatic, cardiac and eventually neurological failure.

Sepsis syndrome. Septic, Gram-negative, bacteraemic or endotoxic shock are names which have been given to a clinical state which may appear following localized or systematic bacterial, fungal or viral infections. The commonest sources of infection are the gastrointestinal tract, particularly after laparotomy, and the urogenital tract, especially after instrumentation. Infections of the respiratory and biliary tracts may also be implicated.

Micro-organisms isolated from patients with this condition are usually Gram-negative gut bacteria, e.g. *Escherichia coli*, *Klebsiella* or *Proteus* species. In a small but significant minority, Gram-positive organisms such as *Staphylococcus aureus* or *Pneumococcus* may be found. Patients who are immunocompromised or receiving chemotherapy are particularly liable to develop septic shock from infection with *Candida* or other fungi.

Sepsis syndrome is extremely rare outside hospital and occurs usually as a complication of existing clinical problems. Its occurrence and mortality are related to the severity of the underlying condition. It is commonest at the extremes of life, in patients in whom resistance to infection is low and after splenectomy (when pneumococcal infection is common).

Characteristically, the patient appears warm and well perfused in early septic shock, with a normal or often elevated cardiac output but a low arterial pressure because of reduced peripheral resistance ('warm phase'). If shock persists, a hypodynamic cardiovascular state develops in which cardiac output and blood volume decrease, systemic and pulmonary resistances increase ('cold phase') and the chances of recovery decrease sharply. In the 'warm phase', the increased

Table 41.5 Cardiovascular indicators. It is often not possible to measure some cardiovascular variables directly, so that it is necessary to use other variables to indicate indirectly what changes are occurring. Changes which are normally undesirable are indicated in the table below. Welcome changes are normally accompanied by alterations in the 'indicator observations' in the opposite direction

Undesirable change	Indicator observations
1. Cardiac output DOWN	Urine flow DOWN. Core–peripheral temperature difference UP
2. Blood volume DOWN	CVP and PCWP DOWN. Inspiratory to expiratory difference in systolic SAP ('paradox') UP (see Fig. 41.4). Dicrotic notch LOWER on arterial pressure waveform (see Fig. 41.4). LARGE SAP fall in response to IPPV, sedatives or analgesics
3. Right ventricular function DETERIORATING	CVP UP. PAP DOWN. Peripheral oedema INCREASING
4. Left ventricular function DETERIORATING	PCWP or left atrial pressure UP. Arterial SAP DOWN. Pulmonary oedema INCREASING. Oxygenation DETERIORATING
5. Peripherial vascular resistance INCREASING	Core–peripheral temperature difference UP. STEEPER pressure decay during diastole
6. Myocardial oxygen demand UP	HR UP. SAP UP. Product of HR × SAP UP
7. Myocardial oxygen supply DOWN	HR UP. Diastolic arterial pressure DOWN

temperature and cardiovascular activity are accompanied by a marked increase in metabolic requirements although, paradoxically, oxygen extraction by the tissues is reduced so that the arteriovenous oxygen content difference is low. Among the factors postulated to contribute to the impaired oxygen utilization are the opening of arteriovenous capillary 'shunts' in tissues and uncoupling of the normal processes that link energy production and oxygenation. In the 'cold phase', the pathophysiological picture more closely resembles that seen in hypovolaemic shock.

Treatment. In shock of all types, the primary aim of treatment is to restore and maintain an adequate flow of well-oxygenated blood. Thus, the initial step in management of the shocked patient is to ensure that arterial blood is well saturated (> 95%). Fluid should be given rapidly through a large i.v. cannula to restore the circulating volume. Most clinicians favour colloid solutions as the main fluid replacement (e.g. human albumin solution (HAS) or Haemaccel), but crystalloids, in larger volumes, are also effective. Whole blood is preferred if blood has been lost. Once circulating blood volume is restored, inotropic support, vasodilators and diuretics may be necessary to maintain circulation and renal function.

In septic shock, blood should be obtained for culture before antibiotics are administered. In this serious condition, large doses of broad-spectrum antibiotics are appropriate (e.g. cefuroxime, gentamicin and metronidazole). It is essential that every appropriate diagnostic technique, including laparotomy, be employed in the search for the source of infection. Collections of pus must be evacuated despite the patient's critical condition, otherwise bacteraemia recurs and progressive multiorgan failure ensues.

Other systems

Many ITU patients are at risk of multiple organ failure and the expert knowledge of many different specialists should be available when required. Bacteriologists, nephrologists and cardiologists, amongst others, are frequent visitors to an ITU to provide advice on patient management. In some hospitals, however, specialist opinions may not be available and it falls to the ITU team to provide care for the more common problems.

Renal failure

The development of renal failure can be prevented in most ITU patients at risk by judicious use of fluids, low-dose dopamine infusion and diuretic therapy. Continuous arteriovenous haemodialysis is now the treatment of choice for established acute renal failure in most ITUs and, in straightforward cases, can be used without the involvement of a nephrologist. If difficulties are encountered, the patient may need to be transferred to a renal unit if specialist support is not available locally. Irreversible renal failure in patients requiring ventilatory support is one of the commonest causes of death in ITU patients.

Nutrition

It is often difficult to maintain an adequate nutritional intake in ITU patients. In acute illness, resuscitation is usually more important than nutrition for the first 24–48 h, but after this time efforts should be made to provide enough food for recovery to occur. Enteral nutrition by nasogastric tube should be used whenever possible but paralytic ileus, other gastrointestinal disturbances or the effects of analgesic and sedative drugs often prevent this in ITU patients. Parenteral nutrition should be undertaken as a planned procedure with the intention of providing a balanced intake of amino acids, carbohydrates, fats, vitamins and trace elements. Parenteral 'diet' in these patients usually requires day-to-day adjustment, and daily monitoring of blood and urinary biochemistry is essential. Hospital pharmacists keep information on preparations available for parenteral nutrition and prepare balanced feeds in a sterile environment.

DEATH IN THE ITU

The mortality rate amongst patients admitted to the ITU is higher than that elsewhere in hospital. This is inevitable in view of the pathological processes which make it necessary to provide artificial assistance for one or more of the vital systems, but it is to be hoped that fewer patients die than if the facilities of the ITU were not available. In order to maintain the morale and sense of purpose of the unit staff, it is essential that the need for therapy, rather than the imminence of death, is the main criterion for admission to the unit.

In a significant proportion of cases, the patient is unable to overcome the pathological processes in spite of maximal therapeutic support and this becomes apparent when the patient fails to improve sufficiently to become independent of the measures employed to support ventilation and/or

perfusion. The prognosis deteriorates markedly in relation to the duration for which IPPV is required and the number of physiological systems which require support. The maintenance of a physiologically satisfactory *status quo* by means of artificial support does not augur well and the appropriate message must be transmitted to the relatives. It must be stressed repeatedly to them that improvement is required to give significant hope of survival, because the patient must be able not only to throw off the effects of the initial insult, but also to resist the infective episodes which often complicate the recovery period. Failure to improve is followed usually by slow deterioration in the efficiency of previously unaffected organs and by a poor response to supportive measures introduced to counteract the effects of this deterioration.

In terms of predicting which patients are unlikely to survive, those who are comatose and

Table 41.6 Recognition of brain stem death. Brain stem death may be assumed if (a) the answer to each of the ten questions is 'NO' and (b) if the assessment is repeated, with the same results, after at least 4 h. If the answer to any of the questions is 'YES' or 'DON'T KNOW', active treatment must be continued

1. Is there any doubt as to the cause of the coma and brain damage (e.g. trauma, cerebrovascular accident, drowning)?
2. Has the patient received (or taken) any drugs which could have either depressed the central nervous system (e.g. alcohol, sedatives, hypnotics, analgesics) or impaired his or her muscular capabilities (e.g. muscle relaxants)?
3. Are there any metabolic or endocrine disturbances which could affect neural function (e.g. blood glucose changes, uraemia, hepatic dysfunction)?
4. Is the patient's temperature less than 35°C? (Midbrain failure is often followed by a rapid fall in temperature, but hypothermia itself may induce coma. If the temperature is below 35°C, active warming must be started and further cooling minimized with 'space blankets')
5. Do the pupils react to light?
6. Are there corneal reflexes?
7. Do the eyes move during or after caloric testing?
8. Are there motor responses in the cranial nerve distribution in response to painful stimulation of the face, trunk or limbs?
9. Does the patient gag, cough or otherwise move following the passage of a suction catheter into the nose, mouth or bronchial tree?
10. Does the patient show any respiratory activity at all when the arterial carbon dioxide tension exceeds 7 kPa (checked on an arterial sample)?

unresponsive after severe brain damage are amongst the easier to distinguish. The signs of 'brain death' are well recognized and a scheme of assessment is included in Table 41.6. Formal assessment must be carried out twice by two consultants.

If 'brain death' is a likely diagnosis, the possibility of organ donation should always be considered and discussed with the patient's family. It is best if these discussions are initiated by ITU staff who are experienced in dealing with bereaved relatives.

FURTHER READING

Hind C J, Watson D 1995 Intensive care: a concise textbook. W B Saunders, London
Tinker J, Rapin M (eds) 1983 Care of the critically ill patient. Springer Verlag, Berlin
Willatts S, Winter R (eds) 1992 Principles and protocols in intensive care. Portland Press, Colchester

42. Management of chronic pain

Considerable advances have been made in recent years in the understanding of the fundamental mechanisms involved in pain transmission and modulation. Contributions from basic scientists and psychologists have significantly extended the range of assessment tools and treatments offered by clinicians to patients in pain. The majority of pain specialists are anaesthetists. For many years anaesthetists have had responsibility for postoperative pain control and this has led to management of acute and ultimately chronic pain. Anaesthetists have acquired skills in percutaneous neural blockade; this expertise, developed originally for local anaesthetics, was then extended to neurolytic agents. Initially, therefore, pain clinics started as nerve-blocking clinics. However, at the instigation of John J. Bonica at the University of Washington Medical School, a multidisciplinary perspective was introduced. This approach, with close interaction between anaesthetists and other specialists, is being increasingly adopted.

DEFINITION OF PAIN

We have all experienced pain, but it has proved difficult to define this sensation satisfactorily. It has been described as 'what the patient says hurts'. The taxonomy committee of the International Association for the Study of Pain defined pain as 'an unpleasant sensory and emotional experience associated with actual or potential tissue damage, or described in terms of such damage'. This definition is important as it states that pain is never only a physical sensation but always ultimately a psychological event. It also accepts that pain can occur in spite of negative physical findings and investigations.

PATHOPHYSIOLOGY

The neural pathways that transmit and modulate pain have been described previously (see Ch. 4). The major function of the pain perception system is to prevent injury. The sensation of pain is usually produced by a noxious stimulus intense enough to be damaging. Protective behaviours, e.g. withdrawal, avoidance and rest, then follow. This protective function of pain is illustrated by the rare condition of congenital insensitivity to pain. Individuals with this condition do not register noxious stimuli and frequently injure themselves without knowing.

However, pain is more than just a physical sensation and responses to a given stimulus are variable. Pain perception threshold is defined as the least experience of pain that a subject can recognize. It is highly reproducible in different individuals and in the same individual at different times. Pain tolerance threshold, defined as the greatest level of pain that the subject is prepared to tolerate, is, in contrast, highly variable. It can vary from person to person and within the same individual on different occasions. It is highly dependent on psychological variables, including cultural factors, past experience and the meaning of the pain for the individual.

Acute pain is easily produced in the laboratory and is a well studied phenomenon. Chronic pain, by contrast, is a more difficult problem. Chronic pain is often not a biological advantage. The link between initial injury and chronic pain can be difficult to elucidate. Peripheral injury produces neurophysiological changes in the spinal cord which themselves can produce further effects. These can persist for much longer than the initial peripheral insult. It also appears that there are sensory neurones present in the periphery which do not respond to transient excessive mechanical and thermal stimuli, but which have a chemical sensitivity that makes them responsive if tissue becomes inflamed. These have been termed 'silent nociceptors'. Their role has not yet been clarified, but it is possible that they may be activated in some chronic pain states.

Further research in this exciting area of neuronal plasticity may help us to understand more fully the link between acute and chronic pain.

CLASSIFICATION OF PAIN

Pain can be classified according to aetiology.

Nociceptive pain

Nociceptive pain results from tissue damage causing continual nociceptor stimulation. It can be either somatic or visceral in origin.

Somatic pain

Somatic pain results from activation of nociceptors in cutaneous and deep tissues, such as bone. Typically it is well localized and described as aching, throbbing or gnawing. Somatic pain is usually sensitive to opioids.

Visceral pain

Visceral pain arises from internal organs. It is characteristically vague in distribution and quality and is often described as deep, dull or dragging. It may be associated with nausea, vomiting and alterations in arterial pressure and heat rate. Stimuli, such as crushing or burning, which are painful in somatic structures usually evoke no pain in visceral organs. Mechanisms of visceral pain include abnormal distension or contraction of smooth muscle, stretching of the capsule of solid organs, hypoxia or necrosis and irritation by algesic substances. Visceral pain is often referred to cutaneous sites distant from the visceral lesion. One example of this is shoulder pain resulting from diaphragmatic irritation.

Neuropathic pain

Neuropathic pain is caused by functional abnormality of the peripheral and/or central nervous system. It is characteristically dysaesthetic in nature and patients complain of unpleasant abnormal sensations. There may be marked allodynia, i.e. a normally non-painful stimulus, such as light touch, provokes pain. Pain may be described as shooting or burning and may occur in areas of numbness. Neuropathic pain may develop immediately after nerve injury or after a variable interval. It is often persistent and relatively resistant to opioids. There is a tendency for a favourable response to centrally modulating medication, such as anticonvulsants and tricyclic antidepressants.

There are many causes for neuropathic pain. Central pain is associated with lesions of the central nervous system, such as infarction and trauma. Lesions in the peripheral nervous system include peripheral nerve injuries, peripheral neuropathies and tumour infiltration.

Sympathetically maintained pain

One type of neuropathic pain which needs special mention is sympathetically maintained pain (SMP). Pain can sometimes be perpetuated by efferent activity in the sympathetic nervous system. Major nerve injury or apparently trivial trauma, such as a sprain, laceration or fracture, may produce this condition. Patients complain of spontaneous burning pain and allodynia. The syndrome termed reflex sympathetic dystrophy (RSD) may develop; in addition to pain, RSD is characterized by a smooth, shiny, sweaty skin with a mottled appearance, muscle wasting, soft tissue swelling and localized osteoporosis. Figure 42.1 shows RSD which developed after a Colles' fracture.

Regional block of the sympathetic nervous system can produce significant pain relief. This can be either by block of the sympathetic chain with a lumbar sympathetic (lower limb) or stellate ganglion (upper limb) block or by an intravenous regional technique using guanethidine. Guanethidine initially releases noradrenaline from nerve endings and then prevents reuptake. The intravenous regional technique is less invasive, appears to last longer and can be more easily repeated. Guanethidine accumulates in the nerve endings

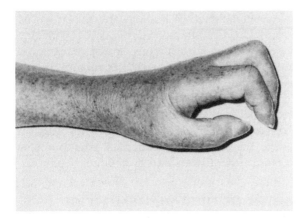

Fig. 42.1 Reflex sympathetic dystrophy following Colles' fracture.

and reduces their ability to respond to autonomic stimulation. Thus, the duration of relief becomes longer with successive blocks. Intravenous guanethidine blocks are usually repeated according to clinical response.

Psychogenic pain

This is an expression that has been used in the past to explain the aetiology of pain in patients whose symptoms do not appear to have an organic basis. It implies that the primary cause of the pain is psychological and that for some reason the patient wants or needs the pain. Chronic pain, however, is usually the cause and not the result of neurotic symptoms. This label has been superseded by more specific terms, for example, somatization disorder or psychogenic pain disorder. Strict diagnostic criteria must be fulfilled before such a diagnosis can be made and this should be done by, or in conjunction with, a psychiatrist.

PAIN MANAGEMENT CLINIC

In the pain management clinic, patients present with pain resulting from many different pathological processes. Common painful conditions include:

Malignant

- Primary tumours
- Metastases
- Treatment-related, e.g. postmastectomy pain.

Non-malignant

- Postherpetic neuralgia
- Trigeminal neuralgia
- Phantom limb
- Stump pain postamputation
- Scar pain
- Ischaemic, e.g. vascular disease, Raynaud's
- Migraine
- Brachial plexus avulsion
- Musculoskeletal
- Pelvic pain
- Sympathetically maintained pain.

Assessment

Comprehensive assessment of patients with pain is a vital first step. Pain is a symptom rather than a disease. Efforts should be made to diagnose and, if possible, treat the underlying cause before using empirical pain relieving techniques. Patients attending a pain management clinic will have been referred by their consultant or general practitioner and this maxim followed. However, it is important that a comprehensive history is taken and many clinics use questionnaires to facilitate this.

Questions with special reference to the pain include:

- Site(s)
- Onset
- Frequency
- Aggravating factors
- Relieving factors
- Quality, e.g. burning, shooting
- Quantity, e.g. verbal rating scale, faces pain scale (children)
- Associated symptoms
- Previous treatments
- Patient's ideas.

Many patients, especially those with malignancy, have more than one site of pain and separate histories should be taken for each complaint as their aetiology may differ. It may be helpful for the patient to draw the sites of pain on a body chart.

A full clinical examination should be performed. Special reference should be made to tender points in muscles and scars, neurological deficit and signs implicating involvement of the sympathetic nervous system including vasomotor, sudomotor and trophic changes.

Psychological assessment can be made informally by the clinician aided by appropriate questionnaires. Levels of anxiety, depression, functional disability and locus of control are some of the variables that can be measured using appropriate tools. However, full psychological assessment should be performed by a clinical psychologist, preferably one who is an integral member of the pain management team.

Pain has been described as a biopsychosocial phenomenon and these dimensions are illustrated in Figure 42.2. Interview of significant friends or relations is often important to ascertain the impact of the pain on lifestyle and the family.

A fully comprehensive assessment of the patient with chronic pain is essential before formulating a treatment plan. It is sometimes helpful to categorize patients into one of the following groups to clarify the position:

1. Well defined pain syndrome – specific effective treatment.

2. Well defined pain problem, origin diagnosed – no effective treatment.

3. Pain problem, no firm diagnosis – no effective treatment.

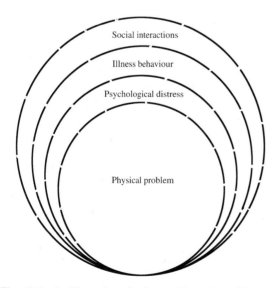

Fig. 42.2 An illustration of pain as a biopsychosocial phenomenon (reproduced with permission from *Spine*).

Full explanation of findings and the proposed treatment plan should be discussed with the patient. Patient expectations should be explored and, if necessary, rationalized. Patients with chronic pain become depressed, anxious and medication-dependent. They lose their jobs, financial security and social status. Their relationships deteriorate. Pain management clinics attempt not only to relieve the physical sensation of pain but also to reduce the distress and disability it produces.

METHODS OF MANAGEMENT OF CHRONIC PAIN

Chronic pain is a complex phenomenon and often multifactorial in aetiology. Several methods of treatment may therefore be used in the same patient, either concomitantly or sequentially.

Medication

Many patients in pain are prescribed analgesic drugs. The pharmacology of these agents is fully discussed elsewhere (Ch. 10) and only aspects of particular relevance to their use in chronic pain are mentioned below.

Non-steroidal anti-inflammatory drugs

Non-steroidal anti-inflammatory drugs (NSAIDs) interfere with the production of prostaglandins and prostacyclins by inhibiting the enzyme cyclo-oxygenase. They are effective for pain associated with tissue damage especially if there is an inflammatory component. They are particularly useful in musculoskeletal pain and dysmenorrhoea. They have a very important role in cancer pain caused by metastatic deposits in bone.

Opioid analgesics

Cancer pain. Approximately 70% of patients with advanced cancer develop significant pain before death. Opioids are the most effective analgesics for the relief of nociceptive pain associated with cancer. Education of the medical and nursing professions and also the general public is still necessary to ensure that adequate doses are prescribed and taken. Addiction, tolerance and respi-

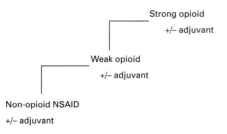

Fig. 42.3 The analgesic ladder.

ratory depression are not problems commonly encountered in this group of patients.

The World Health Organization recommends an 'analgesic ladder' to ensure a logical sequence in prescription (Fig. 42.3).

Treatment is initiated with a non-opioid analgesic for mild pain and a weak opioid alone or in combination with an adjuvant drug for moderate pain. Patients in severe pain are prescribed a strong opioid alone or with an adjuvant. Inadequate pain control at one level requires a move to a drug on the next level, rather than to an alternative of similar efficacy.

Morphine is the most commonly prescribed strong opioid for cancer pain. Cancer pain is continuous and medication must be taken regularly. It is given orally unless intractable nausea and vomiting occur or there is a physical impediment to swallowing. Twycross has succinctly stated the regimen as 'by mouth, by the clock and by the ladder'.

Oral morphine, either elixir or tablets, is given every 4 hours, if necessary in increasing dosage, until pain is controlled. When the required daily dose has been established, it is usual to convert to sustained release morphine tablets which need to be taken only twice daily. In addition, morphine elixir or tablets should be prescribed for breakthrough pain, the dose being approximately one-sixth of the total daily morphine consumption.

There are various alternative routes for opioid administration. Continuous subcutaneous administration is the standard alternative method if oral medication cannot be taken. A small portable battery-operated syringe driver fitted with a 10 ml syringe containing the total daily opioid dose is usually used. Because of its greater solubility, diamorphine is the drug of choice for this route of administration in the United Kingdom. A con-

version ratio of 3 mg oral morphine to 1 mg subcutaneous diamorphine is used.

The rectal route is another alternative for patients unable to take opioids orally and suppositories containing morphine or oxycodone are available.

A transdermal drug delivery system has been developed for fentanyl. Fentanyl patches need to be applied to the skin every 3 days. Steady-state serum fentanyl concentrations may be obtained by the second dose. Fentanyl is absorbed via the skin at the site of application and a reservoir is created which limits fluctuations in serum concentration. As a result of this, the efficacy or toxicity of a change in dose should be obvious within 24 h. This system has been approved in North America for the management of chronic pain in patients requiring opioids but in the United Kingdom it is available only for research purposes at present.

Opioids can also be administered intraspinally, either extradurally or intrathecally. Proposed indications for spinal opioids are as follows:

1. Patients whose pain is effectively controlled by oral opioids but only with unacceptable side-effects, such as drowsiness or vomiting.
2. Patients whose pain cannot be controlled by the use of oral or systemic opioids.

There is still debate regarding these indications. Much smaller doses of drug are required when given spinally and thus side-effects are minimized. Contraindications to the insertion of a spinal catheter are similar to those in the acute situation. Side-effects, such as respiratory depression, itching and urinary retention, that cause such concern in the opioid-naive patient are rare in cancer patients who have been chronically exposed to systemic opioids previously.

There do appear to be situations in which pain is either non-responsive or only partially responsive to morphine. Malignant infiltration of nerves produces excruciating unremitting neuropathic pain which often fits this category. An example of this clinical problem is lumbosacral plexopathy caused by advanced pelvic tumour. The combination of opioid and local anaesthetic administered extradurally has been reported to be of help in this very difficult pain problem. Dosage and concentration are carefully adjusted to provide analgesia with no or only minimal motor and sensory loss and hypotension is not normally a problem.

The field of spinal opioid therapy is sufficiently new that guidelines for selection of route (intrathecal or extradural), choice of drug (opioid or opioid/local anaesthetic combination), administration protocol (intermittent bolus or continuous infusion) and equipment (tunnelled or totally implanted catheter and reservoir) are still being formulated. It is essential to organize a teaching programme for nurses and to devise a formal protocol for administration before introducing the technique into the clinical setting.

Non-cancer pain. Weak opioid drugs, e.g. dihydrocodeine, can be useful for moderate pain. They can be taken excessively by the patient with non-malignant pain and abuse does occur. Treatment in the pain management clinic may involve weaning the patient off such medication.

The use of strong opioids in non-cancer pain is controversial and should not be undertaken lightly. Identifiable painful pathology must exist. Previous psychiatric or current psychological problems or a previous history of drug or alcohol abuse are usually contraindications.

Adjuvant analgesics

These are drugs that have primary indications other than pain but are analgesic in some painful conditions.

Corticosteroids

Corticosteroids have anti-inflammatory actions and also reduce peritumour oedema in neoplastic tissue, thus relieving pain by reducing pressure on adjacent pain-sensitive structures. Recent work has shown that local application reduces transmission in normal unmyelinated C-fibres. Steroids are prescribed in patients with cancer pain for analgesia, for the feeling of well-being they produce and to stimulate appetite. Steroids are also administered by the extradural route for the symptomatic relief of radicular pain resulting from disc prolapse and backache. Randomized controlled double-blind trials in this area are still lacking.

Anticonvulsants

Anticonvulsants have a major role in the management of neuropathic pain, especially when there is a shooting component. These drugs suppress spontaneous neuronal firing. Trigeminal neuralgia is the classic condition for which anticonvulsants are prescribed. Carbamazepine is commonly used as the drug of first choice, though it can cause considerable sedation. Sodium valproate and phenytoin are also used.

Tricyclic antidepressants

Tricyclic antidepressants have an important role in the management of pain. Animal models of acute pain have consistently demonstrated the antinociceptive effect of tricyclic drugs. Controlled clinical trials have shown beneficial results in postherpetic neuralgia, diabetic neuropathy, arthritis, migraine and tension headaches. The effective dose of a tricyclic drug for pain management is lower than that required for depression and analgesia is apparent in 3–4 days compared with 3–4 weeks for the antidepressant effect. Tricyclics reduce the reuptake of the amine neurotransmitters noradrenaline and 5-hydroxytryptamine into the presynaptic terminal, increasing the concentration and duration of action of these substances at the synapse and thereby enhancing activity in the descending inhibitory pain pathway.

Amitryptiline is the tricyclic drug most commonly prescribed for pain. It causes sedation and is usually given as a single dose at night.

Antiarrhythmic drugs

Systemic local anaesthetic infusions have been used diagnostically and therapeutically for chronic neuropathic pain. Lignocaine 5 mg.kg^{-1} given intravenously to patients with painful diabetic peripheral neuropathy in a double-blind cross-over study has been demonstrated to produce analgesia. Unfortunately, the effect is short-lived. Oral mexilitine has been used with some success, but further work in this area is needed.

Capsaicin cream

Capsaicin depletes substance P from sensory

nerve endings in the skin. Local application may alleviate pain in postherpetic neuralgia and postmastectomy pain syndrome.

Neural blockade in pain management

Nerve blocks have been performed for many years in the management of pain. A nerve block comprises injection of a local anaesthetic or a neurolytic agent around a peripheral or central sensory nerve, a sympathetic plexus or a localized tender trigger point. Correct use of nerve blocks in the treatment of pain requires an experienced practitioner with a thorough understanding of pain syndromes. Neural blockade should be undertaken in appropriate locations by clinicians fully acquainted with the anatomy and techniques involved and who are competent to manage complications that may arise. The use of radiological control and contrast media is strongly advocated to confirm accurate needle placement.

Neural blockade is performed for either diagnostic, prognostic or therapeutic indications. The aim of a diagnostic block is to aid localization of the source of pain and the transmission pathway. It can assist in differentiating whether pain is of peripheral or central origin and whether it is somatic, visceral or sympathetic in nature. The duration of pain relief from a local anaesthetic block may far outlast the duration of action of the local anaesthetic agent but the reason for this is unknown.

Several patients obtain long-term relief from neuroablative procedures. A prognostic block enables the patient temporarily to experience the quality of pain relief and any other feelings, such as numbness, that the permanent procedure will produce. Unfortunately, the permanent block does not always produce the same result as the prognostic local anaesthetic block but it is not known why this occurs.

The use of therapeutic neuroablative procedures has diminished in the last two decades. There are many reasons for this, including the improved use of analgesics, the development of neurostimulatory techniques and the appreciation of the contribution of cognitive and behavioural components to pain. Other important factors have been the growing awareness that the effect of neuroablative procedures is often transient, presumably because of plasticity of the nervous system, and that incapacitating side-effects can occur.

Neural destruction can be produced with neurolytic agents, heat or cold. The commonest neurolytic agents employed are phenol and ethyl alcohol. Phenol has local anaesthetic as well as neurolytic effects and this is an advantage as it is painless to inject. However, large systemic doses cause convulsions and then central nervous system depression and cardiovascular collapse.

Radiofrequency lesions

A destructive heat lesion can be produced using a radiofrequency current. The radiofrequency electrode comprises an insulated needle with a small exposed tip. A high-frequency alternating current flows from the electrode tip to the tissues, producing ionic agitation and a frictional heating effect in tissue adjacent to the tip of the probe. The magnitude of this heating effect is monitored by a thermistor in the electrode tip. Damage to nerve fibres sufficient to block conduction occurs at temperatures above 45°C, although in practice most lesions are made with a probe tip of 60–80°C. An integral nerve stimulator is used to ensure accurate placement of the probe.

Cryotherapy

Lesions may be produced in the nervous system by cold using a cryoprobe. Cooling is produced by the Joule–Thompson effect using nitrous oxide as the refrigerant gas. The probe tip may reach a temperature of –75°C. There is complete functional loss after a cryolesion; however, recovery can be expected after several weeks and this may have advantages in certain situations.

Potential sites for neural blockade are shown in Figure 42.4 and indications for commonly performed nerve blocks are shown in Table 42.1. For a full description of the techniques of neural blockade the reader should consult suggested texts in the Further Reading section.

Stimulation-induced analgesia

Stimulation-induced analgesia can be produced

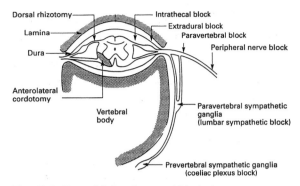

Fig. 42.4 Potential sites for neural blockade.

Table 42.1 Indications for neural blockade

Nerve block	Indications
Trigger point injections	Myofascial pain
Somatic nerve block	Nerve root pain, scar pain
Trigeminal nerve and branches	Trigeminal neuralgia
Intravenous regional sympathetic block (guanethidine)	SMP, RSD
Stellate ganglion block	SMP, RSD, circulatory insufficiency
Lumbar sympathetic block	Circulatory insufficiency Ischaemic rest pain SMP, RSD Phantom pain Amputation stump pain Malignant pelvic pain
Coeliac plexus block	Intra-abdominal malignancy, especially pancreas
Extradural steroids	Nerve root pain, benign or malignant
Intrathecal neurolytics	Malignant pain
Pituitary ablation	Widespread pain from disseminated metastases
Percutaneous cervical cordotomy	Unilateral somatic malignant pain, short life expectancy

by acupuncture, transcutaneous electrical nerve stimulation, dorsal column stimulation or deep brain stimulation.

Acupuncture

The Chinese have known for 4000 years that the insertion of needles at specific points in the body produces analgesia. According to Chinese philosophy, *ch'i*, the life force, circulates around the body in pathways called meridians. Injury and illness can block this passage, causing pain and disease. Acupuncture is believed to release these blocks and balance the energy of the patient. Traditionally, acupuncture points are stimulated by the insertion of fine needles which are then rotated manually or stimulated by heat (moxibustion) or electrically. For acupuncture analgesia to be effective, the patient should experience a numbing heavy sensation, called *te-ch'i*, spreading from the acupuncture site.

It is clear that it is not necessary to use traditional acupuncture sites to obtain analgesia. Several studies have shown that needling provides equally good pain relief whether applied to specified acupuncture sites or to sham sites. Some acupuncture points are over sensitive sites in musculoskeletal tissues that correlate with myofascial trigger points. Acupuncture can be considered to produce high-intensity, low-frequency stimulation. It is thought that this causes the release of enkephalins and endorphins, which are responsible for the analgesic and sedating effects seen. Levels of endogenous opioid peptides in CSF are elevated following acupuncture and naloxone has been shown to reverse acupuncture analgesia. It is postulated that there exists both a segmental and a non-segmental mechanism for acupuncture analgesia, but these have yet to be fully elucidated. However, acupuncture has become an accepted method of treatment in the pain management clinic, especially for musculoskeletal pain.

It has also been shown that single-needle acupuncture to the P6 point on the pericardium meridian is antiemetic in postoperative nausea and vomiting, morning sickness and in patients receiving cytotoxic drugs.

Transcutaneous electrical nerve stimulation

Transcutaneous electrical nerve stimulation has been widely used since Melzack and Wall proposed the gate control theory in 1965. They postulated that large-diameter primary afferents exert a specific inhibitory effect on dorsal horn nociceptive neurones and that stimulation of these fibres would alleviate pain. Conventional TENS

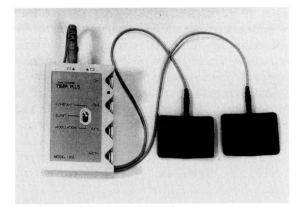

Fig. 42.5 A transcutaneous electrical nerve stimulator.

produces high-frequency, low-intensity stimulation which relieves pain in the area in which it produces paraesthesia. Stimulation variables of TENS can be altered to produce low-frequency acupuncture-like TENS which, unlike conventional TENS, produces analgesia which is reversed by naloxone.

A small battery-powered unit is used to apply the electrical stimulus to the skin via carbon electrodes (Fig. 42.5). These are placed over the painful area, on either side of it or over nerves supplying the region and stimulation is applied at an intensity which the patient finds comfortable. Adverse effects are minimal, with allergy to the electrodes or gel being the commonest problem encountered. TENS is used successfully for a variety of musculoskeletal and neuropathic pains. Unfortunately, tolerance to TENS does sometimes occur, terminating previously effective analgesia. It may be possible to overcome this by changing stimulation variables.

TENS can also be used for postoperative pain and is a useful form of analgesia for the first stage of labour.

Dorsal column stimulation

Electrical stimulation applied to the dorsal columns is effective in relieving pain. Electrodes may be implanted surgically over the dorsal columns or positioned in the extradural space percutaneously. Artificial paraesthesiae are produced in the region of the pain and if relief occurs, the electrode and a receiver for radioactivation permanently implanted. This equipment is expensive and a high proportion of patients obtain good relief initially only to have their pain return after some months.

Dorsal column stimulation has been advocated for deafferentation pain and, more recently, for improving blood flow in vascular disease.

Psychological techniques

Pain is not simply a sensation of tissue damage, but a complex interaction of biochemical, behavioural, cognitive and emotional factors. Chronic pain patients become anxious and depressed, lose self-esteem and their internal locus of control, i.e. the feeling that they can exert control over their situation. These important aspects should be addressed in the pain management clinic. The clinical psychologist is a valuable asset to the pain management team and should be seen as an integral member by staff and patients. The cognitive and behavioural approach investigates how thoughts (often negative) and behaviours (often maladaptive) reinforce the chronic pain state. Cognitive and behavioural techniques are then used to reduce the helplessness and hopelessness of the pain patient and to increase the level of functioning and emotional well-being in spite of the pain. This can be done on an individual or, to optimize efficient use of resources, on a group basis.

Increasingly pain management programmes organized either on an outpatient or inpatient basis are being established. The core team usually consists of an anaesthetist, a clinical psychologist, a physiotherapist, an occupational therapist and a clinical nurse specialist. The sessions are structured to focus on thoughts, feelings and physical activity. Education of the patient regarding the nature of chronic pain and the limitations of medicine in its management are important topics. The patient is taught to identify negative thoughts and to control them using techniques such as imagery, distraction and relaxation therapy. Patients are taught coping strategies that they can use in the future to reduce the feelings of dependence on medical practitioners. Many patients have fallen into the trap of abnormal overactivity/underactivity cycling. Emphasis is placed on activity pacing and the setting of attainable goals.

This type of therapy may represent the only option available to those patients in whom physical treatment has been unsuccessful and its importance in the pain clinic armamentarium should not be underestimated.

Advances in knowledge of pain pathophysiology by scientists and increasingly close cooperation between them and clinicians have led to a better understanding of mechanisms sustaining chronic pain and an increase in therapeutic options. In addition, the increasing acceptance by the medical profession and the general public of the importance of psychological factors in chronic pain of both malignant and non-malignant origin has opened up new treatment opportunities. Further research in the laboratory and audit in the clinical setting is vital to ensure continuing progress.

The recognition by the Royal College of Anaesthetists of chronic pain as a subspeciality within anaesthesia will have an enormous impact on the training of clinicians and the provision of pain management facilities and will thereby significantly benefit the patient suffering chronic pain.

FURTHER READING

Cousins M J, Bridenbaugh P O (eds) 1988 Neural blockade in clinical anaesthesia and management of pain. J B Lippincott, Philadelphia

Diamond A W, Coniam S W 1992 The management of chronic pain. Oxford University Press, Oxford

Fields H L 1987 Pain. McGraw-Hill, New York

Waddell G, Main C J, Morris E W, Di Paola M, Gray I C M 1984 Chronic low back pain, psychological distress and illness behaviour. Spine 9: 209–213

Wildsmith J A W, Armitage E N (eds) 1987 Principles and practice of regional anaesthesia. Churchill Livingstone, Edinburgh

43. Cardiopulmonary resuscitation

Cardiopulmonary resuscitation (CPR) is required when the supply of oxygen to the brain is insufficient to maintain function. Oxygen delivery is dependent upon cardiac output, haemoglobin concentration and saturation of haemoglobin with oxygen, which depends predominantly on respiratory function. CPR is required most commonly after cardiac arrest, respiratory arrest or a combination of the two.

Cerebral hypoxia

The brain is more sensitive to hypoxia than any other organ, including the heart. It has a limited facility for anaerobic metabolism and cannot store oxygen. Hypoxaemia is tolerated remarkably well in the normal individual, as cerebral blood flow (CBF) increases substantially to compensate for reduced oxygen carriage in blood. In contrast, ischaemia (e.g. circulatory arrest) or hypoxaemia in a patient unable to increase CBF (e.g. cerebrovascular atherosclerosis or a low cardiac output state) results in the rapid onset of anaerobic metabolism. The cerebral cortex is damaged permanently by ischaemia of more than 3–4 min duration. Thus, although a patient may survive an episode of circulatory arrest, permanent impairment of cerebral function may result if cerebral oxygen delivery is not restored within 3–4 min of the initial cessation of blood flow. The commonest cause of brain damage after cardiac arrest is delay in starting resuscitation. Therefore, when circulatory arrest has occurred, it is essential to start CPR as rapidly as possible.

SIGNS OF CARDIAC ARREST

These are shown in Figure 43.1. During surgery it

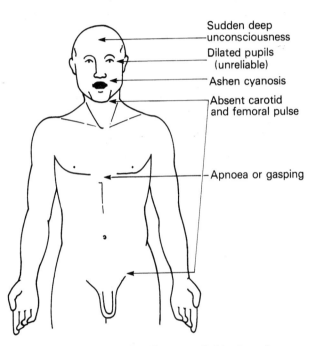

Sudden deep unconsciousness
Dilated pupils (unreliable)
Ashen cyanosis
Absent carotid and femoral pulse
Apnoea or gasping

Fig. 43.1 The signs of cardiac arrest. Sudden loss of consciousness and absence of major pulses are sufficient to justify diagnosis.

may be difficult to distinguish between profound hypotension and circulatory arrest. If neither surgeon nor anaesthetist can find a pulse, external cardiac massage must be instituted.

Guidelines to guide the performance of cardiopulmonary resuscitation have been developed by the European Resuscitation Council (1992) and the American Heart Association (1986). These guidelines are based on the concept of the 'chain of survival'. The chain of survival requires that following an initial clinical assessment of the patient's condition, a telephone call for help is made before starting basic life support. This early call for help decreases the time to the first defibrillation, shortens the time to the delivery of advanced life support, decreases the length of time of performance of basic life support and improves survival from the initial resuscitation event.

ASSESSMENT

Approach the patient ensuring that there is no further danger from the surrounding environment. Assess the level of responsiveness by gently shaking the patient and shouting 'Are you all right?'.

Airway

In the unresponsive patient, open the airway by tilting the head back and lifting the jaw forwards (Fig. 43.2). This displaces the tongue, the most common cause of airway obstruction, from the back of the pharynx. In cases of suspected cervical spine injury, the airway should be opened by using the jaw thrust manoeuvre only whilst maintaining inline cervical spine immobilization. Head tilt and neck extension must never be used in this situation.

Breathing

Look – to see if the chest wall is moving or if the abdominal wall is indicating an obstructed airway by a see-saw movement.

Listen – over the mouth for sounds of air movement or for sounds indicating an obstructed airway.

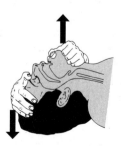

Fig. 43.2 Backward tilt of the head stretches the anterior neck structures and thereby lifts the base of the tongue off the posterior pharyngeal wall.

Feel   – over the mouth with the side of the face for sign of air movement indicating effective breathing.

Circulation

Check the rate and rhythm of the carotid pulse.

Call for help

It is essential to telephone for help as soon as the assessment has been completed.

BASIC LIFE SUPPORT

Cardiac arrest

If breathing and pulse are absent commence basic life support, which is a combination of chest compressions and ventilation.

Chest compressions

Chest compressions are performed on the lower third of the sternum, two fingers breadth above the xiphisternum. The overlapping heels of both hands are used to compress the chest by depressing the sternum approximately 4–5 cm at a rate of 80 compressions per minute (range 60–100 compressions per minute). After 15 compressions open the airway by tilting the head and lifting the chin and give two expired air breaths.

Breathing

This is achieved by expired air ventilation. With the airway held open, pinch the nostrils closed. Take a full breath and seal your lips over the patient's mouth. Blow steadily into the patient's mouth, watching the chest rise as if the patient was taking a deep breath. Each breath should take approximately 2 s for a full inflation. Maintaining the airway, take your mouth off the patient and allow the chest to fall in expiration. Repeat this manoeuvre to give two ventilations.

Continue basic life support, 15 chest compressions with two expired air ventilations, until advanced life support arrives. Do not interrupt basic life support to perform further assessments of the patient unless the patient shows signs of recovery.

Respiratory arrest

If the patient is not breathing but has a pulse, perform 10 expired air breaths before leaving the patient to telephone for help. On returning to the patient recheck the breathing and the pulse. If a pulse is present continue expired air breathing at a rate of 10 breaths per minute but recheck the pulse after every 10 breaths. Commence full basic life support if the pulse stops.

Mechanisms of action of chest compressions

The original theory of the action of chest compressions was that the heart was squeezed between the sternum superiorly and the vertebral column posteriorly with each depression of the sternum. Each compression of the heart pumped blood around the circulation (the heart pump theory).

A later theory, the chest pump theory, is based on the concept that each chest compression raises the intrathoracic pressure. This raised pressure is transmitted to the intrathoracic vessels; the arteries, being thickwalled, retain and transmit this pressure whereas the veins, being thin-walled, collapse. The result is a pressure gradient between the arterial and venous system and thus a forward flow of blood around the circulation. Basic life support only provides 10–15% of normal cardiac output and should be regarded as 'buying time' until the commencement of advanced life support.

ADVANCED LIFE SUPPORT

By following the chain of survival, the early telephone call for help will result in the prompt arrival of the equipment and personnel needed to perform advanced life support. In adult resuscitation, the early use of a defibrillator in ventricular fibrillation has a definitive effect on eventual survival.

In specialized in-hospital areas, for example the operating theatre, the intensive care unit or the coronary care unit, the time to defibrillation is negligible. In these situations it is recommended that if defibrillation is immediately to hand, basic life support is not initiated until defibrillation has been attempted.

There are four underlying disorders of cardiac rhythm associated with cardiac arrest:

1. Ventricular fibrillation
2. Ventricular tachycardia
3. Asystole
4. Electromechanical dissociation (pulseless electrical activity).

Ventricular fibrillation and ventricular tachycardia have identical treatment protocols, thus only three treatment schedules are presented. Of these, the protocol for ventricular fibrillation is the most important as this arrhythmia is the commonest cause of sudden cardiac death and it is also the most amenable to treatment.

Ventricular fibrillation (Fig. 43.3)

Ventricular fibrillation is chaotic electrical activity of the myocardium. In a witnessed or monitored cardiac arrest, a precordial thump should be administered immediately. Early defibrillation is recommended and if the first three defibrillation shocks can be delivered quickly, then this initial defibrillation sequence should not be interrupted for basic life support procedures.

An initial DC shock at 200 J probably causes minimal myocardial damage and is adequate to achieve success in most recoverable situations. This first DC shock decreases the thoracic impedance, thus increasing the amount of energy from the second DC shock at 200 J that reaches the heart. The chance of success of each defibrillation attempt depends on many dynamic variables including the waveform and vectors of myocardial activity. Following two 200 J DC shocks, one defibrillation is attempted at the maximum delivered energy level of 360 J. If all three initial defibrillation attempts (200 J, 200 J, 360 J) are unsuccessful, the prospects of recovery are poor.

Resuscitation should continue with tracheal intubation and lung ventilation with 100% oxygen. Where intubation is not achieved, ventilation with a high inspired oxygen level can be carried out using a self-inflating bag valve and mask, together with an oxygen reservoir system.

Alternatively, a laryngeal mask airway can be inserted. Paramedics, nurses and doctors not experienced in tracheal intubation can learn the technique of insertion of a laryngeal mask airway in a few hours. Whilst the laryngeal mask does

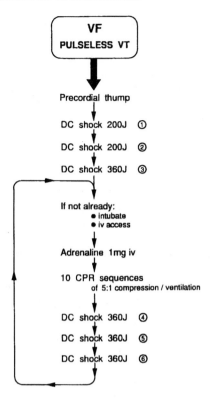

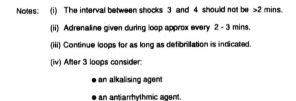

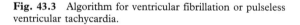

Notes: (i) The interval between shocks 3 and 4 should not be >2 mins.

(ii) Adrenaline given during loop approx every 2 - 3 mins.

(iii) Continue loops for as long as defibrillation is indicated.

(iv) After 3 loops consider:

● an alkalising agent

● an antiarrhythmic agent.

Fig. 43.3 Algorithm for ventricular fibrillation or pulseless ventricular tachycardia.

not provide 100% airway protection it does provide a more secure airway and more effective ventilation compared with an oral Guedel airway and a bag-valve mask system.

At the same time as intubation is being established, another member of the ALS team should be cannulating a vein. Peripheral venous access is the simplest to establish and attempts should be made to cannulate a large peripheral vein with a 14 G or 16 G cannula. Central venous access requires expertise and training but it does provide significant advantages over peripheral access in terms of speed of delivery and action of drugs.

Adrenaline 1 mg (10 ml of 1 in 10 000 solution

or 1 ml of 1 in 1000 solution) is the next action in the protocol. If intravenous access has not been established then 2–3 mg can be given via the tracheal route. This route is definitely second best as the pharmacodynamics of drugs administered via the tracheal route are unpredictable. Adrenaline is used in resuscitation mainly for its α-adrenergic receptor stimulant effects. This α-adrenergic action causes peripheral vasoconstriction, raises the systemic vascular resistance, raises the end-diastolic filling pressure and thus improves coronary perfusion. In addition, adrenaline is believed to 'harden' the major vessels leading away from the heart thus aiding in the transmission of the raised intrathoracic pressure and the forward flow of blood (in the chest pump theory). Adrenaline has a β-adrenergic stimulant activity on the chronotropic and inotropic activity of the myocardium.

Ten sequences of basic life support in the ratio of five compressions to one ventilation should follow the administration of adrenaline. A further three defibrillations at 360 J are then given. Resuscitation in the form of basic life support should not be interrupted for more than 15 s to perform any of the above manoeuvres. Furthermore, there should be no more than a 2 min delay between the third and fourth shock in the algorithm.

If the second set of defibrillation attempts is still unsuccessful then the loop, via intubation and intravenous access, should be repeated. Therefore in any 2 min cycle of resuscitation three defibrillation attempts (360 J), 1 mg of intravenous adrenaline and 10 cycles of basic life support (five compressions: one ventilation) are applied to the patient. The chance of a sucessful resuscitation decreases with an increasing number of shocks and with a prolonged resuscitation time.

Asystole (Fig. 43.4)

Asystole is a flat electrocardiographic trace indicating no ventricular activity. Occasionally there may be P wave electrical activity only.

The results of resuscitation from asystole are extremely poor. It is therefore essential that ventricular fibrillation is not missed. Unless ventricular fibrillation can definitely be excluded the treatment of asystole is started (as in ventricular

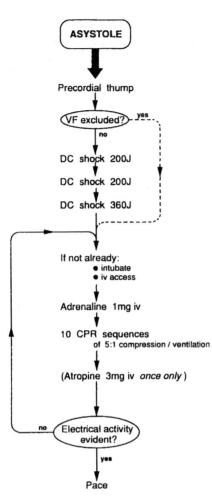

Fig. 43.4 Algorithm for asystole.

depending on the local skills and available equipment. Pacing has not been a great success in the asystole resuscitation situation. This may be a failure in technique or alternatively it may be that pacing is only considered at too late a stage in the resuscitation sequence, probably when the myocardium is beyond electrical situation.

Electromechanical dissociation (EMD) (Fig. 43.5)

EMD or pulseless electrical activity (PEA) has the worst prognosis of all rhythms associated with cardiac arrest. It is diagnosed when the electro-cardiogram shows electrical activity but there is no palpable peripheral pulse (i.e. pulseless electrical activity).

EMD is usually associated with a specific cause and this should be diagnosed and treated as a priority. In some cases cardiac arrest may not be absolute and the circulation may need support by chest compressions. The algorithm for EMD

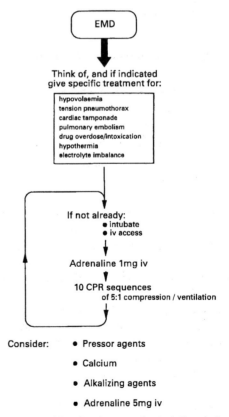

Fig. 43.5 Algorithm for electromechanical dissociation.

fibrillation) by a precordial thump, in a witnessed event, followed by the three initial defibrillations of 200 J, 200 J and 360 J. The sequence continues by establishing tracheal intubation and venous access, the administration of 1 mg of adrenaline and 10 cycles of five compressions to one ventilation. If asystole persists the sequence of further adrenaline and basic life support is continued until an appropriate endpoint. Atropine 3 mg intravenously may be given once during the first cycle of asystole resuscitation. Atropine is a parasympathetic nerve blocker and is used to counter any excess vagal tone.

Electrical pacing of the heart can be attempted where there is P wave activity evident. Percutaneous or pervenous pacing can be attempted

follows the same pattern as previously, only in EMD the cause is diagnosed and treated followed by establishing tracheal intubation and venous access, the administration of adrenaline 1 mg and basic life support at five compressions to one ventilation before the cycle is repeated.

In the EMD situation other additional pressor agents may be considered more advantageous; calcium chloride (10 ml of 10% solution) may be used especially in the diagnosis of an overdose of calcium channel blocking drugs. Adrenaline may be given in a high dose of 5 mg, but this high dose has been associated with post resuscitation renal failure.

ALKALINIZING AGENTS

In prolonged resuscitation the patient may become increasingly acidotic. This is especially so when initial basic life support has been delayed, ventilation has not been performed effectively (respiratory acidosis) or chest compressions have not been successful in achieving a satisfactory flow of blood (metabolic acidosis). In most cases, establishing effective basic life support will maintain the acid–base status quo without further intervention.

Where basic life support procedures have been established and the patient's lungs have been effectively ventilated, any associated acidosis may be reversed pharmacologically by administration of sodium bicarbonate solution. Sodium bicarbonate is usually administered as an intravenous 50 ml bolus of an 8.4% solution (50 mmol of HCO_3 ion). It is best titrated into the circulation in response to the arterial blood gas results by the formula:

$$\left[\frac{\text{Base deficit}}{3} \times \text{body weight (kg)}\right] \begin{array}{l} \text{in mmol of} \\ HCO_3 \text{ solution} \end{array}$$

1 ml of 8.4% $NaHCO_3$ = 1 mmol HCO_3

Following administration of sodium bicarbonate the intravenous line must be carefully flushed as any residual sodium bicarbonate inactivates subsequently administered adrenaline.

Sodium bicarbonate should not be administered without considering that:

- it does not improve ability to defibrillate the heart
- it shifts the oxyhaemoglobin dissociation curve and inhibits the release of oxygen
- it causes hyperosmolality and hypernatraemia
- it produces paradoxical acidosis
- it exacerbates central venous acidosis.

Sodium bicarbonate is only recommended routinely in patients with pre-existing metabolic acidosis, hyperkalaemia, tricyclic antidepressant or phenobarbitone overdosage.

AFTERCARE

For every ten in-hospital resuscitation events, three patients survive the initial resuscitation procedures, two survive the next 24 h, 1.5 survive to discharge from hospital and one patient lives for 1 year after the initial event. These simple statistics illustrate the initial success rate of resuscitation and emphasize the need for careful post resuscitation care.

Following resuscitation, all patients should be cared for on a specialized unit, e.g. an intensive or a coronary care unit. Careful monitoring of vital functions should be established and abnormalities in serum electrolyte concentrations corrected to prevent reoccurrence of the event. In a few patients the event will have been extremely rapid and little additional care is needed. The majority will require further circulatory and respiratory support.

Cardiovascular system

Cardiac output may remain unsatisfactory as a result of cardiogenic shock and may be so poor that unconsciousness persists (see below). A low cardiac output may result from:

1. *Poor myocardial contractility*, e.g. after myocardial infarction or pulmonary embolus. Dopamine $2-10\ \mu g.kg^{-1}.min^{-1}$ by infusion is the treatment of choice. In this dose range, it has little vasoconstrictor effect and causes a preferential increase in renal blood flow. The optimal preload for the failing heart should be ensured by the cautious administration of colloid (Haemaccel, Gelofusine or human albumin solution) as guided by the CVP. A normal CVP does not exclude the possible development of pulmonary oedema.

2. *Hypovolaemia.* This requires further transfusion guided by CVP measurement.

3. *Arrhythmias.* These require treatment if:
    a. cardiac output is compromised; or
    b. they are electrically unstable and therefore predispose to a further episode of circulatory arrest.

All arrhythmias are potentiated by disturbances in blood/gas or potassium homoeostasis. Figure 43.6 summarizes management of important arrhythmias during CPR.

Respiratory system

Lung dysfunction is produced during resuscitation for reasons which may include inhalation of vomit, lung contusion, fractured ribs and pneumothorax. Pulmonary oedema may occur in the presence of heart failure and after head injury,

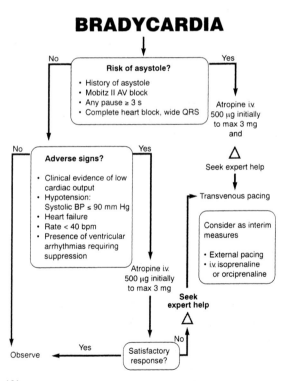

(A)

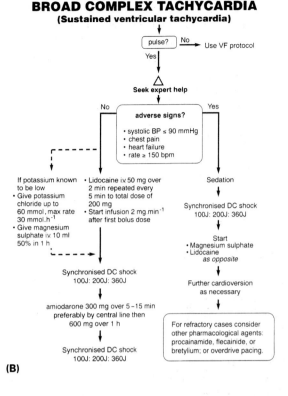

(B)

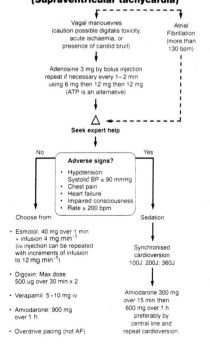

(C)

Fig. 43.6 Emergency treatment for peri-arrest arrhythmias. (**A**) Bradycardia, (**B**) broad complex tachycardia (sustained ventricular tachycardia), (**C**) narrow complex tachycardia (supraventricular tachycardia). If not already done, give oxygen and establish i.v. access. Doses based on adult of average body weight.

drowning or smoke inhalation. Oxygen therapy for 24 h should follow any episode of circulatory arrest. If overt respiratory failure supervenes, more intensive treatment is required, including possibly a period of artificial ventilation. All patients should have a chest X-ray and blood gas analysis after resuscitation.

Central nervous system

Efficient cardiac massage and ventilation provide sufficient oxygen delivery to protect the brain from damage, although not to prevent depression of function. If efficient resuscitation was started immediately after circulatory arrest occurred and was continued until restoration of an adequate spontaneous cardiac output, the patient should regain consciousness fairly quickly. Recovery tends to be delayed after prolonged arrest or when general anaesthesia is involved.

Patients may fail to recover consciousness for the following reasons:

1. Low cardiac output (see above).
2. Brain damage, which may be present if resuscitation was delayed or if the circulatory arrest was precipitated by hypoxaemia.

MANAGEMENT OF BRAIN DAMAGE

The aim of treatment is to provide optimal conditions for recovery of cerebral cells and prevention of secondary neuronal damage.

General measures

Airway obstruction occurs readily in the unconscious patient and leads to hypoxaemia and hypercapnia, which aggravate cerebral damage. In addition, cough and swallowing reflexes are depressed. Continued tracheal intubation protects the lungs, secures the airway and renders it easy to institute mechanical ventilation if respiration becomes inadequate. With the airway secure, epileptiform fits which increase $CMRO_2$ may be treated safely with anticonvulsants. In general, if the patient can tolerate the tracheal tube, it should be left in situ. The unconscious patient whose trachea is not intubated should be nursed in the lateral position to assist drainage of oral secretions. Arterial pressure should be maintained in the normal range to ensure adequate cerebral perfusion pressure and haematocrit in the low normal range to optimize oxygen delivery. Tissue hydration and blood biochemistry should be maintained as normal; there is no evidence that dehydration is beneficial. An increase in body temperature increases $CMRO_2$ and should be avoided. Depth of coma should be assessed regularly.

Specialized treatment

1. *Hyperventilation.* Mild passive hyperventilation to a Pa_{CO_2} of 4 kPa helps to minimize increases in intracranial pressure secondary to cerebral oedema, although there is no evidence that cerebral damage after cardiac arrest is reduced by hyperventilation if the patient is able to achieve adequate gas exchange when breathing spontaneously. Control of ventilation may be achieved with the aid of muscle relaxants or cerebral depressants. A head-up tilt assists cerebral venous drainage.

2. *Osmotherapy.* Increasing the plasma omolality decreases intracranial water content and thus ICP. Mannitol (0.25 g.kg^{-1} initially) is often used. Mannitol increases the circulating blood volume and may be dangerous in the presence of pulmonry oedema or a high CVP. In this situation, frusemide or bumetanide may be more appropriate.

3. *Steroids.* There is no evidence that steroids are beneficial after cardiac arrest.

4. *Barbiturates and CNS depressants.* Thiopentone and diazepam are often used in conventional doses to provide sedation, facilitate control of ventilation and suppress seizures. Both these drugs must be used with care after circulatory arrest. In particular, large loading doses of barbiturates are contraindicated, as they produce profound cardiovascular depression. There is no evidence that they protect the brain after cardiac arrest.

5. *Calcium antagonists.* The role of these drugs after cardiac arrest still awaits clarification. At the present time, there is no evidence that they are of value when administered in the postresuscitation period.

PREVENTION OF CARDIAC ARREST

The commonest causes of cardiac arrest during

surgery are hypoxaemia and haemorrhage. Hypoxaemia may occur with alarming rapidity during periods of apnoea or respiratory obstruction, particularly in obstetric patients and young children; in the latter, bradycardia is an important premonitory sign. Steady haemorrhage may pass unnoticed until the patient deteriorates suddenly. Other causes include overdosage with hypotensive or local anaesthetic agents, exogenously administered adrenaline and the use of i.v. induction agents in the presence of hypovolaemia. Vagal reflexes may be involved in surgery on the eye, rectum, carotid sheath or upper respiratory tract.

Generally, the outcome after abrupt cardiac arrest is good provided that treatment is prompt and effective.

INITIATING AND TERMINATING CPR

In the first instance, all patients should be resuscitated unless the medical or nursing notes indicate that a contrary decision has been reached. If it becomes apparent when resuscitation has started that CPR would be inappropriate (e.g. because the patient is in the terminal stages of an incurable disease), it should cease.

Future cerebral function cannot be predicted accurately during CPR and suspicion of brain damage is no justification for terminating resuscitation. When in doubt, CPR should be continued until there is no doubt that the patient will fail to recover. Good recovery has taken place after 1–2 h of continuous CPR.

FURTHER READING

American Heart Association 1986 Standards and guidelines for cardiopulmonary resuscitation and emergency cardiac care. Journal of the American Medical Association 255: 2843–2989
European Resuscitation Council 1992 ALS guidelines. ERC

Appendices

Appendix Ia: Abbreviations used in text and appendices

α	adrenoceptor type (after Ahlquist)	C_x	clearance of x
ABO	nomenclature for blood groups (after Landsteiner)	C	compliance
		$CaCO_3$	calcium carbonate
ACD	acid citrate dextrose	cAMP	cyclic adenosine monophosphate
ACE	angiotensin-converting enzyme	CaO	calcium oxide
ACh	acetylcholine	CAVG	coronary artery vein graft
ACT	activated clotting time	CBF	cerebral blood flow
ACTH	adrenocorticotrophic hormone	CC	closing capacity
ADH	antidiuretic hormone	CCT	central conduction time
ADP	adenosine diphosphate	CCU	coronary care unit
AHF	antihaemophilic factor (factor VIII)	CDH	Christiansen Douglas Haldane (effect)
AIDS	acquired immunodeficiency syndrome	CFAM	cerebral function analysing monitor
AMP	adenosine monophosphate	CFM	cerebral function monitor
ANP	atrial natriuretic peptide	CHO	carbohydrate
ANS	autonomic nervous system	CI	cardiac index (cardiac output/ body surface area)
ARDS	acute respiratory distress syndrome	CK	creatine kinase
ASA	American Society of Anesthesiologists	Cl	clearance (of drug)
		cm	centimetre (10^{-2} m; not a unit in the SI system)
ATP	adenosine triphosphate		
AV	atrioventricular	cmH_2O	centimetres of water
β	adrenoceptor type (after Ahlquist)	$CMRO_2$	cerebral metabolic rate for oxygen
B	bone marrow dependent (as in B cells)	CMV	cytomegalovirus
		CNS	central nervous system
BCR	British corrected ratio (for oral anticoagulants)	C_0	concentration at time = 0
		CO	cardiac output
BM	Boehringer Mannheim (makers of BM Stix blood glucose testing strips)	CO_2	carbon dioxide
		cp	centipoise
		CPAP	continuous positive airways pressure
BP	boiling point		
BP	*British Pharmacopoeia*	CPB	cardiopulmonary bypass
BSA	body surface area	CPD	citrate phosphate dextrose
BZ	benzodiazepine	CPD–A	citrate phosphate dextrose with adenine
C	cervical or coccygeal vertebra		
°C	degrees Celsius	CPK	creatine phosphokinase

CPP	cerebral perfusion pressure	EUA	examination under anaesthesia
CPPV	continuous positive pressure ventilation	EVR	endocardial viability ratio
		F	Faraday's constant
CPR	cardiopulmonary resuscitation	FDP	fibrin degradation products
^{51}Cr	chromium atom — isotope weight 51 Da (radiolabelled)	$Fe^{2+(3+)}$	iron ionized — ferrous (ferric) ion
CSF	cerebrospinal fluid	FEV_1	forced expiratory volume (in 1 s)
C_{ss}	concentration at steady state	FF	filtration fraction
C_t	concentration at time t	FFP	fresh frozen plasma
CT	computed tomography	$F_{I_{O_2}}$	fractional inspired oxygen concentration
CV	closing volume		
CVP	central venous pressure	FRC	functional residual capacity
Δ	delta — minimal increment (of)	FSH	follicle-stimulating hormone
D	dose (of drug)	FVC	forced vital capacity
d	density	G6PD	glucose-6-phosphate dehydrogenase
D & C	dilatation and curettage (of uterus)		
DAP	diastolic arterial pressure	GABA	γ-aminobutyric acid
DC	direct current	GFR	glomerular filtration rate
DCR	dacrocystorhinostomy	GH	growth hormone
DDAVP	desmopressin	GI	gastrointestinal
DHSS	Department of Health and Social Security	GTN	glyceryl trinitrate
		h	hour
DIC	disseminated intravascular coagulation	H^+	hydrogen ion
		H_1	histamine — type 1 receptor
DNA	deoxyribonucleic acid	H_2	histamine — type 2 receptor
Dopa	Deoxyphenylalanine	HAFOE	high air flow oxygen enrichment
2,3 DPG	2,3-diphosphoglycerate	Hb	haemoglobin
dTC	dextrotubocurarine	HbA	adult haemoglobin
DVT	deep vein thrombosis	Hb_{Barts}	Saint Bartholomew's haemoglobin (γ-thalassaemia)
ECC	extracorporeal circulation (heart bypass)		
		HbF	fetal haemoglobin
ECF	extracellular fluid	HbNH	carbamino haemoglobin
ECG	electrocardiogram	HBsAg	hepatitis B surface antigen
ECM	external cardiac massage	hCG	human chorionic gonadotrophin
ECT	electroconvulsive therapy	HCO_3^-	bicarbonate ion
EDTA	ethylenediaminetetra-acetic acid	H_2CO_3	carbonic acid
EC	European Community	Hct	haematocrit
EEG	electroencephalogram	He	helium
EF	ejection fraction	HFDV	high-frequency forced diffusion ventilation
EMD	electromechanical dissociation		
EMG	electromyogram	HFJV	high-frequency jet ventilation
EMMV	extended mandatory minute ventilation (or volume)	HFOV	high-frequency oscillatory ventilation
EMO	Epstein and Macintosh (of Oxford)	HFPPV	high-frequency positive-pressure ventilation
ENT	ear, nose and throat	HFV	high-frequency ventilation
EP	evoked potential	Hg	mercury
EPI	Eysenck personality inventory	5-HIAA	5-hydroxyindoleacetic acid
EPP	end-plate potential	HIV	human immunodeficiency virus

HLA	human leukocyte antigen	LVEDP	left ventricular end-diastolic pressure
HOCM	hypertrophic obstructive cardio-myopathy	μ	micro (10^{-6})
HPA	hypothalamopituitary axis	μV	microvolts
hPL	human placental lactogen	mA	milliampere
HR	heart rate	MAC	minimum alveolar concentration (for anaesthesia)
5-HT	5-hydroxytryptamine (serotonin)		
Hz	hertz (cycles per second)	MAO	monoamine oxidase
I	infusion rate	MAOI	monoamine oxidase inhibitor
IABP	intra-aortic balloon pump	MAP	mean arterial pressure
ICP	isometric contraction period; intracranial pressure	MC	Mary Caterill (name of pro-prietary mask)
I/E	inspiratory/expiratory	MC	monocomponent — 'free of impurities' (as in insulin)
IgA	immunoglobulin type A (γ-globulin A)		
		MCV	mean corpuscular volume
IgE	immunoglobulin type E (γ-globulin E, reagin)	MEPP	miniature end-plate potential
		mg	milligram
IgG	immunoglobulin type G (γ-globulin G)	Mg^{2+}	magnesium ion
		MI	myocardial infarction
i.m.	intramuscular	min	minute
IMV	intermittent mandatory ventilation	ml	millilitre
IOP	intraocular pressure	mm	millimetre
IPPV	intermittent positive-pressure ventilation	mmHg	millimetres of mercury
		MMPI	Minnesota multiphasic personality inventory
IRP	isometric relaxation period		
ISA	intrinsic sympathomimetic activity	MMV	mandatory minute ventilation
ITU	intensive therapy unit	mN	millinewton
i.v.	intravenous	mol	mole
IVC	inferior vena cava	mosmol	milliosmole
IVRA	intravenous regional anaesthesia	MRI	magnetic resonance imaging
J	joule	ms	millisecond
K	kelvin	mV	millivolt
K^+	potassium ion	MVP	mean venous pressure
KCCT	kaolin cephalin clotting time	MW	molecular weight
kg	kilogram	η	viscosity
K_i^+	potassium ion (inside cell)	N	newton (unit of force)
K_o^+	potassium ion (outside cell)	N/A	not available; not applicable
kPa	kilopascal	N_2O	nitrous oxide
l	length	Na	sodium
L(n)	lumbar vertebra (number n)	Na^+	sodium ion
LAP	left atrial pressure	Na-K-ATPase	sodium and potassium-dependent adenosine triphosphatase
LATS	long-acting thyroid stimulator		
lb/in^2	pounds per square inch	NEEP	negative end-expiratory pressure
LDH	lactate dehydrogenase	NH_3	ammonia
LH	luteinizing hormone	NH_4^+	ammonium ion
LMN	lower motor neurone	NHS	National Health Service (UK)
log	logarithm(ic)	NMR	nuclear magnetic resonance
LOS	lower oesophageal sphincter	NSAID	non-steroidal anti-inflammatory drug
LSCS	lower-segment Caesarean section		

NTD	neural tube defects	PTTK	partial thromboplastin time, kaolin
O_2	oxygen	PVC	polyvinyl chloride
ODC	oxyhaemoglobin dissociation curve	PVR	pulmonary vascular resistance
		$\dot{Q}_t$	total liquid flow in unit time
osmol	osmole	ρ	rho (= density)
π	pi (= 3.14159)	r	radius (of circle or sphere)
π_{BC}	oncotic pressure in Bowman's capsule	R	universal gas constant
		RA_x	renal artery concentration of x
π_{CAP}	oncotic pressure in capillary	RAP	right atrial pressure
P	electrocardiographic nomenclature	RBF	renal blood flow
P_{50}	need for 50% saturation (of haemoglobin)	RDS	respiratory distress syndrome
		Re	Reynolds number (dimensionless)
Pa	pascal (unit of pressure)	REM	rapid eye movement
P_A	alveolar partial pressure (of gas)	Rh(x)	Rhesus blood group (major phenotype x)
Pa	arterial partial pressure (of gas)		
PAH	*para*-aminohippuric acid	RLF	retrolental fibroplasia
PAP	pulmonary artery pressure	RPF	renal plasma flow
PAOP	pulmonary artery occlusion pressure (= PCWP)	RPP	rate–pressure product
		RV	residual volume
P_{BC}	hydrostatic pressure in Bowman's capsule	RV_x	renal vein concentration of x
		s	second
PcA	Patient-controlled analgesia	SA	sinoatrial
P_{CAP}	hydrostatic pressure in capillary	SAB	subarachnoid block
PCWP	pulmonary capillary wedge pressure	SAP	systolic arterial pressure
		s.c.	subcutaneous
PE	pulmonary embolus	SDP	subdural pressure
$P_{\bar{E}}$	mean expired partial pressure	SG	specific gravity
$P_{E'}$	end-expired partial pressure	SI	Système International d'Unités
PEEP	positive end-expiratory pressure	SIMV	synchronized intermittent mandatory ventilation
PEFR	peak expiratory flow rate		
PF	pathological fibrinolysis	SNP	sodium nitroprusside
PG(X)	prostaglandin type (X)	SRS–A	slow-reacting substance of anaphylaxis
pH	hydrogen ion activity (logarithm to base 10 of the measured hydrogen ion concentration)		
		SV	stroke volume
		SVC	superior vena cava
P_I	inspired partial pressure	SVP	saturated vapour pressure
PIFR	peak inspiratory flow rate	T	thymus-dependent (T cells)
pK_a	expression of dissociation constant in an equilibrium (logarithm to base 10 of the dissociation constant)	T	temperature
		$t_{1/2\alpha}$	α half-life (distribution half-time)
		$t_{1/2\beta}$	β half-life (elimination half-time)
PMGV	piped medical gases and vacuum systems	T_3	tri-iodothyronine
		T_4	thyroxine
p.p.m.	parts per million	TA	titratable acid
PRN	pro re nata (as needed)	TBG	thyroxine-binding globulin
PRP	platelet-rich plasma	TLC	total lung capacity
PTA	plasma thromboplastin antecedent (factor IX)	Tm	tubular maximal reabsorption
		TMJ	temporomandibular joint
Ptc_{O_2}	transcutaneous oxygen partial pressure	TNS	transcutaneous nerve stimulation
		TO4	train of four

TPR	total (systemic) peripheral resistance	Vd	dead space (ventilation)
		$V_{d(ANAT)}$	anatomical dead space
TWC	total water content	$V_{d(PHYS)}$	physiological dead space
URT	upper respiratory tract	VF	ventricular fibrillation
V	volt	VFP	ventricular fluid pressure
V	volume	VIC	vaporizer in circuit
$\dot{V}$	volume per unit time (gas flow)	VIE	vacuum insulated evaporator
v	velocity	VOC	vaporizer out of circuit
V4R	mobile chest lead in electrocardiography (position 4 reversed)	VT	ventricular tachycardia
		V_t	tidal volume
VC	vital capacity	W	watt

Appendix Ib: SI system

The Système International d'Unités (SI system) has been developed to reduce the large number of units in everyday physical use to a much smaller number, with standard symbols.

The seven base units are derivatives of the MKS system of physical measurement.

Length	metre	m
Mass	kilogram	kg
Time	second	s
Electric current	amp	A
Thermodynamic temperature	kelvin	K
Amount of substance	mole	mol
Luminous intensity	candela	cd

Any other units are derived units and may be expressed by multiplication or division of base units.

Volume	cubic metre	m^3		
Force	newton	N	$kg.m.s^{-2}$	$= J.m^{-1}$ (J/m)
Work	joule	J	$kg.m^2.s^{-2}$	$= N.m$ (Nm)
Power (rate of work)	watt	W	$kg.m^2.s^{-3}$	$= J.s^{-1}$ (J/s)
Pressure (force/area)	pascal	Pa	$kg.m^{-1}.s^{-2}$	$= N.m^{-2}$ (N/m²)

X^{-1} has been used in preference to the solidus (/), either of which is specified in the standard.

Non-standard units such as the litre, day, hour and minute may be used with SI but are not part of the standard.

Volume

The SI unit of volume is the cubic metre, but for medical purposes the litre (1 dm³) is retained.

Temperature

A temperature difference of 1 kelvin is numerically equivalent to 1 degree Celsius. In everyday use the degree Celsius is retained. The Fahrenheit scale is no longer used medically and is being phased out of use with the general public.

The magnitude of a unit is expressed by the additions of standard prefixes and symbolic prefixes. The magnitude of SI units usually changes by 10^3 per step.

Fraction	SI prefix	Symbol	*Multiple*	SI prefix	Symbol
10^{-1}	deci	d	10	deca	da
10^{-2}	centi	c	10^2	hecto	h
10^{-3}	milli	m	10^3	kilo	k
10^{-6}	micro	μ	10^6	mega	M
10^{-9}	nano	n	10^9	giga	G
10^{-12}	pico	p	10^{12}	tera	T
10^{-15}	femto	f			
10^{-18}	atto	a			

It can be seen that the SI handling of 'kilogram' is non-standard; the name of the base unit already contains a preficacial multiple. Names of decimal multiples and submultiples of the unit of mass are formed by attaching prefixes to the word 'gram'.

Moles

$$\text{Moles} = \frac{\text{weight in g}}{\text{molecular weight}}$$

thus, $1 \text{ mol } H_2O = \dfrac{18 \text{ g}}{18}$

$18 \text{ g } H_2O = 1 \text{ mol}$

For univalent ions, moles and equivalents are

numerically equal, but for multivalent ions the number of equivalents must be divided by the valency to obtain the molar value. Thus 10 mEq Ca^{2+} = 5 mmol Ca^{2+}.

Moles/osmoles

Strictly the SI unit of osmolality should be the mole, this representing the calculated number of particles/molecules in solution. However, the osmole is also used; this is the measured osmolality (the number of osmotically active particles per kilogram of solution). Thus, the molar value for osmolality is theoretical, while the osmolar value is empirical.

Appendix II: Inhaled anaesthetic agents — physical properties

Name	Formula	MW (Da)	BP °C	SVP kPa at 20°C	MAC %	Flammable in O_2	Ostwald solubility coefficients at 37°C			
							Blood/ gas	Fat/ blood	Oil/ gas	Oil/ H_2O
Nitrous oxide	N_2O	44	−88	(5300)	105	0	0.47	2.3	1.4	3.2
Cyclopropane	$CH_2CH_2CH_2$	42	−33	638	9.2	2–60	0.45		11.5	34.4
Halothane	$CF_3CHClBr$	197	50	32	0.75		2.5	51	224	220
Enflurane	$CHFClCF_2\ O\ CF_2H$	184.5	56	23	1.7	6	1.9	36	98	120
Isoflurane	$CF_3CHCl\ O\ CF_2H$	184.5	49	32	1.15	6	1.4	45	91	174
Desflurane	$CF_2H\ O\ CFHCF_3$	168	23.5	89	7.3	18–21	0.42	27	18.7	
Sevoflurane	$CH(CF_3)_2\ O\ CH_2F$	200	58.5	21	2.0		0.59	48	54	
Chloroform	$CHCl_3$	119	61	21.3	0.5		10		260	100
Diethyl ether	$C_2H_5\ O\ C_2H_5$	74	35	56.5	1.9	2–82	12	5	65	3.2
Ethyl chloride	C_2H_5Cl	64.5	13	131	2.0	4–67	3.0			
Fluroxene	$CF_3CH_2\ O\ CHCH_2$	126	43	38	3.5	4	1.4		48	90
Methoxyflurane	$CHCl_2CF_2\ O\ CH_3$	165	105	3	0.2	5–28	13	38	950	400
Trichloroethylene	$CHClCCl_2$	131	87	8	0.17	9–65	9		960	400

MW = molecular weight; BP = boiling point; SVP = saturated vapour pressure; MAC = minimum alveolar concentration. Drugs listed below the line have no product licence in the UK, and are of historical interest only. MAC values are for young adults; MAC is higher in children, and decreases in older adults.

Appendix IIIa: Cardiovascular system — normal values

Blood flows	% of cardiac output	Flow (ml.min^{-1}) (70-kg man)
Heart	4	200
Brain	14	700
Liver	25	1250
Kidneys	24	1200
Lung	3	150
Muscle	19	950
Skin	5	250
Fat	5	250
Remainder	1	50
Total	100	5000

ECg times

P wave	<0.10 s
PR interval	0.12–0.20 s
QRS time	0.05–0.08 s
QT time	0.35–0.40 s
T wave	<0.22 s

Pressures (mmHg)

	Range	Mean
Central venous pressure (CVP)	0–8	4
Right atrial (RA)	0–8	4
Right ventricular (RV)		
Systolic	14–30	25
End-diastolic (RVEDP)	0–8	4
Pulmonary arterial (PA)		
Systolic	15–30	23
Diastolic	5–15	3
Mean ($\overline{\text{PAP}}$)	10–20	15
Pulmonary artery wedge (PAWP)		
Mean	5–15	10
Left atrial (LA)	4–12	7
Left ventricular (LV)		
Systolic	90–140	120
End-diastolic (LVEDP)	4–12	7

Derived haemodynamic variables

Variable		Typical value (70 kg)
Cardiac output (CO)	$SV \times HR$	5 litre.min^{-1}
Cardiac index (CI)	$\dfrac{CO}{BSA}$	3.2 litre.min^{-1}.m^{-2}
Stroke volume (SV)	$\dfrac{CO}{HR} \times 1000$	80 ml
Stroke index (SI)	$\dfrac{SV}{BSA}$	50 ml.m^{-2}
Systemic vascular resistance (SVR)	$\dfrac{MAP - CVP}{CO} \times 80$	1000–1200 dyn.s.cm^{-5} (not SI unit)

Pulmonary vascular resistance (PVR)	$\dfrac{\overline{PAP} - LAP}{CO} \times 80$	60–120 dyn.s.cm^{-5} (not SI unit)
Left ventricular stroke work index (LVSWI)	$\dfrac{1.36\,(MAP - LAP)}{100} \times SI$	50–60 g.m.m^{-2}
Rate–pressure product (RPP)	$SAP \times HR$	9600
Ejection fraction (EF)	$\dfrac{ESV - EDV}{EDV}$	> 0.6

BSA = Body surface area; HR = heart rate; MAP = mean arterial pressure, CVP = central venous pressure; $\overline{PAP}$ = mean pulmonary arterial pressure; LAP = left atrial pressure; SAP = systolic arterial pressure; ESV = end-systolic volume; EDV = end-diastolic volume.

Appendix IIIb: Vasoactive infusions

Drug	Dilution	Typical dosage range
Sympathomimetic drugs		
Adrenaline (low — α, β_{1+2}) (higher — α)	Into glucose 5% 500 ml 5 mg = 10 μg.ml^{-1}	Start at 20–50 ng.kg^{-1}.min^{-1} Most respond to < 200 ng.kg^{-1}.min^{-1} > 500 ng.kg^{-1}.min^{-1} leads to excess vasoconstriction. 500 ng–40 μg.kg^{-1}.min^{-1}
Dobutamine (β_1)	Into glucose 5% 500 ml 250 mg = 500 μg.ml^{-1}	
Dopamine (low — δ) (moderate — δ, β_{1+2}) (high — α, β_1)	Into glucose 5% 500 ml 200 mg = 400 μg.ml^{-1} *or* 800 mg = 1600 μg.ml^{-1}	500 ng–5 μg.kg^{-1}.min^{-1} (low) 5–10 μg.kg^{-1}.min^{-1} (moderate) > 15 μg.kg^{-1}.min^{-1} (high)
Dopexamine (β_2, δ)	Into glucose 5% or saline 0.9% 50 ml 40 mg = 800 μg.ml^{-1}	500 μg.kg^{-1}.min^{-1}
Isoprenaline (β_{1+2})	Into glucose 5% 500 ml 4 mg = 8 μg.ml^{-1}	10–400 ng.kg^{-1}.min^{-1}
Metaraminol (α)	Into glucose 5% 500 ml 50 mg = 100 μg.ml^{-1}	100 ng–1 μg.kg^{-1}.min^{-1} (infrequent use as infusion)
Noradrenaline (α, β_1)	Into glucose 5% 500 ml 4 mg = 8 μg.ml^{-1}	50–200 ng.kg^{-1}.min^{-1}
Phenylephrine (α)	Into glucose 5% 500 ml 25 mg = 50 μg.ml^{-1}	100–500 ng.kg^{-1}.min^{-1}
Miscellaneous		
Amiodarone (Wolff *f*–Parkinson–White syndrome or refractory tachycardias)	Into glucose 5% 250 ml – NOT 0.9% saline 150 mg = 600 μg.ml^{-1}	40 μg.kg^{-1}.min^{-1} for 2 h Max. 1.2 g in 24 h

Disopyramide (membrane stabilization)	Into glucose 5% or saline 0.9% 450 ml 500 mg = 1000 μg.ml⁻¹	5–7 μg.kg⁻¹.min⁻¹ after loading dose — see data sheet or *British National Formulary*
Flecainide (membrane stabilization)	Into glucose 5% or saline 0.9% 500 ml 150 mg = 300 μg.ml⁻¹	4 μg.kg⁻¹.min⁻¹ after loading dose — see data sheet or *British National Formulary*
Glyceryl trinitrate (*venous* and arteriolar dilator)	Into glucose 5% or saline 0.9% to 50 ml (depends upon source) 5–10 mg = 100–200 μg.ml⁻¹ — do not give into Viaflex or other polyvinyl chloride containers — ideally use syringe pump.	10–200 μg.min⁻¹ (0.2–3 μg.kg⁻¹.min⁻¹)
Isosorbide dinitrate (*venous* and arteriolar dilator)	Into glucose 5% or saline 0.9% 45 ml 5 mg = 100 μg.ml⁻¹ — do not give into Viaflex or other polyvinyl chloride — ideally use syringe pump.	30–120 μg.min⁻¹ (0.6–2 μg.kg⁻¹.min⁻¹)
Lignocaine (membrane stabilization)	Into glucose 5% or saline 0.9% 500 ml 1 g = 2 mg.ml⁻¹ = 2000 μg.ml⁻¹	25–50 μg.kg⁻¹.min⁻¹ after loading dose — see data sheet or *British National Formulary*
Mexiletine (membrane stabilization)	Into glucose 5% or saline 0.9% 500 ml 250 mg = 500 μg.ml⁻¹	500 μg.min⁻¹ after loading dose — see data sheet or *British National Formulary*
Sodium nitroprusside (arteriolar and venous) dilator)	Into glucose 5% or saline 0.9% 500 ml 50 mg = 100 μg.ml⁻¹	0.5–8 μg.kg⁻¹.min⁻¹ (for hypertensive crisis) 0.1–1.5 μg.kg⁻¹.min⁻¹ (for hypotensive anaesthesia)

Appendix IIIc: Antibacterial prophylaxis

This appendix gives details of how to prevent endocarditis in patients with a heart valve lesion, septal defect, patent ductus arteriosus or prosthetic valve.

DENTAL PROCEDURES

Dental procedures that require antibiotic prophylaxis are extractions, scaling and surgery involving the gingival tissues. Antibiotic prophylaxis for dental procedures may be supplemented with chlorhexidine gluconate gel 1% or chlorhexidine gluconate mouthwash 0.2% used 5 min before the procedure.

Under local anaesthesia

1. For patients who have not received penicillin more than once in the previous month, including those with a prosthetic valve (but not those who have had endocarditis), oral amoxycillin 3 g 1 h before procedure; child under 5 years, one-quarter the adult dose; 5–10 years, half the adult dose.

2. For patients who are penicillin-allergic or who have received penicillin more than once in the previous month, oral clindamycin 600 mg 1 h before procedure; child under 5 years, one-quarter adult dose; 5–10 years, half the adult dose.

3. For patients who have had endocarditis, amoxycillin + gentamicin, as under general anaesthesia.

Under general anaesthesia

No special risk (including patients who have not received penicillin more than once in the previous month)
Either intramuscular (i.m.) or intravenous (i.v.) amoxycillin at induction then oral amoxycillin 500 mg 6 h later; child under 5 years, one-quarter the adult dose; 5–10 years, half the adult dose
or oral amoxycillin 3 g 4 h before procedure then oral amoxycillin 3 g as soon as possible after the procedure; child under 5 years, one-quarter the adult dose; 5–10 years, half the adult dose
or oral amoxycillin 3 g + oral probenecid 1 g 4 h preoperatively.

Special risk (patients with a prosthetic valve or who have had endocarditis)

i.m. or i.v. amoxycillin 1 g + gentamicin 120 mg at induction, then oral amoxycillin 500 mg 6 h later. Child under 5 years, amoxycillin one-quarter the adult dose, gentamicin 2 mg.kg^{-1}; 5–10 years, amoxycillin, one-half the adult dose, gentamicin 2 mg.kg^{-1}.

Penicillin allergy

For patients who are penicillin-allergic or who have received penicillin more than once in the previous month:
Either i.v. vancomycin 1 g (given over at least 100 min) then i.v. gentamicin 120 mg at induction or 15 min before procedure; child under 10 years, vancomycin 20 mg.kg^{-1}, gentamicin 2 mg.kg^{-1}
or i.v. teicoplanin 400 mg + gentamicin 120 mg at induction or 15 min before procedure; child under *14* years teicoplanin 6 mg.kg^{-1}, gentamicin 2 mg.kg^{-1}
or i.v. clindamycin 300 mg (given over at least 10 min) at induction or 15 min before procedure, then oral or i.v. clindamycin 150 mg 6 h later; child under 5 years, one-quarter the adult dose; 5–10 years, half the adult dose.

Upper respiratory tract procedures

Treatment is as for dental procedures; the post-operative dose may be given parenterally if swallowing is painful.

Genitourinary procedures

Treatment is as for special risk patients undergoing dental procedures under general anaesthesia, except that clindamycin is not given. If urine is infected, prophylaxis should also cover infective organism.

Obstetric, gynaecological and gastrointestinal procedures

Prophylaxis is only required for patients at special risk (with prosthetic valves or who have had endocarditis)

Appendix IV: Chemical pathology — biochemical values

These values are given for example only — each reporting laboratory provides reference values for its own population and method. This is especially true of enzyme assays. Values given are those obtained from Chemical Pathology in Warwick, where these are available. No inference should be made about the molecular weight of a substance by reference to US and SI values

Name	US units	SI units
Adrenaline	100 pg.ml^{-1}	0.55 nmol.litre^{-1}
Amino acid nitrogen	4–8 mg%	3–6 mmol.litre^{-1}
Ammonia	80–110 μg%	<50 μmol.litre^{-1}
Amylase	80–180 Somogyi units%	70–300 i.u. litre^{-1}
Base excess	± 2 mEq.litre^{-1}	± 2 mmol.litre^{-1}
Bicarbonate		
Actual	22–30 mEq.litre^{-1}	22–30 mmol.litre^{-1}
Standard	21–25 mEq.litre^{-1}	21–25 mmol.litre^{-1}
Bilirubin — total	0.3–1.1 mg%	3–18 μmol.litre^{-1}
Buffer base (pH 7.4, Pa_{CO_2} 5.3, Hb 15 g.dl^{-1})	48 mEq.litre^{-1}	48 mmol.litre^{-1}
Calcium		
Total	8.5–10.5 mg% (4.5–5.7 mEq.litre^{-1})	2.25–2.6 mmol.litre^{-1}
Ionized	4–5 mg%	1.0–1.25 mmol.litre^{-1}
Chloride	95–105 mEq.litre^{-1}	95–105 mmol.litre^{-1}
Cholesterol	140–300 mg%	3.6–7.8 mmol.litre^{-1}
Cholinesterase, plasma (pseudocholinesterase)	Dibucaine number >80% usually normal Dibucaine number <20% usually homozygote for atypical cholinesterase	
Copper	80–150 μg%	13–24 nmol.litre^{-1}
Urinary copper	15–50 μg per 24 h	0.2–0.8 μmol per 24 h
Cortisol		
0900 ⎫ radioimmunoassay	9–23 μg.litre^{-1}	250–635 nmol.litre^{-1}
2400 ⎭ technique	<7.2 μg%	<200 nmol.litre^{-1}
Neonatal (competitive protein-binding technique)	30 μg.litre^{-1}	200–650 nmol.litre^{-1} <200 nmol.litre^{-1} 330–1700 nmol.litre^{-1}

Name	US units	SI units
Creatine (phospho)kinase (CK)	100 i.u. litre^{-1} — male	25–200 i.u. litre^{-1}
	60 i.u. litre^{-1} — female	25–150 i.u. litre^{-1}
Creatinine	0.5–1.4 mg%	45–120 μmol.litre^{-1}
Fibrinogen	150–400 mg%	1.5–4.0 g.litre^{-1}
Folate	3–20 ng.ml^{-1}	3–20 μg.litre^{-1}
		2.1–27 nmol.litre^{-1}
Glucose		
Fasting	55–85 mg%	4–6 mmol.litre^{-1}
Postprandial	<180 mg%	<10 mmol.litre^{-1}
γ-Glutamyl transpeptidase	7–25 i.u. litre^{-1}	male: <50 i.u. litre^{-1}
		female: <30 i.u. litre^{-1}
Hydroxybutyrate dehydrogenase (HBD)		100–240 i.u. litre^{-1}
Iodine — total	3.5–8.0 μg.litre^{-1}	273–624 nmol/litre^{-1}
^{131}I uptake	20–50% of administered dose in 24 h	
Iron	80–160 μg%	14–30 μmol.litre^{-1}
Iron-binding capacity	250–400 μg%	45–69 μmol.litre^{-1}
Lactate	0.6–1.8 mEq.litre^{-1}	0.6–1.8 mmol.litre^{-1}
Lactate dehydrogenase	30–90 i.u. litre^{-1}	100–300 i.u. litre^{-1}
Lead		<1.8 μmol/litre^{-1}
Magnesium	1–2 mg%	
	1.5–2.0 mEq.litre^{-1}	0.7–1.0 mmol.litre^{-1}
Methaemoglobin	<3% of total haemoglobin	
Nitrogen (non-protein) (urea + urate + creatinine + creatine)	18–30 mg%	12.8–21.4 mmol.litre^{-1}
Noradrenaline	200 pg.ml^{-1}	1.25 nmol.litre^{-1}
Osmolality	280–300 mosmol.kg^{-1}	280–300 mmol.kg^{-1}
Phosphate	2.0–4.5 mg%	0.8–1.4 mmol.litre^{-1}
	3.0–6.0 mg% (children)	1.0–1.8 mmol.litre^{-1} (children)
	<8.1 mg% (neonatal)	<2.6 mmol.litre^{-1} (neonatal)
Phosphatase		
Acid (total)	1–5 KA units%	1–9 i.u. litre^{-1}
Acid (prostatic)		0–3 i.u. litre^{-1}
Alkaline	3–13 KA units%	17–100 i.u. litre^{-1}
Potassium	3.4–5.3 mEq.litre^{-1}	3.4–5.3 mmol.litre^{-1}
Protein		
Total	6.0–8.0 g%	60–80 g.litre^{-1}
Albumin	3.5–5.0 g%	35–50 g.litre^{-1}
Globulin	1.5–3.0 g%	15–30 g.litre^{-1}
Pyruvate	0.4–0.7 mg%	34–80 μmol.litre^{-1}
Sodium	133–148 mEq.litre^{-1}	133–148 mmol.litre^{-1}
Thyroxine (T$_4$)	4.7–11 μg%	52–140 nmol.litre^{-1}

Name	US units	SI units
Transaminase		
Aspartate transaminase (AST)	5–40 unit.ml^{-1}	5–40 i.u. litre^{-1}
Alanine transaminase (ALT)		2–53 i.u. litre^{-1}
Transferrin	220–400 mg%	2.2–4.0 g.litre^{-1}
Triglycerides (fasting)	71–160 mg%	0.8–1.8 mmol.litre^{-1}
Tri-iodothyronine (T$_3$)	90–170 ng%	0.8–2.5 nmol.litre^{-1}
T$_3$ uptake	95–117%	95–117%
Urea	15–48 mg%	2.5–8.0 mmol.litre^{-1}
Urea nitrogen (BUN)	10–20 mg%	7.1–14.3 mmol.litre^{-1}
Urate		
Men	4–9.5 mg%	225–470 μmol.litre^{-1}
Women	3–7.5 mg%	180–390 μmol.litre^{-1}

Appendix V: Haematology
a. Normal values

Haemoglobin	
Men	13.5–18.0 g.dl^{-1}
Women	11.5–16.5 g.dl^{-1}
10–12 years	11.5–14.8 g.dl^{-1}
12/12	11.0–13.0 g.dl^{-1}
3/12	9.5–12.5 g.dl^{-1}
Full-term	13.6–19.6 g.dl^{-1}
Red blood cell count (RBC)	
Men	4.5–6.0 $\times$ 10^{12} litre^{-1}
Women	3.5–5.0 $\times$ 10^{12} litre^{-1}
White blood cell count (WBC)	4.0–11.0 $\times$ 10^{9} litre^{-1}
Neutrophils	40–70%
Lymphocytes	20–45%
Monocytes	2–10%
Eosinophils	1–6%
Basophils	0–1%
Platelet count	150–400 $\times$ 10^{9} litre^{-1}
Reticulocyte count	0–2% of RBC
Sedimentation rate	
Men	0–15 mm in 1 h
Women	0–20 mm in 1 h
Plasma viscosity	1.50–1.72 cp
Packed cell volume (PCV) and haematocrit (Hct)	
Men	0.4–0.55
Women	0.36–0.47
Mean corpuscular volume (MCV)	76–96 fl
Mean corpuscular haemoglobin concentration (MCHC)	31–35 g.dl^{-1}
Mean corpuscular haemoglobin (MCH)	27–32 pg

Appendix Vb: Coagulation tests

Activated clotting time (ACT; Haemochron type)	80–135 s
Antithrombin III	>80% normal
Bleeding time (platelet function)	2–9 min
Clotting time (largely replaced by ACT)	3–11 min
Fibrinogen — plasma	1.5–4 g.litre^{-1}
Fibrin degradation products	<10 mg.litre^{-1} (μg.ml^{-1})
INR (international normalized ratio; newer warfarin therapy value)	
Therapeutic range for:	
Atrial fibrillation, deep venous thrombosis, pulmonary embolism, tissue heart valves	2–3
Mechanical heart valves	3–4.5
PTTK/APTT (heparin therapy value)	1.5–2.5 times normal
If pregnant	1.5–2.0 times normal
Partial thromboplastin time	35–45 s
Platelet count	150–400 × 10^9 litre^{-1}
Prothrombin time	12–14 s
Thrombin time	circa 15 s
Thrombotest (older warfarin therapy value)	
Normal	70–130%
Therapeutic	5–15%

PTTK = partial thromboplastin time, kaolin
APTT = activated partial thromboplastin time

Appendix Vc: Coagulation screen

What to check?

Prothrombin time (PT)
Partial thromboplastin time (PTT)
Thrombin time (TT)
Fibrinogen
Platelet count

If all are normal, consider checking bleeding time and in neonates factor XIII concentration.

When to check?

Elective patient

1. With suspicious history (bleeding after cuts, previous surgery or dental extractions; easy bruising).
2. With family history of bleeding problems.
3. Receiving anticoagulants — warfarin, heparin or *aspirin*, for example.
4. With intercurrent illness such as obstructive jaundice, liver disease, uraemia or leukaemia.

Emergency or intraoperative patient

With excessive bleeding despite apparent vascular integrity.

What to do?

Possible cause	Treatment
PT and PTT prolonged	
Drug effect (warfarin/coumarin)	Vitamin K
	Fresh frozen plasma (FFP)
	Coagulation concentrates
Obstructive jaundice	Vitamin K
	FFP
Liver disease	Vitamin K
	FFP
Haemorrhagic disease of the newborn	Vitamin K
Factor II, V, X deficiency	FFP
	Coagulation concentrates
If TT is also prolonged	
Fibrinogen deficiency	Cryoprecipitate
	FFP

Possible cause	Treatment
Are D-dimers increased?	
Disseminated intravascular coagulation (DIC)	Treat cause FFP Platelets ? Antithrombin III concentrate
Is PTT prolonged?	
Heparin therapy	Stop therapy ? Reverse effect with protamine
Factor VIII deficiency — haemophilia	Factor VIII concentrate: high purity
Von Willebrand's disease	Vasopressin Factor VIII concentrate: intermediate purity
Factor IX deficiency	Factor IX concentrate
Factor XI or XII deficiency	FFP
Is PT prolonged (with normal PTT)?	
Factor VII deficiency	FFP
Is platelet count decreased (< 100 × 10⁹ litre⁻¹)?	

Peripheral destruction
  ? Immune-mediated
  ? DIC
	Steroids
	Treat cause
	Platelets
	FFP
	? Antithrombin III concentrate

Inadequate production Marrow failure	Platelets
Is bleeding time prolonged?	
Von Willebrand's disease	Factor VIII concentrate: intermediate purity Vasopressin

Functional platelet disorder
  Inherited
  Acquired
Uraemia
	
	Platelets
	Platelets
	Dialysis/haemofiltration
	Cryoprecipitate

Drugs	

If still confused or uncertain, then ask your haematologist or pathologist.

Appendix VIa: Fluid balance

FLUID COMPOSITION OF BODY COMPARTMENTS

Typical blood volume		*Total water content (TWC)*
Infant	90 ml.kg^{-1}	60% male (55% female) of body weight (18–40 years)
Child	80 ml.kg^{-1}	55% male (46% female) of body weight (> 60 years)
Adult male	70 ml.kg^{-1}	Volume of extracellular fluid 35% TWC
Adult female	60 ml.kg^{-1}	Volume of intracellular fluid 65% TWC

Appendix VIb: Intraoperative fluid requirements — adult

(1)	Initial volume	$1.5\ ml.kg^{-1}.h^{-1}$ for duration of preoperative starvation
+ (2)	Maintenance	$1.5\ ml.kg^{-1}.h^{-1}$
+ (3)	Operative insensible loss	e.g. 1–2 litre for abdominal surgery
+ (4)	Blood loss	Replace with blood when loss exceeds 20% of estimated blood volume

Appendix VIc: Fluid, electrolyte and nutritional requirements

Minimum daily requirements per kilogram for adults, and children and infants.

	Adults (per kg)	Children and infants (per kg)		Adults (per kg)	Children and infants (per kg)
Water	30–45 ml	100–150 ml	Mn^{2+}	0.1 μmol	0.3 μmol
Energy	30–50 kcal	90–125 kcal	Zn^{2+}	0.7 μmol	1.0 μmol
	(0.15–0.21 MJ)	(0.38–0.5 MJ)	Cu^+	0.07 μmol	0.3 μmol
Protein	0.7–1.0 g	2.2–2.5 g	Cl^-	1.3–1.9 mmol	1.8–4.3 mmol
Na^+	1–1.4 mmol	1–2.5 mmol			
K^+	0.7–0.9 mmol	2 mmol	*Neonates*		
Ca^{2+}	0.11 mmol	0.5–1 mmol	See Appendix IXc		
Mg^{2+}	0.04 mmol	0.15 mmol			
Fe^{2+}	1 μmol	2 μmol			

Appendix VId: Composition of common intravenous fluids

| Name | pH | Calculated* osmolality | Ions mmol.litre^{-1} | | | | | CHO g.litre^{-1} | Protein g.litre^{-1} | MJ.litre^{-1} |
			Na$^+$	K$^+$	Cl$^-$	HCO$_3^-$	Misc.			
Crystalloids										
Sodium chloride 0.9%	5.0	308	154	0	154	0	0	0	0	0
Glucose 5%	4.0	280	0	0	0	0	0	50	0	0.84
Glucose 4% + saline 0.18%	4.5	286	31	0	31	0	0	40	0	0.67
Glucose 5% + saline 0.45%	4.5	430	77	0	77	0	0	50	0	0.84
Lactated Ringer's (Hartmann's solution)	6.5	280	131	5	112	29 (as lact.)	Mg^{2+} 1 Ca^{2+} 1	0	0	0.038
Sodium bicarbonate 8.4%	8.0	2000	1000	0	0	1000	0	0	0	0

* Calculated value, assuming total dissociation of ions.

Name	pH	Oncotic pressure (mmH$_2$O)	Ionic content (mmol.litre^{-1})			Misc.	CHO (g.litre^{-1})	Protein (g.litre^{-1})	MJ.litre^{-1}	Typical half-life in plasma
			Na$^+$	K$^+$	Cl$^-$					
Colloids										
Gelatin (succinylated, Haemaccel)	7.4	370	145	5.1	145	Ca^{2+} 6.25 PO$_4^{2-}$ Trace SO$_4^{2-}$ Trace	0	35	0	5 h
Gelatin (polygeline, Gelofusine)	7.4	465	154	0.4	125	Ca^{2+} 0.4 Mg^{2+} 0.4	0	40	0	4 h
Dextran 70 in sodium chloride 0.9%	4–7	268	154	0	154	0	0	0	0	12 h
Dextran 70 in glucose 5%	3.5–7	268	0	0	0	0	50	0	0.84	12 h
Hetastarch (Hespan)	5.5	310	154	0	54	0	0	0	0	17 days
Blood products										
Human albumin solution (PPF 4%)	7.4	275	150	2	120					

(20% salt-poor solution also available — ionic content varies with manufacturer)

Whole blood	>6.5	Na$^+$ depends on donor values. K+ increases with storage time				
Plasma-reduced blood	>6.5	Na$^+$ depends on donor value. K$^+$ higher than in whole blood, but total quantity *per unit* similar				
SAGM blood	>6.5		150		150	Adenine 0.6%, glucose 2.6%, mannitol 1.6%

Accepted safe storage times at 4°C

Heparinized blood	Only available for special applications
Acid citrate dextrose	21 days
Citrate phosphate dextrose	28 days
Citrate phosphate dextrose adenine	35 days
SAGM	35 days

SAGM = saline adenine glucose mannitol.

Appendix VII: Renal function tests

Clearance tests

Inulin clearance $\rightleftharpoons$ glomerular filtration $\qquad$ 100–150 ml.min^{-1}
Para-aminohippuric acid clearance $\rightleftharpoons$ renal plasma flow $\qquad$ 560–830 ml.min^{-1}
Creatinine clearance $\rightleftharpoons$ glomerular filtration rate (overestimates low $\qquad$ 104–125 ml.min^{-1}
glomerular filtration rate)

Blood tests

Serum/plasma

Osmolality $\qquad$ 280–300 mosmol.kg^{-1}
Creatinine $\qquad$ 45–120 μmol.litre^{-1}
Urea $\qquad$ 2.7–7.0 mmol.litre^{-1}
Urea nitrogen $\qquad$ 1.6–3.3 mmol.litre^{-1}

Urine tests

Osmolality $\qquad$ 300–1200 mosmol.kg^{-1}
Creatinine $\qquad$ 8.85–17.7 mmol per 24 h
Sodium $\qquad$ 50–200 mmol per 24 h

Comparative urinary values

	SG	Osmolality	U/P urea ratio	U/P osmolality
Normal	1000–1040	300–1200	> 20:1	> 2.0:1
Prerenal failure	> 1022	> 400	> 20:1	> 2.0:1
Renal failure				
Early	1010	< 350	< 14:1	< 1.7:1
Late			< 5:1	< 1.1:1

SG = specific gravity; U = urea; P = plasma.

Appendix VIII: Pulmonary function tests

LUNG SPIROMETRY

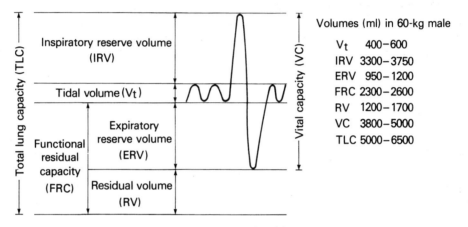

Volumes (ml) in 60-kg male

V_t 400–600
IRV 3300–3750
ERV 950–1200
FRC 2300–2600
RV   1200–1700
VC   3800–5000
TLC 5000–6500

Fig. VIIIa   Lung volumes in an average heathy male adult.

a. SPIROGRAM

Commonly used abbreviations

Primary symbols

C = concentration of gas — blood phase
D = diffusing capacity
F = fractional concentration in the dry gas phase
P = partial pressure — gas
Q = volume of blood
R = respiratory exchange ratio
S = saturation of haemoglobin with oxygen or carbon dioxide
V = volume of gas
$\dot{X}$ = dot above symbol indicates 'per unit time'
$\bar{X}$ = bar above symbol indicates 'mean value'

Example: Pa_{O_2} = partial pressure of arterial oxygen.

Secondary symbols

Usually typed as subscripts, capital letters indicate gaseous phase; lower-case letters indicate liquid phase.

A = alveolar
B = barometric
D = dead space
E = expired
I = inspired
T = tidal
a = arterial
c = capillary (pulmonary capillary)
v = venous

Appendix VIIIb

PULMONARY FUNCTION TESTS — FEMALES

Age (years)	Height (cm)	FEV$_1$ (litres)	FVC (litres)	FEV$_1$/FVC (%)	PEFR (litre.min^{-1})
20	145	2.60	3.13	81.0	377
	152	2.83	3.45	81.0	403
	160	3.09	3.83	81.0	433
	168	3.36	4.20	81.0	459
	175	3.59	4.53	81.0	489
30	145	2.45	2.98	79.9	366
	152	2.68	3.30	79.9	392
	160	2.94	3.68	79.9	422
	168	3.21	4.05	79.9	448
	175	3.44	4.38	79.9	478
40	145	2.15	2.68	77.7	345
	152	2.38	3.00	77.7	371
	160	2.64	3.38	77.7	401
	168	2.91	3.75	77.7	427
	175	3.14	4.08	77.7	457
50	145	1.85	2.38	75.5	324
	152	2.08	2.70	75.5	350
	160	2.34	3.08	75.5	380
	168	2.61	3.45	75.5	406
	175	2.84	3.78	75.5	436
60	145	1.55	2.08	73.2	303
	152	1.78	2.40	73.2	329
	160	2.04	2.78	73.2	359
	168	2.31	3.15	73.2	385
	175	2.54	3.48	73.2	415
70	145	1.25	1.78	71.0	282
	152	1.48	2.10	71.0	308
	160	1.74	2.48	71.0	338
	168	2.01	2.85	71.0	364
	175	2.24	3.18	71.0	394

PULMONARY FUNCTION TESTS — MALES

Age (years)	Height (cm)	FEV$_1$ (litres)	FVC (litres)	FEV$_1$/FVC (%)	PEFR (litre.min^{-1})
20	160	3.61	4.17	82.5	572
	168	3.86	4.53	82.5	597
	175	4.15	4.95	82.5	625
	183	4.44	5.37	82.5	654
	191	4.69	5.73	82.5	679
30	160	3.45	4.06	80.6	560
	168	3.71	4.42	80.6	584
	175	4.00	4.84	80.6	612
	183	4.28	5.26	80.6	640
	191	4.54	5.62	80.6	665
40	160	3.14	3.84	76.9	536
	168	3.40	4.20	76.9	559
	175	3.69	4.62	76.9	586
	183	3.97	5.04	76.9	613
	191	4.23	5.40	76.9	636
50	160	2.83	3.62	73.1	512
	168	3.09	3.98	73.1	534
	175	3.38	4.40	73.1	560
	183	3.66	4.82	73.1	585
	191	3.92	5.18	73.1	608
60	160	2.52	3.40	69.4	488
	168	2.78	3.76	69.4	509
	175	3.06	4.18	69.4	533
	183	3.35	4.60	69.4	558
	191	3.61	4.96	69.4	579
70	160	2.21	3.18	65.7	464
	168	2.47	3.54	65.7	484
	175	2.75	3.96	65.7	507
	183	3.04	4.38	65.7	530
	191	3.30	4.74	65.7	551

FEV$_1$ = Forced expiratory volume in 1 s; FVC = forced vital capacity; PEFR = peak expiratory flow rate.

Appendix VIIIc

LUNG FUNCTION: ADULT AND NEONATAL VALUES

Examples

	Adult (65 kg)	Neonate (3 kg)
V_D	2.2 ml.kg–1	2–3 ml.kg^{-1}
V_T	7–10 ml.kg^{-1}	5–7 ml.kg^{-1}
$\dot{V}_E$	85–100 ml.kg^{-1}.min^{-1}	100–200 ml.kg^{-1}.min^{-1}
Vital capacity	50–55 ml.kg^{-1}	33 ml.kg^{-1}
Respiratory rate	12–18 breath.min^{-1}	25–40 breath.min^{-1}
Pa_{O_2}	12.6 kPa (95 mmHg)	9 kPa (68 mmHg)
Pa_{CO_2}	5.3 kPa (40 mmHg)	4.5 kPa (33 mmHg)

Appendix IX Paediatrics

a. **Tracheal and tracheostomy tube size**

Age (years)	TT and tracheostomy tube size ID (mm)	TT length (cm)		Age (years)	TT and tracheostomy tube size ID (mm)	TT length (cm)	
		Oral	Nasal			Oral	Nasal
0–3 months	3.0	10		9	6.0	16	19
3–6 months	3.5	12	15	10	6.5	17	20
6–12 months	3.5	12	15	11	6.5	17	20
2	4.0	13	16	12	7.0	18	21
3	4.0	13	16	13	7.0	18	21
4	4.5	14	17	14	7.5	21	24
5	5.0	14	17	15	7.5	21	24
6	5.5	15	18	16	8.0	21	24
7	5.5	15	18	17	9.0	22	25
8	6.0	16	19	18	9.5	22	25
				20	9.5	23	26

TT = Tracheal tube; ID = internal diameter.
Below 8–10 years, non-cuffed tubes should be used.
It is always advisable to have available a tube one size smaller than calculated.

Appendix IXb

DOSAGE OF DRUGS IN COMMON
ANAESTHETIC USAGE

Premedication

Atropine	20 µg.kg^{-1}
Hyoscine	20 µg.kg^{-1}
Glycopyrrolate	5 µg.kg^{-1}
Diazepam	200–400 µg.kg^{-1}
Droperidol	100 µg.kg^{-1}
Trimeprazine	2 mg.kg^{-1}

Intravenous induction

Propofol	3 mg.kg^{-1}
Thiopentone	5 mg.kg^{-1}
Methohexitone	1.5 mg.kg^{-1}
Ketamine	2 mg.kg^{-1}

Other induction routes

Ketamine intramuscular	10 mg.kg^{-1}
(Thiopentone rectal	30 mg.kg^{-1})
(Methohexitone rectal	25 mg.kg^{-1})

Neuromuscular blocking drugs

Suxamethonium	2 mg.kg^{-1}
Atracurium	300–500 µg.kg^{-1}
Vecuronium	100 µg.kg^{-1}
Tubocurarine	500 µg.kg^{-1}
Pancuronium	80–100 µg.kg^{-1}

Reversal of neuromuscular blocking drugs

Neostigmine	
Child	50 µg.kg^{-1}
Neonatal	80 µg.kg^{-1}
Atropine	20 µg.kg^{-1}

Analgesics — intravenous/intramuscular

Morphine	200 µg.kg^{-1}
Fentanyl	0.5–1.5 µg.kg^{-1}
Alfentanil	2.5–5 µg.kg^{-1}
Rectal	
Diclofenac	2 mg.kg^{-1} (for acute dosage only)

Appendix IXc: Fluid and electrolyte balance

POSTOPERATIVE FLUID AND ELECTROLYTE REQUIREMENTS IN INFANCY AND CHILDHOOD

Weight	Rate
Up to 10 kg	100 ml.kg^{-1}.day^{-1}
10–20 kg	1000 ml + 50 × [wt (kg) – 10] ml.kg^{-1}.day^{-1}
20–30 kg	1500 ml + 25 × [wt (kg) – 20] ml.kg^{-1}.day^{-1}

FLUID REQUIREMENTS IN THE FIRST WEEK OF LIFE

Day	Rate
1	0
2, 3	50 ml.kg^{-1}.day^{-1}
4, 5	75 ml.kg^{-1}.day^{-1}
6	100 ml.kg^{-1}.day^{-1}
7	120 ml.kg^{-1}.day^{-1}

FLUID AND ELECTROLYTE REQUIREMENTS IN INFANCY AND CHILDHOOD

	Age (years)										
	1 week	1	2	3	4	5	6	7	8	9	10
Weight (kg)	3.5	10	13	15	17	19	21	23	25	28	32
Insensible water loss (ml.kg^{-1}.day^{-1})	30	27.5	27	26.5	26	25	24	23	22	21	20
Water requirement (ml.kg^{-1}.day^{-1})	150	100	100	90	90	90	70	70	70	70	70
Na$^+$ requirement (mmol.kg^{-1}.day^{-1})	4	3	2.5	2	2	1.9	1.9	1.9	1.8	1.75	1.7
K$^+$ requirement (mmol.kg^{-1}.day^{-1})	2.5	2	2	2	2	1.75	1.75	1.5	1.5	1.5	1.5

These are basal requirements. Additional fluid (10–20%) is required during major surgery, in addition to replacement of overt losses. During the postoperative period, fluid requirements are increased in the presence of pyrexia. Fluid and electrolyte balance should be adjusted after measurement of serum electrolyte concentrations and serum osmolality.

Appendix X: Gas flows in anaesthetic breathing systems

System	Spontaneous ventilation	Intermittent positive-pressure ventilation
Mapleson A (Lack or Magill)	Minute ventilation (MV; theoretically V_A) 80 ml.kg^{-1}.min^{-1}	$2.5 \times$ MV 200 ml.kg^{-1}.min^{-1}
Mapleson D (Bain or coaxial Mapleson D)	$2-3 \times$ MV 150–250 ml.kg^{-1}.min^{-1}	70 ml.kg^{-1}.min^{-1} for Pa_{CO_2} of 5.3 kPa 100 ml.kg^{-1}.min^{-1} for Pa_{CO_2} of 4.3 kPa
Mapleson E (Ayre's T-piece)	$2 \times$ MV	As Mapleson D Minimum of 3 litre.min^{-1} fresh gas flow
Mapleson F (Jackson Rees modification of Ayre's T-piece)	As Mapleson E	As Mapleson E

V_A = Alveolar minute volume; Pa_{CO_2} = arterial carbon dioxide tension.

NORMAL VENTILATION VALUES FOR RESTING AWAKE SUBJECTS

Weight		Minute volume (ml)	Tidal volume (ml)	Frequency (breath.min^{-1})
Neonate	2 kg	480	14–16	30–45
	3 kg	600	17–24	25–40
	10 kg	1680	80	21
	20 kg	3040	160	19
	30 kg	4080	240	17
	40 kg	4800	320	15
	50 kg	5200	400	13
	60 kg	5280	480	11
	70 kg	5600	560	10

Index